Evidence-based Emergency Medicine

This book is dedicated to:

Our patients, who have generated the clinical questions proposed in this book and who deserve our best efforts to identify, synthesize, update and disseminate evidence-based care;

The many practitioners from within and outside emergency medicine who have helped advance the field of evidence-based emergency medicine over the past two decades;

And finally to our families, especially our spouses/partners, for their support and encouragement throughout our careers and during the production of this book.

Evidence-based Emergency Medicine

EDITED BY

BRIAN H. ROWE MD, MSc, CCFP(EM), FCCP

Professor and Research Director, Department of Emergency Medicine
University of Alberta, Edmonton, Alberta, Canada

SECTION EDITORS

EDDY S. LANG MDCM, CCFP(EM), CSPQ

Assistant Professor of Emergency Medicine
Department of Family Medicine, McGill University, Montreal
and Attending Physician, Emergency Medicine
SMBD Jewish General Hospital, Montreal, Quebec, Canada

MICHAEL BROWN MD, MSc

Professor of Epidemiology and Emergency Medicine
College of Human Medicine, Michigan State University
Spectrum Health – Butterworth Hospitals
Grand Rapids, Michigan, USA

DEBRA HOURY MD, MPH

Director, Center for Injury Control
Vice Chair for Research
Department of Emergency Medicine, Emory University
Atlanta, Georgia, USA

DAVID H. NEWMAN MD

Assistant Professor
Department of Medicine
Columbia University College of Physicians and Surgeons
New York, USA

PETER C. WYER MD

Associate Clinical Professor, Department of Medicine
Columbia University College of Physicians and Surgeons
New York, USA

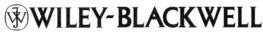

A John Wiley & Sons, Ltd., Publication

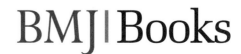

This edition first published 2009, © 2009 by Blackwell Publishing Ltd

BMJ Books is an imprint of BMJ Publishing Group Limited, used under licence by Blackwell Publishing which was acquired by John Wiley & Sons in February 2007. Blackwell's publishing programme has been merged with Wiley's global Scientific, Technical and Medical business to form Wiley-Blackwell.

Registered office: John Wiley & Sons Ltd, The Atrium, Southern Gate, Chichester, West Sussex, PO19 8SQ, UK

Editorial offices: 9600 Garsington Road, Oxford, OX4 2DQ, UK

The Atrium, Southern Gate, Chichester, West Sussex, PO19 8SQ, UK

111 River Street, Hoboken, NJ 07030-5774, USA

For details of our global editorial offices, for customer services and for information about how to apply for permission to reuse the copyright material in this book please see our website at www.wiley.com/wiley-blackwell

Library of Congress Cataloguing-in-Publication Data

Evidence-based emergency medicine / edited by Brian H. Rowe.
  p. ; cm.
  Includes bibliographical references.
  ISBN 978-1-4051-6143-5
  1. Emergency medicine.   2. Evidence-based medicine.   I. Rowe, Brian H.
  [DNLM: 1. Emergency Medicine–methods.   2. Evidence-Based Medicine–methods. WB 105 E935 2008]
  RC86.7.E95 2008
  616.02′5–dc22   2008010823

ISBN: 9781405161435

A catalogue record for this book is available from the British Library.

Set in 9.25/12 Palatino by Aptara Inc., New Delhi, India
Printed & bound in Singapore by Fabulous Printers Pte Ltd

1   2009

Contents

Contents

A companion website with additional resources is available at www.blackwellpublishing.com/medicine/bmj/emergencymedicine/

List of contributors

Riyad B. Abu-Laban MD, MHSc, FRCPC
Assistant Professor
Division of Emergency Medicine
University of British Columbia
Vancouver, British Columbia, Canada *and*
Attending Physician and Research Director
Department of Emergency Medicine
Vancouver General Hospital
Vancouver, British Columbia, Canada

Srikar Adhikari MD, RDMS
Assistant Professor
Department of Emergency Medicine
University of Nebraska
Omaha, Nebraska, USA

Marc Afilalo
Associate Professor
Department of Family Medicine
McGill University
Montreal, Quebec
and Chief of Emergency Medicine
Department of Emergency Medicine
SMBD Jewish General Hospital
Montreal, Quebec, Canada

Robert Bassett DO
Department of Emergency Medicine
Indiana University School of Medicine
Indianapolis, Indiana, USA

Jeffrey J. Bazarian MD, MPH
Associate Professor
Departments of Emergency Medicine
and Neurology
University of Rochester School of Medicine and
Dentistry
Rochester, New York, USA

Steven L. Bernstein MD
Vice Chair for Research
Associate Professor of Clinical Emergency
Medicine

Family/Social Medicine, Epidemiology/
Population Health
Albert Einstein College of Medicine
Montefiore Medical Center
Department of Emergency Medicine
Bronx, New York, USA

Michael Blaivas MD, RDMS
Assistant Professor of Internal Medicine
Department of Internal Medicine
Northside Hospital Forsyth
Cumming, Georgia, USA

Bjug Borgundvaag MD, PhD
Assistant Professor
Schwartz/Reisman Emergency Centre
Mount Sinai Hospital
Toronto, Ontario, Canada

Nicole Bouchard MD
Assistant Clinical Professor
Emergency Medicine Department
New York–Presbyterian Hospital
Columbia University Medical Center
New York
and Director of Medical Toxicology
New York City Poison Control Center
New York, USA

Edwin D. Boudreaux PhD
Research Director
Department of Emergency Medicine
Cooper University Hospital
Camden, New Jersey, USA

Peter Brindley MD
Staff Physician
Division of Critical Care Medicine
University of Alberta Hospital
Edmonton, Alberta, Canada

Robert Brison, MD, MPH, MSc, FRCPC
Professor
Departments of Emergency Medicine
and Community Health and Epidemiology
Queen's University
Kingston, Ontario, Canada

Michael Brown MD, MSc
Professor of Epidemiology and Emergency
Medicine
College of Human Medicine
Michigan State University
Spectrum Health-Butterworth Hospitals
Grand Rapids, Michigan, USA

Michael Bullard MD, CCFP(EM), ABEM,
FRCPC
Professor
Department of Emergency Medicine
University of Alberta
Edmonton, Alberta, Canada

Lisa Cabral MD
Assistant Professor of Clinical Emergency
Medicine
Albert Einstein College of Medicine
Montefiore Medical Center
Department of Emergency Medicine
Bronx, New York, USA

Carlos A. Camargo, Jr., MD, DrPH
Director, EMNet Coordinating Center
Department of Emergency Medicine
Massachusetts General Hospital
Boston, Massachusetts, USA

Sam G. Campbell MB BCh, CCFP(EM),
CHE, Dip PEC(SA)
Associate Professor
Department of Emergency Medicine
Dalhousie University
Halifax, Nova Scotia, Canada

Christopher R. Carpenter MD, MSc
Assistant Professor
Division of Emergency Medicine
St. Louis School of Medicine
Washington University
St. Louis, Missouri, USA

Jenn Carpenter MD, FRCPC
Assistant Professor
Departments of Emergency Medicine
and Community Health and Epidemiology
Queen's University
Kingston, Ontario, Canada

Cheryl K. Chang MD, MPH
Assistant Clinical Professor
Department of Medicine
Columbia University College of Physicians and
Surgeons
New York, USA

Justin Cheung MD, FRCP
Staff Physician
Division of Gastroenterology
Department of Medicine
University of Alberta
Edmonton, Alberta, Canada

Sean P. Collins MD, MSc
Assistant Professor
Department of Emergency Medicine
University of Cincinnati
Cincinnati, Ohio, USA

Matthew Cooke PhD, FCEM, FRCS(Ed)
Professor of Emergency Medicine
Warwick Medical School
University of Warwick, Coventry
and Heart of England NHS Foundation Trust
Birmingham, UK

Liesl A. Curtis MD
Emergency Medicine Physician
Department of Emergency Medicine
Georgetown University
Washington, District of Columbia, USA

Rita K. Cydulka MD, MS
Associate Professor and Vice Chair
Department of Emergency Medicine
MetroHealth Medical Center
Case Western Reserve University School of
Medicine
Cleveland, Ohio, USA

Jerrald Dankoff
Assistant Professor
Department of Emergency Medicine
McGill University
Montreal, Quebec
and Attending Staff

Department of Emergency Medicine
SMBD Jewish General Hospital
Montreal, Quebec, Canada

Richard Dart MD, PhD
Director
Rocky Mountain Poison and Drug Center
Denver, Colorado, USA

Jonathan Davidow MD
Staff Physician
Department of Emergency Medicine
University of Alberta
Edmonton, Alberta
and Division of Critical Care Medicine
University of Alberta Hospital
Edmonton, Alberta, Canada

Linda C. Degutis, DrPH
Associate Professor
Section of Emergency Medicine
Yale University
New Haven, Connecticut, USA

Barry Diner MD, MPH, FACEP
Assistant Professor
Department of Emergency Medicine
Emory University School of Medicine
Emory University
Atlanta, Georgia, USA

Dennis Djogovic MD, FRCPC
Assistant Clinical Professor
Department of Emergency Medicine
University of Alberta
Edmonton, Alberta
and Division of Critical Care Medicine
University of Alberta Hospital
Edmonton, Alberta, Canada

Sandy L. Dong MD, MSc, FRCPC, DABEM
Assistant Clinical Professor and RCPS Assistant
Program Director
Department of Emergency Medicine
University of Alberta
Edmonton, Alberta, Canada

Gail D'Onofrio MD, MS
Professor and Chair
Section of Emergency Medicine
Yale University
New Haven, Connecticut, USA

Marcia L. Edmonds MD, MSc
Staff Physician
Division of Emergency Medicine
University of Western Ontario
London, Ontario, Canada

Marcel Emond MD, MSc, FRCPC
Professor
Departments of Emergency Medicine
and Family Medicine
Laval University
Quebec, Canada

Barnet Eskin MD PhD
Assistant Research Director
Department of Emergency Medicine
Morristown Memorial Hospital
Morristown, New Jersey, USA

Jerome Fan MD, FRCP
Staff Physician
Department of Emergency Medicine
McMaster University
Hamilton, Ontario, Canada

Benjamin W. Friedman MD, MS
Assistant Professor
Department of Emergency Medicine
Albert Einstein College of Medicine
Montefiore Medical Center
Bronx, New York, USA

Theodore Gaeta DO, MPH
Vice-Chairman & Residency Director
Department of Emergency Medicine
New York Methodist Hospital
Brooklyn, New York, USA *and*
Associate Professor of Emergency in Clinical
Medicine
Weill Medical College of Cornell University
New York, USA

Ted Glynn MD, FACEP
Program Director
Michigan State University, Emergency Medicine
Residency, Lansing
and
Assistant Clinical Professor of Emergency
Medicine
Colleges of Human and Osteopathic Medicine
Michigan State University
East Lansing
and
Attending Physician
Ingham Regional Medical Center
Lansing, Michigan, USA

Peter W. Greenwald MD
Visiting Assistant Professor of Medicine
Division of Emergency Medicine
New York–Presbyterian Hospital
Weill Medical College of Cornell University
New York, USA

Stephen R. Hayden MD
Residency Director
Department of Emergency Medicine
University of California at San Diego
San Diego, California, USA

Katherine L. Heilpern MD
Residency Director
Ada Lee and Pete Correll Professor and Chair
Department of Emergency Medicine
Emory University School of Medicine
Emory University
Atlanta, Georgia, USA

Jeremy Hess MD, MPH
Assistant Professor
Departments of Emergency Medicine
and Environmental and Occupational Health
Emory University Schools of Medicine and Public
Health
Emory University
Atlanta, Georgia, USA

Elisabeth Hobden MD, FRCPC, Dip
Sport Med
Department of Emergency Medicine
The Ottawa Hospital
Ottawa, Ontario, Canada

Debra Houry MD, MPH
Director, Center for Injury Control
Vice Chair for Research
Department of Emergency Medicine,
Emory University
Atlanta, Georgia, USA

Andy Jagoda MD
Professor
Department of Emergency Medicine
Mount Sinai School of Medicine
New York, USA

Brett Jones MD, PhD
Staff Physician
Ya vapai Medical Center
Prescott, AZ, USA

Elizabeth B. Jones MD, FACEP
Assistant Professor
Department of Emergency Medicine
University of Texas Health Science Center
Houston, Texas, USA

Barbara M. Kirrane MD
Assistant Professor
Section of Emergency Medicine
Yale University
New Haven, Connecticut, USA

Sunil Kripalani MD, MSc
Assistant Professor
Division of General Internal Medicine and Public
Health
Vanderbilt University
Nashville, Tennessee, USA

Eddy S. Lang MDCM, CCFP(EM), CSPQ
Assistant Professor of Emergency Medicine
Department of Family Medicine
McGill University
Montreal, Quebec
and Attending Physician
Department of Emergency Medicine
SMBD Jewish General Hospital
Montreal, Quebec, Canada

Richard Lappin MD, PhD
Assistant Professor of Clinical Medicine
and Assistant Attending Physician
Department of Emergency Medicine
New York–Presbyterian Hospital
Weill Cornell Medical Center
New York, USA

Joel Lexchin MD
Professor, School of Health Policy and
Management
York University
Toronto, Ontario
and Associate Professor
Department of Family and Community Medicine
University of Toronto, Toronto
and Attending Staff
Emergency Department
University Health Network
Toronto, Canada

Kirk Magee MD, MSc, FRCP(C)
Associate Professor and RCPS Program Director
Department of Emergency Medicine
Dalhousie University
Halifax, Nova Scotia
and QEII Health Sciences Centre
Halifax Infirmary
Halifax, Nova Scotia, Canada

Tom Marrie MD, FRCPC
Professor and Dean
Faculty of Medicine and Dentistry
University of Alberta
Edmonton, Alberta, Canada

Chris McDowell MD
Department of Emergency Medicine
Indiana University School of Medicine
Indianapolis, Indiana, USA

Mary Patricia McKay, MD, MPH
Associate Professor
Department of Emergency Medicine
George Washington University
Washington, District of Columbia, USA

Ann McKibbon PhD
Associate Professor
Department of Clinical Epidemiology and
Biostatistics

McMaster University
Hamilton, Ontario, Canada

David W. Messenger MD
Assistant Professor
Department of Emergency Medicine
Queen's University
Kingston, Ontario, Canada

William J. Meurer MD
Lecturer in Emergency Medicine and Neurology
Department of Emergency Medicine
University of Michigan
Ann Arbor, Michigan, USA

Heather Murray MD, MSc, FRCP(C)
Assistant Professor
Departments of Emergency Medicine
and Community Health and Epidemiology
Queen's University
Kingston, Ontario, Canada

Denise Nassisi MD
Assistant Professor
Department of Emergency Medicine
Mount Sinai School of Medicine
New York, USA

James A. Nelson MD
Assistant Clinical Professor
Department of Emergency Medicine
University of California at San Diego
San Diego, California, USA

David H. Newman, MD
Assistant Professor
Department of Medicine
Columbia University College of Physicians
and Surgeons, New York
and
Director of Clinical Research
Department of Emergency Medicine
St. Luke's/Roosevelt Hospital Center
New York, USA

H. Bryant Nguyen MD, MS
Associate Professor
Departments of Emergency Medicine and
Medicine
Division of Pulmonary and Critical Care Medicine
Loma Linda University
Loma Linda, California, USA

Helen Ouyang MD, MPH
Resident Physician in Emergency Medicine
Department of Emergency Medicine
Brigham and Women's Hospital *and*
Massachusetts General Hospital
Boston, Massachusetts, USA

Linda Papa MD, MSc, CCFP, FRCP(C), FACEP
Director of Academic Clinical Research
Department of Emergency Medicine
Orlando Regional Medical Center
Orlando, Florida
and Adjunct Professor
Department of Emergency Medicine
College of Medicine, University of Florida
Gainsville, Florida
and Clinical Associate Professor
Florida State University College of Medicine
Tallahassee, Florida, USA

Jeffrey J. Perry MD, MSc, CCFP-EM
Assistant Professor
Department of Emergency Medicine
University of Ottawa
Ottawa, Ontario, Canada

Stephen R. Pitts
Associate Professor
Department of Emergency Medicine
Emory University School of Medicine
Emory Crawford Long Hospital
Atlanta, Georgia, USA

Anita Pozgay MD, FRCPC, Dip Sports Med
Assistant Professor
Department of Emergency Medicine
The Ottawa Hospital
Ottawa, Ontario, Canada

James Quinn MD, MS
Associate Professor of Surgery/Emergency Medicine
Division of Emergency Medicine
Stanford University
Stanford, California, USA

Michael S. Radeos MD
Research Director
Department of Emergency Medicine
New York Hospital Queens
Flushing, New York, USA

Ralph J. Riviello MD, MS, FACEP, FAAEM
Associate Professor Director of Clinical Research
and Associate Program Director
Department of Emergency Medicine
Thomas Jefferson University
Philadelphia, Pennsylvania, USA

Brian H. Rowe MD, MSc, CCFP(EM), FCCP
Professor and Research Director
Department of Emergency Medicine
University of Alberta
Edmonton, Alberta, Canada

Arthur B. Sanders MD
Professor
Department of Emergency Medicine
University of Arizona College of Medicine
Tucson, Arizona, USA

Nicola E. Schiebel MD, FRCPC
Assistant Professor
Department of Emergency Medicine
Mayo Clinic
Rochester, Minnesota, USA

Michael Schull MD, MSc, FRCPC
Senior Scientist
Institute for Clinical Evaluative Sciences
Toronto
and Director
Division of Emergency Medicine
Department of Medicine
University of Toronto
Toronto, Canada

Eli Segal
Staff Physician
Department of Family Medicine
McGill University
Montreal, Quebec
and Department of Emergency Medicine
SMBD Jewish General Hospital
Montreal, Quebec, Canada

Rawle A. Seupaul MD
Associate Professor of Clinical Emergency Medicine
Department of Emergency Medicine
Indiana University School of Medicine
Indianapolis, Indiana, USA

Ashley Shreves MD
Attending Physician
Department of Emergency Medicine
St. Luke's–Roosevelt Hospital
New York, USA

Michael Shuster MD, FRCPC
Staff Physician
Department of Emergency Medicine
Mineral Springs Hospital
Banff, Alberta, Canada

Robert Silbergleit MD
Associate Professor
Department of Emergency Medicine
University of Michigan
Ann Arbor, Michigan, USA

Richard Sinert DO
Associate Professor and Research Director
Department of Emergency Medicine
Downstate Medical Center
State University of New York
Brooklyn, New York, USA

Marco L. A. Sivilotti MD, MSc, FRCPC, FACEP, FACMT
Associate Professor
Departments of Emergency Medicine
and Pharmacology and Toxicology
Queen's University
Kingston, Ontario *and*
Consultant
Ontario Poison Centre
Toronto, Ontario, Canada

Errol Stern MDCM, FRCPC, FACEP, CSPQ
Assistant Professor
Department of Family Medicine
McGill University
Montreal, Quebec *and*
Attending Staff
Emergency Medicine
SMBD Jewish General Hospital
Montreal, Quebec, Canada

Michael Stern MD
Assistant Professor of Medicine
Department of Medicine
Division of Emergency Medicine
Weill Cornell Medical Center
New York, USA

Elisha David Targonsky BSc, MSc
Departmental Assistant
Department of Emergency Medicine *and*
Community Health and Epidemiology
Queen's University
Kingston, Ontario, Canada

Will Townend MD, FCEM
Department of Emergency Medicine
Hull Royal Infirmary
Hull, UK

Suneel Upadhye MD, MSc, FRCPC, ABEM
Assistant Clinical Professor
Division of Emergency Medicine
McMaster University
Hamilton, Ontario, Canada

Alain Vadeboncoeur MD, CCFP, CSPQ (EM)
Assistant Professor
Department of Family Medicine
University of Montreal
Montreal, Quebec
and Chief of Emergency Medicine
Montreal Heart Institute
Montreal, Quebec, Canada

Kurt Weber MD
Attending Physician
Department of Emergency Medicine
Orlando Regional Medical Center
Orlando, Florida
and Clinical Assistant Professor
Florida State University College of Medicine
Tallahassee, Florida, USA

Scott Weingart MD
Director
Division of Emergency Critical Care
Department of Emergency Medicine
Mount Sinai School of Medicine
New York, USA

Phil Wells MD, MSc, FRCPC
Professor and Chief
Division of Hematology
Department of Medicine
University of Ottawa
Ottawa, Ontario
and Director of Clinical Research
The Ottawa Hospital
Ottawa, Ontario, Canada

Ursula Whalen MD
Division of General Internal Medicine and Public
Health

Vanderbilt University
Nashville, Tennessee, USA

Andrew Worster MD, CCPF (EM), MSc, FCFP
Associate Professor
Emergency Medicine
Clinical Epidemiology & Biostatistics
McMaster University
Hamilton, Ontario, Canada

Peter C. Wyer MD
Associate Clinical Professor
Department of Medicine
Columbia University College of Physicians and
Surgeons
New York, USA

Mark Yarema MD, FRCPC
Division Chief, Research
Department of Emergency Medicine
Calgary Health Region
Calgary, Alberta, Canada

Benson Yeh MD
Residency Director
Department of Emergency Medicine
Brooklyn Hospital Center
Brooklyn, New York, USA

Luke Yip MD, FACMT, FACEM, FACEP
Consultant
Department of Emergency
The Prince Charles Hospital
Chermside, Queensland, Australia
and Attending Faculty
Rocky Mountain Poison and Drug Center
Denver, Colorado
and Attending Staff Physician
Department of Medicine
Division of Medical Toxicology
Denver Health Medical Center
Denver, Colorado
and Clinical Assistant Professor
School of Pharmacy
University of Colorado Health Sciences Center
Denver, Colorado, USA

Shahriar Zehtabchi MD
Associate Professor
Department of Emergency Medicine
Downstate Medical Center
State University of New York
Brooklyn, New York, USA

Foreword

Although the specialty of emergency medicine is only 40 years old, it has quickly matured into one of the most important arenas of practice in health care. In the United States, half of all hospital admissions and 11% of all outpatient health care encounters take place through emergency departments [1]. In Canada, which has placed a stronger emphasis on primary care, the percentages are smaller, but they are nonetheless substantial. Today, the term "ER" applies to more than a single room in the hospital, or even a popular television show. It is a comprehensive, multifaceted department that provides an astonishing array of advanced medical services, including rapid assessment and stabilization of patients with urgent or life-threatening conditions; medical direction of prehospital emergency medical services (EMS), cost-effective urgent care in specially designated "fast-track" areas, and detailed management of selected patients in emergency-department-based clinical decision units.

Practicing emergency medicine has always been challenging: patients arrive at all hours of the day and night; the range of problems emergency physicians encounter is incredibly broad; and the consequences of error are high. Undaunted, the doctors who established the specialty moved quickly to define its core competencies and teach them to a rapidly expanding circle of colleagues. They also worked diligently to secure recognition for their efforts in the House of Medicine. Almost as quickly, some of their number started figuring out how to make emergency care better.

Forty years later, the tens of millions of patients who annually seek care in hospital emergency departments and the tens of thousands of emergency physicians who treat them owe a debt of gratitude to the specialty's founders. Today, thousands of well-trained emergency physicians annually graduate from over 100 emergency medicine residency training programs in the United States and many more programs internationally. Across the developed world, modern emergency departments conduct comprehensive diagnostic evaluations and provide treatments that used to require a multiday stay in the hospital. In fact, emergency medicine has become such an integral component of modern health care that it is difficult to imagine how the system could function without it.

Concurrent with the growth and maturation of the specialty, emergency physicians have expanded their focus from providing life-saving care to whoever rolls through the door to medical direction of EMS and disaster medicine, education of medical students, residents and other health care professionals, performance of cutting-edge research, administrative leadership of emergency departments, hospitals and health systems, public health surveillance, *and* knowledge translation.

But all is not rosy. In some respects, emergency medicine has become a victim of its own success [2]. Over the past 15 years, society's growing reliance on emergency care has outstripped emergency medicine's capacity to meet this expanding need. In 2006, the Institute of Medicine (IOM) of the National Academies, a highly influential nongovernmental organization in the United States, issued three reports on the future of emergency care in the U.S. health system [3–5]. The picture it painted was troubling—despite dramatic improvements in emergency care, and the unquestioned dedication of those who provide it, the gap between public's need and system's capacity to meet it has grown so wide that hospital-based emergency care is (in the words of the IOM) at the "breaking point."

The IOM emergency care reports explicitly focused on the United States; however, many of its observations were equally germane to the emergency care systems of Canada, Australasia, Europe, and other parts of the developed world. Chief among these is the need to advance the quality, safety, and efficiency of emergency care through research, coupled with rapid translation of new knowledge to bedside care. The arguments for accelerating knowledge translation are compelling. The quickening pace of biomedical research and new developments in biomedical technology have dramatically expanded the diagnostic and treatment options available to emergency physicians. For example, advances in the detection of acute coronary syndrome and the discovery of thrombolytic therapy have given emergency physicians the ability to identify and abort many episodes of acute myocardial infarction before the condition causes death or irreversible harm. Moreover, other diseases that previously required many days of hospitalization (such as deep vein thrombosis, or DVT) can now be diagnosed by emergency physicians and managed in the outpatient setting.

As history has taught us, not every newly developed treatment is a resounding success. Many turn out to be less beneficial than originally claimed. Some tests and treatments are so skillfully marketed that they work their way into standard practice despite inadequate evidence of their effectiveness or an imperfect understanding of their risks. Historic examples include incidents of torsade de pointes following more widespread use of ibutalide for atrial fibrillation and the development of renal failure in some patients receiving nesiritide for heart failure. To add to the modern clinician's dilemma, sometimes a long-established mainstay of emergency care is overturned by new evidence. No one can predict which test or treatment in routine use today will join Ewald tubes, corticosteroids for head trauma, intravenous aminophylline, and military antishock trousers in the dustbin of emergency medicine history.

If old (and time-tested) is not necessarily good, and new (and more expensive) is not necessarily better, where can a busy practitioner turn for guidance? The traditional strategy—asking a senior colleague for advice—does not work anymore. Management by anecdote/experience is unreliable (see "old and time-tested," above). Expert consensus, also known as the BOGGSAT* approach, is little better. It often recycles conventional wisdom or falls for the latest fad. Industry claims should always be viewed with skepticism, especially when accompanied by food or gifts. And the latest peer-reviewed study, even one published in a prestigious journal, may be overturned by subsequent research.

Evidence-based medicine (EBM) was created to meet the clinician's need for objective guidance in patient care. A simple term for a very complex task, EBM is a rigorous approach to finding and analyzing the best available evidence on any clinical question. Because EBM respects the principle of patient autonomy, it does not limit its recommendations to "the best" test or treatment; it presents acceptable alternatives. Moreover, a clinician's experience is also valued in EBM as part of the decision-making process. Championed by international groups such as The Cochrane Collaboration [6], the EBM movement has tackled a growing list of questions. Many of them are relevant to emergency medicine [7].

This book was conceived to place the power and intellectual integrity of the EBM approach into the hands of busy emergency care providers. The brainchild of a group of Canadian and U.S. academic emergency physicians, *Evidence-based Emergency Medicine* (EBEM) takes a different tack than that of traditional textbooks. Rather than providing a detailed review of the pathophysiology of every condition, *EBEM* is designed to answer the direct, give-me-the-bottom-line questions emergency physicians ask in the middle of their shifts—questions like "How useful is D-dimer for detecting DVT, a problem I can't afford to miss?" (answer in Chapter 12) and "What is the best intervention for treating acute migraine headache among the many available to me?" (answer in Chapter 48).

To assemble this compilation, EBEM's chief editor Brian Rowe and his fellow section editors Eddy Lang, Debra Houry, Michael Brown, Dave Newman, and Peter Wyer tapped many of emergency medicine's leading experts in EBM and the book's topics. The result is a practical guide to thoughtful practice, based on the highest level of evidence available. Does this book represent the "final word" on these conditions? Absolutely not. The editors will be the first to acknowledge this. It does represent, however, the best evidence *currently available* from the world's literature on these topics. As more research is published, some of the recommendations may change in future editions. Medicine is not static; it grows and evolves over time. The editors expect that their *EBEM* textbook will do the same.

Will you find answers to every important question in this book? Not yet. This is, after all, a first edition. As the IOM pointed out in its *Future of Emergency Care* series, there is a pressing need for more research in emergency care. If you scour the pages of this book and cannot find an answer for *your* question, do not feel frustrated or give up. Rather, I suggest you contact the editors and volunteer to submit an evidence synthesis for the second edition of *Evidence-Based Emergency Medicine*.

Arthur L. Kellermann, MD, MPH
Professor and Associate Dean for Health Policy
Emory School of Medicine
Atlanta, Georgia, USA

References

1 Pitts SR, Niska RW, Xu J, Burt C. *National Hospital Ambulatory Medical Care Survey: 2006 Emergency Department Summary*. National Health Statistics Reports No. 7. U.S. Department of Health and Human Services, Centers for Disease Control and Prevention, National Center for Health Statistics, Rockville, MD (accessed August 6, 2008). http://www.cdc.gov/nchs/data/nhsr/nhsr007.pdf.

2 Kellermann AL. Crisis in the emergency department. *N Engl J Med* 2006;**355**(13):1300–3.

3 Institute of Medicine Committee on the Future of Emergency Care in the U.S. Health System. *Hospital Based Emergency Care: At the Breaking Point*. The National Academies Press, Washington, DC, 2006.

4 Institute of Medicine Committee on the Future of Emergency Care in the U.S. Health System. *Emergency Medical Services: At the Crossroads*. The National Academies Press, Washington, DC, 2006.

5 Institute of Medicine Committee on the Future of Emergency Care in the U.S. Health System. *Pediatric Emergency Care: Growing Pains*. The National Academies Press, Washington, DC, 2006.

6 The Cochrane Collaboration. Available at http://www.cochrane.org/ (accessed August 5, 2008).

7 Emond SD, Wyer PC, Brown MD, Cordell WH, Spooner CH, Rowe BH. How relevant are the systematic reviews in the Cochrane Library to emergency medical practice? *Ann Emerg Med* 2002;**39**:153–8.

---

* BOGGSAT = "Bunch of guys and gals sitting around a table."

Acknowledgments

The editors would like to acknowledge the publishers Wiley-Blackwell, and especially Ms. Mary Banks, for assisting in the early development of the *Evidence-based Emergency Medicine* idea. We would also like to express our sincerest appreciation to our development editor at Wiley-Blackwell, Ms. Laura Beaumont, for her guidance, patience and friendship during the production of this book. We wish her continued success in her future work. We would also like to thank the *Evidence-based Emergency Medicine* authors for their often Herculean efforts to produce the chapters that have contributed to the success of this book. We are indebted to Mirjana Misina for her careful guidance through production editing. Finally, as the editor, I would like to personally thank the section editors for their time, interest and dedication to the completion of this book.

Brian H. Rowe

List of Abbreviations

ABC	airway, breathing and circulation	ES	effect size
ACE	angiotension-converting enzyme	FAST	focused assessment with sonography for trauma
ACEP	American College of Emergency Physicians	FDA	US Food and Drug Administration
AHRQ	Agency for Healthcare Research and Quality	FEV_1	forced expiratory volume in one second
AP	anteroposterior	GCS	Glasgow Coma Score
ARR	absolute risk reduction	HA	Headache
ASA	acetyl-salicylic acid	HIV	human immunodeficiency virus
BET	best evidence topic	HR	hazard ratio
β_2-agonists	beta-2-receptor agonist agents	ICC	intraclass correlation coefficient
BMJ	*British Medical Journal*	ICD	International Classification of Disease
CADTH	Canadian Agency for Drugs and Technologies in Health	ICU	intensive care unit
		IM	intramuscular
CATS	critically appraised topics	INR	international normalized ratio
CDC	Centers for Disease Control and Prevention	IQR	inter-quartile range
CDSR	Cochrane Database of Systematic Reviews	IV	intravenous
CENTRAL	Cochrane Central Register of Controlled Trials	*JAMA*	*Journal of the American Medical Association*
CI	confidence interval	KT	knowledge translation
CINAHL	Compendium of International Nursing and Allied Health Literature	L	liters
		LMW	low molecular weight
CME	continuing medical education	LOS	length of stay
COPD	chronic obstructive pulmonary disease	LR	likelihood ratio
CPD	continuing professional development	LWBS	left without being seen
CPG	clinical practice guidelines	MDI	metered dose inhaler
CPR	clinical prediction rule	MEDLINE	National Library of Medicine electronic database
CT	computerized tomography	MeSH	medical subject heading
CXR	chest X-ray	mg	milligram
DARE	Database of Abstracts of Reviews of Effects	$MgSO_4$	magnesium sulfate
DSM	*Diagnostic and Statistical Manual of Mental Disorders*, 4th edn	MI	myocardial infarction
		ml	milliliters
DVT	deep vein thrombosis	MMSE	Mini Mental Status Examination
EBEM	evidence-based emergency medicine	MRI	magnetic resonance imaging
EBM	evidence-based medicine	MRSA	methicillin-resistant *Staphylococcus aureus*
ECG	electrocardiogram	NHS	UK National Health Service
ED	emergency department	NICE	National Institute for Health and Clinical Excellence
ELISA	enzyme-linked immunoadsorbent assay		
EMBASE	European-based electronic database maintained by Elsevier	NNH	number needed to harm
		NNT	number needed to treat
EMS	emergency medical services	NSAID	non-steroidal anti-inflammatory drug

O$_2$	oxygen	RRR	relative risk reduction
OR	odds ratio/s	SaO$_2$	oxygen saturation
PBL	problem-based learning	SARS	severe acute respiratory syndrome
PDSA	plan, do, study and act	SC	subcutaneous
PE	pulmonary embolism	SD	standard deviation
PEF	peak expiratory flow	SMD	standardized mean difference
PICO	population, intervention, control and outcome	SR	systematic review
PICO-D	population, intervention, control, outcome and design	STEMI	ST segment elevation myocardial infarction
		SVC	superior vena cava
PO	per oral	TBI	Traumatic brain injury
QI	quality improvement	TIA	transient ischemic attack
RCA	root cause analysis	t-PA	tissue plasminogen activator
RCE	Rational Clinical Examination Series of *JAMA*	VTE	venous thromboembolism
RCT	randomized controlled trial	WBC	white blood cell
ROC	receiver operating curve	WHO	World Health Organization
RR	relative risk/s	WMD	weighted mean difference

Evidence-Based Emergency Medicine: Companion Website

Additional resources to accompany this book are available at:

www.blackwellpublishing.com/medicine/bmj/emergencymedicine

This site provides:

- Useful **evidence-based online calculator**, free to download
- Useful links to **our other evidence-based resources** and to **external websites and information**
- An opportunity to **send us your feedback** on this book and on the Evidence Based series
- **Post-publication updates** added by the authors

1 General Issues

1 Introduction

Brian H. Rowe[1] & Peter C. Wyer[2]

[1]Department of Emergency Medicine, University of Alberta, Edmonton, Canada
[2]Department of Medicine, Columbia University College of Physicians and Surgeons, New York, USA

Case scenario

A 25-year-old woman presented to an emergency department (ED) with an exacerbation of her migraine headaches. Her migraine headaches had previously been well controlled; however, stressful conflicts had recently occurred at work, she had not been able to sleep properly for two nights and she admitted unusually low fluid intake for the previous 2 days. She reported that her headache developed gradually, was associated with nausea and vomiting, and she rated the headache as 9 on a 10-point headache pain scale. She denied fever, syncope or other signs of pathological headaches, and assessed the episode as being "similar to my last migraine headache that brought me to the emergency department 2 years ago".

She improved quickly with intravenous saline and metoclopramide and was ready for discharge home after 90 minutes. Her headache at reassessment was 1 out of 10 and her nausea had resolved. The patient informed you that she was late for an important work meeting that would consume her time for the next 2 days and wondered what she could do to minimize the risk of suffering a recurrence.

Introduction

What is *evidence-based emergency medicine* (EBEM) and why is there such a controversy over the concept and contempt for the phrase? The term evidence-based medicine (EBM) was first coined in the early 1990s by Gordon Guyatt [1] and has now become a stable in the medical lexicon. In addition to EBM's long history, controversy exists regarding its components and value in decision making [2,3]. In most cases, however, it can be described as the combined use of experience, best evidence

Evidence-based Emergency Medicine. Edited by Brian H. Rowe
© 2009 Blackwell Publishing, ISBN: 978-1-4051-6143-5.

and patient's preference and values to develop an approach to a clinical problem, often referred to as *evidence-based medical care.*

The migraine headache example may help readers better understand the concept. The patient's question related to prevention of headache and this topic is well covered in the chapter on migraine headaches in this book (See chapter 48). From an evidence perspective, the well-informed clinician knows that there is evidence that a dose of dexamethasone in the emergency department (ED) (best evidence based on a systematic review (SR) of randomized controlled trials (RCTs)) is helpful [4]. Moreover, experience reminds the clinician that patients with moderate to severe migraine headaches also can deteriorate, re-present to the ED, and/or lose valuable time from work and other activities (clinical experience). The clinician is concerned and wishes to protect the patient from any and all of these events (and so does her employer). Unfortunately, the patient protests this decision because corticosteroids cause her to develop acne, retain water and have insomnia. She also has a major weekend function and feels these medications may create havoc with her social life. Despite the clinician's reassurances, she refuses the intravenous corticosteroid treatment (patient preference and values). Readers in clinical practice will be very familiar with this type of scenario.

What is the evidence-based decision in this case? Some traditionalists may suggest that their decision is final and the patient should accept the corticosteroid treatment. The EBM clinician might further use the available evidence to explain the benefits and risks of treatment options, in conjunction with the patient's preference and his/her experience. In the event that agreement cannot be reached between the clinician and the patient, the EBEM approach would propose an alternative "next-best evidence" and similarly reasonable approach. For example, the clinician may recognize that reduction of pain to less than two out of ten reduces headache relapse [5]. Moreover, the addition of education about triggers and very close follow-up may improve outcomes in such patients. It is this combination of evidence, patient preference and clinical experience that coalesces to form the EBEM decision.

Why EBEM?

The EBM approach may seem intuitive to many emergency practitioners. However, when originally proposed, debate ensued, and in some cases continues [6,7]. This forces the question: why is this being proposed in emergency medicine? In a therapy issue, clinicians must ultimately decide whether the benefits of treatment are worth the costs, inconvenience, and harms associated with the care. This is often a difficult task; however, it is made more difficult by the exponentially increasing volume of literature and the lack of time to search and distill this evidence [8]. Although clinicians of the early 21st century have an urgent need for just-in-time, on-demand clinical information, their time to access such information has likely never been as compressed. Increases in patient volume and complexity, patient care demands, and the lack of access to resources have exacerbated the work frustrations for many clinicians. These concerns often take precedence over seeking the most relevant, up-to-date and comprehensive evidence for patient problems.

Despite the fact that the most common problems posed by patients presenting to emergency rooms are encountered daily around the world, appropriate treatment approaches are often not fully employed and practice variation is impressive. For a variety of reasons, the results from high level evidence such as RCTs are not readily available to busy clinicians and keeping up to date is becoming increasingly difficult. Moreover, a valid, reliable and up-to-date clinical bottom line to guide treatment decisions has been elusive [8].

However, availability of high quality published trials and systematic reviews relevant to an area of practice are not the only components necessary to practicing "best evidence medicine". Clinicians also need rigorously produced, synthesized best evidence information to assist them at the point of care. In emergency care, time is increasingly more precious and the need for this digestible information has never been greater.

Levels of evidence

A wide variety of tools to describe levels of evidence have been developed and employed in clinical medicine to reflect the degree of confidence to which results from research may be accepted as valid. From levels of evidence, strengths of recommendations are generated which are graded according to the strength of the scientific evidence supporting them. These levels of evidence can be criticized for being different with each set of guidelines or report, being overly complex, and being almost universally focused on therapeutic interventions.

Recently, a group of experts in the field of guidelines introduced a grading system as part of an effort to develop a single approach supported by international consensus. The Grades of Recommendation, Assessment, Development and Evaluation (GRADE) Working Group have published their recommendations, which have been adopted by increasing numbers of specialty and health policy organizations [9]. The GRADE system classifies quality of evidence into one of four levels (high, moderate, low and very low) and quality of recommendations in one of two levels (strong and weak).

Once again, an example may be illustrative. In the case scenario described above dealing with therapy, the highest level of evidence (HIGH) is based on RCTs. A single RCT can retain HIGH grading if there are no study limitations, the threats to validity are low, the association is strong and adjustments for all potential confounders have been performed. Although HIGH status is awarded to RCTs, many trials in emergency medicine are not large enough to maintain this evidence status. The evidence would similarly retain its HIGH ranking if meta-analysis of two or more similar trials show consistency of effect and statistically significant relative risk (RR) results (> 2.0 or < 0.5 for reduction) [10]. Fortunately, in this case, the systematic review does support the single clinical trial identified (see Chapter 48).

While considerable debate exists regarding the relative merits of evidence derived from large individual trials versus systematic reviews [11], due to the costs associated with large, multi-centered trials, they remain uncommon across emergency medicine and remain restricted to certain topic areas (e.g., cardiology, rheumatology, stroke, and so forth). While examples of large databases and observational studies do exist in emergency medicine [12], smaller studies are much more common. Consequently, it is likely that systematic reviews will play an increasingly important role in the future decisions made by patients, clinicians, administrators and society in all areas of health care.

MODERATE evidence is based on RCTs that contain flaws that preclude a HIGH evidence rating or observational studies. The RCTs may show either positive trends that are not statistically significant or no trends and are associated with a high risk of false-negative results. The observational studies may be elevated to HIGH evidence (from LOW) in certain cases, such as when a statistically significant relative risk of > 5 (< 0.2) is identified based on direct evidence with no major threats to validity.

Finally, a LOW level of evidence is based on observational studies of any kind (e.g., cohorts, case series, case–control studies or cross-sectional studies). VERY LOW grading can be achieved when evidence is based on observational studies of low quality or the opinion of respected authorities or expert committees as indicated in published consensus conferences or guidelines.

In diagnostic studies, the same rules apply; however, most of the studies in this setting are not RCTs. Given the relatively recent development of the GRADE system, the editors of this text have not required authors to apply this in each chapter; although, given the summary of evidence provided in each chapter, readers should be able to rate the evidence presented using the general guide. Moreover, future editions of the book will focus on GRADE or similar systems of evidence assessment.

Levels of evidence and systematic reviews

As discussed above, one possible solution to the information dilemma for clinicians is to focus on evidence from systematic reviews (SRs) [13]. SRs address a focused clinical question, utilize comprehensive search strategies to avoid publication and selection biases, assess the quality of the evidence and, if appropriate, employ meta-analytic summary statistics to synthesize the results from research on a particular topic with a defined protocol. They represent an important and rapidly expanding body of literature for the clinician dealing with patients presenting to the emergency setting and they are an integral component of EBM.

Although there has been a recent increase in the production of diagnostic testing SRs, the most common application of SRs is in therapeutic interventions in clinical practice. One important exception is the Rational Clinical Examination (RCE) series published in the *Journal of the American Medical Association* (*JAMA*). This series presents SRs in the field of diagnostic testing (especially clinical examination and laboratory/imaging testing). Finally, the Cochrane Collaboration has developed a Diagnostic Methods Working Group and is planning to introduce diagnostic test systematic reviews to their collection of products in the near future. Unfortunately, the methodology of diagnostic SRs lags behind that of the therapeutic SRs; however, there are strong indications that this is changing.

Despite publications illustrating the importance of methodological quality in conducting and reporting both RCTs [14] and SRs [15], not all SRs are created using the same rigorous methods described above. Like most other research, variable methodological quality has been identified in systematic reviews. High-quality SRs of therapies attempt to identify the literature on a specific therapeutic intervention using a structured, *a priori* and well-defined methodology contained in a protocol. Rigorously conducted SRs are recognizable by their avoidance of publication and selection bias. For example, they include foreign language, both published and unpublished literature, and employ well-described comprehensive search strategies to avoid publication bias. Their trial selection includes studies with similar populations, interventions/controls, outcomes and methodologies and use of more than one "reviewer" to select included studies.

Systematic reviews regarding therapy would most commonly combine evidence from RCTs. In the event that statistical pooling is possible and clinically appropriate, the resultant pooled estimate represents the best "summary estimate" of the treatment effect. A systematic review with summary pooled statistics is referred to as a *meta-analysis*, while one is without summary data is referred to as a *qualitative systematic review*. Both of these options represent valid approaches to reporting SRs and both are now increasingly commonly published in the medical literature.

In the field of emergency medicine, SRs have been evaluated and found to contain serious flaws that potentially introduce bias into their conclusions [16]. This is an alarming picture for the profession, and one that needs to be addressed by members as well as authors and journal editors. Most of this research was completed prior to the establishment of the QUOROM (Quality of Reporting of Meta-analyses) statement; however, recent evidence suggests that this situation has not resulted in dramatic improvements in the quality of published SRs [17]. Consequently, ED physicians must be vigilant in their search for and evaluation of SRs as they pertain to this field.

The Cochrane Collaboration

The Cochrane Collaboration, a multinational, volunteer, collaborative effort on the part of researchers, clinicians from all medical disciplines, and consumers, represents one source of high-quality systematic review information available to most clinicians with very little effort [18]. The Cochrane Library is a compendium of databases and related instructional tools. As such, it is the principal product of the large international volunteer effort in the Cochrane Collaboration.

Within the Collaboration, specific review groups are responsible for developing, completing and updating SRs in specific topic areas. For example, the Cochrane Airway Group (CAG: www.cochrane-airways.ac.uk) is responsible for "airway" topics (e.g., asthma, chronic obstructive pulmonary disease, pulmonary embolism). Reviewers within the Cochrane review groups represent consumers, researchers, physicians, nurses, physiotherapists, educators and others interested in the topic areas. Not all review groups have produced acute care reviews; however, ED topics are particularly well covered by some (e.g., CAG) [19]. Recently the relevance of the Cochrane Collaboration effort to emergency medicine has been enhanced through the advent of the Cochrane Prehospital and Emergency Health Field (CPEHF: www.cochranepehf.org), which is expected to substantially increase the number of reviews with direct relevance to this specialty [20].

Systematic reviews produced by members of the Cochrane Collaboration are the products of *a priori* research protocols, meet rigorous methodological standards, and are peer reviewed for content and methods prior to dissemination. Specifically, this process of review production is designed to reduce bias and ensure validity, using criteria discussed in the *JAMA* User's Guide series [21]. As much as possible, this text book will focus on evidence derived from SRs, and as often as possible, those contained within the Cochrane Library.

The Cochrane Library and emergency medicine

The Cochrane Library is comprised of several databases, three of which deserve some description and discussion here as they relate to this EBEM textbook. The Cochrane Central Register of Controlled Trials (CENTRAL) is an extensive bibliographic database of controlled trials that has been identified through structured searches of electronic databases, and hand-searching by Cochrane review groups. Currently, it contains over 300,000 references (Cochrane Library, 2007, Issue 4) and can function as a primary literature searching approach with therapeutic topics. The Database of Abstracts of Reviews of Effects (DARE) consists of critically appraised structured abstracts of non-Cochrane published reviews that meet standards set by the Centre for Reviews and Dissemination at the University of York, England. Currently, DARE contains over 3500 reviews (Cochrane Library, 2007, Issue 4). The last, and possibly most important, resource is the Cochrane Database of Systematic Reviews (CDSR), a compilation of regularly updated SRs with meta-analytic summary statistics. Currently, the CDSR contains over 1200 protocols and 3500 completed reviews (Cochrane Library, 2007, Issue 4). Contents of the CDSR are contributed by Cochrane review groups, representing various medical topic areas (e.g., airways, stroke, heart, epilepsy, etc.). Within the CDSR, "protocols" describe the objectives of SRs that are in the process of being completed; "completed reviews" include the full text, and usually present summary statistics. Both protocols and reviews are produced using a priori criteria, adhere to rigorous methodological standards and undergo peer review prior to publication. Regular "updates" are required to capture new evidence and address criticisms and/or identified errors.

The quality of systematic reviews contained within the Cochrane Library has been shown to be consistently high for individual topic areas as well as throughout the Cochrane Collaboration [22,23]. Recent evidence evaluated the quality of a random selection of SRs published in 2004 and, long after the production of the QUOROM guidelines, found some intriguing results [24]. First and foremost, the volume of SRs identified suggested a rapid proliferation of SRs in health care. Second, 71% of the reviews involved a therapeutic area, recapitulating our previous comment about SRs being less common in diagnostic areas. Finally, there were large differences identified between Cochrane and non-Cochrane reviews in the quality of reporting several important characteristics; Cochrane reviews were rated as higher quality. Overall, the reviewers reiterated the variable quality of some reviews in the literature and the need to be cautious when using these reviews in health care decisions.

Prehospital and emergency medicine involvement has been limited across the Cochrane Collaboration and in many review groups, consequently topics of interest to emergency physicians have perhaps not been a priority. The development of the CPEHF in 2004 was an important milestone for evidence-based prehospital and emergency medicine [25]. CPHEF was registered as an official entity of the Cochrane Collaboration and now has more than 3000 registered members (F. Archer, personal communication). The focus of CPEHF is prehospital (management up to the delivery in the emergency department), emergency (up to hospitalization) and disaster medicine. One of the functions of the field is to develop and maintain a register of studies relevant to the areas of prehospital and emergency health care. CPEHF has developed a validated search strategy to identify SRs and reports of trials in the Cochrane Library that are based on research that was conducted in the prehospital environment [26].

Evidence-based Emergency Medicine format

We are excited about highlighting the approaches to the diagnosis and treatment of common emergency conditions that will be detailed in this book. The editors of *Evidence-based Emergency Medicine* have attempted to select experts in both emergency medicine (content) as well as evidence-based medicine (methodology) to author this text. Following this introductory section, the remainder of the chapters will focus on individual topic areas.

The chapters in this book have all been organized in a similar fashion using the following format:

1 *Case scenario/vignette*: Each chapter author has been asked to describe a patient scenario upon which the remainder of the chapter will be based. Authors have been instructed to provide a real-world clinical problem.

2 *Questions that arise from the case*: Using the PICO methodology described below, questions will be developed from each clinical case. These clinical scenarios will be used to identify important questions relevant to the diagnosis, therapy, adverse effects, and so forth of conditions commonly encountered in emergency practice. While these questions are not all inclusive, they do represent key questions following discussion among the authors and the section editors.

3 *Literature search*: A brief description of the search strategies employed to identify the relevant research used to answer the clinical question will be provided. In general, the evidence from systematic reviews, especially those available in the Cochrane Library, the *JAMA* RCE series and large health technology assessment (HTA) resources (e.g., Agency for Healthcare Research and Quality (AHRQ: www.ahrq.com), Canadian Agency for Drugs and Technologies in Health (CADTH: www.cadth.ca), National Institute for Health and Clinical Excellence (NICE: www.nice.uk)), will be highlighted.

4 *Summary critical appraisal*: A summary of the available evidence will be provided by the authors, focusing on the key results and their implications. Some authors have elected to produce summary of evidence tables.

5 *Answers/conclusions*: A summary approach to the patient will be presented at the end of each chapter.

Question development

Although we have not rigorously followed the methodology of SRs in this book, there is one aspect of that methodology that we have strictly followed. Each chapter is developed around specific clinical questions. Although most chapters include some background discussion of the topic areas, readers will find that these are much more condensed than they would expect from other emergency medicine textbooks and are limited to materials directly relevant to the specific questions.

Patients presenting with many of the signs and symptoms presented in this book represent typical cases commonly encountered in clinical emergency practice. Many potentially important questions arise from these encounters; all of these questions vary based on the perspective or the person asking the question (e.g., clinician, patient, administrators, primary care providers, public health officers and government policy makers). For example, using the example above, what is the *etiology* of this patient's acute migraine headache? What *diagnostic tests* should be performed (if any) and which can the health care system afford? What *therapy* could be prescribed in the ED to treat the headache? What *additional* therapy can be prescribed in order to reduce the chances of continued headache? What is her *prognosis* over the next 3 weeks with respect to her migraine status? Would instituting a prophylactic therapy improve the *long-term prognosis* for this woman? Finally, would educational interventions *prevent* further exacerbations or reduce their severity?

The success of any search for answers to such clinical questions is spelling them out in a detailed and systematic way [27]. While this skill is important for the policy maker in the office, the patient searching for options, and the researcher performing a systematic review, it is perhaps most important for the busy clinician at the bedside. Some have referred to this process as developing an "answerable question". This is because such an approach, among other things, provides an immediate basis for formulating and executing an effective search strategy for locating relevant and high-quality clinical evidence. In this book we report both general and specific search strategies in connection with the specific questions addressed in each chapter.

Components of a good question

Designing an appropriate clinical question includes consideration of the components of a good question (described below), compartmentalizing the topic area and describing the design of studies to be included. All questions should include focused details on the **p**opulation, **i**ntervention, assessment or exposure (and **c**omparison when relevant), and **o**utcomes associated with the question. This approach is often abbreviated as PICO, but these are only part of the components necessary for developing the question. Each component is examined in further detail below and examples illustrated in Table 1.1.

1 *Population*: A clearly defined population under consideration is the first step in developing a successful question; however, this can be a difficult task at times. The selection should be based on the interests and needs of the clinician and the patient's problem.

2 *Intervention, assessment or exposure*: Well-defined interventions must be articulated prior to searching for answers. For example, corticosteroids may be particularly problematic in searches for migraine headaches. Since corticosteroids can be administered via many routes (e.g., intravenous (IV), oral and intramuscular (IM)) in migraine headache treatment, using varying doses and over different duration, these must all be considered when searching for evidence. Moreover, the use of different agents is common (e.g., dexamethasone, prednisone, methylprednisolone, and so forth) and is clearly an important consideration in question development. Diagnostic assessments are also interventions and when the results are compared to a criterion standard for the disease or condition being sought, performance measures such as sensitivity, specificity and likelihood ratios can be derived. Harmful exposures are not quite the same as "interventions" in that we avoid knowingly recommending them to our patients.

3 *Comparisons*: Most therapeutic interventions are compared to a control treatment. In some cases, the comparison is to a placebo; however, in emergency medicine the comparison is often to standard practice at the time or known effective therapies. For example, in the chapter on migraine headaches, the effectiveness of corticosteroids in preventing recurrent headaches is compared to placebo; however, both groups received standard abortive care in the ED. In the chapter on acute asthma, the effectiveness of inhaled corticosteroids to reduce relapse after discharge is compared to placebo; once again, both groups received standard care (7 days of oral prednisone and short-acting β-agonists) at discharge. It is important for researchers to use the correct dose, route of delivery and timing of treatment in order to determine the true benefit (or harm) of the intervention compared to standard care/placebo in drug trials. This is equally important when the intervention is a non-drug treatment (e.g., education, procedure, technology, etc.), since this will ensure valid comparisons of the intervention and the control.

4 *Outcome*: There are a variety of outcomes reported in any emergency or acute care research study. For example, in acute cardiac studies disposition (e.g., death, admission/discharge, relapse, etc.), clinical outcomes (e.g., recurrent angina, myocardial infarction, pericarditis, etc.), interventions (e.g., angioplasty, coronary artery bypass grafting, etc.), physiological parameters (e.g., vital signs, oxygen saturation, etc.), medication use (e.g., β-blocker use, aspirin use, etc.), adverse effects (e.g., tremor, nausea, tachycardia, etc.), complications (e.g., arrhythmia, pneumonia, etc.), and symptoms (e.g., quality of life, specific symptoms, etc.) may all be reported. In other diseases, some of these events would be rare (e.g., intubation in asthma or discharge in myocardial infarction), and seeking evidence for the influence of interventions on these outcomes would be fruitless. The clinician must select appropriate primary and secondary outcomes prior to beginning their evidence search. The primary outcome should reflect the outcome that is most important to the clinicians, patients, policy makers and/or consumers.

Table 1.1 Example of the PICO methodology for developing clinically appropriate questions in emergency medicine (see text for further details).

Population	Intervention/control	Outcome	Design	Topic
Adults with migraine headache in the ED	Metoclopramide vs systemic DHE	Pain relief and relapses after discharge	RCT	Therapy
Adults with new onset COPD	Exposure to work-related or environmental irritants	Development of COPD	Prospective cohort	Etiology
Adults in the ED with acute swollen leg and chest pain	Use of Well's criteria vs unstructured clinical exam	Diagnosis of DVT/PE	Prospective cohort	Diagnosis
ED adult migraine headache patients discharged home	Corticosteroids vs control	Relapse to additional care	RCT	Therapy/prognosis
Adult contacts of a documented case of meningitis	Ciprofloxacin vs hygiene practices	Prevention of meningitis	RCT	Prevention

COPD, chronic obstructive pulmonary disease; DHE, dihydroergotamine; DVT, deep vein thrombosis; ED, emergency department; RCT, randomized controlled trial; PE, pulmonary embolism.

Often the clinician may also be interested in secondary outcomes, side-effects and patient preference. While patient preference is not often reported in clinical trials and therefore SRs, side-effects and secondary outcomes are commonly encountered. The importance of secondary outcomes is that if their pooled results are concordant with that of the primary outcome, this adds corroborating evidence to the conclusion. In addition, side-effect profiles provide the patients, clinician and others with the opportunity to evaluate the risks associated with the treatment. Unfortunately, the lack of uniform reporting of side-effects often precludes these outcomes from being evaluated with any rigor.

Improving efficiency in question development

Two additional components to be considered in the development of an answerable question for a clinical case are the topic area and the study methodology or design [27].

1 *Topic areas*: While selecting between topic areas may initially appear straightforward, there can be confusion. For example, is chest computerized tomography (CT) testing in pulmonary embolism a diagnostic or a prognostic topic? Clearly, the use of chest CT has been examined as a diagnostic tool compared to clinical signs and symptoms, and a review in this area would encompass a diagnostic domain. When CT testing is used to predict outcome (e.g., death, length of stay, etc.) and complications (e.g., pulmonary hypertension) then the topic would be considered a prognostic question. Since there are other domains of systematic reviews (including therapy, prevention and etiology), by selecting the topic of the clinical question, this further clarifies the approach for the clinician.

2 *Design*: The design of the studies to be selected should also be carefully considered in the initial question formulation. For example, if one is interested in a therapeutic topic, the best level of evidence (HIGH) includes results from large RCTs or SRs [28,29]. The next level of evidence might be small RCTs, which are insufficiently powered. Finally, observational studies (e.g., cohort, case–control, case series) would be considered lower levels of evidence for treatment. It is therefore appropriate and efficient for initial searches for therapy answers to be limited to systematic reviews and randomized controlled trials.

Locating the evidence: literature searching

Clearly, we cannot do justice to literature searching in an introductory chapter on evidence-based emergency medicine. Searching for evidence is a complex and time-consuming task, especially with the rapid growth of journals and publications which has increased the body of evidence available in the peer-reviewed published literature. For example, to ensure that one has identified all relevant possible citations pertaining to a clinical problem, simple searching is often ineffective [30]. Search of MEDLINE, the bibliographic database of the National Library of Medicine, for RCTs using a non-comprehensive search strategy will miss nearly half of the relevant publications, depending on the specialty and topic area [31]. In addition, by not adding other electronic searches (e.g., EMBASE, the European-based electronic database maintained by Elsevier), clinicians run the risk of missing considerable evidence [32]. Hand-searching has been shown to increase the yield of RCT searches; however, this is an unreasonable task for busy clinicians and many researchers [32]. Finally, unpublished and foreign language literature may contain important information relevant to your patient's problem and should not be excluded. Given the volume of literature, the search strategies required and the need for multi-lingual translation, it is hardly surprising that clinicians find it difficult to obtain all of the relevant articles on a particular question in a timely fashion. Several strategies can be used to address this issue. One strategy is to target searches, using designated filters (Table 1.2) [8]. Another, and the choice of this text, is to search for high-quality systematic reviews, especially in therapy, to answer important clinical questions [33]. Finally, seeking the advice of a librarian knowledgeable in the various electronic resources, search terms and search strategies is always worthwhile.

Table 1.2 Common search strategies for identifying evidence from electronic databases using search filters.

Topic	Highest level design	Search terms
Therapy	RCT	Publication type: RCT; controlled clinical trial; clinical trial MeSH headings: RCTs; random allocation; double blind; single blind; placebo(s)
Therapy	SR	Publication type: review; SR; meta-analysis MeSH headings: MEDLINE
Diagnosis	Prospective cohort	Publication type: diagnosis MeSH headings: sensitivity and specificity Text word: sensitivity
Prevention	RCT, SR	See above for RCT and SR
Etiology	Prospective cohort	Text word: risk

MeSH, medical subject heading; RCT, randomized controlled trial; SR, systematic review.

Clinical epidemiology terminology

There is a unique lexicon used in clinical epidemiology in general and in systematic reviews in particular. It may be helpful to readers for the editors to describe several of the important terms here (also see the list of abbreviations in the prelims) since they are used frequently in the forthcoming chapters. Publication bias and selection bias are two important terms. Publication bias refers to the publication of positive results faster, in higher impact journals, and to the exclusion of negative results in the medical literature [34]. Publication bias can be reduced when authors search widely and comprehensively for all published and unpublished literature, irrespective of the publication status, journals or language of publication. Bias can occur in the selection of evidence to cite and can be reduced when multiple authors independently decide which articles to select for evidence synthesis. While this is a problem in many areas of medicine, it seems less of an issue in emergency medicine [34].

The reporting of statistical issues in EBM and especially SRs is particularly important to understand. For dichotomous variables (e.g., admit/discharge, relapse/no relapse, event/no event), individual statistics are usually calculated as odds ratios (OR) or relative risks (RR) with 95% confidence intervals (CIs). Pooling of individual trials is accomplished using sophisticated statistical techniques that employ either a fixed or random effects model. The "weight" of each trial's contribution to the overall pooled result is inversely related to the trial's variance. In practical terms, for dichotomous outcomes, this is largely a function of sample size: the larger the trial, the greater contribution it makes to the pooled estimate.

The results of most efforts to quantitatively pool data are represented as Forrest plots and these figures will be used extensively by authors in this textbook. In such displays, the convention is that the effects favoring the treatment in question are located to the left of the line of unity (1.0), while those favoring the control or comparison arm are located to the right of the line of unity. When the 95% CI of the pooled estimate crosses the line of unity, the result is considered non-significant (Fig. 1.1). In addition, tests of statistical significance are also provided.

For continuous outcomes, weighted mean differences (WMDs) or standardized mean differences (SMDs) and 95% CIs are usually reported. The use of the WMD is common in many systematic reviews and is the difference between the experimental and control group outcomes, when similar units of measure are used [35]. The SMD is used when different units of measure are used for the same outcome. For continuous variables with similar units (e.g., airflow measurements), a WMD or effect size (ES) is calculated. The "weight" of each trial's contribution to the overall pooled result is based on the inverse of the trial's variance. In practical terms, for continuous outcomes, this is largely a function of the standard deviation (SD) and sample size: the lower the SD and the larger the sample size, the greater contribution the study makes to the pooled estimate. For continuous measures with variable units (such as quality of life or other functional scales), the use of an SMD is often used. For example, if quality of life were measured using the same instrument in all studies, a WMD would be performed; however, if the quality of life was measured using multiple methods all producing a "score", an SMD would be calculated. For both the SMD and WMD, the convention is the opposite of that for dichotomous variables, that is, effects favoring the treatment in question are located to the right of the line of unity (0) while those favoring the control or comparison arm are plotted to the left. Once again, when the 95% CI crosses the line of no effect, the result is considered non-significant.

Number needed to treat (NNT) is another method of expressing a measure of effect [36]. In the reviews contained in the Cochrane Library, the absolute risk reduction (ARR) is represented by the risk reduction statistic, and the inverse of this (and its 95% CI) provides the NNT estimation. Another convenient method to calculate the NNT is to use on-line calculators (www.nntonline.net). Finally, less exact methods are available to estimate the NNT; however, caution is advised, since these approaches often result in gross approximations of NNT.

Heterogeneity among pooled estimates is usually tested and reported [37]. There are a number of ways of describing

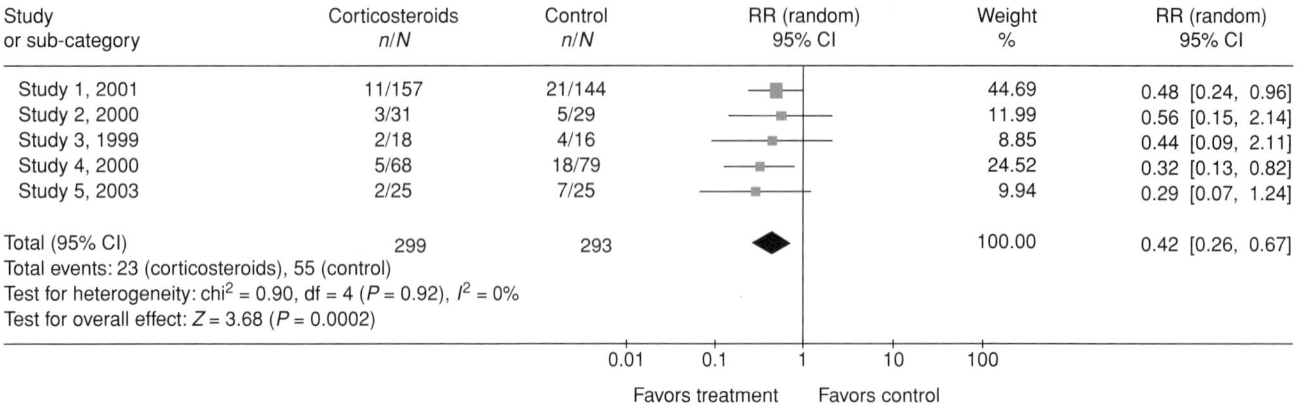

Study or sub-category	Corticosteroids n/N	Control n/N	RR (random) 95% CI	Weight %	RR (random) 95% CI
Study 1, 2001	11/157	21/144		44.69	0.48 [0.24, 0.96]
Study 2, 2000	3/31	5/29		11.99	0.56 [0.15, 2.14]
Study 3, 1999	2/18	4/16		8.85	0.44 [0.09, 2.11]
Study 4, 2000	5/68	18/79		24.52	0.32 [0.13, 0.82]
Study 5, 2003	2/25	7/25		9.94	0.29 [0.07, 1.24]
Total (95% CI)	299	293		100.00	0.42 [0.26, 0.67]

Total events: 23 (corticosteroids), 55 (control)
Test for heterogeneity: chi^2 = 0.90, df = 4 (P = 0.92), I^2 = 0%
Test for overall effect: Z = 3.68 (P = 0.0002)

0.01   0.1   1   10   100

Favors treatment   Favors control

Figure 1.1 Typical systematic review summary figure (referred to as a Forrest plot) used in therapy trials. Note: that in this Forrest plot, five trials have been conducted that compared corticosteroids to placebo to prevent a relapse event. Each study is represented by the point estimate for the outcome in question and by confidence intervals on either side of that value. The vertical line corresponds to a relative risk (RR) of 1.0; studies where the confidence interval crosses the 1.0 line (studies 2, 3 and 5) demonstrate no statistically significant difference between the groups (i.e., those receiving any corticosteroids versus those receiving placebo). Values to the left and *not* crossing the vertical line (studies 1 and 4) indicate a clear benefit of corticosteroids. Values to the right and *not* crossing the vertical line (Study 1 and 4 in this example), indicate that patients receiving placebo had better outcomes than those receiving corticosteroids. The large horizontal black diamond at the bottom of the figure corresponds to the pooled results of the individual studies. The "weight" column represents the percentage contribution of each study to the pooled result. The individual and pooled RR and 95% CIs are displayed to the right of the diagram. Finally, the test for heterogeneity of the pooled result and the overall effect are depicted in the left lower corner as both I^2 and chi-squared statistics (see text for further details).

heterogeneity statistically; the Cochrane reviews often report the I-squared (I^2) statistic [38]. Pooled statistics assessed for heterogeneity using the I^2 statistic are provided with a percentage measurement of heterogeneity; heterogeneity can broadly be classified as limited ($I^2 < 30\%$), moderate ($30\% < I^2 < 75\%$) or severe ($I^2 > 75\%$). Sensitivity and subgroup analyses are often performed to identify sources of heterogeneity, when indicated. Caution has been advised when interpreting subgroup analyses and practical approaches to them have been published [39].

Collecting and interpreting the evidence for clinical practice

Evidence-based medicine relies on the synthesis and reporting of evidence using a format that may be unfamiliar to clinicians (see lexicon above). With multiple publications on a specific topic often identified, some evidence can be summarized statistically as pooled likelihood ratio (LR) for diagnostic test questions or

Organization	Website address
Cochrane Collaboration	http://www.cochrane.org
Cochrane Prehospital and Emergency Health Field (CPEHF)	http://www.cochranepehf.org
Bandolier (various EBM topics)	http://www.jr2.ox.ac.uk/bandolier/
Annals of Emergency Medicine EBEM Section	http://www.annemergmed.com
BestBets	http://www.bestbets.org
ACP Journal / EBM Journal	http://ebm.bmjjournals.com/
Agency for Health Care Policy and Research (AHRQ)	http://www.ahrq.gov
Centre for Evidence-Based Medicine (Oxford, UK)	http://www.cebm.net
Canadian Agency for Drugs and Technologies in Health (CADTH)	http://www.cadth.ca
National Institute for Health and Clinical EXcellence (NICE)	http://www.nice.org.uk
Centre for Reviews and Dissemination (CRD)	http://www.york.ac.uk/inst/crd/
VirtualRx (NNT calculations)	http://www.nntonline.com/ebm/visualrx/nnt.asp

Table 1.3 Selected evidence-based emergency medicine (EBEM) websites.

This list is neither comprehensive nor complete; it represents some of the EBEM resources of use to the authors.

pooled outcome measures (e.g., OR, RR, NNT) in therapy questions. These efforts are made possible when the population, intervention/exposure, control, outcome measure and the designs of the identified studies demonstrate similarities. At other times, these PICO features preclude pooling of evidence and the best possible summary of evidence is descriptive or qualitative. Wherever possible, these approaches will be applied in this text in an effort to distill the evidence for the practicing emergency clinician. There are many text resources as well as internet-based resources available to the reader that can provide additional information, calculations and interpretations of these pooled effect measures (Table 1.3).

Conclusions

Much progress has been made in emergency medicine over the past quarter-century in the areas of diagnosis, therapy, prevention and prognosis. The synthesis of this evidence has been undertaken by many researchers and there is now increasingly valid and reliable evidence for the management of many common conditions presenting to the emergency department. This book attempts to summarize this evidence using a system that values best evidence using relevant examples from clinical practice. We recognize it is not yet comprehensive in all clinical areas; however, as the first evidence-based emergency text, we hope that it is both illustrative and iterative. We anticipate both refinements and substantial expansions of this pilot text in the future. Our goal is to improve the translation of knowledge from the evidence to the bedside in emergency medicine and we hope you will find this approach helpful in improving the clinical care provided at the bedside.

Acknowledgments

The authors would like to thank Mrs. Diane Milette for her secretarial support.

Conflicts of interest

Dr. Rowe is a member of the Cochrane Collaboration, a co-editor of the Cochrane Airways Group, and on the Steering Committee of the Prehospital and Emergency Health Field of the Cochrane Collaboration. Dr. Rowe is supported by a 21st Century Canada Research Chair in Emergency Airway Diseases from the Government of Canada (Ottawa, Canada).

References

1 Guyatt GH. Evidence-based medicine. *ACP J Club* 1991;**114**:A16.

2 Sackett DL, Rosenberg WMC, Gray JAM, Haynes RB. Evidence based medicine: what it is and what it isn't. *BMJ* 1996;**312**:71–2.

3 Haynes RB, Devereaux PJ, Guyatt GH. Physicians' and patients' choices in evidence based practice: evidence does not make decisions, people do. *BMJ* 2002;**324**:1350.

4 Innes GD, Macphail I, Dillon EC, Metcalfe C, Gao M. Dexamethasone prevents relapse after emergency department treatment of acute migraine: a randomized clinical trial. *Can J Emerg Med* 1999;**1**:26–33.

5 Rowe BH, Blitz S, Colman I, Edmonds M. Dexamethasone in migraine relapses: a randomized, placebo-controlled clinical trial. *Acad Emerg Med* 2006;**13**:S16–17.

6 Waeckerle JP, Cordell WH, Wyer PC, Osborn HH. Evidence-based emergency medicine – integrating research into emergency medical practice. *Ann Emerg Med* 1997;**30**:626–8.

7 Edlow JA, Wyer PC. Feedback: computed tomography for subarachnoid hemorrhage: don't throw the baby out with the bath water. *Ann Emerg Med* 2001;**37**:680–85.

8 Haynes RB, Haines A. Barriers and bridges to evidence based clinical practice. *BMJ* 1998;**317**:273–6.

9 Schunemann HJ, Jaeschke R, Cook DJ, et al. An official ATS statement: grading the quality of evidence and strength of recommendations in ATS guidelines and recommendations. *Am J Respir Care Med* 2006;**174**:605–14.

10 Guyatt G, Vist G, Falck-Ytter Y, Kunz R, Magrini N, Schunemann H. An emerging consensus on grading recommendations? (Editorial) *ACP J Club* 2006;**144**:A8–9.

11 LeLorier J, Gregoire G, Benhaddad A, Lapierre J, Derderian F. Discrepancies between meta-analyses and subsequent large randomized, controlled trials. *N Engl J Med* 1997;**337**:536–42.

12 Stiell IG, Clement CM, McKnight RD, et al. The Canadian C-Spine Rule versus the NEXUS low-risk criteria in patients with trauma. *N Engl J Med* 2003;**349**:2510–18.

13 Rowe BH, Alderson P. The Cochrane Library: a resource for clinical problem solving in emergency medicine. *Ann Emerg Med* 1999;**34**:86–90.

14 Moher D, Schulz KF, Altman DG, for the Consort Group. The CONSORT statement: revised recommendations for improving the quality of reports of parallel-group randomized trials. *JAMA* 2001;**285**:1987–91.

15 Moher D, Cook DJ, Eastwood S, et al. Improving the quality of reports of meta-analyses of randomised controlled trials: the QUOROM statement. *Lancet* 1999;**354**:1896–900.

16 Kelly KD, Travers AH, Dorgan M, Slater L, Rowe BH. Evaluating the quality of systematic reviews in the emergency medicine literature. *Ann Emerg Med* 2001;**38**:518–26.

17 Ospina MB, Kelly K, Klassen TP, Rowe BH. Assessing the quality of reports of systematic reviews in emergency medicine: are they improving? *Can J Emerg Med* 2005;**7**:179.

18 Chalmers I, Haynes RB. Reporting, updating, and correcting systematic reviews of the effects of health care. *BMJ* 1994;**309**:862–5.

19 Jadad AR, Moher M, Browman GP, et al. Systematic reviews and meta-analyses on treatment of asthma: critical evaluation. *BMJ* 2000;**320**:537–40.

20 Rowe BH, Brown MD. A primer on the Cochrane Collaboration, its new priorities in out-of-hospital and emergency health, and the role of *Annals of Emergency Medicine*. *Ann Emerg Med* 2007;**49**:351–4.

21 Oxman AD, Cook DJ, Guyatt GH, for the Evidence-Based Medicine Working Group. Users' guides to the medical literature. VI. How to use an overview. *JAMA* 1994;**272**:1367–71.

22 Olsen O, Middleton P, Ezzo J, et al. Quality of Cochrane reviews: assessment of sample from 1998. *BMJ* 2001;**323**:829–32.

23 Jadad AR, Cook DJ, Jones A, et al. Methodology and reports of systematic reviews and meta-analyses. *JAMA* 1998;**280**:278–80.

24 Moher D, Tetzlaff J, Tricco AC, Sampson M, Altman DG. Epidemiology and reporting characteristics of systematic reviews. *PLoS Med* 2007:e78 (doi:10.1371/journal.pmed.0040078).

25 Rowe BH, Brown MD. A primer on the Cochrane Collaboration, its new priorities in out-of-hospital and emergency health, and the role of *Annals of Emergency Medicine. Ann Emerg Med* 2007;**49**:351–4.

26 Smith E, Jennings P, McDonald S, MacPherson C, O'Brien T, Archer F. The Cochrane Library as a resource for evidence on out-of-hospital health care interventions. *Ann Emerg Med* 2007;**49**:344–50.

27 Wyer P, Allen TY, Corrall CJ. How to find evidence when you need it. Part 4: Matching clinical questions to appropriate databases. *Ann Emerg Med* 2003;**42**:136–49.

28 Guyatt GH, Sackett DL, Sinclair JC, et al. Users' guides to the medical literature. IX. A method of grading health care recommendations. *JAMA* 1995;**274**:1800–804.

29 Sackett DL, Richardson WS, Rosenberg W, Haynes RB. *Evidence-based Medicine. How to practice and teach EBM.* Churchill Livingstone, New York, 1992.

30 Dickersin K, Chan S, Chalmers TC, Sacks SH, Smith H. Publication bias and clinical trials. *Control Clin Trials* 1987;**8**:343–53.

31 Dickersin K, Scherer R, Lefebvre C. Identifying relevant studies for systematic reviews. *BMJ* 1994;**309**:1286–91.

32 Suarez-Almazor ME, Belseck E, Homik J, Dorgan M, Ramos-Remus C. Identifying clinical trials in the medical literature with electronic databases: MEDLINE alone is not enough. *Control Clin Trials* 2000;**21**(5):476–87.

33 Hunt DL, McKibbon KA. Locating and appraising systemic reviews. *Ann Intern Med* 1997;**126**:532–8.

34 Ospina MB, Kelly KD, Klassen TP, Rowe BH. Publication bias of randomized controlled trials in emergency medicine. *Acad Emerg Med* 2006;**13**:102–8.

35 Olkin L. Statistical and theoretical considerations in meta-analysis. *J Clin Epidemiol* 1995;**38**:133–46.

36 Laupacis A, Sackett DL, Roberts RS. An assessment of clinically useful measured of the consequences of treatment. *N Engl J Med* 1988;**318**:1728–33.

37 DerSimonian R, Laird N. Meta-analysis in clinical trials. *Control Clin Trials* 1986;**7**:177–88.

38 Higgins JPT, Thompson SG, Deeks JJ, Altman DG. Measuring inconsistency in meta-analyses. *BMJ* 2003;**327**:557–60.

39 Oxman AD, Guyatt GH. A consumer's guide to subgroup analyses. *Ann Intern Med* 1992;**116**:78–84.

2 Knowledge Translation: a Primer for Emergency Physicians*

Eddy S. Lang[1], Peter C. Wyer[2] & Marc Afilalo[1]

[1]Department of Family Medicine, McGill University, Montreal *and* Department of Emergency Medicine, SMBD Jewish General Hospital, Montreal, Canada

[2]Department of Medicine, Columbia University College of Physicians and Surgeons, New York, USA

Clinical scenario

A 23-year-old university student presented to the emergency department (ED) having sustained a left ankle injury while participating in an intramural basketball tournament. She denied ever sustaining a serious musculoskeletal injury or fracture in the past and was in perfectly good health. She was taking oral contraceptives and had just completed her menstrual period. She injured her ankle after landing awkwardly, subsequent to trying to gain control of a jump ball. Upon landing she immediately felt pain and heard what seemed to be a snap in her left ankle prior to falling to the ground. She was able to get on her feet and limp off the court but did not return to play.

In the ED, the patient was ambulating with great difficulty but was able to hobble on the affected foot. Examination of the ankle revealed significant lateral soft tissue swelling but no bony tenderness involving either the anterior or posterior aspects of the lateral malleolus. While not able to recall all of the specific characteristics of the Ottawa Ankle Rule for determining which patients with ankle injuries need radiography, you believed that this patient was actually at very low risk of having suffered a fracture. The ED was extremely busy that day and you sensed the patient's desire to have a radiograph performed after having spent three hours waiting to see a doctor.

*Adapted from an article published in the *Annals of Emergency Medicine* [1] on knowledge translation with the addition of discussions on quality improvement and the role of bedside tools. Research in knowledge translation includes studies that attempt to quantify and understand the discrepancies between what is known and what is done, as well as those that examine the impact and acceptability of interventions designed to narrow or close these gaps. Sentinel examples in this line of research conducted in the emergency department setting are described.

Evidence-based Emergency Medicine. Edited by Brian H. Rowe
© 2009 Blackwell Publishing, ISBN: 978-1-4051-6143-5.

Background

Knowledge translation (KT) is a term that describes activities or processes that facilitate the transfer of high-quality evidence from research into effective changes in health policy and clinical practice. This increasingly important discipline attempts to conceptually combine elements of research, education, quality improvement and electronic systems development to create a seamless linkage between interventions that improve patient care and their routine implementation in daily clinical practice. We outline the gap between research and practice and present a case study of an emergency medicine example of validated evidence that has failed to achieve widespread implementation. We describe a model of organization of evidence and its relationship with the process that links research from the scientific endeavor to changes in practice that affect patient outcomes. Obstacles to evidence uptake are explored, as well as the limitations of current educational strategies. Innovative strategies in realms such as computerized decision support systems designed to enhance evidence uptake are also described. The potential interface between knowledge translation and continuous quality improvement will also be discussed.

Knowledge translation is a relatively new term that has rapidly gained prominence in many health care disciplines, including medicine, public health, and health care policy development and administration. However, the notions underlying KT are not recent and might be recognized by a number of fairly synonymous terms and phrases, including "translating research into practice": getting research into practice, knowledge use, knowledge dissemination, knowledge transfer and evidence translation, research uptake, evidence uptake, and others [2]. The Canadian Institutes of Health Research [3] defines KT as "the exchange, synthesis and ethically sound application of knowledge within a complex system of interactions among researchers and users to accelerate the capture of the benefits of research for patients through improved health, more effective services and products, and a strengthened health care system".

Although KT may be unfamiliar terminology to most emergency physicians, the existing gap between current best evidence and evidence-based practice is a concern that most clinicians can relate to and has been at issue for decades. The members of the Clinical Research Roundtable at the US Institute of Medicine have suggested that the failure to translate new knowledge into clinical practice and decision making in health care is a major barrier preventing human benefit from advances in biomedical sciences [4]. Whether it falls into the realm of acute care, the management of chronic medical conditions or prevention care, it appears that patients often fail to receive recommended standards of care or are receiving potentially harmful or unproven treatments. McGlynn et al. [5] examined more than 400 quality indicators in some 6700 patients drawn from a dozen metropolitan areas and suggested that 45% are not receiving recommended care. This gap in care is also highlighted in the landmark 2001 Institute of Medicine report titled *Crossing the Quality Chasm: A new health system for the 21st century* [6]. The Institute of Medicine report described the "chasm" that exists between medical advances (what we know) and medical care currently in place (what we do). The report emphasized three aspects of quality under achievement: misuse (medical error), underuse (of proven therapies) and overuse (of inappropriate treatments).

The Institute of Medicine report covers a large body of literature that outlines the nature of these deficiencies and outlines how a large proportion of patients in a variety of clinical contexts fail to receive standard care. The recommendations contained within the report outline a number of systems-based changes in the structure and functioning of the health care system designed to close the "quality chasm" in six domains – i.e., care that is safe, effective, patient centered, timely, efficient and equitable. The Institute of Medicine report has played a pivotal role in advancing the knowledge translation agenda in health care policy development, as well as through research initiatives through organizations such as the Agency for Healthcare Research and Quality.

Clinical questions

In this chapter we will deal with the following questions:

1 For practicing emergency physicians (population), what are the barriers (outcome) to the uptake of new, valid and reliable evidence (intervention) compared to usual care practices (control)?

2 For practicing emergency physicians (population), do clinical practice guidelines and their implementation strategies (intervention) improve eventual uptake and patient care (outcomes) compared to usual care (control)?

3 For practicing emergency physicians (population), do knowledge translation methods and innovative continuing medical education / continuing professional development strategies (intervention) improve eventual uptake and patient care (outcomes) compared to usual care (control)?

4 For practicing physicians (population), what models exist for understanding knowledge translation?

5 For practicing physicians (population), does providing research evidence in a validated and organized manner (intervention) increase the sensibility, use and uptake of evidence into patient care (outcome) compared to traditional methods (control)?

6 For practicing physicians (population), are there modalities in place (interventions) that ensure clear evidence for a beneficial or harmful intervention (therapeutic or diagnostic) that translates into management decisions that will impact on patients (outcome) compared to traditional approaches (control)?

7 For practicing physicians (population), what scientific approaches (interventions) can enlighten efforts to close the gap between research and practice (outcome)?

General search strategy

You begin to address the topic of KT by searching for evidence in the common electronic databases such as the Cochrane Library, MEDLINE and EMBASE looking specifically for systematic reviews and meta-analyses. The Cochrane Database of Systematic Reviews includes high-quality systematic review evidence on effective practice and organization of care and includes systematic review evidence on evidence implementation strategies. You also search the Cochrane Central Register of Controlled Trials (CENTRAL), MEDLINE and EMBASE to identify randomized controlled trials (RCTs) that became available after the publication date of the systematic review or, if no systematic reviews were identified, to locate high-quality randomized controlled trials that directly address the clinical question.

Critical review of the literature

Question 1: For practicing emergency physicians (population), what are the barriers (outcome) to the uptake of new, valid and reliable evidence (intervention) compared to usual care practices (control)?

Search strategy

- PubMed: implementation AND barriers AND diffusion of innovation AND guideline adherence

The barriers to evidence uptake have been the subject of extensive study and scholarly work elaborating a number of models describing the obstacles associated with incorporating change

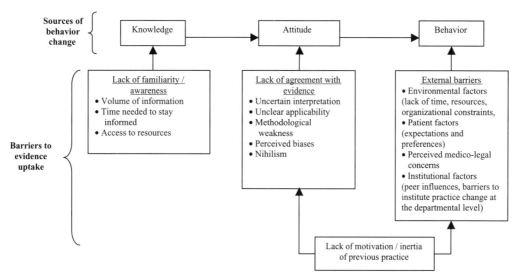

Figure 2.1 Barriers to evidence uptake. Innovation and change in clinical practice both at the individual, departmental and institutional level are contingent on three key sources of behavior change: knowledge, attitudes and behavior. However, a series of complex barriers exist for each of these dimensions, some of which are illustrated here. (Some source material with permission from Cabana et al. [8].)

into professional practice and behavior [7,8]. Much of the work on barriers has involved implementation of practice guidelines but is transferable to all circumstances in which a convincing evidence base is inconsistently applied or ignored in everyday practice.

One of the most comprehensive schemes for considering the barriers to evidence uptake classifies groups of barriers into the three domains of knowledge, attitude and behavior (Fig. 2.1) [8]. The basic premise underlying this schema is that innovation and change in a physician's clinical practice are contingent on some combination of all three domains, each of which may encounter opposing forces. Opposing knowledge acquisition are the increasing volume of new literature relevant to clinical practice, the time investment required to achieve mastery of this information, and barriers to on-line access. Attitudes that encourage change may be hindered by sometimes appropriate skepticism and mistrust of clinical research, as well as by uncertainty about its applicability to practice. Behavioral changes that reflect new evidence and innovation may be impeded by external pressures that favor the inertia of the status quo. These include environmental factors such as the need to commit resources to the process of initiating a new hospital or interdepartmental treatment protocol, medico-legal concerns and patient expectations about the need for diagnostic tests/treatments that may also obstruct change or innovation, and institutional or regulatory issues. Physicians may also be wary of being the first among their peers to introduce significant changes in practice.

In summary, many barriers to evidence uptake exist. Although not insurmountable, specific barriers to change have been addressed with educational approaches that have had less than their desired effects [9].

Question 2: For practicing emergency physicians (population), do clinical practice guidelines and their implementation strategies (intervention) improve eventual uptake and patient care (outcomes) compared to usual care (control)?

Search strategy

- PubMed: clinical practice guidelines AND implementation AND barriers AND diffusion of innovation AND organizational innovation AND guideline adherence.

Guidelines are often deficient in the methodology used for their development and, even when touted as evidence based, may not reflect a systematic methodology. When not developed with rigorous methodology, practice guidelines are vulnerable to the perception of bias from vested interests. Clinical practice guidelines have been greeted with some skepticism in the emergency medicine and wider medical communities, with concerns related to the manner in which recommendations have been reached, the strength of evidence underlying recommendations, and the perspectives and values that have guided the process [10–12]. These issues may partly explain why guideline implementation research has yielded such weak evidence of benefit [13]. A review of 235 studies that examined guideline dissemination and implementation strategies found that these interventions result in no more than a 10% median improvement in health care provider behavior [13].

In summary, clinicians are bombarded with clinical practice guidelines. Although their effect has been shown to be modest, the benefit of guidelines can have important implications at the level of population health.

Question 3: For practicing emergency physicians (population), do knowledge translation methods and innovative continuing medical education / continuing professional development strategies (intervention) improve eventual uptake and patient care (outcomes) compared to usual care (control)?

Search strategy

• PubMed: continuing medical education AND continuing professional development AND diffusion of innovation

Continuing professional development (CPD) initiatives are relied on heavily in the health care system to inform and improve physician practice, making it more compliant with evidence-based strategies. A review of systematic reviews on this topic [14] noted that the most widely used approaches consisting of didactic presentations and the dissemination of printed material are the least effective means for changing physician practice. A systematic review, consisting of randomized trials or well-designed quasi-experimental studies, examined the effect of continuing education meetings (including lectures, workshops and courses) on the clinical practice of health professionals or health care outcomes [15]. This review revealed little or no effect of didactic presentations, in contrast to moderate to large impacts from programs that involved a workshop component. A more recent systematic review confirms the importance of interactive teaching methods, multi-media approaches and repeat exposures as the most promising methods for effecting a change in medical practice through educating professionals [15].

Interactive approaches, such as audit/feedback, academic detailing/outreach and reminders, seem most effective at simultaneously changing physician care and patient outcomes. Audit and feedback is among the best studied of the interactive approaches to changing professional behavior. It refers to analyzing a physician's practice pattern and providing feedback on inconsistencies with evidence-based practice. A systematic review of 72 studies [16] suggested that these approaches can improve physician compliance by as much as 71% but can also have the unintended effect of reducing compliance by 10%. Negligible or paradoxical effects of audit and feedback were seen primarily when the intensity of the intervention was weak (i.e., delayed or anonymous feedback on practice patterns) or when the degree of compliance with the target intervention was already high. Multifaceted interventions that rely on more than one method to remind physicians about following evidence are also generally more effective than simpler approaches, but are also more costly [17].

In summary, continuing professional development initiatives are important methods by which clinicians access and uptake evidence; however, not all continuing medical education (CME)/CPD initiatives are effective. For in-depth discussion of this issue, see Chapter 4.

Question 4: For practicing physicians (population), what models exist for understanding knowledge translation?

Search strategy

• PubMed: knowledge translation AND theoretical models AND diffusion of innovation

The factors that impede the efficient transfer of well-substantiated clinical research into clinical emergency medicine care are myriad and complex. Strategies designed to address them have been categorized by Glasziou and Haynes [18]. They view the research–practice continuum as being divided into two major categories: the first, involving the task of "getting the evidence straight", and the second, related to "getting the evidence used". These concepts are represented as interconnected domains within Fig. 2.2. The pyramid component of this figure was initially proposed as a hierarchical scheme for understanding the different forms in which published research evidence may be presented [19]. The category of "getting the evidence used" is illustrated in the figure by the evidence-to-practice pipeline. The following sections of this chapter will elaborate on and clarify the specific elements of this evidence-to-practice model.

Question 5: For practicing physicians (population), does providing research evidence in a validated and organized manner (intervention) increase the sensibility, use and uptake of evidence into patient care (outcome) compared to traditional methods (control)?

Search strategy

• PubMed: pre-appraised resources AND systematic reviews AND evidence syntheses AND evidence based medicine AND critically appraised topics AND peer review, research AND decision support systems, clinical

Getting the evidence straight: the pyramidal (5S levels) organization of research evidence

Studies

The clinical research upon which evidence-based decision making is informed constitutes the building block for all of the other elements in the model developed by Haynes [20]. Unfortunately, the sheer volume of research that is generated on a weekly basis and which is of relevance to emergency medicine is too overwhelming for most clinicians to keep up with. Hence the need for other approaches to transform the conclusions from this mountain of potentially important research into a format that makes it more clinically applicable.

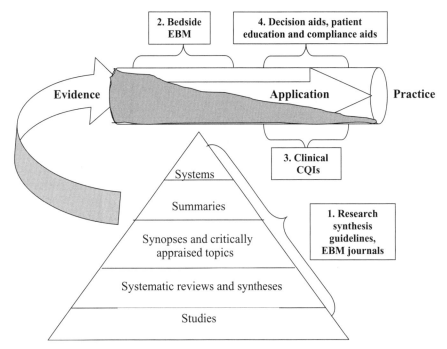

Figure 2.2 A model for closing the evidence-to-practice gap. This schematic demonstrates four stages of moving from research to practice altering outcomes. The first stage involves "getting the evidence straight" illustrated by increasingly more applicable forms of information drawn from valid and important clinical research and represented in the 5S pyramid. The evidence-to-practice pipeline, also shown, reveals the dissipation of useful conclusions from clinical research, thus failing to make it into practice. The three remaining disciplines of knowledge translation can facilitate evidence uptake and help close the gap between research and practice. CQI, continuous quality improvement; EBM, evidence-based medicine. (Adapted with permission from Glasziou & Haynes [18].)

Systematic reviews and syntheses

Keeping emergency physicians up to date requires a filtering process for determining which studies are relevant and could have an influence on their practice. The process of getting the evidence straight is particularly daunting in emergency medicine, which as a broad horizontal specialty might be appropriately influenced by developments from many other fields. Thus, a key component of assimilating the evidence would ideally involve the search, critical appraisal and synthesis of best evidence, using systematic review methodology, to address fundamental questions of diagnosis and management in clinical emergency medicine. The most important feature of systematic reviews is that they use a predetermined methodology for assessing the scope and validity of research evidence and provide an analysis for the application of important findings in clinical practice. Unfortunately, systematic reviews published in the emergency medicine literature during the past several years have been found to be deficient in quality, with gaps evident in the comprehensiveness of search strategies and in the methodology used for evaluating the quality of incorporated studies [21].

The Cochrane Collaboration is recognized for its well-established record in systematic review methodology, with a database of approximately 3000 published systematic reviews to date, covering the gamut of health care interventions and hundreds more protocols for other systematic reviews that are in development. Systematic reviews not prepared under the auspices of the Cochrane Collaboration constitute more than half of all reviews, and both Cochrane and non-Cochrane reviews of relevance to emergency care are included as alerts and for searching through *BMJ Updates* (available at http://bmjupdates.com), a free service

sponsored by the BMJ Publishing Group [22]. PubMed Clinical Queries also provides a search strategy for reviews (available at http://www.ncbi.nlm.nih.gov/entrez/query/static/clinical.shtml).

Synopses and critically appraised topics

Short of fully integrated information systems, clinicians might best be served by readily searchable databases that can provide evidence-based synopses of best evidence specifically designed for bedside use. Perhaps best known of the journals that systematically peruses the biomedical literature for research that is of relevance to the field of internal medicine is the American College of Physicians' *ACP Journal Club*. This bimonthly periodical provides readers with succinct analyses and critical appraisals of published research reports that meet a minimum methodological standard.

The one-page synopses provide information on the citation, research question and study design and include a standardized reporting of results. They also include a relevance and newsworthiness score provided by a network of clinicians, including emergency physicians, who rate each article in advance of the synopses' publication [23]. Unfortunately, the content of *ACP Journal Club*, and even of *Evidence-Based Medicine*, a related publication with a broader clinical focus, overlaps only modestly with the topic interests of an emergency medicine audience. At present, no systematically organized forum for research synopses exists within our specialty.

Some formats for evidence synopses exist within the emergency medicine literature and in on-line databases. These consist of critically appraised topics, or CATs, that provide shortcut reviews of clinical questions based largely on the findings of one or more studies on a given subject. Best evidence topics, or BETs, are a variation on this theme and are summaries of best available research evidence designed to address specific clinical questions of relevance to emergency medicine (available at http://www.bestbets.org). The *Annals of Emergency Medicine* also provides a venue for evidence-based synopses of key questions that are relevant to emergency medicine (available at http://www.annemergmed.com/content/sectII). The other major objective of synopses and critically appraised topics is to provide clinicians with a bottom-line evidence summary in a format that is accessible and readily incorporated into decision making and clinical care. Practice guidelines are rarely able to provide this degree of user friendliness.

In summary, although in its early stages, a growing body of research suggests that ready access to synopses can have various degrees of impact on physician practice and patient outcomes. A systematic review of clinical information retrieval technology suggests that approximately one-third of information retrieval efforts by physicians influence their decision making [24].

Summaries

Next in the hierarchy are the summaries that integrate pertinent information and conclusions from systematic reviews and other rigorously developed synopses and critically appraised topics to provide an overview of evidence-based management options for a single condition (e.g. renal colic). Truly evidence-based textbooks such as this one and *BMJ Clinical Evidence* (http://clinicalevidence.bmj.com), which provide comprehensive overviews of treatment options for a myriad of conditions, are examples of resources for summaries. In theory and in practice, summaries can easily be made universally available through on-line resources and are thus more feasible to keep up to date.

Systems

Located at the peak of the evidence pyramid, "systems" refer to clinical information support instruments such as those that could be seamlessly integrated into a patient's electronic health record. The ideal clinical information system would remind physicians of key relevant actions in both the diagnostic and therapeutic realms that are supported by an existing evidence base. The optimal evidence delivery system would offer recommendations in concise and easily manageable bits of information and would be constantly updated to incorporate recent developments on the research front. Furthermore, this type of system would be automatically activated in the appropriate clinical setting and become seamlessly integrated into workflow for the clinician. Health information systems meeting all of these specifications are still in preliminary stages of development. Early work with expert charting and real-time clinical guidance systems have to date met with only a modicum of success [25].

In summary, increasingly sophisticated hierarchies of evidence are available to the emergency clinician for getting the evidence

straight. Clinicians should look for the highest level of evidence within the evidence pyramid to answer each clinical question.

Question 6: For practicing physicians (population), are there modalities in place (interventions) that ensure clear evidence for a beneficial or harmful intervention (therapeutic or diagnostic) that translates into management decisions that will impact on patients (outcome) compared to traditional approaches (control)?

Search strategy

- PubMed: evidence based medicine AND continuous quality improvement AND decision aids AND physician compliance AND point of care systems

Getting the evidence to patients: the evidence-to-practice pipeline

In the schema adapted from Glasziou and Haynes (see Fig. 2.2) [18], the evidence pipeline represents the trajectory that research evidence (represented as water) must take to be incorporated into clinical practice. The inability of clinical research to influence patient care and affect outcomes is represented as the evaporation of water (research evidence) as it tracks down an evidence pipeline, where a number of factors contribute to its evaporation and dissipation. Knowledge translation is viewed as encompassing four major disciplines (resource development and access, bedside evidence-based medicine, clinical quality improvement and the use of decision aids), all of which improve the path from awareness to adherence. Having considered the relevant categories of resource, the pyramid in Fig. 2.2, we are ready to elaborate on the remaining three steps in the translation process.

Bedside evidence-based medicine

Bedside evidence-based medicine responds to what is commonly a problematic divergence between the questions that arise during clinical encounters and a readily accessible pathway to finding usable answers. Easily searchable databases of clinician-friendly evidence summaries that can be called up quickly would meet this need effectively. Hand-held computers offer the potential to store and make readily available the type of resources that could meet this need. Emergency medicine examples of bedside evidence-based medicine are emerging in the literature on the clinical practice and educational frontiers. Bullard et al. [26] reported a randomized trial comparing a wirelessly networked mobile computer to a traditional desktop version, with both systems providing ready access to a number of decision rules and locally agreed-on clinical practice guidelines. Physicians randomized to the mobile version of the decision support system were more likely to make use of these resources.

In summary, bedside evidence-based medicine also encompasses the large body of evidence that informs the clinical assessment of patients and decision making and guides the ordering and interpretation of any indicated diagnostic tests. Validated instruments that define a patient's probability of a suspected disease (pre-test probability) before undergoing specific diagnostic tests, provide an example of this aspect of bedside evidence-based medicine. An example of such an instrument is the Wells criteria for stratifying the risk of deep venous thrombosis before the performance of a test such as compression ultrasonography [27].

Continuous quality improvement

Continuous quality improvement refers to initiatives that include designing, implementing and monitoring adherence to system-wide changes that facilitate the incorporation of best evidence into patient care. As an example, a quality improvement initiative designed to promote adherence to an evidence-supported management algorithm for suspected pulmonary embolism [28] and a program to monitor compliance by physicians can be viewed as important steps toward ensuring uniformly high-quality care for patients suspected of having this condition. Quality improvement programs designed to improve evidence uptake are new to the emergency medicine literature. Lindsay et al. [29] used a modified Delphi process to develop a series of quality indicators for use in the emergency setting, many of which, such as aspirin use in acute coronary syndromes and corticosteroid use in asthmatic patients being discharged from the ED, address the evidence practice gap.

Emergency care contexts can incorporate quality improvement methodology into evidence-based initiatives. Essential components include planning a strategy to improve adherence to locally agreed-on evidence-based management and monitoring adherence through an "evidence uptake" indicator [30]. For example, such an initiative might use an integrated charting / computerized physician order entry system to require verification of the Ottawa Ankle Rule criteria in the context of radiographic orders for all patients presenting with ankle injuries. Application of the rule occurs within this electronic interface or through selection from a limited number of reasons for bypassing the recommended course of action. Such a system could readily be designed to track quality indicators reflecting uptake of the Ottawa Ankle Rule, impact on the number of radiographs ordered, and specific issues related to non-compliance by members of the clinical team.

Wright et al. [31] describe the creation of a Committee for Procedural Quality and Evidence-Based Practice (CPQE) whose function is to establish evidence-based guidelines for ED health care providers. The CPQE then measures the effect of such guidelines, along with other quality measures, through a pre/post chart auditing exercise and then feeding back the findings to team members in a provider-specific, peer-matched manner. The authors have published the effectiveness of their intervention using asthma care as an example of KT in action.

In summary, continuous quality improvement is a powerful method by which emergency clinicians and departments, hospitals and health regions can improve the flow of evidence down the practice pipeline. For in-depth discussion of this issue, see Chapter 5.

Decision aids, patient education and compliance aids

Computer-based clinical decision support systems would seem to offer important opportunities in the realm of knowledge translation, especially given the traditionally hectic and fast-paced environment of the ED. A review of the effect of these interventions on physician behavior and patient outcomes [32] in 97 eligible studies revealed a significant effect of improving physician compliance, especially in reminder-type systems in which indices of patient care were increased in 76% of the relevant trials. A more recent systematic review identified those features that seem to result in a more significant impact on clinician behavior, namely point-of-care decision support, integration into workflow, and the provision of recommendations rather than just assessments [33].

Increasingly, however, many of the therapeutic interventions that have been proven beneficial in the context of emergency medicine require an integrative and collaborative approach with other specialties. Examples such as early goal-directed therapy in septic shock, therapeutic hypothermia in survivors of cardiac arrest, or timely percutaneous coronary interventions in ST segment elevation acute myocardial infarction all require collaborative clinical pathways developed for local implementation among emergency physicians and other relevant acute care disciplines [34,35]. These interventions also lend themselves to standardized protocols that ensure uniform patient care.

Organizations such as the Agency for Healthcare Quality and Research and the National Guideline Clearing House are actively involved in developing methods for improving the implementation of clinical practice guidelines [36]. This includes anticipation and planning for their implementation from early in their development by involving key stakeholders in the guideline selection and creation process.

Question 7: For practicing physicians (population), what scientific approaches (interventions) can enlighten efforts to close the gap between research and practice (outcome)?

Search strategy

- PubMed: implementation AND cluster analysis AND guideline adherence

Knowledge translation can be viewed as a clinical practice paradigm and a research agenda. Research is relevant to all four of the knowledge translation disciplines illustrated in Fig. 2.2 and needs to address the exigencies and particularities of specific specialties and practice settings.

The common denominator of all knowledge translation research is a measure of practitioner behavior change in the direction of applying evidence-based interventions and strategies to patient care. A second and key objective should be the demonstration that patients benefit, but this is often missing from such studies [30]. Secondary outcomes include tabulation of the financial and manpower resources consumed in the course of achieving change in the primary outcomes.

An aspect of knowledge translation that is largely understudied relates to the impact of evidence summaries and syntheses on patient care. There is no evidence in the realm of emergency medicine that such interventions would be effective. There is, however, evidence that hand-held computers equipped with evidence-based summaries of key research in hypertension can translate into more rational prescribing practices for trainees in family medicine [37]. Another example of practical bedside application of evidence syntheses affecting patient care was described in relation to an inpatient medical service and made use of an evidence cart consisting of textbook and pre-appraised resources [38]. The authors noted that of nearly 100 attempted searches, 90% were effective in uncovering relevant information that informed decision making, and a significant number of these resulted in new or altered management decisions for patients. When the cart was removed from the ward, searches and use of information from research returned to the previous baseline.

Much of knowledge translation research is presented as quality improvement research initiatives. One of the most ambitious examples in emergency medicine is a 32-site cluster randomized trial of the emergency care of pneumonia based on a validated prediction rule for severity [39–41]. This study by Fine et al. [39] and Yealy et al. [40,41] compared three implementation strategies for a clinical practice guideline designed to identify which patients with pneumonia require hospitalization. The guidelines were also meant to ensure that key processes of care, such as antibiotic administration within 4 hours of presentation, were followed. The participating centers were randomly allocated to evidence uptake initiatives according to low-, medium- and high-intensity approaches. The high-intensity approach distinguished itself from the other strategies by incorporating real-time, paper reminders that facilitated scoring and calculation of the severity score, with data provided about predicted mortality by strata. High-intensity centers also incorporated guideline adherence into their center's quality-of-care program, which included audits and feedback on performance. Using discharge of low-risk patients as the primary outcome and adherence to key processes of care as secondary measures, the authors were able to demonstrate that the high intensity and, in some instances, the moderate-intensity approaches were superior to the competing strategies, often achieving a doubling in the outcomes of interest. For example, for discharging low-risk patients, the moderate- and high-intensity sites achieved rates of 61.0% and 61.9%, compared with 37.5% for the low-intensity group ($P = 0.004$).

Although examples of short-term adherence to evidence uptake initiatives are readily available, it is necessary to determine whether these will result in more than brief periods of compliance driven by enthusiasm and novelty. Chouaid et al. [42] describe a 2-year study that examined the implementation of an emergency asthma management guideline. A longitudinal educational and audit/feedback program was effective in achieving a prolonged change in practice.

Conclusions

In the patient described in the scenario, examination using the Ottawa Ankle Rule would suggest no radiograph is required and the patient's pre-test probability of fracture is *less than* 1 in 10,000. Discussing this strategy with the patient, she seemed reassured that a radiograph was unnecessary. She was discharged with instructions to ice the joint, use anti-inflammatories and purchase an ankle brace for ambulation for the next 4–6 weeks (see Chapter 31).

Knowledge translation may best be viewed as the bridge that brings together CME, CPD and quality improvement in the hope of closing the research-to-practice gap [43]. Some important resources already exist for accessing the evidence (in the form of original articles, systematic reviews and evidence-based practice guidelines and systems) that we should be attending to. However, emergency medicine still needs to define the greatest research–practice gaps in its specialty. This compilation of evidence-to-practice deficiencies would constitute a research agenda in knowledge translation as it relates to emergency medicine.

Be it the overuse of antibiotics in bronchitis or the underuse of validated decision rules to guide ordering of radiographs, the field of emergency medicine is replete with opportunities to design and test effective evidence uptake strategies and, in so doing, to bring emergency medicine fully into the era of evidence-based practice.

Conflicts of interest

No conflicts of interest were reported.

References

1 Lang ES, Wyer PC, Haynes RB. Knowledge translation: closing the evidence-to-practice gap. *Ann Emerg Med* 2007;**49**(3):355–63.

2 Graham ID, Logan J, Harrison MB, Straus SE, Tetroe J, Caswell W, Robinson N. Lost in knowledge translation: time for a map? *J Contin Educ Health Prof* 2006;**26**(1):13–24.

3 Canadian Institutes of Health Research. Canadian Institutes of Health Research knowledge translation strategy 2004–2009. Available at http://www.cihr-irsc.gc.ca/e/26574.html# defining (accessed March 26, 2007).

4 Sung NS, Crowley WF, Jr., Genel M, et al. Central challenges facing the national clinical research enterprise. *JAMA* 2003;**289**:1278–87.

5 McGlynn EA, Asch SM, Adams J. The quality of health care delivered to adults in the United States. *N Engl J Med* 2003;**348**:2635–45.

6 Institute of Medicine, Committee on Quality of Health Care in America. Crossing the Quality Chasm: A new health system for the 21st century. Institute of Medicine website, available at http://www.iom.edu/report.asp?id_5432 (accessed March 26, 2007).

7 Grol R, Wensing M. What drives change? Barriers to and incentives for achieving evidence-based practice. *Med J Aust* 2004;**180**(6 Suppl):S57–60.

8 Cabana MD, Rand CS, Powe NR, et al. Why don't physicians follow clinical practice guidelines? A framework for improvement. *JAMA* 1999;**282**:1458–65.

9 Bloom BS. Effects of continuing medical education on improving physician clinical care and patient health: a review of systematic reviews. *Int J Technol Assess Health Care* 2005;**21**:380–85.

10 Fesmire FM, Jagoda A. Are we putting the cart ahead of the horse: who determines the standard of care for the management of patients in the emergency department? *Ann Emerg Med* 2005;**46**:198–200.

11 Hayward RS. Clinical practice guidelines on trial. *Can Med Assoc J* 1997;**156**:1725–7.

12 Laupacis A. On bias and transparency in the development of influential recommendations. *Can Med Assoc J* 2006;**174**:335–6.

13 Grimshaw J, Thomas RE, MacLennan G, et al. Effectiveness and efficiency of guideline dissemination and implementation strategies. *Health Technology Assessment* 2004; **8**(6). Available at http://www.ncchta.org/minisumm/min806.htm.

14 O'Brien MA, Freemantle N, Oxman AD, et al. Continuing education meetings and workshops: effects on professional practice and health care outcomes. *Cochrane Database Syst Rev* 2001;**2**:CD003030.

15 Marinopoulos SS, Dorman T, Ratanawongsa N, et al. *Effectiveness of Continuing Medical Education.* Evidence Report/Technology Assessment No. 149. AHRQ Publication No. 07-E006. Agency for Healthcare Research and Quality, Rockville, MD, 2007.

16 Jamtvedt G, Young JM, Kristoffersen DT, et al. Audit and feedback: effects on professional practice and health care outcomes. *Cochrane Database Syst Rev* 2006;**2**:CD000259.

17 Grimshaw JM, Shirran L, Thomas R. Changing provider behavior: an overview of systematic reviews of interventions. *Med Care* 2001;**39**(8 Suppl 2):II2–45.

18 Glasziou P, Haynes B. The paths from research to improved health outcomes. *ACP J Club* 2005;**142**:A8–10.

19 Haynes RB, Sackett DL, Gray JA, et al. Transferring evidence from research into practice, 2. Getting the evidence straight. *ACP J Club* 1997;**126**:A14–16.

20 Haynes RB. Of studies, syntheses, synopses, summaries, and systems: the "5S" evolution of information services for evidence-based health care decisions. *ACP J Club* 2006;**145**(3):A8.

21 Kelly KD, Travers A, Dorgan M, et al. Evaluating the quality of systematic reviews in the emergency medicine literature. *Ann Emerg Med* 2001;**38**:518–26.

22 Haynes RB, Cotoi C, Holland J, et al., for the McMaster Premium Literature Service (PLUS) Project. Second-order peer review of the medical literature for clinical practitioners. *JAMA* 2006;**295**:1801–8.

23 McMaster Online Rating of Evidence. *About MORE.* McMaster Online Rating of Evidence website, available at http://hiru.mcmaster.ca/more/AboutMORE.htm (accessed March 26, 2006).

24 Pluye P, Grad RM, Dunikowski LG, et al. Impact of clinical information-retrieval technology on physicians: a literature review of quantitative, qualitative and mixed methods studies. *Int J Med Inform* 2005;**74**:745–68.

25 Buller-Close K, Schriger DL, Baraff LJ. Heterogeneous effect of an emergency department expert charting system. *Ann Emerg Med* 2003;**41**:644–52.

26 Bullard MJ, Meurer DP, Colman I, Holroyd BR, Rowe BH. Supporting clinical practice at the bedside using wireless technology. *Acad Emerg Med* 2004;**11**(11):1186–92.

27 Anderson DR, Wells PS, Stiell I, et al. Thrombosis in the emergency department: use of a clinical diagnosis model to safely avoid the need for urgent radiological investigation. *Arch Intern Med* 1999;**159**:477–82.

28 Brown MD, Vance SJ, Kline JA. An emergency department guideline for the diagnosis of pulmonary embolism: an outcome study. *Acad Emerg Med* 2005;**12**:20–25.

29 Lindsay P, Schull M, Bronskill S, et al. The development of indicators to measure the quality of clinical care in emergency departments following a modified-Delphi approach. *Acad Emerg Med* 2002;**9**:1131–9.

30 Bizovi KE, Wears R, Lowe RA. Researching quality in emergency medicine. *Acad Emerg Med* 2002;**9**:1116–23.

31 Wright SW, Trott A, Lindsell CJ, et al. Evidence-based emergency medicine. Creating a system to facilitate translation of evidence into standardized clinical practice: a preliminary report. *Ann Emerg Med* 2008;**51**(1):80–86.

32 Garg AX, Adhikari NK, McDonald H, et al. Effects of computerized clinical decision support systems on practitioner performance and patient outcomes: a systematic review. *JAMA* 2005;**293**:1261–3.

33 Kawamoto K, Houlihan CA, Balas EA, Lobach DF. Improving clinical practice using clinical decision support systems: a systematic review of trials to identify features critical to success. *BMJ* 2005;**330**(7494):765.

34 Green RS, Howes D, for the CAEP Critical Care Committee. Hypothermic modulation of anoxic brain injury in adult survivors of cardiac arrest: a review of the literature and an algorithm for emergency physicians. *Can J Emerg Med* 2005;**7**:42–7.

35 Trzeciak S, Dellinger RP, Abate NL, et al. Translating research into clinical practice: a 1-year experience with implementing early goal-directed therapy for septic shock in the emergency department. *Chest* 2006;**129**:225–32.

36 Agency for Healthcare Research and Quality. Fact Sheet: Translating research into practice (TRIP)-II. Agency for Healthcare Research and Quality website, available at: http://www.ahrq.gov/research/trip2fac.htm (accessed March 24, 2007).

37 Grad RM, Meng Y, Bartlett G, et al. Effect of a PDA-assisted evidence-based medicine course on knowledge of common clinical problems. *Fam Med* 2005;**37**:734–40.

38 Sackett DL, Straus SE. Finding and applying evidence during clinical rounds: the "evidence cart". *JAMA* 1998;**280**:1336–8.

39 Fine MJ, Auble TE, Yealy DM, et al. A prediction rule to identify low-risk patients with community-acquired pneumonia. *N Engl J Med* 1997;**336**:243–50.

40 Yealy DM, Auble TE, Stone RA, et al. The emergency department community-acquired pneumonia trial: methodology of a quality improvement intervention. *Ann Emerg Med* 2004;**43**:770–82.

41 Yealy DM, Auble TE, Stone RA, et al. Effect of increasing the intensity of implementing pneumonia guidelines: a randomized, controlled trial. *Ann Intern Med* 2005;**143**:881–94.

42 Chouaid C, Bal JP, Fuhrman C, et al. Standardized protocol improves asthma management in emergency department. *J Asthma* 2004;**41**:19–25.

43 Davis D, Evans M, Jadad A, et al. The case for knowledge translation: shortening the journey from evidence to effect. *BMJ* 2003;**327**:33–5.

3 Critical Appraisal: General Issues in Emergency Medicine

Suneel Upadhye

Division of Emergency Medicine, McMaster University, Hamilton, Canada

Clinical scenario

As the chief of a busy emergency department (ED), you were asked to generate a new protocol for therapeutic hypothermia in the treatment of post-cardiac arrest survivors, in collaboration with partners in the critical care program. You reviewed the primary trials of this therapeutic modality [1,2], as well as several systematic reviews on the topic [3,4]. You were concerned that the main trials driving this were small and potentially underpowered, and that there may be some concerning methodological flaws in the trials reported and the subsequent meta-analysis. These misgivings were not allayed by a recent position statement by your national emergency medicine organization endorsing this therapy in a recent clinical practice guideline [5]. You decide to investigate further, and bring your concerns to your group.

Background

Physicians are often required to search for the evidence regarding a diagnostic test (e.g., the use of a bedside D-dimer test in diagnosing pulmonary embolism; see Chapter 1), a therapy (e.g., the role of corticosteroids in migraine headaches; see Chapter 48), a policy (e.g., immunization; see Chapter 61) or some other aspect of emergency care. In each case, they are required to pose an answerable question, search widely for the evidence and then, once they identify the evidence, they are expected to critique it. This critiquing is referred to as critical appraisal of the literature.

Critical appraisal of the medical literature remains an integral component of integrating evidence-based medicine into one's clinical practice [6]. For busy clinicians or those who may not have significant training in research methodology, an organized approach to reading, evaluating and integrating new information

is of primary importance. Published critical appraisal tools aim to provide such approaches to readers. There are a number of questions, however, to be asked regarding the definition of "high quality", the performance requirements for appraisal tools that measure quality, the uses of critical appraisal tools in processes of creating and consuming the medical literature, and whether or not critical appraisal tools are able to detect potentially fatal flaws in a study during quality assessment. Finally, one must consider if critical appraisal tools that measure multiple quality domains are better than or equal to a single global evaluation of the report in question. This chapter examines questions around critical appraisal tool evolution and usage, the pitfalls associated with their use, and makes recommendations to emergency clinicians who are trying to use them to improve their clinical practice.

Clinical questions

In order to address the issues of greatest relevance to your assignment and to help in searching the literature for the evidence, a series of questions were structured as recommended in Chapter 1.

1 When evaluating evidence on therapy (population), what are the basic principles (factors) that physicians should understand to assess the quality of a published article (outcome)?

2 When evaluating evidence on therapy (population), what critical appraisal tools (tests) are currently in use and what are their psychometric properties (test properties)?

3 When reading a therapeutic scientific paper (population), what criteria (factors) should a clinician use to identify "high-quality" evidence (outcome)?

4 When reading a systematic review publication (population), what criteria (factors) should a clinician use to identify "high-quality" evidence (outcome)?

5 Could a critical appraisal tool potentially miss a "fatal flaw" in the methodology of a given paper? Could this potentially mislead a reader to change their practice in some inappropriate way?

Evidence-based Emergency Medicine. Edited by Brian H. Rowe
© 2009 Blackwell Publishing, ISBN: 978-1-4051-6143-5.

6 When publishing a scientific paper (populations), what criteria (factors) should editors use to ensure the highest quality of reports (outcome)?

General search strategy

Information was obtained using electronic searches of the PubMed, MEDLINE, CINAHL and EMBASE databases for articles under the following search terms: critical appraisal tools, quality scales, quality checklists, quality assessment, reliability, Jadad scale. Other relevant articles were obtained from the *User's Guide to the Medical Literature* series in the *Journal of the American Medical Association* (*JAMA*) and associated texts [6]. The reference lists of selected articles were also reviewed for any relevant material.

Critical review of the literature:

Question 1: When evaluating evidence on therapy (population), what are the basic principles (factors) that physicians should understand to assess the quality of a published article (outcome)?

Search strategy

- See general search strategy above
- MEDLINE, EMBASE and Cochrane: electronic databases were searched as described in the general search strategy

What is quality?
The concept of "quality" has eluded an accurate definition in the literature. For example, the quality of a controlled clinical trial was first defined as "the confidence that the trial design, conduct, and analysis has minimized or avoided biases in its treatment comparisons" [7]. Another definition of quality was stated as the "likelihood of the trial design to generate unbiased results" [8]. In general, the quality of a study is related to the methods used to collect, analyze and interpret the results of a study. In a way, each study is different, although there are several similarities that indicate higher quality in each domain (e.g., therapeutics, diagnostic testing, prognosis, prevention, and so on).

What is validity?
Both of the above definitions address the notion of internal validity, where the design elements of a trial are consistent with the research question being posed and answered. However, they exclude any reference to the external validity of the trial results (i.e., applicability to practice). It is notoriously difficult for most studies to adequately address external validity, although the final goal of most clinically oriented studies and critical appraisal processes should be to influence clinical practice. There is a surprising lack of attention to the construct of "quality" in published medical

literature and rating tools. Ultimately, the benchmark of "high quality" becomes a floating reference standard, inasmuch as new studies are compared to old studies for relative purposes, but may fail to generate useful certainty. Regardless of how imperfect the definition of "quality" may be, it is still important that critical appraisal tools that evaluate quality be valid and reliable. Properly constructed ratings tools should undergo rigorous scale development and reliability testing, as dictated by psychometric principles [9].

The development of rating tools has enhanced the consumption of medical research by clinicians, researchers, educators, publishers and administrators, by enabling them to evaluate the quality of published studies for their applicability to clinical practice [10]. These tools have taken the form of qualitative checklists and quantitative rating scales. Concerns have been raised about the appropriate use of such rating checklists and scales, inasmuch as they do not necessarily provide valid and reliable measures of quality as applied to critical appraisal of the medical literature [11]. Prior to embarking upon a review of the reliability and validity of the published critical appraisal tools, however, it is useful to review the basic principles of reliability and validity as they apply to measurement scales.

Basic psychometric principles of measurement
Streiner and Norman succinctly review the importance of reliability and validity concepts as applied to measurement scales [9]. Reliability is defined as the ability of a rating tool to provide consistent results when applied under repeated similar testing situations, and validity is the ability of the tool to actually measure the construct which it is supposed to be measuring. To critique published medical literature, this would require critical appraisal tools that would generate similar quality assessment results for the same articles being reviewed by the same reviewer at different times (intra-rater reliability), different reviewers at the same time (inter-rater reliability) and different reviewers at different times (using principles of generalizability theory) [9]. It is in this context that an analysis of current critical appraisal tools can be undertaken.

In summary, quality is an important construct in critical appraisal, and quality tools and checklists exist. Clinicians using them should demand validity and reliability in these tools, and should only use tools where evidence for these are available.

Question 2: When evaluating evidence on therapy (population), what critical appraisal tools (tests) are currently in use and what are their psychometric properties (test properties)?

Search strategy

- See general search strategy above
- MEDLINE, EMBASE and Cochrane: electronic databases were searched as described in the general search strategy

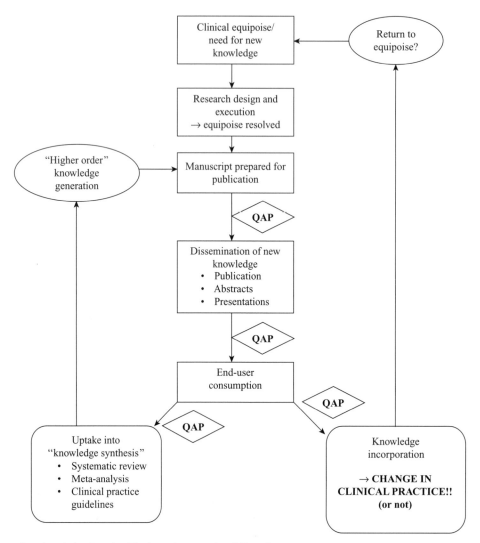

Figure 3.1 The progress of new knowledge through publication and consumption. QAP, quality assessment process.

The processes of critical appraisal/quality assessment can happen at multiple stages in the evolution of a published report, as shown in Fig. 3.1. Prior to publication, a manuscript is scrutinized by journal editors and publishers. After publication, target readers will read and appraise the new information for themselves, and subsequently evaluate its utility in contributing to meaningful clinical practice change. Investigators looking to synthesize old with new knowledge must use critical appraisal tools to evaluate studies for inclusion in their systematic reviews, meta-analyses and clinical practice guidelines. This is a dynamic cyclical process as new questions constantly arise for clinical practice, which need new answers.

Despite the multiple uses of critical appraisal tools in the knowledge dissemination process, there has been very little formal assessment of these tools published in the medical literature. The majority of rating tools fall into the following categories:

1 *Qualitative rating "checklists"*. These tools involve asking a series of methodological questions relating to study design and outcomes, without attempting to quantitatively score any of the components or the article in total. The *User's Guide to the Medical Literature* series is an excellent example of a comprehensive series of ratings checklists [6].

2 *Quantitative rating scales*. These tools involve scoring of specific methodological aspects of a given article, with a summary score at the end. The ratings scale developed by Jadad et al. for randomized controlled trials (RCTs) is one among many such lists [12]. Two major assessments of critical appraisal tools have been published in the literature. The first examined 25 tools for RCTs and found most to have significant deficiencies in methodological rigor during creation and validation [7], the exception being the scale created by Jadad et al. [12]. Less than 25% of scales had a definition of the construct "trial quality", a key component in development of any measurement scale. Less than half reported any measures of reliability. It was unclear whether rating

tools measured the actual methodological quality of the trials, how they were reported, or some combination thereof. One-third of quantitative scales had no information as to how to compute individual and total scores. There was variation as to whether quantitative items were equally weighted, or differentially weighted in item scoring. There was little information as to whether the different tools would agree on comparative scores as applied to the same trial. This could have significant implications when identifying which trials to publish and include in systematic reviews, meta-analyses and clinical practice guidelines (depending upon what scale was used and what quality thresholds were employed).

A follow-up study examined the use of quality ratings by checklists, quantitative scales or individual methodological components of articles, and found that there was no reliable way of using any of these approaches to make valid assessments of quality [11]. Recommendations were made for future scales generation to include common methodological items, ease of use and a focus on items aimed at reducing bias. Uniform guidelines were recommended for systematic reviewers using such scales, as different approaches to quality scoring could affect which studies get included in a systematic review, thereby affecting the final results of a given meta-analysis.

A second review identified 121 different critical appraisal tools from 108 different papers [10]. The authors acknowledge the absence of a gold standard tool with which to critically appraise medical evidence and concluded that the majority of tools (78%) were designed for primary article appraisal, with the remainder being developed for systematic reviews. Regarding psychometric performance, only nine tools (seven experimental, two systematic reviews) established any face validity, one reported some measure of intra-rater reliability during scale development, and nine reported on inter-rater reliability (three during development). It was concluded that there was a distinct lack of information on development processes for most tools, as well as psychometric performance on reliability measures. The authors cautioned that, given the significant volume and variation of tools in print, interpretations of critical analysis must be cautious in the face of the critical appraisal tool used. They also emphasized a need for consensus on important core items for critical appraisal tools to produce a more "standardized environment" in which to conduct critical appraisal of research evidence.

There has been sporadic commentary in the literature regarding quality appraisal issues since these early studies. It has been suggested that quality assessment is a complex construct that encompasses issues of study design, conduct, analysis, reporting and external validity [13]. Another report commented on the elusive metric of quality, stating that quality definitions could relate to design issues generating unbiased results (internal validity) but fail to incorporate issues related to external validity or ethical aspects [14]. The pitfalls of quantitative scales used in meta-analysis were highlighted, where different scales used to score articles lead to different inclusion sets of articles, which could drastically change the magnitude and direction of summary effect estimates produced in a meta-analysis [15]. This supports the position that perhaps an individual component-based approach to quality assessment (compared to total scores) may be more reasonable [14,15].

In summary, emergency physicians should be cautious when using these tools to appraise the literature, with an understanding that these tools may not completely address some important quality domains. If the reader/clinician is unfamiliar with basic design concepts for different studies (e.g., therapy, systematic reviews/meta-analyses, diagnostic tests, etc.), it may be difficult to use critical appraisal tools to see if such studies meet standards of high quality. Emergency physicians should educate themselves in the basic design features of different study designs that meet the requirements for high quality, and apply this knowledge in critical appraisal. Alternatively, they should access second-order review sources that they trust to complete this quality assessment process for them, and filter out the best sources of information for public dissemination.

Question 3: When reading a therapeutic scientific paper (population), what criteria (factors) should a clinician use to identify "high-quality" evidence (outcome)?

Search strategy

- See general search strategy above
- MEDLINE, EMBASE and Cochrane: electronic databases were searched as described in the general search strategy

A number of scales have been developed to critically appraise RCTs with respect to design elements that are considered important. The Jadad scale is the first to have been developed using appropriate psychometric principles (Box 3.1) [9,12]. This scale has been one of the most extensively used in published systematic reviews in paper journals, but less so in the Cochrane Collaboration, which uses a more component-based rating tool [16]. The Jadad scale comprises a simple three-item/five-point scale addressing three key methodological aspects of RCT quality: randomization procedure/appropriateness, blinding procedure/appropriateness, and completeness of follow-up. Although the original authors found the scale to be moderately reliable for critical appraisal, other studies of the scale's reliability have been more variable [17–19]. Overall, the Jadad scale would seem to perform moderately well when trained reviewers understand the items being examined with some expertise. Further validation studies seem to be necessary, and none have been completed in the analysis of emergency medicine literature.

The Cochrane Collaboration uses allocation concealment checklists as an additional method to determine the quality of RCTs [20]. The reason that Jadad et al. did not include this factor in their scoring tool was due to the low frequency of reporting allocation concealment in the literature at the time the scoring system was being developed [12]. This is likely changing with the release of the CONSORT guidelines for reporting RCTs [21]. None the less, the empirical evidence for this factor comes from work performed in

---

Box 3.1 Quality assessment of randomized controlled trials. (From Jadad et al. [12].)

	Score

1. Was the study described as randomized (this includes the use of words such as randomly, random and randomization)?
           Yes = 1   No = 0   ——

2. Was the study described as double blind?
           Yes = 1   No = 0   ——

3. Was there a description of withdrawals and drop-outs?
           Yes = 1   No = 0   ——

Additional points: Add 1 point if:

Method to generate the sequence of randomization was described and was appropriate (e.g., table of random numbers, computer generated, coin tossing, etc.)   ——

Method of double blinding described and appropriate (identical placebo, active placebo, dummy)   ——

Point deduction: Subtract 1 point if:

Method of randomization described and it was **in**appropriate (allocated alternately, according to date of birth, hospital number, etc.)   ——

Method of double blinding described but it was **in**appropriate (comparison of tablet vs injection with no double dummy)   ——

OVERALL SCORE (maximum 5)

---

the past by Schulz and colleagues, which showed that RCTs without concealment of allocation tended to inflate the estimate of treatment effect by as much as 30% [22]. The Cochrane approach is to assign concealment of allocation as follows: clearly concealed (e.g., central randomization, sequential sealed opaque envelopes), unclear (largely due to insufficient reporting), and clearly not concealed (e.g., alteration such as day of the week) (Box 3.2). RCTs that employ concealment of allocation are rated highly since they further reduce the bias(es) associated with research.

Other tools for RCT critical appraisal have also shown variable reliability scores, and this may also be dependent somewhat upon the training and expertise of the rater as well as the tool itself [23,24]. Most scales address only the elements of study design and execution, and do not address issues of external validity; the notable exception to this is the quality index published by Downs et al. [24].

In summary, there are an increasing number of critical appraisal scales for use by readers to examine quality domains of therapy articles; the Jadad scale and the assessment of allocation concealment are two key quality tools in therapy articles. When faced with many scale choices, readers should educate themselves to recognize common quality indicators, and whether or not they have been appropriately addressed in a given study report. It is also important for readers to consider study design features that are *not* commonly addressed by these scales (e.g., outcome measurement, analytical techniques, sample size, funding source and so forth), as any one of them may constitute a "fatal flaw" in the study that may erode confidence in the conclusions the study authors may present.

Question 4: When reading a systematic review publication (population), what criteria (factors) should a clinician use to identify "high-quality" evidence (outcome)?

Search strategy

- See general search strategy above
- MEDLINE, EMBASE and Cochrane: electronic databases were searched as described in the general search strategy

Since systematic reviews (SRs) are an ever increasing component of the emergency medicine literature, and Cochrane reviews are increasingly applicable to ED clinicians [25], it is important to have a clear understanding of the strengths and weaknesses of SRs. In the field of emergency medicine, Kelly et al. examined the scientific quality of 29 SRs published in five leading emergency medicine journals from 1988 to 1998 [26]. Results using the Overview Quality Assessment Questionnaire (OQAQ) total score indicated that the overall scientific quality was low. These authors concluded that the considerable confusion in the design, reporting and description of SRs may limit the validity of the reported results.

The main tool used to assess quality in SRs is the OQAQ developed by Oxman and Guyatt [27]. The OQAQ is a 10-item scale where the first nine questions are rated on a yes/partially/no format to assess how the review was designed and reported (Box 3.3). A final question on the overall scientific quality of the review is rated

---

Box 3.2 Quality assessment of RCTs using concealment of allocation. (From Schulz et al. [22].)

Concealment of treatment allocation:

Adequate
Inadequate
Unclear

Adequate:	e.g., central randomization; numbered/coded containers; drugs prepared by pharmacy; serially numbered, opaque, sealed envelopes
Inadequate:	e.g., alternation, use of case record numbers, dates of birth or day of week; open lists
Unclear:	Allocation concealment approach not reported or fits neither above category

---

on a seven-point Likert scale. The tool consists of questions on how the review is designed and reported; it does not require knowledge about the included trials themselves. The psychometric properties of the OQAQ have been thoroughly tested and clearly validated using a number of different measures [26]. Articles are classified as having serious or extensive flaws if they received a score of 1–3, and as having minimal or minor flaws if they received scores from 4 to 7.

Box 3.3 The Overview Quality Assessment Questionnaire (OQAQ) tool for systematic reviews (from Oxman and Guyatt, 1991 [27]).

Complete form for each study.   Reviewer Initials: _____   Study ID: _____

	Quality features	1	2*	3
1	Were the search methods used to find evidence on the primary question(s) stated?	No	Partially	Yes
2	Was the search for evidence reasonably comprehensive?	No	Can't tell	Yes
3	Were the criteria used for deciding which studies to include in the overview reported?	No	Partially	Yes
4	Was bias in the selection of studies avoided?	No	Can't tell	Yes
5	Were the criteria used for assessing the validity of the included studies reported	No	Partially	Yes
6	Was the validity of all the studies referred to in the text assessed using appropriate criteria?	No	Can't tell	Yes
7	Were the methods used to combine the findings of the relevant studies (to reach a conclusion) reported?	No	Partially	Yes
8	Were the findings of the relevant studies combined appropriately relative to the primary question of the overview?	No	Can't tell	Yes
9	Were the conclusions made by the author(s) supported by the data and/or analysis reported in the overview?	No	Partially	Yes
10	How could you rate the scientific quality of this review?			

Flaw						
Extensive		Minor				
Major					Minimal	
1	2	3	4	5	6	7

Note: If the methods that were used are reported incompletely relative to a specific item, score that item as "partially". Similarly, if there is no information provided regarding what was done relative to a particular question, score it as "can't tell", unless there is information in the overview to suggest either that the criterion was or was not met.

For Question 8, if no attempt has been made to combine findings, and no statement is made regarding the inappropriateness of combining findings, check "no". If a summary (general) estimate is given anywhere in the abstract, the discussion, or the summary section of the paper, and it is not reported how that estimate was derived mark "no", even if there is a statement regarding the limitations of combining the findings of the studies reviewed. If in doubt, mark "can't tell".

For an overview to be scored as "yes" on Question 9, data (not just citations) must be reported that support the main conclusions regarding the primary question(s) that the overview addresses.

The score for Question 10, the overall scientific quality, should be based on your answers to the first 9 questions. The following guidelines can be used to assist with deriving a summary score: if the "can't tell" option is used one or more times on the preceding questions, a review is likely to have minor flaws at best, and it is difficult to rule out major flows (ie, a score ≤4). If the "no" option is used on Questions 2, 4, 6, or 8, the review is likely to have major flaws (ie, a score of ≤3, depending on the number and degree of the flaws).

*A score of 2 for any of the first 9 questions is given if the reviewer's response is "partially" or "can't tell".

Adapted with permission from Annals of Emergency Medicine [26].

As can be seen from Box 3.3, the OQAQ focuses on a variety of components of a systematic review to develop a weighting of the biases associated with the review. First, and foremost, like this textbook, the OQAQ rates SRs highly if they arise from a clear, succinct and relevant clinical question (e.g., population, intervention, control, outcome and design; PICO-D). Second, the OQAQ rates SRs highly if they avoid publication bias and if the search strategy is described and sufficiently comprehensive (e.g., uses a variety of sources for literature related to the topic). For example, if an SR is being completed on RCTs, then publication bias can be a considerable problem. In emergency medicine, recent evidence suggests that publication is not related to the positive nature of results [28]; however, this is not the case in other specialties. Not searching widely for unpublished or hard to find literature will lead to publication bias.

Third, the OQAQ rates SRs highly if they avoid selection bias, by describing their inclusion and exclusion criteria, search strategy, and searching widely through various sources for literature related to the topic. Most high-quality reviews employ various steps in the selection process, use multiple and blinded reviewers, and have a process for resolving disagreement(s). Single authored reviews should be interpreted with caution.

Fourth, the OQAQ rates SRs highly if they describe the method(s) employed to report quality of the included studies. The quality assessment methods for including/excluding trials from meta-analysis play a crucial role in determining the final outcome estimates [13,14]. This was highlighted in a study that examined the use of 25 different quality scales to rate 17 articles on managing deep vein thrombosis with low molecular weight (LMW) heparins [15]. The authors found that using six scales resulted in a selection pool of "high-quality" studies that suggested no significant benefit of LMW heparins compared to standard heparin. However, using seven other scales resulted in a different pool of "high-quality" studies that suggested a statistically significant benefit. The other 12 scales yielded mixed results. The authors concluded that "the type of scale used to assess trial quality can dramatically influence interpretation of meta-analytic studies". They suggest that an approach involving analysis of the relevant key methodological aspects of individual studies (e.g., blinding, randomization, follow-up, etc.) should be the basis of quality assessment of the individual trials included in the systematic review.

The controversy of whether or not there are associations of summary effect estimates with quality scale scores continues. There is uncertainty that effect estimates can be inflated when "poor quality" trials are included in meta-analyses, or that overall effect estimates may not be affected by quality scores or their individual components at all [28–31]. A number of solutions involving differential weighting of quality components to screen studies also yield mixed results; there are many concerns about inappropriate or unjustified weighting, data manipulation and the subsequent risk of increased bias for the final effect estimates, precisely what is ideally avoided during the meta-analytic process [16,29–37].

The most intuitive opinion is that there is no criterion standard for quality assessment, and likely never will be [36]. When rating articles for use in meta-analysis, authors must pay particular attention to potential misclassification, where unreliable "cut-off" thresholds for high versus low quality could lead to inappropriate exclusion of articles from inclusion (eroding the confidence in the precision of the pooled results). A future research agenda proposed would further validate the Delphi criteria for generic quality items and examine the impact of these quality components on assessment procedures [36].

The OQAQ has its weaknesses, and an alternative scoring system has been developed recently by Canadian researchers [38]. It is likely that others will emerge in the near future; however, the important lesson is that clinicians reading SRs and meta-analyses for new information to guide clinical emergency practice should develop strategies to identify the strengths and weakness of the overviews. They should have confidence that the tool being used addresses important study quality domains in the individual studies screened, so that the pooled information and "answers" are valid and reliable.

Question 5: Could a critical appraisal tool potentially miss a "fatal flaw" in the methodology of a given paper? Could this potentially mislead a reader to change their practice in some inappropriate way?

Search strategy

- See general search strategy above
- MEDLINE, EMBASE and Cochrane: electronic databases were searched as described in the general search strategy

None of the previously discussed reviews have heretofore addressed the issue of the ability of critical appraisal tools to detect significant methodological problems in studies, and how one or many of these could seriously impair, or "fatally flaw", the quality of the published report. It is appropriate to explore the shortcomings of critical appraisal tools to detect serious methodological flaws in published trials, given the concerns of poor design methods causing biased effect estimates [37]. It has been suggested that readers focus on reading methods/results sections only, read pre-appraised abstract sources first, and beware faulty comparators, composite endpoints, small treatment effects and subgroup analyses [39]. These topics and others are illustrated in Table 3.1, with reference to published trials relevant to the practice of emergency medicine [40–57]. The examples provided highlight common important domains of trial design that can variably bias results, and that most critical appraisal tools fail to acknowledge appropriately.

In summary, while the OQAQ provides a method to assess fatal flaws in SRs, most critical appraisal tools do not instruct readers in this method. It is likely that no usable tool will be sufficiently comprehensive to detect such flaws, even with experienced readers, so the onus remains on knowledge "consumers" to be alert to

Table 3.1 Summary of fatal flaws missed by critical appraisal tools.

Fatal flaw	Explanation of flaw	Example
Claiming equivalence/non-inferiority in a failed superiority trial	Fundamentally different designs, other conceptual difference [40]	GUSTO III – claimed equivalence of r-Pa to t-PA for STEMI care (failed to prove intended superiority) based on easier use [41]
Active vs placebo comparators	Expect inflated benefits when newer agents compared to placebo vs usual standard treatments [42,43]	CREATE – claimed benefit of adding reviparin to usual myocardial infarction care compared to placebo, not other effective antithrombotics [44]
(Ir)relevant outcomes	Outcomes of interest should be clinically relevant, not just surrogates	Higher doses of mannitol (vs standard dose) showed benefits in reducing pupil size in acute brain injury, but marginal benefit in functional outcome, and no benefit for mortality [45]
Inconsistent co-interventions	Must have otherwise equally treated patients in comparison arms for two specific agents	MERLIN – too many differences in medical care confounding apparent benefits of rescue angioplasty vs medical care after failed STEMI lysis [46]
Blinding	Inconsistent application of the term "double blind;" up to seven different groups can be blinded [47]	Many examples in the literature; most "double blinds" refer to patients and physicians; can also include data analysts, observers, outcome adjudicators, manuscript writers
Multiple tests of comparison/subgroup analyses	Increases the likelihood of finding some significant difference due to chance alone	European multi-country prehospital study found vasopressin superior to epinephrine in asystolic patients; effect negated when reanalyzed with patients lost to follow-up [48,49]
Early stopping of trial	Trials stopped due to some early significant benefit/harm detected; may be negated when trial completed [50–52]	Prevention of CIN with bicarbonate vs saline stopped after 137/260 patients recruited; excess incidence of CIN, but none needed dialysis [53]
Composite endpoints	Used to enhance statistical efficiency or detect rare outcomes; overall effects may confound individual contributions [39]	CLARITY-TIMI 28 added clopidogrel to aspirin-treated STEMI patients; composite benefits driven by restored angiographic blood flow, not reduced recurrent myocardial infarction or death rates [54]
Economic conclusions	Important outcome, yet often ignored (no mention in CONSORT statement) [21,55,56]	Intramuscular methylprednisolone claimed to be cheaper/better compliance vs daily tapered steroids in ED-discharged asthma patients (failed superiority trial) [57]

CIN, contrast-induced nephropathy; ED, emergency department; r-Pa, reteplase; STEMI, ST elevation myocardial infarction; t-PA, tissue plasminogen activator.

such "fatal flaws" when critically appraising and using the reported conclusions.

Question 6: When publishing a scientific paper (populations), what criteria (factors) should editors use to ensure the highest quality of reports (outcome)?

Search strategy

- See general search strategy above

Clinicians often read articles and trust their origin and results, especially publications from major medical journals such as the *Lancet, British Medical Journal* (*BMJ*), *New England Journal of Medicine*, and the *Journal of the American Medical Association* (*JAMA*). Should this be the case? Can readers trust the information released in these and other journals?

The concerns for missing methodological flaws with rating scales/checklists have been addressed in the field of peer review of medical journals. It has been noted that "part of the problem may be that standardized quantitative rating scales are not the right way to gauge a paper's quality ... because they don't capture certain flaws" [6]. The potential disconnect between the peer review process and recognizing good versus bad quality has also been discussed by Enserink [58]. A study involving ratings of manuscripts submitted to the *Annals of Emergency Medicine* demonstrated only moderate agreement (intraclass correlation coefficient (ICC) = 0.44) using a previously validated rating tool [59]. The tool also only detected a mean of 3.4 of 10 potentially "fatal" flaws, and 3.1 "minor" flaws in manuscripts analyzed. The authors noted, however, that there was poor correlation with rates of acceptance recommendations ($R = -0.34$) and "decision congruence" (whether the reviewer recommendation matched the editor's final decision to accept or not; $R = 0.26$). They concluded that, although their rating tool performed reliably, the summary scores did not replace the subjective rating/decision to publish or not. Bordage examined the reliability of manuscript ratings and descriptive comments of referees for medical education articles, and found that it was not possible to distinguish major flaws or reasons to reject from minor ones, using the rating scale they employed [60]. Similarly, 40% of referees recommended rejection of articles after a global assessment, which was contrary to their numeric scores on the rating scale. The diversity of descriptive comments suggested that different referees had focused on different aspects of the manuscripts and had weighted them differentially. They concluded that global ratings seem to be different from the summary score of a quantitative rating scale, and that recommendations for acceptance/rejection seem to be rooted in the global rating. They also acknowledged the notion that certain manuscript deficiencies (e.g., lack of importance, inappropriate study design) were considered "fatal" in their estimation; no comments are given as to whether or not their five-point rating tool captured these deficiencies. It becomes evident that the process of peer review and manuscript acceptance to medical journals is just as fraught with reliability concerns as is primary analysis of published studies and rating for inclusion in systematic reviews.

For emergency medicine referees and editors, this would suggest that there needs to be a close examination of the processes by which submitted manuscripts are reviewed and rated for publication. Readers should have confidence that the papers they read in emergency journals have been rigorously and reliably evaluated, so that only the highest quality information is selected for publication and dissemination (early stages of knowledge progress in Fig. 3.1).

Is there really a difference between the overall gut impression (gestalt) of quality obtained from reading an article compared to critical appraisal with scoring tools? Most individuals will likely rely on their overall impression of a paper regarding the importance and value of the information provided, regardless of whether or not they explicitly use a validated appraisal tool. No studies involving evaluation of the medical literature by comparing overall "gestalt" impressions of quality versus rating scale scores have been published (at the time of this writing). Two Cochrane Collaboration reviews examining peer review processes on study publication and grant review have been completed. Regarding peer review for publishing biomedical studies, only two studies were found that examined the reliability of checklist scoring tools, and these were found to be unreliable [61]. For reviewing grant applications, three studies found high agreement between grant referees, but no impact on the decision to award the grant or not; the authors concluded that some other evaluation process, aside from rating scores, seemed to be predominant in making these decisions [62].

In studies involving performance evaluation on essay examinations and clinical performance of medical students, there were only modest differences in reliability scores generated by global ratings versus checklist ratings [63]. The authors found that despite the perceived subjectivity of global ratings versus objective checklist ratings, both are reliable. In a follow-up study of essay examina-

tion performance rated with global expert ratings versus trained checklist raters, there were high levels of comparable validity between the two ratings, when benchmarked against a standardized National Board Exam test [64]. The global rating was actually more highly correlated with the reference standard. The authors concluded that "objectivity" – defined as the goal for value-free judgment – does not necessarily result from "objectification", the strategies used to reduce measurement error. They also concluded that rating exercises are context-specific, and that different rating strategies may be optimal depending upon the domains being evaluated in subjects.

Both groups of studies suggest that there is disagreement between the quality assessment processes of global rating versus summary checklist scores in various evaluation environments, with the global rating frequently dominating the final decisions involved. This can be extrapolated to the field of critical appraisal, where the studies discussed above suggest that rating scales/checklists may be variably reliable measures of the quality of a study/manuscript. However, they do not necessarily replace the global impression of reviewers using other dimensions of evaluation.

In summary, emergency physicians who are reading the literature should understand that despite many attempts to standardize the assessment process during a manuscript's journey to publication, the tools used for quality assessment may be variably reliable and valid, and that the decision whether to publish a paper may not be related to quality scores at all. Similarly, when deciding whether or not to incorporate new knowledge into their own practices, it may be reasonable for clinicians to trust their overall impression of the scientific quality of a paper, rather than some aggregate score from a critical appraisal tool.

Conclusions

In the scenario described above, the search provided evidence that the use of hypothermia in cardiac arrest is likely a justifiable practice, and can lead to improved patient outcomes. Your group agrees that this can be an important new intervention to offer patients with an otherwise dismal outcome, and that the costs of implementation are minimal. You appoint a group member to "champion" this new intervention, in conjunction with your intensivist colleagues.

The state of the art in critical appraisal tools reveals a field of methodological research that is lacking. There seems to be no definite agreement on what the construct "quality" actually entails. There is an abundance of quality assessment tools in print, most of which are deficient psychometrically. Even the most commonly used rating tools, such as the Jadad scale, reveal equivocal results in terms of their reliability. In areas such as systematic reviews and peer review mechanisms of article publication, the sparse evidence suggests that there are deficiencies in the reliability of tools being used to evaluate studies, and that the ratings generated by such tools may not be influential in decisions to include studies for meta-analysis or publication. It is unlikely that the areas of critical appraisal and scientific overview can progress without some regression to basic principles of defining quality and generating psychometrically sound tools with which to measure them.

For clinicians looking for guidance on how different types of research studies should be reported, a recent summary in the *Archives of Internal Medicine* should provide some direction on the different types of guidelines regarding study reporting, methodological quality assessment, grading systems and ethical information [65]. In addition to randomized trials and systematic reviews discussed earlier, these include study designs such as diagnostic test studies, observational designs, economic evaluations, and so on.

There are a number of biological, social, economic and epidemiological issues that clinicians must consider when deciding whether or not the results of a clinical trial are applicable to their patient populations [66]. It is challenging for time-constrained emergency physicians to know how to approach their reading of the medical literature in the absence of reliable, valid critical appraisal tools. The diversity of activities involving critical appraisal (e.g., peer review for publication, systematic review/meta-analysis, changing clinical practice, and so forth) demands certain baseline knowledge of appropriate definition and reliable measurement of study quality. Given the goal of "knowledge translation" to take high-quality evidence and incorporate it into clinical practice, emergency academicians and clinicians need to understand the different aspects of quality assessment and appraisal, and how to improve patient outcomes with high-quality information [67]. Some of this important work has been undertaken in emergency medicine, but there is much more to be done.

Acknowledgments

The author acknowledges Drs Kevin Eva and Geoffrey Norman in the Program for Education Research and Development at McMaster University, and Dr. Andrew Worster, Division of Emergency Medicine, McMaster University, for their valuable inputs to this chapter.

Conflicts of interest

None were reported.

References

1 The Hypothermia After Cardiac Arrest (HACA) Study Group. Mild therapeutic hypothermia to improve the neurologic outcome after cardiac arrest. *N Engl J Med* 2002;**346**:549–56.

2 Bernard SA, Gray TW, Buist MD, et al. Treatment of comatose survivors of out-of-hospital cardiac arrest with induced hypothermia. *N Engl J Med* 2002;**346**:557–63.

3 Howes D, Green R, Gray S, et al. Evidence for the use of hypothermia after cardiac arrest. *Can J Emerg Med* 2006;**8**(2):109–15.

4 Holzer M, Bernard SA, Hachimi-Idrissi S, et al. Hypothermia for neuroprotection after cardiac arrest: systematic review and individual patient data meta-analysis. *Crit Care Med* 2005;**33**:414–18.

5 Canadian Association of Emergency Physicians and the CAEP Critical Care Committee. Guidelines for the use of hypothermia after cardiac arrest. *Can J Emerg Med* 2006;**8**(2):106–7.

6 Guyatt G, Rennie D, eds. *User's Guide to the Medical Literature. A manual for evidence-based clinical practice.* AMA Press, Chicago, 2002.

7 Moher D, Jadad A, Nichol G, et al. Assessing the quality of randomized controlled trials: an annotated bibliography of scales and checklists. *Controlled Clin Trials* 1995;**16**:62–73.

8 Verhagen AP, de Wet HCW, de Bie RA, et al. The Delphi list: a criteria list for quality assessment of randomized controlled trials for conducting systematic reviews developed by Delphi Consensus. *J Clin Epidemiol* 1998;**51**(12):1235–41.

9 Streiner DL, Norman, GR. *Health Measurement Scales: A practical guide to their development and use.* Oxford University Press, Oxford, 1989.

10 Katrak P, Bialocerkowski AE, Massey-Westropp N, et al. A systematic review of the content of critical appraisal tools. *BMC Med Res Methodol* 2004;**4**:22. Available at www.biomedcentral.com/1471-2288/4/22.

11 Moher D, Jadad A, Tugwell D. Assessing the quality of randomized controlled trials: current issues and future directions. *Int J Tech Assess Health Care* 1996;**12**(2):195–206.

12 Jadad JR, Moore RA, Carroll D, et al. Assessing the quality of reports of randomized clinical trials: is blinding necessary? *Controlled Clin Trials* 1996;**17**:1–12.

13 Ioannidis JPA, Lau J. Can quality of clinical trials and meta-analysis be quantified? *Lancet* 1988;**258**:590–91.

14 Berlin JA, Rennie D. Measuring the quality of trials. *JAMA* 1999;**282**:1083–5.

15 Juni P, Witschi A, Bloch R, et al. The hazards of scoring the quality of clinical trials for meta-analysis. *JAMA* 1999;**282**:1054–60.

16 Moja LP, Telaro D, D'Amico R, et al., for the Metaquality Study Group. Assessment of methodological quality of primary studies by systematic reviews: results of the metaquality cross sectional study. *BMJ* 2005;**330**:1053–7. (doi:10.1136/bmj.38414.515938.8F).

17 Clark HD, Wells GA, Huet C, et al. Assessing the quality of randomized trials: reliability of the Jadad scale. *Controlled Clin Trials* 1999;**20**:448–52.

18 Oremus M, Wolfson C, Perrault A, et al. Interrater reliability of the modified Jadad quality scale for systematic reviews of Alzheimer's disease drug trials. *Dement Geriatr Cogn Disord* 2001;**12**(3):232–6.

19 Bhandari M, Richards RR, Sprague S, et al. Quality in the reporting of randomized trials in surgery: is the Jadad scale reliable? *Controlled Clin Trials* 2001;**22**:687–8.

20 Higgins JPT, et al. *Cochrane Handbook for Systematic Reviews of Interventions 4.2.6* (updated September 2006). Available at http://www.cochrane.org/resources/handbook/hbook.htm (accessed October 6, 2006).

21 Moher D, et al., for the CONSORT Group. The CONSORT statement: revised recommendations for improving the quality of reports of parallel-group randomized trials. *Lancet* 2001;**357**:1191–4.

22 Schulz KF, Chalmers I, Hayes RJ, et al. Empirical evidence of bias: dimension of methodological quality associated with estimates of treatment effects in controlled trials. *JAMA* 1995;**273**:408–12.

23 Verhagen AP, de Wet HCW, de Bie RA, et al. Balneotherapy and quality assessment: interobserver reliability of the Maastricht criteria list and the need for blinded quality assessment. *J Clin Epidemiol* 1998;**51**(4), 335–41.

24 Downs SH, Black N. The feasibility of creating a checklist for the assessment of the methodological quality both of randomized and non-randomised studies of health care interventions. *J Epidemiol Community Health* 1998;**52**:377–84.

25 Zed PJ, Rowe BH, Loewen PS, et al. Systematic reviews in emergency medicine: Part I. Background and general principles for locating and critically appraising reviews. *Can J Emerg Med* 2003;**5**(5):331–5.

26 Kelly KD, Travers A, Dorgan M, et al. Evaluating the quality of systematic reviews in the emergency medicine literature. *Ann Emerg Med* 2001;**38**:518–26.

27 Oxman AD, Guyatt G. Validation of an index of the quality of review articles. *J Clin Epidemiol* 1991;**44**(11):1271–8.

28 Ospina MB, Kelly K, Klassen T, et al. Publication bias of randomized controlled trials in emergency medicine. *Acad Emerg Med* 2006;**13**:102–8.

29 Moher D, Pham B, Jones A, et al. Does quality of reports of randomized trials affect estimates of intervention efficacy reported in meta-analyses? *Lancet* 1998;**352**:609–13.

30 Balk EM, Bonis PAL, Moskowitz H, et al. Correlation of quality measures with estimates of treatment effect in meta-analyses of randomized controlled trials. *JAMA* 2002;**287**(22):2973–82.

31 Greenland S. Invited commentary: A critical look at some popular meta-analytic methods. *Am J Epidemiol* 1994;**140**:290–96.

32 Olkin I. Invited commentary: re: "A critical look at some popular meta-analytic methods". *Am J Epidemiol* 1994;**140**:297–9.

33 Greenland S. Quality scores are useless and potentially misleading. *Am J Epidemiol* 1994;**140**:300–301.

34 Juni P, Altman DG, Egger M. Assessing the quality of randomized controlled trials. In: Egger M, Smith GD, Altman DG, eds. *Systematic Reviews in Health Care: Meta-analysis in context.* BMJ Books, London, 2001.

35 Detsky AS, Naylor CD, O'Rourke K, et al. Incorporating variations in the quality of individual randomized trials into meta-analyses. *J Clin Epidemiol* 1994;**45**:255–65.

36 Greenland S, O'Rourke K. On the bias produced by quality of scores in meta-analysis, and a hierarchical view of proposed solutions. *Biostatistics* 2001;**2**:463–71.

37 Verhagen AP, de West HCW, de Bie RA, et al. The art of quality assessment of RCTs included in systematic reviews. *J Clin Epidemiol* 2001;**54**:651–4.

38 Shea BJ, Grimshaw JM, Wells GA, et al. Development of AMSTAR: a measurement tool to assess the methodological quality of systematic reviews. *BMC Med Res Methodol* 2007;**7**:10.

39 Montori VM, Jaeschke R, Schunemann HJ, et al. Users' guide to detecting misleading claims in clinical research reports. *BMJ* 2005;**329**:1093–6.

40 Ware JH, Antman EM. Equivalence trials. *N Engl J Med* 1997;**337**:1159–61.

41 GUSTO Investigators. A comparison of reteplase with alteplase for acute myocardial infarction. *N Engl J Med* 1997;**337**:1118–23.

42 Rothman KJ, Michels KB. Sounding board: the continuing unethical use of placebo controls. *N Engl J Med* 1994;**331**:394–8.

43 Rothman KJ, Michels KB, Baum M. For and against: declaration of Helsinki should be strengthened. *BMJ* 2000;**321**:442–5.

44 CREATE Trial Group Investigators. Effects of reviparin, a low molecular weight heparin, on mortality, reinfarction and strokes in patients with acute myocardial infarction presenting with St-segment elevation. *JAMA* 2005;**293**:427–36.

45 Cruz J, Minoja G, Okuchi K, et al. Successful use of the new high-dose mannitol treatment in patients with Glasgow Coma Scale scores of 3 and bilateral abnormal pupillary widening: a randomized trial. *J Neurosurg* 2004;**100**:376–83.

46 The MERLIN Trial. A randomized trial of rescue angioplasty versus a conservative approach for failed fibrinolysis in ST-segment elevation myocardial infarction. *J Am Coll Cardiol* 2004;**44**(2):287–96.

47 Devereaux PJ, Bhandari M, Montori VM, et al. Double blind, you are the weakest link – goodbye. *ACP J Club* 2002;**136**:A11–12.

48 Wenzel V, Krismer AC, Arntz HR, et al., European Resuscitation Council Vasopressor during Cardiopulmonary Resuscitation Study Group. A comparison of vasopressin and epinephrine for out-of-hospital cardiopulmonary resuscitation. *N Engl J Med* 2004;**350**(2):105–13.

49 Worster A, Upadhye S, Fermandes CMB. Vasopressin versus epinephrine for out-of-hospital cardiopulmonary resuscitation. *Can J Emerg Med* 2005;**7**(1):48–50.

50 Wheatley K, Clayton CMB. Be skeptical about unexpected large apparent treatment effects: the case of an MRC AML12 randomization. *Controlled Clin Trials* 2003;**24**:66–70.

51 Schoenfeld DA, O'Meade, M. Pro/con clinical debate: it is acceptable to stop large multicentre randomized controlled trials at interim analysis for futility. *Crit Care* 2005;**9**(1):34–6.

52 Slutsky AS, Lavery JV. Data safety and monitoring boards. *N Engl J Med* 2004;**350**(11):1143–7.

53 Merten GJ, Burgess WP, Gray LV, et al. Prevention of contrast-induced nephropathy with sodium bicarbonate: a randomized controlled trial. *JAMA* 2004;**291**(19):2328–34.

54 Sabatine MS, Cannon CP, Gibson CM, et al. Addition of clopidogrel to aspirin and fibrinolytic therapy for myocardial infarction with ST-segment elevation. *N Engl J Med* 2005;**352**(12):1179–89.

55 Drummond MF, O'Brien BJ, Stoddart GL, et al. *Methods for the Economic Evaluation of Health Care Programmes*, 2nd edn. Oxford University Press, Oxford, 1997.

56 Imai K, Zhang P. *Integrating Economic Analysis into Clinical Trials.* Available at www.thelancet.com (published online May 12, 2005; doi: 10.1016/S0140-6736(05) 66390-8 (2005)).

57 Lahn M, Bijur P, Gallagher EJ. Randomized clinical trial of intramuscular vs oral methylprednisolone in the treatment of asthma exacerbations following discharge from an emergency department. *Chest* 2004;**126**:362–8.

58 Enserink M. Peer review and quality: a dubious connection? *Science* 2001;**293**:2187–8.

59 Callaham ML, Baxt WG, Waeckerle JF, et al. Reliability of editors' subjective quality ratings of peer reviews of manuscripts. *JAMA* 1998;**280**:229–31.

60 Bordage G. Reasons reviewers reject and accept manuscripts: the strengths and weaknesses in medical education reports. *Acad Med* 2001;**76**:889–93.

61 Jefferson TO, Alderson P, Davidoff F, et al. Editorial peer-review for improving the quality of reports of biomedical studies (Review). *Cochrane Database Method Rev* 2001;**3**:MR000016 (doi: 10.1002/14651858.MR000016).

62 Demicheli V, Di Peitrantonj C. Peer review for improving the quality of grant applications (Review). *Cochrane Database Method Rev* 2003;**1**:MR000003 (doi: 10.1002/14651858.MR000003).

63 Van der Vleuten CPM, Norman GR, DeGraaf E. Pitfalls in the pursuit of objectivity: issues of reliability. *Med Educ* 1991;**25**:110–18.

64 Norman GR, Van der Vleuten CPM, DeGraaf E. Pitfalls in the pursuit of objectivity: issues of validity, efficiency and acceptability. *Med Educ* 1991;**25**:119–26.

65 Falagas ME, Pitsouni EI. Guidelines and consensus statements regarding the conduction and reporting of clinical research studies. *Arch Intern Med* 2007;**167**:877–8.

66 Dans AL, Dans LF, Guyatt GH, et al., for the Evidence-Based Medicine Working Group. Users' Guide to the Medical Literature XIV: How to decide on the applicability of clinical trial results to your patient. *JAMA* 1998;**279**:545–9.

67 Lang E, Wyer PC, Haynes RB. Knowledge translation: closing the evidence-to-practice gap. *Ann Emerg Med* 2007;**49**:355–63.

4 Continuing Education

Joel Lexchin

School of Health Policy and Management, York University, Toronto *and*
Department of Family and Community Medicine, University of Toronto, Toronto *and*
Emergency Department, University Health Network, Toronto, Canada

Clinical scenario

As the chair of your emergency department's continuing medical education (CME) committee you are approached by a representative of one of the large pharmaceutical companies asking whether or not your department requires additional funding for the emergency medicine conference that it will be staging next year. The representative says that the funding will come in the form of an unrestricted grant but that her company will be glad to help you locate possible speakers for some of your sessions. In addition, the company is interested in sponsoring evening journal clubs at the home of one of the staff or at a local restaurant. Once again, the representative insists she is only interested in providing the funding to support the evening meal (e.g., food, beverages and alcohol); however, she states that her company would be glad to help you locate possible papers for some of your sessions. How should you handle these offers?

Background

Continuing medical education is an important component of professional development and maintenance of competency in a field that is rapidly changing. There are a variety of formats through which CME has traditionally been delivered including: academic rounds, journal clubs, workshops, conferences, journal reading and sponsored events. More innovative methods include self-directed learning using small group, problem-based sessions and web-based learning, to name a few. Despite CME's widely accepted importance, its delivery and format have been the subject of much controversy [1].

Evidence-based Emergency Medicine. Edited by Brian H. Rowe
© 2009 Blackwell Publishing, ISBN: 978-1-4051-6143-5.

All of the emergency medicine specialty accreditation organizations in North America require holders of specialty certificates to participate in yearly CME activities in order to retain their accreditation [2–4]. Running formal CME programs is expensive and there is little money forthcoming from academic institutions or government to subsidize the process. Without outside funding these programs would have to impose high registration fees on individual doctors who might not be willing to pay. High costs would be even more of a burden for medical students and residents, depriving them of the opportunity to attend important national and international events. Physician shortages, increasing work and personal commitments, and lack of time preclude many physicians from traveling to distant CME events. In summary, CME is methodologically complex, time-consuming, costly and an often neglected issue for today's busy practitioner.

In the absence of other sources of money and faced with rising CME costs, event organizers have been increasingly turning to pharmaceutical companies for funding. At the same time, there have been questions raised about commercial biases introduced into CME because of industry funding. Other debates about CME concern the method of delivery, its long-term effectiveness and whether changes in knowledge are predictive of changes in behavior and patient health outcomes. This chapter examines these issues. The definition used for CME is one proposed by Davis as "any attempt to persuade physicians to modify their practice performance by communicating clinical information" [5].

Clinical questions

1 For physicians attending CME events (population), does funding of CME by commercial entities (e.g., pharmaceutical companies, device manufacturers, etc.) (intervention) introduce biases in the content of the course and physicians' knowledge (outcome) compared to events sponsored by non-commercial entities (control)?

2 For physicians seeking CME (population), what are the effects on knowledge uptake and retention (outcome) of CME delivered through multiple interventions (intervention) compared to CME delivered through a single intervention (control)?

3 For physicians seeking CME (population), what are the effects on knowledge uptake and retention (outcome) of CME directed by problem-based education (intervention) compared to other forms of CME (control)?

4 For physicians seeking CME (population), do active formats (e.g., academic detailing) (intervention) improve knowledge uptake and retention (outcome) compared to passive formats (e.g., large group lectures) (control)?

5 For physicians seeking CME (population), does web-based CME (intervention) improve knowledge uptake and retention (outcome) compared to other forms of CME (control)?

6 For physicians attending CME events (population), does the CME (intervention) have a different effect size on patient health outcomes (outcome) compared to physicians' learning and performance (control)?

7 For physicians attending CME events (population), do time factors (longer contact time for each CME program; longer time between the end of the CME program and measurement) (intervention) affect physicians' knowledge (outcome) compared to shorter contact time and shorter time between the end of the CME program and measurement (control)?

8 For physicians who have attended CME events (population), does mandatory CME (intervention) have a larger effect size (outcome) compared to voluntary CME (control)?

General search strategy

The primary search involved a PubMed resource and the Cochrane Library (reviews and other reviews) looking for systematic reviews. Additional articles were identified from the bibliographies of the systematic reviews. In general, the literature tended to explore two separate questions: (i) is CME effective and for what outcomes; and (ii) what kinds of CME are effective [6]? Material from 18 systematic reviews forms the basis for most of the analyses in this chapter. Table 4.1 evaluates their methodology using a validated scale developed by Oxman and Guyatt [7] and shows that the methodological quality of the reviews was highly variable. Although the intent of this chapter was to look at CME both in general and particularly with respect to emergency physicians, there was no literature that specifically identified this group of doctors.

The primary search strategy was:
• PubMed: education, medical, continuing [MeSH] AND English [limitation] AND systematic review [limitation] AND 1985 to present (May 30, 2007) [limitation]
• Cochrane Library (reviews and other reviews): education AND (physician OR doctor)

Critical review of the literature

Question 1: For physicians attending CME events (population), does funding of CME by commercial entities (e.g., pharmaceutical companies, device manufacturers, etc.) (intervention) introduce biases in the content of the course and physicians' knowledge (outcome) compared to events sponsored by non-commercial entities (control)?

Search strategy

• Drug promotion database (http://www.drugpromo.info/): continuing medical education [keyword]
• Healthy Skepticism Library (http://www.healthyskepticism.org/library.php): continuing AND medical AND education [keywords]

Commercial support for CME has increased substantially in developed countries such as the United States. In 1998, industry contributed slightly over a third of the US$ 889 million spent on CME in that year; however by 2005 that had risen to 52% of $2.05 billion [8]. In the past, physicians ranked company-sponsored CME lower than other sources such as journal articles as sources of credible prescribing information [9,10]. More recent surveys have shown a more positive attitude towards commercially sponsored CME, with 70% of Norwegian general practitioners agreeing completely that commercial courses kept high standards [11]. Similarly, industry meetings in Australia were judged to be of good to excellent quality by 81% of generalists, 79% of internists and 87% of psychiatrists [12].

Industry funding appears to limit the number of topics covered in CME events. One paper compared talks developed by Harvard Medical School independent of any commercial influence and pharmaceutical company-funded symposia [13]. The 221 Harvard talks covered 133 topics while the 103 symposia focused on 30 topics, most of which were linked to recently approved new therapeutic agents sold by the funders. Drug therapy was the central topic in 27% of the Harvard talks compared to 66% of the symposia. Both types of courses were highly rated by attendees.

Bowman analyzed the content of two CME events in relation to their source of funding [14]. Both courses were given at a university that had policy guidelines that required the course content to be controlled by the institution. Despite this requirement, in both courses there was a bias in favor of the drug made by the sponsoring company as compared to equally effective drugs made by other companies. Recently, an instrument has been developed to measure bias in individual CME courses but it has not yet been used in practice [15].

Although about 40% of doctors believe that the involvement of pharmaceutical companies in CME can create a conflict of interest, versus just over 50% who felt the opposite, only about half that

Table 4.1 Methodological evaluation of systematic reviews

Study	Item									
	Were the search methods reported?	Was the search comprehensive?	Were the inclusion criteria reported?	Was selection bias avoided?	Were the validity criteria reported?	Was validity assessed appropriately?	Were the methods used to combine studies reported?	Were the findings combined appropriately?	Were the conclusions supported by the reported data?
Beaudry [34]	Yes	Yes	Partial	No	No	No	Yes	Yes	Yes
Bloom [29]	Partial	Yes	Partial	No	No	No	No	No	No
Cauffman et al. [39]	Partial	No	No	No	No	No	No	No	No
Curran & Fleet [36]	Yes	No	Yes	Yes	No	No	No	No	Yes
Davis et al. [5]	Yes	Yes	Yes	No	No	No	No	No	Yes
Davis & Taylor-Vaisey [30]	Yes	Yes	Partial	No	No	No	No	No	Yes
Davis et al. [25]	Yes	Yes	Yes	Yes	Yes	Yes	Yes	Yes	Yes
Figueiras et al. [31]	Yes	Yes	Yes	Yes	Yes	No	No	No	Yes
Hodges et al. [24]	Partial	No	No	No	No	No	No	No	No
Kroenke et al. [21]	Yes	No	Yes	Yes	No	No	Yes	Yes	Yes
Mansouri [19]	Yes	No	Yes	Yes	No	No	Yes	Yes	Yes
Oxman et al. [32]	Yes	Yes	Yes	Yes	Yes	Yes	Yes	Yes	Yes
Pippalla et al. [33]	Partial	No	No	No	No	No	Yes	Yes	No
Smith et al. [22]	Yes	Yes	Yes	Yes	Yes	No	No	No	Yes
Smits et al. [26]	Yes	Yes	Yes	Yes	Yes	Yes	No	No	Yes
Tu & Davis [40]	Yes	Yes	Yes	Yes	No	Yes	No	No	Yes
Wensing et al. [20]	Yes	No	Partial	Yes	No	No	Yes	Yes	Yes
Wutoh et al. [37]	Yes	Yes	Yes	Yes	No	No	Yes	Yes	Yes

number were concerned that their level of industry involvement created a bias in their drug selection [16]. A before and after study of the hospital doctors' prescribing found a dramatic increase in the use of drugs featured at pharmaceutical company symposia despite the fact that the doctors did not believe that their prescribing practices would be influenced by their attendance [17]. Another study surveyed doctors before and 6 months after their attendance at three separate CME courses that were nominally independent of the sponsors [18]. In each case there was a greater increase in prescriptions for the drug made by the sponsoring company than for other drugs in the same class.

In summary, the growing funding of CME events by industry sponsors should be alarming to the health care system for a variety of reasons. First and foremost, despite a lack of concern by physicians about sponsorship influence, it would appear their practice is changed by these sponsored events. Second, the breadth and depth of sponsored CME events likely to be less than required by clinicians. Finally, despite these concerns, physician rating of the quality of sponsored CME is increasing.

Question 2: For physicians seeking CME (population), what are the effects on knowledge uptake and retention (outcome) of CME delivered through multiple interventions (intervention) compared to CME delivered through a single intervention (control)?

Search strategy

- PubMed: education, medical, continuing [MeSH] AND English [limitation] AND systematic review [limitation] AND 1985 to present (May 30, 2007) [limitation]
- Cochrane Library (reviews and other reviews): education AND (physician OR doctor)

Davis and colleagues examined evidence from the randomized controlled trial (RCT) literature on this topic [5]. In their review, interventions that used two or three educational methods were generally positive 64% and 79% of the time, respectively. A positive outcome was defined as either a change in physician performance or in health care outcomes but they did not specify which of these outcomes were affected by multiple interventions.

Subsequent to Davis' systematic review, three further teams have looked at this issue [19–21]. In a review that analyzed both RCTs and controlled before and after studies, some multifaceted interventions lead to changes in clinical behavior (diagnostics, therapy, prevention, or a combination of two or more of these behaviors); in general practice, however, this was not a consistent outcome [20]. Combinations of three or four interventions involving information transfer and learning through social influence or management support were generally effective compared to single interventions [20].

The most recent review that included either RCTs or controlled before and after studies examined the effect of different kinds of CME interventions. The authors found that a multifaceted educational program produced the largest effect size for physician knowledge but the combinations that were examined in the separate studies were not specified [19]. A review of RCTs or quasi-experimental trials in psychiatry did not find multiple interventions superior to single ones but the lack of statistical significance may be the result of small numbers of trials [21].

In summary, the evidence for multifaceted CME interventions appears modestly supportive of this intervention. The ideal combination of interventions that comprise a strategy has yet to be identified, and there is no evidence for any strategies in emergency medicine.

Question 3: For physicians seeking CME (population), what are the effects on knowledge uptake and retention (outcome) of CME directed by problem-based education (intervention) compared to other forms of CME (control)?

Search strategy

- PubMed: education, medical, continuing [MeSH] AND English [limitation] AND systematic review [limitation] AND 1985 to present (May 30, 2007) [limitation]
- Cochrane Library (reviews and other reviews): education AND (physician OR doctor)

Modern learning theory suggests that education should be structured around practical day-to-day concerns and should be relevant to the daily tasks of the learners [22]. According to Mazmanian and Davis, assessment of learning needs is crucial for effective CME: "When gaps are demonstrated and educational resources are extended strategically to help the learner, change occurs more frequently" [23]. There are two broad approaches to identifying learner needs and planning course objectives: (i) deficit based, by which gaps are identified from information gathered about the actual knowledge, skills or attitudes of doctors; and (ii) epidemiologically based, where gaps are identified from epidemiological data [24].

The methodologically strongest review that looked exclusively at RCTs identified four trials that reported the development of an intervention following a needs assessment survey and one that used a six-step process to identify the learning needs. Only one study failed to show a change in either physician performance or health care outcomes [25].

A second review of six controlled trials looked at this same question and defined problem-based learning (PBL) as "a tutor facilitated ... session in which a small, self directed group starts with a brainstorming session. A problem is posed that challenges their knowledge and experience. Learning goals are formulated by consensus, and new information is learnt by self directed study" [26]. There was moderate evidence that doctors were satisfied with this form of learning, but only limited evidence that it actually increased their knowledge and performance and patients' health compared to no intervention at all. Moreover, there was no consistent evidence that it was better than other strategies.

One possible reason why PBL did not perform better may be that doctors are not necessarily adept at identifying their areas of weakness [27]. The self-rated knowledge of two groups of New Zealand general practitioners was compared with their performance on true–false tests on the same topics. Correlations between self-assessments and test scores were poor in all cases. When doctors are given a choice about what CME events to participate in they choose topics that fit into areas they are already comfortable with [28].

In summary, while PBL CME events are considered of the highest quality, they require a reasonable needs assessment, and physicians should be careful to ensure they are focusing on topics of need rather than popularity or familiarity. There is moderate evidence that physicians are satisfied with this form of learning but only limited evidence that it actually changes practice.

Question 4: For physicians seeking CME (population), do active formats (e.g., academic detailing) (intervention) improve knowledge uptake and retention (outcome) compared to passive formats (e.g., large group lectures) (control)?

Search strategy

- PubMed: education, medical, continuing [MeSH] AND English [limitation] AND systematic review [limitation] AND 1985 to present (May 30, 2007) [limitation]
- Cochrane Library (reviews and other reviews): education AND (physician OR doctor)

The general consensus from the nine systematic reviews that have looked at this topic is that active methods of delivering CME are superior to passive formats [5,19,24,25,29–33]. One review that specifically examined this topic analyzed 14 RCTs with 17 separate interventions. Four of six that used interactive techniques had a significant impact on physician performance, whereas none of the four studies using didactic sessions altered performance [25]. Formal CME events and the majority of events using educational materials (e.g., printed information or audiovisual programs) failed to demonstrate any effect [5]. Davis and others have also found that interactive techniques such as case discussions, hands-on practice sessions and outreach visits, including academic detailing, generally demonstrated positive changes [5,22,24]. Likewise, reinforcement strategies such as acknowledgment of correct performances and opportunities whereby education may be translated into practice and reinforced at a later session were found to be quite effective, with an increase in the level of reinforcement related to progressively larger effect sizes [25,34].

The other reviews generally supported these findings, albeit sometimes with differences, so that contrary to Davis, Bloom [29]

showed audit and feedback to be as effective as outreach measures. In one review there was little difference between active and passive methods [31]. Combining active and passive strategies was more likely to be successful in generating positive changes in physician performance and health outcomes than passive methods alone [25,31] and just as effective as active methods alone [19].

Given that traditional passive methods of CME seem to be largely ineffective, the question remains why do doctors attend these events? It is important to acknowledge that doctors:
'. . . attend formal CME events with varying levels of motivation to change, and that the level of their commitment to change may supersede both the immediate clinical value of the information and the method by which it was delivered, as predictors of change in performance . . . Finally, physicians appear to develop their own learning priorities based on external and internal forces: the CME course or conference may be just one of many such forces. [25]'

These observations were explored through six in-depth interviews with family doctors [35]. The informants expressed three main reasons for attending an annual refresher course: to be updated, to be reassured that their practice behavior was within accepted guidelines, and to hear from and interact with the specialists who gave the lectures.

In summary, some active formats for CME, either alone or in combination with passive formats, appear to be the most effective form of CME. However, doctors have a variety of reasons for attending CME events and do not always choose events with active interventions.

Question 5: For physicians seeking CME (population), does web-based CME (intervention) improve knowledge uptake and retention (outcome) compared to other forms of CME (control)?

Search strategy

- PubMed: education, medical, continuing [MeSH] AND English [limitation] AND systematic review [limitation] AND 1985 to present (May 30, 2007) [limitation]
- Cochrane Library (reviews and other reviews): education AND (physician OR doctor)

This question has been examined by two systematic reviews [36,37]. The first of these assessed the results of 14 RCTs and two "modified quasi-experiments". Six of these studies showed positive changes in knowledge compared to traditional formats, three demonstrated a positive change in practices, and the remainder did not find any differences in knowledge levels between internet-based interventions and more traditional forms of CME [37]. The second review included 31 studies but did not assess their methodology. Very few quantitative data were presented; however, the authors concluded "a lack of systematic evidence exists to support the effectiveness of web-based CME in enhancing or improving clinical practice performance and/or patient or health outcomes" [36]. Doctors were generally satisfied with web-based learning.

The lack of any data convincingly demonstrating that web-based learning is superior to other forms of CME may be because it tends to adopt the same deficiencies as traditional CME [37]. Both of the reviews suggest that web-based CME needs to incorporate key principles of adult-based learning and to focus on designing interactive learning environments delivered through the web.

In summary, the evidence for web-based CME is weak, and until more innovation is applied to this form of CME delivery this technique appears no better or worse than traditional CME formats. It may, however, fit the location and lifestyle of some clinicians, so it is reassuring that doctors were generally satisfied with web-based learning when it was employed.

Question 6: For physicians attending CME events (population), does the CME (intervention) have a different effect size on patient health outcomes (outcome) compared to learning and performance (control)?

Search strategy

- PubMed: education, medical, continuing [MeSH] AND English [limitation] AND systematic review [limitation] AND 1985 to present (May 30, 2007) [limitation]
- Cochrane Library (reviews and other reviews): education AND (physician OR doctor)

Continuing medical education can produce three different types of outcomes: changes in physician learning, physician performance and patient health. Table 4.2 provides a definition of these terms. These different types of outcome can be viewed as a hierarchy with the ideal being changes in patient health. Two controlled trials have found that there is a disconnection between increasing physicians' knowledge and changing their practice behavior. General practitioners who received continuing education packages covering common clinical problems showed improvements in knowledge but not overall quality of care [28]. An educational intervention about pharyngitis improved diagnosis compared to a control group but actual treatment decisions did not change [38].

In some cases there is very little literature on performance and patient health outcomes. Sixteen studies of internet-based CME looked at learning outcomes and two examined clinical practice changes. There were no studies that evaluated patient health [36].

Where literature does exist, systematic reviews reinforce the findings from controlled trials that CME has a differential impact on outcomes. Six RCTs found that significant results were more likely to occur in performance outcomes than in patient health care outcomes [39]. However, this review was methodologically very weak. A second higher-quality review examined RCTs and quasi-experimental trials designed to improve the diagnosis and treatment of mental disorders. The majority were able to show an improvement in diagnosis (18/23) and treatment (14/20), but only a minority showed a clinical improvement in either psychiatric symptoms (4/11) or functional status (4/8) [21]. Two more reviews, both of reasonable methodological quality, found a moderate effect size between CME and physician knowledge, compared to a small effect size between CME and both physician performance and patient outcomes [19,34].

Tu and Davis examined the effect of CME on the relatively simple issue of follow-up of hypertension and the more complex problem of managing the disease. They found that it was easier to improve the former than the latter [40].

In summary, the evidence suggests that CME changes physicians' knowledge more frequently than their practice; the evidence for actual improvements in patient care is even more elusive.

Question 7: For physicians attending CME events (population), do time factors (longer contact time for each CME program; longer time between the end of the CME program and measurement) (intervention) affect physicians' knowledge (outcome) compared to shorter contact time and shorter time between the end of the CME program and measurement (control)?

Search strategy

- PubMed: education, medical, continuing [MeSH] AND English [limitation] AND systematic review [limitation] AND 1985 to present (May 30, 2007) [limitation]
- Cochrane Library (reviews and other reviews): education AND (physician OR doctor)

Three reviews have investigated the question of whether the length of the CME intervention makes a difference in terms of its effectiveness [19,25,34]. Beaudry concluded that the average effect size for a 1-day CME course was smaller than that for longer-term courses. The optimal program length was 1–4 weeks [34]. Mansouri found a positive correlation between the effect size and the number of contact hours in a CME event [19].

Table 4.2 Outcomes from CME. (Adapted from Curran & Fleet [36].)

Outcome	Definition
Change in learning	Changes in skills, knowledge or attitudes
Change in performance	Changes in behavior or performance in the practice setting
Change in patient health	Changes in patient health that are a result of participation in CME activity

Different types of events may initiate different changes and therefore assorted activities may lead to changes that a single activity would not. These different activities could either be delivered during the same single event or over a period of time [41]. Davis et al. investigated this question and found that shorter courses (2–6 hours) were less likely to produce positive changes in performance than were interventions held in more than one session [25].

One study in the psychiatric literature has looked at the long-term effectiveness of CME in a rigorous fashion. General practitioners in Sweden were given an educational program on symptoms, etiology, diagnosis, prevention and treatment of depression. At the end of the 20-hour program they were more competent in treating and preventing depressive states and the use of antidepressants increased. The program was associated with decreases in the use of psychiatric inpatient care and there was a slight decline in the suicide rate [42]. However, 3 years later, the inpatient care for depressive disorders increased, the suicide rate returned almost to baseline values and the prescription of antidepressants stabilized [43].

The issue of the sustainability of changes due to CME has been examined in two reviews. In one, the effect size was slightly positive for the correlation between physician knowledge and the measurement interval, while it was negative for performance and health outcomes [19]. This result suggests that outcomes that are the most difficult to modify deteriorate the quickest and are the ones that need reinforcing. These results are contradicted by Beaudry, however, who concluded that physician knowledge was more susceptible to deterioration compared to patient health status [34].

In summary, longer CME courses have larger effect sizes than shorter ones, and reinforcing CME messages through different delivery modalities is more likely to produce positive changes. Outcomes that are the most difficult to change seem to be the ones most in need of reinforcing.

Question 8: For physicians who have attended CME events (population), does mandatory CME (intervention) have a larger effect size (outcome) compared to voluntary CME (control)?

Search strategy

- PubMed: education, medical, continuing [MeSH] AND English [limitation] AND systematic review [limitation] AND 1985 to present (May 30, 2007) [limitation]
- Cochrane Library (reviews and other reviews): education AND (physician OR doctor)

A single review examined this question and found that American states that had mandatory CME legislation in 1984 yielded a significantly lower average effect size compared to states without mandatory CME [34]. Reasons for this finding are unclear. The

kind of CME in each type of state was not described and it might be that the states with mandatory CME offered events less likely to produce a positive change. In addition, "research in states with mandatory CME may have received better funding and measured more complex outcomes" [34].

The self-directed learning components of CME mandated by North American emergency medicine organizations represent traditional, non-innovative approaches to learning. For example, the American College of Emergency Medicine employs an annual reading list for re-certification. In Canada, the Canadian College of Family Physicians had re-certification requirements that were so unpopular that they were dropped prior to the deadline.

In summary, the evidence for re-accreditation through mandatory CME is weak, and the CME policies put forward by emergency medicine accreditation bodies are likely to be ineffective and unpopular.

Conclusions

The emergency physician in the clinical scenario above should not permit the industry sponsor to provide topics, literature or input to the CME events. Unrestricted educational grants from industry for CME must be viewed with caution and strict rules of conduct must be employed. In an ideal setting, the costs of the conference should be borne by the clinicians attending and their needs should be assessed prior to the development of the program. The program should incorporate multiple innovative CME delivery approaches, and reinforce these with later reminder systems.

With the rapid changes in medical knowledge it is essential that doctors, especially those working on the "front lines", ensure that their knowledge and practices are in line with current evidence-based medicine. One of the ways to help accomplish this task is through CME; however, CME is expensive and increasingly the resources to finance CME arise from the pharmaceutical or medical device industries. Doctors appear to be divided in their acceptance of company-sponsored CME and there is evidence that the range of topics is limited when CME is commercially financed and that commercial sponsorship may bias the content.

While there is consensus on some questions regarding CME, on others there is still uncertainty. It appears clear that multiple interventions, active interventions, longer interventions and/or interventions delivered and reinforced over a period of time are superior to short, passive, single event types of CME. What is not clear is how best to incorporate learner-identified problem solving into CME since learners may not be fully cognizant of their own weaknesses. Web-based CME appears to offer potential since it can be delivered without doctors having to travel and it can also be structured to incorporate feedback. Whether or not mandatory CME per se is effective is unproven. Changing doctors' knowledge is relatively easy, but changing behavior and patient outcomes are progressively harder.

While CME should play a central role in the maintenance of competence it is not the only factor that is involved. Allery and colleagues looked at 361 changes in clinical practice. Education was involved in about one-third of changes in clinical practice; other reasons were organizational factors and contact with professionals. Although the contents of CME must be as unbiased as possible, and it should be delivered in a manner that is most likely to produce positive results, the wide range of other factors affecting changes in practice needs to be taken into account in providing and evaluating education [44].

Conflicts of interest

None were reported.

References

1 Van Harrison R. The uncertain future of continuing medical education: commercialism and shifts in funding. *J Contin Educ Health Prof* 2003;**23**:198–209.

2 American Board of Medical Specialties. Maintenance of Certification (MOC). American Board of Medical Specialties, 2006. Available at http://www.abms.org/About_Board_Certification/MOC.aspx (accessed June 10, 2007).

3 College of Family Physicians of Canada. Mainpro® – CME requirements for members. College of Family Physicians of Canada, 2007. Available at http://www.cfpc.ca/English/cfpc/cme/mainpro/maintenance%20of%20proficiency/requirements%20members/default.asp?s=1 (accessed June 10, 2007).

4 Royal College of Physicians and Surgeons of Canada. Maintenance of Certification. Royal College of Physicians and Surgeons of Canada. Available at http://www.royalcollege.ca/index_e.php?submit=maintenance (accessed June 10, 2007).

5 Davis DA, Thomson MA, Oxman AD, Haynes B. Changing physician performance: a systematic review of the effect of continuing medical education strategies. *JAMA* 1995;**274**:700–705.

6 Robertson MK, Umble KE, Cervero RM. Impact studies in continuing education for health professions: update. *J Contin Educ Health Prof* 2003;**23**(3):146–56.

7 Oxman AD, Guyatt GH. Validation of an index of the quality of review articles. *J Clin Epidemiol* 1991;**44**:1271–8.

8 Accreditation Council for Continuing Medical Education. ACCME® Annual Report Data 2005. 2006. Available at http://www.accme.org/dir_docs/doc_upload/9c795f02-c470-4ba3-a491-d288be965eff_uploaddocument.pdf (accessed June 18, 2007).

9 Lexchin J. Interactions between physicians and the pharmaceutical industry: what does the literature say? *Can Med Assoc J* 1993;**149**:1401–7.

10 Wazana A. Physicians and the pharmaceutical industry: is a gift ever just a gift? *JAMA* 2000;**283**:373–80.

11 Andersson SJ, Troein M, Lindberg G. General practitioners' conceptions about treatment of depression and factors that may influence their practice in this area. A postal survey. *BMC Fam Pract* 2005;**6**(1):21.

12 Carney SL, Nair KR, Sales MA, Walsh J. Pharmaceutical industry-sponsored meetings: good value or just a free meal? *Intern Med J* 2001;**31**(8):488–91.

13 Katz HP, Goldfinger SE, Fletcher SW. Academia–industry collaboration in continuing medical education: description of two approaches. *J Contin Educ Health Prof* 2002;**22**(1):43–54.

14 Bowman MA. The impact of drug company funding on the content of continuing medical education. *Mobius* 1986;**6**:66–9.

15 Takhar J, Dixon D, Donahue J, et al. Developing an instrument to measure bias in CME. *J Contin Educ Health Prof* 2007;**27**:118–23.

16 Rutledge P, Crookes D, McKinstry B, Maxwell SR. Do doctors rely on pharmaceutical industry funding to attend conferences and do they perceive that this creates a bias in their drug selection? Results from a questionnaire survey. *Pharmacoepidemiol Drug Saf* 2003;**12**(8):663–7.

17 Orlowski JP, Wateska L. The effects of pharmaceutical firm enticements on physician prescribing patterns: there's no such thing as a free lunch. *Chest* 1992;**102**:270–73.

18 Bowman MA, Pearle DL. Changes in drug prescribing patterns related to commercial company funding of continuing medical education. *J Contin Educ Health Prof* 1988;**8**:13–20.

19 Mansouri M. A meta-analysis of continuing medical education effectiveness. *J Contin Educ Health Prof* 2007;**27**:6–15.

20 Wensing M, van der Weijden T, Grol R. Implementing guidelines and innovations in general practice: which interventions are effective? *Br J Gen Pract* 1998;**48**:991–7.

21 Kroenke K, Taylor-Vaisey A, Dietrich AJ, Oxman TE. Interventions to improve provider diagnosis and treatment of mental disorders in primary care. *Psychosomatics* 2000;**41**:39–52.

22 Smith F, Singleton A, Hilton S. General practitioners' continuing education: a review of policies, strategies and effectiveness, and their implications for the future. *Br J Gen Pract* 1998;**48**(435):1689–95.

23 Mazmanian PE, Davis DA. Continuing medical education and the physician as a learner: guide to the evidence. *JAMA* 2002;**288**:1057–60.

24 Hodges B, Inch C, Silver I. Improving the psychiatric knowledge, skills, and attitudes of primary care physicians, 1950–2000: a review. *Am J Psychiatry* 2001;**158**:1579–86.

25 Davis D, O'Brien MAT, Freemantle N, Wolf FM, Mazmanian P, Taylor-Vaisey A. Impact of formal continuing medical education: do conferences, workshops, rounds, and other traditional continuing education activities change physician behavior or health care outcomes? *JAMA* 1999;**282**:867–74.

26 Smits PB, Verbeek JH, de Buisonje CD. Problem based learning in continuing medical education: a review of controlled evaluation studies. *BMJ* 2002;**324**(7330):153–6.

27 Tracey J, Arroll B, Barham P, Richmond D. The validity of general practitioners' self assessment of knowledge: cross sectional study. *BMJ* 1997;**315**:1426–8.

28 Sibley JC, Sackett DL, Neufeld V, Gerrard B, Rudnick KV, Fraser W. A randomized trial of continuing medical education. *N Engl J Med* 1982;**306**:511–15.

29 Bloom BS. Effects of continuing medical education on improving physician clinical care and patient health: a review of systematic reviews. *Int J Technol Assess Health Care* 2005;**21**(3):380–85.

30 Davis DA, Taylor-Vaisey A. Translating guidelines into practice: a systematic review of theoretic concepts, practical experience and research evidence in the adoption of clinical practice guidelines. *Can Med Assoc J* 1997;**157**:408–16.

31 Figueiras A, Sastre I, Gestal-Otero JJ. Effectiveness of educational interventions on the improvement of drug prescription in primary care: a critical literature review. *J Eval Clin Pract* 2001;**7**(2):223–41.

32 Oxman AD, Thomson MA, Davis DA, Haynes B. No magic bullets: a systematic review of 102 trials of interventions to improve professional practice. *Can Med Assoc J* 1995;**153**:1423–31.

33 Pippalla RS, Riley DA, Chinburapa V. Influencing the prescribing behaviour of physicians: a metaevaluation. *J Clin Pharm Ther* 1995;**20**:189–98.

34 Beaudry JS. The effectiveness of continuing medical education: a quantitative synthesis. *J Contin Educ Health Prof* 1989;**9**:285–307.

35 Harrison C, Hogg W. Why do doctors attend traditional CME events if they don't change what they do in their surgeries? Evaluation of doctors' reasons for attending a traditional CME programme. *Med Educ* 2003;**37**:884–8.

36 Curran VR, Fleet L. A review of evaluation outcomes of web-based continuing medical education. *Med Educ* 2005;**39**:561–7.

37 Wutoh R, Boren SA, Balas EA. eLearning: a review of internet-based continuing medical education. *J Contin Educ Health Prof* 2004;**24**(1):20–30.

38 Poses RM, Cebul RD, Wigton RS. You can lead a horse to water – improving physicians' knowledge of probabilities may not affect their decisions. *Med Decision Making* 1995;**15**:65–75.

39 Cauffman JG, Forsyth RA, Clark VA, et al. Randomized controlled trials of continuing medical education: what makes them most effective? *J Contin Educ Health Prof* 2002;**22**:214–21.

40 Tu K, Davis D. Can we alter physician behavior by educational methods? Lessons learned from studies of the management and follow-up of hypertension. *J Contin Educ Health Prof* 2002;**22**(1):11–22.

41 Gilman SC, Turner JW. Media richness and social information processing: rationale for multifocal continuing medical education activities. *J Contin Educ Health Prof* 2001;**21**(3):134–9.

42 Rutz W, Wålinder J, Eberhard G, et al. An educational program on depressive disorders for general practitioners on Gotland: background and evaluation. *Acta Psychiatr Scand* 1989;**79**:19–26.

43 Rutz W, von Knorring L, Wålinder J. Long-term effects of an educational program for general practitioners given by the Swedish Committee for the Prevention and Treatment of Depression. *Acta Psychiatr Scand* 1992;**85**:83–8.

44 Allery LA, Owen PA, Robling MR. Why general practitioners and consultants change their clinical practice: a critical incident study. *BMJ* 1997;**314**:870–74.

5 Quality Improvement

Andrew Worster[1,2] & Ann McKibbon[2]

[1]Emergency Medicine, Clinical Epidemiology & Biostatistics, McMaster University, Hamilton, Canada
[2]Department of Clinical Epidemiology and Biostatistics, McMaster University, Hamilton, Canada

Clinical scenario

As the newly appointed chief of your emergency department (ED), you are committed to improving the quality of care in your department. To this end, through your years of experience as an emergency physician in this ED and the multiple complaints that you have had to deal with as chief, you have targeted several areas as priorities for evaluation and/or improvement. These include turnaround times for laboratory and diagnostic imaging, staff knowledge and competency assessments and implementation of a chest pain unit in the ED. In order to minimize time and costs, you have also decided to perform chart audits as a first step in your ED performance assessment project.

Background

Medical quality has been defined, as "the care health professionals would want to receive if they got sick" [1]. In business, the quality of a product or service is determined by the degree to which it meets the customer's expectations [1,2]. When we think of customers in the ED, most of us think of patients and their families; however, patients are just one group of customers served by the ED. There are, in fact, many other groups with expectations of ED performance who, therefore, also qualify as customers. These include, but are not limited to, emergency medical services providers, non-ED consultants, hospital administrators, funding organizations and even the various members of the ED staff. While all ED customers have expectations of performance, their priorities may differ [1]. Process times are often a high priority for ED patients. On the other hand, hospital administrators are likely to be more concerned with costs; funding organizations are likely to be more concerned with quality; while ED staff are more concerned with safety and efficiency.

Evidence-based Emergency Medicine. Edited by Brian H. Rowe
© 2009 Blackwell Publishing, ISBN: 978-1-4051-6143-5.

Quality improvement (QI) and similar terms from the business world have only recently become part of the health care vocabulary. While it is beyond the scope of this chapter to explain all that QI encompasses, for the purpose of this narrative, QI has been described as a method of evaluating and improving processes of patient care that emphasizes a multidisciplinary approach to problem solving, and focuses not on individuals, but on systems of patient care which might be the cause of variations [1]. As a first step, it is important to understand that variation is inversely proportional to quality, i.e., as more people do things differently, overall quality of the final product will decrease. Conversely, QI requires reduced variation. In the ED, QI can cover all activities from cleaning floors to triaging patients to inserting arterial lines. These activities are termed processes and, like most ED processes, can be evaluated and improved upon. Methods to accomplish this, also from the business world, include lean six sigma and root cause analysis (RCA).

In health care, the usual method of evaluating efficacy or effectiveness is through experimental designs or, if not feasible, observational studies with controls. Hence, the hierarchy of levels of evidence in evidence-based medicine recognize the N of one randomized controlled trial (RCT) as the highest level of evidence, followed by systematic reviews of RCTs, multi-patient RCTs and then cohort studies. Where clinical research focuses primarily on providing evidence for clinical decision making, QI research focuses on process improvement. Boudreaux et al. describe the two major reasons why QI research does not employ clinical research methods: (i) resources and (ii) feasibility of controls [3]. The objective of QI research is often to maximize effective use of available resources by minimizing error and inefficiency. Unlike clinical research, this precludes large resource investment into research design and analysis. Furthermore, rarely are such resources available for QI research. Controls are often not feasible in QI studies, especially those involving performance improvement, as this involves operating parallel processes simultaneously, which is impossible in a single setting where most QI research is conducted. For this reason, the PICO (patient, intervention, control and outcome) research question format is usually not applicable since there is no control. For those who doubt the validity or effectiveness of

QI study results because of the lack of experimental designs and controls, one only need to look at how the aviation industry has dramatically reduced the morbidity and mortality associated with commercial air travel using only QI research methods and not a single RCT [3].

General search strategy

The power of PubMed has been discussed elsewhere (see Chapter 39). Searching in PubMed for an issue that relates to the care given by emergency clinicians in the ED is not easy. The term "emergency medicine" is not useful to define care given by emergency physicians as the term refers to the medical specialty or profession and has nothing to do with emergency care or the patients with whom these physicians interact. In addition, the single term "emergency" is too broad to use as it gives too many false retrievals. The terms more useful for defining the care that emergency clinicians provide and the term definitions (http://www.nlm.nih.gov/mesh/MBrowser.html) are as follows:
• *Hospital emergency service*: this refers to the hospital department responsible for the administration and provision of immediate care (medical or surgical) to patients coming for emergency attention.
• *Emergency medical services*: this includes services that are designed, staffed and equipped for the emergency care of patients.
• *Emergency treatment*: this may be somewhat less useful. It refers to first aid or other interventions given to persons who have had an accident or require care for medical conditions that need immediate care before definitive medical or surgical management can be procured.
• *Emergencies*: this refers to situations or conditions that require immediate intervention because of a high probability of disabling or immediate life-threatening consequences.

Clinical questions

In order to address the issues of most relevance to QI and to help in searching the literature for the evidence regarding these issues, you should structure your clinical questions as recommended in Chapter 1.

1 In the emergency setting (population), what quality improvement method (intervention) can improve performance (outcome)?

2 Is emergency physician (population) audit and feedback (intervention) effective at improving professional practice (outcome) compared to other forms of continuing medical education (control)?

3 In the emergency setting (population), can medical record reviews (intervention) evaluate quality of care (outcome) compared to other evaluation approaches (control)?

4 In the emergency setting (population), does root cause analysis (intervention) identify causes for delays to turnaround times (outcome)?

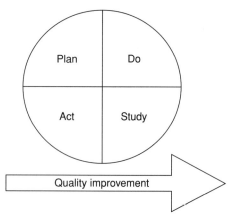

Figure 5.1 Deming's plan, do, study and act (PDSA) cycle to quality improvement.

5 In ED patients with suspected acute coronary syndrome (population), does admission to a chest pain unit (intervention) compared to routine care (control) safely reduce hospital admissions (outcome)?

Critical review of the literature

Question 1: In the emergency setting (population), what quality improvement method (intervention) can improve performance (outcome)?

Search strategy

• PubMed search: quality improvement AND hospital emergency service

One of the most commonly used QI tools was developed by the business guru Deming. Among his many accomplishments, Deming developed a simple, recurring four-step quality improvement method: plan, do, study, act (PDSA; Fig. 5.1) [4]. This approach is referred to by many names including the PDSA cycle and the Deming cycle, although Deming himself apparently referred to it as the Shewhart cycle. There is also some variation in the names of each of the steps, but most commonly they are:
• *Plan*: determine the objective(s) and identify the process change(s) necessary to meet the goal(s).
• *Do*: make the change(s).
• *Study* (or *check*): measure the effect(s) of the change(s) and determine whether the effect(s) meet(s) the objective(s).
• *Act*: apply actions to the outcome for necessary improvement. This means reviewing all steps (plan, do, study, act) and modifying the process to improve it before its next implementation.

Ideally, the PDSA cycle should be repeated as indicated in Fig. 5.1 in close succession with the understanding that each application of the PDSA will yield an incremental improvement in quality. The PDSA method of quality improvement offers many advantages: (i) it can be conducted with available resources; (ii) since no PDSA is too small, sample size is irrelevant; (iii) the short turnaround provides rapid results; (iv) the results are always implemented as part of the process; and (v) PDSA can be used on any process.

The PubMed literature search listed an article by Al Darrab that describes how the PDSA cycle can be applied as part of the lean six sigma approach to improve quality of care for patients presenting to the ED with ST elevation myocardial infarction (STEMI) [5]. The quality improvement model that the authors describe, lean six sigma, employs the PDSA cycle preceded by a systematic process of identifying the process for improvement, which includes RCA [4]. The authors demonstrate how the application of this QI model in conjunction with evidence-based medicine guidelines can "optimize the care of STEMI patients presenting to the ED" [4].

In summary, the ubiquitous utility and genius of the PDSA cycle is that it can be easily implemented in any setting without additional resources or expertise. Furthermore, like the N of one RCT, the results are specific to the setting in which they were conducted.

Question 2: Is emergency physician (population) audit and feedback (intervention) effective at improving professional practice (outcome) compared to other forms of continuing medical education (control)?

Search strategy

- PubMed: clinical queries in systematic review: audit AND feedback

The above search identified multiple potentially relevant studies, almost all of which focused on specific, non-emergency medicine populations. A systematic review published in two journals was an assessment of audit and feedback in general. Audit and feedback is a commonly used method of trying to improve health care professionals' performance. The rationale for audit and feedback is that "healthcare professionals would be prompted to modify their practice if given feedback that their clinical practice was inconsistent with that of their peers or accepted guidelines" [6]. The feedback component can be delivered in a variety of forms including one-on-one interactions and educational meetings. Feedback can also be delivered to allow health care professionals to anonymously compare their performance in specific domains with that of their peers.

The best overall evaluation of the effectiveness of audit and feedback as an intervention can be found in a systematic review of randomized trials [6]. In this review the authors defined audit and feedback as "any summary of clinical performance of health care over a specified period of time" [6]. To be included in the review, the outcome of the study had to be an objective measure of health care outcomes or of provider performance in a health care setting. The authors identified a total of 118 studies that met their criteria, although only 24 were judged to be of high methodological quality. The populations of health care professionals in the studies included physicians, dentists, nurses and pharmacists. Given the

complexity of the topic and the wide spectrum of populations, interventions and outcomes of the included studies, significant heterogeneity should be expected.

The results of the review were variable in that the ranges of outcomes in all comparisons included small negative effects to large positive effects; however, the improvements were generally small and led the authors to conclude that "evidence presented here does not support mandatory use of audit and feedback as an intervention to change practice" [6]. From their review, the authors make several important points:

- It is not possible to determine what, if any, features of audit and feedback have an important impact on its effectiveness.
- There is no empirical basis for deciding how to provide audit and feedback.
- Decisions about how to provide audit and feedback must be guided by pragmatic factors and local circumstances.
- The relative effects of audit and feedback are more likely to be larger when the baseline adherence to recommended practice is low.
- The relative effects of audit and feedback are more likely to be larger when feedback is provided more intensively.
- Audit is commonly used in the context of governance and it is essential to measure practice to know when efforts to change practice are needed.

In summary, it seems intuitive that audit and feedback is an effective intervention for behavior modification and this is supported to varying degrees by published research. However, there does not appear to be a single method or even formula for applying audit and feedback that is applicable to all circumstances. In fact, it might be demonstrated that multiple methods are required in order to achieve the desired outcomes.

Question 3: In the emergency setting (population), can medical record reviews (intervention) evaluate quality of care (outcome) compared to other evaluation approaches (control)?

Search strategy

- PubMed search: medical record review AND emergency medicine

The search term 'emergency medicine' is used in order to identify articles that demonstrate how medical record reviews have been used by the speciality rather than in a specific disorder. The search identified at least three studies of interest published in or since 2004 [7–9]. Two of these assessed the overall quality of published medical record review studies and one describes the methods that should be employed to optimize the reliability of the results. Derived from these three articles are some essential criteria for conducting a quality medical record review study (Table 5.1).

An assessment of the methods of medical record review studies published in emergency medicine journals during a 5-year period used published guidelines and compared the results with those of

Table 5.1 High-quality medical record review criteria

1	Institutional Research Board approval
2	Description of the database from which the data are abstracted
3	Description of the method of sampling from the database
4	Explicit case selection criteria
5	Explicit definitions of dependent and independent variables
6	Training of abstractors
7	Monitoring of abstractor performance
8	Assessment of inter-rater reliability between abstractors
9	Description of statistical management of the missing data

10 years previously [7]. The authors conducted independent, systematic searches and identified all medical record review studies published in 2003. The methodology assessments of each selected study were conducted independently by two other researchers, and disagreements were resolved by arbitration. In all, the authors identified 79 (14%) medical record review studies in 563 original research articles in six emergency medicine journals. The highest adherence to methodological standards was found for sampling method (99%; 95% CI: 93% to 100%), and the lowest was for abstractor blinding to hypothesis (4%; 95% CI: 1% to 11%). A comparison of these results with those of 10 years ago revealed significant improvements in three of the eight original criteria assessed: data abstraction forms, mentioning inter-observer performance and testing inter-observer performance.

In summary, medical record review studies continue to comprise a substantial proportion of original research in the emergency medicine literature. While important improvements have been made in some areas, there remains room for improvement overall and the responsibility for this lies largely with journal editors and authors.

Question 4: In the emergency setting (population), does root cause analysis (intervention) identify causes for delays to turnaround times (outcome)?

Search strategy

- PubMed search: root cause analysis AND turnaround time

The solution for any given problem in a system is not always apparent. In order to improve quality, we must first identify the root cause(s). Rooney and Vanden Heuvel have listed four criteria of a root cause which, in brief, are as follows: (i) specific causes of an event; (ii) identifiable causes of an event; (iii) root causes are controlled by management; and (iv) root causes can be corrected through effective management changes [10].

Root cause analysis (RCA) is a powerful and commonly used industry QI tool that can determine the what, how and why of performance problems [10]. A brief search of the medical literature using RCA as the search term reveals that it is often used to identify the cause of errors and to improve safety. However,

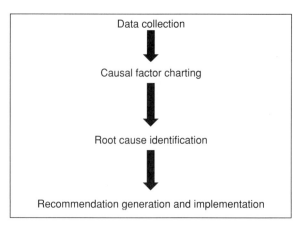

Figure 5.2 Steps in the root cause analysis (RCA) approach to problem solving.

the characteristics of RCA lend it to much wider QI applications. In this chapter, the focus will be on how RCA has been used in emergency medicine studies to improve turnaround times.

Depending on the source that one reads, RCA has any number of steps. In one of the simplest models RCA is a four-step process with striking similarities to Deming's PDSA cycle, explained earlier (Fig. 5.2). Our search for studies of RCA to identify turnaround time delays found three studies: two studies on laboratory turnaround times and one on diagnostic imaging [11–13]. Laboratory and diagnostic imaging are frequently used services in the ED involving multiple steps and coordination of personnel and equipment. Delays can contribute to increased length of stay for ED patients and subsequent ED overcrowding. These studies demonstrate how RCA can be used to identify causes for delays in turnaround times.

1 *Data collection*: the data collection process in all RCAs is typically the most time consuming and labor intensive. In these studies, the investigators held focus group discussions with staff and managers from each of the departments involved to determine the steps involved in the respective processes. Typically in RCA, the starting point is the final event in the process. This is a logical approach when trying to determine the sequence of events and root cause(s) that led to the outcome of concern.

2 *Causal factor charting*: this step is often simultaneous with the data collection process and provides a structure for the investigators to organize the information [10]. It also helps determine what additional information is needed. In each of the identified ED RCA studies, the investigators created flow charts and, in one paper, a cause-and-effect diagram [12]. The causal factor charting for each of the three studies demonstrates that the measurement and collection of times around each event as part of the data collection process is integral to determining the root cause of delay.

3 *Root cause identification*: this process is often accomplished through the use of a root cause map that identifies the reason(s) for each causal factor. This was accomplished in these three studies by using time measurements to identify the points of greatest delay. The cause(s) could then be determined.

4 *Recommendation generation and implementation*: some might argue that this is not part of the RCA process, which is really limited

Table 5.2 Sequence of events for emergency diagnostice imaging

Event time	Individual involved and activity
1	Time emergency physician orders radiograph
2	Time MRT is notified by emergency nurse
3	Time MRT acknowledges request from emergency nurse for radiograph
4	Time of patient departure from emergency department
5	Time radiograph examination is begun by MRT
6	Time radiograph examination is completed by MRT
7	Time patient is returned to emergency department by emergency nurse

MRT, medical radiography technician.

to identifying root causes. However, the RCA results are of no value unless interpreted and transformed into realistic implementation measures that prevent recurrences.

In using RCA to determine laboratory turnaround time delays for ED samples, the authors examined all "stat" hemoglobin and potassium measurements during the study period [11]. The investigators also recorded the hemolysis rate of blood samples as this is a measure of performance: short turnaround times with high hemolysis rates are no better than long turnaround times with low hemolysis rates. Also, hemolysis could require repeat processing thereby doubling the turnaround time. The results of the 147 samples analyzed revealed that 75% of hemoglobin and 10.7% of potassium samples met established benchmark turnaround times. Overall, 5.8% of potassium samples were hemolysed; however, only 1.7% required repeat sample processing. The RCA for turnaround time delays identified by investigators were order-processing times, excessive queue and instrument times, and the high volume of laboratory tests required for admitted patients held in the ED.

A study of the identification of root causes for delays for diagnostic imaging of ED patients used similar methods to the laboratory study [12]. The investigators conducted focus group discussions with staff of the three EDs and diagnostic imaging departments at the academic centre involved to identify and chart key steps in the imaging process from emergency physician ordering to return of patients to the ED. The researchers identified six key steps with corresponding measurable time periods that could be summed for the total turnaround time (Table 5.2). The results of 2297 consecutive cases revealed significant differences in turnaround times between the EDs. The delays in turnaround time identified by RCA included the same order-processing limitations as the laboratory study. Other causes were due to patient transport times and the distance of the diagnostic imaging suite from the ED.

In summary, like the PDSA cycle, RCA is a QI instrument that is easily implemented without utilizing additional resources. RCA also takes an objective approach to problems and, in doing so, effectively and accurately identifies the true cause(s) rather than focusing on the most visible cause(s). Also like the PDSA cycle, the limitation of RCA studies (and many QI studies in general) is that the results have limited external validity. This is because QI studies are often site-specific and the results can only be applied to settings with similar processes.

Question 5: In ED patients with suspected acute coronary syndrome (population), does admission to a chest pain unit (intervention) compared to routine care (control) safely reduce hospital admissions (outcome)?

Search strategy

- PubMed: clinical queries in clinical study category: chest pain AND emergency department

Returning to our ED scenario above, you were wondering about how to deal with patients with chest pain. One possible solution a director may consider is the creation of a chest pain unit or protocol. Chest pain units were created to assess ED patients with suspected acute coronary syndrome (see Chapter 17 for more details). The original objectives were to reduce hospital admissions and, with continued observation and standardized serial investigation protocols, improve the quality of care by also reducing the number of inappropriate discharges. The evidence to date supporting the implementation of chest pain units has been limited to low-risk patients in a limited number of settings.

Our search revealed a multi-centre, cluster RCT involving 14 hospitals with seven randomized to each arm: seven randomly selected hospitals set up chest pain units for the 1-year study period while the other seven continued to provide care without the units [14]. This study also incorporated a before-and-after design in that data collection for all sites began a year prior to the intervention period and continued for 1 year after. The study analyzed data from 43,642 ED visits by 37,319 patients in the pre-intervention year and 47,767 ED visits by 40,951 patients in the post-intervention year. The authors found a slight decrease in the odds of admission for patients presenting to EDs with chest pain units (OR = 0.94; 95% CI: 0.89 to 0.99). However, when this was adjusted for patient age and sex as planned a priori, there was no significant difference in the odds between the two groups (OR = 0.998; 95% CI: 0.94 to 1.06). Similarly, using the hospital as the unit of analysis (as is the norm for cluster RCTs) and the percent of admitted patients in the post-intervention period as the outcome measure, there were no statistically significant differences between the two groups.

In summary, chest pain units have been promoted as the panacea for improved quality of care for the increasing number of patients with suspected acute coronary syndrome presenting to EDs. The current evidence, using randomized study designs, does not support this claim. As the ED director, you and your team are forced to examine alternatives in order to improve and standardize care.

Conclusions

Emergency physicians and their departments are faced with a variety of presentations of a wide array of clinical conditions. Not surprisingly, variability in practice is often demonstrated by audits. Moreover, efforts to standardize practice, especially for common conditions (e.g., chest pain, asthma, pneumonia, heart failure, lacerations, ankle injuries, and so forth), make sense and will likely improve patient outcomes. In order to accomplish this, many EDs will turn to QI strategies, and this chapter offers an opportunity to better understand the theory and process of QI. For example, this chapter has introduced Deming's PDSA approach, the role of high-quality chart reviews and audit and feedback in changing practice, and outlined the contributions that root cause analysis can make in identifying causes of problems. Using these approaches, EDs have the opportunity to standardize and perhaps improve clinical care. The challenge is to convince ED staff not only of the importance of QI initiatives but to become involved themselves in the process. Only by doing so can we expect to provide the highest quality of care in the ED – the care that we would want for ourselves and our family members.

Acknowledgments

Dr. Worster's research is supported in part by the Hamilton Health Sciences Corporation.

References

1 Graff L, Stevens C, Spaite D, Foody J. Measuring and improving quality in emergency medicine. *Acad Emerg Med* 2002;**9**:1091–107.

2 Godfrey AB. A short history of managing for quality in healthcare. In: Caldwell C, ed. *The Handbook for Managing Change in Healthcare.* American Society for Quality, Milwaukee, WI, 1997.

3 Boudreaux ED, Cruz BL, Baumann BM. The use of performance improvement methods to enhance emergency department patient satisfaction in the United States: a critical review of the literature and suggestions for future research. *Acad Emerg Med* 2006;**13**:795–802.

4 Anon. *Continuous Improvement Handbook: A quick reference guide for tools and concepts.* Executive Learning, Inc., Brentwood, TN, 1993.

5 Al Darrab A. Application of lean six sigma for patients presenting with ST-elevation myocardial infarction: the Hamilton Health Sciences experience. *Healthcare Q* 2006;**9**:56–61 (erratum in *Healthcare Q* 2006;**9**:16).

6 Jamtvedt G, Young JM, Kristoffersen DT, O'Brien MA, Oxman AD. Audit and feedback: effects on professional practice and health care outcomes. *Cochrane Database Syst Rev* 2006;**2**:CD000259 (doi: 10.1002/14651858.CD000259).

7 Worster A, Bledsoe RD, Cleve P, Fernandes CM, Upadhye S, Eva K. Reassessing the methods of medical record review studies in emergency medicine research. *Ann Emerg Med* 2005;**45**:448–51.

8 Badcock D, Kelly AM, Kerr D, Reade T. The quality of medical record review studies in the international emergency medicine literature. *Ann Emerg Med* 2005;**45**:444–7.

9 Worster A, Haines T. Advanced statistics: understanding medical record review (MRR) studies. *Acad Emerg Med* 2004;**11**:187–92.

10 Rooney JJ, Vanden Heuvel LN. Root cause analysis for beginners. *Qual Prog* 2004;**37**:45–53.

11 Fernandes CMB, Worster A, Hill S, McCallum C, Eva K. Root cause analysis of delays for laboratory tests on emergency department patients. *Can J Emerg Med* 2004;**6**:116–22.

12 Fernandes CMB, Walker R, Price A, Marsden J, Haley L. Root cause analysis of laboratory delays to an emergency department. *J Emerg Med* 1997;**15**:735–9.

13 Worster A, Fernandes CM, Malcolmson C, Eva K, Simpson D. Identification of root causes for emergency diagnostic imaging delays at three Canadian hospitals. *J Emerg Nurs* 2006;**32**:276–80.

14 Goodacre S, Cross E, Lewis C, Nicholl J, Capewell S, ESCAPE Research Team. Effectiveness and safety of chest pain assessment to prevent emergency admissions: ESCAPE cluster randomised trial. *BMJ* 2007;**335**: 659.

6 Medication Adherence

Ursula Whalen & Sunil Kripalani

Division of General Internal Medicine and Public Health, Vanderbilt University, Nashville, USA

Case scenario

A 50-year-old woman, with a history of asthma since age 20, presented to the emergency department (ED) with a 2-day history of shortness of breath and cough. There was no fever, chest pain or lower extremity swelling. On examination, the patient was diaphoretic and could not speak in complete sentences. She was afebrile, with a pulse rate of 126 beats/min and a blood pressure of 150/94 mmHg. Her respiratory rate was 40 breaths/min, and she was using accessory muscles of respiration. Chest auscultation revealed bilateral inspiratory and expiratory wheezes. Cardiac auscultation revealed tachycardia without evidence of murmur, gallop or rub. The remaining physical examination was unremarkable.

Oxygen saturation was 88% by pulse oximetry on room air. Supplemental oxygen, nebulized albuterol and ipratropium, and intravenous methylprednisolone 80 mg were administered. After 30 minutes of medical treatment, she improved clinically. When asked about her medications, she pulled several inhalers and pill bottles out of her purse and reported not missing any of her doses. When the ED physician noted that several of the pill bottles were for the same medication, the patient reluctantly admitted she was unable to read the labels. He also noted that she had filled the prescriptions 2 months prior to presentation; however, she had approximately 2 weeks of pills remaining in the bottles.

Background

Medication adherence refers to the extent to which patients take their medications as prescribed by their health care providers. Poor medication adherence is an under-recognized, yet major public health problem. Studies have shown that poor medication adherence increases medical costs by an estimated $100 billion yearly in the United States and accounts for approximately 10% of hospitalizations [1].

Factors related to medication adherence are complex. In an attempt to delineate predictors of compliance, more than 200 variables have been studied but no prevailing predictors have been elucidated [2]. For instance, medication adherence is not consistently related to socio-economic status or to pathology-related factors [2]. In fact, studies have shown that patients often choose not to take their medicines as prescribed [3]. Results from 9290 patient surveys showed that of patients who were not adherent to medications, only 24% "forgot to take their medicine" while the others chose not to take their medicine for various reasons [3].

Measuring medication adherence is also complex since no gold standard exists [2]. There are a variety of direct and indirect methods for measuring medication adherence. Direct methods, such as directly observed therapy, measurement of drug metabolites in the blood or urine, and measurement of biological markers added to the drug formulation, are expensive, cumbersome for health care providers, and not feasible in the ED [4]. Indirect methods include asking the patient about adherence to medications, evaluating clinical response, counting pills, determining refill rates of prescriptions, using patient questionnaires, implementing electronic medication monitors, and advising patients to keep a medication diary [3,4]. While perhaps more applicable to the ED setting, many of these also have disadvantages or limitations.

Research has shown that there are problems with each of the indirect methods [4]. For instance, patient self-report tends to overestimate adherence, and pill counting does not account for dose timing, drug holidays, or possible bottle switching [4]. Calculation of refill rates is feasible in closed pharmacy systems but is more challenging for patients who use different pharmacies [4]. While electronic monitors can record the time of opening bottles and thus provide some helpful information about medication usage, they do not account for the patient taking the appropriate number of pills or actually ingesting them at the time of opening [4]. Furthermore, electronic medication monitors are expensive and since insurance companies do not pay for these devices, they are not used routinely [4].

Evidence-based Emergency Medicine. Edited by Brian H. Rowe
© 2009 Blackwell Publishing, ISBN: 978-1-4051-6143-5.

	Adherence status	
Clinical state	Treatment adherence	Treatment non-adherence
No relapse/failure	Option: No changes required (ideal state)	Option: Consider diagnostic error
Relapse/failure	Option: Consider change in management (see assessment of compliance below)	Option: Encourage adherence (see discussion on interventions)

Table 6.1 Two-by-two table of adherence and clinical response associated with each patient seen in medical care.

Epidemiology

Given the complexity of contributing factors and means of measuring non-adherence, it is not surprising that the level of adherence considered acceptable also varies. In certain conditions such as human immunodeficiency virus (HIV) infection, attaining near perfect adherence is critical for long-term response to therapy and avoidance of drug resistance. In most other chronic conditions, an adherence level greater than 80% is considered acceptable. In general, however, medication adherence is poor, with reviews showing rates of 50–75% [2,5]. Medication adherence is highest for acute and symptomatic conditions, which may be somewhat reassuring to emergency physicians [3]. Unfortunately, medication adherence declines over time. For example, after the first 6–12 months of therapy for chronic health problems, medication adherence may drop by 50% [6].

When assessing a patient in the ED, the emergency physician is mainly faced with adherence problems related to drug interventions for chronic disease exacerbations (e.g., asthma, hypertension, coronary artery disease, epilepsy, atrial fibrillation, Crohn's disease, etc.). For example, a seizure in a patient with epilepsy may be the result of non-adherence to medications, while presentations with drug toxicity may result from medication changes, increased patient adherence and/or overuse. Alternatively, non-adherence can be behavioral (failure to comply with alcohol abstinence in alcoholism) or preventive (e.g., failure to comply with helmet legislation for bicycle riders).

In the ED, a clinician needs to decide if a patient presenting with a chronic disease exacerbation represents a failure of treatment and also the state of patient adherence (Table 6.1). The following questions arise from the clinical scenario and this discussion regarding adherence.

Clinical questions

1 In a patient seen in the ED with a chronic disease (population), how sensitive and specific (diagnostic test characteristics) is patient self-report (measure) compared to objective measures (reference standard) in assessing medication adherence (outcome)?

2 In a patient seen in the ED with a chronic disease (population), how sensitive and specific (diagnostic test characteristics) is physician assessment (measure) compared to validated methods (reference standard) in assessing medication adherence (outcome)?

3 In a patient seen in the ED with a chronic disease (population), how sensitive and specific (diagnostic test characteristics) is open-ended physician normalization of non-adherence (measure) compared to closed-ended questioning (reference standard) in detecting medication non-adherence (outcome)?

4 In a patient seen in the ED with a chronic disease (population), what is the relationship (test characteristic) between low literacy (exposure) and medication adherence (outcome)?

5 In a patient seen in the ED with a chronic disease (population), what is the relationship (test characteristic) between medication non-adherence (measure) and return ED visits (outcome)?

6 In a patient seen in the ED with a chronic disease like asthma (population), does a written action plan (intervention) improve medication adherence and reduce ED return visits (outcome) compared to providing a prescription and verbal instructions (control)?

7 In a patient seen in the ED with suspected non-adherence (population), does provision of educational information (intervention) improve compliance and reduce ED return visits (outcomes) compared to referral back to a primary care physician (control)?

8 In a patient seen in the ED with suspected non-adherence (population), do home visits by a trained health professional (intervention) improve compliance and reduce ED return visits (outcomes) compared to referral back to a primary care physician (control)?

9 In a patient seen in the ED with suspected non-adherence (population), does intensive case management (intervention) improve compliance (outcome) compared to referral back to a primary care physician (control)?

10 In a patient seen in the ED with suspected non-adherence (population), what interventions (intervention) improve compliance (outcome) compared to providing a prescription only (control)?

General search strategy

Performing a literature search in electronic databases such as the Cochrane Library and MEDLINE is helpful for finding the evidence available. The Cochrane Library publishes high-quality systematic reviews on medication adherence and is an excellent starting place. MEDLINE is also helpful for finding randomized controlled trials and meta-analyses to answer questions posed.

Critical review of the literature

Question 1: In a patient seen in the ED with a chronic disease (population), how sensitive and specific (diagnostic test characteristics) is patient self-report (measure) compared to objective measures (reference standard) in assessing medication adherence (outcome)?

Search strategy

- MEDLINE: patient compliance/ AND (self-report OR questionnaire OR survey).mp AND (sensitivity and specificity/ OR likelihood ratio$.tw OR reproducibility of results OR exp diagnostic errors/)

Self-report is often used as a measure of adherence because it is inexpensive, simple and can be applied to every patient [7]. Studies have shown conflicting results regarding the reliability of self-reported adherence [8]. For example, a study of medication adherence to antihypertensive treatment compared an electronic medication monitoring system (reference standard) to two different validated measures of self-report [9]. In this study, the electronic monitoring system found 81% adherence, which was identical to the adherence rates for self-report using the Medical Outcomes Study General Adherence Scale (Box 6.1) [9]. There was a discrepancy, however, between the electronic monitoring system and self-report using a visual analog scale, which overestimated adherence at 94% [9]. Another study compared an electronic monitoring system (reference standard) to self-report using an antihypertensive regimen and found a statistically significant association between reported frequency of forgetting to take medication and results from the electronic monitoring system ($P < 0.001$) [10].

Part of the variation among studies can be attributed to diverse methods of assessment, which include medication diaries, structured questionnaires and patient interviews. In a systematic review of 57 studies, medication diaries and questionnaires demonstrated greater concordance with non-self-report measures of adherence than did patient interviews ($P = 0.01$) [8]. Although these techniques may be of interest to emergency physicians, medication diaries and structured questionnaires may be impractical for widespread use in the ED.

In summary, emergency physicians will commonly rely on asking patients about non-adherence; however, to be safe, they should always suspect it is more common than initially reported by their patients.

Question 2: In a patient seen in the ED with a chronic disease (population), how sensitive and specific (diagnostic test characteristics) is physician assessment (measure) compared to validated methods (reference standard) in assessing medication adherence (outcome)?

Search strategy

- MEDLINE: patient compliance/ AND (physician OR clinician OR clinical OR provider).mp AND (medication OR drug OR medicine).mp AND (assess$ OR estimate OR measure$).mp AND (sensitivity and specificity/ OR likelihood ratio$.tw OR reproducibility of results OR exp diagnostic errors/)

A physician can most easily assess patient adherence by asking the patient, estimating adherence clinically, performing pill counts or checking pharmacy dispensing records. In general, physicians do not accurately estimate patients' level of adherence [11–16]. In one study of antiretroviral use, physicians overestimated patient compliance in some cases and inadequately detected poor adherence in others (24–62% sensitivity, depending on the cut-off used) [15]. Another study comparing self-report (reference standard) to physician estimates of antiretroviral adherence demonstrated incorrect estimates for approximately one-third of patients, including overestimation of non-adherence [17]. A similar report comparing physician estimates and

---

Box 6.1 Some validated measures of self-report [9].

Medical Outcomes Study General Adherence Scale
(0–5: 0 = none of the time, 5 = all of the time)
How often was each of the following statements true for you in the past 4 weeks?
1   I had a hard time doing what the health care provider suggested.
2   I followed the health care provider's suggestions exactly.
3   I was unable to do what was necessary to follow my health care provider's suggestions.
4   I found it easy to do the things my health care provider suggested.
5   How often were you able to do what the health care provider told you to?

Visual analog scale
Over the past 6 months, what percent of the time would you estimate that you took your study medications?
(Place an X on the line between 0 and 100 percent)

patient self-report found that self-report of non-adherence predicted the non-response of HIV RNA, but physician estimates did not [18].

In another investigation, physicians estimated adherence in 245 patients with uncontrolled hypertension. These estimates correlated poorly with other measures of adherence, including self-report, electronic monitoring and urine drug levels (Spearman's rho = 0.02 to 0.16) [9]. The low performance was observed in spite of the patients being well known to the physicians, a feature that has been associated with more accurate clinical assessment of adherence in other studies [15].

Because physician estimates of medication adherence are unreliable, clinicians may more accurately assess medication adherence by pill counts and verification of pharmacy records [14]. In a study of 286 patients on antihypertensive medication, adherence assessed by pill counts and pharmacy dispensing records moderately correlated with electronic monitoring systems (absolute value of correlations = 0.17 to 0.52) [10]. In another study evaluating medication adherence to oral agents for diabetes, return pill counts and prescription refill data overestimated adherence when compared to electronic monitoring [7].

In summary, emergency physicians should not attempt to estimate patients' medication adherence, even when the patient is familiar to them or their ED. While inaccuracies with pill counting and verifying pharmacy records exist, these techniques can be useful general ways to determine medication adherence.

Question 3: In a patient seen in the ED with a chronic disease (population), how sensitive and specific (diagnostic test characteristics) is open-ended physician normalization of non-adherence (measure) compared to closed-ended questioning (reference standard) in detecting medication non-adherence (outcome)?

Search strategy

- MEDLINE: patient compliance/ AND (physician OR clinician OR clinical OR provider).mp AND (medication OR drug OR medicine).mp AND (assess$ OR estimate OR measure$).mp AND (sensitivity and specificity/ OR likelihood ratio$.tw OR reproducibility of results OR exp diagnostic errors/)

Quantitative evidence about how to assess medication use during a physician–patient interview is limited [19]. One qualitative study showed that asking patients about medication use in an open-ended manner generates more discussion than does a closed-ended or leading approach [20]. This should provide the physician with a better understanding of patients' actual medication use. An example of an open-ended question is "How often are you taking your medication?" By contrast, a closed-ended question is, "Are you taking your medication as prescribed?" and a leading question is, "So, you're taking your medication, right?" [20].

Normalizing the likelihood of non-adherence may also be an effective technique to encourage patients to more accurately describe their medication use. This can be done by appropriately framing the question (e.g., "People often miss taking their medications. In the past week, on how many days did you forget to take a pill?"). Questions structured in this manner were more highly associated with electronic measures of adherence [21].

In summary, emergency physicians should employ normalized statements and open-ended questions to estimate a patient's medication adherence.

Question 4: In a patient seen in the ED with a chronic disease (population), what is the relationship (test characteristic) between low literacy (exposure) and medication adherence (outcome)?

Search strategy

- MEDLINE: patient compliance/ AND literacy.mp

Health literacy is a term used to describe a patient's ability to understand and use basic health information in order to make appropriate health decisions [22]. In the United States, 36% of adults have "basic" or "below basic" levels of health literacy [23]. These patients have difficulty comprehending most health-related materials, including the instructions commonly found on prescription drug labels [24].

The largest investigation that has evaluated the association of health literacy with medication adherence was a study of 1549 Medicare patients. Overall, 40% of patients in this investigation had low refill adherence, defined as not having medications available at least 20% of the time [25]. In unadjusted analyses, patients with inadequate health literacy had greater odds of poor adherence to medication refills, compared to patients with adequate health literacy skills (OR = 1.37; 95% CI: 1.08 to 1.74). In multivariable analyses that adjusted for age, race, gender and education, health literacy was not statistically associated with low refill adherence (OR = 1.21; 95% CI: 0.91 to 1.62) [25]. Other reports have shown a significant association between inadequate literacy and poor adherence [26,27]; however, not all studies have demonstrated this relationship [28,29].

Improper use of medications is another form of medication non-adherence. Low health literacy is associated with improper use of medications, such as metered dose inhalers (MDIs) [30,31]. In a study of 483 patients with asthma that was conducted in part at an inner city emergency department, literacy was the strongest predictor of MDI technique. Poor technique, which meant correctly performing less than half of six steps in inhaler usage, was present among 89% of patients who read at or below a third grade level, compared with 48% of patients who read at a high school level [31]. In a subsequent study of 73 patients hospitalized with asthma exacerbation, inadequate health literacy was significantly associated with worse medication knowledge and MDI technique

[30]. Following one educational session, however, 59% of those with inadequate health literacy exhibited mastery of MDI technique [30]. Inadequate literacy was not associated with the ability to learn or retain medication instructions. Thus, while low health literacy is strongly associated with improper MDI technique, educational interventions are effective in improving skills.

In summary, low literacy is a potential risk factor for poor medication adherence and should be considered when evaluating patients in the ED setting.

Question 5: In a patient seen in the ED with a chronic disease (population), what is the relationship (test characteristic) between medication non-adherence (measure) and return ED visits (outcome)?

Search strategy

- MEDLINE: patient compliance AND (emergency treatment/ OR emergency service, hospital)

Multiple studies have shown that medication non-adherence is associated with higher rates of ED visits and hospital admissions for patients with chronic medical conditions such as congestive heart failure, diabetes and asthma [1,32]. A retrospective cohort analysis of 137,277 patients under age 65 years found that higher rates of medication non-adherence were associated with higher rates of hospitalization for diabetes, hypertension, hypercholesterolemia and congestive heart failure [1]. For example, this study found that patients with diabetes who had high rates of non-adherence (taking medications appropriately 1–19% of the time) had a hospitalization risk of 30%, while those taking their medications 80–100% of the time had a hospitalization risk of 13% ($P < 0.05$).

A study of almost 68,000 patients with diabetes showed that higher rates of medication adherence (measured by prescription refill data) were linked to significantly fewer ED visits and inpatient admissions [32]. Surprisingly, while this study found decreased utilization of medical care services amongst patients with higher adherence rates, the authors found a shift in costs toward pharmaceutical agents but not lower costs overall [32]. Other studies have found a large and significant association between overall costs and adherence [1].

In summary, non-adherence is important to suspect and detect since it has an impressive influence on outcomes. These findings illustrate the importance of considering potential interventions for improving medication adherence.

Question 6: In a patient seen in the ED with a chronic disease like asthma (population), does a written action plan (intervention) improve medication adherence and reduce ED return visits (outcome) compared to providing a prescription and verbal instructions (control)?

Search strategy

- Cochrane database: asthma AND action plan

Interventions are needed to improve medication adherence in an effort to improve outcomes from chronic diseases such as asthma, especially after an ED visit for an exacerbation. A Cochrane review summarized the results of seven, small, randomized controlled trials to determine whether written individualized management plans alone are effective in improving adherence and decreasing emergency department return visits for asthma [33]. The written action plans used in the studies were individualized according to the patient's asthma severity and treatment and included information about the following: (i) when and how to modify medication in response to worsening asthma; and (ii) how to access the medical system in response to worsening asthma. There was no consistent evidence that written action plans alone improved adherence or clinical outcomes. Three of the seven studies evaluated emergency department utilization and did not find benefit (RR = 0.86; 95% CI: 0.44 to 1.67) [33].

Another Cochrane review combined the results of 15 studies comparing optimal self-management, which included written action plans in addition to self-management and regular medical review, to usual care [34]. The authors found a statistically significant reduction in emergency department visits (RR = 0.78; 95% CI: 0.67 to 0.91) and hospitalizations for asthma (RR = 0.56; 95% CI: 0.43 to 0.77).

In summary, it appears that written action plans alone may be insufficient to change clinical outcomes; however, when used in combination with other management strategies, they reduce health care utilization. The pressing question for emergency physicians is how these might be incorporated successfully and efficiently into ED practice, especially in chronic diseases other than asthma.

Question 7: In a patient seen in the ED with suspected non-adherence (population), does provision of educational information (intervention) improve compliance and reduce ED return visits (outcomes), compared to referral back to a primary care physician (control)?

Search strategy

- MEDLINE: patient compliance/ AND patient education/Cochrane database: (medication adherence OR medication compliance) AND education

A recent systematic review summarized 37 randomized controlled trials designed to enhance adherence in chronic medical conditions [35]. It was based on a broader Cochrane review [36]. Among the 37 trials were 12 studies that tested the effect of educating patients through additional information. Six of the 12 educational interventions showed some improvement in adherence, and four of 12 had some positive impact on clinical outcomes. The most successful educational interventions involved fairly intensive counseling that was reinforced over time. Most of the included interventions took place in the setting of outpatient chronic disease management; however, a few were directly relevant to the ED. One such study among patients with asthma provided structured education that addressed beliefs, knowledge, attitudes and social support; it was successful in improving peak expiratory flow and in reducing urgent visits for asthma exacerbation [37]. Two other similar interventions, however, were not as successful [38,39].

Other Cochrane reviews have summarized the evidence in the context of specific diseases, such as asthma [40], hypertension [41] and hypercholesterolemia [42]. In a review of 12 studies that tested the effect of information-only education programs on asthma outcomes, clinical outcomes did not improve significantly, though some improvement was noted in perceived symptoms [40]. Most of the included studies did not measure medication adherence, but one of the trials reported an increase in bronchodilator and corticosteroid usage, which was interpreted to indicate better adherence [43]. Four of the studies reported a reduction in ED visits; only one provided complete information about the effect size [44]. In that study, information-only education to high-risk patients reduced ED visits by a mean of 2.8 per year (95% CI: 1.18 to 4.34). In another review on antihypertensive medication adherence, education alone was not effective in improving adherence [41]. In the context of lipid-lowering therapy, modest benefit was found from education alone [42].

Overall, the evidence would suggest education may be beneficial in some cases, but it does not appear as effective as behavioral interventions or more intensive combined interventions [35]. Another issue for emergency physicians is how that education is delivered and by whom in an already chaotic and overcrowded setting.

Question 8: In a patient seen in the ED with suspected non-adherence (population), do home visits by a trained health professional (intervention) improve compliance and reduce ED return visits (outcomes) compared to referral back to a primary care physician (control)?

Search strategy

- MEDLINE: patient compliance/ AND (house calls/ OR home visit)

Home visits are rarely offered or available for emergency patients; however, in some chronic diseases (e.g., asthma, heart failure, chronic obstructive pulmonary disease) they offer the potential for a health care professional to provide education and evaluate patients' exposure to health risks. Most trials of home visits have focused on hard-to-reach populations, such as inner city children with asthma, and difficulties have been noted in program implementation and completion [45]. One study of Medicaid-managed care patients aged 2 to 56 years used two evaluative approaches to assess the effectiveness of a home-based teaching program [46].

In a pre/post evaluation, a significant reduction in ED utilization was noted ($P < 0.001$). When outcomes were compared against a concurrent control group, however, no significant difference was found ($P = 0.51$).

Another trial randomized 104 children with asthma to active home visits, placebo home visits or control [47]. The emphasis of the active home visits was allergen avoidance through practices such as dust mite and cockroach control. In this study, the active home visit group had a 33% reduction in ED visits ($P < 0.001$ for comparison to control), but the placebo home visit group had a similar reduction (30%, $P < 0.001$ for comparison to control).

A third study enrolled 239 adults and children with moderate to severe asthma who presented to the ED [48]. Patients were randomized to usual care or to a facilitated office visit with the primary care physician followed by a home visit. During 6 months' follow-up, the reduction in urgent asthma-related visits was not statistically significant (hazard ration (HR) = 0.79; 95% CI: 0.48 to 1.29). Subgroup analyses indicated that the program might be more effective in children (HR = 0.62; 95% CI: 0.33 to 1.19) than in adults (HR = 1.08; 95% CI: 0.50 to 2.33).

One study was identified that assessed the utility of home visits in a broader population of adults following hospitalization [49]. Almost 900 adults over the age of 80 were randomized to usual care or home visits by a pharmacist, who focused on safe medication management and adherence. Unexpectedly, the intervention group experienced a significantly higher rate of hospital readmission during the 6-month follow-up (rate ratio = 1.30; 95% CI: 1.07 to 1.58).

Overall, this evidence suggests that home visits may not be an effective approach for adult ED patients and until further evidence is available, the strategy is not recommended.

Question 9: In a patient seen in the ED with suspected non-adherence (population), does intensive case management involvement (intervention) improve compliance (outcome) compared to referral back to a primary care physician (control)?

Search strategy

- MEDLINE: patient compliance/ AND case management AND (emergency treatment/ OR emergency service, hospital)
- MEDLINE: patient compliance/ AND case management
- MEDLINE: case management/ AND (emergency treatment/ OR emergency service, hospital)

Although case management has been shown to positively influence adherence in outpatient settings [50,51], searching identified no studies that reported the effect of case management on adherence in the ED. Other literature was identified that supports the utility of ED case management for different outcomes. One review summarized the beneficial effect of case management on satisfaction and perhaps costs [52]. The effect on ED utilization is less clear. One study of patients who frequently used the ED found a large decrease in utilization with the implementation of a case management model [53]. However, three other studies did not find a reduction in ED utilization [54–56], although two of them demonstrated better primary care linkages through the case management approach [54,56].

Three pediatric studies were identified that also may shed some light on the current state of the science. Several randomized studies have evaluated the effect of case management on control of asthma among children [57–60]. One study was based in the ED and randomized children to usual care (patient education, written action plan, and instructions to follow-up with the primary care physician within 7 days), usual care plus assistance with scheduling follow-up, or these interventions plus enrolment in a case management program [59]. No significant differences were observed in ED visits during the next 6 months, quality of life scores or use of controller medications.

Another investigation among 57 children enrolled in a managed care plan found that a case management intervention reduced ED visits by 57% ($P < 0.05$) and hospitalizations by 75% ($P < 0.05$) [60]. A school-based program led by nurses also demonstrated reductions in ED visits ($P < 0.001$), hospital days ($P < 0.05$) and school absences (mean 4.38 days vs 8.18 days in control group) [58]. However, an investigation among inner city children that compared case management to two educational strategies found no significant incremental benefit as a result of case management [57]. These three studies did not measure medication adherence.

In summary, there is limited evidence supporting the effectiveness of case management in the ED.

Question 10: In a patient seen in the ED with suspected non-adherence (population), what interventions (intervention) improve compliance (outcome) compared to providing a prescription only (control)?

Search strategy

- Cochrane: (medication adherence OR medication compliance) AND intervention$
- MEDLINE: patient compliance/ AND intervention$.mp

A Cochrane review summarized the effect of randomized controlled trials designed to enhance medication adherence and clinical outcomes [36]. Based on the included studies, it appears relatively easy to improve short-term adherence through interventions such as verbal counseling, written information and changes in medication packaging. Studies in the setting of chronic illness management, however, were less likely to be positive [36].

A subsequent analysis [35], based on the Cochrane review, demonstrated that the most consistently effective interventions to enhance long-term adherence appeared to be those that reduced dosing demands (three of three studies), or those that provided monitoring of adherence and feedback (three of four studies).

Several multi-session informational interventions were also effective, as were many interventions that combined informational and behavioral elements. However, few of these interventions were able to demonstrate better clinical outcomes, and the relationship between clinical outcomes and improvements in adherence was inconsistent.

In summary, evidence suggests that ED physicians should attempt to provide the simplest dosing schedule (once or twice daily), and encourage the use of feedback to enhance adherence.

Conclusions

The patient in the case above was treated with systemic and inhaled corticosteroids, education about her medication and asthma in the ED, provided with a written action plan, and advised to closely follow-up with her primary care provider. Literacy was addressed since this seemed to be an issue for this patient.

Non-adherence to a health care provider's prescriptions and advice is common. No consistent predictors of medication non-adherence have been elucidated. The most feasible methods of measuring medication adherence include self-report, physician assessment, pill count and prescription refill records. Though problems exist with using each of these methods, self-report, pill counts and prescription refill records have been proven to be reliable sources of determining medication adherence. Physician assessment, however, is unreliable.

Increased medication adherence has been proven to be associated with fewer ED visits and inpatient admissions for chronic diseases like asthma, congestive heart failure, hypertension, hypercholesterolemia and diabetes. Interventions targeting patients who are non-adherent are critical to improve health outcomes.

Conflicts of interest

Dr. Kripalani is a consultant to and holds equity in PictureRx, LLC, which makes a patient education aid to promote appropriate medication use. The terms of this arrangement have been reviewed and approved by Emory University in accordance with its conflict of interest policies.

References

1 Sokol MC, McGuigan KA, Verbrugge RR, Epstein RS. Impact of medication adherence on hospitalization risk and healthcare cost. *Med Care* 2005;**43**(6):521–30.

2 Vermeire E, Hearnshaw H, Van Royen P, Denekens J. Patient adherence to treatment: three decades of research. A comprehensive review. *J Clin Pharm Ther* 2001;**26**(5):331–42.

3 Boston Consulting Group. *The Hidden Epidemic: Finding a cure for unfilled prescriptions and missed doses.* Boston Consulting Group, Boston, 2003. Available at http://www.bcg.com/publications/publications-splash.jsp.

4 Osterberg L, Blaschke T. Adherence to medication. *N Engl J Med* 2005;**353**(5):487–97.

5 DiMatteo MR. Variations in patients' adherence to medical recommendations: a quantitative review of 50 years of research. *Med Care* 2004;**42**(3):200–209.

6 Benner JS, Glynn RJ, Mogun H, Neumann PJ, Weinstein MC, Avorn J. Long-term persistence in use of statin therapy in elderly patients. *JAMA* 2002;**288**(4):455–61.

7 MacLaughlin EJ, Raehl CL, Treadway AK, Sterling TL, Zoller DP, Bond CA. Assessing medication adherence in the elderly: which tools to use in clinical practice? *Drugs Aging* 2005;**22**(3):231–55.

8 Garber MC, Nau DP, Erickson SR, Aikens JE, Lawrence JB. The concordance of self-report with other measures of medication adherence: a summary of the literature. *Med Care* 2004;**42**(7):649–52.

9 Hamilton GA. Measuring adherence in a hypertension clinical trial. *Eur J Cardiovasc Nurs* 2003;**2**(3):219–28.

10 Choo PW, Rand CS, Inui TS, et al. Validation of patient reports, automated pharmacy records, and pill counts with electronic monitoring of adherence to antihypertensive therapy. *Med Care* 1999;**37**(9):846–57.

11 Du Pasquier-Fediaevsky L, Tubiana-Rufi N. Discordance between physician and adolescent assessments of adherence to treatment: influence of HbA1c level. The PEDIAB Collaborative Group. *Diabetes Care* 1999;**22**(9):1445–9.

12 Gross R, Bilker WB, Friedman HM, Coyne JC, Strom BL. Provider inaccuracy in assessing adherence and outcomes with newly initiated antiretroviral therapy. *AIDS* 2002;**16**(13):1835–7.

13 Farley J, Hines S, Musk A, Ferrus S, Tepper V. Assessment of adherence to antiviral therapy in HIV-infected children using the Medication Event Monitoring System, pharmacy refill, provider assessment, caregiver self-report, and appointment keeping. *J AIDS* 2003;**33**(2):211–18.

14 Farmer KC. Methods for measuring and monitoring medication regimen adherence in clinical trials and clinical practice. *Clin Ther* 1999;**21**(6):1074–90; discussion 1073.

15 Miller LG, Liu H, Hays RD, et al. How well do clinicians estimate patients' adherence to combination antiretroviral therapy? *J Gen Intern Med* 2002;**17**(1):1–11.

16 Butler JA, Peveler RC, Roderick P, Horne R, Mason JC. Measuring compliance with drug regimens after renal transplantation: comparison of self-report and clinician rating with electronic monitoring. *Transplantation* 2004;**77**(5):786–9.

17 Murri R, Ammassari A, Trotta MP, et al. Patient-reported and physician-estimated adherence to HAART: social and clinic center-related factors are associated with discordance. *J Gen Intern Med* 2004;**19**(11):1104–10.

18 Haubrich RH, Little SJ, Currier JS, et al. The value of patient-reported adherence to antiretroviral therapy in predicting virologic and immunologic response. California Collaborative Treatment Group. *AIDS* 1999;**13**(9):1099–107.

19 Steele DJ, Jackson TC, Gutmann MC. Have you been taking your pills? The adherence-monitoring sequence in the medical interview. *J Fam Pract* 1990;**30**(3):294–9.

20 Bokhour BG, Berlowitz DR, Long JA, Kressin NR. How do providers assess antihypertensive medication adherence in medical encounters? *J Gen Intern Med* 2006;**21**(6):577–83.

21 Choo PW, Rand CS, Inui TS, et al. Validation of patient reports, automated pharmacy records, and pill counts with electronic monitoring of adherence to antihypertensive therapy. *Med Care* 1999;**37**(9):846–57.

22 Selden CR, Zorn M, Ratzan S, Parker RM. *Current Bibliographies in Medicine: Health Literacy*. National Library of Medicine, Bethesda, MD, 2000.

23 Kutner M, Greenberg E, Jin Y, Paulsen C. *The Health Literacy of America's Adults: Results from the 2003 National Assessment of Adult Literacy (NCES 2006-483)*. US Department of Education, National Center for Education Statistics, Washington, DC, 2006.

24 Davis TC, Wolf MS, Bass PF, III, et al. Low literacy impairs comprehension of prescription drug warning labels. *J Gen Intern Med* 2006;**21**(8):847–51.

25 Gazmararian JA, Kripalani S, Miller MJ, Echt KV, Ren J, Rask K. Factors associated with medication refill adherence in cardiovascular-related diseases: a focus on health literacy. *J Gen Intern Med* 2006;**21**(12):1215–21.

26 Kalichman S, Ramachandran B, Catz S. Adherence to combination antiretroviral therapies in HIV patients of low health literacy. *J Gen Intern Med* 1999;**14**:267–73.

27 Raehl CL, Bond CA, Woods TJ, Patry RA, Sleeper RB. Screening tests for intended medication adherence among the elderly. *Ann Pharmacother* 2006;**40**(5):888–93.

28 Golin CE, Liu H, Hays RD, et al. A prospective study of predictors of adherence to combination antiretroviral medication. *J Gen Intern Med* 2002;**17**(10):756–65.

29 Paasche-Orlow MK, Cheng DM, Palepu A, Meli S, Faber V, Samet JH. Health literacy, antiretroviral adherence, and HIV-RNA suppression: a longitudinal perspective. *J Gen Intern Med* 2006;**21**(8):835–40.

30 Paasche-Orlow MK, Riekert KA, Bilderback A, et al. Tailored education may reduce health literacy disparities in asthma self-management. *Am J Respir Crit Care Med* 2005;**172**(8):980–86.

31 Williams MV, Baker DW, Honig EG, Lee TM, Nowlan A. Inadequate literacy is a barrier to asthma knowledge and self-care. *Chest* 1998;**114**(4):1008–15.

32 Hepke KL, Martus MT, Share DA. Costs and utilization associated with pharmaceutical adherence in a diabetic population. *Am J Manag Care* 2004;**10**(2/2):144–51.

33 Toelle BG, Ram FS. Written individualised management plans for asthma in children and adults. *Cochrane Database Syst Rev* 2004;**2**:CD002171.

34 Gibson PG, Powell H, Coughlan J, et al. Self-management education and regular practitioner review for adults with asthma. *Cochrane Database Syst Rev* 2007;**1**:CD001117.

35 Kripalani S, Yao X, Haynes RB. Interventions to enhance medication adherence in chronic medical conditions: a systematic review. *Arch Intern Med* 2007;**167**(6):540–50.

36 Haynes RB, Yao X, Degani A, Kripalani S, Garg A, McDonald HP. Interventions to enhance medication adherence. *Cochrane Database Syst Rev* 2005;**4**:CD000011.

37 Cote J, Bowie DM, Robichaud P, Parent JG, Battisti L, Boulet LP. Evaluation of two different educational interventions for adult patients consulting with an acute asthma exacerbation. *Am J Respir Crit Care Med* 2001;**163**(6):1415–19.

38 Levy ML, Robb M, Allen J, Doherty C, Bland JM, Winter RJ. A randomized controlled evaluation of specialist nurse education following accident and emergency department attendance for acute asthma. *Respir Med* 2000;**94**(9):900–908.

39 Morice AH, Wrench C. The role of the asthma nurse in treatment compliance and self-management following hospital admission [see comment]. *Respir Med* 2001;**95**(11):851–6.

40 Gibson PG, Powell H, Coughlan J, et al. Limited (information only) patient education programs for adults with asthma. *Cochrane Database Syst Rev* 2002;**1**:CD001005.

41 Schroeder K, Fahey T, Ebrahim S. Interventions for improving adherence to treatment in patients with high blood pressure in ambulatory settings. *Cochrane Database Syst Rev* 2004;**2**:CD004804.

42 Schedlbauer A, Schroeder K, Peters TJ, Fahey T. Interventions to improve adherence to lipid lowering medication. *Cochrane Database Syst Rev* 2004;**4**:CD004371.

43 Soondergaard B, Davidsen F, Kirkeby B, Rasmussen M, Hey H. The economics of an intensive education programme for asthmatic patients: a prospective controlled trial. *Pharmacoeconomics* 1992;**1**(3):207–12.

44 Bolton MB, Tilley BC, Kuder J, Reeves T, Schultz LR. The cost and effectiveness of an education program for adults who have asthma. *J Gen Intern Med* 1991;**6**(5):401–7.

45 Brown JV, Demi AS, Celano MP, Bakeman R, Kobrynski L, Wilson SR. A home visiting asthma education program: challenges to program implementation. *Health Educ Behav* 2005;**32**(1):42–56.

46 Catov JM, Marsh GM, Youk AO, Huffman VY. Asthma home teaching: two evaluation approaches. *Dis Manag* 2005;**8**(3):178–87.

47 Carter MC, Perzanowski MS, Raymond A, Platts-Mills TA. Home intervention in the treatment of asthma among inner-city children. *J Allergy Clin Immunol* 2001;**108**(5):732–7.

48 Brown MD, Reeves MJ, Meyerson K, Korzeniewski SJ. Randomized trial of a comprehensive asthma education program after an emergency department visit. *Ann Allergy Asthma Immunol* 2006;**97**(1):44–51.

49 Holland R, Lenaghan E, Harvey I, et al. Does home based medication review keep older people out of hospital? The HOMER randomised controlled trial. *BMJ* 2005;**330**(7486):293.

50 Vlasnik JJ, Aliotta SL, DeLor B. Using case management guidelines to enhance adherence to long-term therapy. *Case Manager* 2005;**16**(3):83–5.

51 Nyamathi A, Stein JA, Schumann A, Tyler D. Latent variable assessment of outcomes in a nurse-managed intervention to increase latent tuberculosis treatment completion in homeless adults. *Health Psychol* 2007;**26**(1):68–76.

52 Bristow DP, Herrick CA. Emergency department case management: the dyad team of nurse case manager and social worker improve discharge planning and patient and staff satisfaction while decreasing inappropriate admissions and costs: a literature review. *Lippincott's Case Manag* 2002;**7**(3):121–8.

53 Pope D, Fernandes CM, Bouthillette F, Etherington J. Frequent users of the emergency department: a program to improve care and reduce visits. *Can Med Assoc J* 2000;**162**(7):1017–20.

54 Phillips GA, Brophy DS, Weiland TJ, Chenhall AJ, Dent AW. The effect of multidisciplinary case management on selected outcomes for frequent attenders at an emergency department. *Med J Aust* 2006;**184**(12):602–6.

55 Lee KH, Davenport L. Can case management interventions reduce the number of emergency department visits by frequent users? *Health Care Manager* 2006;**25**(2):155–9.

56 Horwitz SM, Busch SH, Balestracci KM, Ellingson KD, Rawlings J. Intensive intervention improves primary care follow-up for uninsured emergency department patients. *Acad Emerg Med* 2005;**12**(7):647–52.

57 Karnick P, Margellos-Anast H, Seals G, Whitman S, Aljadeff G, Johnson D. The pediatric asthma intervention: a comprehensive cost-effective approach to asthma management in a disadvantaged inner-city community. *J Asthma* 2007;**44**(1):39–44.

58 Levy M, Heffner B, Stewart T, Beeman G. The efficacy of asthma case management in an urban school district in reducing school absences and hospitalizations for asthma. *J Sch Health* 2006;**76**(6):320–24.

59 Gorelick MH, Meurer JR, Walsh-Kelly CM, et al. Emergency department allies: a controlled trial of two emergency department-based follow-up interventions to improve asthma outcomes in children. *Pediatrics* 2006;**117**(4/2):S127–34.

60 Greineder DK, Loane KC, Parks P. A randomized controlled trial of a pediatric asthma outreach program. *J Allergy Clin Immunol* 1999;**103**(3/1):436–40.

7 Emergency Department Triage

Sandy L. Dong & Michael Bullard

Department of Emergency Medicine, University of Alberta, Edmonton, Canada

Clinical scenario

A 50-year old male walks to the emergency triage desk and states that he has just finished a 6-day drinking binge and needs to "dry out". He appears tremulous and diaphoretic. He has a past history of alcohol withdrawal seizures. The vital signs are: pulse 120 beats/min, blood pressure 158/90 mmHg, and respirations 16 breaths/min.

While the triage nurse is assessing the first patient, an ambulance arrives with a 20-year old female patient responding only to painful stimuli. She is breathing at 40 breaths/min with poor air entry throughout. The paramedic reports that the patient is asthmatic. The paramedics have administered oxygen using a bag-valve mask and 0.3 mg of intramuscular epinephrine.

Meanwhile, a 30-year-old female is brought in by her friends. She has taken a "large amount" of acetaminophen an hour and a half ago. She is awake and alert. Her vital signs are: pulse 88 beats/min, blood pressure 110/62 mmHg, and respirations 14 breaths/min.

It is a typically busy day in the emergency department (ED). There is one resuscitation stretcher and one non-monitored bed available in the department. Which of these patients should be seen first?

Background

In an ideal ED, each patient arriving would be immediately assessed and treated by an available nurse and physician. In most EDs this does not occur, and each patient accessing the ED starts with the triage process. ED triage staff prioritize patients for the urgency with which they need medical care through a process that includes a "quick look" assessment, evaluation of the chief complaint, vital signs and the collection of other physical or historical features in a necessarily limited examination. For obviously unsta-

Evidence-based Emergency Medicine. Edited by Brian H. Rowe
© 2009 Blackwell Publishing, ISBN: 978-1-4051-6143-5.

ble patients, the "quick look" is all that is required to complete the triage. Despite the brevity of the encounter, triage staff need to be as focused and accurate as possible. Under-triage (underestimating the severity of a patient's condition) can compromise patient safety and delay time-sensitive care, while over-triage (assigning a triage level higher than the patient's acuity) can misdirect scarce ED resources and potentially divert those resources from another more needy patient.

Triage is derived from the French word "trier", meaning "to sort". Its origins have been attributed to the Napoleonic wars, where battlefield victims were triaged based on medical need and not rank or social class. In today's spirit of egalitarianism and ever-expanding demands on resources, triaging patients based on need for care continues in modern EDs. Triage systems do exist in a variety of other settings such as the prehospital setting, surgical queues, etc.; however, this chapter is confined to triage as it applies to the assessment and treatment of ED patients.

Clinical questions

1 In ED settings (population), what are the common ED triage systems (intervention)? What are the major differences between the systems?

2 In ED settings (population), how are emergency triage systems evaluated (outcome)? What are the measurements of reliability and validity?

3 In ED settings (population), can triage (intervention) produce reliable results (outcome) when different nurses are compared?

4 In ED settings (population), can triage (intervention) produce valid results (outcome)?

5 In ED settings (population), what is the role of triage (intervention) in relieving ED overcrowding (outcome)?

6 In ED settings (population), what impact does ED overcrowding (intervention) have on triage (outcome)?

Table 7.1 A review of common ED triage systems.

System	Scale	Grades
CTAS [4,13]	Five points	CTAS 1: resuscitation, immediage physician assessment
		CTAS 2: emergent, physician assessment within 15 minutes
		CTAS 3: urgent, physician assessment within 30 minutes
		CTAS 4: less urgent, physician assessment within 60 minutes
		CTAS 5: non-urgent, physician assessment within 120 minutes
ESI [6]	Five points	ESI 1: requires immediate life-saving intervention
		ESI 2: high-risk situation
		ESI 3: two or more resources needed
		ESI 4: one resource needed
		ESI 5: no resources
ATS [3,41]	Five points	Category 1: immediately life-threatening, requires immediate simultaneous assessment
		Category 2: important time-critical treatment, assessment and treatment within 10 minutes
		Category 3: potentially life-threatening or situational urgency, assessment and treatment within 30 minutes
		Category 4: potentially serious or situational urgency or significant complexity or severity, assessment and treatment within 60 minutes
		Category 5: less urgent, assessment and treatment within 120 minutes
MTS [1]	Five points	Category 1: immediate = red
		Category 2: very urgent = orange
		Category 3: urgent = yellow
		Category 4: standard = green
		Category 5: non-urgent = blue

CTAS, Canadian Triage and Acuity Scale; ESI, Emergency Severity Index; MTS, Manchester Triage Scale; ATS, Australasian Triage Scale.

7 In ED settings (population), what is the role of electronic triage (intervention) compared to memory or paper-based triage (control) on reliability (outcome)?

General search strategy

Our search for triage literature will start with electronic medical databases, namely MEDLINE and EMBASE. We do not expect many randomized controlled trials (RCTs) or systematic reviews related to triage, so the Cochrane Library would not be as valuable a resource for triage literature as it would be for therapy questions. We would anticipate, however, that "gray literature" on triage, such as administrative reports and other non-indexed publications, would be common and helpful. To increase our chances of capturing these references, a search on the Google website could prove useful. Furthermore, searching the bibliographies of identified articles may yield some more useful references.

Critical review of the literature

Question 1: In ED settings (population), what are the common ED triage systems (intervention)? What are the major differences between the systems?

Search strategy

- MEDLINE and EMBASE: triage AND (emergency medicine OR emergency nursing)
- Google: emergency department triage [bend]

Numerous triage systems have been developed for use in the ED. The Manchester Triage Scale (MTS) is in use in the United Kingdom [1], the Australasian Triage Scale (ATS, formerly known as the National Triage Scale) in Australia [2,3] and the Canadian Triage Scale (CTAS) in Canada [4]. There are numerous triage systems in use in the United States, owing to the absence of a national health system that can mandate a single triage system [5]. The most studied system in the United States is the Emergency Severity Index (ESI) [6]. While the above mentioned systems differ in many ways, they all use a five-level triage system in which level 1 is the most emergent and level 5 the least emergent. The triage systems are summarized in Table 7.1.

The MTS and CTAS are complaint-based triage systems in which the clinical user selects from a number of complaint types and applies various modifiers to determine the appropriate triage level. The National Triage Scale was introduced in 1994 and modified to become the ATS in 2000 and associates a time to medical intervention as a goal for each level. In some jurisdictions, ED performance in meeting these goals is published on-line [7].

The CTAS was developed in the late 1990s and is loosely based on the National Triage Scale. The CTAS also designates a recommended time to physician assessment for each triage level and proposes a fractile response rate for each acuity level that can be used to evaluate an ED's ability to meet those requirements. The MTS was developed in the 1990s and uses flow chart diagrams that present key discriminators for each chief complaint that assist the user to assign triage level.

By contrast, ESI users first identify those patients requiring resuscitation (level 1) then those who are critically ill or high-risk situations (level 2). Levels 3, 4 and 5 are then assigned not based on acuity but rather the number of resources the nurse expects the patient to require. The ESI does not mandate a time to physician assessment or suggest a fractile response time.

The CTAS has published separate pediatric triage criteria [8] and the ESI has integrated pediatric vital signs into its algorithm. Neither the ATS nor the MTS have specific pediatric components.

In summary, there are a variety of well established triage scoring systems available and most use a 5-level scoring system that assigned the sickest patients a score of 1. Other parochial triage systems have operated in the past (e.g., urgent, emergent, deferrable, etc.); however, they have not been reported widely in the medical literature and are generally not commonly used.

Question 2: In ED settings (population), how are emergency triage systems evaluated (outcome)? What are the measurements of reliability and validity?

Search strategy

- MEDLINE and EMBASE: triage AND emergency medicine AND reproducibility of results
- Google: emergency triage reliability AND emergency triage validity

The psychometric properties of a triage system of interest to emergency medicine are reliability and validity. Reliability (also referred to as reproducibility or consistency), is commonly reported as the statistical measurement of agreement between two or more users of a triage system [5]. For example, *intra-rater reliability* refers to the comparison of scores recorded for the same patient by the same nurse using the same triage scoring system at different times. *Inter-rater reliability* refers to the comparison of triage scores recorded for the same patient by different nurses using the same triage scoring system or the same nurse using different triage scoring systems. Because patients' conditions can change rapidly in the acute setting, inter-rater reliability is the most commonly reported reliability measure.

The ideal triage system would allow different users to arrive at the same triage level for each patient, regardless of non-patient factors, such as the triage nurse, the acuity of patients in the ED or the time of day, to name a just a few variables. There are a range of agreement metrics used to describe agreement including within one level agreement, simple agreement (SA), kappa (κ) and weighted kappa (κ_w). Simple agreement can be misleading when the cell sizes are imbalanced, and more sophisticated statistics are

often required. Inter-rater reliability is most commonly reported using the κ statistic [9–15]. The κ statistic measures agreement beyond what would be observed by chance, and ranges from less than 0 (worse than by chance alone) to 1 (perfect agreement). Common qualitative descriptions for κ scores are "excellent" ($\kappa \geq 0.8$), "good" ($0.6 \leq \kappa < 0.8$), "moderate" ($0.4 \leq \kappa < 0.6$), "fair" ($0.2 \leq \kappa < 0.4$) and "poor" ($\kappa < 0.2$) [16].

There are variations to the κ statistic. Unweighted κ treats any disagreement, regardless of the magnitude, equally. For example, if one observer assigns a triage score of 3 to a patient and another observer assigns a triage score of 5, unweighted κ calculates this situation the same way as if the two scores were 3 and 4, respectively. Weighted κ gives partial credit for closer agreement (scores of 3 and 4 would create a greater κ_w score than 3 and 5). Some authors feel that κ_w overestimates the agreement [17] while others feel that the magnitude of disagreement needs to be considered in κ calculations [18].

There are further variations to the κ_w statistic. A quadratically weighted κ penalizes the "near misses" less harshly than linearly weighted κ. When specified, most triage reliability studies report quadratic κ_w [13–15,19,20], but many studies do not specify the weighting method [10,11,21–25].

From the literature review, there are clearly a large number of studies that report on triage reliability (Table 7.2). Few triage reliability studies are conducted in an ED using real patients [14,15,21], instead simulated patient scenarios are used. Neither a patient's general appearance nor the often chaotic activity of a busy ED environment is recreated in scenario studies. A study in a live setting may intuitively be a more valid study; however, logistics and concerns for patient safety (a second triage assessment may delay patient care) make such studies difficult to conduct. The value of live patient studies compared to studies of case scenarios has not been determined.

Validity refers to the ability of a triage system to correctly stratify each patient's need for medical care. There is no standard to measure the validity of a triage system. Surrogate measures of need for medical care include hospital admission, intensive care admission, use of investigations, human and physical resource utilization and length of stay in the ED [11,21,22,26–33]. One study used 60-day all-cause mortality as a measure of validity [34]. However, an individual patient's need for medical attention does not necessarily correlate with any of these outcomes. For example, a patient with severe anaphylaxis may meet "emergent" or "resuscitation" criteria, but may not need hospital admission, investigations or have a prolonged ED stay. On the other hand, an elderly patient may present after a fall with an inability to ambulate. This patient may require a prolonged course in the ED, detailed imaging and eventual admission to hospital despite a lower triage score. There are numerous clinical scenarios in which the need for urgent medical assessment may not correlate with any reported outcomes in triage validity studies.

Instead of using measurable outcomes to estimate validity, other studies use a blinded expert panel to retrospectively assign a "gold standard" triage score and compare the "live" triage score

Table 7.2 A review of research of triage reliability.

System	Study	Live environment study	Outcomes
MTS	Goodacre et al. [9]	No	$\kappa = 0.31$ to 0.63
NTS	Jelinek & Little [42]	No	86% within one level of agreement
NTS	Considine et al. [23]	No	$\kappa = 0.42$ to 0.56
NTS	Dilley & Standen [43]	No	$\kappa = 0.25$
CTAS	Beveridge et al. [13]	No	$\kappa_q = 0.80$
CTAS (in Sweden)	Göransson et al. [44]	No	$\kappa_u = 0.46$, $\kappa_w = 0.71$
CTAS	Grafstein et al. [14]	Yes; computer-assisted triage	$\kappa_u = 0.66$, $\kappa_q = 0.75$
CTAS	Manos et al. [19]	No	$\kappa_q = 0.77$
CTAS	Worster et al. [20]	No	$\kappa_q = 0.91$
CTAS	Dong et al. [15]	Yes; computer-assisted triage	$\kappa_l = 0.52$, $\kappa_q = 0.66$
ESI	Wuerz et al. [11]	No	$\kappa_w = 0.80$
ESI	Eitel et al. [21]	Yes	$\kappa_w = 0.69$ to 0.87
ESI	Tanabe et al. [22]	No	$\kappa_w = 0.89$
ESI	Worster et al. [20]	No	$\kappa_q = 0.89$
ESI (on pediatric patients)	Baumann & Strout [25]	Yes; also included a scenario phase	$\kappa_w = 0.84$ to 1.00 for scenarios; $\kappa_w = 0.82$ for live setting

CTAS, Canadian Triage and Acuity Scale; ESI, Emergency Severity Index; MTS, Manchester Triage Scale; NTS, National Triage Scale (the former name of the Australasian Triage Scale).

κ, unspecified kappa statistic; κ_l, linear weighted kappa; κ_q, quadratic weighted kappa; κ_u, unweighted kappa; κ_w, unspecified weighted kappa.

[10,24,35]. In these studies, validity was measured by using a reliability score, comparing the "live" triage score to the "gold standard".

In summary, the psychometric properties of a triage tool are important and users should demand evidence of both reliability and validity.

Question 3: In ED settings (population), can triage (intervention) produce reliable scores (outcome) when different nurses are compared?

Search strategy

- MEDLINE and EMBASE: triage AND emergency medicine AND reproducibility of results
- Google: emergency triage reliability

Table 7.2 summarizes the reliability research of the common triage systems. Most studies report the κ statistic, and more recent studies specify the type of κ statistic. Most triage systems have been evaluated to have at least moderate reliability, and most of these studies report good reliability. As stated above, the designs of the studies vary; in general, paper-based scenarios report higher agreement than clinical scenarios. There does not seem to be any important difference among the various scoring systems; however, direct comparisons are rare. One study directly compared ESI and CTAS, showing similar agreement statistics [36].

In summary, the currently available tools appear to provide moderate to good reliability. The lack of head-to-head comparisons precludes a decision on the most reliable triage system.

Question 4: In ED settings (population), can triage (intervention) produce valid results (outcome)?

Search strategy

- MEDLINE and EMBASE: triage AND emergency medicine AND validity
- Google: emergency triage validity

Validity is a complex term that implies a tool measures what it purports to represent. For example, a peak flow meter used in assessment of airway diseases such as asthma is valid because it is low in severe dyspnea (as reported by the patient) and generally high when the patient has responded to therapy or is at their baseline state. There are a number of ways that validity may be measured including face (appearance), content (especially in quality of life measures), discriminant, divergent, predictive, and so forth. Most validity assessments use a variety of comparisons with known and accepted measures to define validity.

Table 7.3 summarizes research published on the validity of the most common triage systems. A number of surrogate measures of triage validity have been reported. The most common was admission to hospital [22,25–27,30–33], followed by resource utilization [25,27,29,32,33], length of stay in the ED [25,27,29,32,33] and agreement with a retrospectively applied "gold standard" triage score [10,24,25,35]. Eitel et al. [21] and Wuerz [34] evaluated the ESI by correlating triage scores with all-cause mortality at 60 days and 6 months, respectively. Due to the rarity of mortality in the ED and the difficulty correlating ED presentations to remote death, this approach is commonly not performed. Other reported measures of triage score validity were admission to the intensive

Table 7.3 A review of research of triage validity.

System	Study	Outcomes
MTS	Cooke & Jinks [28]	67% patients admitted to critical care area in hospital received initial triage scores of 1 and 2 (medical attention within 10 minutes); 18 cases of under-triage were attributed to incorrect coding by the triage nurse
CTAS	Spence et al. [26]*	CTAS scores correlated with admission to hospital
CTAS	Stenstrom et al. [27]*	CTAS scores correlated with ED length of stay, admission to hospital, use of imaging (CT, ultrasound, X-ray) and use of a complete blood count
CTAS	Dong et al. [35]	Compared to a triage level assigned retrospectively by a blinded expert panel, scores given by nurses using CTAS had an unweighted $\kappa = 0.26$ and quadratically weighted $\kappa = 0.53$. When using computer-assisted CTAS, agreement improved to 0.43 and 0.65, respectively
CTAS	Dong et al. [32,33]	CTAS scores from nurses using computer-assisted triage correlated with resource utilization (specialist consultation, CT scan, ED length of stay), patient acuity (hospitalization, death) and hospital costs
ESI	Wuerz et al. [11]	Hospitalization was strongly associated with triage level. ESI demonstrated good predictive validity for resource use (cardiac monitoring, specialty consultation, diagnostic testing, therapeutic procedures). ED length of stay and charges (professional and facility fees) were moderately associated with ESI level
ESI	Wuerz et al. [30]*	ESI level correlated with hospital admission, ED length of stay and charges to the patient
ESI	Wuerz et al. [31]	ESI level was strongly associated with hospitalization and ED length of stay
ESI	Wuerz [34]	Severity based on ESI score was associated with 6-month all-cause mortality
ESI	Eitel et al. [21]	ESI demonstrated good predictive value for hospitalization and 60-day all-cause mortality
ESI	Tanabe et al. [22]	ESI level was associated with hospitalization, admission to intensive care and admission to telemetry
ESI	Tanabe et al. [29]	Nurses using ESI were able to predict resource consumption. ED or hospital length of stay did not correlate with ESI level
ESI	Travers et al. [10]	Compared to a triage score retrospectively assigned by two experts, nurses using ESI had a 12% under-triage rate; weighted $\kappa = 0.68$; Spearman correlation between ESI and resource intensity $= 0.57$
ESI	Travers et al. [24]*	Compared to a triage score retrospectively assigned by an expert panel, the under-triage rate for nurses using ESI was 60% for ESI level 2. Spearman correlation between ESI and resource intensity $= 0.57$
ESI (on pediatric patients)	Baumann & Strout [25]	ESI level correlated with hospitalization, ED length of stay and resource utilization

*Published abstract.

CT, computerized tomography; CTAS, Canadian Triage and Acuity Scale; ESI, Emergency Severity Index; ED, emergency department; MTS, Manchester Triage Scale.

care unit [22], need for specialist consultation [32,33], hospital costs [32,33] and length of hospital stay for admitted patients [29]. Overall, the five- and four-level triage scoring systems demonstrate validity in the reported measures. There are some concerns with these data, since validation has only been completed on large numbers of heterogeneous patients. There are limited complaint-specific triage studies. In addition, the evidence base may be influenced by publication bias.

In summary, the currently available tools appear to be valid based on the measures reported. The lack of head-to-head comparisons precludes a decision on the most valid triage system.

Question 5: In ED settings (population), what is the role of triage (intervention) in relieving ED overcrowding (outcome)?

Search strategy

- MEDLINE and EMBASE: triage AND emergency medicine AND crowding
- Google: emergency overcrowding AND systematic reviews

A recent report on ED overcrowding for the Canadian Agency for Drugs and Technologies in Health included a review of published literature on emergency overcrowding and a survey of ED physicians, nurses and administrators on the topic [37]. The survey identified that the time interval between the triage assessment and physician contact as a measure to document ED overcrowding. The report examined the role of a number of different interventions, including triage, on reducing ED overcrowding. While many of the interventions studied had a "positive" impact on reducing length of stay and left-without-being-seen patients in overcrowded EDs, triage was found to produce variable effects [37]. For example, in six studies triage failed to provide clear evidence of improvement in ED overcrowding. The report concluded that the influence of triage on overcrowding remains inconclusive and that the overall quality of research was poor.

In summary, since triage was instituted as a result of overcrowding and not as a method *to reduce* overcrowding, these findings are not surprising. Until further evidence is available to the contrary, triage should not be looked upon as a means of reducing ED overcrowding. These results are perhaps not surprising, since triage was instituted as a result of overcrowding and not as a method *to reduce* overcrowding. Until further evidence is available to the contrary, triage should not be looked upon as a means of reducing ED overcrowding.

Question 6: In ED settings (population), what impact does ED overcrowding (intervention) have on triage (outcome)?

Search strategy

- MEDLINE and EMBASE: triage AND emergency medicine AND crowding
- Google: emergency overcrowding AND triage

The question addresses whether overcrowding, which tends to intensify the already chaotic environment of the ED, can affect the triage process; namely, if triage staff are influenced by the level of activity in the ED. Two studies attempted to answer this question. The first study found a downward shift (less acuity) in the triage distribution scores during periods of high ED volume [38]. A second study found no significant differences in agreement between two nurses using a computerized CTAS tool through periods of varying levels of ED overcrowding [15].

In summary, there are two studies from Canada that indicate the role of ED overcrowding on triage reliability and validity remains unclear. These studies are both from Canada and provide divergent results, which suggests that the evidence for the role of ED overcrowding on triage reliability and validity remains unclear.

Question 7: In ED settings (population), what is the role of electronic triage (intervention) compared to memory or paper-based triage (control) on reliability (outcome)?

Search strategy

- MEDLINE and EMBASE: triage AND emergency medicine AND information technology
- Google: computerized emergency triage AND electronic emergency triage

There are a number of published electronic decision support tools for emergency triage. In Canada, an estimated 39% of EDs use a computerized ED information system and an estimated 19% of EDs use some form of electronic triage [37]. Electronic triage may be as simple as an electronic system for recording the triage decision and as complicated as an electronic decision aide with decision support capabilities and educational interactions.

The Soterion Rapid Triage System is a proprietary computerized five-level triage system and has been recently studied in both pediatric and adult patients [39,40]. Investigators found high reliability

($\kappa_w = 0.87$ to 0.90) and significant ability to predict hospitalization, resource utilization and costs.

Two electronic triage systems based on CTAS have been reported. Grafstein examined inter-rater reliability in a live setting (quadratically weighted $\kappa = 0.75$) of a PC-linked triage system based on CTAS [14]. Predictive validity was not reported. Another CTAS-based software, eTRIAGE©, was found to have good reliability (quadratically weighted $\kappa = 0.66$) [15] and good predictive validity for hospitalization, resource utilization and cost [32,33].

In summary, electronic triage systems are growing in availability and popularity. Despite the promising results associated with electronic triage, only two Canadian and one American single-centered studies have been produced and employed at the site of development, which suggests that the evidence for the role of electronic triage in improving the psychometric properties of triage remains unclear.

Conclusions

Using the eTRIAGE® tool, the 20-year-old asthmatic in severe respiratory distress was classified as CTAS 1 and assigned the only available monitored bed. The 30-year-old overdose was classified as CTAS 2 due to her "high-risk" ingestion, and assigned the remaining bed (although monitoring would be appropriate in the setting of a mixed drug overdose). Finally, the male with what appeared to be alcohol withdrawal, was assigned a CTAS score of 3 and asked to wait until a treatment space became available.

Triage is an important process within the emergency department. A number of triage systems are used worldwide, with many countries adopting a standardized system within their borders. Despite this variability, most triage systems are four- or five-level categorizations designed to stratify patients by acuity level, with physician response time recommendations for each level. Current research suggests that the triage system employed may be less important than the process of triage itself, and each system has its own pros and cons.

The published literature generally reports favorable psychometric properties of these triage systems, although there is no current accepted measure of accuracy or validity of a triage system. Additional reliability and validity research may better define the most important characteristics and components of successful triage scales. Finally, the use of true electronic triage with decision support capabilities remains uncommon, although its psychometric properties are encouraging.

In today's climate of ED overcrowding, the triage process will need to be as reliable and accurate as ever. The few studies examining the relationship between overcrowding and triage do not demonstrate an adverse effect on the triage process, but little is known about how triage can alleviate overcrowding. Computerization and ED information systems will likely become more common in the future, and the current literature on computerized decision support tools is favorable.

Acknowledgments

The authors would like to thank Mr. David Meurer and Dr. Brian Rowe for providing helpful suggestions on the manuscript.

Conflicts of interest

SLD and MJB are authors of studies examining eTRIAGE©. They receive no compensation from its use or deployment nor derive any other financial benefits from this software.

References

1 Mackway-Jones K, Marsden J, Windle J, Manchester Triage Group. *Emergency Triage*, 2nd edn. Blackwell Publications, Oxford, 2006.

2 Australasian College for Emergency Medicine. National Triage Scale. *Emerg Med* 1994;**6**:145–6.

3 Australasian College for Emergency Medicine. *P06 Policy on the Australasian Triage Scale*. West Melbourne, Australia, revised 2006. Available at http://www.acem.org.au (accessed April 9, 2007).

4 Beveridge R, Clarke B, Janes L, et al. Canadian Emergency Department and Triage Scale: implementation guidelines. *Can J Emerg Med* 1999;**1**(3 Suppl):S1–24.

5 Fernandes CM, Tanabe P, Gilboy N, et al. Five-level triage: a report from the ACEP/ENA Five-level Triage Task Force. *J Emerg Nurs* 2005;**31**(1):39–50.

6 Gilboy N, Tanabe P, Travers D, Rosenau A, Eitel DR. *Emergency Severity Index, Version 4: Implementation Handbook*. Agency for Healthcare Research and Quality, Rockville, MD, 2005.

7 Health N. *Hospital Information*. Available at www.healthinfo.nsw.gov.au/hospitalinfo, 2006 (accessed March 26, 2007).

8 Canadian Association of Emergency Physicians. Implementation of Canadian Paediatric Triage and Acuity Scale. *Can J Emerg Med* 2001; **3**(4 Suppl):1–32.

9 Goodacre SW, Gillett M, Harris RD, Houlihan KP. Consistency of retrospective triage decisions as a standardised instrument for audit. *J Accid Emerg Med* 1999;**16**(5):322–4.

10 Travers DA, Waller AE, Bowling JM, Flowers D, Tintinalli J. Five-level triage system more effective than three-level in tertiary emergency department. *J Emerg Nurs* 2002;**28**(5):395–400.

11 Wuerz RC, Milne LW, Eitel DR, Travers D, Gilboy N. Reliability and validity of a new five-level triage instrument. *Acad Emerg Med* 2000;**7**(3):236–42.

12 Fernandes CM, Wuerz R, Clark S, Djurdjev O. How reliable is emergency department triage? *Ann Emerg Med* 1999;**34**(2):141–7.

13 Beveridge R, Ducharme J, Janes L, Beaulieu S, Walter S. Reliability of the Canadian emergency department triage and acuity scale: interrater agreement. *Ann Emerg Med* 1999;**34**(2):155–9.

14 Grafstein E, Innes G, Westman J, Christenson J, Thorne A. Inter-rater reliability of a computerized presenting-complaint-linked triage system in an urban emergency department. *Can J Emerg Med* 2003;**5**(5):323–9.

15 Dong SL, Bullard MJ, Meurer DP, et al. Reliability of computerized emergency triage. *Acad Emerg Med* 2006;**13**(3):269–75.

16 Kramer MS, Feinstein AR. Clinical biostatistics. LIV. The biostatistics of concordance. *Clin Pharmacol Ther* 1981;**29**(1):111–23.

17 Grafstein E. Close only counts in horseshoes and . . . triage? *Can J Emerg Med* 2004;**6**(4):288–9.

18 Fan J, Upadhye S, Woolfrey K. ESI and CTAS. *Can J Emerg Med* 2004;**6**(6):395–6.

19 Manos D, Petrie DA, Beveridge R, Walter S, Ducharme J. Inter-observer agreement using the Canadian Emergency Department Triage and Acuity Scale. *Can J Emerg Med* 2002;**4**(1):16–22.

20 Worster A, Gilboy N, Fernandes CM, et al. Assessment of inter-observer reliability of two five-level triage and acuity scales: a randomized controlled trial. *Can J Emerg Med* 2004;**6**(4):240–45.

21 Eitel DR, Travers DA, Rosenau AM, Gilboy N, Wuerz RC. The emergency severity index triage algorithm version 2 is reliable and valid. *Acad Emerg Med* 2003;**10**(10):1070–80.

22 Tanabe P, Gimbel R, Yarnold PR, Kyriacou DN, Adams JG. Reliability and validity of scores on the Emergency Severity Index version 3. *Acad Emerg Med* 2004;**11**(1):59–65.

23 Considine J, LeVasseur SA, Villanueva E. The Australasian Triage Scale: examining emergency department nurses' performance using computer and paper scenarios. *Ann Emerg Med* 2004;**44**(5):516–23.

24 Travers DA, Waller AE, Bowling JM, Flowers DF. Comparison of 3-level and 5-level triage acuity systems. *Acad Emerg Med* 2000;**7**(5):522–52a.

25 Baumann MR, Strout TD. Evaluation of the Emergency Severity Index (version 3) triage algorithm in pediatric patients. *Acad Emerg Med* 2005;**12**(3):219–24.

26 Spence JM, Beaton DE, Murray MJ, Morrison LJ. Does the Canadian emergency department triage and acuity scale correlate with admission to the hospital from the emergency department? *Can J Emerg Med* 2003;**6**(3):180.

27 Stenstrom R, Grafstein GE, Innes G, Christenson J. The predictive validity of the Canadian Triage and Acuity Scale (CTAS). *Can J Emerg Med* 2003;**5**(3):184.

28 Cooke MW, Jinks S. Does the Manchester triage system detect the critically ill? *J Accid Emerg Med* 1999;**16**(3):179–81.

29 Tanabe P, Gimbel R, Yarnold PR, Adams JG. The Emergency Severity Index (version 3) 5-level triage system scores predict ED resource consumption. *J Emerg Nurs* 2004;**30**(1):22–9.

30 Wuerz R, Milne L, Eitel D, Wiencek J, Simonds W. Outcomes are predicted by a new five-level triage algorithm. *Acad Emerg Med* 1999;**6**(5):398.

31 Wuerz RC, Travers D, Gilboy N, Eitel DR, Rosenau A, Yazhari R. Implementation and refinement of the emergency severity index. *Acad Emerg Med* 2001;**8**(2):170–76.

32 Dong SL, Bullard MJ, Meurer D, et al. Predictive validity of a computerized triage tool. *Can J Emerg Med* 2006;**8**(3 Suppl):S17–18.

33 Dong SL, Bullard MJ, Meurer DP, et al. Predictive validity of a computerized emergency triage tool. *Acad Emerg Med* 2007;**14**(1):16–21.

34 Wuerz R. Emergency severity index triage category is associated with six-month survival. ESI Triage Study Group. *Acad Emerg Med* 2001;**8**(1):61–4.

35 Dong SL, Bullard MJ, Meurer DP, et al. Emergency triage: comparing a novel computer triage program with standard triage. *Acad Emerg Med* 2005;**12**(6):502–7.

36 Worster A, Gilboy N, Fernandes CM, et al. Inter-rater reliabilities of the Emergency Severity Index (ESI) vs. the Canadian Triage Acuity Scale (CTAS): a randomized controlled trial. *Can J Emerg Med* 2003;**5**(3):183.

37 Rowe BH, Bond K, Ospina MB, et al. *Emergency Department Overcrowding in Canada: What are the issues and what can be done*. Technology

Overview No. 21. Canadian Agency for Drugs and Technology in Health, Ottawa, 2006.

38 Spence JM, Murray MJ, Morrison LJ. Does emergency department activity level affect triage categorization and admission to hospital? *Acad Emerg Med* 2005;**11**(5):457.

39 Maningas PA, Hime DA, Parker DE. The use of the Soterion Rapid Triage System in children presenting to the emergency department. *J Emerg Med* 2006;**31**(4):353–9.

40 Maningas PA, Hime DA, Parker DE, McMurry TA. The Soterion Rapid Triage System: evaluation of inter-rater reliability and validity. *J Emerg Med* 2006;**30**(4):461–9.

41 Australasian College for Emergency Medicine. *Guidelines on the Implementation of the Australasian Triage Scale in Emergency Departments*. Australasian College for Emergency Medicine, West Melbourne, 2005.

42 Jelinek GA, Little M. Inter-rater reliability of the National Triage Scale over 11,500 simulated occasions of triage. *Emerg Med* 1996;**8**:226–30.

43 Dilley S, Standen P. Victorian nurses demonstrate concordance in the application of the National Triage Scale. *Emerg Med* 1998;**10**:12–18.

44 Goransson K, Ehrenberg A, Marklund B, Ehnfors M. Accuracy and concordance of nurses in emergency department triage. *Scand J Caring Sci* 2005;**19**(4):432–8.

8 Emergency Department Overcrowding

Michael Schull[1] & Matthew Cooke[2]

[1] Institute for Clinical Evaluative Sciences, Toronto *and* Division of Emergency Medicine, Department of Medicine, University of Toronto, Toronto, Canada
[2] Warwick Medical School, University of Warwick, Coventry *and* Heart of England NHS Foundation Trust, Birmingham, UK

Case scenario

As the director of a busy community emergency department (ED), you are aware that your patient census has risen in recent years, and, adding to the challenge, patients seem to be getting older. In departmental meetings, distressed clinical staff complain about severe overcrowding in your department. Most written patient complaints focus on prolonged waiting, and seriously ill patients frequently spend many hours in the waiting room. Several near-disaster cases have been averted in the last year or so; however, just last week you received a call at home that a 53-year-old woman had collapsed in the waiting room 2 hours after being triaged with chest pain. Her first electrocardiogram (ECG) was performed following her collapse, and it showed an anterior ST elevation acute myocardial infarction (MI). In an urgent meeting you set up with the hospital Chief Executive Officer (CEO) and risk management staff, you argue that overcrowding in your ED is a serious problem that requires immediate attention from the hospital. The hospital CEO is sympathetic, but she asks for data to demonstrate that the problem is really worsening, and for evidence that quality of care is suffering. You reply that overcrowding is a complex construct to measure, but that every emergency physician and nurse knows it when they see it. As for evidence, you point to the 53-year-old woman who collapsed in the waiting room with an acute MI. However, your CEO reminds you of a similar case a number of years ago of a chest pain patient suffering a cardiac arrest from an undiagnosed acute MI only minutes after being discharged from the ED, and wonders if the recent event was truly a consequence of overcrowding.

Background

Emergency department overcrowding is generally defined as a mismatch between patient care needs and the available resources of a department to safely meet those needs in timely fashion. ED overcrowding is a new or worsening problem in many modern health care systems. At the same time, the evidence base has grown from one largely based on surveys and professional association consensus statements to one which includes high-quality observational studies and even some randomized controlled trials. However, the absence of a clear and measurable definition of the problem from the outset has meant some difficulty in accurately describing the problem (or comparing it between settings). In addition, the complexity of some of the health system changes instituted to address ED overcrowding have been difficult to evaluate using rigorous experimental designs. None the less, the expanding evidence base and increasing attention paid to the problem merit a careful review focusing on the questions below.

Clinical questions

In order to address the issues of most relevance to your patients and to help in searching the literature for the evidence regarding these issues, you structure your clinical questions as recommended in Chapter 1.

1 In hospital EDs (setting), how is overcrowding (outcome) defined?
2 In hospital EDs (setting), does overcrowding (comparison) impact on patient care (increased morbidity and/or mortality) (outcomes) compared to periods when no crowding exists (control)?
3 In hospital EDs experiencing overcrowding (setting), do interventions to reduce overcrowding (intervention) improve patient flow and care (outcomes) compared to status quo (control)?
4 In hospital EDs experiencing overcrowding (setting), do fast-track systems (intervention) reduce overcrowding and improve patient care (outcomes) compared to status quo (control)?

Evidence-based Emergency Medicine. Edited by Brian H. Rowe
© 2009 Blackwell Publishing, ISBN: 978-1-4051-6143-5.

5 In hospital EDs experiencing overcrowding (setting), do system-wide interventions (intervention) reduce overcrowding and improve patient care (outcomes) compared to status quo (control)?

6 In hospital EDs experiencing overcrowding (setting), does the 4-hour rule (intervention) reduce overcrowding and improve patient care (outcomes) compared to status quo (control)?

7 In hospital EDs experiencing overcrowding (setting), does a full-capacity protocol (intervention) reduce overcrowding and improve patient care (outcomes) compared to status quo (control)?

General search strategy

Emergency department overcrowding can be described using a variety of terms (such as crowding, over capacity, access block, and so on). Consequently, searching can be difficult and strategies need to be employed to be sure to include all ED overcrowding-related articles. You begin to address these questions by searching for evidence in the common electronic databases such as the Cochrane Library and MEDLINE (through OVID) looking specifically for systematic reviews and meta-analyses. The Cochrane Database of Systematic Reviews includes high-quality systematic review evidence on many emergency topics and issues related to professional practice; however, there are no specific systematic reviews on ED overcrowding. You also search MEDLINE to identify randomized controlled trials (RCTs) that have been published on the specific interventions (fast track, 4-hour rule, and so on). In addition, access to relevant health technology assessments and systematic reviews are available through international agency websites such as the Canadian Agency for Drugs and Technologies in Health (CADTH), Agency for Healthcare Research and Quality (AHRQ) and National Institute for Health and Clinical Evidence (NICE). Much of the ED overcrowding literature exists in the gray literature, much of which is beyond the scope of this chapter; however, gray literature searches in health technology assessments and systematic reviews were considered to enhance the quality of the evidence reviewed. Details of an extensive literature search methodology are included in the systematic review by Cooke et al. [1].

Critical review of the literature

Question 1: In hospital EDs (setting), how is overcrowding (outcome) defined?

Search strategy

- MEDLINE: (ED OR emergency department) AND (overcrowding OR crowding) AND definition

The understanding of ED overcrowding has been hampered by the absence of a single, widely accepted definition of the problem. Medical organizations have tended to define overcrowding in de-scriptive terms, such as "a situation in which the demand for emergency services exceeds the ability to provide quality care within a reasonable time" [2], proposed by the Canadian Association of Emergency Physicians, or "a situation in which the identified need for emergency services outstrips available resources in the ED" [3], proposed by the American College of Emergency Physicians.

These definitions have intuitive appeal; however, they are difficult to express in terms that can be measured and studied, and may have very different interpretations in different settings. To address this problem, a variety of metrics and scales have been proposed, usually based on mathematical formulae consisting of selected ED factors, often measured in real time. Examples include the Emergency Department Work Index (EDWIN) [4], the National Emergency Department Overcrowding Scale (NEDOCS) [5], the Demand Value of the Real-time Emergency Analysis of Demand Indicators (READI) [6] and the Work Score [7]. The feasibility of calculating such scales varies in different settings, as does their performance, and one study suggested that none of these scales was superior to an occupancy measure consisting simply of the number of patients in treatment spaces in the ED over the number of licensed treatment spaces [8].

In a survey [9] of US emergency department directors, multiple possible implicit definitions were suggested: (i) patients waiting more than 60 minutes to see a physician; (ii) all ED beds filled more than 6 hours a day; (iii) patients placed in corridors more than 6 hours a day; (iv) emergency physicians feel rushed more than 6 hours a day; and (v) waiting room filled more than 6 hours a day. These definitions have not been operationalized, and their relationship to other measures of overcrowding is not known.

Studies of overcrowding have mostly used proxy or related measures, such as "access block" or the "boarding" of patients (both of which refer to delays getting admitted patients out of the ED and onto wards), ambulance diversion (the practice by some hospitals of temporarily refusing to accept ambulance patients due to overcrowding), "left-without-being-seen" (LWBS) rates (patients leaving prior to being assessed by a physician), and ED length of stay (LOS) or waiting time (usually expressed as the total time a patient spends in the ED, from the point of first contact to physical departure from the ED). Some of these proxy measures of overcrowding could equally be considered contributors to (e.g., boarded patients) or outcomes of (e.g., LWBS rates) overcrowding.

Emergency department overcrowding is a multi-factorial problem that strikes hospital systems, not patients, and hospital systems vary substantially across jurisdictions. So it is not surprising that no single satisfactory definition has emerged within the literature. Yet one thing is the same everywhere: patients have a measurable LOS, or waiting time, from ED arrival to departure, and this tends to be longer in overcrowded EDs reflecting poor patient flow [10]. Thus ED LOS represents a simple, readily measured, patient-focused and comparable metric that is available to document and study the problem of ED overcrowding. In England, the National Health Service (NHS) Plan [11] has defined an excessive wait as more than 4 hours total time in the ED (measured from the time

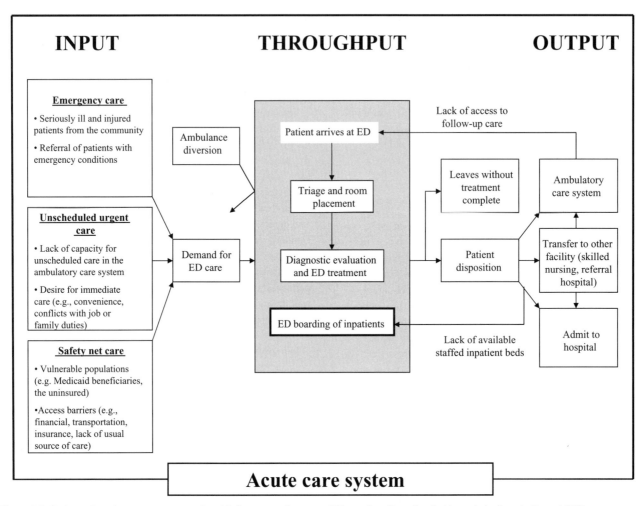

Figure 8.1 The input–throughput–output conceptual model of emergency department (ED) crowding. (Reproduced with permission from Asplin et al. [12].)

a patient arrives until they leave the ED). The NHS concentrates on time spent in the ED, rather than "overcrowding" per se.

Despite definitional difficulties, our understanding of over-crowding has been aided by conceptual models that help to explain factors which are at the root of the problem. The most widely cited is the input–throughput–output model shown in Fig. 8.1. Input factors include any condition, event or system characteristic that contributes to the demand for ED services. Throughput refers to timing and delays in ED patient care from triage to disposition decision. Output refers to actual disposition of ED patients (to home, ward or other in-hospital location, or transfer to another institution), and factors which may slow this phase, such as the inability to move admitted patients from the ED to an inpatient bed [12].

This model reflects what have been called "micro" level factors, i.e., those within a given ED or hospital, and is useful since it demonstrates that overcrowding should be seen as a hospital, not an ED, problem. It provides a framework for understanding and studying causes of overcrowding, though it cannot estimate their relative importance. Yet the model does not address broader "macro" level factors in a region's health system, policy and

demographic context that can contribute to crowding, such as the availability of primary health care, changes in public health policy including financing, demographic trends, or evolving clinical care trends and patient expectations [13].

In summary, definitions for ED overcrowding vary within and between health systems, and even within institutions in the same health system, adding to the complexity of describing and studying the problem.

Question 2: In hospital EDs (setting), does overcrowding (comparison) impact on patient care (increased morbidity and/or mortality) (outcomes) compared to periods when no crowding exists (control)?

Search strategy

- MEDLINE: (ED OR emergency department) AND (overcrowding OR crowding) AND outcome (mortality OR morbidity)

Despite substantial evidence that the problem of ED overcrowding is widespread, there is relatively little high-quality evidence regarding the adverse effects associated with overcrowding [14]. In a national survey of Canadian ED directors, a large majority of respondents felt overcrowding was associated with increased stress and reduced satisfaction for medical staff, as well as worsened ED waiting times for patients. However, only about half believed it was associated with worsened patient outcomes, delays in care or the risk of medical errors [15].

A small number of studies have examined how mortality is associated with ED overcrowding. One single-center study examined the ecological association between weekly ED volume and ED mortality in a Spanish hospital, and found that there was an association ($P < 0.01$) between increased ED visits and higher mortality [16]. An Australian study examined the association between hospital overcrowding (based on inpatient occupancy level) and mortality among patients admitted from the ED; compared with an occupancy rate of < 90%, they found absolute increases in mortality rates at 7 days post admission of 0.4% with occupancy rates of 90–99%, and 1.0% with occupancy rates > 99%, representing relative increases of 18% (95% CI: 0.5% to 38%) and 46% (95% CI: 14% to 85%), respectively [17]. A second Australian study found increased odds of in-hospital death for patients presenting during overcrowded ED shifts (based on patient-hours in each shift) versus non-overcrowded shifts (OR = 1.34; 95% CI: 1.04 to 1.72) [18]. Another study of mortality among trauma patients found no increase in mortality during periods of ambulance diversion [19]. Such observational studies offer evidence of a possible relationship; however, they must be interpreted with caution since confounding due to variations in severity of illness among patients presenting for care in EDs may be difficult to exclude.

Several studies have examined the association between overcrowding and ED quality of care, with mixed results. One study of thrombolysis for acute ST elevation myocardial infarction in 25 Canadian hospitals found that median door-to-needle time increased from 40 to 47 minutes ($P < 0.001$) during periods of high ED overcrowding versus none (based on ambulance diversion); the adjusted odds of major delay in thrombolysis (> 60 minute door-to-needle time) were also increased (OR = 1.40; 95% CI: 1.1 to 1.8) [20]. Another study of non-ST elevation myocardial infarction found that prolonged ED LOS was associated with a reduced likelihood of receiving five evidence-based therapies, including acetyl-salicylic acid (OR = 0.76; 95% CI: 0.67 to 0.87) [21]. In a case–control study of the effect of ED LOS among intubated trauma patients on the development of pneumonia, each hour in the ED was associated with a small increase in the risk of developing pneumonia while in hospital (OR = 1.20; 95% CI: 1.04 to 1.39) [22]. Several studies have examined the effect of overcrowding on time to antibiotic administration for pneumonia patients. One found that for each additional patient present in the ED at the time of a community-acquired pneumonia patient's arrival, the odds of receiving antibiotics within 4 hours decreased by 4% (adjusted OR = 0.96; 95% CI: 0.93 to 0.99) [23]. In another

study, increasing ED overcrowding was associated antibiotic delays for pneumonia patients; under non-crowded conditions, the predicted probability of delayed antibiotic administration was 31% (95% CI: 21% to 42%) versus 72% (95% CI: 61% to 81%) under crowded conditions [24].

A study of analgesia given to older patients with hip fracture found that ED overcrowding (defined as ED census > 120% capacity) at the time of patient arrival was associated with a lower odds of pain assessment documentation (OR = 0.46; 95% CI: 0.21 to 0.98) and an increase in time to pain assessment (+6.1 minutes, $P = 0.01$); however, there was no difference in time to delivery of analgesic or opioid prescribing [25]. A second study looked at analgesia administration in a heterogeneous population of more than 13,000 ED patients complaining of severe pain for any reason at a single center [26]. Only 49% of these patients received any analgesia regardless of crowding levels, but the odds of non-receipt of analgesics (OR = 1.03; 95% CI: 1.02 to 1.03) or delay in receipt (OR = 1.05; 95% CI: 1.04 to 1.06) increased significantly during periods of ED crowding.

Several studies have examined mortality associated with ambulance diversion and found either no association or a reduced mortality among diverted ambulance patients, likely as a result of a reluctance to divert critically ill patients [27]. Other studies have assessed prehospital ambulance transport delays associated with ambulance diversion. In a Canadian study comparing ambulance transport of chest pain patients, a significant increase in the transport time to hospital was seen in a period of high ambulance diversion versus a period of low diversion (13.4 vs 17.2 minutes, $P < 0.001$; a 28% relative increase) [28]. Another study by the same group again found transport delays for chest pain patients associated with ambulance diversion, but only when all EDs within a given geographic area were simultaneously diverting ambulances [29].

Finally, several studies have examined the association between overcrowding and patients who leave the ED without being seen. In one single-center study in the USA, the odds of a patient leaving the ED without being seen almost doubled (OR = 1.96; 95% CI: 1.22 to 3.17) when ED occupancy was > 140% [30]. In another study from Canada, the most common reason behind a decision to leave without being seen was being "fed up with waiting"; the authors also found that 60% of LWBS patients sought medical attention within 1 week of their aborted ED visit [31].

In summary, there is increasing evidence that ED overcrowding negatively affects process of care and quality of care measures, some of which are known to be important predictors of patient outcome. There is some evidence that hospital and ED overcrowding may also increase mortality.

Question 3: In hospital EDs experiencing overcrowding (setting), do interventions to reduce overcrowding (intervention) improve patient flow and care (outcomes) compared to status quo (control)?

Although a variety of interventions have both been described and attempted in EDs to address the issue of ED overcrowding, many have not been scientifically studied. Studies that do examine interventions to address ED overcrowding have mostly been single-site intervention studies and therefore the interaction of a complex array of changes cannot be assessed. It is likely that individual changes are introduced in study hospitals because of a perceived need and they may therefore not be generalizable. Three major reviews [1,32,33] of interventions were located; their results are included in the text below.

Triage may cause delays in care and does not reduce overall waits [34]. The staff undertaking triage have an influence on waits [35]; for example, triage psychiatric support can reduce waits [36]. Triaging out of the ED (whereby patients are redirected to an alternative source of care) can reduce ED patient numbers [37,38] but more work is required to assess the safety of such systems, due to conflicting evidence [39], and to assess whether they have any impact on overcrowding or waiting times for other ED patients. Differential payment systems may reduce ED visits [40], but may equally reduce attendances by those requiring emergency care [41].

Waiting for results of tests is one of the commonest causes of patient delays. Point-of-care testing and satellite laboratories produce quicker results [42] and may reduce LOS [43] although some studies failed to demonstrate this [44]. Nurse ordering of X-rays may speed up processes where fast track does not operate [45], although other studies have found conflicting results [46]. ED staff undertaking ultrasounds may reduce delays for those having this procedure [47]. Results delivery needs further investigation but there are suggestions that electronic reporting may delay results delivery.

There are very few studies looking at the impact of differing staffing levels, skill mix or systems of work. Availability of senior staff may reduce admissions and delays as may increased staffing levels [48]. Having an emergency physician at night also reduces length of stay in the ED [49]. Having a system that allocates patients to ED staff may be better at reducing waits than allowing ED staff to determine allocation [50]. Allowing ED staff to admit to wards will reduce delays. Nurse practitioners are safe and effective but their effect on waits is unknown. The role of other health care professionals in ED care needs evaluation.

A study of extensive restructuring and staff reorganization resulted in an increase in the number of discharges and decreased overcrowding in the ED [51]. Teams of staff available for unpredicted surges in activity may reduce delays [52], but the simple physical expansion of the department does not improve overcrowding [53].

In summary, within the ED changes in staffing numbers and processes can reduce waits. The impact of triage systems on waiting times is still contentious. Improving access to diagnostic tests does improve waits.

Question 4: In hospital EDs experiencing overcrowding (setting), do fast-track systems (intervention) reduce overcrowding and improve patient care (outcomes) compared to status quo (control)?

Fast-track systems can be applied to the ED, to specific acuity levels of patients in the ED, or to a specific injury or illness seen in the ED. A review of fast-track systems for minor injury and illness concluded that ED fast-track systems appeared efficient, cost-effective, safe and satisfactory for patients. Low acuity patients were confirmed as being seen quicker [54].

Some systems simply placed a senior doctor in the triage area. A Canadian RCT demonstrated a reduction in overall LOS in the ED (4 hours 21 minutes vs 4 hours 57 minutes per patient, $P = 0.001$) as well as a decrease in those leaving before completion of treatment [55]. A UK study demonstrated that the average time for all the patients triaged was "about 50 minutes", compared to 1 hour 8 minutes without the consultant at triage [56]. A similar American interrupted time series study showed that on days when faculty triage was undertaken there was a significant decrease in total time in the ED of 82 minutes against the original background of 445 minutes across all patients ($P = 0.005$). It was also noticed that the number of patients leaving without being seen halved to 8% [57]. A Saudi Arabian study reduced the mean waiting time from 58 minutes to 25 minutes ($P < 0.005$) [58].

Other systems used a completely separate stream of care for minor injuries. In one RCT comparing fast-track to regular care, the waiting times to be seen by a doctor showed no difference in triage category 2 and 3 patients, with a difference of several minutes for triage category 4 and 5 patients. The time spent in the ED showed no difference in categories 2 and 3, but showed a 20–25 minute advantage in categories 4 and 5 for those using the rapid assessment clinic [59]. In an interrupted time series study, a similar system resulted in more rapid initial assessment of the patient across all triage categories (59% within target compared to 39% when no team was working, $P < 0.001$) except for category 1 patients [60]. A UK study showed that the risk of waiting more than 1 hour to see the doctor decreased by 30% to 50% with increased presence of consultants in the department [61], and a second study demonstrated an increase in the patients seen within 1 hour from 52% to 75% without an increase in staffing [62]. In another study the median length of stay was 36 minutes for fast-tracked patients compared with 63 minutes for the control group [63]. This has worked equally well in pediatric units [64]. A recent study [65] of a fast-track unit also demonstrated an improvement in length of stay from 127 to 53 minutes ($P < 0.001$). However, Saywell et al. [66] undertook an economic evaluation of fast-track systems and found that it did not cover all related costs in their hospital.

Fast-track systems have also been developed for patients with specific injuries or illnesses (e.g., fractured neck of femur). A review [67] of 104 patients with a fractured neck of femur showed that after introducing a fast-track system the transfer time was reduced from 2 hours 45 minutes $\pm$ 57 minutes to 1 hour 32 minutes $\pm$ 41 minutes ($P < 0.001$). Another system resulted in a decrease in the admission time from 4.5 to 2.5 hours; however, patients were excluded if there was no identifiable orthopedic bed [68], and subsequent non-availability of beds caused the LOS of patients to increase by 40%. In a similar system [69], Finlayson found the major delays lay in performing the X-ray and in junior orthopedic staff resisting admission directly to the ward. A group of 50 patients with hip fractures admitted to a hospital via the ED in Manchester were studied prior to the introduction of a fast-track hip fracture protocol. The median ED-to-ward transfer time was reduced following its introduction by 43%, from 7 hours 4 minutes (range 2 hours 46 minutes to 11 hours 50 minutes) to 4 hours (range 1 hour 8 minutes to 11 hours 58 minutes, $P < 0.0001$) [70]. A major limitation of these studies of hip fracture-specific fast-track systems is that none studied their effect on waiting times for other patients in the ED. Another fast-track system for psychiatric patients only, consisting of a small cadre of nurses specifically trained to undertake psychiatric assessments, resulted in the ED waiting times for psychiatric patients dropping by 44% [71].

In conclusion, fast-track systems have been tested in a variety of environments and most have been shown to be effective as a means to reduce waiting times and overcrowding. Research, including some RCTs, supports the fast tracking of minor illnesses and injuries, though many studies had significant weaknesses. For example, few studies have looked at the influence on other patients, although those that did found no detrimental effects and no study showed any adverse patient effects. Moreover, reported outcomes were mainly related to time, and an effect (either positive or negative) was not demonstrated on important outcomes such as quality of care and/or patient outcomes. Finally, fast tracks may potentially be less effective, inefficient and costly in institutions where such patients are uncommon.

Question 5: In hospital EDs experiencing overcrowding (setting), do system-wide interventions (intervention) reduce overcrowding and improve patient care (outcomes) compared to status quo (control)?

Search strategy

- MEDLINE: (ED OR emergency department) AND (overcrowding OR crowding OR waits) AND system solutions. Followed by using the "find similar" facility
- Google Scholar: waits, emergency departments, fast track

Three major reviews of interventions were located; their results are included in the text below [32,33,72].

Input to the ED comes from self-referral, emergency medical services (EMS) and referrals from other health professionals. Since EMS patients are often complex and time consuming, the reduction in EMS traffic could be a partial solution to ED overcrowding. Evidence of impact on overcrowding of ambulance dispatch and prioritization systems, including diverting 999 or 911 calls to advice lines, is generally poor. Some 999 or 911 calls can be diverted to advice lines but the safety of such systems is still questioned. Although it has been shown that 36.6% of calls could be diverted to other sources of care, 9% of callers were subsequently admitted to hospital [73]. Physician staffing in ambulance control (dispatch) may have a beneficial effect [74].

Ambulance crews often bring patients to ED by default. Alternatives may include taking patients to the nearest appropriate source of health care, including primary care centers, walk-in centers and minor injury units. The impact of introducing such services has been small or absent [75–78]. The role of paramedics in either discharging patients from the scene or deciding on appropriate destinations has not been adequately studied to confirm its safety and effectiveness and is likely to be highly dependent on training [79].

While interpretation of some evidence suggests that many patients in the ED can be deferred due to their ambulatory nature [80], other evidence contradicts this [81]. Moreover, while some suggest better primary care access may reduce ED utilization [82,83], other studies suggest the opposite, and access to walk-in clinics does not appear to affect ED visits [77,84]. None the less, efforts on the part of health regions to reduce the influx of these patients have been common. Introduction of primary care out-of-hours centers has been shown to have a deleterious effect in some studies and no effect in others [85]. Telephone advisory services have not been demonstrated to reduce attendances at EDs [86] and may increase the attendance of some groups [87]. Primary care gatekeeping (i.e., requiring a referral from a primary care physician for a patient to see a specialist) can reduce ED attendance but its safety is unknown. Gadomski et al. demonstrated that gatekeeping did not influence future ED usage [88]. Easier access to primary care can decrease ED visits by up to 40% [89] and in children by up to 24% [90]. There is no evidence about the effects on waiting times of general practitioners working in EDs. The benefits of creating primary care alternatives to ED care are unclear in terms of reducing visits by low acuity patients, and at least one study demonstrated that such reductions would have little to no effect on the waiting times of other ED patients [91].

Inappropriate or preventable admissions may account for 4.7–37% of hospital admissions, depending on the criteria used. A recent systematic review has defined effective admission avoidance schemes [92], but reduction of admissions can have a variable effect on overcrowding and has not been studied in most admission avoidance research.

No trials of variations in bed management strategies have been discovered, although there is a wealth of advice on good practice in bed management. Two studies [93,94] showed that performance against the 4-hour rule was linked to bed occupancy, however subsequent work failed to demonstrate that changes in bed occupancy were associated with a change in the 4-hour performance. Several studies [95–97] describe whole hospital changes including new policies, bed management and other broad changes that decreased ED LOS for discharged patients.

There is a lack of evidence regarding innovations to reduce delays in discharge from hospital for patients awaiting placement in long-term care facilities, such as social care or complex continuing care. Informal evidence from the UK suggests that reducing discharge delays has improved inpatient flow through the hospital, but this has never been formally studied.

In conclusion, there are few system-wide interventions that have been shown to reduce overcrowding in a safe and persistent manner. While some system-wide efforts have been reported, many report short-term outcomes that may not be sustainable. Moreover, most studies simply cannot identify which of the many interventions may have had a critical role on the observed outcomes. Further research is urgently required in this field.

Question 6: In hospital EDs experiencing overcrowding (setting), does the 4-hour rule (intervention) reduce overcrowding and improve patient care (outcomes) compared to status quo (control)?

Search strategy

- MEDLINE: (ED OR emergency department) AND (overcrowding OR crowding OR waits) AND four hour. Followed by using the "find similar" facility
- Google Scholar: waits, emergency departments, four hour

The 4-hour rule ("By 2004 no one should be waiting more than 4 hours in accident and emergency from arrival to admission, transfer or discharge") was announced in England in 2000 to be gradually implemented until 2005 when all hospitals had to achieve this rule [98]. Strategies to achieve this goal were multi-factorial, and were unique to institutions; however, the goals were incentive based. Most institutions addressed this problem through ED interventions with some system-wide interventions including, but not limited to, nurse practitioners, fast-track systems, development of specialist assessment units, full-capacity protocols for inpatients, improved discharge processes, and increased chronic and social care capacity.

Over this period, patient waiting times in UK EDs gradually decreased. By 2007, 98% of ED patients had waiting times of less than 4 hours, compared to 77% in 2002 [99]. It is recognized that patient waiting time is a major determinant of satisfaction [100], but direct study of the impact of the 4-hour rule has not been undertaken. The impact on quality of care is not well studied, though a survey suggested that patients' lives were on occasions put at risk in order to achieve the rule [101]. A study by the English National Audit Office [102] concluded that the rule had resulted in improvement in waiting times and environment for patients and staff. It did, however, note that changes were mainly in EDs and that changes across the whole system were required to achieve sustainability. It noted the lack of evidence to support or refute issues of quality of care and outcome. One small study suggested that while the rule resulted in better patient care satisfaction and improved staff morale, there may also have been unintended consequences, such as increased staff workload, concerns over the quality of care, pressure on support systems and training, and increased staff turnover [103].

In conclusion the 4-hour rule introduced in England appears to have improved patient satisfaction and the number of patients in EDs; however, there is no convincing evidence regarding its effect on quality of care or patient outcomes.

Question 7: In hospital EDs experiencing overcrowding (setting), does a full-capacity protocol (intervention) reduce overcrowding and improve patient care (outcomes) compared to status quo (control)?

Search strategy

- MEDLINE: (ED OR emergency department) AND (overcrowding OR crowding OR waits) AND full capacity protocol. Followed by using the "find similar" facility
- Google Scholar: full capacity, protocol

Full-capacity protocols (FCPs) represent efforts to decant the ED by placing patients in the halls or rooms on inpatient floors even when a bed is unavailable. Such innovations have be employed only during certain times (e.g., severe overcrowding) or at all times (e.g., the UK 4-hour rule described above). Overall, despite extensive searching, limited evidence exists upon which to base a decision regarding the implementation of the FCP to address the issue of ED overcrowding.

There is one published study, two websites and one report accessed through personal communication where the FCP has been evaluated (Table 8.1). There were no cost-evaluation studies of the FCPs that we could identify in the published or unpublished literature. The variation in the actual FCP strategies is impressive, as no two FCPs were similar and several were part of a system-wide change. The evidence that does exist, however, demonstrates that the FCP is an effective measure to rapidly reduce LOS for admitted patients, to reduce ambulance diversion, and to increase efficiency within the hospital system.

Table 8.1 Available evidence for the implementation of full-capacity protocols to reduce ED overcrowding.

Location	Intervention/ design	Description	Source/outcome	Results
Regina, Canada 2005	FCP Design unclear	Seven beds available for "full capacity" in two hospitals that would be opened in the event of reaching FC	Regina Health Region website pdf document, http://www.rqhealth.ca (accessed November 10, 2006); outcomes not reported	"The strategy improves the flow of admitted patients through the emergency by transferring them to unit where they will receive care, thus allowing the emergency department staff to continue working efficiently and effectively"
Vancouver, Canada 2006	FCP Unpublished before–after controlled clinical trial	2 hours (ED assessment) + 2 hours (decision to admit) + 2 hours (to transfer to the floor)	Grant Innes (personal communication, November 10, 2006); emergency department length of stay for medical (M), surgical (S) and psychiatric (P) admitted patients with active intervention (SP) and control (C)	LOS M_{SP} = 30.2 to 11.2 hours (−69%) M_C = 19.5 to 15.5 hours (−21%) S_{SP} = 9.2 to 7.6 hours (−17%) S_C = 10.3 to 11.1 hours (+8%) P_{SP} = 56.3 to 47.1 hours (−69%) P_C = 12.2 to 11.1 hours (−9%)
New York, USA 2001	FCP Uncontrolled study	2-hour rule whereby patients would be transferred to the floor after 2 hours from the decision to admit; no more than two patients/unit; must be stable	Dr. Vicellio's website http://www.hospitalovercrowding.com (accessed November 10, 2006)	"Positive effect despite increased volumes"; LOS = 6.2 hours (in ED hall) vs 5.4 hours on floor (FCP)
Maryland, USA 2006	FCP+ Before–after controlled clinical trial	N/A	*Journal of Quality and Patient Safety* The absolute and percentage change in ambulance diversions	"From 2003 to 2004, the hospital reduced ambulance diversion hours from 2365 to 655 – a 72% reduction"

FC, full capacity; FCP, full-capacity protocol; FCP+, full-capacity protocol in addition to other interventions within the health care system; LOS, length of stay; N/A, not available.

In summary, the introduction of an FCP may improve ED LOS for admitted patients and improve flow in the ED; however, there is no convincing evidence regarding its effect on quality of care or patient outcomes. Moreover, what are the effects of an FCP policy on patient outcomes, medical staff morale and interactions, infection control, and patient satisfaction remains to be answered.

Conclusions

Using the evidence outlined above, the ED director met with the hospital staff. A task force was created which included representation from senior administration, the ED and internal medicine. A triage liaison physician was introduced, and a fast-track area was created to help decant the ED and improve flow. In addition, the task force identified delays in getting internal medicine patients admitted to a hospital bed after the decision to admit as a key objective to reduce ED overcrowding and improve patient care. Finally, they contacted their regional health authority to begin discussions on developing a region-wide approach to reducing ED overcrowding.

Overall, ED overcrowding is a common problem in many EDs around the world. The causes of the problem are multi-factorial; however, there has been a reluctance to address this issue due to the perceived complexity and the lack of examples of successful interventions. However, worsening overcrowding, combined with increasing evidence of adverse effects on patients and impressive emerging evidence from the UK and other jurisdictions that highly effective interventions exist, has prompted some hospital and regional health system level efforts to tackle the issue. Successful interventions that achieve substantial and sustained improvements in ED overcrowding are likely to be characterized by being site-specific, having a focus on patient flow across the continuum (from prehospital to ED to inpatient care through to discharge), being innovative and involving broad collaboration.

Conflicts of interest

None were reported.

References

1 Cooke M, Fisher J, Dale J, et al. *Reducing Attendances and Waits in Emergency Departments: A systematic review of present innovations.* Report to the NHS Service Delivery and Organisation R&D Programme, London. University of Warwick, Warwick, 2005.

2 Canadian Association of Emergency Physicians (CAEP), National Emergency Nurses Affiliation (NENA). Joint Position Statement on Emergency Department Overcrowding. Available at http://caep.ca/template.asp?id=1d7c8feb2a7c4a939e4c2fe16d654e39 (accessed September 9, 2007).

3 ACEP Crowding Resources Task Force. *Responding to Emergency Department Crowding: A guidebook for chapters.* American College of Emergency Physicians, Dallas, 2002.

4 Bernstein SL, Verghese V, Leung W, Lunney AT, Perez I. Development and validation of a new index to measure emergency department crowding. *Acad Emerg Med* 2003;**10**:938–42.

5 Weiss SJ, Derlet R, Arndahl J, et al. Estimating the degree of emergency department overcrowding in academic medical centers: results of the National ED Overcrowding Study (NEDOCS). *Acad Emerg Med* 2004;**11**:38–50.

6 Reeder TJ, Garrison HG. When the safety net is unsafe: real-time assessment of the overcrowded emergency department. *Acad Emerg Med* 2001;**8**:1070–74.

7 Epstein SK, Tian L. Development of an emergency department work score to predict ambulance diversion. *Acad Emerg Med* 2006;**13**:421–6.

8 Hoot NR, Zhou C, Jones I, Aronsky D. Measuring and forecasting emergency department crowding in real time. *Ann Emerg Med* 2007;**49**:747–55.

9 Derlet RW, Richards JR, Kravitz RL. Frequent overcrowding in U.S. emergency departments. *Acad Emerg Med* 2001;**8**:151–5.

10 Asplin BR. Measuring crowding: time for a paradigm shift. *Acad Emerg Med* 2006;**13**:459–61.

11 Department of Health UG. *The NHS Plan. A plan for investment. A plan for reform.* Stationery Office, London, 2000.

12 Asplin BR, Magid DJ, Rhodes KV, et al. A conceptual model of emergency department crowding. *Ann Emerg Med* 2003;**42**:173–180.

13 American College of Emergency Physicians. Emergency Department Crowding Information Paper. Available at http://www.acep.org/NR/rdonlyres/IFDC6583-A6F6-4022-95DF-92FCFFEE77F3/0/empcCrowdingPPR.pdf (accessed September 9, 2007).

14 Magid DJ, Asplin BR, Wears RL. The quality gap: searching for the consequences of emergency department crowding. *Ann Emerg Med* 2004;**44**:586–8.

15 Bond K, Ospina MB, Blitz S, et al. Frequency, determinants and impact of overcrowding in emergency departments in Canada: a national survey. *Healthcare Q* 2007;**10**:32–40.

16 Miro O, Antonio MT, Jimenez S, et al. Decreased health care quality associated with emergency department overcrowding. *Eur J Emerg Med* 1999;**6**:105–7.

17 Sprivulis PC, Da Silva JA, Jacobs IG, Frazer AR, Jelinek GA. The association between hospital overcrowding and mortality among patients admitted via Western Australian emergency departments. *Med J Aust* 2006;**184**:208–12.

18 Richardson DB. Increase in patient mortality at 10 days associated with emergency department overcrowding. *Med J Aust* 2006;**184**:213–16.

19 Begley CE, Chang Y, Wood RC, Weltge A. Emergency department diversion and trauma mortality: evidence from Houston, Texas. *J Trauma* 2004;**57**:1260–65.

20 Schull MJ, Vermeulen M, Slaughter G, Morrison LJ, Daly P. Emergency department overcrowding and thrombolysis delays in acute myocardial infarction. *Ann Emerg Med* 2004;**44**:577–85.

21 Diercks DB, Roe MT, Chen AY, et al. Prolonged emergency department stays of non-ST-segment-elevation myocardial infarction patients are associated with worse adherence to the American College of Cardiology/American Heart Association guidelines for management and increased adverse events. *Ann Emerg Med* 2007;**50**:489–96.

22 Carr BG, Kaye AJ, Wiebe DJ, et al. Emergency department length of stay: a major risk factor for pneumonia in intubated blunt trauma patients. *J Trauma* 2007;**63**:9–12.

23 Fee C, Weber EJ, Maak CA, Bacchetti P. Effect of emergency department crowding on time to antibiotics in patients admitted with community-acquired pneumonia. *Ann Emerg Med* 2007;**50**:501–9.

24 Pines JM, Localio AR, Hollander JE, et al. The impact of emergency department crowding measures on time to antibiotics for patients with community-acquired pneumonia. *Ann Emerg Med* 2007;**50**:510–16.

25 Hwang U, Richardson LD, Sonuyi TO, Morrison RS. The effect of emergency department crowding on the management of pain in older adults with hip fracture. *J Am Geriatr Soc* 2006;**54**:270–75.

26 Pines JM, Hollander JE. Emergency department crowding is associated with poor care for patients with severe pain. *Ann Emerg Med* 2008;**51**(1):1–5.

27 Pham JC, Patel R, Millin MG, Kirsch TD, Chanmugam A. The effects of ambulance diversion: a comprehensive review. *Acad Emerg Med* 2006;**13**:1220–27.

28 Schull MJ, Morrison LJ, Vermeulen M, Redelmeier DA. Emergency department overcrowding and ambulance transport delays for patients with chest pain. *Can Med Assoc J* 2003;**168**:277–83.

29 Schull MJ, Morrison LJ, Vermeulen M, Redelmeier DA. Emergency department gridlock and out-of-hospital delays for cardiac patients. *Acad Emerg Med* 2003;**10**:709–16.

30 Polevoi SK, Quinn JV, Kramer NR. Factors associated with patients who leave without being seen. *Acad Emerg Med* 2005;**12**:232–6.

31 Rowe BH, Channan P, Bullard M, et al. Characteristics of patients who leave emergency departments without being seen. *Acad Emerg Med* 2006;**13**:848–52.

32 Guo B, Harstall C. *Strategies to Reduce Emergency Department Overcrowding.* HTA Report No. 38. Alberta Heritage Foundation for Medical Research, Edmonton, 2006.

33 Bond K, Ospina MB, Blitz S, et al. *Interventions to Reduce Overcrowding in Emergency Departments.* Technology Report No. 67.4. Canadian Agency for Drugs and Technologies in Health, Ottawa, 2006.

34 George S, Read S, Westlake L, et al. Evaluation of nurse triage in a British accident and emergency department. *BMJ* 1992;**304**:876–8.

35 Paulson DL. A comparison of wait times and patients leaving without being seen when licensed nurses versus unlicensed assistive personnel perform triage. *J Emerg Nurs* 2004;**30**:307–11.

36 Holroyd BR, Bullard MJ, Latoszek K, et al. Impact of a triage liaison physician on emergency department overcrowding and throughput: a randomized controlled trial. *Acad Emerg Med* 2007;**14**:702–8.

37 Kelly KA. Referring patients from triage out of the emergency department to primary care settings: one successful emergency department experience. *J Emerg Nurs* 1994;**20**:458–63.

38 Washington DL, Stevens CD, Shekelle PG, et al. Safely directing patients to appropriate levels of care: guideline-driven triage in the emergency service. *Ann Emerg Med* 2000;**36**:15–22.

39 Derlet RW, Nishio D, Cole LM, Silva J, Jr. Triage of patients out of the emergency department: three-year experience. *Am J Emerg Med* 1992;**10**:195–9.

40 Selby JV, Fireman BH, Swain BE. Effect of a copayment on use of the emergency department in a health maintenance organization. *N Engl J Med* 1996;**334**:635–41.

41 Young GP, Lowe RA. Adverse outcomes of managed care gatekeeping. *Acad Emerg Med* 1997;**4**:1129–36.

42 Kendall J, Reeves B, Clancy M. Point of care testing: randomised controlled trial of clinical outcome. *BMJ* 1998;**316**:1052–7.

43 Murray RP, Leroux M, Sabga E, Palatnick W, Ludwig L. Effect of point of care testing on length of stay in an adult emergency department. *J Emerg Med* 1999;**17**:811–14.

44 Parvin CA, Lo SF, Deuser SM, et al. Impact of point-of-care testing on patients' length of stay in a large emergency department. *Clin Chem* 1996;**42**:711–17.

45 Lindley-Jones M, Finlayson BJ. Triage nurse requested X rays – are they worthwhile? *J Accid Emerg Med* 2000;**17**:103–7.

46 Parris W, McCarthy S, Kelly AM, Richardson S. Do triage nurse-initiated X-rays for limb injuries reduce patient transit time? *Accid Emerg Nurs* 1997;**5**:14–15.

47 Burgher SW, Tandy TK, Dawdy MR. Transvaginal ultrasonography by emergency physicians decreases patient time in the emergency department. *Acad Emerg Med* 1998;**5**:802–7.

48 Vilke GM, Brown L, Skogland P, Simmons C, Guss DA. Approach to decreasing emergency department ambulance diversion hours. *J Emerg Med* 2004;**26**:189–92.

49 Bucheli B, Martina B. Reduced length of stay in medical emergency department patients: a prospective controlled study on emergency physician staffing. *Eur J Emerg Med* 2004;**11**:29–34.

50 Hirshon JM, Kirsch TD, Mysko WK, Kelen GD. Effect of rotational patient assignment on emergency department length of stay. *J Emerg Med* 1996;**14**:763–8.

51 Miro O, Sanchez M, Espinosa G, et al. Analysis of patient flow in the emergency department and the effect of an extensive reorganisation. *Emerg Med J* 2003;**20**:143–8.

52 Shaw KN, Lavelle JM. VESAS: a solution to seasonal fluctuations in emergency department census. *Ann Emerg Med* 1998;**32**:698–702.

53 Han JH, Zhou C, France DJ, et al. The effect of emergency department expansion on emergency department overcrowding. *Acad Emerg Med* 2007;**14**:338–43.

54 Yoon P. *Emergency Department Fast-track System*. Alberta Heritage Foundation for Medical Research, Canada, 2003.

55 Holroyd BR, Bullard MJ, Latoszek K, et al. Impact of a triage liaison physician on emergency department overcrowding and throughput: a randomized controlled trial. *Acad Emerg Med* 2007;**14**:702–8.

56 Redmond AD, Buxton N. Consultant triage of minor cases in an accident and emergency department. *Arch Emerg Med* 1993;**10**:328–30.

57 Partovi SN, Nelson BK, Bryan ED, Walsh MJ. Faculty triage shortens emergency department length of stay. *Acad Emerg Med* 2001;**8**:990–95.

58 Bond PA. A staffed ED assessment room: impact on wait times for nonurgent patients at a Saudi Arabian hospital. *J Emerg Nurs* 2001;**27**:394–5.

59 Ardagh MW, Wells JE, Cooper K, et al. Effect of a rapid assessment clinic on the waiting time to be seen by a doctor and the time spent in the department, for patients presenting to an urban emergency department: a controlled prospective trial. *NZ Med J* 2002;**115**:U28.

60 Grant S, Spain D, Green D. Rapid assessment team reduces waiting time. *Emerg Med* 1999;**11**:72–7.

61 Cooke MW, Wilson S, Pearson S. The effect of a separate stream for minor injuries on accident and emergency department waiting times. *Emerg Med J* 2002;**19**:28–30.

62 Shrimpling M. Redesigning triage to reduce waiting times. *Emerg Nurse* 2002;**10**:34–7.

63 Kilic YA, Agalar FA, Kunt M, Cakmakci M. Prospective, double-blind, comparative fast-tracking trial in an academic emergency department during a period of limited resources. *Eur J Emerg Med* 1998;**5**:403–6.

64 Hampers LC, Cha S, Gutglass DJ, Binns HJ, Krug SE. Fast track and the pediatric emergency department: resource utilization and patient outcomes. *Acad Emerg Med* 1999;**6**:1153–9.

65 Rodi SW, Grau MV, Orsini CM. Evaluation of a fast track unit: alignment of resources and demand results in improved satisfaction and decreased length of stay for emergency department patients. *Qual Manag Health Care* 2006;**15**:163–70.

66 Saywell RM, Jr., Cordell WH, Nyhuis AW, et al. The use of a break-even analysis: financial analysis of a fast-track program. *Acad Emerg Med* 1995;**2**:739–45.

67 Rajmohan B. Audit of the effect of a fast tracking protocol on transfer time from A&E to ward for patients with hip fractures. *Injury* 2000;**31**:585–9.

68 Ryan JM, Singh S, Bryant G, Edwards S, Staniforth P. Fast tracking patients with a proximal femoral fracture – more than a broken bone. *J Accid Emerg Med* 2000;**17**:76.

69 Finlayson BJ. Fast tracking patients with a proximal femoral fracture. *J Accid Emerg Med* 1996;**13**:367.

70 Charalambous CP, Yarwood S, Paschalides C, et al. Reduced delays in A&E for elderly patients with hip fractures. *Ann R Coll Surg Engl* 2003;**85**:200–203.

71 Dunn J. Psychiatric intervention in the community hospital emergency room. *J Nurs Admin* 1989;**19**:36–40.

72 Guo B, Harstall C. *Strategies to Reduce Emergency Department Overcrowding*. HTA Report No. 38. Alberta Heritage Foundation for Medical Research, Edmonton, 2006.

73 Dale J, Higgins J, Williams S, et al. Computer assisted assessment and advice for "non-serious" 999 ambulance service callers: the potential impact on ambulance dispatch. *Emerg Med J* 2003;**20**:178–83.

74 Shah MN, Fairbanks RJ, Maddow CL, et al. Description and evaluation of a pilot physician-directed emergency medical services diversion control program. *Acad Emerg Med* 2006;**13**:54–60.

75 Heaney D, Paxton F. *First Year Interim Report – Minor injuries clinic*. Western General Hospital, Edinburgh, 1995.

76 Hsu RT, Lambert PC, Dixon-Woods M, Kurinczuk JJ. Effect of NHS walk-in centre on local primary healthcare services: before and after observational study. *BMJ* 2003;**326**:530.

77 Salisbury C, Chalder M, Manku-Scott T, et al. *National Evaluation of NHS Walk-in Centres*. University of Bristol, Bristol, 2002.

78 Salisbury C, Hollinghurst S, Montgomery A, et al. The impact of co-located NHS walk-in centres on emergency departments. *Emerg Med J* 2007;**24**:265–9.

79 Cooke M. Emergency care practitioners: a new safe effective role? *Qual Saf Health Care* 2006;**15**:387.

80 Canadian Institute for Health Information. *Understanding Emergency Department Wait Times*. Canadian Institute for Health Information, Toronto, 2005.

81 Vertesi L. Does the Canadian Emergency Department Triage and Acuity Scale identify non-urgent patients who can be triaged away from the emergency department? *Can J Emerg Med* 2004;**6**:337–342.

82 van Uden CJ, Crebolder HF. Does setting up out of hours primary care cooperatives outside a hospital reduce demand for emergency care? *Emerg Med J* 2004;**21**:722–3.

83 van Uden CJ, Winkens RA, Wesseling GJ, Crebolder HF, van Schayck CP. Use of out of hours services: a comparison between two organisations. *Emerg Med J* 2003;**20**:184–7.

84 Oterino-de-la-Fuente, D. Banos Pino JF, Blanco VF, Alvarez AR. Does better access to primary care reduce utilization of hospital accident and emergency departments? A time-series analysis. *Eur J Public Health* 2007;**17**:186–92.

85 Stoddart D, Ireland AJ, Crawford R, Kelly B. Impact on an accident and emergency department of Glasgow's new primary care emergency service. *Health Bull (Edinb)* 1999;**57**:186–91.

86 Lattimer V, George S, Thompson F, et al. Safety and effectiveness of nurse telephone consultation in out of hours primary care: randomised controlled trial. *BMJ* 1998;**317**:1054–9.

87 Richards DA, Meakins J, Tawfik J, et al. Nurse telephone triage for same day appointments in general practice: multiple interrupted time series trial of effect on workload and costs. *BMJ* 2002;**325**:1214.

88 Gadomski AM, Perkis V, Horton I, Cross S, Stanton B. Diverting managed care Medicaid patients from pediatric emergency department use. *Pediatrics* 1995;**95**:170–78.

89 Sjonell G. Effect of establishing a primary health care centre on the utilization of primary health care and other out-patient care in a Swedish urban area. *Fam Pract* 1986;**3**:148–54.

90 Franco SM, Mitchell CK, Buzon RM. Primary care physician access and gatekeeping: a key to reducing emergency department use. *Clin Pediatr (Phila)* 1997;**36**:63–8.

91 Schull MJ, Kiss A, Szalai J. The effect of low-complexity patients on emergency department waiting times. *Ann Emerg Med* 2007;**49**:257–64.

92 Health Services Management Centre. *Reducing Unplanned Hospital Admissions: What does the literature tell us?* Health Services Management Centre, University of Birmingham, Birmingham. Available at http://www.hsmc.bham.ac.uk/ltcnetwork/howtoreduceemergencyhospitaladmissions.pdf (accessed June 1, 2008).

93 Cooke MW, Wilson S, Halsall J, Roalfe A. Total time in English accident and emergency departments is related to bed occupancy. *Emerg Med J* 2004;**21**:575–6.

94 Cooke M, Black S, Fletcher A, Jennings M. Flows through beds not occupancy. Available at http://emj.bmj.com/cgi/eletters/21/5/575.

95 Cardin S, Afilalo M, Lang E, et al. Intervention to decrease emergency department crowding: does it have an effect on return visits and hospital readmissions? *Ann Emerg Med* 2003;**41**:173–85.

96 Hoffenberg S, Hill MB, Houry D. Does sharing process differences reduce patient length of stay in the emergency department? *Ann Emerg Med* 2001;**38**:533–40.

97 Cameron P, Scown P, Campbell D. Managing access block. *Aust Health Rev* 2002;**25**:59–68.

98 Department of Health. *The NHS Plan. A plan for investment. A plan for reform.* Stationery Office, London, 2000.

99 Anon. *Hospital Activity Statistics. Total time in A & E.* NHS National Activity Statistics. Available at www.performance.doh.gov.uk/hospitalactivity/data_requests/total_time_ae.htm.

100 Hedges JR, Trout A, Magnusson AR. Satisfied Patients Exiting the Emergency Department (SPEED) Study. *Acad Emerg Med* 2002;**9**:15–21.

101 British Medical Association. *British Medical Association Survey of Accident and Emergency Waiting Times.* Available at www.bma.org.uk/ap.nsf/content/aandewaiting.

102 National Audit Office. *Improving Emergency Care in England. Report by the Controller and Auditor General.* National Audit Office, London, 2004.

103 Mortimore A, Cooper S. The "4-hour target": emergency nurses' views. *Emerg Med J* 2007;**24**:402–4.

2   Respiratory

9 Emergency Management of Asthma Exacerbations

Brian H. Rowe[1] & Carlos A. Camargo, Jr.[2]
[1]Department of Emergency Medicine, University of Alberta, Edmonton, Canada
[2]EMNet Coordinating Center, Department of Emergency Medicine, Massachusetts General Hospital, Boston, USA

Case scenario

A 21-year-old woman presents to the emergency department (ED) with a 3-day history of cough, shortness of breath and wheezing which began after symptoms of a common cold. She is alert and oriented but talking in short phrases only, with a respiratory rate of 32 breaths/min, heart rate of 150 beats/min and oxygen saturation of 85%. Examination reveals severe intercostal and subcostal retractions and she is too dyspneic to perform peak expiratory flow (PEF) measurements. On auscultation, there is diffuse expiratory wheezing throughout all lung fields with prolongation of the expiratory phase. The heart sounds are tachycardic but otherwise normal. The remainder of the physical examination is within normal limits. You diagnose her with an asthma exacerbation and commence inhaled salbutamol (5 mg) therapy in addition to IV methyl-prednisolone (125 mg). The medical student asks whether you would consider using an inhaled short-acting anticholinergic agent as well.

The patient improves marginally over the first 20 minutes but remains dyspneic. The patient reports that she had previously received IV magnesium sulfate ($MgSO_4$). You ask the nurse to continue with nebulized salbutamol and infuse 2 g of IV $MgSO_4$ in a 100 cm^3 mini-bag over 20 minutes. The medical student is relieved when the magnesium infusion appears to improve her respiratory symptoms after another hour; however, she asks what other agents might have been useful had this not been the case?

After 4 hours, the patient has improved to the point that her PEF is 71% predicted for her age, sex, race and height. The patient asks you what can be done to prevent her from relapsing back to the ED over the next 2–3 weeks. Review of history reveals that this young woman has had several asthma exacerbations in the past 12 months, with one requiring an ED visit. Most recently, these have been the result of upper respiratory tract infections. The patient describes her asthma as being worse with exertion and at night, and it has stopped her from socializing with friends. She describes using a salbutamol puffer several times per day before and after exertion and often in the middle of the night when she awakes with coughing episodes. After reviewing these details, the patient asks if there is any way for her to decrease her chances of having another severe asthma exacerbation and whether she really requires the daily inhaled corticosteroid she has recently re-started.

Background

Asthma is a common chronic condition and is characterized by intermittent exacerbations followed by variable degrees of "stability". The prevalence of asthma varies widely with demographics (more common in boys, adult women and some racial groups), geography (regional variation is often noted) and socio-economic status. The hallmark of exacerbation includes a history of asthma, increasing symptoms of dyspnea, wheeze and/or cough, and an increasing need for short-acting β-agonists. Asthma exacerbations are common presentations to the ED in many parts of the world [1] and the costs associated with the care of asthma are enormous [2–4]. For example, in the United States approximately $14 billion per year is spent on asthma [2]. Twenty-five percent of all asthma expenses are related to acute exacerbations (ED visits, hospitalizations) [4]. As a result, it is clear that asthma, and acute asthma in particular, is a very important health problem.

Given this importance, it is not surprising that there are a number of guidelines that have been developed to direct the management of this problem [5–7]. Despite the availability of these guidelines there is a "care gap" between what is known and what is practiced and the dissemination of evidence often does not reach the patient in the ED or other acute care settings. This is due, in part, to the rapidly changing understanding of the pathophysiology and treatment of asthma and the introduction of new management strategies in this field. Moreover, basic economics (patients often cannot afford the appropriate medicines) and education (patients do not know that it is possible to live a normal

Evidence-based Emergency Medicine. Edited by Brian H. Rowe
© 2009 Blackwell Publishing, ISBN: 978-1-4051-6143-5.

life with asthma) continue to complicate the management of asthma.

Clinical questions

In order to address the issues of most relevance to your patient and to help in searching the literature for the evidence regarding these issues, you should structure your clinical questions as recommended in Chapter 1.

1 In adults with acute asthma presenting to the ED (population), does the measurement of pulmonary function or oxygen saturation (tests) have sufficient sensitivity and specificity (diagnostic test characteristics) to predict the need for hospital admission (outcome)?

2 In adults with acute asthma presenting to the ED (population), does the use of β_2-agonist inhalers with holding chambers (intervention) result in similar bronchodilation and admission to hospital (outcome) compared to treatment using nebulized medication (control)?

3 In adults with acute asthma presenting to the ED (population), does the addition of nebulized ipratropium bromide (intervention) to nebulized β-agonist decrease the risk of admission to hospital (outcome) compared to treatment with β-agonist therapy alone (control)?

4 In adults with acute asthma presenting to the ED (population), does the use of intravenous corticosteroids (intervention) in the ED reduce the admissions to hospital (outcome) compared to standard care (control)?

5 In adults with *severe* acute asthma presenting to the ED (population), does intravenous magnesium sulfate (intervention) in addition to nebulized salbutamol and systemic corticosteroids (control) reduce admissions to hospital (outcome)?

6 In adults with acute asthma discharged from the ED (population), does treatment with systemic corticosteroids (intervention) compared to standard care (control) reduce relapses to additional care (outcome)?

7 In adults with acute asthma discharged from the ED (population), does the addition of inhaled corticosteroids (intervention) to routine therapy (control) after discharge reduce relapse events (outcomes)?

8 In adults with acute asthma seen in the ED (population), what is the role of long-acting β-agonists (intervention) in addition to inhaled corticosteroids in reducing admissions or relapses of asthma (outcomes) compared to inhaled corticosteroids alone (control)?

9 In adults with acute asthma seen in the ED (population), do systemic leukotriene antagonists (intervention) reduce admissions to hospital (outcome) compared to standard care (control)?

10 In adults with acute asthma discharged from the ED (population), what is the role of patient education (intervention) compared to standard care (control) in reducing relapse and future exacerbations of asthma (outcomes)?

General search strategy

You begin to address these questions by searching for evidence in the common electronic databases such as the Cochrane Library,

MEDLINE and EMBASE looking specifically for systematic reviews and meta-analyses. The Cochrane Library is particularly rich in high-quality systematic review evidence on numerous aspects of acute asthma [8]. When a systematic review is identified, you also search for recent updates on the Cochrane Library and also search MEDLINE and EMBASE to identify randomized controlled trials (RCTs) that became available after the publication date of the systematic review. In addition, access to relevant, updated and evidence-based clinical practice guidelines (CPGs) on acute asthma are accessed to determine the consensus rating of areas lacking evidence.

Searching for evidence synthesis: primary search strategy

- Cochrane Library: asthma AND (topic)
- MEDLINE: asthma AND MEDLINE AND (systematic review OR meta-analysis OR metaanalysis) AND adult AND (topic)
- EMBASE: asthma AND MEDLINE AND (systematic review OR meta-analysis OR metaanalysis) AND adult AND (topic)

Critical review of the literature

Question 1: In adults with acute asthma presenting to the ED (population), does the measurement of pulmonary function or oxygen saturation (tests) have sufficient sensitivity and specificity (diagnostic test characteristics) to predict the need for hospital admission (outcome)?

Search strategy

- MEDLINE and EMBASE: asthma AND (pulmonary functions OR spirometry OR PEF OR PEFR OR FEV1 OR FEV) AND emergency AND sensitivity and specificity

Physicians' estimates of exacerbation severity, response to therapy, and risk of relapse following discharge are often inaccurate in acute asthma. The assessment of asthma severity is recommended by all major acute asthma guidelines; however, the method of assessing severity is widely debated. Some guidelines recommend that severity be determined objectively using spirometry, PEF or both, for all patients over 5 years of age [5]. Despite a general lack of evidence of the sensitivity or specificity of individual measures [9], the use of a pulmonary function measure has been encouraged. Most emergency departments measure PEF, rather than forced expiratory volume in 1 second (FEV_1), and follow this marker over the course of treatment during the acute visit. Not surprisingly, the cut-points for severity vary among the different guidelines; however, all suggest < 40–50% predicted of either PEF or FEV_1 indicates severe disease, where adjunctive therapy is effective. Perhaps the more important consideration for ED physicians relates to the change in pulmonary function over the acute treatment period. For example, blunted improvement in either the FEV_1 or PEF rate following initial bronchodilator therapy is predictive of a more prolonged ED course or the need for actual hospital admission [10]. Finally, most guidelines suggest the ED target for discharge should be 70% predicted.

Pulse oximetry measurements (oxygen saturation or SaO_2) have been used extensively in children; however, researchers question whether this measurement alone is a clinically useful predictor of hospital admission in children who present to the ED with acute asthma [11]. Although low SaO_2 may indicate a need for admission to hospital, other clinical factors may be more helpful. Moreover, normal or near-normal levels do not exclude severe asthma or the possibility of post-ED relapse. Measurement of SaO_2 may help to guide treatment in adult patients; however, no studies were identified that clearly demonstrated that SaO_2 predicted admission or relapse in adult asthmatic patients.

In summary, acute asthma severity is a multi-factorial assessment in the emergency setting. The use of pulse oximetry, pulmonary function tests, vital signs, history, physical examination, response to therapy and current medications are all required to determine the need for hospital admission and the risk of relapse after discharge [12,13].

Question 2: In adults with acute asthma presenting to the ED (population), does the use of β_2-agonist inhalers with holding chambers (intervention) result in similar bronchodilation and admission to hospital (outcome) compared to treatment using nebulized medication (control)?

Search strategy

- Cochrane Library: asthma AND (holding chambers OR aerochamber OR spacer) AND (emergency department OR exacerbation)

Early treatment of acute asthma has generally focused on the use of inhaled (usually via a nebulizer) short-acting β_2-agonists because of their undisputed and generally rapid bronchodilation effect. Whether the drug is most effective when delivered via a nebulizer or a metered dose inhaler (MDI) with a holding chamber (or spacer) device has been an area of intense research. A Cochrane Library systematic review, updated in 2006, involves 2066 children and 614 adults from 25 trials from emergency room and community settings. This review suggests that the use of either delivery method yields similar outcomes [14]. In adults, the relative risk of admission or poor outcome for holding chamber versus nebulizer was 0.97 (95% CI: 0.63 to 1.47). The ED length of stay for adults and FEV_1 or PEF measures were also similar for the two delivery methods. Finally, the use of an MDI with holding chamber was associated with fewer side-effects (e.g., tachycardia, tremor) than nebulizers, especially in children. Economic evaluations of these competing approaches demonstrate an advantage favoring

β_2-agonist treatments by MDIs with holding chambers as compared to nebulizers [15].

An important caveat is that these data do not include patients with severe or near-fatal asthma. For patients with severe asthma, the benefits and ease of continuous nebulization [16], and the need to focus on other management issues, may make nebulization a more attractive choice for emergency bronchodilation. Nevertheless, for patients with mild to moderate exacerbations, the Cochrane Library systematic review supports using an MDI with a holding chamber instead of a nebulizer. Another advantage of using an MDI and holding chamber in the acute setting is that it affords a potential opportunity to assess inhaler technique and educate patients about appropriate self-care.

Attempts to identify optimal doses or treatment intervals to achieve maximal bronchodilation or symptom relief have not been successful [17]. Continuous nebulization treatment may have an advantage over intermittent treatment in severe asthma exacerbations [16]. In addition, lower β_2-agonist doses appear to be equivalent to higher nebulizer doses (up to 5–10 mg/nebulization dose) with regard to maximizing bronchodilation or clinical outcome [18]. A substantial number of patients achieve a bronchodilation "plateau" and in these people additional β_2-agonist therapy only seems to cause more side-effects. Some guidelines now recommend that β-agonists be titrated to plateau using an objective assessment of airway obstruction with pulmonary function measures [5].

Despite this very strong evidence supporting the use of MDIs and holding chambers for bronchodilation in mild to moderate exacerbations, the convenience and patient acceptance of nebulized salbutamol is fairly entrenched [19]. The recent worldwide severe acute respiratory syndrome (SARS) outbreak and its apparent spread following nebulization [20] has discouraged routine treatment by nebulizer; in some settings, these recent events may facilitate conversion to MDIs with holding chambers.

Question 3: In adults with acute asthma presenting to the ED (population), does the addition of nebulized ipratropium bromide (intervention) to nebulized β-agonist decrease the risk of admission to hospital (outcome) compared to treatment with β-agonist therapy alone (control)?

Search strategy

- Cochrane Library and MEDLINE (OVID): *explode* asthma AND (anticholinergic OR atrovent OR ipratropium bromide) AND emergency services, hospital AND EBM reviews

There is increasing support, particularly in respect of children, for adding anticholinergic agents (most commonly ipratropium bromide) to β_2-agonist therapy in moderate to severe acute asthma; one systematic review in children [21] and two in adults form the basis of this conclusion [22,23]. The adult reviews identified a modest beneficial effect of adding ipratropium bromide to inhaled β_2-agonists. After 45–90 minutes of treatment, the absolute increase in FEV_1 and PEF, respectively, was 7.3% (95% CI: 4% to 11%) and 22.1% (95% CI: 11% to 33%). The risk of admission was decreased by 27% (RR = 0.73; 95% CI: 0.53 to 0.99). A large RCT has since been completed that confirms the systematic review evidence [23]. The study observed a 21% (95% CI: 3% to 38%) improvement in PEF rate and a 48.1% (95% CI: 20% to 76%) improvement in FEV_1 over the control group. Multiple doses of ipratropium bromide reduced the risk of hospital admission by 49% (RR = 0.51; 95% CI: 0.31 to 0.83); the number needed to treat (NNT) to prevent a single admission was five (95% CI: 3 to 17). Although questions still need to be resolved regarding anticholinergic therapy in the ED setting (such as the dose–response relationship), evidence supports adding this to β_2-agonists for patients with moderate to severe acute asthma.

Question 4: In adults with acute asthma presenting to the ED (population), does the use of intravenous corticosteroids (intervention) in the ED reduce the admissions to hospital (outcome) compared to standard care (control)?

Search strategy

- Cochrane Library and MEDLINE (OVID): *explode* asthma AND (adrenal cortex hormones OR corticosteroids) AND emergency services, hospital AND EBM reviews

The airway edema and increased secretions associated with acute asthma are the result of inflammation and can be effectively treated with systemic corticosteroids. The early use (i.e., within 90 minutes of arrival) of corticosteroids delivered by either oral or IV routes is a principal treatment choice in published guidelines [5–7]. A Cochrane meta-analysis investigating this issue identified 12 RCTs involving 863 patients with acute asthma and concluded that the early use of systemic corticosteroids significantly reduced admissions (OR = 0.50; 95% CI: 0.31 to 0.81); the NNT was eight (95% CI: 5 to 20) [24]. This benefit was more pronounced for those not already receiving corticosteroids (OR = 0.37; 95% CI: 0.19 to 0.70) and those experiencing a severe exacerbation (OR = 0.35; 95% CI: 0.21 to 0.59). The effects of corticosteroids on pulmonary function were variable in the short term, mainly due to insufficient reporting of results in the individual trials. Side-effect profiles were similar between all corticosteroid treatment routes and placebo, suggesting that early treatment with corticosteroid is safe.

Current treatment options for physicians include using IV and/or oral corticosteroids in the ED; however, there is little support on the part of patients and physicians to use the IV route on all (or even most) presentations. The current evidence-based approach would be to use oral agents (prednisone or dexamethasone) on most patients and attempt to identify patients who require the IV route of administration. There is no evidence from controlled

trials or meta-analyses to suggest the advantage offered by corticosteroids in moderate to severe asthma is related to the route of administration [24]. Further systematic review evidence on dosing suggests that high-dose corticosteroids, at least in hospitalized patients, are no more effective than moderate and low doses [25].

Applying this information to practice requires a clear understanding that not all levels of severity have been assessed with sufficient rigor to confirm equivalency of systemic routes. Until further evidence is available, it seems reasonable to select oral agents as the first-line choice while reserving IV corticosteroids for those who are too dyspneic to swallow, are obtunded or intubated, or are unable to tolerate oral medications (e.g., vomiting). The agent and dose of corticosteroid administered should be based on cost, availability and patient factors. The main issue to remember is the need to start systemic corticosteroids early and consistently for patients with moderate to severe acute asthma.

Question 5: In adults with *severe* acute asthma presenting to the ED (population), does intravenous magnesium sulfate (intervention) in addition to nebulized salbutamol and systemic corticosteroids (control) reduce admissions to hospital (outcome)?

Search strategy

- Cochrane Library and MEDLINE (OVID): *explode* asthma AND (magnesium sulfate OR MgSO4) AND emergency services, hospital AND EBM reviews

Intravenous $MgSO_4$ is a treatment option for a variety of diseases such as eclampsia, cardiac arrhythmia and asthma. In asthma, it has both a direct effect on smooth muscles, through its influence on cellular calcium homeostasis, and a proposed airway anti-inflammatory effect. The use of intravenous and inhaled $MgSO_4$ in unresponsive acute asthma has gained support over the past decade. There have been a number of systematic reviews which all conclude that IV magnesium sulfate is not only safe but effective in those patients with severe disease [26,27]. In the updated Cochrane review, 13 studies (eight with adults, five with children) involving 965 patients have examined the addition of IV $MgSO_4$ to β-agonists and systemic corticosteroids. When all studies were considered, the addition of $MgSO_4$ reduced hospitalization; however, moderate heterogeneity was identified ($I^2 = 47.6\%$) (Fig. 9.1). When the analysis was restricted to only adults the treatment did not appear to reduce admissions (RR = 0.91; 95% CI: 0.77 to 1.09). In the severe asthma subgroup, $MgSO_4$ did reduce hospitalization when all studies were considered (RR = 0.60; 95% CI: 0.48 to 0.74), and also improved pulmonary function (PEF: 26.8 L/min; 95% CI: 7.3 to 45) [26]. Overall, adverse effects and side-effects with this treatment were rare or minor, although these outcomes are poorly reported in most clinical trials.

Adult patients with clinically severe asthma, pulmonary function testing of less than 30% predicted, and/or who exhibit a poor

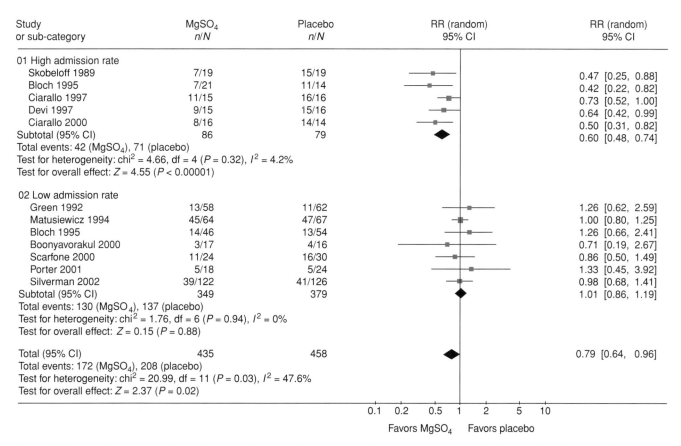

Study or sub-category	MgSO$_4$ n/N	Placebo n/N	RR (random) 95% CI	RR (random) 95% CI
01 High admission rate				
Skobeloff 1989	7/19	15/19		0.47 [0.25, 0.88]
Bloch 1995	7/21	11/14		0.42 [0.22, 0.82]
Ciarallo 1997	11/15	16/16		0.73 [0.52, 1.00]
Devi 1997	9/15	15/16		0.64 [0.42, 0.99]
Ciarallo 2000	8/16	14/14		0.50 [0.31, 0.82]
Subtotal (95% CI)	86	79		0.60 [0.48, 0.74]
Total events: 42 (MgSO$_4$), 71 (placebo)				
Test for heterogeneity: chi^2 = 4.66, df = 4 (P = 0.32), I^2 = 4.2%				
Test for overall effect: Z = 4.55 (P < 0.00001)				
02 Low admission rate				
Green 1992	13/58	11/62		1.26 [0.62, 2.59]
Matusiewicz 1994	45/64	47/67		1.00 [0.80, 1.25]
Bloch 1995	14/46	13/54		1.26 [0.66, 2.41]
Boonyavorakul 2000	3/17	4/16		0.71 [0.19, 2.67]
Scarfone 2000	11/24	16/30		0.86 [0.50, 1.49]
Porter 2001	5/18	5/24		1.33 [0.45, 3.92]
Silverman 2002	39/122	41/126		0.98 [0.68, 1.41]
Subtotal (95% CI)	349	379		1.01 [0.86, 1.19]
Total events: 130 (MgSO$_4$), 137 (placebo)				
Test for heterogeneity: chi^2 = 1.76, df = 6 (P = 0.94), I^2 = 0%				
Test for overall effect: Z = 0.15 (P = 0.88)				
Total (95% CI)	435	458		0.79 [0.64, 0.96]
Total events: 172 (MgSO$_4$), 208 (placebo)				
Test for heterogeneity: chi^2 = 20.99, df = 11 (P = 0.03), I^2 = 47.6%				
Test for overall effect: Z = 2.37 (P = 0.02)				

0.1 0.2 0.5 1 2 5 10

Favors MgSO$_4$ Favors placebo

Figure 9.1 Reduction in hospital admissions with early administration of intravenous magnesium sulfate compared to placebo in acute asthma. (Reprinted with permission from Rowe et al. [26], © Cochrane Library.)

response to initial bronchodilator therapy, appear to benefit most from IV MgSO$_4$ treatment. Since the publication of the original Cochrane Library review, additional studies have been published; however, the results do not change with review update. Since this agent has been shown to be easy to use, extremely safe and inexpensive, its early use in severe acute asthma should be considered. Currently, the recommended dose is 2 g IV over 20 minutes in adults, and this approach has been widely accepted by emergency physicians surveyed in North America [28].

Question 6: In adults with acute asthma discharged from the ED (population), does treatment with systemic corticosteroids (intervention) compared to standard care (control) reduce relapses to additional care (outcome)?

Search strategy

- Cochrane Library and MEDLINE (OVID): *explode* asthma AND (corticosteroids OR prednisone OR dexamethasone OR glucocorticoids) AND (relapse OR failure).

While most patients (~80–90%) with acute asthma will respond to treatment and meet the criteria for discharge [19], approxi-

mately 12–16% of those discharged will relapse within 2 weeks of ED discharge, many because of unresolved inflammation that leaves the airways sensitive to inhaled irritants [13,29]. Guidelines strongly encourage treatment with systemic corticosteroids following ED discharge for an asthma exacerbation to reduce the risk of relapse [5–7]. Compelling evidence for this approach is found in a Cochrane systematic review of six trials, involving approximately 350 patients, comparing corticosteroid therapy to placebo following discharge (Fig. 9.2) [29]. Significantly fewer patients in the corticosteroid group relapsed in the first week (RR = 0.38; 95% CI: 0.20 to 0.74). This reduced risk continued over the 21-day follow-up period (RR = 0.47; 95% CI: 0.25 to 0.89). The corticosteroid group also had less need for β_2-agonists (mean difference: 3 activations/day; 95% CI: −5.5 to −1.0). Changes in pulmonary function tests and side-effects, while rarely reported, showed no differences between the treatment groups. Nine (95% CI: 6 to 25) patients would need to be treated to prevent one relapse after an exacerbation of asthma [30].

There are now six RCTs involving 601 patients comparing intramuscular (IM) corticosteroids to a 7–10-day tapering course of corticosteroids following discharge from the ED. When pooled in a meta-analysis these results reveal a statistically non-significant trend favoring the IM route over the oral route at 7–10 days' follow-up (RR = 0.73; 95% CI: 0.73 to 1.09); however, this trend

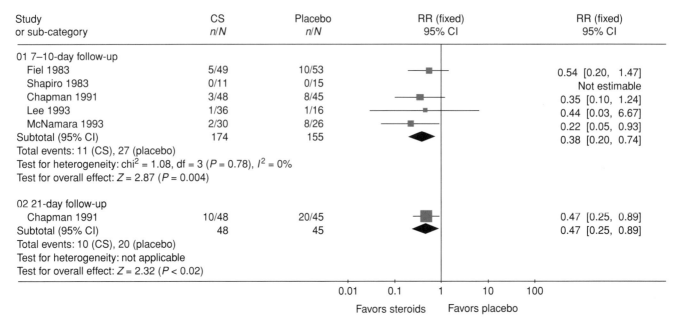

Study or sub-category	CS n/N	Placebo n/N	RR (fixed) 95% CI	RR (fixed) 95% CI
01 7–10-day follow-up				
Fiel 1983	5/49	10/53		0.54 [0.20, 1.47]
Shapiro 1983	0/11	0/15		Not estimable
Chapman 1991	3/48	8/45		0.35 [0.10, 1.24]
Lee 1993	1/36	1/16		0.44 [0.03, 6.67]
McNamara 1993	2/30	8/26		0.22 [0.05, 0.93]
Subtotal (95% CI)	174	155		0.38 [0.20, 0.74]

Total events: 11 (CS), 27 (placebo)
Test for heterogeneity: chi^2 = 1.08, df = 3 (P = 0.78), I^2 = 0%
Test for overall effect: Z = 2.87 (P = 0.004)

02 21-day follow-up				
Chapman 1991	10/48	20/45		0.47 [0.25, 0.89]
Subtotal (95% CI)	48	45		0.47 [0.25, 0.89]

Total events: 10 (CS), 20 (placebo)
Test for heterogeneity: not applicable
Test for overall effect: Z = 2.32 (P < 0.02)

0.01   0.1   1   10   100

Favors steroids   Favors placebo

Figure 9.2 Reduction in relapses with the addition of systemic corticosteroids (CS) after discharge from the emergency setting with acute asthma. (Reprinted with permission from Rowe et al. [29], © Cochrane Library.)

evaporates at the 3–4-week assessment periods (RR = 1.02; 95% CI: 0.73 to 1.42). These results cannot be interpreted as indicating equivalence since the 95% confidence intervals are wide. Consequently, IM therapy may be best reserved for those patients with questionable adherence to prescribed medications, inability to afford an oral corticosteroid prescription, or those who are otherwise unreliable (cognitive impairment, intoxication, etc.).

For a variety of reasons, examination of the relative effectiveness of various regimens and dosing protocol(s) cannot be provided. Given the enhanced compliance associated with once-daily dosing, however, and the availability of 40 or 50 mg tablets in many parts of the world, the use of oral corticosteroids for a short period (5–10 days) seems appropriate for most patients discharged after ED treatment of acute asthma. The need to "taper" these oral corticosteroids over that period appears unnecessary [31,32], especially in the presence of concurrent inhaled corticosteroids [33].

Question 7: In adults with acute asthma discharged from the ED (population), does the addition of inhaled corticosteroids (intervention) to routine therapy (control) after discharge reduce relapse events (outcomes)?

Search strategy

- Cochrane Library and MEDLINE (OVID): *explode* asthma AND (adrenal cortex hormones OR corticosteroids) AND emergency services, hospital AND EBM reviews

Many ED-based reviews suggest that the majority of patients with acute asthma are prescribed a short course (5–7 days) of oral corticosteroids at discharge [13,34]. Less information exists regarding the use of inhaled corticosteroids (ICSs); however, the data that exist indicate impressive practice variation with respect to this treatment. For example, in US sites associated with a large North American emergency medicine research network, only 10% of discharged asthmatic patients were prescribed an ICS if they were not regularly taking one, whereas in Canadian sites, more than 50% of similar patients were treated with an ICS at discharge [35].

There is mounting evidence that examines using a combination of inhaled and oral corticosteroids after discharge from the ED. There are two published RCTs [33,36] and one published as an abstract [37] that individually provide somewhat conflicting evidence for the addition of ICSs; however, when combined in a systematic review the studies favor the combination [38]. The pooled effect suggests that the ICS plus oral corticosteroid group has fewer relapses after discharge than the group on oral corticosteroids alone (RR = 0.72; 95% CI: 0.50 to 1.02).

While the test for heterogeneity in the pooled result was not statistically significant (I^2 = 0%), it did appear that the results of the three trials were sufficiently different to warrant further scrutiny. None the less, the prospect of an RR as high as 50% favoring ICS use cannot be ignored. Since the publication of the review, further non-RCT evidence has been published supporting the role of ICSs at discharge. Administrative research examining low-income patients who were discharged from EDs suggested that a prescription for an ICS significantly reduced future relapses with no difference between high and low doses (Table 9.1) [39].

Table 9.1 Estimated comparative daily dose for inhaled corticosteroid.

Drug	Low daily dose		Medium daily dose		High daily dose	
	Adult	Child*	Adult	Child*	Adult	Child*
Beclomethasone CFS 42 or 84 μg/puff	168–504 μg	84–336 μg	504–840 μg	336–672 μg	>840 μg	>672 μg
Beclomethasone HFA 40 or 80 μg/puff	80–210 μg	80–160 μg	240–180 μg	160–320 μg	>480 μg	>320 μg
Budesonide DPI 200 μg/inhalation	200–600 μg	200–400 μg	600–1200 μg	400–800 μg	>1200 μg	>800 μg
Inhalation suspension for nebulization (child dose)		0.5 mg		1.0 mg		2.0 mg
Flunisolide 250 μg/puff	500–1000 μg	500–750 μg	1000–2000 μg	1000–1250 μg	>2000 μg	>1250 μg
Fluticasone MDI 44, 110, or 220 μg/puff	88–261 μg	88–176 μg	264–660 μg	176–440 μg	>660 μg	>440 μg
DPI 50, 100, or 250 μg/inhalation	100–300 μg	100–200 μg	300–600 μg	200–400 μg	>600 μg	>400 μg
Triamcinolone acetonide 100 μg/puff	400–1000 μg	400–800 μg	1000–2000 μg	800–1200 μg	>2000 μg	>1200 μg

* Children 12 years of age and younger.

From Reference #6; National Asthma Education and Prevention Program (NAEPP). Expert Panel Report II: Guidelines for the Diagnosis and Management of Asthma. National Institutes of Health; Bethesda, MD, 1997.

Clinically, the results of this review indicate patients already receiving an ICS should be counseled by the ED staff regarding adherence-enhancing interventions [40,41]. Many patients with acute asthma presenting to the ED exhibit features associated with poorly controlled chronic asthma and represent vulnerable patients who are ideal candidates for ICSs. Consequently, those patients not already on ICS agents should be considered for short- or long-term ICS therapy in conjunction with oral prednisone after discharge [42]. The dose and duration of ICS agents should be based on recent history of symptom control, health care utilization and quality of life indicators. For those patients with more severe illness, this clearly would be the optimal treatment strategy.

There are also several recent publications examining the effect of replacing oral corticosteroids with ICSs. These studies generally compare oral prednisone to very high doses of ICSs in mild asthma exacerbations after discharge. While the systematic review failed to demonstrate a significant difference in asthma relapse between the two treatments (RR = 1.0; 95% CI: 0.71 to 1.41), these results need to be interpreted cautiously [38]. It must be stressed that these results do not imply equivalence due to the width of the confidence intervals and the inclusion of only patients with mild asthma exacerbations. Moreover, given the limited data on this issue to date, use of an ICS alone for treating asthma exacerbations should be discouraged. Compared to the traditional short course of prednisone, ICSs are expensive and more difficult for patients and families to use. Given the potential for added benefit with combined therapy (i.e., ICS plus long-acting β-agonist (LABA)), future research should focus on this important comparison.

Question 8: In adults with acute asthma seen in the ED (population), what is the role of long-acting β-agonists (intervention) in addition to inhaled corticosteroids in reducing admissions or relapses of asthma (outcomes) compared to inhaled corticosteroids alone (control)?

Search strategy

- Cochrane Library and MEDLINE (OVID): *explode* asthma AND (long-acting beta-agonists OR LABA OR Advair OR Symbicort OR Seritide) AND emergency services, hospital AND discharged, patients

Systematic review evidence supports the use of add-on therapies, such as LABA and leukotriene receptor antagonists (LTRAs), for chronic asthma management. Moreover, despite the use of anti-inflammatory agents in acute asthma, relapses after discharge occur at an unacceptably high rate. Overall, acute asthma highlights the fact that many patients are unstable and out of control. Consequently, the use of these add-on agents may seem reasonable, especially in the case where patients are already receiving ICSs. Efforts to reduce these statistics may involve these new agents, which are enjoying widespread use in chronic asthma therapy.

To date, limited research has been conducted on the use of LABAs in the acute setting. Only two RCTs reported as abstracts could be located in which improvements in quality of life were not observed by adding LABAs to systemic and inhaled corticosteroids in patients discharged from the ED [43,44]. Overall, 206 patients receiving ICS/LABA and prednisone have been compared to ICS alone and prednisone regimens. The influence on relapse in all patients is unclear (RR = 0.57; 95% CI: 0.28 to 1.18); however, in the subgroup of patients who were concurrently receiving ICS agents, quality of life was higher in those who were taking the combination agents [43]. A possible interpretation would be to use ICS/LABA combination therapy in patients who present with an exacerbation, are already receiving ICS agents and who are discharged from the ED. This issue requires further study.

For the increasing proportion of patients presenting to the ED already receiving ICS plus LABA combination agents, treatment options have been infrequently studied. Use of short-course systemic corticosteroids, encouraging adherence with current inhaler therapy, and close follow-up seem appropriate until clinical trials clarify the management for this group of patients.

Question 9: In adults with acute asthma seen in the ED (population), do systemic leukotriene antagonists (intervention) reduce admissions to hospital or relapses following discharge (outcomes) compared to standard care (control)?

Search strategy

- Cochrane Library and MEDLINE (OVID): *explode* asthma AND (montelukast OR accolade OR LTRA OR LKTRA OR leukotrienes) AND emergency services, hospital AND discharge, patients

The best evidence for the use of LTRA in acute asthma was provided in an RCT of 201 patients treated with placebo, 7 or 14 mg of IV montelukast [45]. The results suggested a clinically significant improvement in FEV_1 within 10 minutes of administration; however, ipratropium bromide and corticosteroids were not administered to all patients. Moreover, the intravenous formulation is not yet available for patient care. Another study examined treatments in the ED and after discharge [46]. The effect of LTRA in chronic asthma has been summarized in a Cochrane review, and the authors suggest that these agents have limited benefit compared to inhaled corticosteroids [47].

While LTRA research on acute asthma is encouraging, whether intravenous LTRAs should be added to the in-ED asthma treatment or oral LTRA should be added after discharge remains uncertain. As the evidence for and against the use of both LTRA and LABA accumulates, readers of this text are encouraged to search for updates in the Cochrane Library.

Question 10: In adults with acute asthma discharged from the ED (population), what is the role of patient education (intervention) compared to standard care (control) in reducing relapse and future exacerbations of asthma (outcomes)?

Search strategy

- Cochrane Library and MEDLINE (OVID): *explode* asthma AND education AND EBM review

Providing asthma education is one of the key recommendations contained in many asthma guidelines. Moreover, when surveyed, emergency physicians felt it was an important component of asthma care and rated many educational items as necessary [41]. In a narrative review of asthma education, authors have emphasized the need to educate asthma patients [48]. However, the results of individual trials and systematic reviews involving education delivered in the acute setting have been somewhat disappointing.

A recent Cochrane review examined the impact of ED-based education on asthma relapses and subsequent hospitalization [49]. From 13 studies, a total of 2004 adults with asthma exacerbations were enrolled in studies comparing education to standard care. The interventions were considered mixed; however, 54% included education on symptoms and trigger control, 38% provided an asthma booklet, 38% taught the use of medication and inhalers, 38% attempted to reinforce the importance of follow-ups, and one study provided a 24-hour hotline. Over a mean follow-up of 7.4 months, the evidence suggests that ED visits were not decreased significantly in the group receiving education (RR = 0.72; 95% CI: 0.47to 1.14) although hospitalizations were reduced (RR = 0.49; 5% CI: 0.29 to 0.84).

In other reviews, limited asthma education programs (information only) for adults with asthma has been shown to improve asthma symptoms (OR = 0.40; 95% CI: 0.18 to 0.86) but not health outcomes [50]. Another review assessed the effects of adult asthma self-management programs coupled with regular medical review [51]. Self-management education reduced hospitalizations, emergency visits, unscheduled doctor visits, missed work/school days and nocturnal asthma by approximately 50%. If a written action plan was added to this program there was an even greater reduction in hospitalization (OR = 0.35; 95% CI: 0.18 to 0.68). Patients who could self-adjust their medications using an individualized written plan had better lung function than those whose medications were adjusted by a doctor.

Overall, asthma education results to date have been variable and some of the most encouraging data arise from the ED delivery of a variety of educational interventions. The challenge for EDs is to deliver this treatment in an efficient and cost-effective manner.

Conclusions

Emergency physicians have an important role in both acute and chronic asthma management. The patient mentioned above was treated with systemic corticosteroids and inhaled corticosteroids, and was provided with education in the ED. Moreover, she was encouraged to maintain adherence to the regimen prescribed and to be in close contact with her family physician. She recovered without incident and was motivated to continue to explore ways to reduce her asthma severity and the frequency of her ED visits. One year later, she remained adherent with her ICS regimen, was exercising regularly and had lost weight, and had avoided asthma exacerbations requiring ED visits.

Asthma is a common, chronic and often debilitating disease that frequently presents to the ED in most developed countries. The new treatment approaches to control bronchial inflammation summarized herein provide hope for an early return to activities, reduced symptoms and improved quality of life in the post-ED period. Combining self-management skills and simple educational interventions with appropriate preventive medication provides patients with the best opportunity to maintain excellent health status (without recurrent exacerbations or acute asthma relapse) in the future.

Acknowledgments

The authors would like to thank Mrs. Diane Milette for her secretarial support. In addition the authors would like to acknowledge the work of the Airway Review Group staff (Mr. Stephen Milan and Mr. Toby Lasserson) and the Review Group Editor (Professor Paul Jones: 1995–2003; Dr. Christopher Cates: 2003 to present) at the St. George's Hospital Medical School in London, UK for their support with the completion of the acute asthma reviews.

Conflicts of interest

Dr. Rowe is supported by a 21st Century Canada Research Chair in Emergency Airway Diseases from the Government of Canada (Ottawa, Canada). Dr. Rowe has received financial support from a variety of groups for participation in conferences, consulting and medical research. These groups include government agencies, private foundations, professional organizations and industry. In the past 5 years, industry sponsors with an interest in asthma included AstraZeneca and GlaxoSmithKline. Dr. Rowe does not own stocks or other ownership interest in any of these companies.

Dr. Camargo has received financial support from a variety of groups for participation in conferences, consulting and medical research. These groups include government agencies, private foundations, professional organizations and industry. In the past 5 years, industry sponsors with an interest in asthma were AstraZeneca, Dey, GlaxoSmithKline, Merck, Novartis and Schering-Plough. Dr. Camargo does not own stocks or other ownership interest in any of these companies.

References

1 Mannino DM, Homa DM, Pertowski CA, et al. Surveillance for asthma – United States, 1960–1995. *MMWR CDC Surveill Summ* 1998;**47**(1):1–28.

2 Weiss KB, Sullivan SD, Lyttle CS. Trends in the cost of illness for asthma in the United States, 1985–1994. *J Allergy Clin Immun* 2000;**106**:493–9.

3 Weiss KB, Sullivan SD. The health economics of asthma and rhinitis. I. Assessing the economic impact. *J Allergy Clin Immun* 2001;**107**:3–8.

4 Krahn MD, Berka C, Langlois P, Detsky AS. Direct and indirect costs of asthma in Canada. *Can Med Assoc J* 1996;**154**:821–31.

5 Boulet L-P, Becker A, Berube D, Beveridge RC, Ernst P, on behalf of the Canadian Asthma Consensus Group. Canadian asthma consensus report, 1999. *Can Med Assoc J* 1999;**161**:S1–61.

6 National Asthma Education and Prevention Program (NAEPP). *Expert Panel Report II: Guidelines for the Diagnosis and Management of Asthma.* National Institutes of Health, Bethesda, MD, 1997.

7 Network BTSSIG. British guideline on the management of asthma. *Thorax* 2003;**58**:1–94.

8 Jadad AR, Moher M, Browman GP, et al. Systematic reviews and meta-analyses on treatment of asthma: critical evaluation. *BMJ* 2000;**320**:537–40.

9 Worthington JR, Ahuja J. The value of pulmonary function tests in the management of acute asthma. *Can Med Assoc J* 1989;**140**:153–6.

10 Rodrigo G, Rodrigo C. Early prediction of poor response in acute asthma patients in the emergency department. *Chest* 1998;**114**(4):1016–21.

11 Keahey L, Bulloch B, Becker AB, et al. Initial oxygen saturation as a predictor of admission in children presenting to the emergency department with acute asthma. *Ann Emerg Med* 2002;**40**(3):300–307.

12 Beveridge B, Rowe BH, Boulet L-P, et al. What is new since the last (1999) Canadian Asthma Consensus Guidelines? *Can Respir J* 2001;**8**(Suppl A):5A–27A.

13 Emerman CL, Woodruff PG, Cydulka RK, et al. Prospective multicenter study of relapse following treatment for acute asthma among adults presenting to the emergency department. *Chest* 1999;**115**:919–27.

14 Cates CJ, Crilly JA, Rowe BH. Holding chambers (spacers) versus nebulisers for beta-agonist treatment of acute asthma. *Cochrane Database Syst Rev* 2006;**2**:CD000052 (doi: 10.1002/14651858.CD000052.pub2).

15 Turner MO, Gafni A, Swan D, Fitzgerald JM. A review and economic evaluation of bronchodilator delivery methods in hospitalized patients. *Arch Intern Med* 1996;**156**:2113–18.

16 Camargo CA, Jr., Spooner CH, Rowe BH. Continuous versus intermittent beta-agonists for acute asthma (Cochrane review). *Cochrane Database Syst Rev* 2003;**4**:CD001115 (doi: 10.1002/14651858.CD001115).

17 Emerman CL, Cydulka RK, McFadden ER. Comparison of 2.5 vs 7.5 mg of inhaled albuterol in the treatment of acute asthma. *Chest* 1999;**115**:92–6.

18 Stauss L, Hejal R, Galan G, Dixon L, McFadden ER, Jr. Observations on the effects of aerosolized albuterol in acute asthma. *Am J Resp Crit Care* 1997;**155**:454–8.

19 Weber EJ, Silverman RA, Callaham ML, et al. A prospective multicenter study of factors associated with hospital admission among adults with acute asthma. *Am J Med* 2002;**113**(5):371–8.

20 Varia M, Wilson S, Sarwal S, et al. Investigation of a nosocomial outbreak of severe acute respiratory syndrome (SARS) in Toronto, Canada. *Can Med Assoc J* 2003;**169**(4):285–92.

21 Plotnick LH, Ducharme FM. Combined inhaled anticholinergics and beta2-agonists for initial treatment of acute asthma in children (Cochrane review). *Cochrane Database Syst Rev* 2000;**3**:CD000060 (doi: 10.1002/14651858.CD000060).

22 Stoodley RG, Aaron SD, Dales RE. The role of ipratropium bromide in the emergency management of acute asthma exacerbation: a meta-analysis of randomized clinical trials. *Ann Emerg Med* 1999;**34**(1):8–18.

23 Rodrigo GJ, Rodrigo C. First-line therapy for adult patients with acute asthma receiving a multiple-dose protocol of ipratropium bromide plus albuterol in the emergency department. *Am J Resp Crit Care* 2000;**161**:1862–8.

24 Rowe BH, Spooner C, Ducharme FM, Bretzlaff JA, Bota GW. Early emergency department treatment of acute asthma with systemic corticosteroids (Cochrane review). *Cochrane Database Syst Rev* 2001;**1**:CD002178 (doi: 10.1002/14651858.CD002178).

25 Manser R, Reid D, Abramson M. Corticosteroids for acute severe asthma in hospitalised patients (Cochrane review). *Cochrane Database Syst Rev* 2001;**1**:CD001740 (doi: 10.1002/14651858.CD001740).

26 Rowe BH, Bretzlaff JA, Bourdon C, Bota GW, Camargo CA, Jr. Magnesium sulfate for treating exacerbations of acute asthma in the emergency department (Cochrane review). *Cochrane Database Syst Rev* 2000;**1**:CD001490 (doi: 10.1002/14651858.CD001490).

27 Alter HJ, Koepsell TD, Hilty WM. Intravenous magnesium as an adjunct in acute bronchospasm: a meta-analysis. *Ann Emerg Med* 2000;**36**:191–7.

28 Rowe BH, Camargo CA, Jr., Multicenter Airway Research Collaboration (MARC) Investigators. The use of magnesium sulfate in acute asthma: rapid uptake of evidence in North American emergency departments. *J Allergy Clin Immunol* 2006;**117**(1):53–8.

29 Rowe BH, Spooner CH, Ducharme FM, Bretzlaff JA, Bota GW. Corticosteroids for preventing relapses following acute exacerbations of asthma. *Cochrane Database Syst Rev* 2007, Issue 3. Art. No.: CD000195.DOI: 10.1002/14651858.CD000195.pub2.

30 Laupacis A, Sackett DL, Roberts RS. An assessment of clinically useful measures of the consequences of treatment. *N Engl J Med* 1988;**318**:1728–33.

31 Verbeek PR, Gerts WH. Nontapering versus tapering prednisone in acute exacerbations of asthma: a pilot study. *J Emerg Med* 1995;**13**:715–19.

32 O'Driscoll BR, Karla S, Wilson M, Pickering CAC, Carrol KB, Woodcock AA. Double-blind trial of steroid tapering in acute asthma. *Lancet* 1993;**341**:324–7.

33 Rowe BH, Bota GW, Fabris L, Therrien SA, Milner RA, Jacono J. Inhaled budesonide in addition to oral corticosteroids to prevent relapse following discharge from the emergency department: a randomized controlled trial. *JAMA* 1999;**281**:2119–26.

34 Salmeron S, Liard R, Elkharrat D, Muir J, Neukirch F, Ellrodt A. Asthma severity and adequacy of management in accident and emergency departments in France: a prospective study. *Lancet* 2001;**358**(9282):629–35.

35 Rowe BH, Bota GW, Clark S, Camargo CA, Jr., for the MARC Investigators. Comparison of Canadian versus US Emergency Department visits for acute asthma. *Can Respir J* 2007;**14**:331–7.

36 Brenner BE, Chavda KK, Camargo CA, Jr. Randomized trial of inhaled flunisolide versus placebo among asthmatics discharged from the emergency department. *Ann Emerg Med* 2000;**36**:417–26.

37 Camargo CA, Jr., for the MARC Investigators. Randomized trial of medium-dose fluticasone vs placebo after an emergency department visit for acute asthma (Abstract). *J Allergy Clin Immunol* 2000;**105**(1/2): S262.

38 Edmonds ML, Camargo CA, Jr., Brenner B, Rowe BH. Inhaled steroids in acute asthma following emergency department discharge (Cochrane review). *Cochrane Database Syst Rev* 2000;**3**:CD002316 (doi: 10.1002/14651858.CD002316).

39 Sin DD, Man SFP. Low-dose inhaled corticosteroid therapy and risk of emergency department visits for asthma. *Arch Intern Med* 2002;**162**:1591–5.

40 Haynes RB, Xao X, Degani A, Kripalani S, Garg A, McDonald HP. Interventions for enhancing medication adherence (Cochrane review). *Cochrane Database Syst Rev* 2005;**4**:CD000011 (doi: 10.1002/14651858.CD000011.pub2).

41 Emond SD, Reed CR, Graff LG, Clark S, Camargo CA, Jr., on behalf of the MARC Investigators. Asthma education in the emergency department. *Ann Emerg Med* 2000;**36**:204–11.

42 Rowe BH, Edmonds ML. Inhaled corticosteroids for acute asthma after emergency department discharge. *Ann Emerg Med* 2000;**36**:477–80.

43 Rowe BH, Wong E, Blitz S, et al. Addition of long-acting beta-agonists to corticosteroid therapy after discharge for acute asthma. *Acad Emerg Med* 2004;**11**:436.

44 Rowe BH, Travers A, Brown JB, et al. Long-acting beta-agonists following ED discharge: a randomized controlled trial. *Acad Emerg Med* 2001;**8**(5):531.

45 Camargo CA, Jr., Smithline HA, Malice MP, Green SA, Reiss TF. A randomized controlled trial of intravenous montelukast in acute asthma. *Am J Respir Crit Care Med* 2003;**167**:528–33.

46 Silverman RA, Nowak RM, Korenblat PE, et al. Zafirlukast treatment for acute asthma: evaluation in a randomized, double-blind, multicenter trial. *Chest* 2004;**126**(5):1480–89.

47 Ducharme FM, Di Salvio F. Anti-leukotriene agents compared to inhaled corticosteroids in the management of recurrent and/or chronic asthma in adults and children (Cochrane review). *Cochrane Database Syst Rev* 2004;**1**:CD002314 (doi: 10.1002/14651858.CD002314.pub2).

48 Clark NM, Gotsch A, Rosenstock IR. Patient, professional and public education on behavioral aspects of asthma: a review of strategies for change and needed research. *J Asthma* 1993;**30**:241–55.

49 Tapp S, Lasserson TJ, Rowe BH. Education interventions for adults who attend the emergency room for acute asthma. *Cochrane Database Syst Rev* 2007;**3**:CD003000 (doi: 10.1002/14651858.CD003000).

50 Gibson PM, Powell J, Coughlan J, et al. Limited (information only) patient education programs for adults with asthma (Cochrane review). *Cochrane Database Syst Rev* 2002;**1**:CD001005 (doi: 10.1002/14651858.CD001005).

51 Gibson PM, Powell H, Coughlan J, et al. Self-management education and regular practitioner review for adults with asthma (Cochrane review). *Cochrane Database Syst Rev* 2002;**3**:CD001117 (doi: 10.1002/14651858.CD001117).

10 COPD Exacerbations

Brian H. Rowe[1] & Rita K. Cydulka[2]

[1]Department of Emergency Medicine, University of Alberta, Edmonton, Canada
[2]Department of Emergency Medicine, MetroHealth Medical Center, Case Western Reserve University School of Medicine, Cleveland, USA

Case scenario

A 76-year-old man presented to the emergency department (ED) with a history of increased shortness of breath, sputum production and wheezing which began after attending a social event 7 days previously. He reported a long history of emphysema following a 45 pack/year history of smoking. He was alert and oriented although only talking in short phrases, with a respiratory rate of 32 breaths/min, heart rate of 110 beats/min and an oxygen saturation of 88%. Visual examination of the chest revealed a wasted man with a barrel chest, and moderate intercostal and subcostal retractions. On auscultation, there was decreased air entry to the bases and diffuse expiratory wheezing throughout all lung fields with prolongation of the expiratory phase. The heart sounds were distant but seemed normal. The remainder of the physical examination was within normal limits. A diagnosis of *COPD exacerbation* was entertained and bronchodilator therapy in addition to intravenous methyl-prednisolone was commenced.

The patient improved minimally with treatment using salbutamol and corticosteroids and the senior house staff asked whether you would consider using antibiotics or non-invasive ventilation in this patient. Review of symptoms revealed that this patient had several previous episodes of acute COPD in the past 12 months presenting to the ED, usually as a result of upper respiratory tract infections. The patient believed that his COPD had been getting worse since he stopped smoking 2 years previously and since his last flu vaccination. He described using his salbutamol puffer several times per day before and after exertion and often in the middle of the night when he woke with coughing episodes. He stated that he does not wish to be intubated and wanted to know if you could give him something else to help his breathing (he was once given a sleeping pill).

Evidence-based Emergency Medicine. Edited by Brian H. Rowe
© 2009 Blackwell Publishing, ISBN: 978-1-4051-6143-5.

Background

Chronic obstructive pulmonary disease (COPD) is one of the few major chronic diseases in which mortality has been increasing over the past decade [1]. Global mortality due to COPD is forecast to more than double over 30 years [2], making it the third leading cause of death worldwide by 2020. Individuals with COPD are prone to exacerbations of their illness which are characterized clinically by symptoms of worsening dyspnea, cough, sputum production and sputum purulence, as well as by worsening of airflow obstruction [3]. It is difficult to predict expected exacerbation rates for individual patients; however, most patients with COPD experience one to four exacerbations per year. As airflow obstruction becomes more severe, exacerbations tend to occur more frequently. In the United States in 2000, there were 8 million physician office or hospital outpatient visits for COPD, 1.5 million ED visits and 673,000 hospitalizations [4].

Patients with COPD commonly present to the ED or other acute care settings with exacerbations, and disease severity is often high. For example, in a recent North American study, over 59% of patients presenting to the ED with COPD symptoms required hospitalization. ED length of stay was nearly 6 hours, and mechanical ventilation was higher than in other acute respiratory presentations such as asthma [5–9]. Given the severe nature and high mortality rates of acute COPD it is not surprising that there are a number of guidelines that have been developed to direct the management of this problem [1,6–10]. Despite the availability of these guidelines, there exists a chasm between what is known and what is practiced. This is in part due to the rapidly changing understanding of the pathophysiology and treatment of COPD and partly due to the difficulty of keeping up with the medical literature and rapidly multiplying number of guidelines in medicine.

Management of acute COPD is aimed at relieving bronchospasm, treating infection/inflammation, maintaining adequate oxygenation, and identifying the cause(s) of the exacerbation. This is usually achieved with diagnostic work-up and concomitant treatment with bronchodilators, corticosteroids, antibiotics and low-dose oxygen therapy.

Clinical questions

In order to address the issues of most relevance to your patient with COPD exacerbation and to help in searching the literature for the evidence regarding these, you structure your questions as recommended in Chapter 1.

1 In adults with exacerbations of COPD assessed in the ED (population), does the treatment with inhaled β-agonist alone (intervention) improve pulmonary function (outcome) compared to treatment with inhaled ipratropium bromide alone (control)?

2 In adults with exacerbations of COPD assessed in the ED (population), does the combination of inhaled β-agonist and anticholinergic agents (intervention) improve pulmonary function (outcome) compared to treatment with inhaled β-agonist or ipratropium bromide alone (control)?

3 In adults with exacerbations of COPD assessed in the ED (population), does the use of intravenous aminophylline (intervention) reduce admission to hospital or improve pulmonary function (outcome) compared to standard care (control)?

4 In adults with exacerbations of COPD assessed in the ED (population), does the use of systemic corticosteroids (intervention) reduce the admissions to hospital or reduce length of stay (outcome) compared to standard care (control)?

5 In adults with exacerbations of COPD assessed in the ED (population), does the use of non-invasive ventilation (intervention) in the ED reduce complications (e.g., admissions, intubation, etc.) compared to standard care (control)?

6 In adults with exacerbations of COPD assessed in the ED (population), do systemic antibiotics (intervention) improve the rate of recovery (outcome) compared to standard care (control)? Who benefits most?

7 In adult COPD patients discharged from the ED (population), does treatment with systemic corticosteroids (intervention) reduce relapse to additional care (outcome) compared to standard care (control)?

8 In adult COPD patients discharged from the ED (population), what is the role of patient education, smoking cessation and immunization (interventions) in reducing further relapses and exacerbations of COPD (outcome) compared to standard care (control)?

General search strategy

You begin to address these questions by searching for evidence in the common electronic databases such as the Cochrane Library, MEDLINE and EMBASE looking specifically for systematic reviews and meta-analyses. The Cochrane Library is particularly rich in high-quality systematic review evidence on numerous aspects of acute COPD. When a systematic review is identified, you also search for recent updates on the Cochrane Library and also search MEDLINE and EMBASE to identify randomized controlled trials

(RCTs) that became available after the publication date of the systematic review. In addition, relevant, updated and evidence-based clinical practice guidelines (CPGs) on acute COPD are accessed to determine the consensus rating of areas lacking evidence.

Searching for evidence synthesis: primary search strategy

- Cochrane Library: COPD AND (topic)
- MEDLINE: COPD AND MEDLINE AND (systematic review OR meta-analysis OR metaanalysis) AND adult AND (topic)

Critical review of the literature

Question 1: In adults with exacerbations of COPD assessed in the ED (population), does the treatment with inhaled β-agonist alone (intervention) improve pulmonary function (outcome) compared to treatment with inhaled ipratropium bromide alone (control)?

Search strategy

- Cochrane Library and MEDLINE: COPD AND (beta-agonists OR ipratropium bromide)

The two most common medication types used to treat the acute bronchospasm associated with COPD exacerbation are short-acting β-agonists, such as albuterol or salbutamol and anticholinergic agents, such as ipratropium bromide. Few studies comparing bronchodilating agents in patients with COPD exacerbation have been performed, thus there is limited data available to help guide the clinician in choosing between these treatment options.

Most guidelines recommend initiating treatment of COPD exacerbation with short-acting β-agonists, such as albuterol or salbutamol [1,6–10]. Although these agents are accepted worldwide as the initial treatment for both asthma and COPD exacerbation, the reversibility of bronchospasm in patients with COPD exacerbation is quite limited compared to that seen in patients with asthma exacerbations. Nevertheless, early treatment focuses on bronchodilation as the short-acting β-agonists and the anticholinergic agents provide rapid – albeit incomplete – relief of bronchospasm.

The authors of a Cochrane review originally designed to assess the benefit of short-acting β_2-agonists alone versus placebo in the treatment of acute COPD exacerbation were unable to find any trials of this kind so the authors analyzed trials comparing the use of inhaled β_2-agonists with that of anticholinergic agents in acute COPD exacerbations [11]. Both β_2-agonists and ipratropium produce small improvements in forced expired volume in 1 second (FEV_1); however, neither agent proved to be superior to the other (weighted mean difference (WMD) = 0.01; 95% CI: −0.22 to 0.23). Minimal side-effects, such as tremor and dry mouth, were reported in the trials included in this review. Clinically important

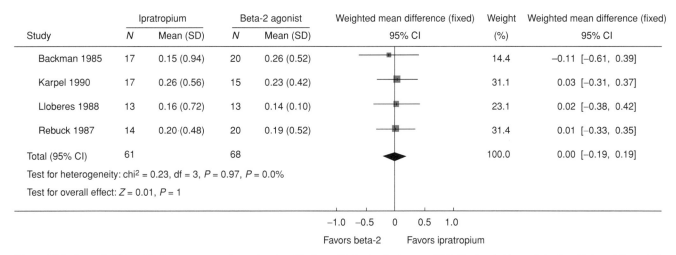

Study	Ipratropium N	Ipratropium Mean (SD)	Beta-2 agonist N	Beta-2 agonist Mean (SD)	Weighted mean difference (fixed) 95% CI	Weight (%)	Weighted mean difference (fixed) 95% CI
Backman 1985	17	0.15 (0.94)	20	0.26 (0.52)		14.4	−0.11 [−0.61, 0.39]
Karpel 1990	17	0.26 (0.56)	15	0.23 (0.42)		31.1	0.03 [−0.31, 0.37]
Lloberes 1988	13	0.16 (0.72)	13	0.14 (0.10)		23.1	0.02 [−0.38, 0.42]
Rebuck 1987	14	0.20 (0.48)	20	0.19 (0.52)		31.4	0.01 [−0.33, 0.35]
Total (95% CI)	61		68			100.0	0.00 [−0.19, 0.19]

Test for heterogeneity: chi^2 = 0.23, df = 3, P = 0.97, P = 0.0%

Test for overall effect: Z = 0.01, P = 1

−1.0 −0.5 0 0.5 1.0

Favors beta-2   Favors ipratropium

Figure 10.1 Change in FEV$_1$ at 90 minutes comparing ipratropium bromide alone with β$_2$-agonists in acute COPD. (Reprinted with permission from McCrory & Brown [12], © Cochrane Library.)

clinical outcomes, such as symptom or dyspnea scores or need for hospitalization, were not reported.

Another review, which included five studies involving 129 patients, compared the short-term effects of β$_2$-agonists with ipratropium bromide [12]. Again, the authors reported no difference in FEV$_1$ outcomes between the two medications in the treatment of acute exacerbation of COPD within the first 90 minutes (WMD = 0.00; 95% CI: −0.19 to 0.19) (Fig. 10.1).

In summary, clinicians may choose either a β$_2$-agonist or an anticholinergic agent as the initial treatment agent in acute COPD exacerbation. While most clinicians use nebulized agents as their preferred route of administration, a Cochrane systematic review in acute asthma demonstrates similar outcomes (admissions and pulmonary functions) using either nebulizers or inhalers with spacer devices [13]. It seems reasonable to substitute nebulizers in the acute setting, although elderly patients with COPD may have difficulty coordinating an inhaler and spacer during exacerbation (Table 10.1). Concerns regarding transmissibility of airborne pathogens may limit the use of nebulizer therapy in the future.

Question 2: In adults with exacerbations of COPD assessed in the ED (population), does the combination of inhaled β-agonist and anticholinergic agents (intervention) improve pulmonary function (outcome) compared to treatment with inhaled β-agonist or ipratropium bromide alone (control)?

Search strategy

• Cochrane Library and MEDLINE: COPD AND ipratropium bromide AND β-agonists

A frequent and important clinical question in the treatment of acute COPD exacerbation is whether there is an *additive benefit*

of using ipratropium bromide with inhaled β$_2$-agonists, as seen in acute asthma. Meta-analysis in adults with asthma demonstrated a modest beneficial effect (reduced admissions, improved pulmonary functions) when ipratropium bromide was added to inhaled β$_2$-agonists in the acute setting [14]. A Cochrane systematic review has examined the issue of combining bronchodilators in exacerbations of COPD [12]. Three studies involving 118 patients, looking at short-term effects, found no advantage of adding ipratropium bromide to β$_2$-agonist treatment on FEV$_1$ outcomes at 90 minutes (WMD = 0.02 L; 95% CI: −0.08 to 0.12) (Fig. 10.2). No additional differences were noted at 24 hours (WMD = 0.05 L; 95% CI: −0.14 to 0.05). Side-effects were minimal (dry mouth and tremor for ipratropium bromide-treated patients) and there were no significant hemodynamic concerns or reported adverse events. The degree of bronchodilation achieved with ipratropium bromide was similar to that reported with short-acting β$_2$-agonists. The combination of a β$_2$-agonist and ipratropium did not increase the effect on FEV$_1$ over either intervention used alone. Even in the setting of stable COPD, there is only minimal evidence of additional bronchodilation with combination therapy [15–17].

In summary, physician and/or patient preference will likely guide the treatment approach used. Clinicians should be cautioned to observe patients for signs of β-agonist toxicity (tremor and tachycardia).

Question 3: In adults with exacerbations of COPD assessed in the ED (population), does the use of intravenous aminophylline (intervention) reduce admission to hospital or improve pulmonary function (outcome) compared to standard care (control)?

Search strategy

• Cochrane Library: COPD AND aminophylline

Drug	Admitted	Discharged
Methyl-prednisolone	80–125 mg IV	N/A
Hydrocortisone	250–500 mg IV	N/A
Prednisone	40–60 mg/dose	40–60 mg/day (for outpatients: 7–10 days; tapering not generally required)
Methyl-xanthines	Not recommended in the ED	Continue oral agents if patients receiving prior to ED visit
Albuterol/salbutamol	Single treatment: 2.5–5.0 mg nebulized (0.5–1.0 ml of 0.5% solution) every 20 minutes	
	Inhaled: 4–6 activations using a holding chamber every 20 minutes	Inhaled: 1–2 activations via a holding chamber qid
Ipratropium bromide	Nebulizer: 250–500 mg every 20 minutes	Inhaled: 1–2 activations using a holding chamber qid
	Inhaled: 4–6 activations via a holding chamber every 20 minutes	
Antibiotics	First-line agents recommended to be started for severe cases	First-line agents recommended to be continued in hospital for 7–10 days
NIV	Respiratory failure (see text)	N/A
Supplemental oxygen	Low flow titrated to SaO_2	Variable guidelines for chronic domiciliary oxygen

Table 10.1 Summary of typical dosing recommendations for effective treatments of exacerbations of COPD.

ED, emergency department; IV, intravenous; N/A, not applicable; NIV, non-invasive ventilation; SaO_2, oxygen saturation; qid, four times daily.

Methyl-xanthines act as non-selective phosphodiesterase inhibitors, although they also have been reported to have a range of non-bronchodilator actions. Despite aminophylline's widespread clinical use in the past, the role of methyl-xanthines in the treatment of exacerbations of COPD is that of a distant second-line intravenous therapy, only to be considered when there is inadequate response to short-acting inhaled bronchodilators.

A Cochrane systematic review of four trials involving 169 subjects suggests that intravenous aminophylline yields no additional benefits during acute exacerbation of COPD [18]. The mean change in FEV_1 at 2 hours was similar in aminophylline- and placebo-treated groups; however, at 3 days, FEV_1 was briefly increased. Non-significant reductions in hospitalization (RR = 1.15; 95% CI: 0.17 to 7.85) and length of stay were offset by a non-significant increase in relapses at 1 week. Changes in symptom scores were neither statistically or clinically significant. Adverse effects were dramatically increased with the use of methyl-xanthines. Nausea and vomiting were increased five fold over patients given

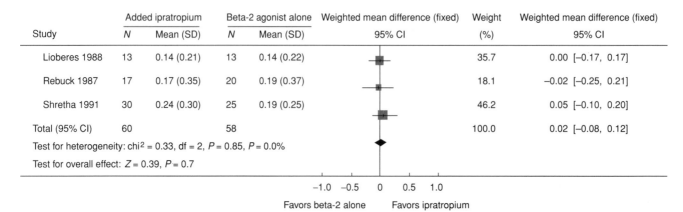

Figure 10.2 Change in FEV_1 at 90 minutes comparing ipratropium bromide combined with β_2-agonists with β_2-agonists alone in acute COPD. (Reprinted with permission from McCrory & Brown [12], © Cochrane Library.)

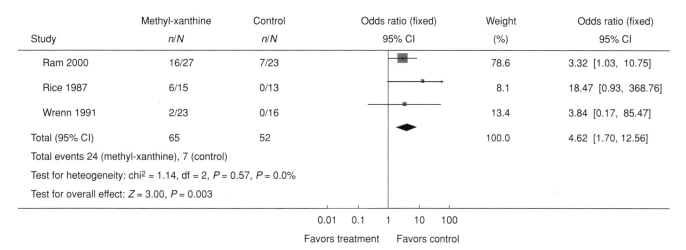

Study	Methyl-xanthine n/N	Control n/N	Odds ratio (fixed) 95% CI	Weight (%)	Odds ratio (fixed) 95% CI
Ram 2000	16/27	7/23		78.6	3.32 [1.03, 10.75]
Rice 1987	6/15	0/13		8.1	18.47 [0.93, 368.76]
Wrenn 1991	2/23	0/16		13.4	3.84 [0.17, 85.47]
Total (95% CI)	65	52		100.0	4.62 [1.70, 12.56]

Total events 24 (methyl-xanthine), 7 (control)

Test for heteogeneity: chi2 = 1.14, df = 2, P = 0.57, P = 0.0%

Test for overall effect: Z = 3.00, P = 0.003

0.01   0.1   1   10   100

Favors treatment   Favors control

Figure 10.3 Adverse events (nausea/vomiting) comparing methyl-xanthines with standard care in COPD exacerbations. (Reprinted with permission from Barr et al. [18], © Cochrane Library.)

placebo (OR = 4.62; 95% CI: 1.7 to 12.56) (Fig. 10.3). Non-significant increases in tremor, palpitations and arrhythmias were also noted.

Overall, while still recommended in some recent literature [2], available clinical trial data have failed to demonstrate the efficacy of methyl-xanthines for the treatment of COPD exacerbations. Theoretical benefits of methyl-xanthines on lung function and symptoms were not demonstrated and clinically important adverse effects were significantly increased.

Question 4: In adults with exacerbations of COPD assessed in the ED (population), does the use of systemic corticosteroids (intervention) reduce the admissions to hospital or reduce length of stay (outcome) compared to standard care (control)?

Search strategy

- Cochrane Library and MEDLINE: COPD AND corticosteroids

Evidence for the effectiveness of corticosteroids in the treatment of acute COPD exacerbation is not as compelling as the evidence for their effectiveness in the treatment of acute asthma. A Cochrane review examined 10 trials that involved over 900 adult patients in RCTs in acute COPD [19]. Six of the studies specifically examined patients admitted to hospital, two involved outpatients and two involved ED patients. Outcomes reported varied, and few were common to all studies. The most commonly reported airway measurement was the FEV_1 between 6 and 72 hours after treatment and this showed a significant treatment benefit for corticosteroids (WMD = 40 ml; 95% CI: 80 to 200) although this difference was not sustained. The number needed to treat (NNT) to prevent one treatment failure was nine (95% CI: 7 to 14). One adverse outcome was reported for every six patients treated (95% CI: 4 to 10). Adverse outcomes associated with corticosteroid use included hyperglycemia (OR = 5.48; 95% CI: 1.58 to 8.96), increased appetite

(OR = 3.09; 95% CI: 1.47 to 6.47), weight gain (OR = 10.18; 95% CI: 1.25 to 82.68) and insomnia (OR = 3.53; 95% CI: 1.65 to 7.53). There were also half as many treatment failures within 30 days for patients treated with corticosteroids (OR = 0.48; 95% CI: 0.34 to 0.68); however, only seven trials reported this outcome and there was significant heterogeneity among them ($I^2 = 43.7\%$). Others have demonstrated reduced admission rates with the administration of systemic corticosteroids [20,21], decreased hospital length of stay [20,21] and reduced treatment failure in hospitalized patients [19]. There were no demonstrated differences for other outcomes, including mortality (RR = 0.85; 95% CI: 0.47 to 1.54), quality of life and exercise tolerance [19].

Despite the fact that there was significant heterogeneity among the studies, the data support the administration of corticosteroids in the treatment of acute exacerbations of COPD, especially in patients requiring hospitalization. The current data do not address whether the improved outcomes outweigh the increased likelihood of adverse drug reactions. Since oral corticosteroids are as effective as intravenous agents, intravenous corticosteroids should be reserved for patients who are too dyspneic to swallow or those who have been intubated. Most physicians treating acute COPD select intravenous methyl-prednisolone to avoid the mineralo-corticoid effects of the steroid treatment, although the evidence for both dosing and route of administration is anecdotal.

Question 5: In adults with exacerbations of COPD assessed in the ED (population), does the use of non-invasive ventilation (intervention) in the ED reduce complications (e.g., admissions, intubation, etc.) compared to standard care (control)?

Search strategy

- Cochrane Library and MEDLINE: COPD AND (non-invasive ventilation OR NIV OR NIPPV)

Non-invasive ventilation (NIV), also referred to as non-invasive positive pressure ventilation (NPPV), uses a full facial or nasal mask that administers ventilatory support from a flow generator. It enhances ventilation by unloading fatigued ventilatory muscles. NIV has been used increasingly over the past decade as adjunct therapy for patients with acute dyspnea in the ED, especially for exacerbations of heart failure [22], asthma [23] and COPD [24].

Evidence from 14 studies with 758 patients shows that the use of NIV results in decreased mortality (RR = 0.52; 95% CI: 0.35 to 0.76) (Fig. 10.4), decreased need for intubation (RR = 0.41; 95% CI: 0.33 to 0.53), reduction in treatment failure (RR = 0.48; 95% CI: 0.37 to 0.63), and rapid improvement within the first hour in pH (WMD = 0.03; 95% CI: 0.02 to 0.04), $PaCO_2$ (WMD = -0.40 kPa; 95% CI: -0.78 to -0.03) and respiratory rate (WMD = -3.08 breaths/min; 95% CI: -4.26 to -1.89) [24]. In addition, complications associated with treatment (RR = 0.38; 95% CI: 0.24 to 0.60) and length of hospital stay (WMD = -3.24 days; 95% CI: -4.42 to -2.06) was also reduced in this group. The NNT to avoid one treatment failure was five (95% CI: 4 to 6).

All patients in these studies were treated in hospital settings and received aggressive medical management for their condition in addition to NIV. The expiratory pressure setting was kept constant and ranged from 2 to 6 cmH$_2$O, and the inspiratory pressure ranged from 9 to 30 cmH$_2$O. There is strong evidence supporting the use of NIV as an early intervention along with usual medical care in all suitable patients for the management of respiratory failure secondary to an acute exacerbation of COPD. A trial of

NIV should be considered early in the course of respiratory failure and before severe acidosis ensures, as a means of reducing the risk of endotracheal intubation, treatment failure and mortality. It is important to keep in mind that NIV has some limitations: 13–29% of patients are unable to tolerate the mask and facial skin ulcers are caused by mask pressure. In addition, NIV initiation requires a conscious and cooperative patient who can protect his or her airway, is hemodynamically stable and does not have life-threatening hypoxemia. In cases where NIV is not appropriate, rapid sequence endotracheal intubation by a physician experienced at securing an airway in emergency conditions should be employed. As a side note, the transmission of severe acute respiratory syndrome (SARS) during the 2003 outbreak due to respiratory droplets created by nebulization, NIV and mechanical ventilation temporarily discouraged NIV use in some centers. Moreover, respiratory isolation precautions for special populations may be warranted.

In summary, NIV is an effective treatment for patients with severe COPD exacerbations and impending respiratory failure in order to reduce intubations, length of stay and complications.

Question 6: In adults with exacerbations of COPD assessed in the ED (population), do systemic antibiotics (intervention) improve the rate of recovery (outcome) compared to standard care (control)? Who benefits most?

Study	NPPV n/N	UMC n/N	Relative risk (fixed) 95% CI	Weight (%)	Relative risk (fixed) 95% CI
Avdeev 1998	7/29	12/29		10.6	0.58 [0.27, 1.27]
Barbe 1996	4/14	0/10		0.5	6.60 [0.39, 110.31]
Bott 1993	5/30	13/30		11.4	0.38 [0.16, 0.94]
Brochard 1995	12/43	33/42		29.4	0.36 [0.21, 0.59]
Celikel 1998	1/15	6/15		5.3	0.17 [0.02, 1.22]
Dikensoy 2002	4/19	7/17		6.5	0.51 [0.18, 1.45]
Plant 2000	22/118	35/118		30.8	0.63 [0.39, 1.00]
Thys 2002	0/7	5/5		5.5	0.07 [0.00, 1.01]
Total (95% CI)	275	266		100.0	0.48 [0.37, 0.63]

Total events 55 (NPPV), 111 (UMC)

Test for heteogeneity: chi^2 = 9.55, df = 7, P = 0.22, P = 26.7%

Test for overall effect: Z = 5.23, P = 0.00001

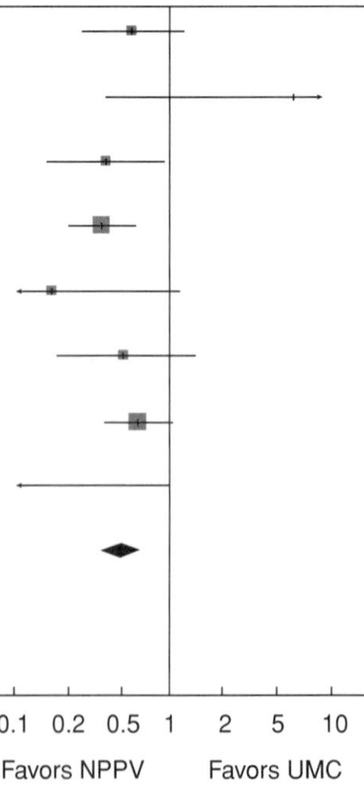

0.1 0.2 0.5 1 2 5 10

Favors NPPV   Favors UMC

Figure 10.4 Reduction in clinical failures with NIV plus standard care versus standard care alone in acute COPD. NPPV, non-invasive positive pressure ventilation; UMC, usual medical care. (Reprinted with permission from Ram et al. [23], © Cochrane Library.)

Bronchoscopic studies have shown that at least 50% of patients with COPD have bacteria in high concentrations in their lower airways during exacerbations. The most common cause of exacerbation is infection. Although a significant number of COPD patients have bacterial colonization of their lower airways while in the stable phase of their disease, studies indicate that the bacterial burden increases during exacerbation [25–27]. Three bacterial pathogens, namely *Streptococcus pneumoniae*, *Haemophilus influenzae* and *Moraxella catarrhalis*, are frequently implicated in flare-ups of COPD; however, these bacteria can be found in the upper respiratory tracts of healthy people and are often found in the sputum of patients with COPD during periods of clinical quiescence [28]. Determining whether these bacteria are responsible for clinical deterioration is therefore often difficult.

A meta-analysis of nine randomized trials and 1101 patients compared the outcomes in patients treated with antibiotics compared to placebo for exacerbation of COPD [29]. The meta-analysis revealed a modest overall summary effect size (ES) when comparing antibiotics with placebo (ES = 0.22; 95% CI: 0.10 to 0.34), indicating a clinical benefit (reduction in "clinical failures") in the antibiotic-treated group. A modest summary ES for changes in peak expiratory flow (PEF) was also demonstrated (ES = 0.19; 95% CI: 0.03 to 0.35) in favor of the antibiotic group. This translates to a difference in PEF of only 11 L/min (95% CI: 4.96 to 16.54). This evidence is based on trials using first-line, older and less expensive antibiotics in acute COPD such as amoxicillin, trimethoprim/sulfamethoxazole and tetracycline.

A more recent meta-analysis of 11 trials with 917 patients demonstrated significantly lower mortality (RR = 0.23; 95% CI: 0.10 to 0.52) with a NNT of eight (95% CI: 6 to 17), fewer treatment failures (RR = 0.47; 95% CI: 0.36 to 0.62) with a NNT of three (95% CI: 3 to 5), and reduced sputum purulence (RR = 0.56; 95% CI: 0.41 to 0.77) with a NNT of eight (95% CI: 6 to 17) associated with antibiotic use over placebo. These results did not appear to be influenced by the antibiotic choice. Antibiotic use was not associated with improvement in either arterial blood gases or PEF, and diarrhea among patients using antibiotics was triple that of patients not using antibiotics (RR = 2.86; 95% CI: 1.06 to 7.76). This review demonstrates that in exacerbations of COPD associated with increased cough and sputum purulence, antibiotic therapy, regardless of choice, significantly decreases short-term mortality, treatment failure and sputum purulence. This effect was greatest in the sickest group of patients who are hospitalized. In fact analysis restricted to community-based studies did not identify differences between antibiotic and placebo. Caution is advised as the included trials had important differences in selection of patients, choice of

antibiotic and only a small number of trials were included in the review.

The general recommendations from guidelines [30] are to choose an antibiotic that reflects local antibiotic sensitivity patterns to the three most common pathogens, *S. pneumoniae*, *H. influenzae* and *M. catarrhalis*. All patients requiring hospitalization should receive antibiotics; first-line agents are indicated in most cases (see Table 10.1). In patients with mild COPD exacerbations, *S. pneumoniae* is predominant. In patients with severely diminished FEV$_1$, more frequent exacerbations and/or co-morbid diseases, *H. influenzae* and *M. catarrhalis* may be more frequent [6]. *Pseudomonas aeruginosa* should be considered in patients with severe airway limitation, recent hospitalization, frequent administration of antibiotics (four courses in the last year), severe COPD exacerbations, and isolation of *P. aeruginosa* during a previous exacerbation or colonization during a stable period [1].

According to the Anthonisen criteria for classification of COPD exacerbations, patients with exacerbations of COPD not requiring hospitalization should be treated with antibiotics if they have a combination of increased dyspnea, increased sputum volume and increased sputum purulence, or if they have two of these three symptoms [3]. Newer guidelines downplay the role of antibiotics in this presentation, so emergency physicians need to carefully consider and individualize their management approaches [31].

Question 7: In adult COPD patients discharged from the ED (population), does treatment with systemic corticosteroids (intervention) reduce relapse to additional care (outcome) compared to standard care (control)?

Approximately 50–60% of all patients seen in large-volume North American EDs will require admission to hospital [5]. Even when discharged, approximately 20–30% of patients treated for acute COPD will relapse within 4 weeks of ED discharge, likely due to unresolved inflammation and infection [5]. There exists evidence to support the prescription of systemic corticosteroids following ED discharge for an acute exacerbation to reduce the risk of relapse (Fig. 10.5) [19]. A Cochrane review included studies with patients from a variety of settings (admitted patients, ED patients and outpatients), with a wide range of severity, and has been summarized above. The most impressive RCT included in this analysis examined the effect of adding corticosteroids to standard care in 147 patients discharged after treatment for acute COPD [32]. Patients were treated with first-generation antibiotics and bronchodilators and were randomized to oral prednisone (40 mg daily for 10 days) or placebo. Patients discharged with systemic corticosteroids had fewer relapses/episodes of unscheduled care (43%

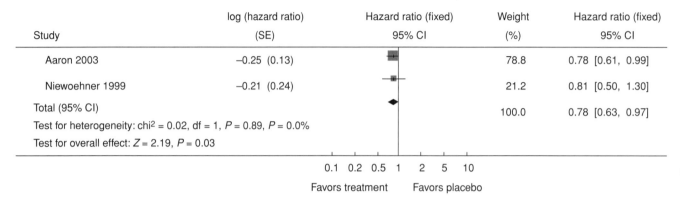

Study	log (hazard ratio) (SE)	Hazard ratio (fixed) 95% CI	Weight (%)	Hazard ratio (fixed) 95% CI
Aaron 2003	−0.25 (0.13)		78.8	0.78 [0.61, 0.99]
Niewoehner 1999	−0.21 (0.24)		21.2	0.81 [0.50, 1.30]
Total (95% CI)			100.0	0.78 [0.63, 0.97]

Test for heterogeneity: chi² = 0.02, df = 1, *P* = 0.89, *P* = 0.0%
Test for overall effect: *Z* = 2.19, *P* = 0.03

0.1 0.2 0.5 1 2 5 10
Favors treatment   Favors placebo

Figure 10.5 Reduction in clinical failures with corticosteroids plus standard care versus standard care alone in acute COPD. (Reprinted with permission from Wood-Baker et al. [19], © Cochrane Library.)

vs 27%, *P* = 0.05), representing an absolute risk reduction of 16% and a NNT of six. In addition, the use of corticosteroids significantly improved pulmonary function and dyspnea at 10 days, and quality of life up to 30 days.

In summary, a short course of corticosteroids should be prescribed to patients after an acute exacerbation of COPD requiring a visit to the emergency department. While short-term corticosteroids are generally well tolerated, adverse effects associated with these agents are not uncommon, as described above [19]. As always, the beneficial short-term effects of oral corticosteroids on the rate of relapse, dyspnea and pulmonary function should be balanced against the risk of adverse effects.

Data that elucidate the relative effectiveness of various regimens do not exist. It seems reasonable to prescribe a fixed once- or twice-daily dose of 40–60 mg of oral corticosteroids for 7–10 days (see Table 10.1).

Question 8: In adult COPD patients discharged from the ED (population), what is the role of patient education, smoking cessation and immunization (interventions) in reducing further relapses and exacerbations of COPD (outcome) compared to standard care (control)?

Search strategy

- Cochrane Library and MEDLINE: COPD AND education
- Cochrane Library: COPD AND (influenza immunization OR smoking cessation)

The ED visit for COPD is an opportunity to re-evaluate a patient's ongoing chronic care plan. Communication between the emergency physician and the primary care physician will facilitate this process. The evidence in this section arises from the chronic stable literature since limited research in the area of patient education, smoking cessation and respiratory rehabilitation has been performed in the setting of COPD exacerbations. Encouraging smoking cessation [33], influenza vaccination [34] and educat-

ing patients [35] seem like reasonable and cost-effective strategies for decreasing the number of COPD exacerbations. In addition, encouraging adherence to prescribed, evidence-based medication regimens is another important factor associated with treatment success [36].

Influenza vaccination is an effective and cost-effective public health intervention. The Cochrane review on this subject included six studies specifically addressing influenza vaccination in patients with COPD. Vaccination in COPD patients resulted in a significant reduction in the total number of exacerbations compared with those who received placebo (WMD = −0.37; 95% CI: −0.64 to −0.11) [34]. Given this evidence, all patients who present with exacerbation of COPD who have not yet been immunized should be advised to receive influenza immunization as soon as feasible.

The Cochrane review specifically addressing smoking cessation for patients with COPD examined all RCTs in which smoking cessation was compared with placebo or standard care [33]. The authors reported evidence that a combination of psychosocial interventions and pharmacological interventions is superior to no treatment or to psychosocial interventions alone. All patients who present for treatment of exacerbations of COPD and continue to smoke should be encouraged to stop smoking and seek assistance from their regular physician.

Educational interventions – with a focus on self-management – have only been studied in the stable disease state in COPD. Self-management education reduced the need for rescue medication, and led to an increased use of courses of oral steroids and antibiotics for respiratory symptoms [37]. The studies showed no effect of self-management education on hospital admissions, emergency room visits, days lost from work and lung function. Inconclusive results were observed on health-related quality of life, COPD symptoms and use of other health care resources such as doctor and nurse visits. Another Cochrane review demonstrated evidence of a positive effect of action plans on self-management knowledge in the areas of recognition of a severe exacerbation (mean difference (MD) = 2.50; 95% CI: 1.04 to 3.96), self-action in severe exacerbations (MD = 1.50; 95% CI: 0.62 to 2.38), and the use of antibiotics (MD = 6.00; 95% CI: 2.68 to 9.32) [38]. Patients with an action plan were more likely to initiate antibiotics (OR = 10.16; 95% CI: 2.02 to 51.09) and/or oral steroids (OR = 6.58; 95% CI: 1.29 to 33.62) when needed. However, there was no significant effect of an action plan on health care utilization, health-related quality of life, lung function, functional capacity, symptom scores, mortality, anxiety or depression. No trials studied the number of exacerbations, length of exacerbations or days lost from work as an outcome.

In summary, pulmonary rehabilitation for patients with COPD is effective in reducing further exacerbations and improving quality of life [39]. Emergency physicians should consider referral for rehabilitation for patients with severe COPD after their exacerbation stabilizes. Finally, compliance assessment and efforts to enhance adherence to medications and lifestyle modifications remain important issues for patients with COPD [36].

Conclusions

The patient in the aforementioned case was treated with non-invasive ventilation for 9 hours and admitted to the hospital. Intubation was not required; and he recovered without incident, albeit slowly. After hospital discharge, the patient was referred for pulmonary rehabilitation and returned to baseline function within several weeks of hospital admission.

COPD is a chronic and frequently debilitating disease. Despite the high morbidity and increasing mortality from this disease, the evidence base for acute therapeutic options is based on a limited number of trials. Many of the trials included in systematic reviews in this area are small or methodologically flawed. In some cases, multiple, similar, small trials have been combined appropriately in systematic reviews to produce clarity (e.g., NIV in acute respiratory failure). In many areas of study, the resultant wide confidence intervals suggest insufficient sample size to draw appropriate conclusions. Moreover, in some areas of study, (e.g., the additive benefit of ipratropium bromide to β_2-agonists) the evidence remains scant. Overall, therapeutic options during acute COPD exacerbation remain an area that is under-studied. More research is required to better guide the complex management decisions that these patients require. Future studies should focus on clinically meaningful issues and endpoints.

The treatment approaches outlined above to control bronchial inflammation and infection provide an approach for expediting return to activities, reduced symptoms and improved quality of life in the sub-acute period following an exacerbation. In addition, referral to smoking cessation programs, immunization and prevention programs, and rehabilitation programs, along with prescribing with appropriate preventive medication will provide patients with the best opportunity possible to maintain a reasonable lifestyle.

Summary for clinicians
• Bronchodilators (short-acting β-agonists and anticholinergics) produce small and clinically similar increases in FEV_1.

• Evidence does not support the combination of short-acting β-agonists and anticholinergics in the acute care setting.
• Methyl-xanthines increase adverse effects, without evidence of clinical benefit.
• Systemic corticosteroids reduce treatment failure in severe COPD.
• NIV decreases the likelihood of intubation and intensive care admissions in selected patients.
• Oral corticosteroids after discharge increase FEV_1 and reduce treatment failure but increase the likelihood of adverse effects.
• Antibiotics during exacerbation decrease clinical failures and increase PEF rate, although the overall effect is small. Use should be reserved for patients requiring hospitalization or patients with two or more Anthonisen criteria.
• Secondary preventive measures, such as patient education, smoking cessation and immunization, are considered important in preventing future exacerbations in spite of limited supporting evidence.

Conflicts of interest

Dr. Rowe is supported by a 21st Century Canada Research Chair in Emergency Airway Diseases from the Government of Canada (Ottawa, Canada). Dr. Rowe has received financial support from a variety of groups for participation in conferences, consulting and medical research. These groups include government agencies, private foundations, professional organizations and industry. Since 2000, industry sponsors with an interest in COPD included AstraZeneca, Abbott and GlaxoSmithKline, and Boehringer-Ingelheim. Dr. Rowe does not own stocks or other ownership interest in any of these companies.

Dr. Cydulka has received financial support from a variety of groups for participation in conferences, consulting and medical research. These groups include government agencies, private foundations, professional organizations and industry. Since 2000, industry sponsors with an interest in COPD included Boehringer-Ingelheim. Dr. Cydulka does not own stocks or other ownership interest in this company.

References

1 NHLBI WHO Workshop Report. *Global Strategy for the Diagnosis, Management, and Prevention of Chronic Obstructive Pulmonary Disease.* 2006:1–88.

2 Stoller JK. Clinical practice. Acute exacerbations of chronic obstructive pulmonary disease. *N Engl J Med* 2002;**346**(13):988–94.

3 Anthonisen N, Manfreda J, Warren P, Hershfield E, Harding G, Nelson N. Antibiotic therapy in exacerbation of chronic obstructive pulmonary disease. *Ann Intern Med* 1987;**106**:196–204.

4 Mannino DM, Homa DM, Akinbami LJ, Ford ES, Redd SC. Chronic obstructive pulmonary disease surveillance – United States, 1971–2000. *MMWR CDC Surveill Summ* 2002;**51**(SS-6):1–16.

5 Cydulka RK, Rowe BH, Clark S, Emerman CL, Camargo CA, Jr. Emergency department management of acute exacerbations of chronic obstructive pulmonary disease in the elderly: the Multicenter Airway Research Collaboration. *J Am Geriatr Soc* 2003;**51**(7):908–16.

6 Balter MS, LaForge J, Low DE, Mandell L, Grossman RF, the Chronic Bronchitis Working Group on behalf of the Canadian Thoracic Society and the Canadian Infectious Disease Society. Canadian guidelines for the management of acute exacerbations of chronic bronchitis. *Can Respir J* 2003;**10**(Suppl B):3B–32B.

7 Roche N, Lepage T, Bourcereau J, Terrioux P. Guidelines versus clinical practice in the treatment of chronic obstructive pulmonary disease. *Eur Respir J* 2001;**18**(6):903–8.

8 Laitinen LA, Koskela K. Chronic bronchitis and chronic obstructive pulmonary disease: Finnish National Guidelines for Prevention and Treatment 1998–2007. *Respir Med* 1999;**93**(5):297–332.

9 The COPD Guidelines Group of the Standard of Care Committee of the BTS. BTS guidelines for the management of chronic obstructive pulmonary disease. *Thorax* 1997;**52**(Suppl 5):S1–28.

10 American Thoracic Society. Standards for the diagnosis and care of patients with chronic obstructive pulmonary disease. *Am J Resp Crit Care* 1995;**152**(Suppl):S77–120.

11 Brown CD, McCrory D, White J. Inhaled short-acting beta2-agonists versus ipratropium for acute exacerbations of chronic obstructive pulmonary disease. *Cochrane Database Syst Rev* 2001;**1**:CD002984 (doi: 10.1002/14651858.CD002984).

12 McCrory DC, Brown CD. Anticholinergic bronchodilators versus beta2-sympathomimetic agents for acute exacerbations of chronic obstructive pulmonary disease (Cochrane review). *Cochrane Database Syst Rev* 2003;**1**: CD003900 (doi: 10.1002/14651858.CD003900).

13 Cates CJ, Crilly JA, Rowe BH. Holding chambers (spacers) versus nebulisers for beta-agonist treatment of acute asthma. *Cochrane Database Syst Rev* 2006;**2**:CD000052 (doi: 10.1002/14651858.CD000052.pub2).

14 Stoodley RG, Aaron SD, Dales RE. The role of ipratropium bromide in the emergency management of acute asthma exacerbation: a meta-analysis of randomized clinical trials. *Ann Emerg Med* 1999;**34**(1):8–18.

15 Easton PA, Jadue C, Dhingra S, Anthonisen NR. A comparison of the bronchodilating effects of a beta-2 adrenergic agent (albuterol) and an anticholinergic agent (ipratropium bromide), given by aerosol alone or in sequence. *N Engl J Med* 1986;**315**:735–9.

16 The COMBIVENT Inhalation Solution Study Group. Routine nebulized ipratropium and albuterol together are better than either alone in COPD. *Chest* 1997;**112**:1514–21.

17 Appleton S, Jones T, Poole P, et al. Ipratropium bromide versus short acting beta-2 agonists for stable chronic obstructive pulmonary disease (Cochrane review). *Cochrane Database Syst Rev* 2006;**2**:CD001387 (doi: 10.1002/14651858.CD001387.pub2).

18 Barr RG, Rowe BH, Camargo CA, Jr. Methylxanthines for exacerbations of chronic obstructive pulmonary disease (Cochrane review). *Cochrane Database Syst Rev* 2003;**2**:CD002168 (doi: 10.1002/14651858.CD002168).

19 Wood-Baker RR, Gibson PG, Hannay M, Walters EH, Walters JAE. Systemic corticosteroids for acute exacerbations of chronic obstructive pulmonary disease (Cochrane review). *Cochrane Database Syst Rev* 2005;**1**:CD001288 (doi: 10.1002/14651858.CD001288.pub2).

20 Bullard MJ, Liaw SJ, Tsai YH, Min HP. Early corticosteroid use in acute exacerbations of chronic airflow obstruction. *Am J Emerg Med* 1996;**14**(2):139–43.

21 Niewoehner D, Erbland M, et al. Effect of systemic glucocorticoids on exacerbations of chronic obstructive pulmonary disease. *N Engl J Med* 1999;**340**:1941–7.

22 Collins SP, Mielniczuk LM, Whittingham HA, Boseley ME, Schramm DR, Storrow AB. The use of noninvasive ventilation in emergency department patients with acute cardiogenic pulmonary edema: a systematic review. *Ann Emerg Med* 2006;**48**(3):260–69.

23 Ram FSF, Wellington SR, Rowe BH, Wedzicha JA. Non-invasive positive pressure ventilation for treatment of respiratory failure due to severe acute exacerbations of asthma. *Cochrane Database Syst Rev* 2005;**1**:CD004360 (doi: 10.1002/14651858.CD004360.pub2).

24 Ram FSF, Lightowler JV, Wedzicha JA. Non-invasive positive pressure ventilation for treatment of chronic obstructive pulmonary disease (Cochrane review). *Cochrane Database Syst Rev* 2004;**3**:CD004104 (do: 10.1002/14651858.CD004104.pub3).

25 Varia M, Wilson S, Sarwal S, et al. Investigation of a nosocomial outbreak of severe acute respiratory syndrome (SARS) in Toronto, Canada. *Can Med Assoc J* 2003;**169**(4):285–92.

26 Sethi S, Evans N, Grant BJB, Murphy TF. New strains of bacteria and exacerbations of chronic obstructive pulmonary disease. *N Engl J Med* 2002;**347**:465–71.

27 Monso ERJ, Rosell A, Manterola J, et al. Bacterial infection in chronic obstructive pulmonary disease. A study of stable and exacerbated outpatients using the protected specimen brush. *Am J Respir Crit Care Med* 1995;**152**(4):1316–20.

28 Murphy TF, Brauer AL, Schiffmacher AT, Sethi S. Persistent colonization by *Haemophilus influenzae* in chronic obstructive pulmonary disease. *Am J Respir Crit Care Med* 2004;**170**(3):266–72.

29 Saint S, Bent S, Vittinghoff E, Grady D. Antibiotics in chronic obstructive pulmonary disease exacerbations. *JAMA* 1995;**273**:957–60.

30 Global Initiative for Chronic Obstructive Lung Disease. *Global Strategy for the Diagnosis, Management, and Prevention of Chronic Obstructive Pulmonary Disease.* Copyright © 2006 MCR VISION Inc., 2006.

31 O'Donnell DE, Hernandez P, Aaron S, et al. Canadian Thoracic Society recommendations for management of chronic obstructive pulmonary disease – 2007 update. *Can Respir J* 2003;**10**:183–5.

32 Aaron S, Vandemheen K, Hebert P, et al. Outpatient oral prednisone after emergency treatment of chronic obstructive pulmonary disease. *N Engl J Med* 2003;**348**:2618–25.

33 van der Meer RM, Wagena EJ, Ostelo RWJG, Jacobs JE, van Schayck CP. Smoking cessation for chronic obstructive pulmonary disease (Cochrane review). *Cochrane Database Syst Rev* 2001;**1**:CD002999 (doi: 10.1002/14651858.CD002999).

34 Poole PJ, Chacko E, Wood-Baker R, Cates CJ. Influenza vaccine for patients with chronic obstructive pulmonary disease (Cochrane review). *Cochrane Database Syst Rev* 2006;**1**:CD002733 (doi: 10.1002/14651858.CD002733.pub2).

35 Blackstock F, Webster KE. Disease-specific health education for COPD: a systematic review of changes in health outcomes. *Health Educ Res* 2006; **22**(5): 703–717.

36 Haynes RB, Xao X, Degani A, Kripalani S, Garg A, McDonald HP. Interventions for enhancing medication adherence (Cochrane review). *Cochrane Database Syst Rev* 2005;**4**:CD000011 (doi: 10.1002/14651858.CD000011.pub2).

37 Monninkhof EM, van der Valk P, van der Palen J, et al. Self-management education for chronic obstructive pulmonary disease (Cochrane review). *Cochrane Database Syst Rev* 2002;**4**:CD002990 (doi: 10.1002/14651858.CD002990).

38 Turnock AC, Walters EH, Walters JAE, Wood-Baker R. Action plans for chronic obstructive pulmonary disease (Cochrane review). *Cochrane Database Syst Rev* 2005;**4**:CD005074 (doi: 10.1002/14651858. CD005074.pub2).

39 Lacasse Y, Goldstein R, Lasserson TJ, Martin S. Pulmonary rehabilitation for chronic obstructive pulmonary disease (Cochrane review). *Cochrane Database Syst Rev* 2006;**4**:CD003793 (doi: 10.1002/14651858. CD003793.pub2).

11 Diagnosis and Treatment of Community-Acquired Pneumonia

Sam G. Campbell[1] & Tom Marrie[2]

[1]Department of Emergency Medicine, Dalhousie University, Halifax, Canada
[2]Faculty of Medicine and Dentistry, University of Alberta, Edmonton, Canada

Clinical scenario

A 59-year-old man presented with a 3-day history of cough productive of yellow sputum, fever and pleuritic pain in his right axilla. The illness began with rigors, and had been accompanied by poor appetite and fatigue. He had been unable to work and his oral intake had been restricted to fluids due to anorexia and mild nausea. His past medical history included hypertension, non-insulin-dependent diabetes and gout, and he had a 30 pack/year smoking history. He denied recurrent respiratory symptoms or morning cough at his baseline state.

On clinical examination, he appeared to be in no acute distress, although he was coughing intermittently. His vital signs were temperature 38.2°C (oral), pulse rate 128 beats/min, blood pressure 146/90 mmHg and respiratory rate 24 breaths/min. His oxygen saturation (SaO_2) on room air at sea level was 91%. His blood glucose via a glucometer reading was 16 mmol/L. Auscultation of his chest revealed rhonchi throughout his lung fields and inspiratory crackles on the right side of his chest, with no dullness to percussion. He had no history of malignancy, immunocompromise or renal or liver impairment.

Background

Pneumonia is a common illness of the respiratory system resulting from inflammation of lung tissue (excluding bronchi). Although it may be caused by a number of non-infectious pulmonary irritants (in which case it is termed pneumonitis), the majority of cases of pneumonia presenting to the emergency department (ED) result from microbial infection. Infecting agents may be intracellular or extracellular bacteria, viruses, fungi or protozoa; however, differentiation between offending organisms is clinically unreliable.

Evidence-based Emergency Medicine. Edited by Brian H. Rowe
© 2009 Blackwell Publishing, ISBN: 978-1-4051-6143-5.

Following a breach in the pulmonary defense system, microbial invasion of the lower respiratory tract allows proliferation of microorganisms in the alveoli. Infective organisms may spread via the bronchial tree, causing multiple areas of involvement (bronchopneumonia), or via the interalveolar pores (of Kohn) to involve adjacent lung segments (lobar pneumonia). When the filling of alveoli (consolidation) with infective organisms, plasma constituents, pneumocytes and inflammatory cells is extensive enough to be detected radiographically, pneumonia is said to be present. Infection confined to the lung tissue without filling the airspaces may also be visible radiologically (interstitial pneumonia).

Community-acquired pneumonia (CAP) refers to pneumonia acquired outside hospitals or extended-care facilities (at least 14 days since residence in either), and affects nearly 4 million adults a year. Pneumonia occurs at all stages of life, although older individuals are at particular risk for pneumonia and associated mortality. In the USA, pneumonia is the sixth leading cause of death and the foremost cause of infectious death [1].

The most common organisms implicated include *Streptococcus pneumoniae*, *Hemophilus influenzae* or "atypical" organisms like *Chlamydophila* species or *Mycoplasma pneumoniae*. Viral pneumonia is relatively common, yet with the exception of the influenza virus, which can cause severe pneumonia, the majority of viral pneumonias in immunocompetent adults are mild. In contrast to CAP, hospital-acquired pneumonia, or "nosocomial" pneumonia, suggests a much higher likelihood of Gram-negative bacteria and staphylococci, which can be difficult to treat and are more dangerous to the patient.

Typical symptoms of CAP include cough, fever, chills, chest pain and shortness of breath, although in older or immune-suppressed patients, symptoms may be very subtle and pulmonary disease may not be apparent, with symptoms such as confusion, weakness, abdominal pain or falls being predominant. Clinical signs, which may also be subtle in older patients, include fever, tachypnea, tachycardia or crackles on pulmonary auscultation. Although patients with mild CAP may appear quite well, in severe cases patients may be cyanosed and hypotensive. The differential diagnosis of patients with suspected CAP includes non-infectious illnesses like pulmonary embolism, congestive heart failure and malignancy, or infectious causes outside of the lower respiratory tract.

From an emergency clinician's perspective, one challenge is to differentiate CAP from acute bronchitis, with which it shares some features. The latter is usually caused by viruses, and has been found not to benefit from antibiotic treatment [2–4], so stable patients with features of a chest infection but a clear chest X-ray (CXR) should ideally have CAP confirmed by definite clinical signs or another means of diagnostic imaging before antibiotic treatment is prescribed [5].

The prevalence of CAP, and the variations in treatment among care givers, has led to recognition of the need for guidelines to direct appropriate management, and several of these have been produced [6–10]. Variable perceptions of the importance of certain aspects of CAP have led to significant differences in the recommendations of North American guidelines [6,7] compared to those proposed by European or Australasian authorities with reference to antibiotic choices [8–10]. This chapter will review some of the important ED decisions for CAP patients.

Clinical questions

1 In patients presenting to the ED with acute respiratory symptoms suggestive of pneumonia (population), what is the sensitivity and specificity (diagnostic test characteristics) of historical criteria and clinical findings (test) in detecting pneumonia (outcome)?

2 In patients presenting to the ED with acute respiratory symptoms suggestive of pneumonia (population), what is the sensitivity and specificity (diagnostic test characteristics) of chest radiography (test) in detecting pneumonia (outcome)?

3 In patients diagnosed with pneumonia (population), what is the utility (diagnostic test characteristics) of blood cultures (test) in improving clinical outcomes (outcomes)?

4 In ED patients with documented pneumonia (population), what is the utility (diagnostic test characteristics) of pneumonia clinical decision rules (test) in determining the need for hospital admission (outcome)?

5 In patients with documented pneumonia requiring admission (population), does treatment with intravenous antibiotics (intervention) increase clinical cures and reduce relapse (outcomes) compared to oral antibiotics (control)?

6 In patients diagnosed with CAP in the ED (population), do second- and third-line antibiotics (intervention) improve clinical outcomes (outcomes) compared to first-generation antibiotics (control)?

7 In patients with documented pneumonia (population), what is the clinical outcome (prognosis) following standard treatment with antibiotics (intervention)?

8 In ED patients with documented pneumonia treated with antibiotics (population), does routine follow-up (intervention) reduce relapse and improve quality of life (outcomes) compared to symptomatic follow-up (control)?

9 In patients with documented pneumonia treated with antibiotics (population), does avoiding the antibiotic class(es) prescribed within 3 months (intervention) improve cure rates and reduce relapse (outcomes) compared to following guideline recommendations (control)?

General search strategy

You begin to address these questions by searching for evidence in the common electronic databases such as the Cochrane Library, MEDLINE and EMBASE looking specifically for systematic reviews and meta-analyses. Unfortunately, the Cochrane Database of Systematic Reviews includes few high-quality systematic reviews on therapy for pneumonia. You also search the Cochrane Central Register of Controlled Trials (CENTRAL), MEDLINE and EMBASE to identify randomized controlled trials (RCTs) that became available after the publication date of the systematic review or, if no systematic reviews were identified, to locate high-quality RCTs that directly address the therapy questions. In addition, relevant, updated, evidence-based clinical practice guidelines (CPGs) on pneumonia are accessed to determine the consensus rating of areas lacking evidence.

Searching for evidence synthesis: primary search strategy
- Cochrane Library: pneumonia AND (topic)
- MEDLINE: pneumonia AND (systematic review OR meta-analysis OR metaanalysis) AND (topic)
- EMBASE: pneumonia AND (systematic review OR meta-analysis OR metaanalysis) AND (topic)

Critical review of the literature

Question 1: In patients presenting to the ED with acute respiratory symptoms suggestive of pneumonia (population), what is the sensitivity and specificity (diagnostic test characteristics) of historical criteria and clinical findings (test) in detecting pneumonia (outcome)?

Search strategy

- Cochrane Library: pneumonia AND (history OR physical) AND diagnosis
- MEDLINE: pneumonia AND (systematic review OR meta-analysis OR metaanalysis) AND (history OR physical OR diagnosis)

The baseline prevalence of CAP in unselected patients suspected of having the infection is approximately 5% [11]. Missing the diagnosis exposes patients to the risks of untreated bacterial illness, while "over-diagnosis" presents the risk of unnecessary treatment to the patient and to society, as well of the risk of the real cause of the symptoms remaining unaddressed.

The tradition of clinical assessment of patients suspected of having CAP is long established, with the elicitation of "typical" symptoms including cough, dyspnea, pleuritic chest pain, fatigue, anorexia and myalgias, with enquiry for more subtle symptoms, especially in older patients. The search for physical findings generally follows a structured, four-stepped approach through inspection, palpation, percussion and auscultation [12].

Two review articles discussed the limitations of history and physical examination in the diagnosis of CAP [11,12]. Symptoms at presentation were found to distinguish poorly between CAP and other respiratory illness. With reference to physical examination, clinical signs typically attributed to pneumonia were found to be of limited value in ruling the diagnosis in or out [11]. Auscultatory findings have been found to be absent in up to 25% of patients with CAP [13]. A post hoc evaluation of two controlled intervention trials published subsequently to the above reviews confirmed the limitations of clinical findings in diagnosing CAP [14].

Since individual symptoms and signs are inadequate to rule CAP in or out, various combinations of these findings have been assessed and some have been found to increase or decrease the pre-test probability of pneumonia. The simplest and most objective of these is the absence of abnormalities in the vital signs of: respiratory rate <30 breaths/min, heart rate <100 beats/min and temperature <37.8°C, which was found to have a likelihood ratio of 0.18 (95% CI: 0.07 to 0.46) in one study [12]. Significant inter-observer variability in the elicitation of clinical signs further complicates any assessment of their utility [12].

In conclusion, there is no evidence supporting the use of history and physical examination alone to include or exclude the diagnosis of CAP. In a patient who is suspected of having CAP, further testing (usually a chest radiograph) is generally required.

Question 2: In patients presenting to the ED with acute respiratory symptoms suggestive of pneumonia (population), what is the sensitivity and specificity (diagnostic test characteristics) of chest radiography (test) in detecting pneumonia (outcome)?

Search strategy

- Cochrane Library: pneumonia AND diagnosis AND (chest x-ray OR chest xray)
- MEDLINE and EMBASE: pneumonia AND (systematic review OR meta-analysis)

Chest radiography or CXR has long been considered the gold standard for the diagnosis of CAP [15,16], and contemporary guidelines for CAP state that patients suspected of having CAP should undergo CXR to confirm or refute the diagnosis [6,7]. This gold standard, however, is not without flaws. For example, CXR is prone to significant inter- and intra-observer variability,

and rates of agreement among radiologists regarding the interpretation of CXRs of patients with pneumonia are, at best, 80% – whilst amongst trainees or non-radiologist practitioners, they are considerably lower [17–22].

With regard to the diagnosis of CAP resulting from "over-interpretation" of CXR findings, two studies comparing emergency physician diagnoses of CAP with subsequent radiologist reports have shown that in 20% and 18.9%, respectively, of "pneumonia" diagnoses, the radiologist interpreted the CXR findings as "normal" [23,24]. In a study that also evaluated 144 cases with an emergency physician diagnosis of "possible pneumonia", the radiologist reported "normal" or an opinion other than pneumonia in 72.2% of cases [24]. Regarding the incidence of missed diagnosis of positive CXR findings by emergency physicians, rates reported range from 0.35% in a British study [25] to 3.1% (2.8% considered clinically significant) in an American series [26].

One group of investigators simultaneously obtained CXRs and high-resolution computerized tomography (CT) in patients with clinical presentations suggestive of CAP. They reported that 30.8% of pneumonias seen on high-resolution CT were not seen on CXR (18 of 26 cases of CAP in 47 patients were identified by CXR). CXR showed bilateral involvement in only six of 16 such cases identified by high-resolution CT [5].

It would appear that further studies on the sensitivity and specificity of CXR in CAP are needed, and that the "gold standard" status of CXRs has been called into question. Clinicians with a high index of suspicion for CAP, but with a normal or equivocal CXR, should consider obtaining high-resolution CT for the patient after weighing the potential benefits of a clearer diagnosis against the risk of the significantly higher radiation dose [27]. Failing this, the choices include treating the patient empirically for pneumonia or, in the case of less "sick" patients, repeating the CXR in 24–48 hours if the patient fails to respond to supportive therapy.

Question 3: In patients diagnosed with pneumonia (population), what is the utility (diagnostic test characteristics) of blood cultures (test) in improving clinical outcomes (outcomes)?

Search strategy

- Cochrane Library: pneumonia AND diagnosis AND blood cultures
- MEDLINE and EMBASE: pneumonia AND (systematic review OR meta-analysis OR metaanalysis) AND diagnosis AND blood cultures

Blood cultures (BCs) have traditionally been recommended as part of the work-up of patients admitted to hospital for CAP. Although a positive result can be of great assistance to the clinician in optimizing the management of pneumonia, and in ensuring that the most cost-effective antimicrobial regimen is used, the yield of clinically significant positive results of BCs ranges from 1.4–2.1% in outpatients [28,29] to 5–14% in hospitalized patients, with over 60% of positive cultures growing *S. pneumoniae* [7], which is empirically covered by all recommended regimens [6–10]. Moreover, physician response to positive results is commonly inappropriate [30,31]. Positive results are often neglected and negative results have not been shown to indicate less severe disease [32]. Cost of the treatment of CAP is increased by false-positive results [33].

Although the vast majority of quantitative studies have cast doubt on the clinical value of BCs [34–43], no systematic reviews on the subject of BCs in CAP exist, nor have RCTs evaluated the clinical impact of BCs. Clinical variables reliably predicting bacteremia have not been found [44]. The most recent North American guidelines [7] recommend the use of BC in patients with severe CAP or with any of the following criteria: intensive care unit admission, cavitary infiltrate, leucopenia, alcohol abuse, severe liver disease, asplenia, pleural effusion or positive pneumococcal urinary antigen test. The use of BCs in other patients is listed as "optional" [7].

In conclusion, the utility of BC in CAP patients needs further study. At this stage it seems that the best option is to restrict their use to patients with severe CAP or with any of the above guidelines' criteria [7].

Question 4: In ED patients with documented pneumonia (population), what is the utility (diagnostic test characteristics) of pneumonia clinical decision rules (test) in determining the need for hospital admission (outcome)?

Search strategy

- Cochrane Library: pneumonia AND clinical decision rules; pneumonia AND severity index; pneumonia AND CURB-65

- MEDLINE and EMBASE: pneumonia AND (systematic review OR meta-analysis OR metaanalysis) AND clinical decision rules; pneumonia AND severity index; pneumonia AND CURB-65

The majority of patients with CAP can be treated as outpatients, although hospital admission is advisable in certain cases, especially those in which intensive therapy might be needed to prevent poor clinical outcome. The responsibility for deciding the appropriate venue for a patient with CAP to undergo treatment (hospital or outpatient) falls primarily on the shoulders of the emergency physician. This decision has significant implications both in terms of patient outcome, and cost to the health care system [45], and it has been shown that physicians tend to overestimate the risk of death in their CAP patients [7,46]. Considering that one of the chief reasons to admit patients with CAP to the hospital is to reduce the risk of death, scoring systems designed to estimate the risk of mortality in CAP patients have been adapted to guide the "admit or discharge" decision. The two tools in common use for this purpose are the pneumonia severity index (PSI), developed in the USA [46], and the CURB-65 rule adapted from the British Thoracic Society [47].

The PSI, introduced in 1997, consists of 20 variables predictive of adverse outcome in CAP, derived from and validated in more than 50,000 patients, the largest database ever studied in the history of pneumonia research [48]. Using the PSI, patients younger than 50 years of age with none of the historical or vital sign features specified in the PSI checklist can be selected for outpatient therapy. For other patients, the clinician tallies the scores of each variable that a patient has, and assigns the patient to one of five classes of pneumonia severity (Table 11.1). The first three PSI classes have been deemed suitable for outpatient treatment. In the fourth and fifth classes (with predicted mortalities of 9% and 27%, respectively) admission is recommended [46]. Critics of the PSI have noted its complexity, its emphasis on age and defined cut-points for certain variables, and its neglect of the social needs of patients with reference to the need for admission. Further objections include the PSI's capacity to seriously underestimate the severity of disease in younger patients without co-morbidities [48].

The CURB-65 rule consists of the following elements: confusion, urea >7 mmol/L, respiratory rate >30 breaths/min, low systolic (<90 mmHg) or diastolic (<60 mmHg) blood pressure, and age (>65 years), with one point being assigned for the presence of each. This rule appears to function comparably to the PSI [49] and is very simple to remember and use, yet it fails to take into account the effect of co-morbidities that may be destabilized by even mild episodes of CAP.

One prospective observational study of 3181 CAP patients in the ED compared the PSI with CURB-65. It found that the PSI appeared to be more selective in identifying patients with a low risk of mortality, and could thus be considered the better of the two for avoiding unnecessary hospitalization [49]. The 30-day mortality in the 68% of patients determined to be low risk by PSI (classes I–III) was 1.4%, compared to 1.7% of the 61% deemed low risk by the CURB-65 (score of 0–1). The CURB-65, however, did appear to be more discriminating between the risks of death among sicker patients, because it defined high-risk patients as those with a score of 2, 3, 4 or 5, with each of these classes having a progressively increasing risk of death (3%, 17% and 43%, respectively, for groups 3, 4 and 5). The PSI, on the other hand, defined only two groups (IV and V) as severely ill with mortalities of 8.1% and 24%, respectively. Both systems, however, predicted mortality with a similar level of accuracy, and were thus comparable in identifying patients in need of admission.

In conclusion, the evidence does suggest that the use of decision rules is likely to identify patients who can safely be treated as outpatients more reliably than clinical judgment alone, and in this sense the PSI is the better of the two. The CURB-65, however, is far easier to remember and apply, and is also useful for making disposition decisions. Using the two systems in combination, as suggested by some authors [50], may allow each to avoid the pitfalls of the other in making safe decisions regarding the site of care. In any deliberation of prediction rules, it is imperative to recognize their limitations with reference to social factors that indicate admission, hypoxia (which may be present in patients with low

Table 11.1 Point scoring system for the pneumonia severity index for assignment to risk classes II, III, IV and V. (Reprinted with permission from Fine et al. [46].)

Characteristic	Points assigned*
Demographic factor	
Age	
Men	Age (yr)
Women	Age (yr)–10
Nursing home resident	+10
Coexisting illnesses[†]	
Neoplastic disease	+30
Liver disease	+20
Congestive heart failure	+10
Cerebrovascular disease	+10
Renal disease	+10
Physical examination findings	
Altered mental status[‡]	+20
Respiratory rate ≥30 breaths/min	+20
Systolic blood pressure <90 mmHg	+20
Temperature <35°C or ≥40°C	+15
Pulse ≥125 beats/min	+10
Laboratory and radiographic findings	
Arterial pH <7.35	+30
Blood urea nitrogen ≥30 mg/dl	
(11 mmol/L)	+20
Sodium <130 mmol/L	+20
Glucose ≥250 mg/dl (14 mmol/L)	+10
Hematocrit <30%	+10
Partial pressure of arterial oxygen	
<60 mmHg[§]	+10
Pleural effusion	+10

*A total point score for a given patient is obtained by summing the patient's age in years (age minus 10 for women) and the points for each applicable characteristic. The points assigned to each predictor variable were based on coefficients obtained from the logistic-regression model used in step 2 of the prediction rule.

[†]Neoplastic disease is defined as any cancer except basal or squamous cell cancer of the skin that was active at the time of presentation or diagnosed within 1 year of presentation. Liver disease is defined as a clinical or histological diagnosis of cirrhosis or another form of chronic liver disease, such as chronic active hepatitis. Congestive heart failure is defined as systolic or diastolic ventricular dysfunction documented by history, physical examination, and chest radiography, echocardiogram, multiple-gated acquisition scan or left ventriculogram. Cerebrovascular disease is defined as a clinical diagnosis of stroke or transient ischemic attack or stroke documented by magnetic resonance imaging or computed tomography. Renal disease is defined as a history of chronic renal disease or abnormal blood urea nitrogen and creatinine concentrations documented in the medical record.

[‡]Altered mental status is defined as disorientation with respect to person, place or time that is not known to be chronic, stupor or coma.

[§]In the Pneumonia PORT cohort study, an oxygen saturation of less than 90% on pulse oximetry or intubation before admission was also considered abnormal.

scores) or marginal vital signs in young patients – the rules should be used to augment, rather than supersede, clinical judgment.

Question 5: In patients with documented pneumonia requiring admission (population), does treatment with intravenous antibiotics (intervention) increase clinical cures and reduce relapse (outcomes) compared to oral antibiotics?

Search strategy

- Cochrane Library: pneumonia AND (antibiotics OR antibacterial OR antimicrobial) AND oral
- MEDLINE and EMBASE: pneumonia AND (systematic review OR meta-analysis OR metaanalysis) AND (antibiotics OR antibacterial OR antimicrobial) AND oral

Most episodes of CAP in adults are caused by bacteria sensitive to antibiotics, so antimicrobial treatment is considered "standard care" for patients with CAP. Parenteral administration of antibiotics is widely considered to be more effective, and especially appropriate, in patients with CAP sick enough to be admitted. This mode of administration, however, is more expensive and invasive and is associated with longer hospital stays [51]. Newer, highly bio-available oral formulations provide the choice for exclusively oral treatment of CAP.

A meta-analysis that identified seven studies involving 1366 patients that compared exclusively oral to parenteral antibiotic therapy for CAP [51] concluded that oral therapy is effective in terms of clinical success and mortality in patients with "non-severe" CAP (Fig. 11.1). The author's conclusion, which is further limited by several methodological flaws, is that exclusive oral antibiotic therapy for patients with CAP was effective, although they found insufficient evidence to identify appropriate candidates for such treatment.

In summary, it appears that the clinical threshold for exclusively oral treatment of CAP in admitted patients has yet to be determined, although clinicians should feel comfortable treating stable CAP patients exclusively with oral antibiotics.

Question 6: In patients diagnosed with CAP in the ED (population), do second- and third-line antibiotics (intervention) improve clinical outcomes (outcomes) compared to first-generation antibiotics (control)?

Search strategy

- Cochrane Library: pneumonia AND (macrolide OR cephalosporin OR beta-lactam OR fluoroquinolone)
- MEDLINE and EMBASE: pneumonia AND (systematic review OR meta-analysis OR metaanalysis) AND (macrolide OR cephalosporin OR beta-lactam OR fluoroquinolone)

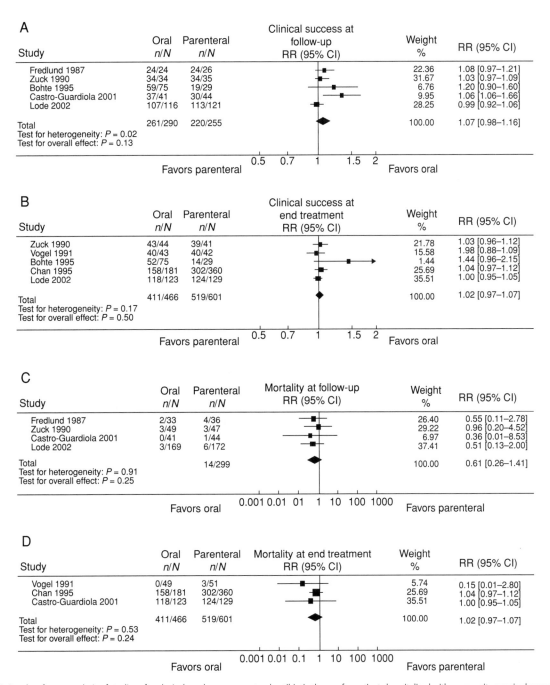

Figure 11.1 Results of meta-analysis of studies of exclusively oral versus parenteral antibiotic therapy for patients hospitalized with community-acquired pneumonia. A: Clinical success at follow-up. B: Clinical success at end of treatment. C: Mortality at follow-up. D: Mortality at the end of treatment. Results were considered heterogeneous if $P < 0.2$. Reprinted with permission from Marras et al. [51].

Once a diagnosis has been confirmed and a decision has been made to prescribe antibiotics, the decision of what agent to use is influenced by numerous factors. Microbiological tests to determine the offending organism are slow and because delay in the institution of treatment is associated with poorer outcome, rapidly instituted empirical treatment is the current standard of care. While guidelines tend to use the chosen site of care and presence of chronic

obstructive pulmonary disease (COPD) to steer antibiotic selection, numerous other factors – such as local resistance patterns, clinical experience and the marketing efforts of the pharmaceutical industry – all undoubtedly play a part. The "atypical" organisms, *Chlamydophila pneumoniae* and *Mycoplasma pneumoniae*, are known to be a common cause of mild CAP, and a less common cause of severe CAP. *Legionella pneumophila* is a less common, but more dangerous, 'atypical' microbe. In earlier years, β-lactam and cephalosporin antimicrobial agents were considered "first line" for the treatment of CAP. However, resistance to these agents by "atypicals" as well as concerns about rising levels of penicillin resistance in *Streptococcus pneumoniae* have driven recommendations in North American guidelines. These guidelines recommend macrolide antibiotics as the first-line choice for outpatients, and a macrolide/β-lactam combination or "respiratory fluoroquinolone" for inpatients with CAP, in order to ensure adequate coverage of atypical organisms [6,7]. Several non-randomized, unblinded, retrospective studies supported this view by showing a positive impact on mortality in bacteremic streptococcal CAP [52].

European and Australasian guidelines [8–10], on the other hand, in recognition of the facts that intermediate resistant *S. pneumoniae* can still be effectively treated by β-lactams, that macrolide resistance rates are rising [53], and that "atypical" pneumonias in outpatients are usually mild, recommend β-lactams (usually amoxicillin) for this purpose.

Outpatient antibiotic selection

A systematic review of high-quality RCTs comparing different antibiotics for outpatients with CAP [54], found only three studies involving 622 patients that met their selection criteria. They concluded that there was insufficient evidence from RCTs to make evidence-based recommendations for the choice of antibiotic to be used for the treatment of CAP in ambulatory patients.

A meta-analysis of RCTs comparing a macrolide, β-lactam or doxycycline antibiotic with a newer oral fluoroquinolone for the treatment of CAP requiring oral treatment found a modest therapeutic benefit of fluoroquinolone in mainly younger patients with mild CAP and no co-morbidities (quoting a number needed to treat (NNT) of 33) [55]. No deaths were reported, and the benefit of fluoroquinolones was limited to faster resolution of symptoms. No studies were found comparing doxycycline with a fluoroquinolone.

In summary, there is little evidence to help clinicians decide on what agent to use in outpatients with CAP. This issue undoubtedly requires further study – however, in the light of the risks of furthering resistance to second- or third-line antibiotics, and the increased cost of the latter, it would appear that monotherapy with a first-line agent remains a good choice for patients treated for CAP on an ambulatory basis.

Inpatient antibiotic choices

In a meta-analysis of 18 double-blind RCTs involving 6749 patients, little evidence was identified to support the use of antibiotic monotherapy active against atypical pathogens (fluoroquinolones, macrolides, ketolides) over β-lactam antibiotics (penicillins, cephalosporins) for patients with undifferentiated, non-severe CAP [56] (Fig. 11.2). Interestingly, they found no significant treatment effect in patients with *M. pneumoniae* or *C. pneumoniae*. The authors conclude that β-lactam antibiotics should remain the first choice for the management of non-severe CAP in adults. In applying these conclusions, it should be noted

that studies included in this review involved younger patients than in observational studies [46,56], with mostly non-severe CAP. Furthermore, although *L. pneumophila* was rarely identified in patients in the included trials, antibiotics against atypicals were found to be superior in the subgroup with *Legionella*-related pneumonia. Finally, it should be noted that in four of the 18 studies the drug in the "β-lactam" arm was amoxicilin/clavulanic acid, which, although indeed a β-lactam, can overcome β-lactamase-producing bacteria and is thus not strictly a first-line agent.

In an effort to evaluate the evidence for the North American antimicrobial recommendations for inpatients with CAP, Oosterheert et al. performed a limited systematic review of the literature examining whether β-lactam plus macrolide antibiotics or quinolone monotherapy reduce mortality or length of stay, compared with β-lactams alone, in hospitalized adults with CAP, and identified only one prospective and seven retrospective cohort studies [57]. Although reductions in mortality and length of stay were found with treatment consisting of a macrolide plus a β-lactam antibiotic, or monotherapy with quinolone, the authors acknowledge that the non-experimental design of the studies reviewed make the results unreliable. They conclude that, pending the results of an RCT to circumvent the methodological flaws in the designs of the currently available studies, there is insufficient evidence to support the addition of a macrolide, or monotherapy with one of the newer fluoroquinolones as standard care. A subsequently published narrative review echoed these conclusions [58].

A Cochrane review specifically examined the efficacy of adding "atypical" coverage in CAP inpatients. After a review of 24 RCTs, they found no significant difference compared to patients without such coverage (RR = 1.13; 95% CI: 0.82 to 1.54), although there was a trend to improved outcomes in the patients whose coverage included antibiotics with efficacy against atypical microbes [59]. Cases of *L. pneumophila* in the atypical coverage arm had a significantly better clinical outcome, while that of patients with pneumococcal pneumonia was non-significantly worse. The rates of (total) adverse events were similar in both groups, although gastrointestinal events were more common in the non-atypical arm (RR = 0.73; 95% CI: 0.54 to 0.99). This conclusion relates mostly to the comparison of quinolone monotherapy to non-atypical monotherapy.

A well-conducted review of RCTs of orally administered fluoroquinolones versus other current antibiotics, published in 2001, showed no statistically significant difference in clinical success in intention-to-treat analyses [60]. In all evaluable subjects, however, orally administered new fluoroquinolones were slightly more successful (RD = 2.9%; 95% CI: 0.5 to 5.3) and when initially administered intravenously, new fluoroquinolones were more successful (RD = 5.4%; 95% CI: 2.1 to 8.6) than non-fluoroquinolone antibiotics. The authors conclude that the new fluoroquinolones are at least as effective as and may be slightly more effective than comparator antibiotics for the treatment of empirical CAP. No difference in adverse effects was found.

Finally, with regard to the contribution of bacterial resistance to CAP outcomes, a systematic review of available evidence regarding the effect of initial discordant therapy with β-lactam antibiotics for

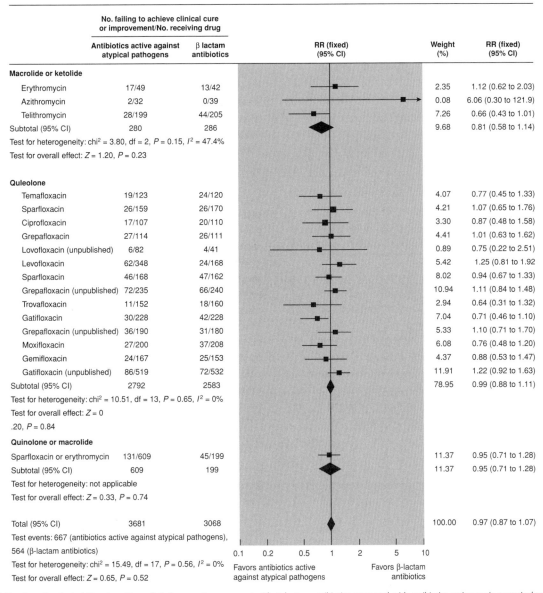

	No. failing to achieve clinical cure or improvement/No. receiving drug		RR (fixed) (95% CI)	Weight (%)	RR (fixed) (95% CI)
	Antibiotics active against atypical pathogens	β lactam antibiotics			
Macrolide or ketolide					
Erythromycin	17/49	13/42		2.35	1.12 (0.62 to 2.03)
Azithromycin	2/32	0/39		0.08	6.06 (0.30 to 121.9)
Telithromycin	28/199	44/205		7.26	0.66 (0.43 to 1.01)
Subtotal (95% CI)	280	286		9.68	0.81 (0.58 to 1.14)
Test for heterogeneity: chi² = 3.80, df = 2, *P* = 0.15, *I²* = 47.4%					
Test for overall effect: *Z* = 1.20, *P* = 0.23					
Quleolone					
Temafloxacin	19/123	24/120		4.07	0.77 (0.45 to 1.33)
Sparfloxacin	26/159	26/170		4.21	1.07 (0.65 to 1.76)
Ciprofloxacin	17/107	20/110		3.30	0.87 (0.48 to 1.58)
Grepafloxacin	27/114	26/111		4.41	1.01 (0.63 to 1.62)
Lovofloxacin (unpublished)	6/82	4/41		0.89	0.75 (0.22 to 2.51)
Levofloxacin	62/348	24/168		5.42	1.25 (0.81 to 1.92)
Sparfloxacin	46/168	47/162		8.02	0.94 (0.67 to 1.33)
Grepafloxacin (unpublished)	72/235	66/240		10.94	1.11 (0.84 to 1.48)
Trovafloxacin	11/152	18/160		2.94	0.64 (0.31 to 1.32)
Gatifloxacin	30/228	42/228		7.04	0.71 (0.46 to 1.10)
Grepafloxacin (unpublished)	36/190	31/180		5.33	1.10 (0.71 to 1.70)
Moxifloxacin	27/200	37/208		6.08	0.76 (0.48 to 1.20)
Gemifloxacin	24/167	25/153		4.37	0.88 (0.53 to 1.47)
Gatifloxacin (unpublished)	86/519	72/532		11.91	1.22 (0.92 to 1.63)
Subtotal (95% CI)	2792	2583		78.95	0.99 (0.88 to 1.11)
Test for heterogeneity: chi² = 10.51, df = 13, *P* = 0.65, *I²* = 0%					
Test for overall effect: *Z* = 0.20, *P* = 0.84					
Quinolone or macrolide					
Sparfloxacin or erythromycin	131/609	45/199		11.37	0.95 (0.71 to 1.28)
Subtotal (95% CI)	609	199		11.37	0.95 (0.71 to 1.28)
Test for heterogeneity: not applicable					
Test for overall effect: *Z* = 0.33, *P* = 0.74					
Total (95% CI)	3681	3068		100.00	0.97 (0.87 to 1.07)
Test events: 667 (antibiotics active against atypical pathogens), 564 (β-lactam antibiotics)					
Test for heterogeneity: chi² = 15.49, df = 17, *P* = 0.56, *I²* = 0%					
Test for overall effect: *Z* = 0.65, *P* = 0.52					

0.1   0.2   0.5   1   2   5   10

Favors antibiotics active against atypical pathogens   Favors β-lactam antibiotics

Figure 11.2 Number of patients failing to achieve clinical cure or improvement with β-lactam antibiotics compared with antibiotics active against atypical pathogens in all-cause CAP. (Reprinted with permission from Mills et al. [56].)

the treatment of pneumococcal pneumonia showed no association between initial discordant treatment and unfavorable treatment outcomes [61].

In conclusion, reliable evidence does not support the routine use of newer macrolides or fluoroquinolones for the empirical treatment of CAP. Caveats include sicker patients (who are not well represented in prospective studies) and those in whom *L. pneumophila* is a reasonable possibility.

Question 7: In patients with documented pneumonia (population), what is the outcome (prognosis) following standard treatment with antibiotics (intervention)?

Search strategy:

- Cochrane Library: pneumonia AND (prognosis OR outcome)
- MEDLINE and EMBASE: pneumonia AND (systematic review OR meta-analysis OR metaanalysis) AND (prognosis OR outcome)

Studies of mortality in pneumonia conducted before the advent of antibiotics reported a mortality for pneumonia that ranged from 12% in patients younger than 20 years to 72% in those over 60, with mortality for patients with bacteremic pneumococcal pneumonia of 62% [62]. Antibiotics have changed this dire picture dramatically. In 1964, Austrian and Gold reported a mortality of 19.5% in

Table 11.2 Prognostic variables associated with death in patients with CAP. (Reprinted with permission from Kaplan et al. [65], © American Medical Association. All rights reserved.)

Prognostic factor	Odds ratio (95% CI)
Hypothermia	5.0 (2.4 to 10.4)
Systolic hypotension	4.8 (2.8 to 8.3)
Neurological disease	4.6 (2.3 to 8.9)
Multi-lobar radiographic pulmonary infiltrate	3.1 (1.9 to 5.1)
Tachypnea	2.9 (1.7 to 4.9)
Neoplastic disease	2.8 (2.4 to 3.1)
Bacteremia	2.8 (2.3 to 3.6)
Leucopenia	2.5 (1.6 to 3.7)
Diabetes mellitus	1.3 (1.1 to 1.5)
Male sex	1.3 (1.2 to 1.4)
Pleuritic chest pain	0.5 (0.3 to 0.8)

adults with uncomplicated bacteremic pneumococcal pneumonia treated with penicillin, increasing to over 25% in the elderly or in those with chronic systemic illness [63].

A reasonable question for patients, their care givers and clinicians is "How should I expect the clinical course of this episode of CAP to proceed?" Logically, one would expect the course to be determined by a number of factors, including the patient's age and pre-existing health, the organism responsible for the infection, and the extent of the infection at the time that treatment is initiated.

With reference to factors associated with mortality, Fine et al. systematically reviewed the medical literature on the prognosis and outcomes of patients with CAP [64]. In 33,148 CAP patients they found a mortality of 13.7%, ranging from 5.1% for hospitalized and ambulatory patients (in six study cohorts) to 36.5% for the intensive care unit patients (in 13 cohorts). Eleven prognostic factors were significantly associated with mortality (Table 11.2).

Mortality varied by pneumonia etiology, ranging from less than 2% for *Chlamydia psittaci, Coxiella burnetii* and *Mycoplasma pneumoniae* to as high as 61.1% for *Pseudomonas aeruginosa* pneumonia. In patients with an unknown etiological agent, mortality was 12.8%. Subsequently, in the PORT study, Fine et al. described CAP mortality in terms of the PSI score (Tables 11.3, 11.4) [46].

In patients aged 65 or older, hospitalization with pneumonia was found, in analysis of a large Medicare database cohort study [65], to be associated with double the in-hospital mortality than hospitalized controls (11.0% vs 5.5%, P <0.001). One year after discharge of survivors, mortality rates in the pneumonia and control cohorts were 33.6% and 24.9%, respectively (P <0.001). Standardized against the general population, the risk of death for both cohorts decreased monthly but was still elevated 1 year after hospital discharge. The standardized mortality ratio was 2.69 (95% CI: 2.47 to 2.93) for CAP patients and 1.93 (95% CI: 1.79 to 2.08) for hospital controls.

A long-term (median 9.2 years) follow-up study [66] of patients over the age of 60 showed that the high risk of subsequent mortality in elderly patients treated for CAP persists for several years (RR of

pneumonia-related mortality = 2.1; 95% CI: 1.3 to 3.4; P = 0.004; RR for total mortality = 1.5; 95% CI: 1.2 to 1.9; P = 0.001).

With regard to short-term outcome in admitted patients, a Spanish prospective, multi-center, observational study designed to identify factors that influence the time to clinical stability (defined as a temperature of <37.2°C, a heart rate of <100 beats/min, a respiratory rate of <24 breaths/min, a systolic blood pressure of >90 mmHg, and oxygen saturation >90% or arterial oxygen partial pressure of >60 mmHg) in patients with CAP found a median time to stability of 4 days [67]. Overall, six independent variables recorded during the first 24 hours after hospital admission were found to be associated with a longer time to stability: dyspnea (hazard ratio (HR) = 0.76), confusion (HR = 0.66), pleural effusion (HR = 0.67), multi-lobar CAP (HR = 0.72), high PSI (HR = 0.73) and adherence to the Spanish guidelines for treatment of CAP (HR = 1.22).

With reference to symptom resolution in patients in whom mortality is not expected, no systematic review was found. Recent evidence for outcomes in this group includes the prospective multi-center cohort study by Metlay et al. to determine the rates of resolution of five symptoms (cough, fatigue, dyspnea, sputum, chest pain) and return to premorbid health status. They found in 576 adults with low PSI scores that all symptoms, except pleuritic chest pain, were still commonly reported at 30 days, and the prevalence of each symptom at 90 days was still nearly twice pre-pneumonia levels [68].

Using data from a randomized trial involving 102 adults with mild-to-moderate-severe CAP [69], another study found that respiratory symptoms resolved within 14 days, while the well-being symptoms resolved more slowly. Full recovery, taking the pre-pneumonia status into account, could be expected by 6 months. The authors concluded that the presence of symptoms beyond 28 days and any impairment in health-related quality of life were found to reflect age and co-morbidity rather than the persistent effects of the pneumonia itself. Overall, the evidence suggests that patients should be warned about slow resolution of CAP and that a group of factors (e.g., diabetes mellitus, age, gender, etc.) can predict these poor outcomes. This information is critically important for patients in order to protect them against subsequent costly, needless and potentially harmful antibiotic treatment.

Question 8: In ED patients with documented pneumonia treated with antibiotics (population), does routine follow-up (intervention) reduce relapse and improve quality of life (outcomes) compared to symptomatic follow-up (control)?

Search strategy

- Cochrane Library: pneumonia AND (follow-up)
- MEDLINE and EMBASE: pneumonia AND (systematic review OR meta-analysis OR metaanalysis) AND follow-up

Table 11.3 Comparisons of mortality* using the PSI risk stratification method. (Reprinted with permission from Fine et al. [46].)

| | Medisgroups derivation cohort | | Medisgroups validation cohort | | Pneumonia PORT validation cohort | | | | | |
| | | | | | Inpatients | | Outpatients | | All patients | |
Risk class (No. of points)†	No. of patients	% who died	No. of patients	% who died	No. of patients	% who died	No. of patients	% who died	No. of patients	% who died
I	1,372	0.4	3,034	0.1	185	0.5	587	0.0	772	0.1
II (≤70)	2,412	0.7	5,778	0.6	233	0.9	244	0.4	477	0.6
III (71–90)	2,632	2.8	6,790	2.8	254	1.2	72	0.0	326	0.9
IV (91–130)	4,697	8.5	13,104	8.2	446	9.0	40	12.5	486	9.3
V (>130)	3,086	31.1	9,333	29.2	225	27.1	1	0.0	226	27.0
Total	14,199	10.2	38,039	10.6	1343	8.0	944	0.6	2287	5.2

*There were no statistically significant differences in overall mortality or mortality within risk class among patients in the MedisGroups derivation, MedisGroups validation or overall pneumonia PORT validation cohort. The P values for the comparisons of mortality across risk classes are as follows: class I, $P = 0.22$; class II, $P = 0.67$; class III, $P = 0.12$; class IV, $P = 0.69$; and class V, $P = 0.09$.

†Inclusion in risk class I was determined by the absence of all predictors identified in step 1 of the prediction rule. Inclusion in risk classes II, III, IV and V was determined by a patient's total risk score, which was compounded according to the scoring system shown in Table 11.1.

Although specific follow-up recommendations are frequently absent in CAP guidelines, those that exist range from the British Thoracic Society's suggestion to "review of patients in the community with CAP after 48 hours or earlier if clinically indicated" [9] to the Canadian guidelines' recommendation for follow-up "by telephone with the patient or a return clinic visit" in 48–72 hours [6]. None of these is based on more than the weakest evidence (e.g., "expert opinion"), and few organizations have this capacity or protocol. The only study to evaluate an early follow-up strategy was a retrospective observational study, which found poor physician compliance with the Canadian Infectious Diseases Society/Canadian Thoracic Society's approach and no benefit to patients followed up as prescribed [70]. In view of the limitations of this study, however, it appears that good evidence to guide early follow-up is lacking. At this stage, it seems prudent to instruct discharged patients to return for reassessment if clear improvement is not evident within 48–72 hours of discharge, with closer follow-up in cases where the treating physician is especially concerned about the risk of poor outcome or non-compliance.

With reference to radiological follow-up, the lag between clinical improvement and radiological clearing has long been recognized [9]. One study investigated the practice of performing bronchoscopy before discharge from hospital on patients admitted with CAP [71]. Fourteen percent of patients aged over 50 or those who were current or ex-smokers, were found to have an abnormality at bronchoscopy (bronchial carcinoma was diagnosed in 11%), leading to recommendations that a CXR be performed after about 6 weeks for patients with persistent symptoms or physical signs

Table 11.4 Comparisons of health outcomes using the PSI risk stratification method. (Reprinted with permission from Fine et al. [46].)

Medical outcome	Class I	Class II	Class III	Class IV	Class V	Total	P value
Outpatient							
No. of patients	587	244	72	40	1	944	
Subsequent hospitalization (% of patients)	5.1	8.2	16.7	20.0	0	7.4	<0.001
Inpatient							
No. of patients	185	233	254	446	225	1343	
Admission to intensive care unit (% of patients)*	4.3	4.3	5.9	11.4	17.3	9.2	<0.001
Length of hospital stay†	5.0	6.0	7.0	9.0	11.0	7.0	<0.001
Median no. of days							
≤3 days (% of patients)	26.1	22.1	13.1	5.9	3.7	13.1	<0.001
4–7 days (% of patients)	48.9	44.2	41.0	31.3	23.8	37.3	
>7 days (% of patients)	25.0	33.8	45.8	62.8	72.6	49.6	

*This category includes all patients admitted to an intensive care unit for hemodynamic instability, respiratory failure or mechanical ventilation during their index hospitalization.

†The assessment of the length of hospital stay was restricted to 1236 inpatients who were discharged after the index hospitalization.

or who are at higher risk of underlying malignancy (especially smokers and those over 50 years), whether or not they have been admitted to hospital [9,71]. Further investigations, which may include bronchoscopy, should be considered in patients with persisting signs, symptoms and radiological abnormalities at around 6 weeks after completing treatment [9].

In summary, although a 6-week follow-up for all CAP patients is commonly recommended, there is no evidence on which to base any "routine" follow-up recommendation in patients at low risk for underlying lung cancer [9].

Question 9: In patients with documented pneumonia treated with antibiotics (population), does avoiding the antibiotic class(es) prescribed within 3 months (intervention) improve cure rates and reduce relapse (outcomes) compared to following guideline recommendations (control)?

Search strategy

- Cochrane Library: pneumonia AND (antibiotic OR antimicrobial) AND (rotation OR cycling)
- MEDLINE and EMBASE: pneumonia AND (systematic review OR meta-analysis OR metaanalysis) AND (antibiotic OR antimicrobial) AND (rotation OR cycling)

A large study of invasive pneumococcal isolates showed the association between recent antibiotic use and resistance to the class of antibiotic used, spawning suggestions that knowledge of antimicrobial use during the 3 months before infection is crucial to determine appropriate therapy for patients who may be infected with *Streptococcus pneumoniae* [72]. The clinical impact of avoiding recently used classes of antimicrobials has yet to be investigated. The idea of cycling antibiotic use in the community has been considered and is not likely practical. A meta-analysis of antibiotic cycling studies based in hospitals concluded that methodological flaws and lack of standardization in the existing literature do not permit any conclusions as to the utility of this concept [73].

In conclusion, it seems sensible that, until outcome studies are conducted, an attempt is made to avoid the use of classes of drugs in patients who have received these similar classes (within the past 3 months) wherever possible. While the study cited [72] examined a 3-month time interval, the minimum time period before safely using the same antibiotics again remains unknown.

Conclusions

The patient described at the beginning of this chapter demonstrated a slight pleural effusion and a uni-lobar infiltrate on chest radiograph. Through these clinical and radiographic criteria, the patient had a PSI score of 79 calculated (59 {age} + 10 {hyperglycemia} + 10 {pleural effusion}); these class III pa-

tients occasionally require a short hospitalization (or observation unit stay). Clinically, the patient appeared reasonably well, had an adequate social support system and was likely to comply with the antibiotic prescription. Oral antibiotic and antipyretic therapy was initiated in the ED (acetaminophen and doxycycline 100 mg). After a period of observation, the patient was noted to have tolerated the antibiotic, was eating a bland diet and was discharged home with a 7-day prescription for doxycycline. He was advised to stop smoking and referred to an appropriate support service. He followed with his family doctor, and was able to return to work within a few days. He received both pneumococcal and influenza vaccination, and was advised to receive the latter annually. Because of his age (>50 years) and the fact that he is a smoker, he was referred for a follow-up CXR in 6 weeks, which showed almost total resolution of the pneumonic opacity.

CAP is a common ED diagnosis, and many recent advances have increased our understanding of the management of this disease. Diagnosis is generally based on symptoms and signs and is confirmed with CXR. A severity score calculation can improve the appropriateness of hospital/discharge disposition decisions and identify patients who have a high risk of complications. Most patients can be managed with oral monotherapy, even when hospitalized. The agents of choice should be dictated by recent antibiotic use and national guidelines; however, first-line agents appear to be sufficient. Adequate short- and long-term primary care follow-up is recommended for most patients.

Conflicts of interest

Sam Campbell has served on advisory boards and/or received speaking fees from Abbott, Bayer, Hoffmann la Roche, Janssen-Ortho, Pfizer and Wyeth. Tom Marrie currently has no conflicts. Neither author is an employee of any pharmaceutical company nor owns shares in pharmaceutical companies.

References

1 Marrie TJ. Community-acquired pneumonia: epidemiology, etiology, treatment, *Infect Dis Clin North Am* 1998;**12**(3):723–40.

2 Bent S, Saint S, Vittinghoff E, Grady D. Antibiotics in acute bronchitis: a meta-analysis. *Am J Med* 1999;**107**:62–7.

3 Smucny J, Fahey T, Becker L, Glazier R. Antibiotics for acute bronchitis. *Cochrane Database Syst Rev* 2004;**4**:CD000245.

4 Wenzel RP, Fowler AA, III. Acute bronchitis. *N Engl J Med* 2006;**355**: 2125–30.

5 Syrjala H, Broas M, Suramo I, et al. High-resolution computed tomography for the diagnosis of community-acquired pneumonia. *Clin Infect Dis* 1998;**27**:358–63.

6 Mandell LA, Marrie TJ, Grossman RF, et al. Canadian guidelines for the initial management of community-acquired pneumonia: an evidence-based update by the Canadian Infectious Diseases Society and the Canadian Thoracic Society. *Clin Infect Dis* 2000;**31**:383–421.

7 Mandell LA, Wunderink RG, Anzueto A, et al. Infectious Diseases Society of America/American Thoracic Society guidelines on the management of community-acquired pneumonia in adults. *Clin Infect Dis* 2007;**44**:S27–72.

8 Woodhead M, Blasi F, Ewig S, et al. European Society of Clinical Microbiology and Infectious Diseases guidelines for the management of adult lower respiratory tract infections. *Eur Respir J* 2005;**26**(6):1138–80.

9 British Thoracic Society Standards of Care Committee. BTS guidelines for the management of community acquired pneumonia in adults. *Thorax* 2001;**56**(Suppl 4):IV1–64.

10 Johnson PDR, Irving LB, Turnidge JD. Community-acquired pneumonia. *Med J Aust* 2002;**176**: 341–7.

11 Metlay JP, Fine MJ. Testing strategies in the initial management of patients with community-acquired pneumonia. *Ann Intern Med* 2003;**138**(2):109–18.

12 Metlay JP, Kapoor WN, Fine MJ. Does this patient have community-acquired pneumonia? Diagnosing pneumonia by history and physical examination. *JAMA* 1997;**278**:1440–45.

13 Marrie TJ. Community-acquired pneumonia. *Clin Infect Dis* 1994;**18**:501–15.

14 Muller B, Harbarth S, Stolz D, et al. Diagnostic and prognostic accuracy of clinical and laboratory parameters in community-acquired pneumonia. *BMC Infect Dis* 2007;**7**:10.

15 Katz DS, Leung AN. Radiology of pneumonia. *Clin Chest Med* 1999;**3**:549–62.

16 Bartlett JG, Mundy LM. Community-acquired pneumonia. *N Eng J Med* 1995;**333**:1618–24.

17 File TM, Tan JS. Incidence, etiologic pathogens, and diagnostic testing of community-acquired pneumonia. *Curr Opin Pulmon Med* 1997;**3**:89–97.

18 Young M, Marrie TJ. Interobserver variability in the interpretation of chest roentgenograms of patients with possible pneumonia. *Arch Intern Med* 1994;**154**:2729–32.

19 Albaum MN, Hill LC, Murphy M, et al. Interobserver reliability of the chest radiograph in community-acquired pneumonia. *Chest* 1996;**110**:342–50.

20 Melbye H, Dale K. Interobserver variability in the radiographic diagnosis of adult outpatient pneumonia. *Acta Radiol* 1992;**33**:79–81.

21 Robinson PJ, Wilson D, Coral A, et al. Variation between experienced observers in the interpretation of accident and emergency radiographs. *Br J Radiol* 1999;**2**:323–30.

22 Herman PG, Gerson DE, Hessel SJ, et al. Disagreements in chest roentgen interpretation. *Chest* 1975;**68**:278–82.

23 Malcolm C, Marrie TJ. Antibiotic therapy for ambulatory patients with community-acquired pneumonia in an emergency department setting. *Arch Intern Med* 2003;**163**:797–802.

24 Campbell SG, Murray DD, Hawass A, et al. Agreement between emergency physician diagnosis and radiologist reports in patients discharged from an emergency department with community-acquired pneumonia. *Emerg Radiol* 2005;**11**:242–6.

25 Benger JR, Lyburn ID. What is the effect of reporting all emergency department radiographs? *Emerg Med J* 2003;**20**:40–43.

26 Gratton MC, Salomone JA, III, Watson WA. Clinically significant radiograph misinterpretations at an emergency medicine residency program. *Ann Emerg Med* 1990;**19**:497–502.

27 Katz DS, Leung AN. Radiology of pneumonia. *Clin Chest Med* 1999;**20**(3):549–62.

28 Marrie TJ, Poulin-Costello M, Beecroft MD, et al. Etiology of community-acquired pneumonia treated in an ambulatory setting. *Respir Med* 2005;**99**:60–65.

29 Campbell SG, Marrie TJ, Anstey R, et al. Utility of blood cultures in the management of adults with community acquired pneumonia discharged from the emergency department. *Emerg Med J* 2003;**20**:521–3.

30 Chang NN, Murray CK, Houck PM, et al. Blood culture and susceptibility results and allergy history do not influence fluoroquinolone use in the treatment of community-acquired pneumonia. *Pharmacotherapy* 2005;**25**:59–66.

31 Campbell SG, Marrie TJ, Anstey R, et al. The contribution of blood cultures to the clinical management of adult patients admitted to hospital with community-acquired pneumonia: a prospective observational study. *Chest* 2003;**123**:1142–50.

32 Mountain D, Bailey PM, O'Brien D, Jelinek GA. Blood cultures ordered in the adult emergency department are rarely useful. *Eur J Emerg Med* 2006;**13**:76–9.

33 Bates DW, Goldman L, Lee TH. Contaminant blood cultures and resource utilization. The true consequences of false-positive results. *JAMA* 1991;**25**:365–9.

34 San Pedro GS, Campbell GD. Limitations of diagnostic testing in the initial management of patients with community-acquired pneumonia. *Semin Resp Infect* 1997;**12**:300–307.

35 Levy M, Dromer F, Brion N, et al. Community-acquired pneumonia: importance of initial noninvasive bacteriologic and radiographic investigations. *Chest* 1988;**92**:43–8.

36 Chalasani NP, Valdecanas MAL, Gopal AK, et al. Clinical utility of blood cultures in adult patients with community-acquired pneumonia without defined underlying risks. *Chest* 1995;**108**:932–8.

37 Woodhead MA, Arrowsmith J, Chamberlain-Webber R, et al. The value of routine microbiological investigation in community-acquired pneumonia. *Respir Med* 1991;**85**:313–17.

38 Ewig S, Bauer T, Hasper E, et al. Value of routine microbial investigation in community-acquired pneumonia treated in a tertiary care centre. *Respiration* 1996;**63**:164–9.

39 Waterer GW, Wunderink RG. The influence of the severity of community-acquired pneumonia on the usefulness of blood cultures. *Respir Med* 2001;**95**:78–82.

40 Theerthakarai R, El-Halees W, Ismail M, et al. Non value of the initial microbiological studies in the management of nonsevere community-acquired pneumonia. *Chest* 2001;**119**:181–4.

41 Sanyal S, Smith PR, Saha AC, et al. Initial microbiologic studies did not affect outcome in adults hospitalized with community-acquired pneumonia. *Am J Respir Crit Care Med* 1999;**160**:346–8.

42 Ramanujam P, Rathlev NK. Blood cultures do not change management in hospitalized patients with community-acquired pneumonia. *Acad Emerg Med* 2006;**13**:740–45.

43 Kennedy M, Bates DW, Wright SB, et al. Do emergency department blood cultures change practice in patients with pneumonia? *Ann Emerg Med* 2005;**46**:393–400.

44 Marrie TJ, Low DE, De Carolis E, et al. A comparison of bacteremic pneumococcal pneumonia with nonbacteremic community-acquired pneumonia of any etiology – results from a Canadian multicentre study. *Can Respir J* 2003;**10**:368–74.

45 Pomilla PV, Brown RB. Outpatient treatment of community-acquired pneumonia in adults. *Arch Intern Med* 1994;**154**:1793–802.

46 Fine MJ, Auble TE, Yealy DM, et al. A prediction rule to identify low-risk patients with community-acquired pneumonia. *N Engl J Med* 1997;**336**:243–50.

47 Lim WS, van der Eerden MM, Laing R, et al. Defining community acquired pneumonia severity on presentation to hospital: an international derivation and validation study. *Thorax* 2003;**58**:377–82.

48 Ewig S, Torres A, Woodhead M. Assessment of pneumonia severity: a European perspective. *Eur Respir J* 2006;**27**:6–8.

49 Aujeski D, Auble TE, Yealy DM, et al. Prospective validation of three validated prediction rules for prognosis in community-acquired pneumonia. *Am J Med* 2005;**118**:384–92.

50 Niederman MS, Feldman C, Richards GA. Combining information from prognostic scoring tools for CAP: an American view on how to get the best of all worlds. *Eur Respir J* 2006;**27**:9–11.

51 Marras TK, Nopmaneejumruslers C, Chan CK. Efficacy of exclusively oral antibiotic therapy in patients hospitalized with nonsevere community-acquired pneumonia: a retrospective study and meta-analysis. *Am J Med* 2004;**116**(6):385–93.

52 Weiss K, Tillotson GS. The controversy of combination vs monotherapy in the treatment of hospitalized community-acquired pneumonia. *Chest* 2005;**128**:940–46.

53 Lonks JR, Garau J, Medeiros AA. Implications of antimicrobial resistance in the empirical treatment of community-acquired respiratory tract infections: the case of macrolides. *J Antimicrob Chemother* 2002;**50**(S2):87–92.

54 Bjerre LM, Verheij TJM, Kochen MM. Antibiotics for community acquired pneumonia in adult outpatients. *Cochrane Database Syst Rev* 2004;**2**:CD002109 (doi: 10.1002/14651858.CD002109.pub2).

55 Salkind AR, Cuddy PG, Foxworth JW. Fluoroquinolone treatment of community-acquired pneumonia: a meta-analysis. *Ann Pharmacother* 2002;**36**:1938–43.

56 Mills GD, Oehley MR, Arrol B. Effectiveness of beta lactam antibiotics compared with antibiotics active against atypical pathogens in non-severe community acquired pneumonia: meta-analysis. *BMJ* 2005;**330**:456.

57 Oosterheert JJ, Bonten MJ, Hak E, et al. How good is the evidence for the recommended empirical antimicrobial treatment of patients hospitalized because of community-acquired pneumonia: a systematic review. *J Antimicrob Chemother* 2003;**52**:555–63.

58 Kolditz M, Halank M, Hoffken G. Monotherapy versus combination therapy in patients hospitalized with community-acquired pneumonia. *Treat Respir Med* 2006;**5**:371–83.

59 Shefet D, Robenshtok E, Paul M, Leibovici L. Empiric antibiotic coverage of atypical pathogens for community acquired pneumonia in hospitalized adults. *Cochrane Database Syst Rev* 2005;**2**:CD004418 (doi: 10.1002/14651858.CD004418.pub2).

60 Metge CJ, Vercaigne L, Carrie A, Zhanel GG. *New Fluoroquinolones in Community-acquired Pneumonia: A clinical and economic evaluation.* Canadian Coordinating Office for Health Technology Assessment (CCOHTA), Ottawa, 2001:75.

61 Falagas ME, Siempos II, Bliziotis IA, Panos GZ. Impact of initial discordant treatment with beta-lactam antibiotics on clinical outcomes in adults with pneumococcal pneumonia: a systematic review. *Mayo Clin Proc* 2006;**81**:1567–74.

62 Heffron R. *Pneumonia with Special Reference to Pneumococcus Lobar Pneumonia.* Harvard University Press, Cambridge, MA, 1939:656–726.

63 Austrian R, Gold J. Pneumococcal bacteremia with especial reference to bacteremic pneumococcal pneumonia. *Ann Intern Med* 1964;**60**:759–76.

64 Fine MJ, Smith MA, Carson CA, et al. Prognosis and outcomes of patients with community-acquired pneumonia. *JAMA* 1996;**12**:134–41.

65 Kaplan V, Clermont G, Griffin MF, et al. Pneumonia – still the old man's friend? *Arch Intern Med* 2003;**163**:317–23.

66 Koivula I, Stén M, Mäkelä PH. Prognosis after community-acquired pneumonia in the elderly – a population-based 12-year follow-up study. *Arch Intern Med* 1999;**159**:1550–55.

67 Menendez R, Torres A, Rodriguez de Castro F, et al. Reaching stability in community-acquired pneumonia: the effects of the severity of disease, treatment, and the characteristics of patients. *Clin Infect Dis* 2004;**39**:1783–90.

68 Metlay JP, Fine MJ, Schulz R, et al. Measuring symptomatic and functional recovery in patients with community-acquired pneumonia. *J Gen Intern Med* 1997;**12**:423–30.

69 El Moussaoui R, Opmeer BC, de Borgie CA, et al. Long-term symptom recovery and health-related quality of life in patients with mild-to-moderate-severe community-acquired pneumonia. *Chest* 2006;**130**:1165–72.

70 Campbell SG, Murray DD, Urquhart DG, et al. Utility of follow-up recommendations for patients discharged with community-acquired pneumonia. *Can J Emerg Med* 2004;**6**:97–103.

71 Gibson SP, Weir DC, Burge PS. A prospective audit of the value of fibreoptic bronchoscopy in adults admitted with community acquired pneumonia. *Respir Med* 1993;**87**:105–9.

72 Vanderkooi OG, Low DE, Green K, et al. Predicting antimicrobial resistance in invasive pneumococcal infections. *Clin Infect Dis* 2005;**40**:1288–97.

73 Brown EM, Nathwani D. Antibiotic cycling or rotation: a systematic review of the evidence of efficacy. *J Antimicrob Chemother* 2005;**55**:6–9.

12 Deep Vein Thrombosis

Eddy S. Lang[1] & Phil Wells[2]

[1]Department of Family Medicine, McGill University, Montreal *and* Department of Emergency Medicine, SMBD Jewish General Hospital, Montreal, Canada
[2]Division of Hematology, Department of Medicine, University of Ottawa, Ottawa *and* The Ottawa Hospital, Ottawa, Canada

Case scenario

An 82-year-old male presents to the emergency department (ED) at 10 p.m. on a Friday evening with complaints of a swollen and tender left lower extremity of 3 days' duration. The symptoms seem to have developed after a vigorous tennis match, which he enjoys with a group of players three times a week. He first noticed calf soreness at that time but was surprised to note marked swelling tenderness and some redness the morning after his symptoms first appeared.

The patient's past medical history is significant for remote prostate cancer for which he was treated with a radical prostatectomy 3 years ago as well as hormonal therapy, which he discontinued 2 years ago. Nothing in his history or exam suggests recurrence. The patient also recently returned (1 week prior to this presentation) home after taking a 3-hour plane ride from the Bahamas. The patient is taking a small dose of aspirin on a daily basis for "cardio-protection" and an angiotension-converting enzyme (ACE) inhibitor to treat his hypertension. The patient is otherwise healthy, has no history of thromboembolic disease and denies fever, chills or any respiratory symptoms.

On examination the patient appears in no significant distress but is limping. His vital signs reveal a heart rate of 80 beats/min, blood pressure of 140/90 mmHg (right arm), respiratory rate of 16 breaths/min and a temperature of 36.9°C (oral). The left leg appears diffusely swollen and mildly erythematous from the level of the upper calf down to the ankle. There is a 3 cm difference in calf circumference as measured 10 cm below the tibial tuberosity in comparison to the unaffected side and mild pitting edema. There is no evidence of either varicose or superficial collateral veins or ecchymosis. There is diffuse tenderness of the calf muscles but this is not limited to the distribution of the deep venous system. Posterior tibial and dorsalis pedis arterial pulses are palpable,

regular and strong. The remainder of the physical examination is unremarkable.

Background

Suspected and confirmed deep vein thrombosis (DVT) is a commonly encountered diagnostic and therapeutic challenge in the emergency department (ED). DVTs can mimic a wide variety of conditions including cellulitis, Baker's cyst, mixed connective tissue disease, ischemic limb, musculoskeletal trauma and extrinsic venous compression from various causes. Consequently, suspected cases require a thorough diagnostic approach searching for alternative diagnoses. The incidence of DVT in the general population is believed to be 67 in 100,000 [1]. This translates to an individual lifetime risk of one in 20 for any given individual [2]. An imbalance between clot formation and degradation, favoring the former, is believed to lie at the heart of the development of DVT. The classic triad of venous injury, impaired blood flow and hypercoagulability, described by Virchow in the 19th century, are the major factors associated with the development of DVT. The management of the patient with a swollen leg has been refined with epidemiological and robust clinical decision rule research over the last 10–15 years and is one of the success stories of evidence-based emergency medicine decision making.

The venous anatomy of the lower extremity consists of both a deep and superficial system. The superficial system consists primarily of the greater and short saphenous veins, the perforating veins and the muscle veins of the gastrocnemius and soleus. The deep venous system includes the anterior tibial, posterior tibial and peroneal veins, collectively called the *calf veins*. The calf veins join together at the knee to form the popliteal vein, which extends proximally and becomes the femoral vein at the adductor canal. Although part of the deep venous system, the femoral vein is sometimes called the *superficial femoral vein*, and this nomenclature may contribute to some confusion when interpreting imaging reports. The femoral vein joins with the deep femoral vein to form the common femoral vein, which subsequently becomes the external

Evidence-based Emergency Medicine. Edited by Brian H. Rowe
© 2009 Blackwell Publishing, ISBN: 978-1-4051-6143-5.

iliac vein at the inguinal ligament. Proximal DVT refers to clot in the popliteal vein or higher, whereas *distal clot* refers to an isolated calf vein thrombosis. The majority of DVTs (70–80%) involve proximal veins, namely the popliteal and superficial femoral veins, whereas the remaining 20–30% involve the calf veins, consisting of the peroneal, posterior tibial or anterior tibial veins [3]. Proximal DVTs carry a significantly greater risk of embolization than calf DVTs.

Increasingly, DVT is recognized as a continuum of a spectrum of illness, known as venous thomboembolism (VTE), and includes the embolic manifestation of DVT, pulmonary embolism (PE), which itself carries a mortality of up to 8% even in adequately treated patients [4,5]. The overlap between DVT and PE is supported by the observation that approximately 50% of patients with documented DVT have high probability V/Q scans or filling defects on spiral computerized tomography (CT), and coexistent venous thrombosis is found in approximately 70% of patients with confirmed PE [6]. With its high risk of death, PE can be considered the major complication of DVT that timely diagnosis and treatment seeks to avoid [4,5]. Another important complication, post-phlebitic syndrome, will develop in 20–50% of patients with DVTs, one-quarter of these acquiring the severe form characterized by lower extremity ulcerations [7].

General search strategy

You begin to address these questions by searching for evidence in the common electronic databases such as the Cochrane Library, MEDLINE and EMBASE looking specifically for systematic reviews and meta-analyses. The Cochrane Database of Systematic Reviews includes high-quality systematic review evidence on therapy for DVT and the Database of Abstracts of Reviews of Effects (DARE) includes systematic review evidence on the diagnosis of DVT. You also search the Cochrane Central Register of Controlled Trials (CENTRAL), MEDLINE and EMBASE to identify randomized controlled trials (RCTs) that became available after the publication date of the systematic review or, if no systematic reviews were identified, to locate high-quality RCTs that directly address the clinical question. In addition, access to relevant, updated, evidence-based clinical practice guidelines (CPGs) on DVT are accessed to determine the consensus rating of areas lacking evidence.

Clinical questions

1 In patients with suspected DVT (population), are there valid and reliable clinical criteria (clinical decision rules) that can accurately define a patient's (prior) probability of suffering from a DVT (outcome)?
2 In patients with suspected DVT (population), are the odds ratios (diagnostic test characteristics) for uncommon risk factors (e.g., genetic predispositions, rare suspected side-effects of medications, prolonged flight) sufficiently powerful to assist in the diagnosis of a DVT (outcome)?

3 In patients with a low or moderate pre-test probability of DVT (population), are the likelihood ratios (diagnostic test characteristics) of a D-dimer assay sufficiently powerful to exclude a DVT (outcome) without the need for imaging modalities?
4 In patients with suspected DVT who undergo compression ultrasonography (population), are the likelihood ratios (diagnostic test characteristics) associated with a positive and negative result sufficiently powerful to cross test and treatment thresholds (outcome)?
5 In patients with a confirmed diagnosis of calf DVT (population), does anticoagulation with heparin (adjusted dose UFH or LMWH) (intervention) reduce the incidence of recurrent venous thromboembolism and proximal extension of deep vein thromboses (outcome) compared to placebo or non-steroidal anti-inflammatory agents?
6 In patients with a confirmed diagnosis of proximal DVT (population), does anticoagulation with a LMWH (intervention) reduce the incidence of subsequent thromboembolic events (outcome) compared to adjusted dose UFH administered either subcutaneously or intravenously (control)?
7 In patients with a confirmed diagnosis of proximal DVT (population), does inpatient anticoagulation therapy (intervention) reduce morbidity and recurrent VTE (outcome) compared to at-home treatment with similar agents (control)?
8 In patients with a confirmed diagnosis of proximal DVT (population), does the early utilization of compressive stockings (intervention) reduce the incidence and severity of post-phlebitic syndrome (outcome) compared to standard care (control)?
9 In patients with a confirmed diagnosis of proximal DVT (population), does anticoagulation with one LMWH (intervention) lead to lower subsequent VTE events (outcome) compared with others (control)?
10 In patients with suspected DVT can treatment be safely initiated in the ED if diagnostic testing will be delayed?

Question 1: In patients with suspected DVT (population), are there valid and reliable clinical criteria (clinical decision rules) that can accurately define a patient's (prior) probability of suffering from a DVT (outcome)?

Search strategy

- Cochrane Library, MEDLINE and EMBASE: (venous thrombosis OR thrombophlebitis) AND (fibrin OR fibrinogen degradation products) AND predictive value of tests. Also used keywords: DVT, D-dimer, diagnosis, clinical prediction rules, clinical probability, clinical model, decision rules, sensitivity, specificity

Clinical decision rule (CDR) development is perhaps more advanced in the realm of DVT than in any other area of clinical medicine. CDRs use standardized and easily determined elements of the clinical examination, generally those that are most discriminating, to define a patient's likelihood of suffering from a DVT. The rationale for the development and application of a CDR for suspected DVT is that it empowers clinicians who may have variable

Table 12.1 Wells' prediction rule for deep venous thrombosis: clinical evaluation table for predicting pre-test probability of deep vein thrombosis.

Clinical characteristic	Score
Active cancer (treatment ongoing, within previous 6 months or palliative)	1
Paralysis, paresis or recent plaster immobilization of the lower extremities	1
Recently bedridden > 3 days or major surgery within 12 weeks requiring general or regional anesthesia	1
Localized tenderness along the distribution of the deep venous system	1
Entire leg swollen	1
Calf circumference 3 cm or larger than asymptomatic side (measured 10 cm below tibial tuberosity)	1
Pitting edema confined to the symptomatic leg	1
Collateral superficial veins (non-varicose)	1
Alternative diagnosis at least as likely as deep venous thrombosis	−2

Note: a score of 3 or higher indicates a high probability of deep vein thrombosis; 1 or 2, a moderate probability; and 0 or lower, a low probability.

degrees of clinical experience and acumen to determine, based on objective criteria, the likelihood of a given patient suffering a DVT. Moreover, these CDRs have the potential to significantly reduce practice variation and improve patient flow in the ED setting. Armed with this accurate assessment of clinical probability the emergency physician is then able to confidently decide on the need for diagnostic testing or serial diagnostic testing in the event that first results are negative. Similarly, the likelihood of DVT will determine the need for empirical anticoagulant therapy when imaging studies are not readily available. Finally, an appreciation of this pre-test probability is essential to the interpretation of subsequent laboratory and imaging tests, achieving an informed and accurate post-test probability of disease.

Among existing CDRs to define likelihood of DVT, the Wells criteria are both the most validated and widely studied instrument [8]. Outlined in Table 12.1, the Wells simplified CDR for DVT has been consistently shown to accurately discriminate between patients at low, moderate and high probability of DVT. In a systematic review performed to examine the properties of the Wells clinical probability model for determining the likelihood of DVT, the combined findings of 14 studies recruiting over 8000 patients were presented [8]. The prevalence of DVT in the low, moderate and high clinical probability groups, based on the Wells score, was 5.0% (95% CI: 4.0% to 8.0%), 17% (95% CI: 13% to 23%) and 53% (95% CI: 44% to 61%), respectively. The overall prevalence of DVT in this population was 19% (95% CI: 16% to 23%). Some authors have suggested that this prevalence reflects a referral bias and that the prevalence in most primary care and ED settings would be even lower. If true, this would argue for the safety of strategies that use CDR-driven determination of low pre-test probability in combination with other tests to exclude DVT. The Wells rule has been compared against alternative models and empirical clinical judgment in a number of studies and, while determined to be equivalent, the robustness of this evidence is limited and may only apply to more experienced clinicians [9,10].

In summary, the Wells criteria CDR is a valid, reliable and sensible tool to assign pre-test probability to patients in the ED with suspected lower limb DVT. Emergency physicians using this tool, in conjunction with other diagnostic modalities, can safely and reliably manage patients with suspected DVT.

Question 2: In patients with suspected DVT (population), are the odds ratios (diagnostic test characteristics) for uncommon risk factors (e.g., genetic predispositions, rare suspected side-effects of medications, prolonged flight) sufficiently powerful to assist in the diagnosis of a DVT (outcome)?

Search strategy

- Cochrane Library, MEDLINE and EMBASE: (venous thrombosis OR thrombophlebitis) AND predictive value of tests. Also used keywords: DVT, diagnosis, risks, genetics, predisposition, sensitivity, specificity

While Virchow's triad describes the three global factors that predispose to DVT, there is an emerging literature identifying a myriad of other factors that are associated with an increased risk of DVT and VTE. Well-established associations with an increased risk of DVT are features such as advancing age and sex. Specifically epidemiological research suggests that VTE is more common in men and that for each 10-year increase in age, the incidence is doubled [11].

As demonstrated by individual elements within the highly validated Wells CDR, prolonged immobility – as one might observe after prolonged bed rest related to major surgery or illness – carries a strong association with the development of DVT. Similarly, active malignancy, defined as diagnosed or actively treated within the previous 12 months, is recognized as a predisposing factors for DVT. However, the nature of CDR development is that risk factor that are either unknown, difficult to measure or occur very rarely might not readily get incorporated as one of the elements of the CDR.

Fortunately, additional work has established rarer and lesser known risk factors that appear to increase a patient's risk of DVT and which merit consideration in the ED evaluation of the patient. Of note, a history of previous DVT is well described as an important risk factor in the evaluation of patients suspected of an acute thrombosis. This feature was not among the factors in the original Wells model as it constituted an exclusion criteria for entry into the studies that derived and validated this rule. Recent data suggest it can be incorporated into the model and be scored as +1 when present [11]. In a comprehensive review of 42 established risk factors for VTE a number of features that can be either asked about or suspected in the ED setting are described in Table 12.2, presented as both acquired and inherited elements [12]. Among the more uncommon risk factors that an emergency physician can elicit on history are the inherited or genetic thrombophilias, listed in Table 12.3, that are becoming increasingly recognized as important and surprisingly prevalent risk factors for the development of VTE.

Table 12.2 Acquired risk factors for venous thromboembolism. (Adapted from Anderson & Spencer [12].)

Strong risk factors (odds ratio > 10)
Fracture (hip or leg)
Hip or knee replacement
Major general surgery
Major trauma
Spinal cord injury

Moderate risk factors (odds ratio 2 to 9)
Arthroscopic knee surgery
Central venous lines
Chemotherapy
Congestive heart or respiratory failure
Hormone replacement therapy, although recent evidence suggests no
 increased risk with estradiol patches
Active malignancy
Oral contraceptive therapy, especially in the first year of use
Paralytic stroke
Pregnancy/postpartum
Previous venous thromboembolism
Thrombophilia

Weak risk factors (odds ratio <2)
Bed rest >3 days
Immobility due to sitting (e.g., prolonged car or air travel)
Increasing age
Laparoscopic surgery (e.g., cholecystectomy)
Obesity
Pregnancy/antepartum
Varicose veins

Table 12.3 Frequency (%) of inherited thrombophilic syndromes in the general population and in patients with venous thrombosis syndrome. (Adapted with permission from Anderson & Spencer [12], © 2003 *Circulation*.)

	General population	Unselected patients with venous thrombosis
AT deficiency	0.02–0.17	1.1
PC deficiency	0.14–0.5	3.2
PS deficiency	2.2	1.4–7.5
APC resistance (factor V Leiden)	3.6–6.0	21.0, up to 30%
Prothrombin G20210A81	1.7–3.0	6.2, up to 8%

APC, activated protein C; AT, anti-thrombin; PC, protein C; PS, protein S.

Question 3: In patients with a low or moderate pre-test probability of DVT (population), are the likelihood ratios (diagnostic test characteristics) of a D-dimer assay sufficiently powerful to exclude a DVT (outcome) without the need for imaging modalities?

Search strategy

- Cochrane Library, MEDLINE and EMBASE: (venous thrombosis OR thrombophlebitis) AND (fibrin OR fibrinogen degradation products) AND predictive value of tests. Also used keywords: DVT, D-dimer, diagnosis, clinical prediction rules, clinical probability, clinical model, decision rules, sensitivity, specificity

D-dimers are the degradation products of a cross-linked fibrin clot and are generally elevated in patients with acute VTE. D-dimer elevation is not, however, specific to VTE and is elevated in a number of inflammatory conditions, chronic diseases and patients that are both sedentary and elderly. The value of a sensitive D-dimer assay in the setting of low-to-moderate pre-test probability of DVT, as established by an instrument such as the Wells CDR, is that it can render post-test probability low enough to exclude the diagnosis of DVT without the need to arrange imaging studies.

There are a variety of D-dimer assays available and these have been the focus of extensive clinical investigation. The question has been the object of extensive research since the practice implications are significant. Systematic reviews have specifically examined whether the addition of a D-dimer (either highly sensitive or not) can be combined with pre-test probability to exclude an acute DVT. For the purpose of this review we will consider D-dimers in three categories. The first being the highly sensitive assays such as the enzyme-linked immunosorbent assay (e.g., VIDAS™, Biomerieux), the second being moderately sensitive tests such as those that employ quantitative immunoturbimetric and latex methods, and the third being the qualitative agglutination assays such as the SimpliRED® D-dimer.

In their review of 11 high-quality studies that recruited over 5600 patients Wells et al. determined the summary likelihood ratios (LRs) of high-sensitivity D-dimer assays according to clinical probability [8]. As demonstrated in Table 12.4, the summary negative LR (–LR) for patients in all ranges of clinical probability based on decision rule criteria is 0.1 or lower. However, only patients in low and moderate pre-test probability strata will have a post-test probability of < 1%, allowing the clinician reasonable confidence in excluding that diagnosis. When examining moderate-sensitivity D-dimer assays, including the SimpliRED® whole-blood agglutination assay, in the context of varying levels of pre-test probability, this review reported that the summary –LR associated with a low Wells score was 0.20 (95% CI: 0.12 to 0.31), which enables exclusion of only low probability patients [8].

A *Health Technology Assessment* (*HTA*) report also determined that a diagnostic strategy based on Wells clinical criteria in combination with D-dimer testing was both the most effective and cost-effective diagnostic algorithm to employ when evaluating patients suspected of an acute proximal DVT [9]. Yet another systematic review included 12 trials that examined the question of combining Wells criteria and D-dimer assays to exclude DVTs and reached similar conclusions [13]. The combination of clinical probability testing and D-dimer assay has also been subjected to the rigor of a randomized controlled trial of over 1000 patients with suspected DVT. Patients were randomized to one of two groups: (i) where a D-dimer assay was combined

Table 12.4 Accuracy measures in high-sensibility ᴅ-dimer studies. (Reprinted with permission from Wells et al. [8], © 2006 American Medical Association.)

Clinical probability before testing	Study	Sensitivity, %	Specificity, %	NPV, %	LR (95% CI)	−LR (95% CI)
Low	Bates et al. 2003	97	69	100	3.3 (2.7/3.9)	0.04 (0/0.65)
	Schutgens et al. 2003	96	51	99	2.0 (1.7/2.4)	0.07 (0.01/0.5)
	Bucek et al. 2002	83	53	99	2.1 (1.7/2.6)	0.32 (0.03/3.9)
	Weighted average (95% CI)	95 (82–99)	58 (45–71)	99 (97–100)	2.4 (1.7/3.3)	0.10 (0.03/0.3)
Moderate	Bates et al. 2003	94	52	99	2.0 (1.6/2.4)	0.11 (0.02/0.7)
	Schutgens et al. 2003	100	40	99	1.7 (1.5/1.9)	0.01 (0/0.16)
	Aguilar et al. 2002	98	32	99	1.5 (1.3/1.7)	0.06 (0/0.85)
	Weighted average (95% CI)	98 (91–100)	41 (31–52)	99 (96–100)	1.7 (1.5/1.9)	0.05 (0.01/0.2)
High	Bales et al. 2003	98	40	98	1.7 (1.3/2.1)	0.06 (0/0.85)
	Schutgens et al. 2003	98	34	90	1.5 (1.3/1.7)	0.07 (0.03/0.2)
	Weighted average (95% CI)	97 (94–99)	36 (29–43)	92 (81–97)	1.5 (1.4/1.7)	0.07 (0.03/0.1)

LR, Positive likelihood ratio; −LR, negative likelihood ratio; NPV, negative predictive value.

with clinical probability, with the ultrasound dependent on the ᴅ-dimer result; or (ii) where clinical probability with ultrasound was used in all patients approached. In the former group no compression ultrasonography was performed if DVT-unlikely patients (score = 1 by the Wells model) had negative ᴅ-dimer assays (using moderate-sensitivity ᴅ-dimer assays). Results of this trial revealed that both strategies were equally safe in regard to subsequently diagnosed (and presumed missed) VTE, while ultrasound imaging was reduced by 39% in the ᴅ-dimer arm [11].

In conclusion, patients with low or moderate probability of DVT can forego imaging if they are deemed to have a negative result on a highly or moderately sensitive ᴅ-dimer assay.

Question 4: In patients with suspected DVT who undergo compression ultrasonography (population), are the likelihood ratios (diagnostic test characteristics) associated with a positive and negative result sufficiently powerful to cross test and treatment thresholds (outcome)?

Search strategy

- Cochrane Library, MEDLINE and EMBASE: (venous thrombosis OR thrombophlebitis) AND (diagnosis OR ultrasonography). Also used keywords: DVT, ᴅ-dimer, diagnosis, sensitivity, specificity

The most widely used modality for the imaging of patients with suspected DVT involves ultrasound. Ultrasound has largely replaced other modalities such as venography and impedence plethysmography for reasons of patient comfort and safety as well as improved diagnostic accuracy. Ultrasound-mediated modalities for DVT diagnosis consist largely of compression ultrasonography whereby the incompressibility of a deep vein is considered diagnostic (except in cases of recurrent DVT). Color or continuous wave Doppler are also helpful in identifying veins and may delineate thrombus and abnormal venous flow suggestive of DVT.

In the most comprehensive systematic review on this topic, Goodacre in concert with the National Health Service (NHS) HTA agency identified 151 studies that reported the diagnostic properties of ultrasound in the diagnosis of DVT [9]. The following techniques were used: 22 used compression ultrasonography alone, five used color Doppler alone, 16 used continuous wave Doppler alone, 28 used duplex (compression and color Doppler), 25 used triplex (compression, color Doppler and continuous wave Doppler) and four used other techniques. Among 100 cohorts of patients with symptoms of DVT, ultrasound proved to be both fairly sensitive and highly specific for the diagnosis of DVT. Pooled sensitivity for detecting proximal DVT was 94.2% (95% CI: 93.2 to 95.0); however, for distal DVT it was only as good as 63.5% (95% CI: 59.8 to 67.0). Pooled specificity, calculated using data from all 98 studies, was 93.8% (95% CI: 93.1 to 94.4). These values would equate to crude positive and negative likelihood ratios of 15 and 0.06, respectively.

In summary, ultrasound imaging of the deep veins, using the criterion of non-compressibility, is the diagnostic modality of first choice for detecting proximal vein DVT.

Question 5: In patients with a confirmed diagnosis of calf DVT (population), does anticoagulation with heparin (adjusted dose UFH or LMWH) (intervention) reduce the incidence of recurrent venous thromboembolism and proximal extension of deep vein thromboses (outcome) compared to placebo or non-steroidal anti-inflammatory agents?

Search strategy

- Cochrane Library, MEDLINE and EMBASE: (venous thrombosis OR thrombophlebitis) AND (treatment OR management). Also used keywords: DVT, heparin, low molecular weight heparin, nonsteroidal anti-inflammatory agents, anticoagulation and anticoagulants

The goal of therapy in proximal DVT is to prevent the extension and embolization of thrombus to the lungs. In addition, therapy should attempt to reduce the incidence of local complications of DVT (i.e., post-phlebitic syndrome). Anticoagulation with heparin and heparinoid agents has been advocated as the treatment for proximal DVT for over four decades and has developed into a standard of care incorporated into a number of clinical practice guidelines. This has occurred despite an absence of high-quality evidence from RCTs comparing heparin against placebo or anti-inflammatories [14]. One study, however, demonstrated superiority of unfractionated heparin (UFH) followed by oral anticoagulants when compared to oral anticoagulants alone for proximal DVT [14]. Less evident is the optimal management of patients with calf DVTs, which are not only more difficult to diagnose but are thought to carry a much better prognosis than proximal DVTs. Nevertheless, calf DVTs are associated with eventual proximal extension in about 20% of cases [15].

A systematic review of the treatment of DVT conducted by the Agency for Healthcare Research and Quality (AHRQ) concluded that anticoagulation is beneficial for symptomatic calf DVT, based primarily on two studies of isolated calf thromboses [16]. These findings were based on two RCTs that included less than 250 patients in total and suggested that warfarin treatment for 3 months significantly reduced recurrence, extension and pulmonary embolism at 3 months. A study by Pinede et al. suggests 6 weeks of therapy is as effective as 3 months' therapy, and that overall recurrence risk is much less than with proximal DVT [17].

In the Seventh Conference on Antithrombotic and Thrombolytic Therapy, the American College of Chest Physicians recommended treating symptomatic isolated calf DVT with anticoagulation for 3 months (international normalized ratio (INR) 2–3) [18]. They explicitly place higher value on "preventing recurrent thromboembolic events . . . [than] on bleeding and cost". Another systematic review notes that searching for distal DVT entails a risk of over-treatment, since data in support of anticoagulant therapy for distal DVT are limited [19].

In summary, calf vein DVT is a difficult diagnosis to make. In practice, many physicians do treat distal DVT symptomatically with non-steroidal anti-inflammatory agents and perform serial ultrasound testing to rule out proximal extension. Further study is clearly indicated in this group of patients.

Question 6: In patients with a confirmed diagnosis of proximal DVT (population), does anticoagulation with a LMWH (intervention) reduce the incidence of subsequent thromboembolic events (outcome) compared to adjusted dose UFH administered either subcutaneously or intravenously (control)?

Search strategy

- Cochrane Library, MEDLINE and EMBASE: (venous thrombosis OR thrombophlebitis) AND (treatment OR management). Also used keywords: DVT, recurrence, heparin, low molecular weight heparin, nonsteroidal anti-inflammatory agents, anticoagulation and anticoagulants

The introduction of low molecular weight heparins (LMWHs) has revolutionized the treatment of VTE. The Cochrane group reported findings from nine high-quality trials involving 4451 participants with proximal DVT and reported lower recurrent VTEs at follow-up (generally 3–6 months) in the LMWH group (OR = 0.57; 95% CI: 0.44 to 0.75) [20]. In the same Cochrane review involving eight trials and 4157 patients, LMWH use resulted in fewer deaths (OR = 0.62; 95% CI: 0.46 to 0.84), less heparin-induced thrombocytopenia, and less major bleeding (OR = 0.50; 95% CI: 0.29 to 0.85) compared to UFH. Thus the Cochrane group concluded that in patients with proximal DVT, weight-based, fixed-dose, subcutaneous LMWH is more effective than adjusted dose UFH for reducing the incidence of symptomatic recurrent VTE, major hemorrhage and all-cause mortality.

A number of systematic reviews have been performed on this question and have reached remarkably similar conclusions. Specifically, systematic reviews published by the AHRQ in 2003 and a review performed by the American College of Physicians and the American Academy of Family Physicians are all consistent with the Cochrane group conclusion [16,21]. This literature suggests that LMWH is advantageous in comparison to adjusted dose intravenous UFH in the treatment of proximal DVT both in terms of efficacy and safety outcomes. These publications also emphasize the safety, convenience and cost-effectiveness associated with LMWH.

In summary, patients with uncomplicated proximal DVTs should be started on LMWH by emergency physicians and assessed for home-based treatment (see below). The benefit associated with LMWH treatment does not appear to be specific to any one LMWH; this appears to be a class effect (see Question 9 below). The selection of the LMWH agent should be left to the institution or the treating physician.

Question 7: In patients with a confirmed diagnosis of proximal DVT (population), does inpatient anticoagulation therapy (intervention) reduce morbidity and recurrent VTE (outcome) compared to at-home treatment with similar agents (control)?

Search strategy

- Cochrane Library, MEDLINE and EMBASE: (venous thrombosis OR thrombophlebitis) AND (treatment OR management). Also used keywords: DVT, recurrence, outpatient, home therapy, heparin, low molecular weight heparin, nonsteroidal anti-inflammatory agents, anticoagulation, anticoagulants

Schraibman et al. addressed this question within the context of a Cochrane review of home versus inpatient treatment of patients with VTE [22]. The review incorporates three RCTs involving 1101 participants. All three had fundamental problems including high exclusion rates, partial hospital treatment of many in the LMWH arms, and comparison of UFH in hospital with LMWH at home. The trials showed that home treatment was no more likely to result in complications than hospital treatment. For instance, recurrence of VTE (RR = 0.78; 95% CI: 0.48 to 1.26), minor bleeding (RR = 1.57; 95% CI: 1.03 to 2.39), major bleeding (RR = 0.90; 95% CI: 0.35 to 2.31) and crude death rate (RR = 0.72; 95% CI: 0.44 to 1.18) were not statistically significantly different. The authors concluded that limited evidence suggests that home management is cost-effective, and likely to be preferred by patients. Several cohort studies have demonstrated the safety and efficacy of home treatment [23–25].

Furthermore, all the recent large RCTs of therapy have allowed treatment of patients on an outpatient basis. Home treatment has become the standard in many countries and it is likely that further research will be directed to resolving practical issues. Consideration for hospitalization should be given to patients in extreme pain or with iliofemoral DVTs. The AHRQ review of this question reached similar conclusions; the review also included nine relevant trials including cost-effectiveness studies [16]. The authors of this work also found that in comparisons between LMWH in the hospital or at home there was no difference in outcomes, but found a major savings in hospitalization costs.

In summary, most patients with uncomplicated proximal DVTs can be treated in the outpatient setting with LMWH and oral anticoagulants. The follow-up and monitoring of these patients is critical and the emergency medicine physician must ensure not only that patients are candidates for outpatient therapy, but also identify and communicate with the primary care provider.

Question 8: In patients with a confirmed diagnosis of proximal DVT (population), does the early utilization of compressive stockings (intervention) reduce the incidence and severity of post-phlebitic syndrome (outcome) compared to standard care (control)?

Search strategy

- Cochrane Library, MEDLINE and EMBASE: (venous thrombosis OR thrombophlebitis) AND (treatment OR management); post phlebitic AND post thrombotic syndrome. Also used keywords: DVT, heparin, low molecular weight heparin, complications, compression stockings, nonsteroidal anti-inflammatory agents, anticoagulation, anticoagulants

One out of every three people with DVT will develop post-phlebitic syndrome within 5 years. Although there is no consensus on the definition in the literature, the main item in all definitions is a documented DVT preceding the development of chronic leg complaints. These may include subjective symptoms of the legs, e.g., pain, cramps, heaviness, pruritus and paraesthesias as well as signs of stasis (pre-tibial edema, redness, induration (hardening) of the skin, hyperpigmentation, new venous ectasia (dilation) and pain during calf compression) and venous leg ulceration.

The pathophysiology of post-thrombotic syndrome is not entirely understood. Contributing factors are thought to be deep vein obstruction, venous reflux (back flow of blood in the veins) and calf muscle pump dysfunction. In the acute phase of DVT, a fresh thrombus in the deep vein produces an obstruction. In the first few months following deep venous thrombosis, recanalization, a complex process, occurs involving fibrinolysis, thrombus organization and neovascularization (proliferation of blood vessels). This process can result in valve destruction. Damaged valves, insufficient closure and/or occlusion of the veins increase pressure in the veins (venous hypertension). It is postulated that this venous hypertension disturbs the normal flow in small capillaries, resulting in increased capillary filtration leading to ankle flare, edema (swelling of the tissue caused by excessive fluid in the subcutaneous tissue) in the lower leg, and a number of skin changes which include dermatitis and, in severe cases, ulceration.

Kolbach et al. identified three trials reviewed through the Cochrane Collaboration which examined the benefit of compressive elastic stockings for the prevention of post-phlebitic syndrome [26]. These trials, with a composite recruitment of 421 patients, suggest a marked reduction in the risk of both the incidence and severity of post-phlebitic syndrome through the use of compression stockings. Specifically, the reviewers report that in the treatment group at 2 years, the use of elastic compression stockings was associated with a significant reduction in the incidence of post-phlebitic syndrome (OR = 0.31; 95% CI: 0.20 to 0.48). In addition, the incidence of severe post-phlebitic syndrome was reduced (OR = 0.39; 95% CI: 0.20 to 0.76). In most trials the intervention consisted of made-to-measure below-knee elastic compression stockings, with an ankle pressure of 40 mmHg. In all three trials compression stockings were initiated within 1 month of diagnosis and hence one could argue the limited relevance of this intervention for the ED. In light of the suggested effectiveness offered by this intervention, however, it certainly seems reasonable to recommend compression stockings early in the course of a patient's post-emergency care.

A more recent review on the same topic, which included four RCTs, reached the same conclusion as the Cochrane review [27]. Note that all these studies are limited by lack of blinding to treatment assignment and the subjective nature of the diagnosis of post-thrombotic syndrome. Furthermore, and perhaps most importantly, none of these studies evaluated patients after discontinuation of the graduated compression stockings. It is possible graduated compression stockings only treat, not prevent, PTS. The definitive trial to evaluate this is in progress (www.clinicaltrials.gov) [28].

In summary, evidence is unclear regarding the role emergency physicians can play in preventing post-phlebitis in patients with DVT. At the very least, patients likely should be fitted for compression stockings.

Question 9: In patients with a confirmed diagnosis of proximal DVT (population), does anticoagulation with one LMWH (intervention) lead to lower subsequent VTE events (outcome) compared with others (control)?

Search strategy

- Cochrane Library, MEDLINE and EMBASE: (venous thrombosis OR thrombophlebitis) AND (treatment OR management). Also used keywords: DVT, heparin, low molecular weight heparin, nonsteroidal anti-inflammatory agents, anticoagulation, anticoagulants

Only one RCT presents the results of a head-to-head comparison between two LMWHs. Wells et al. randomized 505 patients with proximal DVT and PE to a regimen based on either tinzaparin or dalteparin as the initial anticoagulant prior to switching to warfarin therapy [29]. The study's primary efficacy endpoint was recurrent VTE and a composite safety endpoint examining bleeding was also considered. The incidence of adverse outcomes was equivalent in both study arms, leading the authors to conclude that the agents were equivalent in the treatment of VTE. Although the Wells trial may not have been sufficiently powered to detect small differences in outcome based on those two agents, it has been suggested that it may be impractical to conduct the very large trials required to establish what may ultimately prove to be very small differences in outcomes [30].

Other evidence for a similar class effect among LMWHs is suggested by the effect size noted among the various LMWH agents examined in the Cochrane Collaboration review of these agents in the management of VTE [20]. This review compiled efficacy and safety data on six unique LMWH compounds, all revealing similar benefit and no statistical evidence of heterogeneity. Similarly, no differences between compounds have been identified when used for prophylaxis of venous thromboembolism [31]. While not technically a LMWH, fondaparinux (a synthetic factor Xa inhibitor) was compared to enoxaparin in an international multi-center RCT [31,32]. The Matisse trial enrolled 2022 patients with symptomatic DVT to a minimum 5-day regimen with one of the two molecules [33]. The trial reported similar 3-month rates of recurrent VTE, bleeding and mortality, leading the authors to conclude that fondaparinux was not inferior to twice-daily enoxaparin.

The benefit associated with LMWH treatment does not appear to be specific to any one LMWH; this appears to be a class effect. The selection of the LMWH agent should be left to the institution or the treating physician.

Question 10: In patients with suspected DVT can treatment be safely initiated in the ED if diagnostic testing will be delayed?

Search strategy

- Cochrane Library, MEDLINE and EMBASE: (venous thrombosis OR thrombophlebitis) AND (treatment OR management). Also used keywords: emergency department, diagnostic delay, DVT, heparin, low molecular weight heparin, nonsteroidal anti-inflammatory agents, anticoagulation, anticoagulants

As a result of the limited availability of imaging resources, emergency physicians are frequently faced with a patient in whom a DVT is suspected but the means of establishing an immediate definitive diagnosis are lacking. The question posed in this section has not been assessed with the rigor of a randomized controlled trial; however, a number of prospective cohort studies (i.e., management trials have reported outcomes with a practice of empirical LMWH in patients with suspected DVT) have been completed [34–37]. Specifically, these trials administered anywhere from 1 to 3 days of LMWH to patients with either a high pre-test probability of DVT as established by valid criteria, an elevated D-dimer, or both. All of these studies reported very low complication rates in what appears to be an extremely well-tolerated treatment and imaging strategy.

In summary, armed with valid clinical assessment instruments and D-dimer testing it appears that empirical initiation of LMWH until definitive imaging with ultrasonography can be performed is a safe and well-tolerated strategy in patients who do not have high bleeding risks or contraindications to anticoagulation.

Conclusions

A swollen limb is a common and important presentation in emergency medicine and consideration of DVT in the differential diagnosis is an important step to identifying this potentially deadly disease. Over the past decade, improvement in the diagnostic approach and treatment of DVT has been impressive. An organized approach using clinical decision rules, D-dimer testing and LMWH will lead clinicians to a more accurate and timely diagnosis of DVT.

The 82-year-old male who presented to the ED with a complaint of a swollen leg described in the clinical scenario had a moderate pre-test probability of DVT using the Wells clinical decision tool (pitting edema (+1), 3 cm swelling differential swelling (+1)). Having no alternative diagnosis to explain his symptoms, muscle tear is considered but there is no ecchymosis and the swelling is considered excessive (did not lose 2 points), and presenting at an inconvenient time, he underwent D-dimer testing which was positive. He was given a subcutaneous shot of LMWH and returned the next day for a venous ultrasound, which demonstrated a proximal DVT. On the basis of this, a diagnosis of DVT was made. He was treated at home with therapeutic doses of LMWH and concomitant oral anticoagulant therapy with warfarin.

Acknowledgments

Dr. Wells' research is supported by the Government of Canada through the 21st Century Canada Research Chairs Program.

References

1 White RH. The epidemiology of venous thromboembolism. *Circulation* 2003;**107**(Suppl 1):I4–8.

2 Schreiber D. Deep venous thrombosis and thrombophlebitis. eMedicine. WebMD, available at http://www.emedicine.com/emerg/topic122.htm (accessed May 20, 2008).

3 Scarvelis D, Wells PS. Diagnosis and treatment of deep-vein thrombosis. *Can Med Assoc J* 2006;**175**(9):1087–92.

4 Kearon C. Excluding pulmonary embolism with helical (spiral) computed tomography: evidence is catching up with enthusiasm. *Can Med Assoc J* 2003;**168**(11):1430–1.

5 Kearon C. Natural history of venous thromboembolism. *Circulation* 2003;**107**(23 Suppl 1):I22–30.

6 Moser KM, Fedullo PF, LitteJohn JK, Crawford R. Frequent asymptomatic pulmonary embolism in patients with deep venous thrombosis. *JAMA* 1994;**271**(3):223–5 (erratum in *JAMA* 1994;**271**(24):1908).

7 Kahn SR, Ginsberg JS. Relationship between deep venous thrombosis and the postthrombotic syndrome. *Arch Intern Med* 2004;**164**:17–26.

8 Wells PS, Owen C, Doucette S, Fergusson D, Tran H. Does this patient have deep vein thrombosis? (Review). *JAMA* 2006;**295**(2):199–207.

9 Goodacre S, Sampson F, Stevenson M, et al. Measurement of the clinical and cost-effectiveness of non-invasive diagnostic testing strategies for deep vein thrombosis. *Health Technology Assessment* 2006;**10**(15).

10 Subramaniam RM, Snyder B, Heath R, Tawse F, Sleigh J. Diagnosis of lower limb deep venous thrombosis in emergency department patients: performance of Hamilton and modified Wells scores. *Ann Emerg Med* 2006;**48**(6):678–85.

11 Wells PS, Anderson DR, Rodger M, et al. Evaluation of D-dimer in the diagnosis of suspected deep-vein thrombosis. *N Engl J Med* 2003;**349**:1227–35.

12 Anderson FA, Jr., Spencer FA. Risk factors for venous thromboembolism. *Circulation* 2003;**107**(23, Suppl 1):I9–16.

13 Fancher TL, White RH, Kravitz RL. Combined use of rapid D-dimer testing and estimation of clinical probability in the diagnosis of deep vein thrombosis: systematic review. *BMJ* 2004;**329**(7470):821.

14 Cundiff DK, Manyemba J, Pezzullo JC. Anticoagulants versus non-steroidal anti-inflammatories or placebo for treatment of venous thromboembolism. *Cochrane Database Syst Rev* 2006;**1**:CD003746.

15 Hull R, Delmore T, Carter C, et al. Adjusted subcutaneous heparin versus warfarin sodium in the long-term treatment of venous thrombosis. *N Engl J Med* 1982;**306**(4):189–94.

16 Agency for Healthcare Research and Quality. Evidence Report/Technology Assessment No. 68. AHRQ Publication No. 03-E012. Agency for Healthcare Research and Quality, Rockville, MD, 2003. Available at http://www.ahrq.gov/clinic/epcsums/dvtsum.htm (accessed March 6, 2007).

17 Pinede L, Ninet J, Duhaut P, et al., Investigators of the "Duree Optimale du Traitement AntiVitamines K" (DOTAVK) Study. Comparison of 3 and 6 months of oral anticoagulant therapy after a first episode of proximal deep vein thrombosis or pulmonary embolism and comparison of 6 and 12 weeks of therapy after isolated calf deep vein thrombosis. *Circulation* 2001;**103**(20):2453–60.

18 Buller HR, Agnelli G, Hull RD, Hyers TM, Prins MH, Raskob GE. Antithrombotic therapy for venous thromboembolic disease: the Seventh ACCP Conference on Antithrombotic and Thrombolytic Therapy (Review). *Chest* 2004;**126**(Suppl 3):401S–428S (erratum in *Chest* 2005;**127**(1):416).

19 Righini M, Paris S, Le Gal G, Laroche JP, Perrier A, Bounameaux H. Clinical relevance of distal deep vein thrombosis. Review of literature data. *Thromb Haemost* 2006;**95**(1):56–64.

20 Den Belt AG, Prins MH, Lensing AW, et al. Fixed dose subcutaneous low molecular weight heparins versus adjusted dose unfractionated heparin for venous thromboembolism. *Cochrane Database Syst Rev* 2000;**2**:CD001100 (update in *Cochrane Database Syst Rev* 2004;**4**:CD001100).

21 Segal JB, Streiff MB, Hoffman LV, Thornton K, Bass EB. Management of venous thromboembolism: a systematic review for a practice guideline. *Ann Intern Med* 2007;**146**(3):211–22.

22 Schraibman IG, Milne AA, Royle EM. Home versus in-patient treatment for deep vein thrombosis (Review). *Cochrane Database Syst Rev* 2001;**2**:CD003076.

23 Harrison L, McGinnis J, Crowther M, Ginsberg J, Hirsh J. Assessment of outpatient treatment of deep-vein thrombosis with low-molecular-weight heparin. *Arch Intern Med* 1998;**158**(18):2001–3.

24 Wells PS, Kovacs MJ, Bormanis J, et al. Expanding eligibility for outpatient treatment of deep venous thrombosis and pulmonary embolism with low-molecular-weight heparin: a comparison of patient self-injection with homecare injection. *Arch Intern Med* 1998;**158**(16):1809–12.

25 Rymes NL, Lester W, Connor C, Chakrabarti S, Fegan CD. Outpatient management of DVT using low molecular weight heparin and a hospital outreach service. *Clin Lab Haematol* 2002;**24**(3):165–70.

26 Kolbach DN, Sandbrink MW, Hamulyak K, Neumann HA, Prins MH. Non-pharmaceutical measures for prevention of post-thrombotic syndrome. *Cochrane Database Syst Rev* 2004;**1**:CD004174.

27 Kakkos SK, Daskalopoulou SS, Daskalopoulos ME, Nicolaides AN, Geroulakos G. Review on the value of graduated elastic compression stockings after deep vein thrombosis. *Thromb Haemost* 2006;**96**(4):441–5.

28 The SOX Trial: Compression Stockings to Prevent the Post-Thrombotic Syndrome. PI – Dr. Susan R. Kahn. Available at http://www.clinicaltrials.gov/ct/show/NCT00143598?order=1.

29 Wells PS, Anderson DR, Rodger MA, et al. A randomized trial comparing 2 low-molecular-weight heparins for the outpatient treatment of deep vein thrombosis and pulmonary embolism. *Arch Intern Med* 2005;**165**(7):733–8.

30 Zakarija A, Bennett CL. Low-molecular-weight heparins: do we have the GUSTO to identify differences between alternative formulations? *Arch Intern Med* 2005;**165**(7):722–3.

31 Agnelli G, Bergqvist D, Cohen AT, Gallus AS, Gent M, PEGASUS Investigators. Randomized clinical trial of postoperative fondaparinux versus perioperative dalteparin for prevention of venous thromboembolism in high-risk abdominal surgery. *Br J Surg* 2005;**92**(10):1212–20.

32 Turpie AG, Bauer KA, Eriksson BI, Lassen MR. Fondaparinux vs enoxaparin for the prevention of venous thromboembolism in major orthopedic surgery: a meta-analysis of 4 randomized double-blind studies. *Arch Intern Med* 2002;**162**(16):1833–40.

33 Buller HR, Davidson BL, Decousus H, et al., Matisse Investigators. Fonda-parinux or enoxaparin for the initial treatment of symptomatic deep venous thrombosis: a randomized trial. *Ann Intern Med* 2004;**140**(11):867–73.

34 Bauld DL, Kovacs MJ. Dalteparin in emergency patients to prevent admission prior to investigation for venous thromboembolism. *Am J Emerg Med* 1999;**17**(1):11–15.

35 Anderson DR, Wells PS, Stiell I, et al. Management of patients with suspected deep vein thrombosis in the emergency department: combining use of a clinical diagnosis model with D-dimer testing. *J Emerg Med* 2000;**19**(3):225–30.

36 Imberti D, Ageno W, Dentali F, Giorgi Pierfranceschi M, Croci E, Garcia D. Management of primary care patients with suspected deep vein thrombosis: use of a therapeutic dose of low-molecular-weight heparin to avoid urgent ultrasonographic evaluation. *J Thromb Haemost* 2006;**4**(5):1037–41.

37 Siragusa S, Anastasio R, Porta C, et al. Deferment of objective assessment of deep vein thrombosis and pulmonary embolism without increased risk of thrombosis: a practical approach based on the pretest clinical model, D-dimer testing, and the use of low-molecular-weight heparins. *Arch Intern Med* 2004;**164**(22):2477–82.

13 Pulmonary Embolism

Phil Wells[1] & Michael Brown[2]

[1]Division of Hematology, Department of Medicine, University of Ottawa, Ottawa *and* The Ottawa Hospital, Ottawa, Canada
[2]College of Human Medicine, Michigan State University, Spectrum Health-Butterworth Hospitals, Hospitals, Grand Rapids, Michigan, USA

Case scenario

A 55-year-old male presented to emergency department (ED) with complaints of right-sided pleuritic chest pain. He was previously healthy with no medical problems and indicated to you that the prior evening the pain developed after engaging in a game of ice hockey. He wears good equipment. He was not aware of sustaining any injury to his chest wall. In the locker room after the game, he had noted that his right leg was feeling painful in the calf region and there was some slight swelling around his ankle after the game. He denied having shortness of breath during the game. Today, however, he felt somewhat short of breath walking the four flights of stairs that he usually walks effortlessly every morning to his job. He denied cough, palpitations and history of recent illness. He was not an any medication.

On exam, he appeared well. His vital signs revealed a heart rate of 96 beats/min, blood pressure of 120/78, respiratory rate of 18 breaths/min and temperature of 37.5°C (oral). His right calf was mildly swollen, painful and he had +1 edema around his ankle. He had mild discomfort to deep palpation of his calf. Examination of his chest revealed no abnormalities on auscultation but slight tenderness over the ribcage in the region of complaint of pleuritic pain. This was in the mid-axillary line. Cardiac exam other than the tachycardia was normal. The monitor revealed an oxygen saturation (SaO_2) of 96%. You chose to walk him up and down the hallway a few times and his saturation dropped to 93%, his heart rate increased to 140 and he exhibited mild shortness of breath. His chest X-ray (CXR) and electrocardiogram (ECG) were normal.

Background

Venous thromboembolism (VTE), manifesting as deep vein thrombosis (DVT) or pulmonary embolism (PE), is one of the most common cardiovascular disorders in industrialized countries, affecting about 5% of people in their lifetime [1]. PE is the third leading cause of cardiovascular mortality in North America with an age- and sex-adjusted incidence rate of 21–69 per 100,000 per year in population-based studies. Fatal PE is not uncommon and in 22% of cases is not diagnosed before causing death [2,3]. PE is estimated to cause 5–10% of all deaths in American hospitals [4,5].

Mismanagement of PE has been a frequent problem [6], which is at least in part due to such factors as atypical presentations, lack of physician recognition and the limitations of diagnostic tests. While imaging tests still have limitations, these patients can be better managed since the diagnostic work-up for suspected PE has now evolved. This currently uses an integrated approach that includes clinical pre-test probability assessment and D-dimer testing in combination with imaging. In fact, we are currently observing an encouraging decrease in mortality from PE, which may reflect both more accurate diagnosis and the use of diagnostic algorithms [7,8].

PE originates in the deep veins of the extremities or from pelvic and abdominal deep veins; however, the lower extremities are by far the most common source. PE from the lower extremity is felt to most frequently arise from proximal DVT (i.e., DVT in the popliteal veins and above). Pooling data from six large diagnostic studies demonstrates that over 50% of patients with PE had proximal DVT.

Among patients presenting with PE, the rate of fatal PE during anticoagulant therapy is low (1.5–4%); however, the case fatality rate of recurrent VTE is 26% [9]. The all-cause mortality at 3 months was 17% in the ICOPER registry study, and 45% of deaths were ascribed to PE [10]. Predictive variables and models have consistently demonstrated that co-morbidities (e.g., cancer, chronic obstructive pulmonary disease, heart failure) increase mortality rates [10,11].

Several studies have documented that resolution of emboli after acute PE occurs progressively over time but often remains incomplete. A recent systematic review by Nijkeuter et al. showed that residual pulmonary thrombi were identified in 87% of patients at

Evidence-based Emergency Medicine. Edited by Brian H. Rowe
© 2009 Blackwell Publishing, ISBN: 978-1-4051-6143-5.

8 days, 57% at 6 months, and 52% at 11 months after PE [12]. Documentation of these residual defects at follow-up may help to establish the diagnosis of subsequent recurrent PE. Furthermore, all patients who developed symptomatically significant chronic thromboembolic pulmonary hypertension (CTPH) had residual pulmonary vascular obstruction ranging from 40% to 70% of the vascular bed [13]. In the past, CTPH was considered a rare complication of PE, albeit one with very significant mortality. More recently, in a prospective, long-term study the cumulative incidence of CTPH was 1% at 6 months, 3.1% at 1 year, and 3.8% at 2 years – rates that were much higher than previously recognized.

In summary, the available short- and long-term data indicate that:

1 Management (diagnosis and therapy) of PE could be improved.

2 The likelihood of dying in the year following PE is substantial, even if PE is not the direct cause of death.

3 Recurrent VTE events are low in treated patients but common after anticoagulants are stopped, especially in those with idiopathic events or persistent risk factors such as cancer.

4 In at least 50% of cases, residual thrombi are still visible on ventilation-perfusion (V/Q) scan or computerized tomographic pulmonary angiography (CTPA) 6 months to 1 year after the initial event.

5 Pulmonary hemodynamics may be altered to a greater degree and with greater chronicity than previously appreciated.

This chapter examines ways in which emergency physicians can improve their diagnostic approach to PE, establish evidence-based treatment approaches and reduce the complications associated with this illness.

Clinical questions

1 In patients with suspected PE (population), are there valid and reliable clinical criteria (clinical prediction guides) that can accurately determine a patient's pre-test probability of PE (outcome)?

2 In patients with suspected PE (population), what are the likelihood ratios (diagnostic test characteristics) of D-dimer assays (test) for the diagnosis of PE (outcome)? In what clinical scenario is a negative D-dimer assay sufficient to exclude a diagnosis of PE without the need for imaging modalities (outcome)?

3 In patients with suspected PE (population) in whom the diagnostic imaging modality is a V/Q scan (test), what diagnostic approach is appropriate in order to safely rule out PE (outcome)?

4 In patients with suspected PE (population), what are the likelihood ratios (diagnostic test characteristics) of CTPA (test) for the diagnosis of PE (outcome)? When is additional imaging of the lower extremities (by ultrasound or computerized tomographic venography) necessary?

5 In patients with confirmed PE (population), does anticoagulation with low molecular weight heparin (treatment) result in lower mortality and morbidity (outcome) than treatment with adjusted dose unfractionated heparin (control)?

6 In patients with confirmed PE (population), is anticoagulation with discharge home (treatment) less expensive, more convenient and as safe (outcome) as similar care within the hospital (control)?

7 In patients with confirmed PE (population), does thrombolytic therapy in addition to heparin (treatment) result in lower mortality and morbidity (outcome) than treatment with heparin alone (control)?

8 In patients with confirmed PE (population), have other anticoagulant drugs (treatment) resulted in lower mortality and morbidity (outcome) compared to heparin or thrombolytic agents (control)?

9 In patients with suspected PE (population), does the use of diagnostic algorithms (treatment) result in higher diagnostic accuracy and lower morbidity and mortality (outcome) compared to clinical gestalt (control)?

General search strategy

You begin to address these questions by searching for evidence in the common electronic databases such as the Cochrane Library, MEDLINE and EMBASE looking specifically for systematic reviews and meta-analyses. The Cochrane Database of Systematic Reviews includes high-quality systematic review evidence on therapy for PE and the Database of Abstracts of Reviews of Effects (DARE) includes systematic review evidence on diagnosis of PE. You also search the Cochrane Central Register of Controlled Trials (CENTRAL), MEDLINE and EMBASE to identify randomized controlled trials (RCTs) that became available after the publication date of the systematic review or, if no systematic reviews were identified, to locate high-quality randomized controlled trials that directly address the clinical question. In addition, access to relevant, updated, evidence-based clinical practice guidelines (CPGs) on PE are accessed to determine the consensus rating of areas lacking evidence.

Searching for evidence synthesis: primary search strategy

- Cochrane Library: pulmonary embolism AND (topic)
- MEDLINE: pulmonary embolism AND (systematic review OR meta-analysis OR metaanalysis) AND (topic)
- EMBASE: pulmonary embolism AND (systematic review OR meta-analysis OR metaanalysis) AND (topic)

Critical review of the literature

Question 1: In patients with suspected PE (population), are there valid and reliable clinical criteria (clinical prediction guides) that can accurately determine a patient's pre-test probability of PE (outcome)?

Search strategy

- MEDLINE and EMBASE: pulmonary embolism AND (sensitivity and specificity OR likelihood ratio OR LR) AND (clinical decision rules OR CDR OR clinical signs).

Table 13.1 Variables used to determine patient pre-test probability for pulmonary embolism.*

Clinical variable	Score
Clinical signs and symptoms of DVT (minimum of leg swelling and pain with palpation of the deep veins)	3
PE as or more likely than an alternative diagnosis	3
Heart rate greater than 100	1.5
Immobilization or surgery in the previous 4 weeks	1.5
Previous DVT/PE	1.5
Hemoptysis	1
Malignancy (on treatment, treated in the last 6 months, or palliative)	1

*Scoring: >4 probability of PE is "likely"; ≤4 probability for PE is "unlikely". Alternatively, <2 is low probability, moderate is 2–6, and high is >6.
DVT, deep vein thrombosis; PE, pulmonary embolism.

PE is suspected in many patients with respiratory or chest complaints due to the non-specific nature of the presenting signs and symptoms. Despite the limitations of the individual clinical predictors [14,15], the PIOPED investigators and others have demonstrated that the clinicians' overall diagnostic impression could be useful in management [16,17]. Several explicit clinical models have been described to determine pre-test probability for PE using clinical findings, ECG and CXR. The most widely applied model has been used in at least 12 studies, over 10,000 patients have been evaluated including five studies, and over 5800 patients using the dichotomous scoring system of PE unlikely (score ≤4) or PE likely (score of >4) (Table 13.1) [18–31]. The two main limitations of this model are the complexity of the model and hence accurate recall, and the need for the physician to consider an alternative diagnosis, which may be dependent on the physician's experience.

The first problem can be overcome with diagnostic decision aides (e.g., pocket cards, computerized clinical support tools, hand-held computer devices, etc.). Despite the second concern, the kappa for inter-observer variability has been reported to be in an acceptable range [30]. At least three studies have demonstrated moderate to substantial inter-rater agreement and reproducibility of the Wells et al. model; however, one study noted only moderate agreement. The latter study reported a higher inter-observer agreement for the Charlotte Rule, which has only safe and unsafe categories [32]. Our search did not find evidence of inter-rater agreement and reproducibility for other clinical assessment/prediction rules. Wicki et al. devised a model in emergency room patients (subsequently revised and designated the Geneva Rule), which in comparison to the Wells model seems to be equally effective [33,34].

In the ED setting, researchers developed the following Charlotte Rule strategy:

A patient aged 50 years or older or any [patient with] a pulse rate greater than the systolic blood pressure, *and* either (i) unexplained hypoxemia (SaO_2 on pulse oximetry <95% while breathing room air) or (ii) unilateral leg swelling or recent surgery or hemoptysis, was unsafe

and required a V/Q scan or CTPA. In a further study, they suggested that if all the above factors were negative *and* the patient had no

prior VTE *and* was not on hormone therapy, the patient was at low risk for PE [35].

In summary, there are several prediction rules to choose from, and not much evidence exists to advise one over the other. However, the use of these rules appears to help categorize patient pre-test probability and should improve the diagnostic process as we will outline below. All these rules have limitations, predominantly the fact that they have several variables and complex scoring systems. Efforts to simplify the rules are ongoing.

Question 2: In patients with suspected PE (population), what are the likelihood ratios (diagnostic test characteristics) of D-dimer assays (test) for the diagnosis of PE (outcome)? In what clinical scenario is a negative D-dimer assay sufficient to exclude a diagnosis of PE without the need for imaging modalities (outcome)?

Search strategy

- Cochrane Library: PE AND D-dimer

Three systematic reviews assessing the test characteristics of D-dimers for the diagnosis of PE were identified in DARE, two of which included only studies that enrolled predominantly outpatient populations [36,37]. The pooled summary estimate across all 11 studies ($n = 2126$) using an enzyme-linked immunoadsorbent assay (ELISA) D-dimer test produced a sensitivity of 0.95 (95% CI: 0.90 to 0.98) and a specificity of 0.45 (95% CI: 0.38 to 0.52). Thus, the negative likelihood ratio (–LR) is approximately 0.1 and the positive LR (+LR) is 1.7. The subgroup analysis based on age showed a dramatic decrease in specificity to 0.14 based on one study that included only elderly patients >70 years [36]. The meta-analysis of immunoturbidimetric latex D-dimer tests included nine studies ($n = 1901$) and yielded similar pooled results [36]; with a sensitivity of 0.93 (95% CI: 0.89 to 0.96) and specificity 0.51 (95% CI: 0.42 to 0.59), resulting in a –LR of 0.14 and +LR of 1.8. The sensitivity analysis in both reviews assessing the effects of study quality on the results showed no significant change in these estimates.

A search of CENTRAL in the Cochrane Library yielded only a few randomized controlled trials comparing a management strategy based on D-dimer results versus a standard evaluation using radiological imaging [27,38]. In the most recent study, the Wells prediction rule was used to stratify patients. The low pre-test probability arm of the study ($n = 373$) included predominantly outpatients (73%), while the moderate-high–pre-test probability arm ($n = 83$) included only 43 outpatients (53%). The overall recurrence of VTE indicated no difference between groups (one event in each group; difference −0.5%; 95% CI: −3 to 1.6%) [27].

The results of this trial, which used an erythrocyte agglutination D-dimer assay yielding a −LR of 0.2, combined with the −LR derived in the systematic reviews for ELISA (0.1) and immunoturbidimetric D-dimer (0.14) tests provide consistent results. Therefore, it is safe and efficient to avoid additional diagnostic testing in patients who present to the ED with a low pre-test probability or are "PE unlikely" (score <4.5 by the Wells model) and who have a negative D-dimer test result.

Question 3: In patients with suspected PE (population) in whom the diagnostic imaging modality is a V/Q scan (test), what diagnostic approach is appropriate in order to safely rule out PE (outcome)?

Search strategy

- MEDLINE and EMBASE: pulmonary embolism AND (sensitivity and specificity OR likelihood ratio OR LR) AND (nuclear scan OR lung scan OR V/Q).

The safety of a protocol for the diagnosis of PE is primarily defined by the rate of eventually detected PE in patients in whom the protocol excluded the diagnosis (i.e., the false-negative rate). A threshold of approximately 1–2% is comparable to the rate of PE or DVT at follow-up after a normal pulmonary angiogram, a negative CTPA [39] or a normal result on a V/Q scan [40]. To strive for a post-test probability of less than 1% would lead to an unacceptable trade-off in increased imaging, and increased false-positive diagnosis of PE. If the imaging modality is V/Q scan, it is recommended to use one of the validated prediction rules to stratify patients into "PE unlikely" or "PE likely" groups. Subsequently, if patients are less than 80 years old and are considered to fall into the PE unlikely risk group, then a D-dimer is performed using a D-dimer test with a −LR of ≤0.20. Patients who are PE unlikely or low probability can have PE excluded with a negative D-dimer.

If patients are designated as PE likely using a clinical decision rule or they have a positive D-dimer, then V/Q scanning has long been considered the first test option in many centers. If the V/Q scan result is non-diagnostic (i.e., neither normal nor high probability; Figs 13.1, 13.2), then lower extremity venous ultrasound is recommended as an additional confirmatory test. An initially normal ultrasound result is reassuring but should be repeated 1 week later in PE likely patients with a positive D-dimer.

High-probability V/Q scans can usually be considered diagnostic if pre-test probability is high or PE likely. When the pre-test clinical probability is low or PE unlikely, high-probability V/Q scans cannot be considered diagnostic of PE. In this case, the results should be reviewed with the radiologist for consideration of a false-positive result, and confirmatory ultrasound or conventional pulmonary angiography should be considered [41].

Question 4: In patients with suspected PE (population), what are the likelihood ratios (diagnostic test characteristics) of CPTA (test) for the diagnosis of PE (outcome)? When is additional imaging (by ultrasound or computerized tomographic venography) of the lower extremities necessary?

Search strategy

- MEDLINE and EMBASE: pulmonary embolism AND (sensitivity and specificity OR likelihood ratio OR LR) AND (CT scan OR CTPA OR chest computerized tomography).

Over the past decade, CTPA has emerged as the imaging test of choice for the investigation of most patients with suspected PE. There were initial concerns about lack of sensitivity with CTPA [42]; however, in a more recent meta-analysis the pooled sensitivity and specificity of CTPA were 86% and 93.7%, respectively [43]. Furthermore, a recent study supports a higher sensitivity with multi-detector row CTPA [44], although accurate estimates of specificity (and likelihood ratios) are not available since there is no gold standard to confirm or refute positive findings. Since the imaging resolution of CTPA has rapidly increased with the advent of multi-detector row scanners, it is difficult to interpret earlier studies and it may not be possible to determine true accuracy at this point. Moreover, concerns over sensitivity have been assuaged by a number of management studies that have shown that it is safe to withhold treatment in patients with suspected PE in whom the CTPA result is negative [21,44,45]. Several features make CTPA more attractive than V/Q scanning: (i) the number of indeterminate CTPAs is much lower than for V/Q (5% vs 60–70%); (ii) CTPA may identify alternative causes for a patient's presentation whereas V/Q has no such benefit; and (iii) CTPA is more widely accessible and more often available after hours.

Notwithstanding these advantages, some questions in the management of patients using CTPA remain unanswered. One issue is the conflicting data on the need for ultrasound when the CTPA is negative. Two large prospective CTPA studies combined clinical probability and ultrasound with single row detector CTPA [26,46]. Patients with a negative CTPA, negative ultrasound and low or moderate pre-test probability had PE excluded (follow-up event rates 0.4–1.8%). Importantly, 15–18% of patients had negative CTPA but positive ultrasound studies. Two large, more recent studies in which many patients underwent multi-detector

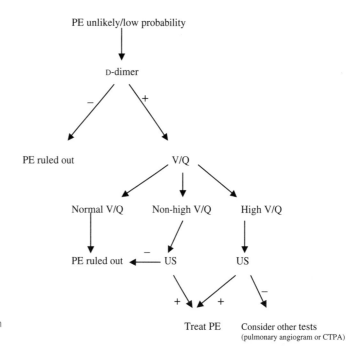

Figure 13.1 Strategy for the diagnosis of PE using V/Q in patients who are PE unlikely or low probability. CTPA, computerized tomographic pulmonary angiography; PE, pulmonary embolism; US, ultrasound; V/Q, ventilation-perfusion lung scan; −, negative test result; +, positive test result.

row CTPA suggested very little additional yield from ultrasound with only 0.9–1.4% of patients with a negative CTPA having a positive ultrasound result [20,44]. As further evidence, three large studies totaling over 4600 patients, have now demonstrated that the combination of clinical probability, D-dimer testing and CTPA results in a strategy that safely excludes PE without ultrasound imaging [21,22,45]. With the lack of direct comparison of the two strategies, it does not seem unreasonable to perform ultrasound

if clinical suspicion remains high despite a normal CTPA, if the patient has leg symptoms (indeed ultrasound could be performed first due to its high +LR and thereby spare radiation exposure), or if single detector row CTPA is employed (Fig. 13.3).

The other concern regarding CTPA is false positives. In Hayashino's meta-analysis, the post-test probability of PE with a positive CTPA was only 30% (70% false positive) in low pre-test probability patients and 84% in patients with moderate pre-test

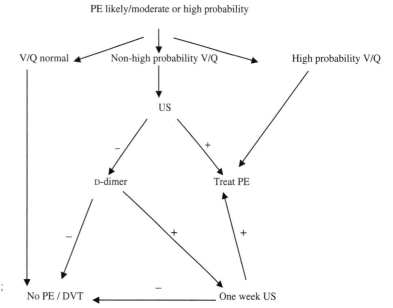

Figure 13.2 Strategy for diagnosis of PE using V/Q in patients who are PE likely or moderate–high probability. Abbreviations as in Fig. 13.1; DVT, deep vein thrombosis.

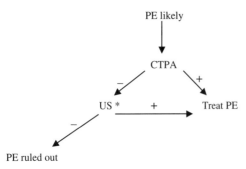

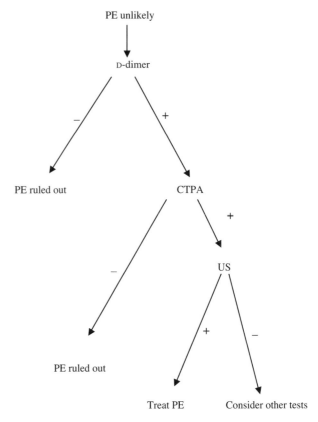

Figure 13.3 Strategy for diagnosis of PE using single row detector CTPA in patients who are PE likely.* If multi-detector CTPA is used, in most cases PE is ruled out without the need for ultrasound, however, consider ultrasound if the patient has leg symptoms or clinical suspicion is high. Abbreviations as in Fig. 13.1.

probability. Furthermore, in a large accuracy study of CTPA, the positive predictive values for PE detected by CTPA in the lobar, segmental and sub-segmental vessels were 97%, 68% and 25%, respectively [47]. A recent accuracy study comparing multi-detector row CTPA to pulmonary angiography demonstrated a false-positive CTPA rate of 30% with most false computerized tomography results incorrectly detecting PE in isolated segmental vessels or sub-segmental vessels [48]. Therefore, clinical probability assessment enables a strategy to deal with potentially false-positive results. Strategies with CTPA are in shown in Figs 13.3 and 13.4.

Figure 13.4 Strategy for diagnosis of PE using CTPA in patients who are PE unlikely. Abbreviations as in Fig. 13.1

Question 5: In patients with confirmed PE (population), does anticoagulation with low molecular weight heparin (treatment) result in lower mortality and morbidity (outcome) than treatment with adjusted dose unfractionated heparin (control)?

Search strategy

- Cochrane Library: pulmonary embolism AND low molecular weight heparin

From the discussions above, it is clear that a diagnosis of PE is imperative before patients are committed to anticoagulation. Emergency physicians and consultants involved in difficult cases must ensure that patients receive an accurate diagnostic work-up to confirm the presence or absence of a PE. The consequences of misdiagnosis may be catastrophic, false reassurance may result in fatal PE and a false-positive diagnosis can change a person's employment, insurance and associated risks of anticoagulation.

A high-quality meta-analysis of four randomized controlled trials comparing fixed dose subcutaneous low molecular weight heparins (LMWHs) to adjusted dose unfractionated heparin (UFH) showed no difference in the rate of recurrent VTE (Fig. 13.5;

OR = 0.88; 95% CI: 0.48 to 1.63) [49]. Recently updated, evidenced-based clinical practice guidelines support these conclusions [50,51]. Overall, the decision to use LMWH versus UFH is based less on efficacy and more on patient stability, patient preference, ability to inject the agent in a non-hospital environment, and other related considerations.

Question 6: In patients with confirmed PE (population), is anticoagulation with discharge home (treatment) less expensive, more convenient and as safe (outcome) as similar care within the hospital (control)?

Search strategy

- Cochrane Library, MEDLINE and EMBASE: pulmonary embolism AND low molecular weight heparin AND outpatient

No trial was identified that randomized subjects to outpatient versus inpatient management; however, if we consider the outcomes of patients selected for outpatient therapy in recent drug trials we can estimate the event rates in select populations with PE. In

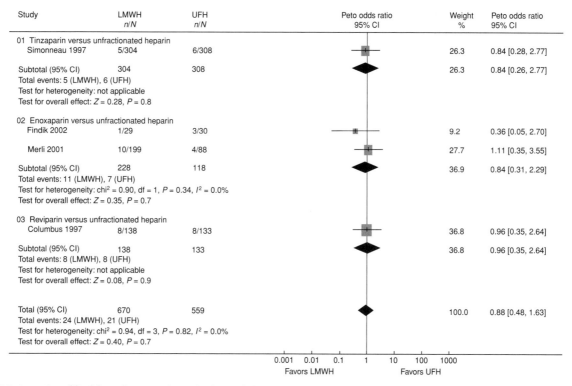

Figure 13.5 Comparison of fixed dose subcutaneous low molecular weight heparin (LMWH) to adjusted dose unfractionated heparin (UFH) for PE. (Reprinted with permission from van Dongen CJ et al. [49], © Cochrane Library.)

a single-blind randomized trial designed to compare two forms of LMWH, the rates of death, recurrent PE and bleeding complications among the 90 patients with PE treated as outpatients were similar to previous inpatient trials [52]. There were a number of exclusions, including patients presenting with hypotension, hypoxia or severe pain requiring narcotics. Another recent open-label randomized trial designed to compare subcutaneous UFH to LMWH had similar outcomes among the 52 patients with PE that were treated as outpatients [53].

It has been established that outpatient treatment for DVT is safe and cost-effective [54]. Recent PE guidelines conclude that little evidence exists regarding outpatient treatment of PE but this approach can be considered in selected patients with appropriate support services [50,55]. Cohort studies support the safety of outpatient therapy; however, a lack of comparator groups limits the generalizability of these results. For emergency physicians, such a decision cannot be made lightly and close follow-up for monitoring treatment compliance, routine lab testing and surveillance for complications must be in place prior to considering this approach.

Question 7: In patients with confirmed PE (population), does thrombolytic therapy in addition to heparin (treatment) result in lower mortality and morbidity (outcome) than treatment with heparin alone (control)?

> ### Search strategy
>
> • Cochrane Library: pulmonary embolism AND thrombolysis

Theoretically, lysis of clot should restore perfusion to the injured lung tissue in acute PE. However, a high-quality meta-analysis of eight randomized controlled trials comparing thrombolysis followed by heparin to UFH alone did not demonstrate a decrease in mortality (OR = 0.89; 95% CI: 0.45 to 1.78) or recurrence of PE (OR = 0.63; 95% CI: 0.33 to 1.20) [56]. There was also no difference in the risk of major hemorrhage with thrombolysis, but the largest study in the analysis (contributing about 40% of the patients) used an unconventional definition of major hemorrhage and was the only study not to suggest increased bleeding risks with thrombolytics. The authors of the Cochrane review were unable to determine if there was benefit in a subgroup of unstable patients. Only one randomized controlled trial of patients with massive PE was identified and this trial did not meet their inclusion criteria. There may be subgroups of patients with acute PE who would benefit from thrombolysis but this remains unproven. Overall, emergency physicians should not consider thrombolysis of patients with PE without consultation with their inpatient critical care colleagues.

Question 8: In patients with confirmed PE (population), have other anticoagulant drugs (treatment) resulted in lower mortality and morbidity (outcome) compared to heparin or thrombolytic agents (control)?

Search strategy

- Cochrane Library, MEDLINE and EMBASE: pulmonary embolism AND (treatment OR therapy OR anticoagulants)

The only other drug studied, and published, specifically in patients with PE is the specific factor Xa inhibitor fondaparinux. This study compared 1110 patients initially treated with intravenous UFH to 1103 patients treated with fondaparinux (5–10 mg, depending on weight) subcutaneously once daily. Overall, 158 patients received at least some of their fondaparinux therapy on an outpatient basis. Recurrence rates were 3.8% in the fondaparinux group versus 5.0% in the heparin groups. Major hemorrhage rates were 1.3% and 1.0%, respectively. This study confirms once-daily fondaparinux is at least as effective and safe as heparin in the initial treatment of PE.

Question 9: In patients with suspected PE (population), does the use of diagnostic algorithms (treatment) result in higher diagnostic accuracy and lower morbidity and mortality (outcome) compared to clinical gestalt (control)?

Search strategy

- MEDLINE and EMBASE: pulmonary embolism AND (algorithms OR care maps) AND (morbidity OR mortality).

In the PIOPED study, patients were stratified into risk categories using the clinical judgment of individual clinicians, but in the other studies physicians also used a predefined clinical decision tool or practiced in centers in which the rules were developed. As such, it is unclear if empirical assessment would be generalizable. In addition, with empirical assessment, the exact methods used by each clinician to estimate pre-test probability are difficult to measure or reproduce [57], clinicians often disagree (even for broad categories) on the pre-test probability of PE [58], the clinician's experience level appears to influence the accuracy of his or her pre-test assessment [59], and probability estimates often tend to follow a middle road, so that fewer patients are categorized into the more useful low- or high-probability groups. While using clinical gestalt is the easiest method as there is no requirement to memorize criteria, it has a variety of drawbacks and its use is discouraged.

It is possible that the use of diagnostic algorithms increases the number of patients "screened" for PE; Goldstein et al. implemented a D-dimer-based screening system and found a 40% increase in the rate of V/Q scanning [60]. Conversely, the percentage of V/Q scans that were read as positive for PE increased and the diagnosis of PE almost doubled using a D-dimer algorithm.

Another group of investigators did not find an increase in imaging when D-dimer testing and algorithms were employed [60,61]. Additionally, at hospitals where imaging is not available at night, algorithms may offer a rational method to decide which patients should receive temporary anticoagulation until imaging is available. Finally, it has been demonstrated that following algorithms improves patient care, since more diagnostic failures occurred if algorithms were not followed [7,8,18]. Overall, a diagnostic algorithm is recommended to improve the diagnostic accuracy of PE in the emergency setting. Emergency physicians and administrators should implement and evaluate their use as part of quality assurance programs.

Conclusions

In summary, there are other agents being investigated for the treatment of VTE. Emergency physicians should base their treatment decisions on local practice, the published evidences and the agents they feel most comfortable using.

The 55-year-old male who presented to the ED with complaint of right-sided pleuritic chest pain and a swollen leg described in the clinical scenario had a high pre-test probability of PE using the Wells et al. PE clinical decision tool (leg symptoms suggestive of DVT, no alternative diagnosis to explain his pulmonary symptoms). Having a normal chest radiograph, and presenting at a convenient time, he underwent V/Q scanning and was found to have a non-diagnostic result and intermediate probability by the PIOPED criteria. His D-dimer was positive and his subsequent leg vein ultrasound demonstrated a proximal DVT. On the basis of this a diagnosis of DVT with probable PE was made. He was admitted to hospital and treated with therapeutic doses of LMWH with concomitant oral anticoagulant therapy with warfarin.

Dyspnea is a common and important presentation in emergency medicine and consideration of PE in the differential diagnosis is an important step to identifying this potentially deadly disease. Over the past decade, improvement in the diagnostic approach and treatment of PE has been impressive. An organized approach using clinical decision rules, D-dimer testing and advanced imaging will lead clinicians to a more accurate and timely diagnosis of PE.

Acknowledgments

Dr. Wells' research is supported by the Government of Canada through the 21st Century Canada Research Chairs Program.

References

1 Spencer FA, Emery C, Lessard D, et al. The Worcester Venous Thromboembolism Study. A population-based study of the clinical epidemiology of venous thromboembolism. *J Gen Intern Med* 2006;**21**:722–7.

2 Heit JA, Silverstein MD, Mohr DN, et al. Risk factors for deep vein thrombosis and pulmonary embolism: a population-based case-control study. *Arch Intern Med* 2000;**160**:809–15.

3 Heit JA, O'Fallon WM, Petterson TM, et al. Relative impact of risk factors for deep vein thrombosis and pulmonary embolism: a population-based study. *Arch Intern Med* 2002;**162**:1245–8.

4 Silverstein MD, Heit JA, Mohr DN, et al. Trends in the incidence of deep vein thrombosis and pulmonary embolism: a 25-year population-based study. *Arch Intern Med* 1998;**158**:585–93.

5 Nordstrom M, Lindblad B. Autopsy-verified venous thromboembolism within a defined urban population – the city of Malmo, Sweden. *Acta Pathol Microbiol Immunol Scand* 1998;**106**:378–84.

6 Schluger N, Henschke C, King T, et al. Diagnosis of pulmonary embolism at a large teaching hospital. *J Thorac Imaging* 1994;**9**:180–84.

7 Berghout A, Oudkerk M, Hicks SG, et al. Active implementation of a consensus strategy improves diagnosis and management in suspected pulmonary embolism. *Q J Med* 2000;**93**:335–40.

8 Roy PM, Meyer G, Vielle B, et al. Appropriateness of diagnostic management and outcomes of suspected pulmonary embolism. *Ann Intern Med* 2006;**144**:157–64.

9 Douketis JD, Kearon C, Bates SM, et al. Risk of fatal pulmonary embolism in patients with treated venous thromboembolism. *JAMA* 1998;**279**:458–62.

10 Goldhaber SZ, Visani L, De Rosa M, ICOPER. Acute pulmonary embolism: clinical outcomes in the international cooperative pulmonary embolism registry (ICOPER). *Lancet* 1999;**353**:1386–9.

11 Aujesky D, Obrosky DS, Stone RA, et al. A prediction rule to identify low-risk patients with pulmonary embolism. *Arch Intern Med* 2006;**166**:169–75.

12 Nijkeuter M, Hovens MM, Davidson BL, Huisman MV. Resolution of thromboemboli in patients with acute pulmonary embolism: a systematic review. *Chest* 2006;**129**:192–7.

13 Pengo V, Lensing AW, Prins MH, et al. Incidence of chronic thromboembolic pulmonary hypertension after pulmonary embolism. *N Engl J Med* 2004;**350**:2257–64.

14 Stein PD, Terrin ML, Hales CA, et al. Clinical, laboratory, roentgenographic, and electrocardiographic findings in patients with acute pulmonary embolism and no pre-existing cardiac or pulmonary disease. *Chest* 1991;**100**:598–603.

15 Rodger MA, Carrier M, Jones GN, et al. Diagnostic value of arterial blood gas measurement in suspected pulmonary embolism. *Am J Respir Crit Care Med* 2000;**162**:2105–8.

16 PIOPED Investigators. Value of the ventilation/perfusion scan in acute pulmonary embolism. Results of the prospective investigation of pulmonary embolism diagnosis (PIOPED). *JAMA* 1990;**263**:2753–9.

17 Perrier A, Desmarais S, Miron MJ, et al. Non-invasive diagnosis of venous thromboembolism in outpatients. *Lancet* 1999;**353**:190–95.

18 Wells PS, Anderson DR, Rodger MA, et al. Excluding pulmonary embolism at the bedside without diagnostic imaging: management of patients with suspected pulmonary embolism presenting to the emergency department by using a simple clinical model and D-dimer. *Ann Intern Med* 2001;**135**:98–107.

19 Wells PS, Anderson DR, Rodger MA, et al. Derivation of a simple clinical model to categorize patients' probability of pulmonary embolism: increasing the models' utility with the SimpliRED D-dimer. *Thromb Haemost* 2000;**83**:416–20.

20 Anderson DR, Wells PS, Kahn SR, et al. Computerized-tomographic pulmonary angiography compared with ventilation-perfusion lung scanning as initial diagnostic modality for patients with suspected pulmonary embolism: a randomized controlled trial. *Blood* 2005;**106**:463.

21 van Belle A, Buller HR, Huisman MV, et al. Effectiveness of managing suspected pulmonary embolism using an algorithm combining clinical probability, D-dimer testing, and computed tomography. *JAMA* 2006;**295**:172–9.

22 Goekoop RJ, Steeghs N, Niessen RW, et al. Simple and safe exclusion of pulmonary embolism in outpatients using quantitative D-dimer and Wells' simplified decision rule. *Thromb Haemost* 2007;**97**:146–50.

23 Penaloza A, Melot C, Dochy E, et al. Assessment of pretest probability of pulmonary embolism in the emergency department by physicians in training using the Wells model. *Thromb Res* 2007;**120**:173–9.

24 Sohne M, Kamphuisen PW, van Mierlo PJ, Buller HR. Diagnostic strategy using a modified clinical decision rule and D-dimer test to rule out pulmonary embolism in elderly in- and outpatients. *Thromb Haemost* 2005;**94**:206–10.

25 Bosson JL, Barro C, Satger B, et al. Quantitative high D-dimer value is predictive of pulmonary embolism occurrence independently of clinical score in a well-defined low risk factor population. *J Thromb Haemost* 2005;**3**:93–9.

26 Anderson DR, Kovacs MJ, Dennie C, et al. Use of spiral computed tomography contrast angiography and ultrasonography to exclude the diagnosis of pulmonary embolism in the emergency department. *J Emerg Med* 2005;**29**:399–404.

27 Kearon C, Ginsberg JS, Douketis J, et al. An evaluation of D-dimer in the diagnosis of pulmonary embolism: a randomized trial. *Ann Intern Med* 2006;**144**:812–21.

28 Leclercq MGL, Lutisan JG, van Marwijk Kooy M, et al. Ruling out clinically suspected pulmonary embolism by assessment of clinical probability and D-dimer levels: a management study. *Thromb Haemost* 2003;**89**:97–103.

29 Kruip MJ, Slob MJ, Schijen JH, van der Heul C, Buller HR. Use of a clinical decision rule in combination with D-dimer concentration in diagnostic workup of patients with suspected pulmonary embolism: a prospective management study. *Arch Intern Med* 2002;**162**:1631–5.

30 Rodger MA, Maser E, Stiell I, Howley HE, Wells PS. The interobserver reliability of pretest probability assessment in patients with suspected pulmonary embolism. *Thromb Res* 2005;**116**:101–7.

31 Wolf SJ, McCubbin TR, Feldhaus KM, Faragher JP, Adcock DM. Prospective validation of Wells criteria in the evaluation of patients with suspected pulmonary embolism. *Ann Emerg Med* 2004;**44**:503–10.

32 Runyon MS, Webb WB, Jones AE, Kline JA. Comparison of the unstructured clinician estimate of pretest probability for pulmonary embolism to the Canadian score and the Charlotte rule: a prospective observational study. *Acad Emerg Med* 2005;**12**:587–93.

33 Chagnon I, Bounameaux H, Aujesky D, et al. Comparison of two clinical prediction rules and implicit assessment among patients with suspected pulmonary embolism. *Am J Med* 2002;**113**:269–75.

34 Le Gal G, Righini M, Roy PM, et al. Prediction of pulmonary embolism in the emergency department: the revised Geneva score. *Ann Intern Med* 2006;**144**:165–71.

35 Kline JA, Mitchell AM, Kabrhel C, Richman PB, Courtney DM. Clinical criteria to prevent unnecessary diagnostic testing in emergency department patients with suspected pulmonary embolism. *J Thromb Haemost* 2004;**2**:1247–55.

36 Brown MD, Rowe BH, Reeves MJ, Bermingham JM, Goldhaber SZ. The accuracy of the enzyme-linked immunosorbent assay D-dimer test in

the diagnosis of pulmonary embolism: a meta-analysis. *Ann Emerg Med* 2002;**40**:133–44.

37 Brown MD, Lau J, Nelson RD, Kline JA. Turbidimetric D-dimer test in the diagnosis of pulmonary embolism: a metaanalysis. *Clin Chem* 2003;**49**:1846–53.

38 Rodger MA, Bredeson CN, Jones G, et al. The Bedside Investigation of Pulmonary Embolism Diagnosis Study: a double-blind randomized controlled trial comparing combinations of 3 bedside tests vs ventilation-perfusion scan for the initial investigation of suspected pulmonary embolism. *Arch Intern Med* 2006;**166**:181–7.

39 Tillie-Leblond I, Mastora I, Radenne F, et al. Risk of pulmonary embolism after a negative spiral CT angiogram in patients with pulmonary disease: 1-year clinical follow-up study. *Radiology* 2002;**223**:461–7.

40 Hull RD, Raskob GE, Coates G, Panju AA. Clinical validity of a normal perfusion lung scan on patients with suspected pulmonary embolism. *Chest* 1990;**97**:23–6.

41 Wells PS, Ginsberg JS, Anderson DR, et al. Use of a clinical model for safe management of patients with suspected pulmonary embolism. *Ann Intern Med* 1998;**129**:997–1005.

42 Rathbun SW, Raskob G, Whitsett TL. Sensitivity and specificity of helical computed tomography in the diagnosis of pulmonary embolism: a systematic review. *Ann Intern Med* 2000;**132**:227–32.

43 Hayashino Y, Goto M, Noguchi Y, Fukui T. Ventilation-perfusion scanning and helical CT in suspected pulmonary embolism: meta-analysis of diagnostic performance. *Radiology* 2005;**234**:740–48.

44 Perrier A, Roy PM, Sanchez O, et al. Multidetector-row computed tomography in suspected pulmonary embolism. *N Engl J Med* 2005;**352**:1760–68.

45 Ghanima W, Almaas V, Aballi S, et al. Management of suspected pulmonary embolism (PE) by D-dimer and multi-slice computed tomography in outpatients: an outcome study. *J Thromb Haemost* 2005;**3**:1926–32.

46 Musset D, Parent F, Meyer G, et al. Diagnostic strategy for patients with suspected pulmonary embolism: a prospective multicentre outcome study. *Lancet* 2002;**360**:1914–20.

47 Stein PD, Fowler SE, Goodman LR, et al. Multidetector computed tomography for acute pulmonary embolism. *N Engl J Med* 2006;**354**:2317–27.

48 Winer-Muram HT, Rydberg J, Johnson MS, et al. Suspected acute pulmonary embolism: evaluation with multi-detector row CT versus digital subtraction pulmonary arteriography. *Radiology* 2004;**233**:806–15.

49 van Dongen CJ, van den Belt AGM, Prins MH, Lensing AWA. Fixed dose subcutaneous low molecular weight heparins versus adjusted dose un-fractionated heparin for venous thromboembolism. *Cochrane Database Syst Rev* 2004;**4**:CD001100 (doi: 10.1002/14651858.CD001100.pub2).

50 Snow V, Qaseem A, Barry P, et al. Management of venous thromboembolism: a clinical practice guideline from the American College of Physicians and the American Academy of Family Physicians. *Ann Intern Med* 2007;**146**:204–10.

51 Segal JB, Streiff MB, Hoffman LV, Thornton K, Bass EB. Management of venous thromboembolism: a systematic review for a practice guideline. *Ann Intern Med* 2007;**146**:211–22.

52 Wells PS, Anderson DR, Rodger MA, et al. A randomized trial comparing 2 low-molecular-weight heparins for the outpatient treatment of deep vein thrombosis and pulmonary embolism. *Arch Intern Med* 2005;**165**:733–8.

53 Kearon C, Ginsberg JS, Julian JA, et al. Comparison of fixed-dose weight-adjusted unfractionated heparin and low-molecular-weight heparin for acute treatment of venous thromboembolism. *JAMA* 2006;**296**:935–42.

54 Rodger MA, Bredeson CN, Wells PS, et al. Cost-effectiveness of low-molecular-weight heparin and unfractionated heparin in treatment of deep vein thrombosis. *Can Med Assoc J* 1998;**159**:931–8.

55 Segal JB, Bolger DT, Jenckes MW, et al. Outpatient therapy with low molecular weight heparin for the treatment of venous thromboembolism: a review of efficacy, safety, and costs. *Am J Med* 2003;**115**:298–308.

56 Dong B, Jirong Y, Liu G, Wang Q, Wu T. Thrombolytic therapy for pulmonary embolism. *Cochrane Database Syst Rev* 2006;**2**:CD004437 (doi: 10.1002/14651858.CD004437.pub2).

57 Richardson WS. Where do pretest probabilities come from? *ACP J Club* 1999;**4**:68–9.

58 Jackson RE, Rudoni RR, Pascual R. Emergency physician assessment of the pretest probability of pulmonary embolism. *Acad Emerg Med* 1999;**4**:891–7.

59 Rosen MP, Sands DZ, Morris J, Drake W, Davis RB. Does a physician's ability to accurately assess the likelihood of pulmonary embolism increase with training? *Acad Med* 2000;**75**:1199–205.

60 Goldstein NM, Kollef MH, Ward S, Gage BF. The impact of the introduction of a rapid D-dimer assay on the diagnostic evaluation of suspected pulmonary embolism. *Arch Intern Med* 2001;**161**:567–71.

61 Kline JA, Webb WB, Jones AE, Hernandez-Nino J. Impact of a rapid rule-out protocol for pulmonary embolism on the rate of screening, missed cases, and pulmonary vascular imaging in an urban US emergency department. *Ann Emerg Med* 2004;**44**:490–502.

14 Prevention and Treatment of Influenza

Stephen R. Pitts

Department of Emergency Medicine, Emory University School of Medicine, Emory Crawford Long Hospital, Atlanta, USA

Case scenario

A 34-year-old third grade school teacher with a history of mild asthma presented to the emergency department (ED) in the evening complaining that she woke up with a sore throat and clear nasal discharge yesterday, and then developed a frequent cough now productive of clear mucus. In the last 12 hours she experienced worsening subjective fever, chills, muscle aches and fatigue. Because of severe ED crowding, she had waited over 30 minutes in the waiting room before vital signs were taken. Temperature was $39.2°C$, respirations were increased to 24 breaths/min at rest but not labored, heart rate was 105 beats/min and blood pressure is 115/70 mmHg. Oxygen saturation (SaO_2) was 92% on room air. On examination she appeared healthy but acutely ill. She had bilateral mild expiratory wheezes, but was not using accessory muscles nor was her speech limited by dyspnea. No crackles or diminished breath sounds were noted. A chest radiograph revealed small, bilateral, patchy infiltrates confined to the lower lung fields.

The emergency physician was aware that influenza A was currently circulating in the community, based on regionalized weekly Centers for Disease Control and Prevention (CDC) surveillance reports and local news reports of increased absenteeism in schools for acute respiratory illness. In order to confirm the suspicion of acute influenza, a nasopharyngeal swab was sent for a rapid antigen test for influenza A and B, and returned negative. The patient was treated for a mild exacerbation of asthma with nebulized salbutamol and for bacterial pneumonia with an oral macrolide (azithromycin).

The patient lived at home with her husband and two small children, and with her husband's mother who has oxygen-dependent emphysema. All were currently asymptomatic. She worried that they will also become infected and wonders whether oral medication may prevent disease among her family contacts. After

treatment for wheezing her dyspnea had improved and her fever had decreased.

Background

Influenza is the most important of the many causes of seasonal respiratory illness because of its global distribution and relative severity. Clinical symptoms begin after an incubation period of 2 days and last 4 days on average in otherwise healthy persons. Infection can spread to others from 1 day before to 5 days after the onset of clinical symptoms, mainly by respiratory droplet transmission [1]. The annual global epidemics are usually restricted to one or two predominant influenza subtypes. Although influenza infection can be asymptomatic, it is on average more severe than the "common cold" and there are several distinctive symptoms and signs that differentiate the two (Table 14.1).

Hemagglutinin and neuraminidase surface glycoprotein antigens are the target of natural immunity to influenza A, and are also used to classify subtypes [1]. The major strain circulating in the 2006–2007 season, for example, was classified as influenza type A, subtype H1N1, though subtype H3N2 was also circulating at lower rates. These antigens experience genetic drift, so that natural immunity wanes between seasons. Influenza B, which was also transmitted during this season, causes less severe illness and undergoes little genetic drift. In the last 30 US flu seasons, the national prevalence of influenza peaked in February 43% of the time, though this peak has occurred in each of the months between November and May [1] and local peak prevalence may vary considerably from the national average. The annual epidemic is driven largely by transmission among children and teenagers: subjects <18 years old in longitudinal community cohorts experience both a much higher rate of seasonal respiratory illness and, among these, a higher prevalence and severity of influenza, but are less likely to be diagnosed with influenza [2,3].

Inter-pandemic influenza is an intense, self-limited illness with little lasting health impact among otherwise healthy persons, but with massive indirect societal costs due to decreased productivity,

Evidence-based Emergency Medicine. Edited by Brian H. Rowe
© 2009 Blackwell Publishing, ISBN: 978-1-4051-6143-5.

Table 14.1 Likelihood ratios for clinical predictors of culture-proven influenza in patients with influenza-like illness. Ranges represent range-of-point estimates from individual trials.

Finding	Likelihood ratio	
	Present	Absent
Systematic review of non-ED studies [15]		
Fever	1.1–3.8	0.21–0.72
History fever	1.0–2.1	0.68–0.70
Cough	1.0–2.9	0.11–0.85
Myalgia	0.81–2.7	0.64–1.7
Malaise	0.98–2.6	0.55–1.1
Headache	1.0–2.1	0.62–0.81
Sore throat	0.91–2.1	0.61–1.2
Sneezing	0.47–1.2	0.85–2.1
Nasal congestion	0.95–1.1	0.47–1.0
Chills	1.1–2.6	0.66–0.68
Vaccine history	0.11–0.63	1.1–1.2
Fever and cough together	1.9–5.0	0.54–0.75
Fever, cough, and acute onset	2.0–5.4	0.54–0.77
Single study of adult ED patients [27]		
All patients		
Fever and cough together	3.8	0.7
Clinical judgment	5.1	0.8
Influenza test	28.2	0.7
Symptoms <48 hours		
Fever and cough together	17.3	0.3
Clinical judgment	6.5	0.4
Influenza test	15.2	0.4

absenteeism and overcrowding of health care facilities. Complications of acute influenza include bacterial pneumonia and exacerbation of underlying illness, especially in patients aged ≥65, who account for 90% of the 30000–40000 influenza-associated deaths in the United States annually [1].

Severe respiratory complications in young healthy persons do not occur on a large scale except during influenza pandemics, which have accompanied antigenic shifts to a new hemagglutinin type (1918, 1957 and 1968) [4]. During pandemic years even relatively young persons are at risk of viral pneumonia, immune-mediated acute respiratory distress syndrome and multiple organ failure. Recent clusters of severe human influenza have been caused by avian subtypes, especially H5N1, after avian contact [5]. There has been little evidence of efficient human-to-human transmission, but the reassortment of avian and human viruses might one day cause severe illness to spread rapidly [6]. The potential of such an epidemic has led to coordinated international planning, and a sense of urgency was imparted by the unrelated but highly lethal 2003 outbreak of severe acute respiratory syndrome (SARS) due to a novel coronavirus [7]. SARS was particularly devastating to hospital personnel, and transmission of fatal disease occurred within the ED [8].

The World Health Organization (WHO), the CDC and other professional organizations have developed clinical guidelines for the management of specific serious causes of respiratory disease such as avian influenza, SARS and tuberculosis, but the National Guideline Clearinghouse reports no evidence-based guidelines for ED patients with undiagnosed seasonal respiratory illness, or even for inter-pandemic influenza. Some of the component questions that would support such guidelines have been the subject of previous research, which is reviewed below.

Unlike other illnesses, influenza-like illness is so common and familiar that a large body of folklore and commercial product promotion may strongly affect patient expectations and distract the physician who wishes to manage the disease rationally. Because a large variety of non-influenza infections may be considered "flu" or "grippe" by self-referred patients, this chapter begins with diagnostic questions, followed by questions on the effectiveness of therapy and prevention.

Clinical questions

1 In ED patients with an acute influenza-like illness (population), does regional surveillance (intervention) accurately predict a virological diagnosis of influenza in individual ED patients (outcome)?
2 In ED patients with an acute influenza-like illness during the peak weeks of virologically proven influenza transmission (population), do clinical criteria (intervention) predict a virological diagnosis of influenza (outcome)?
3 In ED patients with an acute influenza-like illness during the peak weeks of virologically proven influenza transmission (population), do positive rapid diagnostic tests (intervention) predict a virological diagnosis of influenza (outcome) compared to negative tests?
4 In ED patients with influenza-like illness (population), do antiviral drugs (intervention) reduce duration of symptoms (outcome) compared to conservative treatment (control)?
5 In ED patients with influenza at high risk of complications (population), do antiviral drugs (intervention) reduce serious adverse events (outcome) compared to conservative treatment (control)?
6 In exposed family members of influenza patients (population), does prophylaxis with antiviral drugs (intervention) reduce the likelihood of getting clinical influenza (outcome) compared with usual care?
7 In immuno competent adults (population), does influenza vaccination (intervention) reduce the severity of subsequent influenza infection (outcome) compared to not receiving vaccination (control)?

General search strategy

Influenza can be described using a variety of terms (such as as "flu", "influenza" and "influenza-like illness"). Consequently, searching can be difficult and a controlled-vocabulary hierarchy can be employed using OVID's thesaurus results for "influenza" to be sure to include all influenza-related articles. You begin to address these questions by searching for evidence in the common electronic databases such as the Cochrane Library and MEDLINE (through OVID) looking specifically for systematic reviews and meta-analyses. The Cochrane Database of Systematic Reviews includes high-quality systematic review evidence on therapy for influenza and the Database of Abstracts of Reviews of Effects (DARE) includes systematic review evidence on the diagnosis of influenza. You also search OVID to identify randomized controlled trials (RCTs) that became available after the publication date of the systematic review or, if no systematic reviews were identified, to locate high-quality randomized controlled trials that directly address the clinical question. In addition, access to relevant, updated, evidence-based clinical practice guidelines (CPGs) and CDC/WHO guidelines on influenza are accessed to determine the consensus rating of areas lacking evidence.

Critical review of the literature

Question 1: In ED patients with an acute influenza-like illness (population), does regional surveillance (intervention) accurately predict a virological diagnosis of influenza in individual ED patients (outcome)?

Search strategy

- OVID: (explode influenza A virus OR influenza, human) AND diagnosis filter [9] AND explode population surveillance

The diagnosis of influenza is always initially uncertain because other respiratory illnesses present with similar symptoms. These patients should be considered to have "influenza-like illness" (ILI). A consensus definition used by the CDC in its sentinel surveillance network is the presence of fever > 100°F (37.7°C), plus a cough or sore throat in the absence of a known cause other than influenza [10]. As with many ED complaints, the physician's first task is diagnostic: Which of these patients actually has influenza? Clinical examination and laboratory tests can help discriminate, but unlike most other diseases the pre-test probability of influenza changes dramatically over calendar time, since influenza occurs in unpredictable outbreaks against a variable background of other respiratory viral infections. Therefore local status of the influenza epidemic strongly affects the pre-test probability (prevalence) of influenza among ED patients with ILI. A systematic, real-time surveillance program using a network of 130 collaborating laboratories and 1200 volunteer sentinel outpatient providers is operated by the CDC in the United States, which assembles a national estimate of "percent of specimens positive for influenza" and subtype analysis of a proportion of positive specimens. Results are published during the flu season weekly on Fridays for the week ending on the previous Saturday on the following public internet site, http://www.cdc.gov/flu/weekly/fluactivity.htm. Figure 14.1 shows that during the 2006–2007 season, influenza prevalence among submitted samples nationally peaked at 28% in week 6 of 2007

in mid-February. Subtype composition is indicated in a superimposed bar graph. However, influenza was not evenly distributed by geography, as the week 6 map of influenza activity illustrates (Fig. 14.2). A similar website for the WHO reports international human influenza activity [11].

No published studies have compared the CDC reported "percent positive" with local prevalence of influenza among ILI cases in the ED. Historically the prevalence of virologically proven influenza among samples submitted for analysis to the participating laboratories during the peak week of the epidemic has been quite low, between 24% and 35% since surveillance began in 1995. Local ILI surveillance by an ED's hospital laboratory, if available, would provide a more accurate estimate of pre-test probability than regional influenza prevalence in principle, since the latter must average the results of several sites. Many state health departments and federal agencies also report influenza activity on updated web pages.

Although virus isolation defines the onset of the epidemic, a surrogate is an increase in the percent of office visits for ILI [12], a statistic also reported weekly by the CDC (Fig. 14.3). Like virological surveillance, however, there has been no systematic research investigating the usefulness of this information in estimating pre-test probability of influenza for individual ED patients with ILI.

In summary, the pre-test probability of influenza in patients with ILI varies dramatically with the local status of the epidemic. Emergency physicians need to remain aware of this status using the resources at hand, which may include local, regional or national surveillance systems.

Question 2: In ED patients with an acute influenza-like illness during the peak weeks of virologically proven influenza transmission (population), do clinical criteria (intervention) predict a virological diagnosis of influenza (outcome)?

Search strategy

- OVID: (explode influenza A virus OR influenza, human) AND diagnosis filter [9] AND (explode physical examination OR explode history taking OR examination.tw)

Compared to other causes of ILI, influenza more consistently causes cough, fever and systemic symptoms. Can this distinction be used to make a diagnosis in ED practice? One systematic review concluded that the presence of rigors, fever and presentation soon after symptom onset (within 3 days) were the best predictors of influenza, while absence of fever or cough, or not being confined to bed, were each individual predictors of a non-influenza cause of ILI [13]. None of these individual associations was very strong, i.e., no single test had a likelihood ratio of >10 or <0.1. Furthermore, a single study of pooled drug trials dominated the results, and none of the studies included any ED patients [14]. A subsequent systematic review similarly concluded that no single clinical finding can be used to reliably diagnose influenza among patients

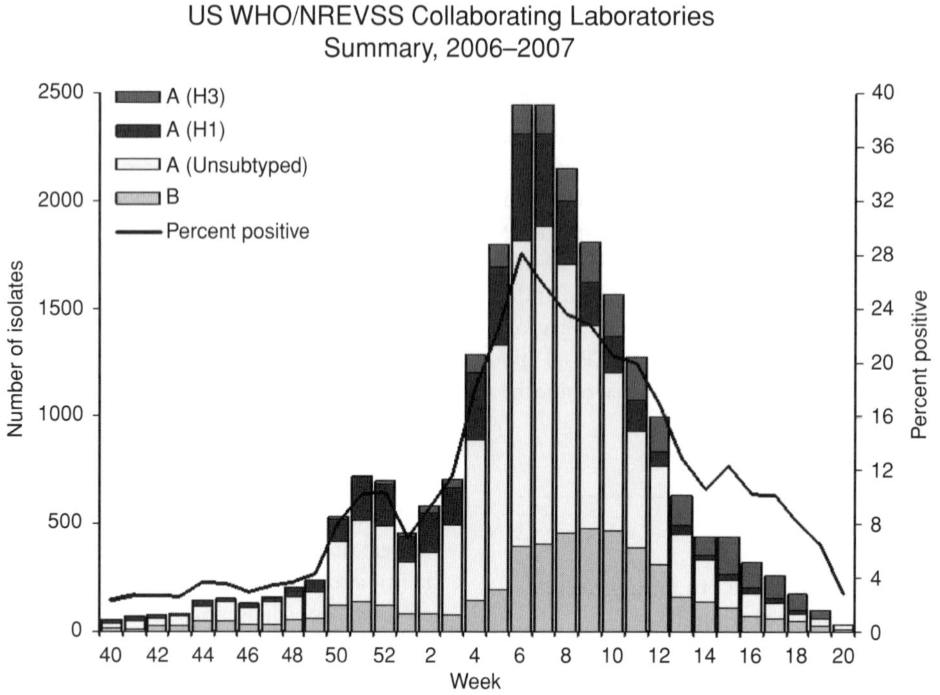

US WHO/NREVSS Collaborating Laboratories
Summary, 2006–2007

Figure 14.1 CDC influenza surveillance website screenshot, June 2007, showing the percent of submitted respiratory specimens positive for influenza (line) with the distribution of influenza subtypes (bars), by week of the year. Influenza prevalence (all ages and regions combined) peaked at 28% during week 6 of 2007, with most specimens of the H1 subtype, but with co-circulation of influenza B and an H3 subtype. The latter had been dominant since the 2003–2004 season. (Reproduced from http://www.cdc.gov/flu/weekly/weeklyarchives2006-2007/images/WhoLab20.gif.)

with ILI [15]. Clinical trials are able to recruit populations with a high likelihood of influenza by delaying enrollment until influenza is definitely circulating and requiring strict inclusion criteria, such as measured fever combined with multiple symptoms. Case definitions for such trials are intentionally very specific, often recruiting populations with >50% influenza cases, but thereby also excluding many cases. Such patient samples have a higher prevalence and severity of influenza than adult ED patients with ILI (spectrum bias) and are likely to distort the diagnostic value of clinical findings, e.g., cough and fever, by using them as inclusion criteria for the trial (work-up bias) [16].

Even during the peak of the flu season most adult ED visitors with ILI usually do not have influenza. Furthermore, changes in the composition of the non-influenza cases can influence the discriminating power of the clinical examination as much as variation in influenza cases. For example, respiratory syncytial virus often occurs in winter epidemics of severe illness very similar to influenza, unlike common rhinovirus, coronavirus and parainfluenza virus infections [17], thereby reducing the discriminating power of fever and systemic symptoms.

Though individual clinical findings have little predictive power, combinations of findings from the history and physical examination may yet prove useful, but no studies to date have had sufficient sample size to derive a valid clinical decision rule. If such a study were to evaluate 15 potential discriminators (e.g., cough, fever, rapid onset, nasal discharge, CDC surveillance variables,

local surveillance variables, immunization status, etc.) then 10 times as many influenza cases would need to be enrolled to generate a predictive model that is likely to be valid i.e., a multi-center study is needed [18]. In a season with 25% influenza prevalence over a 3-month data collection period, (this represents a total enrollment of 600 ILI patients). Smaller studies may generate accurate rules, but such rules are less likely to prove valid in other settings.

In summary, the clinical examination is of limited value in defining which ED patients with ILI have influenza in inter-pandemic years, though future collaborative studies may help resolve this problem.

Question 3: In ED patients with an acute influenza-like illness during the peak weeks of virologically proven influenza transmission (population), do rapid diagnostic tests (intervention) predict a virological diagnosis of influenza (outcome) compared to history alone?

Search strategy

- OVID: (explode influenza A virus OR influenza, human) AND diagnosis filter [9] AND explode laboratory techniques and procedures

More than 10 different point-of-care rapid antigen tests for influenza have been tested against a viral culture gold standard,

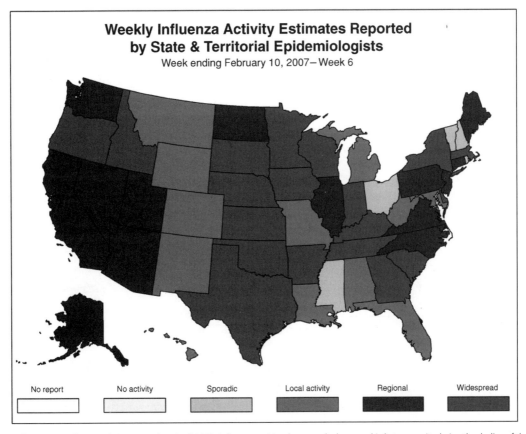

Figure 14.2 CDC influenza surveillance website screenshot, April 2007. Influenza activity shows marked geographic heterogeneity during the decline of the epidemic. (Reproduced from http://www.cdc.gov/flu/weekly/weeklyarchives2006-2007/weekly06.htm.)

and distributed commercially [19]. Some of these discriminate between influenza A and B, others do not. The promise of such tests is their ability to identify patients with influenza early, even during their ED stay, allowing targeted antiviral therapy. Such tests have also reduced the intensity of diagnostic testing, length of ED stay, and antibiotic use for ILI patients in some [20–23] but not all [24] settings; however, these have been conducted mostly in pediatric patients. Other studies have shown decreased use of antibiotics in hospitalized adults, and improved influenza surveillance [25,26]. Influenza tests yield more positives with nasopharyngeal swabs or washings compared with throat specimens. A limitation of all antigen tests is the reduction in viral yield after 2–4 days of symptoms. In one study of adult ED patients with ILI, just 25% arrived in the ED within 2 days of symptom onset [27]. Children with ILI are more likely to have influenza, have more severe symptoms and higher viral loads, thus increasing the sensitivity of antigen tests. In addition, one study of UK general practice found that 64% of children arrived within 48 hours of the onset of symptoms [28].

Only one study has characterized adult ED patients with ILI. This study was performed during the peak of the 2001–2002 flu season (January through March) and found an influenza prevalence of 21% [27]. The sensitivity of the Quickvue rapid antigen

test was 33% (95% CI: 22% to 47%) and specificity was 92% (95% CI: 87% to 95%). Another study evaluated the feasibility of rapid testing for sentinel surveillance (adults and children) in Hawaii during the 1998–2001 flu seasons using the Biostar OIA test and found a sensitivity of 41% and specificity of 88% (calculated from a results table). This test was considerably less sensitive than the preliminary studies performed by the test manufacturer [25].

Two authors have reviewed multiple point-of-care diagnostic test kits [15,29]. One review included six mostly pediatric studies [15], and another reviewed 28 exclusively pediatric studies of rapid antigen tests [29]. Summarization is difficult since samples differed in many ways, including test technology, test manufacturer, site of patient recruitment, influenza prevalence and specimen source. One pediatric study overcame this difficulty by comparing four test kits on the same patient specimens in a study sample with a 49% prevalence of influenza, and found similar predictive power for each test, with a summary likelihood ratio of 4.7 for positive results and 0.06 for negative results, excluding the ZStat Flu kit, which had significantly lower sensitivity [30].

In summary, point-of-care tests for influenza have been widely evaluated in children but not adults. Since these tests have moderate sensitivity and high specificity, they are useful for ruling in

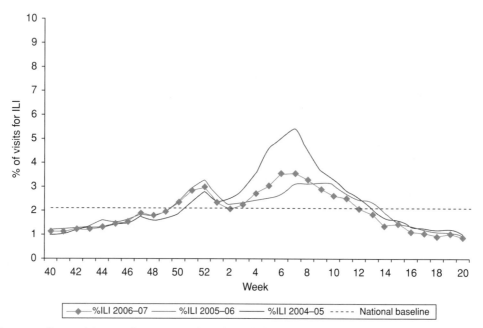

Figure 14.3 CDC influenza surveillance website screenshot, June 2007. The incidence of influenza-like illness (ILI) coincides with the peak of influenza prevalence in Fig. 14.1, and matches the pattern of previous years closely. (Reproduced from http://www.cdc.gov/flu/weekly/weeklyarchives2006-2007/images/picILI20.gif.)

influenza when other serious diseases are under consideration, but are less reliable for excluding influenza.

Question 4: In ED patients with influenza-like illness (population), do antiviral drugs (intervention) reduce duration of symptoms (outcome) compared to conservative treatment (control)?

Search strategy

- OVID: (explode influenza A virus OR influenza, human) AND explode antiviral agents AND review filter [9]

Two antiviral drug classes have been used to treat influenza: the adamantanes include amantadine and rimantadine, and the neuraminidase inhibitors (NIs) include oseltamivir and zanamivir, the latter only available as an inhaled spray. While systematic reviews have shown these drugs to be effective in previous years for treatment, prevention and post-exposure prophylaxis in adults [31,32], over 95% of isolates of influenza A abruptly developed resistance to the adamantanes in the last 2 years in the United States. They should currently be excluded from consideration for this reason alone [1]. In addition, the adamantanes are ineffective against influenza B, which has co-circulated with influenza A in the most recent epidemics.

In systematic reviews both oseltamivir and zanamivir reduce the time to alleviation of symptoms for this 4-day illness by about 1.5 days in adults with virologically proven influenza (efficacy analysis), and by 1 day in all patients with ILI recruited for these trials (effectiveness analysis). This minor benefit is likely to be even smaller in unselected ED patients with a lower prevalence and severity of influenza. Side-effects of NIs were minimal in these trials, including nausea with oseltamivir. For healthy adults with an acute ILI, NIs have moderate efficacy but no effectiveness in preventing bronchitis and pneumonia [32].

In a separate Cochrane review of ILI in children, NIs were found to have a similar impact on time to alleviation of symptoms, and in addition oseltamivir (but not zanamivir) reduced the rate of otitis media in patients with positive viral cultures. The number needed to treat (NNT) was 11 (95% CI: 6 to 40) for ages 1 to 12, and for children aged 1 to 5 years the NNT was 5 (95% CI: 3 to 14), with no effectiveness analysis reported. Children with asthma, who account for most pediatric influenza hospitalizations, may have benefited less in terms of alleviation of symptoms, but NIs produced better peak flow rates after 6 days than placebo [33].

As with the adamantanes, resistance develops to NIs during treatment, though transmission of resistant viruses has not been observed [34]. Furthermore, viral shedding continues even as clinical symptoms abate. Because of the possibility of provoking large-scale resistance, the authors of the Cochrane review suggest that the use of NIs should not be routine during a typical inter-pandemic influenza season, unless documented influenza is causing high rates of severe disease locally. Even then, public health measures may be of greater importance than antivirals in containing the outbreak [32].

There are no placebo-controlled trials of NIs for avian influenza, given the high likelihood of serious adverse outcomes. Indirect evidence suggests some efficacy: the development of resistance to oseltamivir was accompanied by rapid worsening in one report [35], and exposed persons given prophylaxis had better outcomes in one non-randomized outbreak investigation [36].

In summary, treatment of influenza with NIs should be reserved for early presentations, and should not be routine during a typical inter-pandemic influenza season, unless documented influenza is causing high rates of severe disease locally.

Question 5: In ED patients with influenza at high risk of complications (population), do antiviral drugs (intervention) reduce serious adverse events (outcome) compared to conservative treatment (control)?

Search strategy

- OVID: (explode influenza A virus OR influenza, human) AND explode antiviral agents AND review filter [9]

As noted above, a meta-analysis of antiviral drug trials demonstrated efficacy for preventing relatively common complications of bronchitis and pneumonia, and otitis media in children, but very little if any effectiveness, i.e., NIs are unlikely to prevent these complications in undifferentiated ED patients with ILI. However, few studies of antiviral drugs have been able to assess outcomes in a sufficiently large subgroup of high-risk adults. One study pooled seven zanamivir trials to evaluate high-risk patients and found an even greater reduction in time to symptom alleviation (2.5 days) than in healthy adults [37]. A single open-label trial compared oseltamivir with placebo in adults with chronic lung diseases, similarly finding a return of symptoms to baseline 5 days earlier than placebo and also a reduced rate of complications and antibiotic use [38]. No serious adverse events such as death or respiratory failure occurred in either of these trials. Similarly, one trial could not demonstrate a difference in hospitalization rates between trial limbs [39].

The immediate cause of death in patients with influenza is often a bacterial infection, especially staphyloccocal pneumonia [40]. In summary, monotherapy with antiviral drugs should not be considered in influenza victims who are seriously ill. Tailored antibiotic coverage is strongly recommended as in any patient with suspected sepsis.

Question 6: In exposed family members of influenza patients (population), does prophylaxis with antiviral drugs (intervention) reduce the likelihood of getting clinical influenza (outcome)?

Search strategy

- OVID: (explode influenza A virus OR influenza, human) AND explode antiviral agents AND review filter [9]

Post-exposure prophylaxis (PEP) is the prevention of influenza among asymptomatic contacts of a person who has been diagnosed with influenza and is still infectious (i.e., between disease onset and 5 days later). A typical prophylaxis regimen is a 7-day course of antiviral drugs at a lower dose than the treatment dose. Even if treated, a clinically ill person will continue to shed virus for variable periods of time, especially children. Unlike a physician's office, the ED does not normally care for patients without symptoms, but in this case the ED physician is caring for the index case and has the opportunity to prevent spread within the patient's family, of particular concern when the patient might expose a high-risk contact. Health care personnel themselves are potential beneficiaries of PEP.

Prevention differs from treatment in that drug side-effects are more likely to be noticed since the patient is not suffering from influenza, and benefits are less tangible since the subject does not "get better". In the case of influenza, however, there is also the potential societal benefit of reducing transmission and containing the epidemic, particularly important in a pandemic year [41].

Four placebo-controlled trials of PEP in adults – two for each NI – were reviewed by Jefferson et al. [32]. All four trials demonstrated a marked reduction in clinical influenza infection. For example, oseltamivir yielded a relative reduction for symptomatic influenza of 59% (95% CI: 16% to 80%) for households and 68% (95% CI: 35% to 84%) for individuals, though there was no reduction in asymptomatic infection [42]. Similar results were noted for oseltamivir in the only PEP trial in children: relative risk reduction was 64% (95% CI: 16% to 85%) [43].

In summary, post-exposure influenza prophylaxis for asymptomatic exposed family members at high risk of complications should be considered when the ED identifies an index case with a high likelihood of influenza.

Question 7: In immunocompetent adults (population), does influenza vaccination (intervention) reduce the severity of subsequent influenza infection (outcome) compared to not receiving vaccination (control)?

Search strategy

- OVID: (explode influenza A virus OR influenza, human) AND explode immunization AND review filter [9]

One recent case–control study reported reduced hospitalization and death rates in healthy adults who received vaccine [44]. However, death and hospitalization are rare outcomes in this age category. A recently updated Cochrane review of 25 methodologically more rigorous randomized trials involving 59,566 subjects concludes that while influenza vaccination is efficacious in preventing serologically confirmed influenza in healthy adults, it is much less effective in preventing clinical influenza or reducing work-days lost. Therefore, the authors conclude that universal immunization of healthy adults is not worthwhile [45]. No studies addressed the issue of disease severity among those patients who contracted influenza despite vaccination, nor were any subjects systematically recruited from an ED population.

Vaccine trials in patients with asthma were pooled in a similar review, which found no reduction in asthma exacerbations; nor was there an increase in exacerbations immediately after vaccination [46]. A separate review of randomized placebo-controlled trials of vaccination in chronic obstructive pulmonary disease (COPD) patients did show a reduced number of exacerbations after 3 weeks, and a reduced incidence of clinical influenza [47].

Immunization of patients aged > 65 years is strongly recommended by the CDC, based on the conclusion that vaccination reduces the high rate of death in this population [1]. These studies have also been systematically reviewed in the Cochrane Library, which pooled the results of 96 trials [48]. Because ethical consideration discourages the use of an unvaccinated control group, most of these are observational studies without random assignment, potentially biased by imbalances in baseline health status favoring vaccination. Among these studies the evidence of reduced complications, including pneumonia, hospitalization, influenza-associated mortality and all-cause mortality is most robust in long-term care facilities.

Should the ED consider vaccinating asymptomatic patients who happen to be in the ED during the flu season? Opportunistic case finding of this sort has been suggested for other prevention strategies such as cervical cancer screening, and is somewhat attractive since chronically ill and elderly patients are increasingly encountered in EDs rather than physician offices. A similar strategy of vaccinating injured patients against the vanishing disease tetanus remains an ED ritual. However, not only would inter-pandemic flu vaccination require a seasonal system change at a time of increased stress in the ED, its practicality and cost-effectiveness needs to be documented in a group randomized trial before national resources are committed on a large scale.

In summary, seasonal population-based vaccination against influenza is probably life-saving and cost-effective in high-risk patients, and is a formal policy for the CDC and many governmental organizations. It is possible that an ED-based strategy of identifying and vaccinating eligible patients is a useful adjunct to such a strategy; however, this needs to be formally investigated before widespread implementation.

Conclusions

The diagnosis of influenza by clinical examination is not supported by large clinical ED studies, and antigen tests of nasal swab specimens are insensitive in adults. Positive local surveillance or reference to the CDC weekly flu activity website can demonstrate that influenza is circulating in a community, but has not been evaluated as a diagnostic test. Nevertheless, in this scenario the presence of multiple positive factors during a documented influenza epidemic in a teacher exposed to the cauldron of disease activity typical among children suggests that she probably has the disease. Antivirals have a weak effect on alleviation of symptoms in effectiveness trials, and from the societal perspective are cost-effective only when the probability of disease is very high (i.e., in patients with multiple symptoms during local epidemics documented by viral culture [49]). The simultaneous presence of pneumonia in this scenario does not imply a viral etiology, thus antibiotics should be used. In this case, the fact that she was a teacher, arrived early in the course of infection, and was on a drug plan suggests that antivirals are also indicated. Antiviral drugs reduce the risk of clinical influenza in the household contacts of a symptomatic ED patient. High-risk family members, such as this patient's mother-in-law, stand to benefit most from post-exposure prophylaxis. High-risk patients who become ill with influenza have longer disease courses but also benefit more from antiviral drugs than healthy adults.

The teacher's long wait in an ED crowded by patients with respiratory complaints is a seasonal, global, public health problem affecting the efficiency of care for all diseases. This can only become worse in an influenza pandemic. One narrative review details the evidence for respiratory hygiene in ED waiting rooms [50]. During the flu season this should include the barrier and distance elements of droplet precautions when feasible: 1 m minimum segregation, access to tissues, cough etiquette posters, handwashing stations and surgical masks for patients with respiratory complaints. The pandemic potential of influenza creates an exceptional public health opportunity for a specialty usually oriented to the diagnosis and treatment of acute illness. Attention to ED systems during seasonal inter-pandemic flu may help blunt the impact of a pandemic.

References

1 Center for Disease Control. Prevention and control of influenza: recommendations of the Advisory Committee on Immunization Practices (ACIP). *MMWR* 2007;**56**(RR06):1–54.

2 Monto AS, Kioumehr F. The Tecumseh study of respiratory illness. I. Occurrence of influenza in the community, 1966–1971. *Am J Epidemiol* 1975;**102**:553–63.

3 Poehling KA, Edwards KM, Weinberg GA, et al. The underrecognized burden of influenza in young children. *N Engl J Med* 2006;**355**(1):31–40.

4 Belshe RB. The origins of pandemic influenza – lessons from the 1918 virus. *N Engl J Med* 2005;353(21):2209–11.

5 The Writing Committee of the World Health Organization Consultation on Human Influenza AH. Avian influenza A (H5N1) infection in humans. *N Engl J Med* 2005;**353**(13):1374–85.

6 Hien TT, Liem NT, Dung NT, et al. Avian influenza A (H5N1) in 10 patients in Vietnam. *N Engl J Med* 2004;**350**(12):1179–88.

7 Holmes KV. SARS-associated coronavirus. *N Engl J Med* 2003;**348**(20):1948–51.

8 Poutanen SM, Low DE, Henry B, et al. Identification of severe acute respiratory syndrome in Canada. *N Engl J Med* 2003;**348**(20):1995–2005.

9 Health Information Research Unit, McMaster University. Search strategies for MEDLINE in Ovid syntax and the PubMed translation. 2000. Available at http://hiru.mcmaster.ca/hedges/ (accessed April 8, 2007).

10 Center for Disease Control. Overview of influenza surveillance in the United States. 2006. Available at http://www.cdc.gov/flu/weekly/pdf/flu-surveillance-overview.pdf (accessed March 29 2007).

11 World Health Organization. Seasonal influenza activity in the world. 2007. Available at http://www.who.int/csr/disease/influenza/update/en/ (accessed April 6, 2007).

12 Monto AS, Ohmit SE, Margulies JR, Talsma A. Medical practice-based influenza surveillance: viral prevalence and assessment of morbidity. *Am J Epid* 1995;**141**:502–6.

13 Ebell MH, White LL, Casault T. A systematic review of the history and physical examination to diagnose influenza. *J Am Board Fam Prac* 2004;**17**(1):1–5.

14 Monto AS, Gravenstein S, Elliott M, Colopy M, Schweinle J. Clinical signs and symptoms predicting influenza infection. *Arch Intern Med* 2000;**160**(21):3243–7.

15 Call SA, Vollenweider MA, Hornung CA, Simel DL, McKinney WP. Does this patient have influenza? *JAMA* 2005;**293**(8):987–97.

16 Jaeschke R, Guyatt G, Sackett DL. Users' guides to the medical literature. III. How to use an article about a diagnostic test. A. Are the results of the study valid? Evidence-Based Medicine Working Group. *JAMA* 1994;**271**(5):389–91.

17 Zambon MC, Stockton JD, Clewley JP, Fleming DM. Contribution of influenza and respiratory syncytial virus to community cases of influenza-like illness: an observational study. *Lancet* 2001;**358**:1410–16.

18 Peduzzi P, Concato J, Kemper E, Holford TR, Feinstein AR. A simulation study of the number of events per variable in logistic regression analysis. *J Clin Epid* 1996;**49**(12):1373–9.

19 Center for Disease Control. Influenza symptoms and laboratory diagnostic procedures. 2007. Available at http://www.cdc.gov/flu/professionals/diagnosis/labprocedures.htm (accessed April 2, 2007).

20 Bonner AB, Monroe KW, Talley LI, Klasner AE, Kimberlin DW. Impact of the rapid diagnosis of influenza on physician decision-making and patient management in the pediatric emergency department: results of a randomized, prospective, controlled trial. *Pediatrics* 2003;**112**(2):363–7.

21 Noyola DE, Demmler GJ. Effect of rapid diagnosis on management of influenza A infections. *Pediatr Infect Dis J* 2000;**19**:303–7.

22 Sharma V, Dowd MD, Slaughter AJ, Simon SD. Effect of rapid diagnosis of influenza virus type A on the emergency department management of febrile infants and toddlers. *Arch Pediatr Adolesc Med* 2002;**156**(1):41–3.

23 Falsey AR, Murata Y, Walsh EE. Impact of rapid diagnosis on management of adults hospitalized with influenza. *Arch Intern Med* 2007;**167**:354–60.

24 Iyer SB, Gerber MA, Pomerantz WJ, Mortensen JE, Ruddy RM. Effect of point-of-care influenza testing on management of febrile children. *Acad Emerg Med* 2006;**13**(12):1259–68.

25 Effler PV, Ieong M-C, Tom T, Nakata M. Enhancing public health surveillance for influenza virus by incorporating newly available rapid diagnostic tests. *Emerg Infect Dis* 2002;**8**(1):23–8.

26 Turner KS, Shaw KA, Coleman DJ, Misrachi A. Augmentation of influenza surveillance with rapid antigen detection at the point-of-care: results of a pilot study in Tasmania, 2004. *Commun Dis Intell* 2006;**30**(2):201–4.

27 Stein J, Louie J, Flanders S, et al. Performance characteristics of clinical diagnosis, a clinical decision rule, and a rapid influenza test in the detection of influenza infection in a community sample of adults. *Ann Emerg Med* 2005;**46**(5):412–19.

28 Ross AM, Kai J, Salter R, Ross J, Fleming DM. Presentation with influenza-like illness in general practice: implications for use of neuraminidase inhibitors. *Commun Dis Pub Health* 2000;**3**(4):256–60.

29 Uyeki TM. Influenza diagnosis and treatment in children: a review of studies on clinically useful tests and antiviral treatment for influenza. *Pediatr Infect Dis J* 2003;**22**(2):164–77.

30 Rodriguez WJ, Schwartz RH, Thorne MM. Evaluation of diagnostic tests for influenza in a pediatric practice. *Pediatr Infect Dis J* 2002;**21**(3):193–6.

31 Jefferson T, Demicheli V, Di Pietrantonj C, Rivetti D. Amantadine and rimantadine for influenza A in adults. *Cochrane Database Syst Rev* 2006;**2**:CD001169.

32 Jefferson TO, Demicheli V, DiPietrantonj C, Jones M, Rivetti D. Neuraminidase inhibitors for preventing and treating influenza in healthy adults. *Cochrane Database Syst Rev* 2006;**3**:CD001265.

33 Glezen WP. Asthma, influenza, and vaccination. *J Allergy Clin Imm* 2006;**118**(6):1199–206

34 Monto AS, McKimm-Breschkin JL, Macken C, et al. Detection of influenza viruses resistant to neuraminidase inhibitors in global surveillance during the first 3 years of their use. *Antimicrob Agents Chem* 2006;**50**(7):2395–402.

35 de Jong MD, Tran TT, Truong HK, et al. Oseltamivir resistance during treatment of influenza A (H5N1) infection. *N Engl J Med* 2005;**353**(25):2667–72.

36 Koopmans M, Wilbrink B, Conyn M, et al. Transmission of H7N7 avian influenza A virus to human beings during a large outbreak in commercial poultry farms in the Netherlands. *Lancet* 2004;**363**(9409):587–93.

37 Monto AS, Webster A, Keene O. Randomized, placebo-controlled studies of inhaled zanamivir in the treatment of influenza A and B: pooled efficacy analysis. *J Antimicrob Chem* 1999;**44**(Suppl B):23–9.

38 Lin J-T, Yu X-Z, Cui D-J, et al. A multicentre, randomized, controlled trial of oseltamivir in the treatment of influenza in a high-risk Chinese population. *Curr Med Res Opin* 2006;**22**(1):75–82.

39 Kaiser L, Wat C, Mills T, Mahoney P, Ward P, Hayden F. Impact of oseltamivir treatment on influenza-related lower respiratory tract complications and hospitalizations. *Arch Intern Med* 2003;**163**:1667–72.

40 Hageman JC, Uyeki TM, Francis JS, et al. Severe community-acquired pneumonia due to *Staphylococcus aureus*, 2003–04 influenza season. *Emerg Infect Dis* 2006;**12**(6):894–9.

41 Longini I, Halloran M, Nizam A, Yang Y. Containing pandemic influenza with antiviral agents. *Am J Epidemiol* 2004;**159**(7):623–33.

42 Hayden FG, Belshe R, Villanueva C, Lanno R, Hughes C, Small I. Management of influenza in households: a prospective, randomized comparison of oseltamivir treatment with or without postexposure prophylaxis. *J Infect Dis* 2004;**189**:440–49.

43 Matheson NJ, Symmonds-Abrahams M, Sheikh A, Shepperd S, Harnden A. Neuraminidase inhibitors for preventing and treating influenza in children. *Cochrane Database Syst Rev* 2003;**3**:CD002744.

44 Herrera GA, Iwane MK, Cortese M, et al. Influenza vaccine effectiveness among 50–64-year-old persons during a season of poor antigenic match between vaccine and circulating influenza virus strains: Colorado, United States, 2003–2004. *Vaccine* 2007;**25**:154–60.

45 Demicheli V, Rivetti D, Deeks JJ, Jefferson TO. Vaccines for preventing influenza in healthy adults. *Cochrane Database Syst Rev* 2004;**3**: CD001269.

46 Cates CJ, Jefferson TO, Bara AI, Rowe BH. Vaccines for preventing influenza in people with asthma. *Cochrane Database Syst Rev* 2004;**2**:CD000364.

47 Poole PJ, Chacko E, Wood-Baker RWB, et al. Influenza vaccine for patients with chronic obstructive pulmonary disease. *Cochrane Database Syst Rev* 2006;**1**:CD002733.

48 Rivetti D, Jefferson T, Thomas R, et al. Vaccines for preventing influenza in the elderly. *Cochrane Database Syst Rev* 2006;**3**:CD004876.

49 Rothberg MB, He S, Rose DN. Management of influenza symptoms in healthy adults: cost-effectiveness of rapid testing and antiviral therapy. *J Gen Intern Med* 2003;**18**:808–15.

50 Rothman RE, Irvin CB, Moran GJ, et al. Respiratory hygiene in the emergency department. *Ann Emerg Med* 2006;**48**(5):570–82.

15 Anaphylaxis

Theodore Gaeta

Department of Emergency Medicine, New York Methodist Hospital, Brooklyn *and* Weill Medical College of Cornell University, New York, USA

Case scenario

A 19-year-old woman presented to the emergency department (ED) with acute onset of dyspnea. An accompanying friend reported that the patient developed generalized flushing and pruritis minutes after eating a chocolate chip cookie while at school. En route to the ED the patient had one episode of vomiting and began complaining of difficulty breathing. Her vitals signs were pulse 124 beats/min, respiration 30 breaths/min, blood pressure 90/60 mmHg (right arm), temperature 37.1°C (98.8°F) and pulse oximetry 94% SaO_2 on room air. The patient was placed on a cardiac monitor and given supplemental oxygen. Intravenous access was established and an IV fluid bolus of normal saline was administered.

On physical examination, she was lethargic but responsive to verbal stimuli. Her airway was patent and there was no stridor; however, diminished breaths sounds at the bases and end-expiratory wheezing in the upper fields were detected. Her pulses were weak bilaterally and there was delayed capillary refill. Inspection of her skin revealed a diffuse, maculo-papular erythematous rash and a MedicAlert® bracelet indicating a history of peanut allergy. The remainder of the physical examination was within normal limits. The primary diagnosis was anaphylaxis secondary to severe peanut allergy. Initial treatment consisted of the administration of 0.3 ml of 1:1000 dilution epinephrine intramuscularly and 50 mg diphenhydramine intravenously.

Background

Anaphylaxis is an immediate and life-threatening systemic reaction to an exogenous stimulus, characterized by either hypotension or airway compromise. Anaphylaxis therefore lies at the far end of the gradient of hypersensitivity reactions (a continuum of the acute allergic reaction). The simplest and least threatening allergic reactions include urticarial skin eruptions which occur locally or, in more severe cases, systemically. Generalized allergic reactions involving bronchospasm or throat symptoms represent an intermediate severity between the skin manifestations and true anaphylaxis. Often, it is clinically difficult to distinguish between this intermediate stage and true anaphylaxis due to prehospital and early interventions that abort the progression of the allergic reaction.

Despite the emergent nature and potential for morbidity and mortality, limited data are available on the frequency and management of anaphylaxis in the ED. The true incidence and prevalence of anaphylaxis is unclear. For many years there has been no universally accepted working definition of anaphylaxis or criteria for diagnosis. In 2005, the National Institute of Allergy and Infectious Disease and Food Allergy and Anaphylaxis Network recommended the following brief and broad definition: "anaphylaxis is a serious allergic reaction that is rapid in onset and may cause death" [1].

The coding and classification of allergic reactions and anaphylaxis has also evolved over the past several years. New codes to describe fatal anaphylactic reactions including "anaphylactic shock due to adverse food reaction" and "anaphylactic shock, unspecified" were developed in 2003. Research has indicated, however, that these codes are widely underused and also has suggested that International Classification of Disease (ICD) codes might be limited in their ability to retrospectively identify specific allergic reactions in the ED [2,3].

Despite a formal definition and the newly introduced allergen-specific codes (such as those categorizing food allergies), the study of anaphylaxis in the ED remains complicated. In practice, clinicians often do not account for other patient characteristics, such as the complexity or severity of the reaction. Failure to differentiate between the singular presence of mucocutaneous signs (i.e., urticaria or angioedema) and the additional occurrence of respiratory and cardiovascular symptoms (i.e., wheezing, hypotension, arrhythmias) is a potential source of misclassification. Similarly, when symptoms do not appear imminently life-threatening or

Evidence-based Emergency Medicine. Edited by Brian H. Rowe
© 2009 Blackwell Publishing, ISBN: 978-1-4051-6143-5.

respond to initial ED therapy, physicians may classify the presentation as an acute allergic reaction, de-emphasizing and under-reporting the diagnosis of anaphylaxis.

An equally difficult task is to determine the standard treatment practices in ED patients with anaphylaxis. Recent multi-center studies and a large national database review suggest great variability in the ED management approach [4–6]. Historically, the standard of care for severe allergic reactions has revolved around epinephrine and supportive care. In addition, agents such as H_1-blockers and corticosteroids have enjoyed some popularity in treating the mucocutaneous effects, while inhaled β-agonists have been used to treat respiratory symptoms. Other agents, such as H_2-blockers, have been used but their effectiveness has yet to be fully elucidated. Therapeutic recommendations are based largely on clinical observations, interpretation of underlying pathophysiology and animal models. Given the paucity of controlled trials, the best evidence we are left with often comes from published consensus guidelines [7].

Clinical questions

In order to address the issues of most relevance to your patient and to help in searching the literature for the evidence regarding these, you should structure your questions as recommended in Chapter 1.

1 In patients with anaphylaxis presenting to the ED (population), does the administration of intramuscular epinephrine (intervention) decrease the risk of admission to hospital (outcome) compared to subcutaneous epinephrine (control)?

2 In hypotensive patients with anaphylaxis presenting to the ED (population), does the administration of intravenous epinephrine (intervention) decrease the risk of death (outcome) compared to intramuscular epinephrine (control)?

3 In patients with anaphylaxis presenting to the ED (population), does the addition of H_2-antagonist agents (intervention) to H_1-antagonists decrease the risk of admission to hospital (outcome) compared to treatment with H_1-antagonist therapy alone (control)?

4 In patients with anaphylaxis presenting to the ED (population), does the use of intravenous corticosteroids (intervention) in the ED reduce admissions to the hospital (outcome) compared to standard care (control)?

5 In patients with treatment-refractory anaphylaxis presenting to the ED (population), does intravenous glucagon (intervention) in addition to epinephrine and systemic antihistamines (control) improve hemodynamic parameters (outcome)?

6 In patients with anaphylaxis in the ED (population), will 6 hours of clinical observation (intervention) identify relapses related to "biphasic" allergic reactions (outcome)?

7 In patients with acute allergic reactions (population), does the out-of-hospital use of self-injectable epinephrine (intervention) reduce admissions to the hospital (outcome) compared to supportive care alone (control)?

General search strategy

You begin to address these questions by searching for evidence in the common electronic databases such as the Cochrane Library, MEDLINE and EMBASE looking specifically for systematic reviews and meta-analyses. The Cochrane Library is particularly rich in high-quality systematic review evidence; however, in the field of allergy and anaphylaxis, the Cochrane Database of Systematic Reviews and Database of Abstracts of Reviews of Effects (DARE) do not yield many relevant reviews. Other resources (MEDLINE, EMBASE) yield more systematic reviews. When a systematic review is identified, you also search for recent updates in CENTRAL, MEDLINE and EMBASE to identify randomized controlled trials (RCTs) that may have been published after the publication date of the systematic review. Finally, access to relevant, updated and evidence-based clinical practice guidelines (CPGs) on anaphylaxis are accessed to determine the consensus rating of areas lacking evidence.

Searching for evidence synthesis: primary search strategy
- Cochrane Library: (anaphylaxis OR allergic reaction) AND (topic)
- MEDLINE: (anaphylaxis OR allergic reaction) AND MEDLINE AND (systematic review OR meta-analysis OR metaanalysis) AND (topic)
- EMBASE: (anaphylaxis OR allergic reaction) AND MEDLINE AND (systematic review OR meta-analysis OR metaanalysis) AND (topic)

Critical review of the literature

Your search strategy for the Cochrane Library identified two systematic review products addressing your clinical questions. There was a protocol for review to assess the benefits or harms related to epinephrine in the treatment of anaphylaxis [8], and a review performed to assess the benefits and harm of H_1-antihistamines which found no studies that satisfied the inclusion criteria [9]. Your MEDLINE search identified several relevant articles including evidence-based CPGs. Again, there were no systematic reviews or meta-analyses.

Question 1: In patients with anaphylaxis presenting to the ED (population), does the administration of intramuscular epinephrine (intervention) decrease the risk of admission to hospital (outcome) compared to subcutaneous epinephrine (control)?

Search strategy
- MEDLINE and EMBASE: (anaphylaxis OR allergic reaction) AND (adrenaline OR epinephrine)

Like many severe illnesses, the primary assessment in the ED requires assessment of **a**irway, **b**reathing and **c**irculation (ABC). Current recommendations for the ED treatment of anaphylaxis include ensuring a patent airway, administrating supplemental oxygen, establishing intravenous access and, most critically, administering parenteral epinephrine [1].

Epinephrine is the treatment of choice and the first drug to be administered in the therapy of anaphylaxis. This has been confirmed in every guideline issued worldwide dating back to at least 1973 [10]. Although the benefits of epinephrine in the treatment of anaphylaxis have been cited, its particular indications, dosing requirements and route of administration remain a source of controversy and have been known to hinder its appropriate use among health care providers [6,11,12]. For example, no large-scale studies or systematic reviews were identified to clarify the role of epinephrine in anaphylaxis using the search above.

The α-adrenergic, vasoconstrictive effect reverses peripheral vasodilation, which alleviates hypotension and also reduces angioedema and urticaria. It may also minimize further absorption of antigen from the sting or injection. The β-adrenergic properties of epinephrine cause bronchodilation, increase myocardial output and contractility, and suppress further mediator release from mast cells and basophils [10,13].

Practice parameters suggest that aqueous epinephrine 1:1000 dilution, 0.2–0.5 ml (0.01 mg/kg in children; maximum dose 0.3 mg), administered intramuscularly or subcutaneously every 5 minutes, as necessary, should be used to control symptoms and increase blood pressure (noting that if the clinician deems it appropriate, the 5-minute interval between injections can be liberalized to permit more frequent injections) [7].

Comparisons of intramuscular to subcutaneous injections have not been performed during anaphylaxis. However, there have been studies that compare systemic absorption based on the route of administration. Absorption is complete, more rapid and associated with higher plasma levels in asymptomatic adults and children who receive epinephrine intramuscularly [14,15]. Intramuscular injection into the anterolateral thigh (vastus lateralis) is superior to intramuscular injection into the arm (deltoid) [15]. Administration with the use of a 1-inch (2.5 cm) needle is preferred since patients with accentuated subcutaneous fat may prevent or complicate intramuscular access [16]. Whether the injection site or method translates into improved clinical outcomes has not been demonstrated. Subcutaneous administration of medication is highly dependent on cutaneous blood flow, which may already be compromised in anaphylaxis and further aggravated by epinephrine's potent local vasoconstrictor activity.

In summary, intramuscular epinephrine injection in the vastus lateralis muscle of either thigh has theoretical benefit over subcutaneous injection; however, the benefit on clinical outcomes in general, and in anaphylaxis specifically, remains unclear. ED management reviews have indicated that less than 25% of all patients with allergies receive epinephrine (regardless of route; Fig. 15.1), and in US emergency departments epinephrine usage is on a decline (19% to 7% over a 12-year interval) [4–6]. Current international consensus panels and practice guidelines for emergency cardiovascular care and anaphylaxis recommend intramuscular epinephrine injections [2,7,17].

Question 2: In hypotensive patients with anaphylaxis presenting to the ED (population), does the administration of intravenous epinephrine (intervention) decrease the risk of death (outcome) compared to intramuscular epinephrine (control)?

Search strategy

- MEDLINE and EMBASE: (anaphylaxis OR allergic reaction) AND (adrenaline or epinephrine)

The search described above failed to identify any high-quality direct effect of intravenous epinephrine on the outcomes associated with anaphylaxis compared to intramuscular epinephrine. There are no critically appraised guidelines or established dosage for intravenous epinephrine in anaphylaxis. There is evidence that suggests, however, that the initial management of hypotension in anaphylaxis may be successful using intravenous epinephrine [18]. In this prospective evaluation of patients with insect sting anaphylaxis, all 19 patients enrolled responded rapidly to treatment with no appreciable adverse reactions attributed to epinephrine. This study demonstrated that a carefully titrated epinephrine infusion combined with volume resuscitation is effective, and perhaps opens the doors for a comparison between intramuscular and intravenous epinephrine. Caution is warranted, since evidence suggests that complications associated with intravenous use of epinephrine are not insignificant.

An intravenous preparation can be prepared by diluting 0.1 ml (100 μg) of 1:1000 (1 mg/ml) aqueous epinephrine solution in 10 ml normal saline. The 10 ml dose can be infused over 5–10 minutes, resulting in a total dose of 100 μg at a rate of 10–20 μg/min. This could be repeated depending on the response [13]. The side-effects of intravenous epinephrine are considerable and can be serious (e.g., arrhythmia); they have been examined in a retrospective ED cohort of patients with asthma [19]. While these patients did not all have allergic asthma, the similarity between this young, healthy population suffering an inflammatory crisis and those with anaphylaxis, makes extrapolation of these results to allergy appealing. Overall, these investigators reported approximately 31% minor and 4% major side-effects from 220 episodes of care that met the inclusion criteria. Since there is a potential for lethal arrhythmias, continuous low-dose epinephrine infusions might represent the safest and most effective form of delivery because the dose can be titrated to the desired effect (avoiding the potential for accidental administration of large boluses of epinephrine) [2,7].

In summary, the evidence for the use of intravenous epinephrine is limited. Its use may be warranted in some cases, but should be reserved for the most extreme conditions, such as when the

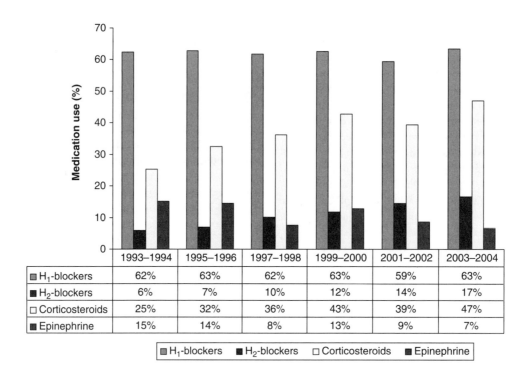

	1993–1994	1995–1996	1997–1998	1999–2000	2001–2002	2003–2004
▨ H_1-blockers	62%	63%	62%	63%	59%	63%
■ H_2-blockers	6%	7%	10%	12%	14%	17%
□ Corticosteroids	25%	32%	36%	43%	39%	47%
■ Epinephrine	15%	14%	8%	13%	9%	7%

▨ H_1-blockers   ■ H_2-blockers   □ Corticosteroids   ■ Epinephrine

Figure 15.1 Trends in medication use. ED staff prescribed medications in 87% of visits. Across the 11-year period, the most commonly prescribed medications were H_1-blockers (overall = 62%, P for trend = 0.47), corticosteroids (37%, P = 0.02) and H_2-blockers (11%, P = 0.01). Epinephrine was also used in 11% of all cases, and use appeared to be declining over time (P = 0.02).

patient has been unresponsive to intramuscular injection or when the initial presentation includes shock or cardiovascular collapse.

Question 3: In patients with anaphylaxis presenting to the ED (population), does the addition of H_2-antagonist agents (intervention) to H_1-antagonists decrease the risk of admission to hospital (outcome) compared to treatment with H_1-antagonist therapy alone (control)?

Search strategy

- MEDLINE and EMBASE: (anaphylaxis OR allergic reaction) AND (antihistamines OR histamine blockers OR histamine antagonists)

Histamine plays a pivotal role in acute allergic inflammation and during anaphylaxis a number of inflammatory mediators are released. In an attempt to minimize the impact of histamine release, H_1-antihistamines are often given. These agents are slow in onset of action and have little effect on blood pressure. Therefore, when discussing anaphylaxis, antihistamines should be considered supportive and second-line therapy.

Historical trends reveal an over-reliance on antihistamines (both H_1- and H_2-antagonists) in patients presenting to the ED with acute allergic reactions and anaphylaxis [6]. Antihistamines are useful in the treatment of symptomatic manifestations of an anaphylactic reaction (pruritis or urticaria/angioedema). Diphen-

hydramine, 25–50 mg for adults and 1 mg/kg (up to 50 mg) for children, has been recommended by practice guidelines [2,7]. It may be administered as a slow intravenous push in anaphylaxis and can be given orally in less severe reactions. The evidence for these treatments is limited and, as mentioned earlier, the Cochrane review on this topic failed to identify any randomized controlled trials on the topic.

Several reports have demonstrated that a treatment with a combination of H_1- and H_2-antagonists is more effective in anaphylactic and anaphylactoid reactions than treatment with H_1 agents alone [20–24]. There is increasing support that the combination of H_1- and H_2-antagonists is more effective in attenuating both the cutaneous manifestations and the hemodynamic instability of anaphylaxis than treatment with H_1 agents alone [25–28].

There are no data available regarding which specific H_2-antagonist is most efficacious. Cimetidine and ranitidine have been most commonly studied. The advantages of ranitidine over cimetidine include fewer potential adverse drug events (cimetidine affects the P450 system), and a good safety profile [27,28]. The recommended administration of ranitidine is 1 mg/kg in adults and 12.5–50 mg in children, infused over 10–15 minutes. Cimetidine, 4 mg/kg in adults, should be administered slowly because rapid intravenous administration has been associated with hypotension. No dosing is currently available for children [7].

In summary, although the evidence is weak or indirect, consensus guidelines now favor the use of antihistamine agents. Given their potential benefit, combined with a low propensity for adverse events, the adjunct administration of H_1 agents with H_2 agents is reasonably warranted. ED management reviews have indicated that 62% of all patients with allergies receive antihistamines; however, only 11% use the combination H_1 agents with H_2 agents (see Fig. 15.1) [6]. Although practice patterns reveal increasing use, care could be improved in this area.

Question 4: In patients with anaphylaxis presenting to the ED (population), does the use of intravenous corticosteroids (intervention) in the ED reduce admissions to the hospital (outcome) compared to standard care (control)?

Search strategy

- MEDLINE and EMBASE: (anaphylaxis OR allergic reaction) AND (steroids OR corticosteroids)

The effectiveness of corticosteroids in anaphylaxis has never been determined in placebo-controlled trials. However, their efficacy in other allergic diseases (including asthma) has led to their incorporation into anaphylaxis management. The Joint Task Force on Practice Parameters in Allergy, Asthma and Immunology states that "systemic corticosteroids have no role in the acute management of anaphylaxis because they might have no effect for 4–6 hours, even when administered intravenously" [7]. Despite this statement, systemic corticosteroids have been shown to work effectively and quickly in acute asthma seen in the ED [29]. Moreover, there is emerging pathophysiological evidence that this effect can be measured. Consequently, the validity of this guideline's claim is questionable.

Although the current literature does not support any specific dose, route of administration or particular corticosteroid formulation, it has been suggested that corticosteroid use might prevent protracted or biphasic reactions [30], and may be an essential part of the prevention of frequent idiopathic anaphylaxis [31]. At least in asthma, no differences have been identified between oral and intravenous delivery routes.

In summary, there are no direct data available that support the use of intravenous corticosteroids in anaphylaxis; however, the literature supporting the use of systemic corticosteroids in acute exacerbations of asthma is robust [29]. This information has been extrapolated to this patient population. Reviews of ED management reveal that use of corticosteroids in acute allergic reactions is on the rise, with up to 50% of all patients with allergies receiving therapy while in the ED (see Fig. 15.1) [6]. If given, intravenous corticosteroids should be administered early in the treatment of anaphylaxis and the dosing should be equivalent to 1.0–2.0 mg/kg of methyl-prednisolone every 6 hours [2]. Currently there are no data describing the prevalence of after-care prescriptions for corticosteroids, representing another area for future research and education.

Question 5: In patients with treatment-refractory anaphylaxis presenting to the ED (population), does intravenous glucagon (intervention) in addition to epinephrine and systemic antihistamines (control) improve hemodynamic parameters (outcome)?

Search strategy

- MEDLINE and EMBASE: (anaphylaxis OR allergic reaction) AND glucagons

There are no epidemiological studies that demonstrate increased frequency of anaphylaxis in patients receiving β-adrenergic blockers; however, there are reported cases of increased severity or treatment-refractory anaphylaxis in these patients [32]. Glucagon may have a role to play in anaphylaxis that is refractory to standard treatments, especially in patients receiving beta-blockers [33].

Patients taking β-adrenergic antagonists might be more likely to experience severe anaphylactic reactions, characterized by paradoxical bradycardia, profound hypotension and severe bronchospasm [34]. Epinephrine administered to these patients might be ineffective, requiring both fluid expansion and intravenous glucagons [35]. Although there is a physiological rationale for the use of glucagon in patients with refractory anaphylaxis receiving β-adrenergic blocker therapy, the best evidence of efficacy is limited to case reports [32].

In summary, despite the limited quality of the supporting evidence, the evidence from case reports suggest that glucagon might benefit patients who are taking β-adrenergic blockers when all other treatments for anaphylaxis have failed. A worldwide shortage of this agent has precluded its use in many centers, and this supply concern may persist.

Question 6: In patients with anaphylaxis in the ED (population), will 6 hours of clinical observation (intervention) identify relapses related to "biphasic" allergic reactions (outcome)?

Search strategy

- MEDLINE and EMBASE: (anaphylaxis OR allergic reaction) AND (relapse OR biphasic reaction OR multiphasic OR refractory OR recurrence)

Recurrent anaphylaxis, the reappearance of allergic symptoms following complete resolution of the original reaction (without re-exposure), may be characterized by mucocutaneous symptoms or physiological derangements leading to respiratory or hemodynamic compromise [36]. Therefore, after treatment of an anaphylactic reaction, an observation period should be considered for all patients. The rate of multiphasic reactions in anaphylaxis have been reported to be as high as 20% [37–39].

The reported time interval between the initial reaction and the onset of the second phase has ranged from 1 to 72 hours, and no reliable clinical predictors have been identified to define those at risk for biphasic reations [17]. ED management reviews suggest that admission for anaphylaxis is rare (4%) [6] and the majority of patients can be discharged from the ED after a period of observation.

In summary, based on the evidence to date, the observation period for patients with acute anaphylactic reactions should be based on the severity of the initial reaction, reliability of the patient and access to future care. The suggested observation periods for those with anaphylaxis who receive epinephrine and remain stable is 24 hours. A reasonable approach would be to observe all others for 12 hours [40]. In addition, emergency physicians should be particularly cautious with patients with reactive airway disease or asthma because most anaphylaxis-related fatalities occur in this population [2].

Question 7: In patients with acute allergic reactions (population), does the out-of-hospital use of self-injectable epinephrine (intervention) reduce admissions to the hospital (outcome) compared to supportive care alone (control).

Search strategy

- MEDLINE and EMBASE: (anaphylaxis OR allergic reaction) AND (adrenaline OR epinephrine) AND self-injectable

Anaphylaxis often occurs outside of the hospital setting. Optimizing prevention of anaphylaxis is crucial, because future anaphylactic episodes may be fatal despite appropriate management. Prompt self-administration of epinephrine is critical to effective management in these cases. There is little disagreement that self-injectable epinephrine should be prescribed to individuals who have a prior history of anaphylaxis involving respiratory distress or shock [2]. However, there are no evidence-based guidelines on this topic and no data related to patient outcomes. It is also unclear as to who else should be given a prescription for self-injectable epinephrine.

Patients who are prescribed self-injectable epinephrine should also have an emergency action plan detailing its use and the follow-up management. Patients discharged from the ED should receive information about how to avoid the precipitating allergen, contact information for national resources and educational material, and prompt follow-up with an allergist (where available). Prescribed self-injectables, patient education and follow-up referrals are infrequently performed in the ED setting [4–6] and represent a unique opportunity for care improvement.

In summary, while evidence for this practice is lacking, consensus guidelines suggest that prescribing self-injectable epinephrine and discussing an emergency action plan should be part of follow-up management for most ED patients with a diagnosis of anaphylaxis.

Conclusions

Following the initial treatment, an additional dose of epinephrine was administered, and albuterol 0.5% inhalation solution was administered via a nebulizer. Methyl-prednisolone (125 mg) was also administered intravenously and the patient's blood pressure improved after an additional bolus of intravenous fluids. She was observed for 4 hours, and at reassessment her lungs were clear and her vital signs were: pulse 90 beats/min, respiration 16 breaths/min, blood pressure 120/70 mmHg (right arm), temperature 37.1°C (98.8°F) and pulse oximetry 98% SaO_2 on room air. The patient was treated with antihistamine and a short course of corticosteroids. A new Epi-pen prescription was provided and she was referred to an anaphylaxis website for additional information about anaphylaxis.

Anaphylaxis is a severe, immediate-type hypersensitivity reaction characterized by life-threatening upper airway obstruction, bronchospasm and hypotension. The patient presented here served to elucidate several potential problems related to the treatment of patients presenting with anaphylaxis. There is a great deal of variability in the ED approach to these patients. A variety of contributory factors have been identified, including a lack of consensus regarding anaphylaxis diagnosis and management, gaps in knowledge among physicians and patients, and limitations in research.

Therapeutic strategies for the management of anaphylaxis have been suggested largely on the basis of "clinical experience", and are based largely on extrapolation from other populations and physiological assumptions. Although virtually all authorities agree that epinephrine is the drug of choice for the treatment of acute anaphylaxis, there are limited data on the appropriate dose, timing and route of administration. In addition, common second-line therapies have virtually no data demonstrating their effectiveness in improving anaphylaxis outcomes. Bridging the gap between clinical research and clinical practice requires a concerted effort on the part of leaders in both groups, and this is clearly the case in the management of anaphylaxis. Treatment protocols must be evidence based and validated by appropriate, high-quality clinical studies; the treatment of anaphylaxis in the acute setting is a topic in which research evidence is urgently needed.

Acknowledgments

The author would like to thank the section editor for his assistance.

Conflicts of interest

Dr. Gaeta declares no conflicts of interest in the preparation of this chapter.

References

1 Sampson HA, Munoz-Furlong A, Block SA, et al. Symposium on the definition and management of anaphylaxis: summary report. *J Allergy Clin Immunol* 2005;**115**:584–91.

2 Sampson HA, Munoz-Furlong A, Campbell RL, et al. Second symposium on the definition and management of anaphylaxis: summary report – Second National Institute of Allergy and Infectious Disease/Food Allergy and Anaphylaxis Network symposium. *J Allergy Clin Immunol* 2006;**117**:391–97 (reprint in *Ann Emerg Med* 2006;**47**:373–80).

3 Clark S, Gaeta TJ, Kamarthi GS, Camargo CA, Jr. ICD-9-CM coding of emergency department visits for food and insect sting allergy. *Ann Epidemiol* 2006;**16**:696–700.

4 Clark S, Block SA, Gaeta TJ, et al. Multicenter study of emergency department visits for food allergy. *J Allergy Clin Immunol* 2004;**113**:347–52.

5 Clark S, Long AA, Gaeta TJ, Camargo CA, Jr. Multicenter study of emergency department visits for insect sting allergy. *J Allergy Clin Immunol* 2005;**116**:643–9.

6 Gaeta TJ, Clark S, Pellettier AJ, Camargo CA, Jr. National study of US emergency department visits for acute allergic reactions, 1993–2004. *Ann Allergy Asthma Immunol* 2007;**98**:360–65.

7 Lieberman P, Kemp SF, Oppenheimer J, et al. The diagnosis and management of anaphylaxis: an updated practice parameter. *J Allergy Clin Immunol* 2005;**115**:S483–523.

8 Sheikh A, Shehata Y, Brown SGA, Simons FER. Adrenaline for the treatment of anaphylaxis with and without shock (Cochrane protocol). In: *The Cochrane Library*, Issue 3. Update Software, Oxford, 2007.

9 Sheikh A, ten Broek VM, Brown SGA, Simons FER. H1-antihistamines for the treatment of anaphylaxis with and without shock (Review). In: *The Cochrane Library*, Issue 3. Update Software, Oxford, 2007.

10 Lieberman P. Use of epinephrine in the treatment of anaphylaxis. *Curr Opin Allergy Clin Immunol* 2003;**3**:313–18.

11 Anchor J, Settipane R. Appropriate use of epinephrine in anaphylaxis. *Am J Emerg Med* 2004;**22**:488–90.

12 Oswalt ML, Kemp SF. Anaphylaxis: office management and prevention. *Immunol Allergy Clin North Am* 2007;**27**:177–91.

13 Barach EM, Nowak RM, Lee TG, et al. Epinephrine for the treatment of anaphylaxic shock. *JAMA* 1984;**251**:2118–22.

14 Simons FER, Roberts JR, Gu X, et al. Epinephrine absorption in children with a history of anaphylaxis. *J Allergy Clin Immunol* 1998;**101**:33–7.

15 Simons FER, Gu X, Simons KJ. Epinephrine absorption in adults: intramuscular versus subcutaneous injection. *J Allergy Clin Immunol* 2001;**108**:871–3.

16 Song TT, Nelson MR, Chang JH, et al. Adequacy of the epinephrine auto-injector needle length in delivering epinephrine to the intramuscular tissues. *Ann Allergy Asthma Immunol* 2005;**94**:539–42.

17 Project Team of the Resuscitation Council (UK). Emergency medical treatment of anaphylactic reactions. *J Accid Emerg Med* 1999;**16**:243–7.

18 Brown SGA, Blackmean KE, Steniake V, et al. Insect sting anaphylaxis: prospective evaluation of treatment with intravenous adrenaline and volume resuscitation. *Emerg Med J* 2004;**21**:149–54.

19 Putland M, Kerr D, Kelly AM. Adverse events associated with the use of intravenous epinephrine in emergency department patients presenting with severe asthma. *Ann Emerg Med* 2006;**47**(6):564–6.

20 Vidivich RR, Heiselman DE, Hudock D. Treatment of urokinase-related anaphylactoid reaction with intravenous famotidine. *Ann Pharmacother* 1992;**26**: 782–3.

21 Kambam J, Merrill WH, Smith BE. Histamine receptor blocker in the treatment of protamine related anaphylactoid reactions: two case reports. *Can J Anaesth* 1989;**36**:463–5.

22 Mayumi H, Kimura S, Asano M, et al. Intravenous cimetidine as an effective treatment for systemic anaphylaxis and acute allergic skin reactions. *Ann Allergy* 1987;**58**:447–50.

23 DeSoto H, Turk M. Cimetidine in anaphylactic shock refractory to standard therapy. *Anesth Anal* 1989;**69**:264–5.

24 Yarbrough JA, Moffitt JE, Brown DA, et al. Cimetidine in the treatment of refractory anaphylaxis. *Ann Allergy* 1989;**63**:235–8.

25 Simon FE. Advances in H1-antihistamines. *N Engl J Med* 2004;**351**:2203–17.

26 Lin RY, Schwartz LB, Curry A, et al. Histamine and tryptase levels in patients with acute allergic reactions: an emergency department-based study. *J Allergy Clin Immunol* 2000;**106**:65–71.

27 Runge JW, Martinez JC, Caravati EM, et al. Histamine antagonists in the treatment of acute allergic reactions. *Ann Emerg Med* 1992;**21**:237–42.

28 Lin RY, Curry A, Pesola G, et al. Improved outcomes in patients with acute allergic syndromes who are treated with combines H1 and H2 antagonists. *Ann Emerg Med* 2000;**36**:462–8.

29 Rowe BH, Spooner C, Ducharme FM, et al. Early emergency department treatment of acute asthma with systemic corticosteroids. (Cochrane review). In: *The Cochrane Library*, Issue 4. Update Software, Oxford, 2003.

30 Lieberman P. Biphasic anaphylactic reactions. *Ann Allergy Asthma Immunol* 2005;**95**:217.

31 Lieberman P. Anaphylaxis and anaphylactoid reactions. In: Adkinson NF, Jr., Yunginger JW, Busse WW, et al., eds. *Middleton's Allergy: Principles and practice*, 6th edn. Mosby-Year Book, St. Louis, 2003:1497–522.

32 Thomas M, Crawford I. Best evidence topic report. Glucagon infusion in refractory anaphylactic shock in patients on beta-blockers. *Emerg Med J* 2005;**22**:272–3.

33 Pollack CV, Jr. Utility of glucagon in the emergency department. *J Emerg Med* 1993;**11**:195–205.

34 Lang DM, Alpern MB, Visintainer PF, Smith ST. Increased risk for anaphylactoid reaction from contrast median in patients on beta-adrenergic blockers or with asthma. *Ann Intern Med* 1991;**115**:270–76.

35 Zaloga GP, Delacey W, Holmboe E, et al. Glucagon reversal of hypotension in a case of anyphylactoid shock. *Ann Intern Med* 1986;**105**:65–6.

36 Stark BJ, Sullivan BJ. Biphasic and prolonged anaphylaxis. *J Allergy Clin Immunol* 1986;**78**:76–83.

37 Sampson HA, Mendelson LM, Rosen JP. Fatal and near-fatal anaphylactic reactions to food in children and adolescents. *N Engl J Med* 1992;**327**:380–84.

38 Douglas DM, Sukenick E, Andrade WP, et al. Biphasic systemic anaphylaxis – an inpatient and outpatient study. *J Allergy Clin Immunol* 1994;**93**:977–85.

39 Lee JM, Greenes DS. Biphasis anaphylactic reactions in pediatrics. *Pediatrics* 2000;**106**:762–76.

40 de Smit V, Cameron PA, Rainer TH. Anaphylaxis presentations to the emergency department in Hong Kong: incidence and predictors of biphasic reactions. *J Emerg Med* 2005;**28**(4):381–8.

3 Cardiology

16 Chest Pain

Alain Vadeboncoeur[1], Jerrald Dankoff[2] & Eddy S. Lang[2]

[1]Department of Family Medicine, University of Montreal, Montreal *and* Montreal Heart Institute, Montreal, Canada
[2]Department of Family Medicine, McGill University, Montreal *and* Department of Emergency Medicine, SMBD Jewish General Hospital, Montreal, Canada

Case scenario

A 56-year-old man presented to the emergency department (ED) with a chief complaint of chest pain. He began to feel the pain while at work, where as the senior partner in an accounting firm, he still worked 6 full days a week. His symptoms began as a central chest pain, dull but pronounced in nature, soon after a heated meeting where the company financial problems were reviewed. This was the first time he had experienced such symptoms. The pain lasted for over 45 minutes with irradiation to the left and right shoulders, some mild shortness of breath and a sense of panic. There was mild diaphoresis and transient nausea but no vomiting. The pain seemed to abate after the ambulance technicians applied an oxygen mask.

His past medical history was significant for type 2 diabetes controlled by diet and hypercholesterolemia for which prescription medication was prescribed by his internist. He had not smoked in years, regularly attended a gym and denied significant family history of coronary disease. The patient also detailed a history of panic attacks that occurred several years ago but these seemed not to be associated with severe chest pain; they were well controlled with medication, which he stopped taking 3 years ago.

The physical examination revealed an anxious appearing gentleman with a heart rate of 80 beats/min, blood pressure of 120/80 mmHg in both arms and respiratory rate of 16 breaths/min. The patient appeared slightly pale but his skin was warm and dry. His examination was normal, including chest, abdominal and neurological examination. Specifically, the cardiac examination demonstrated normal heart sounds but no murmur. There was no evidence of jugular venous distension or peripheral edema.

Background

Chest pain is a common presentation, accounting for 5% of all ED presentations, and carries a differential diagnosis that consists of numerous life-threatening conditions. Acute coronary syndrome (ACS), aortic dissection and pulmonary embolism are the most serious conditions that are likely to present with chest pain as a chief complaint and all present diagnostic challenges in the ED setting. This chapter will address key questions related to the evaluation of suspected ACS and aortic dissection while pulmonary embolism is addressed in Chapter 13.

Acute coronary syndrome has evolved as a useful operational term to refer to any constellation of clinical symptoms that are compatible with acute or evolving myocardial ischemia. It encompasses acute myocardial ischemia (AMI) (ST segment elevation and depression, Q wave and non-Q wave) as well as unstable angina and non-ST segment elevation myocardial infarction (NSTEMI). For the purposes of this chapter unstable angina/NSTEMI will be considered as a single entity as has been suggested by the American Heart Association (AHA) guidelines [1]. According to the AHA and numerous other authorities these entities share a similar clinical profile with the exception of the release of cardiac biomarkers, which is the hallmark of NSTEMI. Because of its high incidence and high potential lethality, ACS is the most significant potential chest pain diagnosis in the ED. Atherosclerotic heart disease accounts for 35% of all deaths in the United States and, reflecting the diagnostic challenge often associated with the evaluation of suspected ACS, emergency physicians reportedly miss anywhere from 0.4% to 5% of myocardial infarctions that present to the ED and this in turn results in a significant contributor to medico-legal liability [2,3].

With over 15,000 patients and 17,000 visits, the Internet Tracking Registry of Acute Coronary Syndromes (i*trACS) is the largest registry of patients suspected of this diagnosis. A breakdown of final diagnoses reveals that more than 82% of the patients in this registry obtained a final diagnosis of non-cardiac chest pain, reflecting the challenge in identifying which patients have a truly cardiac origin to their symptoms. Thus, most patients with chest pain presenting to the ED have a benign origin of their pain; the challenge is in separating out and appropriately treating patients with serious causes [3].

Clinical questions

In order to address the issues of most relevance to chest pain patients and to help in searching the literature for the evidence regarding these issues, you structure your clinical questions as recommended in Chapter 1.

1 In patients who present to the ED with chest pain (population), what is the likelihood (prior probability) of a given final diagnosis (outcome) established either at the index visit or during hospitalization and follow-up, i.e., a probabilistic differential diagnosis?

2 In patients with chest pain suspected of being ischemic in origin (population), can the likelihood ratios (diagnostic test characteristics) of historical and physical examination features (tests) help in either excluding or ruling in cardiac ischemia as the cause of the patient's symptoms (outcome)?

3 In patients with chest pain suspected of being ischemic in origin (population), can the likelihood ratios (diagnostic test characteristics) of a collection of valid and reliable clinical criteria (clinical prediction guides) accurately define a patient's post-test probability of having acute coronary syndrome (outcome)?

4 In patients with chest pain suspected of being caused by a thoracic aortic dissection (population), can the likelihood ratios (diagnostic test characteristics) of historical and physical examination features and radiography (tests) help in either excluding or ruling in a dissection as the cause of the patient's symptoms (outcome)?

5 In patients with chest pain suspected of being ischemic in origin (population), can the likelihood ratios (diagnostic test characteristics) of electrocardiographic features (tests) help either exclude or rule in acute myocardial infarction as the cause of a patient's symptoms (outcome)?

6 In patients with chest pain suspected of being ischemic in origin and with electrocardiograms (ECGs) demonstrating a left bundle branch block (LBBB) (population), can the likelihood ratios (diagnostic test characteristics) of specific features in these ECGs (tests) help either exclude or rule in myocardial infarction as the cause of a patient's symptoms (outcome)?

7 In patients with chest pain suspected of being ischemic in origin (population), can the likelihood ratios (diagnostic test characteristics) of symptomatic relief with sublingual nitroglycerine (test) help either exclude or rule in cardiac ischemia as the cause of a patient's symptoms (outcome)?

8 In patients with atypical chest pain suspected of being either gastrointestinal or cardiac in origin (population), can the likelihood ratios (diagnostic test characteristics) of symptomatic relief with antacid with or without a liquid anesthetic therapy (test) help either exclude or rule out a gastrointestinal or cardiac cause for a patient's symptoms (outcome)?

9 In patients with chest pain presenting to the ED (population), does treatment with aspirin (treatment) reduce acute myocardial infarction and the need for procedures (outcomes) compared to standard care with oxygen and pain relief (control)?

General search strategy

You begin to address the topic of chest pain, ACS and AMI by searching for evidence in the common electronic databases such as the TRIP database MEDLINE and EMBASE looking specifically for systematic reviews and large cohort studies. These three topics create a large body of evidence, and to increase efficiency systematic reviews such as the Rational Clinical Examination (RCE) series and Cochrane Library are also examined. In addition, access to relevant, updated, evidence-based clinical practice guidelines (CPGs) on chest pain and ACS and AMI are accessed to determine the consensus rating of areas lacking evidence.

Critical appraisal of the literature

Question 1: In patients who present to the ED with chest pain (population), what is the likelihood (prior probability) of a given final diagnosis (outcome) established either at the index visit or during hospitalization and follow-up, i.e., a probabilistic differential diagnosis?

Search strategy

- PubMed: chest pain AND emergency department AND differential diagnosis AND clinical probability AND clinical queries filter: prognosis

There are no large registries of adult ED patients who present to the ED with a primary complaint of chest pain. However, as outlined above, the i*trACS registry is the largest ED-based registry of an undifferentiated population of patients presenting with suspected ACS. The i*trACS data registry prospectively collected data on patients presenting to one of eight EDs in the United States as well as one in Singapore, from June 1, 1999 to August 1, 2001. Potential study subjects were evaluated for enrollment if they presented with a complaint of chest pain consistent with an ACS or other symptoms prompting the performance of a 12-lead electrocardiogram (ECG). Thus, most enrolled patients had a chief complaint of chest pain, but others with symptoms such as syncope or dyspnea could also be enrolled.

In i*trACS final diagnoses were established according to the final ED diagnosis and were obtained by medical record review, and were thus defined as the discharge diagnosis for patients discharged home or the admitting diagnosis for patients admitted to an inpatient setting. ACS was defined by 30-day revascularization,

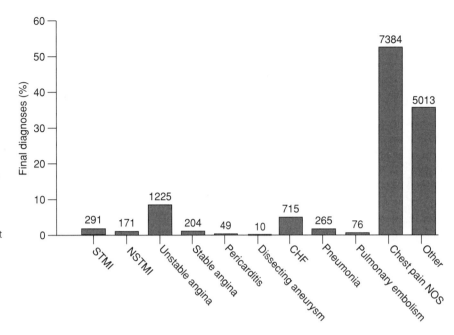

Figure 16.1 Relative frequency of final diagnoses in the ED from the i*trACS registry. Data were prospectively collected on 17,000 patients presenting to one of eight EDs in the USA as well as one in Singapore, from June 1, 1999 to August 1, 2001. Most enrolled patients had a chief complaint of chest pain. CHF, congestive heart failure; NOS, not otherwise specified; NSTEMI, non-ST segment elevation myocardial infarction; STEMI, ST segment elevation myocardial infarction. (Reproduced with permission from Lindsell et al. [3].)

diagnostic-related group codes or death within 30 days, with positive cardiac biomarkers at index hospitalization. Among all comers with chest pain, i.e., 17,000 visits, the relative frequency of final diagnoses as established in the ED are demonstrated in Fig. 16.1, revealing unstable angina/NSTEMI as the most likely cardiac diagnosis followed by congestive heart failure as a primary diagnosis and ST segment elevation MI (STEMI) as the third most common entity [3].

In a more focused analysis of 7742 patients admitted to hospital, the final cardiac diagnosis at discharge was STEMI in 287 (3.7%) patients, unstable angina/NSTEMI in 1327 (17%) and stable angina in 128 (1.6%). Even among admitted patients, noncardiac diagnoses were assigned to the vast majority of hospitalized patients (6066; 78%). This reflects the conservative admitting practices and utilization of chest pain units in many American hospitals. Thus, from a practical perspective the emergency physician can estimate that among patients who present to the ED with chest pain, even of those of sufficient gravity to merit hospitalization in a US context, less than 5% will be suffering from a STEMI, 15–20% will fulfill criteria for a diagnosis of unstable angina or NSTEMI, and the majority will have non-cardiac diagnoses, most of which are benign (i.e., musculoskeletal, functional, anxiety). Among dangerous diagnoses, however, pulmonary embolism and aortic dissection are particularly rare making up only 1% or less of patients with a chest pain presentation to the ED.

Question 2: In patients with chest pain suspected of being ischemic in origin (population), can the likelihood ratios (diagnostic test characteristics) of historical and physical examination features (tests) help in either excluding or ruling in cardiac ischemia as the cause of the patient's symptoms (outcome)?

The clinical assessment of suspected ACS is an important emergency physician skill. A carefully crafted history and, to a lesser degree, elements of the physical assessment are in some ways the emergency physician's most important instruments in defining which patients with chest pain are harboring either a cardiac cause, another life-threatening etiology or a benign etiology. There is a limited body of evidence to inform the clinician about the individual contribution of historical elements and clinical findings and their discriminative abilities in the assessment of patients with suspected ACS.

A systematic review published as part of the RCE series addressed this question based on literature of patients evaluated for myocardial infarction [4]. In this paper, data from over a dozen trials were collected to provide estimates of diagnostic performance and agreement for a variety of clinical elements. Likelihood ratios for the most discriminating components are shown in Table 16.1.

Panju's work suggests there are no clinical features with sufficient diagnostic performance to rule in or rule out the diagnosis of myocardial infarction. What is perhaps notable is that radiation of chest pain to the right shoulder is actually suggestive of a cardiac etiology and that radiation in both arms should make the emergency physician suspect ACS. Another general observation is that clinical features that argue against a cardiac etiology to a patient's chest pain are actually better at ruling out than other features are at ruling in ACS. As such, chest pain that is positional,

Table 16.1 Features that increase or decrease the probability of an acute myocardial infarction in patients presenting with acute chest pain. (Reproduced with permission from Panju et al. [4], © American Medical Association.)

Clinical feature	Likelihood ratio (95% CI)
Features that increase probability	
Pain in chest or left arm	2.7*
Chest pain radiation	
Right shoulder	2.9 (1.4 to 6.0)
Left arm	2.3 (1.7 to 3.1)
Both left and right arm	7.1 (3.6 to 14.2)
Chest pain most important symptom	2.0*
History of myocardial infarction	1.5 to 3.0[†]
Nausea or vomiting	1.9 (1.7 to 2.3)
Diaphoresis	2.0 (1.9 to 2.2)
Third heart sound on auscultation	3.2 (1.6 to 6.5)
Hypotension (systolic blood pressure ≤80 mmHG)	3.1 (1.8 to 5.2)
Pulmonary crackles on auscultation	2.1 (1.4 to 3.1)
Features that decrease probability	
Pleuritic chest pain	0.2 (0.2 to 0.3)
Chest pain sharp or stabbing	0.3 (0.2 to 0.5)
Positional chest pain	0.3 (0.2 to 0.4)
Chest pain reproduced by palpation	0.2 to 0.4[†]

*Data not available to calculate confidence intervals.

[†]In heterogeneous studies the likelihood ratios are reported as ranges.

sharp, pleuritic and reproduced by palpation effectively reduces the likelihood of myocardial ischemia as the cause. A comprehensive review by the National Health Service (NHS) found that very few clinical features were useful in ruling in unstable angina or myocardial infarction as the cause of a patient's symptoms (Table 16.2) [5]. In keeping with Panju's work certain features are, however, useful in ruling out a cardiac etiology (i.e., sharp, pleuritic, positional and reproducible pain).

Risk factor profiling is also believed to be an integral aspect of the ED evaluation of patients with chest pain presentations. In a secondary analysis of the i*trACS database the diagnostic value of defining risk value profile was addressed [6]. Cardiac risk factors included diabetes, hypertension, smoking, hypercholesterolemia and family history of coronary artery disease. For the purpose of analysis, risk factor, burden was defined as the number of risk factors present. A stratified analysis was performed for three age categories. In patients younger than 40 years, having no risk factors had a negative likelihood ratio (−LR) of 0.17 (95% CI: 0.04 to 0.66), while having four or more risk factors had a positive likelihood ratio (+LR) of 7.39 (95% CI: 3.09 to 17.67). Among patients between 40 and 65 years of age, having no risk factors had a −LR of 0.53 (95% CI: 0.40 to 0.71), and having four or more risk factors had a +LR of 2.13 (95% CI: 1.66 to 2.73). Remarkably, in patients older than 65 years, having no risk factors was associated with a −LR of 0.96 (95% CI: 0.74 to 1.23), and having four or more risk factors had a +LR of 1.09 (95% CI: 0.64 to 1.62).

In summary, in contrast to conventional teaching, it would seem that isolated cardiac risk factor profiling has limited clinical value in diagnosing acute coronary syndromes in the ED setting, especially in patients older than 40 years of age. Emergency physicians should thus limit risk factor profiling to patients under 65 years of age and be especially cognizant of the diagnostic value of these elements in patients under 40 years.

Question 3: In patients with chest pain suspected of being ischemic in origin (population), can the likelihood ratios (diagnostic test characteristics) of a collection of valid and reliable clinical criteria (clinical prediction guides) accurately define a patient's post-test probability of having acute coronary syndrome (outcome)?

Search strategy

- PubMed: chest pain AND emergency department AND clinical prediction rule AND acute coronary syndromes AND risk stratification

For a patient with chest pain suspected to be of ischemic origin, a central question to be addressed in the ED is whether any given patient can be identified as suffering from a high-risk ACS, i.e., what is the probability that they will have a bad outcome (death or ACS) in the next month? A month is a reasonable time limit to consider in that it corresponds to the timeframe required to complete a patient's outpatient work-up and determine whether they have coronary heart disease or perhaps some other non-cardiac process. This section will review prediction guides that can in some way establish the pre-test probability of low- and high-risk ACS after the initial history, physical and laboratory assessment. Unfortunately, there are currently no sufficiently sensitive prediction tools that can effectively rule out the possibility of a bad outcome; however, a highly discriminative instrument can establish a pre-test probability that can be used to interpret other tests, such as the 8–12-hour levels of cardiac biomarkers, exercise stress test, and so forth.

The most notable of these are the Thrombolysis in Myocardial Infarction (TIMI) and Global Registry of Acute Coronary Events (GRACE) risk scores (Table 16.3) [7,8]. The TIMI score was derived from a study of a population of patients with known unstable angina/NSTEMI. Through a multivariate analysis of the Efficacy and Safety of Subcutaneous Enoxaparin in Unstable Angina and Non-Q-wave MI (ESSENCE) and TIMI 11B databases, Antman et al. [7] identified seven factors that were independently predictive of the adverse outcomes of death, AMI or recurrent ischemia at 14 days and documented increased risk with the addition of each positive risk factor (Fig. 16.2). Similarly, the more recent GRACE score was developed from that registry, with a population of patients across the entire spectrum of ACS. All these scores

Table 16.2 Likelihood ratios associated with various historical features that are included in the clinical assessment of chest pain. (From Mant et al. 2004 [5].)

Symptom		MI only				MI or unstable angina		
		Number of studies	LR	95% CI	P for heterogeneity	Number of studies	LR	95% CI
Pleuritic pain	+LR	3	0.19	0.14 to 0.25	0.5	0		
	−LR		1.17	1.15 to 1.19	0.003			
Sharp pain	+LR	2	0.32	0.21 to 0.50	0.3	1	0.41	0.29 to 0.57
	−LR		1.36	1.26 to 1.46	0.4		132	1.20 to 1.45
Positional pain	+LR	2	0.27	0.21 to 0.36	0.3	1	0.27	0.17 to 1.42
	−LR		1.12	1.11 to 1.14	0.09		1.35	1.25 to 1.47
Pain on palpation	+LR	3	0.23	0.08 to 0.30	0.15	1	0.17	0.11 to 0.27
	−LR		1.18	1.16 to 1.20	0.001		1.56	1.42 to 1.71
Crushing pain	+LR	6	1.44	1.39 to 1.49	0.14	2	1.56	1.36 to 1.78
	−LR		0.63	0.60 to 0.67	0.9		0.63	0.55 to 0.73
Central pain	+LR	3	1.24	1.2 to 1.27	0.01	1	1.12	1.07 to 1.17
	−LR		0.49	0.43 to 1.56	0.002		0.31	0.19 to 0.50
Left-sided radiation of pain	+LR	2	1.45	1.36 to 1.55	0.004	2	1.22	1.15 to 1.30
	−LR		0.78	0.73 to 0.82	0.02		0.58	0.49 to 0.69
Right-sided radiation of pain	+LR	2	2.59	1.85 to 3.70	0.7	1	6.68	2.95 to 15.2
	−LR		0.8	0.72 to 0.88	0.01		0.73	0.65 to 0.81
Any radiation of pain	+LR	2	1.43	1.33 to 1.55	0.7	1	1.26	1.13 to 1.40
	−LR		0.8	0.75 to 0.84	0.01		0.27	0.13 to 0.53
Pain duration >1 hour	+LR	1	1.3	1.15 to 1.47		1	1.05	0.92 to 1.21
	−LR		0.35	0.19 to 0.64		1	0.84	0.56 to 1.27
Previous myocardial infarction	+LR	4	1.29	1.22 to 1.36	0.001	1	1.22	1.09 to 1.37
	−LR		0.84	0.81 to 0.88	0.001	1	0.77	0.67 to 0.90
Nausea/vomiting	+LR	4	1.88	1.58 to 2.23	0.5	1	1.78	1.16 to 2.74
	−LR		0.77	0.71 to 0.84	0.001		0.82	0.72 to 0.95
Sweating	+LR	5	2.06	1.96 to 2.16	0.07	0		
	−LR		0.65	0.62 to 0.67	0.001			

were developed for short-term prognosis: events in-hospital for the GRACE risk score; at 14 days for the TIMI score.

The TIMI and GRACE scores, both developed as prognostic instruments in patients with unstable angina/NSTEMI, are the two best studied clinical prediction guides in the undifferentiated chest pain population presenting to the ED [9–13]. In the study by Chase et al., the TIMI score was evaluated in all adult patients older than 30 years, presenting to the ED with a primary complaint of non-traumatic chest pain – in all, 1458 emergency patients [9]. The score correlated quite well with the rate of all-cause mortality, AMI or revascularization by percutaneous coronary intervention or coronary artery bypass surgery at 30 days after presentation. Even with a TIMI score of 0, however, there was a 1.7% (95% CI: 1% to 4%) rate of adverse events in 30 days. Consequently, the score can be used to establish a pre-test probability but cannot rule out the possibility of adverse events. Similarly, the GRACE score has undergone prospective evaluation in the ED and performs as well as the TIMI [12,13].

For example, assume that a 58-year-old male presents to the ED for assessment of atypical chest pain. The patient describes multiple risk factors for ischemic heart disease: hypertension, smoker, elevated cholesterol and a positive family history (his brother had percutaneous coronary intervention at age 50). His exam is normal, chest X-ray is normal and multiple ECG without pain remains normal. Without any formal calculation of pre-test probability of disease, most ED doctors would say the pre-test probability of ACS is too high to send him home without extensive work-up. When you calculate the TIMI risk score he scores 2, which is approximately a 12% risk of "bad" outcome over 30 days. A negative cardiac biomarker at 8 hours (sensitivity 94%, specificity 81%) lowers this probability to ∼1%. This level of risk may be the best achievable level of certainty that can realistically be attained [5].

Table 16.3 TIMI risk score for patients presenting with chest pain suggestive of an acute coronary syndrome. (From Eagle et al. [8].)

TIMI (0–7)		
	Age ≥65 years	1
	≥3 risk factors for CAD	1
	Use of ASA (last 7 days)	1
	Known CAD (stenosis ≥50%)	1
	>1 episode rest angina in <24 h	1
	ST segment deviation	1
	Elevated cardiac markers	1

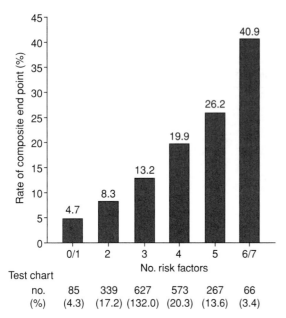

Test chart

no.	85	339	627	573	267	66
(%)	(4.3)	(17.2)	(132.0)	(20.3)	(13.6)	(3.4)

Figure 16.2 Rates of all-cause mortality, myocardial infarction and severe recurrent ischemia prompting urgent revascularization for 14 days after randomization. These rates were calculated for various patient subgroups based on the number of risk factors present in the test cohort (the unfractionated heparin group in the TIMI 11B trial (*n* = 1957). (From Antman et al. [7].)

Question 4: In patients with chest pain suspected of being caused by a thoracic aortic dissection (population), can the likelihood ratios (diagnostic test characteristics) of historical and physical examination features and radiography (tests) help in either excluding or ruling in a dissection as the cause of the patient's symptoms (outcome)?

Search strategy

- PubMed: aortic dissection AND emergency department AND clinical assessment AND physical examination AND chest radiography AND clinical queries filter: diagnosis

Thoracic aortic dissection has an incidence of 0.5–1 per 100,000 population with a mortality rate exceeding 90% if misdiagnosed [14]. It is a rare cause of chest pain in the ED setting, although it is the most immediately life-threatening in many cases. Misdiagnosis of acute thoracic aortic dissection as a thrombotic condition such as pulmonary embolism, unstable angina or myocardial infarction can have disastrous iatrogenic consequences should the patient receive anticoagulants or thrombolytic therapy. Physicians are therefore acutely dependent upon the clinical history, examination and plain chest radiograph to determine which patients are at increased risk and require further study. As part of the RCE series, Klompas conducted a systematic review of 21 eligible studies to quantify the contribution of major elements of the history and physical examination in predicting the presence of an aortic dissection [14]. The classic clinical history for thoracic aortic dissection

consists of the sudden onset of severe tearing or ripping chest pain radiating to the interscapular region or mid-back, occurring in late middle-aged men with a history of hypertension. Both the sudden and/or severe nature of aortic dissection pain are borne out by the Klompas review as being important elements in dissection, carrying pooled sensitivities of 84% and 95%, respectively. These two elements exceed any other historical feature including tearing pain as being important indicators of dissection. Additional findings that are outlined in Table 16.4 reinforce the contribution of tearing chest pain to a clinical diagnosis of dissection and suggest that focal neurological deficits and pulse deficits are of use as well for their specificity and thus high positive likelihood ratios.

The value of pulse deficits was reviewed by a best evidence topic that presented the findings from three studies addressing the diagnostic value of this feature [15]. All the reports point to a sensitivity of merely 30%, which reinforces the notion that pulse differentials do not represent a sensitive test whereby a negative result is useful for ruling out disease (SnOut) and that the absence of this finding cannot be relied upon to exclude a dissection. Moreover, there are very few clinical features which possess negative likelihood ratios that are sufficient to exclude a diagnosis of aortic dissection. None the less, the most potentially worthy of these is the absence of a mediastinal abnormality on chest X-ray and the absence of sudden pain.

Von Kodolitsch developed a clinical prediction rule in 250 patients that may hold promise in the evaluation of suspected aortic dissection. It suggests that in combination the presence or absence of either tearing, sudden onset pain, a pulse differential and an abnormal mediastinum on chest radiography can dramatically increase or reduce the likelihood of dissection (Table 16.5) [16].

The specific role of chest radiography was addressed by Hogg and Teece in the context of a best evidence topic. Reviewing evidence from four trials, the authors report a maximum sensitivity of 90%, albeit from studies with significant methodological limitations. In summary, aortic dissection is a life-threatening disease that is difficult to diagnose. The clinical implication of this evidence summary is that in patients who have a high clinical index of suspicion for aortic dissection, advanced imaging (computerized tomography (CT) scan or magnetic resonance imaging) are called for to rule out this life-threatening diagnosis [17].

Question 5: In patients with chest pain suspected of being ischemic in origin (population), can the likelihood ratios (diagnostic test characteristics) of electrocardiographic features (tests) help either exclude or rule in acute myocardial infarction as the cause of a patient's symptoms (outcome)?

Search strategy

- PubMed: chest pain AND emergency department AND clinical assessment AND electrocardiography AND clinical queries filter: diagnosis

Table 16.4 The accuracy of clinical findings of aortic dissection. (From Klompas [14].)

Symptom or sign	Source	Postive likelihood ratio (95% CI)	Negative likelihood ratio (95% CI)
History of hypertension	Chan, 1991[*]	1.5 (0.8 to 3.0)	0.7 (0.4 to 1.3)
	Enia et al. 1989[†]	1.1 (0.7 to 1.6)	0.7 (0.4 to 2.4)
	Von Kodolitsch et al. 2000[‡]	1.8 (1.4 to 2.3)	0.4 (0.3 to 0.6)
	Summary	1.6 (1.2 to 2.0)	0.5 (0.3 to 0.7)
Sudden chest pain	Chan, 1991[*]	1.0 (0.7 to 1.4)	0.98 (0.3 to 3.1)
	Armstrong et al. 1998[§]	1.5 (1.1 to 1.9)	0.3 (0.1 to 0.8)
	Von Kodolitsch et al. 2000[‡]	2.6 (2.0 to 3.5)	0.3 (0.2 to 0.4)
	Summary	1.6 (1.0 to 2.4)	0.3 (0.2 to 0.5)
"Tearing" or "ripping" pain	Armstrong et al. 1998[§]	1.2 (0.2 to 8.1)	0.99 (0.9 to 1.1)
	Von Kodolitsch et al. 2000[‡]	10.8 (5.2 to 22.0)	0.4 (0.3 to 0.5)
Migrating pain	Chan, 1991[*]	1.1 (0.5 to 2.4)	0.97 (0.6 to 1.6)
	Von Kodolitsch et al. 2000[‡]	7.6 (3.6 to 16.0)	0.6 (0.5 to 0.7)
Pulse deficit	Armstrong et al. 1998[§]	2.4 (0.5 to 12.0)	0.93 (0.8 to 1.1)
	Enia et al. 1989[†]	2.7 (0.7 to 9.8)	0.63 (0.4 to 1.0)
	Von Kodolitsch et al. 2000[‡]	47.0 (6.6 to 333.0)	0.62 (0.5 to 0.7)
	Summary	5.7 (1.4 to 23.0)	0.7 (0.6 to 0.9)
Focal neurological deficit	Armstrong et al. 1998[§]	6.6 (1.6 to 28.0)	0.71 (0.6 to 0.9)
	Von Kodolitsch et al. 2000[‡]	33.0 (2.0 to 549.0)	0.87 (0.8 to 0.9)
Diastolic murmur	Chan, 1991[*]	4.9 (0.6 to 40.0)	0.8 (0.6 to 1.1)
	Armstrong et al. 1998[§]	1.2 (0.4 to 3.8)	0.97 (0.8 to 1.2)
	Enia et al. 1989[†]	0.9 (0.5 to 1.7)	1.1 (0.6 to 1.7)
	Von Kodolitsch et al. 2000[‡]	1.7 (1.1 to 2.5)	0.79 (0.6 to 0.9)
	Summary	1.4 (1.0 to 2.0)	0.9 (0.8 to 1.0)
Enlarged aorta or wide mediastinum	Chan, 1991[*]	1.6 (1.1 to 2.3)	0.13 (0.02 to 1.00)
	Armstrong et al. 1998[§]	1.6 (1.1 to 2.2)	0.42 (0.2 to 0.9)
	Von Kodolitsch et al. 2000[‡]	3.4 (2.4 to 4.8)	0.31 (0.2 to 0.4)
	Summary	2.0 (1.4 to 3.1)	0.3 (0.2 to 0.4)
Left ventricular hypertrophy on admission electrocardiogram	Chen, 1991[*]	0.2 (.03 to 1.9)	1.2 (0.9 to 1.6)
	Von Kodolitsch et al. 2000[‡]	3.2 (1.5 to 6.8)	0.84 (0.7 to 0.9)

[*] CI indicates confidence interval.
[†] A total of 18 ($n = 40$) patients with thoracic aortic dissection.
[‡] A total of 35 ($n = 46$) patients with thoracic aortic dissection.
[§] A total of 128 ($n = 250$) patients with thoracic aortic dissection.
[‖] A total of 34 ($n = 75$) patients with thoracic aortic dissection.

In a comprehensive review of 53 studies, the specific ECG features useful in diagnosing AMI were outlined [5]. Given the unpredictable and often transient nature of ECG abnormalities in the setting of unstable angina/NSTEMI, as well as the variability in the contribution that the ECG makes to that diagnosis, the review addressed their value in the setting of AMI. As demonstrated in Table 16.6, ST segment elevation is a convincing component of a diagnosis of AMI with a +LR of 13.1 as suggested by a robust body of evidence. Similarly, a normal ECG is a very useful indication of the absence of an AMI (−LR = 0.14; 95% CI: 0.11 to 0.2).

Specific attention has also been paid to the diagnostic value of the first ECG in chest pain patients presenting with a possible myocardial infarction. A best bet review of this topic, incorporating

Table 16.5 Positive likelihood ratio of aortic dissection in patients with combined findings. (From von Kodolitsch et al. [16].)

Number of findings	Positive likelihood ratio (95% CI)
0	0.1 (0.0 to 0.2)
1	0.5 (0.3 to 0.8)
2	5.3 (3.0 to 9.4)
3	66.0 (4.1 to 1062.0)

10 trials that could specifically address this question, revealed that the sensitivity of the first ECG was no greater than 69% and potentially as low as 13% [18]. This finding was included in the American College of Emergency Physicians (ACEP) policy on the evaluation of chest pain patients, which advocated for serial ECGs in patients suspected of ischemic chest pain. Specifically, the policy designates repeating an ECG within 30–60 minutes of the patient's arrival in the ED as a management strategy that reflects moderate clinical certainty [19].

Question 6: In patients with chest pain suspected of being ischemic in origin and with electrocardiograms (ECGs) demonstrating a left bundle branch block (LBBB) (population), can the likelihood ratios (diagnostic test characteristics) of specific features in these ECGs (tests) help either exclude or rule in myocardial infarction as the cause of a patient's symptoms (outcome)?

Search strategy

- PubMed: chest pain AND emergency department AND clinical assessment AND left bundle branch block AND clinical queries filter: diagnosis

Current American College of Cardiology (ACC)/AHA guidelines recommend fibrinolytic therapy in AMI patients with "new or presumably new LBBB" as a class I indication (cited as level A evidence) [20] There is controversy, however, over the optimal approach to identify AMI in those patients with LBBB. LBBB is characterized by repolarization changes whereby the ST segments are usually discordant (deviated in the opposite direction) to the major direction of the QRS complex. This baseline pattern of repolarization renders the diagnosis of ischemia and AMI in LBBB notoriously difficult and contributes to delays in diagnosis and time to revascularization. In an effort to derive criteria to facilitate the diagnosis of AMI in patients with LBBB, Sgarbossa et al. compared ECG findings from patients with LBBB and AMI who were enrolled in the Global Utilization of Streptokinase and Tissue Plasminogen Activator for Occluded Coronary Arteries trial (GUSTO-1) to those of a control group of patients with LBBB derived from an outpatient ECG database [21]. Using the presence of abnormal ST deviation at the J-point to delineate three ECG cri-

teria (termed the Sgarbossa criteria), his research group derived and validated a scoring system for the prediction of AMI in the presence of LBBB in which a score of ≥3 had a +LR of 7.8 and a −LR of 0.2 (Table 16.7).

A systematic review of the diagnostic accuracy of the Sgarbossa criteria in detecting AMI was identified in the search [22]. The authors identified 11 studies involving over 2200 patients in whom ECGs with LBBBs were compared against a reference standard. A Sgarbossa ECG algorithm score of ≥2 had a sensitivity of 41% (95% CI: 37% to 45%) and specificity of 86% (95% CI: 84% to 89%), yielding a +LR of 3.0 (95% CI: 2.4 to 3.7) and a −LR of 0.6 (95% CI: 0.6 to 0.7). A score of ≥3 had a sensitivity of 20% (95% CI: 18% to 23%) and specificity of 98% (CI, 97% to 99%), yielding a +LR of 10.8 (95% CI: 6.5 to 17.8) and a −LR of 0.8 (95% CI: 0.8 to 0.8). Intra- and inter-observer agreement was substantial. The analysis of only the highest quality studies yielded similar results.

In summary, the practical implications of this work suggest that the presence of either two or three Sgarbossa criteria are useful for ruling in AMI in the appropriate clinical context but their absence cannot be relied upon to exclude AMI in the setting of LBBB.

Question 7: In patients with chest pain suspected of being ischemic in origin (population), can the likelihood ratios (diagnostic test characteristics) of symptomatic relief with sublingual nitroglycerine (test) help either exclude or rule in cardiac ischemia as the cause of a patient's symptoms (outcome)?

Search strategy

- PubMed: chest pain AND emergency department AND clinical assessment AND nitroglycerin AND clinical queries filter: diagnosis

Nitroglycerin (North American spelling) or nitroglycerine (UK spelling) (NTG) is a potent coronary vasodilator with a well-established role in the treatment of both stable and unstable coronary artery disease. What is less certain is whether it has a diagnostic role in patients who present to the ED with undifferentiated chest pain. A commonly held belief is that NTG-responsive pain is predictive of cardiac ischemia. Henrikson et al. conducted a prospective study of 459 patients who received NTG for chest pain in the ED and then were admitted for further evaluation and followed for a period of 4 months [23]. NTG relieved pain in 39% of all patients. It was effective in 35% of the 141 patients with subsequent evidence of active coronary disease, and in 41% of the 275 patients with no subsequent evidence of active coronary disease. Such weak discriminative ability corresponded to a +LR and −LR of 0.85 and 1.13, respectively. In a similar study of 270 patients, Steele et al. reported a +LR and −LR of 1.1 and 0.8, respectively [24]. A third trial, which used a quantitative analysis to measure degrees of pain relief, reached remarkably similar conclusions as

Table 16.6 Resting ECG findings in patients with acute chest pain. (From Mant et al. [5].)

Findings			Studies	LR	95% CI	P for heterogeneity
	MI only					
Normal ECG	+LR		11	0.14	0.11 to 0.20	0.007
	−LR			1.58	1.42 to 1.76	<0.001
Sinus rhythm	+LR		0			
	−LR					
Atrial fibrillation	+LR		1	0.57	0.13 to 2.49	
	−LR			1.02	0.98 to 1.05	
ST elevation (STe)	+LR		17	13.1	8.28 to 20.6	<0.001
	−LR			0.47	0.47 to 0.54	<0.001
ST depression (STd)	+LR		2	3.13	2.50 to 3.92	0.6
	−LR			0.60	0.25 to 1.43	<1.001
T waves	+LR		1	1.87	1.41 to 2.48	
	−LR			0.66	0.50 to 0.87	
Q waves	+LR		1	5.01	3.56 to 7.06	
	−LR			0.45	0.32 to 0.64	
Left BBB	+LR		1	0.49	0.15 to 1.60	
	−LR			1.03	0.99 to 1.08	
Right BBB	+LR		1	0.28	0.04 to 2.12	
	−LR			1.03	1.00 to 1.06	
STe/STd/Q/T	+LR		5	5.30	3.66 to 7.70	<0.001
	−LR			0.38	0.21 to 0.65	<0.001
STe/STd/Q/T/BBB	+LR		3	4.34	2.46 to 7.67	0.08
	−LR			0.36	0.33 to 0.38	0.7
STe/STd/Q/T/BBB	+LR		2	2.11	1.17 to 3.78	<0.001
or other rhythm	−LR			0.28	0.16 to 0.50	0.003

to the markedly limited utility of NTG in determining if a patient's symptoms are cardiac in origin [25].

In conclusion, NTG performs poorly as a diagnostic test and emergency physicians should not be falsely reassured that relief of chest pain by NTG confirms ischemic heart disease and angina.

Question 8: In patients with atypical chest pain suspected of being either gastrointestinal or cardiac in origin (population), can the likelihood ratios (diagnostic test characteristics) of symptomatic relief with antacid with or without a liquid anesthetic therapy (test) help either exclude or rule out a gastrointestinal or cardiac cause for a patient's symptoms (outcome)?

Search strategy

- PubMed: chest pain AND emergency department AND clinical assessment AND antacids AND clinical queries filter: diagnosis

A significant overlap exists between the symptomatology of ischemic chest pain and gastro-esophageal reflux [26]. Unfortu-

nately many patients have been known to interpret the symptomatology of cardiac ischemia with a gastrointestinal (GI) process with disastrous consequences. Since the symptom profiles of cardiac and GI pain overlap, the notion of using an agent that can be used to relieve the symptoms of acid reflux in the esophagus with an antacid or a topical anesthetic have been considered as a viable diagnostic strategy. Unfortunately, there is a paucity of research that has examined this strategy with any reasonable degree of rigor and none conducted in the last 15 years. In a best bet review from 2003, Teece and Crawford could identify only two poorly designed trials that pertained to this issue and concluded that antacids are useful in the relief of pain that is clearly esophageal in origin; however, the effect is insufficiently specific to be of value in confirming a diagnosis [27].

Table 16.7 Criteria for the Sgarbossa ECG algorithm*

ST segment elevation >1 mm in lead with concordant QRS complex	5 points
ST segment depression >1 mm in leads V1, V2, or V3	3 points
ST segment deviation >5 mm in lead with discordant QRS complex	2 points

*ST segment deviation measured at the J-point.

In a case report and review Dickinson cites other studies on GI cocktails and chest pain [28]. He describes an observational case series that concluded that antacids relieved chest pain due to esophagitis in 39% of cases and relieved cardiac chest pain in 7%, using esophagoscopy and ECG criteria for diagnosis. He also noted that most of the rest of the literature on the topic is poor in quality and conflicting in conclusions [28]. In a letter to the editor, Castrina cites the results of an assessment of a medical malpractice carrier database and states that misdiagnosis of myocardial infarction occurred frequently when the GI cocktail (liquid antacid and viscous xylocaine) was used to distinguish between the various causes of chest pain [29].

In summary, high-quality studies are lacking to characterize the likelihood ratios associated with relief of chest pain using antacids and viscous xylocaine and until these are available clinicians should not use this as a valid diagnostic test.

Question 9: In patients with chest pain presenting to the ED (population), does treatment with aspirin (treatment) reduce acute myocardial infarction and the need for procedures (outcomes) compared to standard care with oxygen and pain relief (control)?

Search strategy

- PubMed: chest pain AND emergency department AND aspirin AND acute myocardial infarction AND clinical queries filter: therapy

There are no randomized controlled trials (RCTs) that specifically address this question for all comers presenting to an ED with chest pain. There is, however, an extensive body of evidence to support the notion that aspirin provides important benefits for the subgroup of these patients who prove to be suffering from an ACS, be it either unstable angina/NSTEMI or AMI. A collaborative meta-analysis conducted by the Antithrombotic Trialists' Collaboration (search date 1997: 287 RCTs with 135,000 people at high risk of vascular events) compared antiplatelet treatment versus placebo. Twelve of these trials included a total of 5031 people with unstable angina [30]. The review found that, in people with unstable angina, antiplatelet treatment (mostly medium dose aspirin, 75–325 mg/day) reduced the combined outcome of vascular death, myocardial infarction or stroke at up to 12 months compared with placebo (8% with antiplatelet treatment vs 13% with placebo; $P < 0.0001$).

An earlier version of that systematic review (search date 1990: nine RCTs with 18,773 people), compared antiplatelet agents begun soon after the onset of AMI and for at least 1 month afterwards versus placebo [31]. Almost all (>95%) of the people in these studies were randomized to either aspirin or placebo. That review found that aspirin significantly reduced mortality, reinfarction and stroke at 1 month compared with control. The largest of the RCTs identified by that review (17,187 people with suspected AMI) compared aspirin 162.6 mg versus placebo chewed and swal-

lowed on the day of the AMI and continued daily for 1 month [32]. There was a 2.4% absolute reduction in vascular death at 35 days. The survival benefit was maintained for up to 10 years [33]. In the systematic review, the most widely tested aspirin regimens were 75–325 mg daily.

With regard to harm, these reviews found no increase in non-vascular mortality with antiplatelet treatment compared with placebo (OR = 0.92; 95% CI: 0.82 to 1.03). There was an increase in major extracranial bleeding with antiplatelet treatment compared with placebo, but the absolute risk was low (OR = 1.6; 95% CI: 1.4 to 1.8). The review concluded that the weight of the evidence suggests no added cardiovascular benefit, and greater incidence of adverse effects, for aspirin doses greater than 325 mg daily. In the light of impressive benefit (number needed to treat to prevent major cardiovascular adverse event is 25) and minimal risk associated with short-term aspirin therapy, it is entirely appropriate to recommend this treatment empirically in non-aspirin allergic patients who present to the ED with chest pain.

Conclusions

The aforementioned patient underwent serial ECGs over a 2-hour observation period, none of which revealed evidence of ischemic abnormalities. The patient reported some relief with sublingual nitroglycerin and received 160 mg of aspirin to chew. Initial troponin levels were normal and a D-dimer was only slightly greater than the normal range for the hospital laboratory. A portable X-ray revealed a widened mediastinum prompting a request for a CT scan of the chest to rule out an aortic dissection. Prior to transport to CT, the patient's pain increased considerably and developed pronounced radiation to the back. A differential blood pressure was now detectable between both arms and intravenous labetolol was initiated to control the blood pressure. Transesophageal echocardiography confirmed a type A thoracic aortic dissection and the patient was transferred to the operating room for successful surgical repair.

Chest pain is both a common and challenging presentation for the emergency physician. It is a high-risk and high-stakes chief complaint with the life-threatening differentials of acute coronary syndromes, pulmonary embolism and thoracic aortic dissection constituting the major preoccupation for the clinician. The diagnostic approach, while well informed with high-quality research evidence, remains imperfect and a high index of suspicion coupled with validated approaches to clinical assessment and a reasonable and judicious use of diagnostic test strategies remains elusive. The possible initial treatment of some of the most worrisome differential diagnoses (e.g., anticoagulation) can prove to be fatal for other conditions on this list. Equally troubling is the knowledge that the clinical response to therapy and a reduction in pain may not necessarily prove to be very useful as a diagnostic strategy or in reducing the patient's risk of experiencing an adverse outcome.

A carefully executed history focused on the most discriminating elements of the clinical presentation and the optimal utilization of validated decision rules, which incorporate serial serum biomarkers and electrocardiograms, remain the emergency physician's most potent ally in the evaluation of the patient with chest pain.

References

1 Braunwald E, Antman EM, Beasley JW, et al., American College of Cardiology, American Heart Association, Committee on the Management of Patients with Unstable Angina. ACC/AHA 2002 guideline update for the management of patients with unstable angina and non-ST-segment elevation myocardial infarction – summary article: a report of the American College of Cardiology/American Heart Association task force on practice guidelines (Committee on the Management of Patients with Unstable Angina). *J Am Coll Cardiol* 2002;**40**:1366–74.

2 Pope JH, Aufderheide TP, Ruthazer R, et al. Missed diagnoses of acute cardiac ischemia in the emergency department. *N Engl J Med* 2000;**342**:1163.

3 Lindsell CJ, Anantharaman V, Diercks D, et al., EMCREG-International i*trACS Investigators. The Internet Tracking Registry of Acute Coronary Syndromes (i*trACS): a multicenter registry of patients with suspicion of acute coronary syndromes reported using the standardized reporting guidelines for emergency department chest pain studies. *Ann Emerg Med* 2006;**48**:666–77.

4 Panju AA, Hemmelgarn BR, Guyatt GH, Simel DL. Is this patient having a myocardial infarction? *JAMA* 1998;**280**:1256.

5 Mant J, McManus RJ, Oakes RA, et al. Systematic review and modelling of the investigation of acute and chronic chest pain presenting in primary care. *Health Technology Assessment* 2004;**8**(2).

6 Han JH, Lindsell CJ, Storrow AB, et al., EMCREG i*trACS Investigators. The role of cardiac risk factor burden in diagnosing acute coronary syndromes in the emergency department setting. *Ann Emerg Med* 2007;**49**:145–52.

7 Antman EM, Cohen M, Bernink PJ, et al. The TIMI risk score for unstable angina/non-ST elevation MI: a method for prognostication and therapeutic decision making. *JAMA* 2000;**284**:835–42.

8 Eagle KA, Lim MJ, Dabbous OH, et al., GRACE Investigators. A validated prediction model for all forms of acute coronary syndrome: estimating the risk of 6-month postdischarge death in an international registry. *JAMA* 2004;**291**:2727–33.

9 Chase M, Robey JL, Zogby KE, Sease KL, Shofer FS, Hollander JE. Prospective validation of the Thrombolysis in Myocardial Infarction Risk Score in the emergency department chest pain population. *Ann Emerg Med* 2006;**48**:252–9.

10 Pollack CV, Jr., Sites FD, Shofer FS, Sease KL, Hollander JE. Application of the TIMI risk score for unstable angina and non-ST elevation acute coronary syndrome to an unselected emergency department chest pain population. *Acad Emerg Med* 2006;**13**:13–18.

11 Soiza RL, Leslie SJ, Williamson P, Wai S, Harrild K, Peden NR, Hargreaves AD. Risk stratification in acute coronary syndromes – does the TIMI risk score work in unselected cases? *Q J Med* 2006;**99**:81–7.

12 Ramsay G, Podogrodzka M, McClure C, et al. Risk prediction in patients presenting with suspected cardiac pain: the GRACE and TIME risk scores versus clinical examination. *Q J Med* 2007;**100**:11–18.

13 Lyon R, Morris AC, Caesar D, et al. Chest pain presenting to the emergency department – to stratify risk with GRACE or TIMI? *Resuscitation* 2007;**74**(1):90–93.

14 Klompas M. Does this patient have an acute thoracic aortic dissection? *JAMA* 2002;**287**:2262.

15 Teece S, Hogg K. Related articles, best evidence topic report. Peripheral pulses to exclude thoracic aortic dissection. *Emerg Med J* 2004;**21**:589.

16 Von Kodolitsch Y, Schwartz AG, Nienaber CA. Clinical prediction of acute aortic dissection. *Arch Intern Med* 2000;**160**:2977–82.

17 Hogg K, Teece S. Related articles, best evidence topic report. The sensitivity of a normal chest radiograph in ruling out aortic dissection. *Emerg Med J* 2004;**21**:199–200.

18 Speake D, Terry P. Towards evidence based emergency medicine: best BETs from the Manchester Royal Infirmary. First ECG in chest pain. *Emerg Med J* 2001;**18**:61–2.

19 Fesmire FM, Decker WW, Diercks DB, et al. American College of Emergency Physicians Clinical Policies Subcommittee (Writing Committee) on Non-ST-Segment Elevation Acute Coronary Syndromes. Clinical policy: critical issues in the evaluation and management of adult patients with non-ST-segment elevation acute coronary syndromes. *Ann Emerg Med* 2006;**48**:270–301.

20 Antman EM, Anbe DT, Armstrong PW, et al. ACC/AHA guidelines for the management of patients with ST-elevation myocardial infarction: executive summary: a report of the ACC/AHA Task Force on Practice Guidelines (Committee to Revise the 1999 Guidelines on the Management of Patients with AMI). *Circulation* 2004;**100**:1–49.

21 Sgarbossa EB, Pinski SL, Barbagelata A, et al. Electrocardiographic diagnosis of evolving acute myocardial infarction in the presence of left bundle-branch block. GUSTO-1 (Global Utilization of Streptokinase and Tissue Plasminogen Activator for Occluded Coronary Arteries) Investigators. *N Engl J Med* 1996;**334**:481–7.

22 Tabas JA, Rodriguez RM, Seligman HK, Goldschlager NF. Electrocardiographic criteria for detecting acute myocardial infarction in patients with left bundle branch block: a meta-analysis. Manuscript No. 2006-928R1. *Ann Emerg Med* (e-published 14 March 2008).

23 Henrikson CA, Howell EE, Bush DE, et al. Chest pain relief by nitroglycerin does not predict active coronary artery disease. *Ann Intern Med* 2003;**139**:979–86.

24 Steele R, McNaughton T, McConahy M, Lam J. Chest pain in emergency department patients: if the pain is relieved by nitroglycerin, is it more likely to be cardiac chest pain? *Can J Emerg Med* 2006;**8**:164–9.

25 Diercks DB, Boghos E, Guzman H, Amsterdam EA, Kirk JD. Changes in the numeric descriptive scale for pain after sublingual nitroglycerin do not predict cardiac etiology of chest pain. *Ann Emerg Med* 2005;**45**:581–5.

26 Ros E, Armengol X, Grande L, Toledo-Pimentel V, Lacima G, Sanz G. Chest pain at rest in patients with coronary artery disease. Myocardial ischemia, esophageal dysfunction, or panic disorder? *Dig Dis Sci* 1997;**42**:1344–53.

27 Teece S, Crawford I. Towards evidence based emergency medicine: best BETs from the Manchester Royal Infirmary. Antacids and diagnosis in patients with atypical chest pain. *Emerg Med J* 2003;**20**:170–71.

28 Dickinson MW. The "GI cocktail" in the evaluation of chest pain in the emergency department. *J Emerg Med* 1996;**14**(2):245–6.

29 Castrina, FP. Unexplained noncardiac chest pain. *Ann Intern Med* 1997;**126**:663.

30 Antithrombotic Trialists' Collaboration. Collaborative meta-analysis of randomised trials of antiplatelet therapy for prevention of death, myocardial infarction, and stroke in high risk patients. *BMJ* 2002;**324**:71–86.

31 Antiplatelet Trialists' Collaboration. Collaborative overview of randomised trials of antiplatelet therapy – I: Prevention of death, myocardial

infarction, and stroke by prolonged antiplatelet therapy in various categories of patients. *BMJ* 1994;**308**:81–106.

32 ISIS-2 (Second International Study of Infarct Survival) Collaborative Group. Randomised trial of intravenous streptokinase, oral aspirin, both, or neither among 17,187 cases of suspected acute myocardial infarction: ISIS-2. *Lancet* 1988;**2**:349–60.

33 Baigent C, Collins R, Appleby P, Parish S, Sleight P, Peto R. ISIS-2: 10 year survival among patients with suspected acute myocardial infarction in randomised comparison of intravenous streptokinase, oral aspirin, both, or neither. The ISIS-2 (Second International Study of Infarct Survival) Collaborative Group. *BMJ* 1998;**316**:1337–43.

17 Acute Coronary Syndromes

Kirk Magee

Department of Emergency Medicine, Dalhousie University, Halifax *and* QEII Health Sciences Centre, Halifax Infirmary, Halifax, Canada

Case scenario

A 43-year-old male presented to the emergency department (ED) after 90 minutes of ongoing chest pain associated with shortness of breath which started while he was mowing the lawn. Over the previous several weeks, he reported having had new episodic chest pain on exertion which was relieved with rest. On examination, he was mildly diaphoretic with a heart rate of 96 beats/min and a blood pressure of 142/86 mmHg. Examination of the chest revealed no evidence of adventitious breath sounds and normal heart sounds. The remainder of the physical exam was within normal limits. An electrocardiogram (ECG) and cardiac markers were ordered. The ECG showed ST segment depression in the anterior leads (V1–4). You diagnose him with an acute coronary syndrome (ACS) and treat him with oxygen, acetyl-salicylic acid (ASA), a β-blocker and nitroglycerin. The resident asked you whether it is possible to differentiate between patients at low and high risk for subsequent cardiovascular events.

The patient improves rapidly and, after treatment with ASA, sublingual nitroglycerin and intravenous metoprolol, he is pain free. You consulted the patient to cardiology for admission and further diagnostic work-up. The patient described how his neighbor recently had angioplasty with stenting, and he wonders whether he would benefit from this treatment.

Background

Acute coronary syndromes represent a spectrum of disease ranging from unstable angina (UA) to non-ST segment elevation myocardial infarction (NSTEMI) and ST segment myocardial infarction (STEMI). NSTEMI may be differentiated from UA by the presence of elevated cardiac enzymes indicating actual myocardial necrosis and infarction. Clinical manifestations of ACS are secondary to atherosclerotic plaque rupture with endovascular thrombus formation. Patients with ACS experience chest pain associated with other symptoms such as dyspnea, diaphoresis, weakness/presyncope and/or nausea. These symptoms are reported variably in patients with ACS, and some patients may present without the cardinal feature of chest pain.

A potentially life-threatening disorder, more than 5.3 million patients per year present to EDs in the United States with chest pain or related symptoms [1] and 1.4 million are admitted to hospital [2]. Direct medical costs for treating patients with ACS in the United States are over $51 billion per year and pharmaceutical costs are the fastest growing sector in health care [3]. In Canada, there has been a substantial increase in both the utilization and expenditures for cardiovascular medications [4]. Despite the abundance of clinical practice guidelines and positive randomized controlled trials (RCTs) in the cardiology literature, one review of four major drug trials estimated that only nine out of 100 patients actually benefited from receiving the drugs [5]. There is a need not only to search for new therapies, but to also better define which patients with ACS will most benefit from existing therapies.

Clinical questions

In order to address the issues of most relevance to your patient and to help in searching the literature for the evidence regarding these, you should structure your questions as recommended in Chapter 1.

1 In patients with UA/NSTEMI (population), do risk stratification instruments (intervention) accurately differentiate between patients at low risk and high risk for subsequent cardiovascular events (outcome)?

2 In patients with UA/NSTEMI (population), does the use of aspirin in the ED setting (intervention) decrease mortality and morbidity (outcome) compared to placebo or routine care (control)?

3 In patients with UA/NSTEMI (population), does the use of clopidogrel in the ED setting (intervention) decrease mortality and morbidity (outcome) compared to routine care with ASA (control)?

Evidence-based Emergency Medicine. Edited by Brian H. Rowe
© 2009 Blackwell Publishing, ISBN: 978-1-4051-6143-5.

	Clinical predication tool		
	TIMI	PURSUIT	GRACE
Derivation cohort	1957 subjects	9641 subjects	17,142 patients
Number of predictor variables	7	7	9
C statistic with 95% CI*	0.68 (0.59 to 0.77)	0.80 (0.71 to 0.88)	0.81 (0.73 to 0.89)

Table 17.1 Comparison of various clinical prediction tools.

*Data in bottom row from Yan et al. [66].

4 In patients with UA/NSTEMI (population), does the use of nitroglycerin in the ED setting (intervention) decrease mortality and morbidity (outcome) compared to placebo or routine care (control)?

5 In patients with UA/NSTEMI (population), does the use of β-blockers in the ED setting (intervention) decrease mortality and morbidity (outcome) compared to placebo or routine care (control)?

6 In patients with UA/NSTEMI (population), does the use of heparins (low molecular weight heparin (LMWH) or unfractionated heparin (UFH)) in the ED setting (intervention) decrease mortality and morbidity (outcome) compared to placebo or routine care (control)?

7 In patients with ACS (population), does the use of LMWH in the ED setting (intervention) decrease mortality and morbidity (outcome) compared to UFH (control)?

8 In patients with ACS (population), does the use of IIb/IIIa inhibitors in the ED setting (intervention) decrease mortality and morbidity (outcome) compared to routine care (control)?

9 In patients with ACS (population), does an immediate invasive strategy (intervention) improve mortality and morbidity (outcome) compared to a selective (conservative) strategy (control)?

General search strategy

You begin to address these questions by searching for evidence in the common electronic databases such as the Cochrane Library, MEDLINE and EMBASE looking specifically for systematic reviews and meta-analyses. When a systematic review is identified, you also search for recent updates in the Cochrane Library and also search MEDLINE and EMBASE to identify RCTs that became available after the publication date of the systematic review. In addition, relevant, updated and evidence-based clinical practice guidelines (CPGs) on UA/NSTEMI are accessed.

Searching for evidence synthesis: primary search strategy

- Cochrane Library: (acute coronary syndrome OR unstable angina) AND (topic)
- MEDLINE: (acute coronary syndrome OR unstable angina) AND MEDLINE AND (systematic review OR meta-analysis OR metaanalysis) AND (topic)

- EMBASE: (acute coronary syndrome OR unstable angina) AND MEDLINE AND (systematic review OR meta-analysis OR meta-analysis) AND (topic)

Critical review of the literature

Question 1: In patients with UA/NSTEMI (population), do risk stratification instruments (intervention) accurately differentiate between patients at low risk and high risk for subsequent cardiovascular events (outcome)?

Search strategy

- MEDLINE and EMBASE: (acute coronary syndrome OR unstable angina) AND (validation OR validate)

Patients with ACS are a diverse group with disease severity ranging from unstable angina to completed myocardial infarction. Some patients, initially suspected of ACS, will even be ultimately diagnosed with a non-cardiac cause for their chest pain. Prognostication of risk is important to help physicians identify which patients will be best served by therapies that are often expensive and not without significant risk. Numerous prediction tools have been developed to aid in risk stratification [6]. At least three of these instruments have been prospectively validated (Table 17.1) [7–9].

The Platelet Glycoprotein IIb/IIIa in Unstable Angina: Receptor Suppression Using Integrilin Therapy (PURSUIT) model was derived from 9461 trial patients. The best independent predictors of 30-day mortality included: advanced age, female sex, increased heart rate, lower systolic blood pressure, severity of prior angina, ST segment depression, signs of heart failure and elevated cardiac markers [9]. When retrospectively validated against 2925 patients in the Canadian ACS Registry, the PURSUIT model demonstrated good discriminatory performance in predicting in-hospital deaths (C statistic = 0.84; 95% CI: 0.79 to 0.89) but tended to overestimate the risk [10]. The C (for concordance) statistic defines how well a prediction rule discriminates between patients who will and will not have an event [11]. A C statistic of 0.84 means that the PURSUIT model accurately discriminates those patients who will die in hospital 84% of the time. With completely random prediction, the value would be 0.50.

Derived from a cohort of 1957 patients the Thrombolysis in Myocardial Infarction 11B (TIMI) tool identifies seven dichotomous variables that predict risk: 65 years of age or older, three or more cardiac risk factors, prior coronary stenosis of at least 50%, ST segment deviation, severe anginal symptoms (greater than two anginal events in the last 24 hours), aspirin use in the previous week, and elevated serum cardiac markers [7]. Prior revascularization procedure or myocardial infarction (MI) is often used as a proxy for significant coronary stenosis. With each characteristic given a value of 1, the total TIMI score is predictive of mortality at 14 days (C statistic = 0.72 to 0.78). Rates of the triple endpoint of all-cause mortality, MI and severe recurrent ischemia prompting urgent revascularization ranged from 4.7% for the lowest score (0 or 1) to 40.9% for the highest (6 or 7). The TIMI score has been validated retrospectively in several trials and registries [12–16] consistently demonstrating its ability to discriminate between patients with a low risk and those with a high risk of having UA/NSTEMI. Of note, the TIMI risk score has also been prospectively validated in the ED setting in over 5000 patients presenting with undifferentiated chest pain syndromes or suspected ACS [17,18] (see Chapter 16 for more details).

Unlike the PURSUIT model and the TIMI risk score, which were derived from patients in the highly controlled environment of a clinical trial, the Global Registry of Acute Coronary Events (GRACE) risk calculator is derived from a multinational registry of 17,142 patients with ACS which more closely reflects everyday clinical practice [8]. Several factors were predictive for all-cause mortality at 6 months after discharge: increasing age, history of MI, history of congestive heart failure, elevated heart rate, decreased systolic blood pressure, elevated serum creatinine, elevated cardiac enzymes, ST segment depression, and no hospital percutaneous coronary intervention (PCI) (Fig. 17.1). The GRACE model accurately predicts 6-month mortality for all patients across the entire spectrum of ACS (unstable angina, NSTEMI and STEMI) (C statistic = 0.71). It has been retrospectively validated in several populations [10,19] and prospectively validated in 1000 ED patients [20].

With the ready accessibility of hand-held computers, more complex and accurate scoring systems are now available to the clinician at the bedside. With further research, these prediction tools will aid physicians in determining which patients with ACS will most benefit from specific therapies and management strategies.

Question 2: In patients with UA/NSTEMI (population), does the use of aspirin in the ED setting (intervention) decrease mortality and morbidity (outcome) compared to placebo or routine care (control)?

Search strategy

- MEDLINE and EMBASE: (acute coronary syndrome OR unstable angina) AND MEDLINE AND (systematic review OR meta-analysis OR metaanalysis) AND aspirin

Acetyl-salicylic acid (or aspirin) irreversibly inhibits cyclooxygenase-1 within platelets preventing the formation of thromboxane A_2 thereby inhibiting platelet aggregation. The evidence for the use of ASA in ACS arises from a meta-analysis which included 287 studies totaling 135,000 patients [21]. Twelve of the trials representing 5031 subjects specifically examined patients with unstable angina. Patients receiving ASA had significantly reduced combined outcomes of vascular death, MI or stroke at 12 months compared to those receiving placebo (8.0% vs 13.3%, $P < 0.0001$) with a number needed to treat (NNT) of 19. Although this was accompanied by a significant increase in major extracranial bleeding in those patients treated with ASA (OR = 1.6; 95% CI: 1.4 to 1.8), the absolute risk was low (1.13% compared to 0.71%). The review concluded that there was no significant difference in cardiovascular benefit with different daily dosing regimes of ASA, but cautioned that there was less evidence for doses of <75 mg/day and greater risk of adverse effects with doses >325 mg/day.

In summary, given the favorable risk–benefit profile and the minimal costs associated with treatment, ASA should be considered as the standard of care in patients with UA/NSTEMI.

Question 3: In patients with UA/NSTEMI (population), does the use of clopidogrel in the ED setting (intervention) decrease mortality and morbidity (outcome) compared to routine care with ASA (control)?

Search strategy

- MEDLINE and EMBASE: (acute coronary syndrome OR unstable angina) AND MEDLINE AND (clopidogrel OR ticlopidine)

Thienopyridines are antiplatelet agents that inhibit the platelet aggregation induced by adenosine diphosphate, thus reducing ischemic events [22]. There was no systematic review that addressed the use of thienopyridines in ACSs; however, one RCT comparing clopidogrel to placebo or conventional treatment was identified [23]. The CURE trial randomized 12,562 patients to receive a loading dose of clopidogrel (300 mg) followed by a daily dose of 75 mg for 3–12 months compared to placebo. All patients received daily aspirin. Clopidogrel significantly reduced the composite primary outcome of death from cardiovascular causes, non-fatal MI or stroke compared to placebo at 9 months (RR = 0.80; 95% CI: 0.72 to 0.90), with a NNT of 47. This was accompanied by a significantly increased incidence of major bleeding (RR = 1.38; 95% CI: 1.13 to 1.67) with a number needed to harm (NNH) of 100. In the PCI-CURE sub-study, 2658 patients undergoing PCI in the CURE study were randomly treated with clopidogrel or placebo in addition to ASA 6 days prior to PCI and continued for a median of 10 days overall followed by an open-label thienopyridine. Fewer patients in the clopidogrel group experienced cardiovascular death, MI or urgent target-vessel revascularization compared to the placebo group (RR = 0.70; 95% CI: 0.50 to 0.97). Interestingly,

Risk calculator for 6-month post-discharge mortality after hospitalization for acute coronary syndrome

Record the points for each variable at the bottom left and sum the points to calculate the total risk score. Find the total score on the *x*-axis of the nomogram plot. The corresponding probability on the *y*-axis is the estimated probability of all-cause mortality from hospital discharge to 6 months

Medical history

① Age in years

Age in years	Points
≤29	0
30–39	0
40–49	18
50–59	36
60–69	55
70–79	73
80–89	91
≥90	100

② History of congestive heart failure 24

③ History of myocardial infarction 12

Findings at initial hospital presentation

④ Resting heart rate, beats/min

Resting heart rate, beats/min	Points
≤49.9	0
50–69.9	3
70–89.9	9
90–109.9	14
110–149.9	23
150–199.9	36
≥200	43

⑤ Systolic blood pressure, mmHg

Systolic blood pressure, mmHg	Points
≤79.9	24
80–99.9	22
100–119.9	18
120–139.9	14
140–159.9	10
160–199.9	4
≥200	0

1

⑤ ST segment depression 11

Findings during hospitalization

⑦ Initial serum creatinine, mg/dl

Initial serum creatinine, mg/dl	Points
0–0.39	1
0.4–0.79	3
0.8–1.19	5
1.2–1.59	7
1.6–1.99	9
2–3.99	15
≥4	20

⑧ Elevated cardiac enzymes 15

⑨ No in-hospital percutaneous coronary invervention 14

Points

① ________

② ________

③ ________

④ ________

⑤ ________

⑥ ________

⑦ ________

⑧ ________

⑨ ________

Total risk score ________ (sum of points)

Mortality risk ________ (From plot)

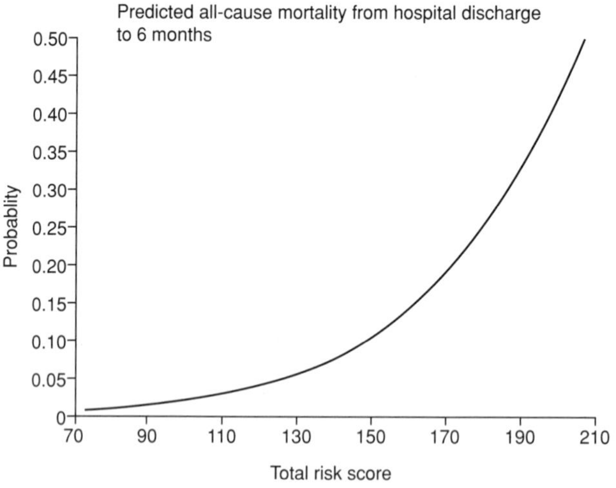

Figure 17.1 GRACE prediction score card and nomogram for all-cause mortality from discharge to 6 months. (Reproduced with permission from Eagle et al. [8], courtesy of the *Journal of the American Medical Association.*)

treatment with clopidogrel was as beneficial in those patients who received coronary stents as in those who did not [24].

A much smaller trial ($n = 652$) that compared ticlopidine to conventional treatment in patients recruited within 48 hours of admission to cardiac care units with high-risk unstable angina demonstrated similar results [25]. Patients treated with ticlopidine experienced fewer MIs and vascular deaths compared to those treated with placebo (RR = 0.5; 95% CI: 0.2 to 0.9). Bleeding complications were not reported in this non-placebo, open-label study.

Clearly the benefits of clopidogrel must be weighed against the increased risk of significant hemorrhagic complications. Patients in the CURE study in whom clopidogrel was stopped less than 5 days before coronary artery bypass graft (CABG) surgery, experienced a non-significant excess in major bleeding that was consistent with the duration of the effects of clopidogrel on platelets in the circulation. This translates to one additional patient with life-threatening bleeding per 100 undergoing CABG surgery compared to placebo. Though some have advocated that clopidogrel is safe immediately prior to CABG surgery [26] based on the results of the CLARITY-TIMI 28 trial [27], others have argued against this [28].

In summary, current guidelines recommend that a loading dose of 300 mg of clopidogrel should be added to standard aspirin therapy for patients with UA/NSTEMI when it is clear that CABG surgery will not be scheduled within the next few days, followed by 75 mg/day. Typically, patients whose ECGs show large territories of ischemia, thus reflecting multi-vessel disease, are at increased likelihood for undergoing CABG surgery. Otherwise, CABG surgery should be delayed for 5–7 days following the discontinuation of clopidogrel [29].

Question 4: In patients with UA/NSTEMI (population), does the use of intravenous nitroglycerin in the ED setting (intervention) decrease mortality and morbidity (outcome) compared to placebo or routine care (control)?

Search strategy

- MEDLINE and EMBASE: (acute coronary syndrome OR unstable angina) AND MEDLINE AND nitroglycerin

Nitroglycerin is an endothelium-independent vasodilator that reduces myocardial oxygen demand while enhancing myocardial oxygen delivery. Rationale for the traditional use of nitroglycerin in the treatment of unstable angina was based on an overview of 10 studies with approximately 2000 patients with suspected acute MI in the pre-thrombolytic era where intravenous nitroglycerin was associated with a reduction in mortality [30]. Despite this, two large prospective trials that examined the use of nitrates in patients with acute MI in the thrombolytic era found no evidence for benefit [31,32], although the "control" groups were confounded by frequent prehospital and hospital use of nitroglycerin.

The best evidence for the use of nitroglycerin in the treatment of ACS comes from two small placebo-controlled RCTs [33,34]. The first trial compared a 48-hour intravenous infusion of nitroglycerin to placebo in 162 patients with unstable angina (11 patients were excluded from the final analysis because they were felt to have non-ST segment MI at randomization). Patients treated with nitroglycerin had significantly less ongoing MI, defined as more than two episodes of recurrent angina or one episode lasting longer than 20 minutes (RR = 0.50; 95% CI: 0.28 to 0.89; NNT = 6). In the second trial, 200 patients admitted with unstable angina 2 weeks to 6 months after coronary angioplasty were randomized

to one of four groups: nitroglycerin, heparin, nitroglycerin plus heparin, or placebo. In the combined analysis intravenous nitroglycerin significantly reduced the rate of recurrent angina (RR = 0.56; 95% CI: 0.43 to 0.73; NNT = 3). Although recurrent angina is admittedly a "soft" outcome, both studies only included patients with high-risk chest pain making it likely that the etiology of this outcome was indeed ischemic. This is consistent with the known pathophysiological properties of nitrates.

In summary, provided the patient has not taken a phosphodiesterase inhibitor, such as sildenafil (Viagra®), in the previous 24 hours and that the medication is titrated to avoid hypotension, it is reasonable to consider the use of intravenous nitroglycerin to prevent recurrent ischemia in patients diagnosed with ACS.

Question 5: In patients with UA/NSTEMI (population), does the use of β-blockers in the ED setting (intervention) decrease mortality and morbidity (outcome) compared to placebo or routine care (control)?

Search strategy

- MEDLINE and EMBASE: (acute coronary syndrome OR unstable angina) AND MEDLINE AND (systematic review OR meta-analysis OR metaanalysis) AND beta-blocker

Beta-blockers work to decrease cardiac work and myocardial oxygen demand. Despite the fact that they have long been considered a mainstay in the treatment of ischemic cardiac disease, the evidence for their use in UA/NTEMI in the ED setting is less vigorous than that for other drug classes. Four small RCTs conducted in inpatient units have examined the use of β-blockers in UA/NSTEMI [35]. The first (n = 338) found that oral metoprolol significantly reduced the composite outcome of recurrent angina and MI within 48 hours compared to oral nifedipine (RR = 0.66; 95% CI: 0.43 to 0.98); however, it was not significantly better than placebo (RR = 0.76; 95% CI: 0.49 to 1.16) [35]. In the second study (n = 81), oral propranolol was no better than placebo in preventing death, MI or the need for a revascularization procedure [36]. Patients in the propranolol group, however, experienced fewer episodes of recurrent angina over 4 weeks. When oral carvedilol was compared to placebo in another RCT (n = 116), there was a similar reduction in the total ischemic burden over 48 hours although there was no difference in the primary endpoint [37]. A final trial comparing intravenous esmolol to placebo (n = 113) found no significant difference in the two study groups over a 72-hour period though there was a trend towards less ischemia in the intervention group [38].

COMMIT, a Chinese trial which enrolled 45,852 patients, indicated that β-blockade in acute MI reduced fatal arrhythmias and reinfarction but increased deaths from cardiogenic shock [39]. However, COMMIT included patients with moderate heart failure where the early use of β-blockers may be contraindicated.

In summary, when considered with evidence from other large RCTs in acute MI [40], oral β-blockers should be considered a routine part of care in patients with UA/NSTEMI who do not have contraindications (e.g., heart failure, reactive airway diseases, diabetes mellitus, and so forth) to their use [29].

Question 6: In patients with UA/NSTEMI (population), does the use of heparins (low molecular weight heparin (LMWH) or unfractionated heparin (UFH)) in the ED setting (intervention) decrease mortality and morbidity (outcome) compared to placebo or routine care (control)?

Search strategy

- Cochrane Library: (unstable angina OR acute coronary syndrome) AND heparin

Heparins inhibit factors in the coagulation cascade that are activated as a result of the disruption of unstable atherosclerotic plaque in ACS. A number of reviews have concluded that heparins are efficacious in the treatment of ACS [41,42]. A Cochrane systematic review identified eight studies involving a total of 3110 patients. There was a trend towards fewer deaths in the heparin group compared to the placebo group, but this was not statistically significant (RR = 0.84; 95% CI: 0.36 to 1.98). Patients treated with heparins had a lower incidence of MI (RR = 0.40; 95% CI: 0.25 to 0.63) with a NNT of 33 (95% CI: 25 to 100). There were no statistically significant differences in the rates of recurrent angina, revascularization procedures or thrombocytopenia. There was a trend towards more major bleeds in the heparin groups (RR = 2.05; 95% CI: 0.91 to 4.60); however, this did not reach the level of statistical significance. Only three studies ($n = 1931$) reported minor bleeding and there was heterogeneity in this outcome ($I^2 = 66.9\%$). Patients treated with heparins experienced significantly more minor bleeds than those receiving placebo (RR = 6.80; 95% CI: 1.23 to 37.49) such that the NNH was 17 (95% CI: 9 to 50).

Only two studies ($n = 1602$) included in the review compared LMWH to placebo [43,44]. In subgroup comparisons, the LMWH subgroup was alone in showing benefit over the control group in any of the outcomes reported. Because of the relative scarcity of events, the point estimates had relatively wide confidence intervals. Nevertheless, the upper CI did not cross the null value and the benefits were statistically and likely clinically significant. Patients treated with LMWH had a lower incidence of MI (RR = 0.28; 95% CI: 0.14 to 0.55), recurrent angina (RR = 0.52; 95% CI: 0.36 to 0.74) and revascularization procedures (RR = 0.26; 95% CI: 0.09 to 0.78) compared to those treated with placebo, with no significant increase in complications.

In summary, given in addition to ASA to patients with a history of typical angina accompanied by either a past medical history of coronary artery disease or ECG/cardiac enzyme changes, heparins reduce the rate of MI, but not mortality.

Question 7: In patients with ACS (population), does the use of LMWH in the emergency department setting (intervention) decrease mortality and morbidity (outcomes), compared to UFH (control)?

Search strategy

- Cochrane Library: (unstable angina OR acute coronary syndrome) AND low molecular weight heparin

Low molecular weight heparins, which are produced from the depolymerization of standard UFH into smaller fragments, lack some of the shortcomings of UFH [45]. They have a fixed dose anticoagulation effect, fewer bleeding complications and a lower incidence of heparin-induced thrombocytopenia compared to UFH (Fig. 17.2) [46]. A Cochrane review which compared the treatment of LMWH versus UFH in patients with ACS identified seven studies with 11,128 participants [47]. Overall, LMWH did not reduce mortality compared to UFH (RR = 1.00; 95% CI: 0.69 to 1.44). LMWH was superior to UFH in preventing MI when data were pooled from all follow-up time periods (RR = 0.83; 95% CI: 0.70 to 0.99). The NNT to prevent one MI was 125. Similarly, patients treated with LMWH experienced fewer revascularization procedures compared to UFH (RR = 0.88; 95% CI: 0.82 to 0.95), with the NNT being 50. Although LMWH was associated with more minor bleeding than UFH (RR = 1.40; 95% CI: 0.68 to 2.90), this trend was not statistically significant. There was no evidence of an increased rate of major bleeding in patients receiving LMWH (RR = 1.00; 95% CI: 0.80 to 1.24). Thrombocytopenia was a relatively rare outcome with only four of the seven trials reporting this. Significantly less thrombocytopenia was reported in patients receiving LMWH compared to UFH (RR = 0.64; 95% CI: 0.44 to 0.94) such that the NNT was 125.

A similar meta-analysis that reported a composite endpoint of mortality and MI as its primary outcome concluded that "there is no convincing difference in efficacy or safety between LMWH and UFH" [42]. This review did not include two smaller studies contained in the Cochrane review [43,48]. Comparing the two reviews reinforces the view that the benefit of LMWH over UFH is driven by the prevention of MI and not mortality. Point estimates between the two reviews were actually quite similar with the 95% CIs accounting for most of the differences. This suggests that the difference in interpretation may be based on different modeling used to calculate the pooled effect, and it is unclear which of these analyses took a more conservative approach.

Current guidelines support the use of LMWH or UFH for patients with intermediate to high-risk UA or NSTEMI [29]. It is impossible to recommend a particular dosing regimen, although enoxaparin was the only individual LMWH to show benefit over UFH in the Cochrane review. To date, the only head-to-head

Review: Low molecular weight heparins versus unfractionated heparin for acute coronary syndromes

Comparison: 01 LMWH vs unfractionated heparin in acute coronary syndromes.

Outcome: 08 Incidence of MI over all periods

Study	Treatment	Control	Relative risk (fixed)	Weight	Relative risk (fixed)
	n/N	n/N	95% CI	(%)	95% CI
01 Enoxaparin vs unfractionated heparin					
ESSENCE 1997	62/1607	81/1564		29.5	0.74 [0.54, 1.03]
TIMI 11B 1999	81/1938	103/1936		37.0	0.79 [0.59, 1.04]
Subtotal (95% CI)	3545	3500		66.5	0.77 [0.62, 0.95]
Total events: 143 (treatment), 184 (control)					
Test for heterogeneity: chi² = 0.06, df = 1, P = 0.81, I² = 0.0%					
Test for overall effect: Z = 2.43, P = 0.02					
02 Dalteparin vs unfractionated heparin					
FRIC 1997	19/751	23/731		8.4	0.80 [0.44, 1.46]
Subtotal (95% CI)	751	731		8.4	0.80 [0.44, 1.46]
Total events: 19 (treatment), 23 (control)					
Test for heterogeneity: not applicable					
Test for overall effect: Z = 0.71, P = 0.5					
03 Nadroparin vs unfractionated heparin					
FRAXIS 1999	71/1166	64/1151		23.1	1.10 [0.79, 1.52]
Godoy 1998	0/30	1/40		0.5	0.44 [0.02, 10.46]
Grrfinkel 1995	0/68	4/70		1.6	0.11 [0.01, 2.08]
Subtotal (95% CI)	1264	1261		25.2	1.02 [0.74, 1.41]
Total events: 71 (treatment), 69 (control)					
Test for heterogeneity: chi² = 2.63, df = 2, P = 0.27, I² = 24.0%					
Test for overall effect: Z = 13, P = 0.9					
04 Tinzaparin vs unfractionated heparin					
x Suvarna 1997	0/20	0/20		0.0	Not estimable
Subtotal (95% CI)	20	20		0.0	Not estimable
Total events: 0 (treatment), 0 (control)					
Test for heterogeneity: not applicable					
Test for overall effect: not applicable					
Total (95% CI)	5580	5512		100.0	0.83 [0.70, 0.99]
Total events: 233 (treatment), 276 (control)					
Test for heterogeneity: chi² = 5.26, df = 5, P = 0.39, I² = 4.9%					
Test for overall effect: Z = 2.09, P = 0.04					

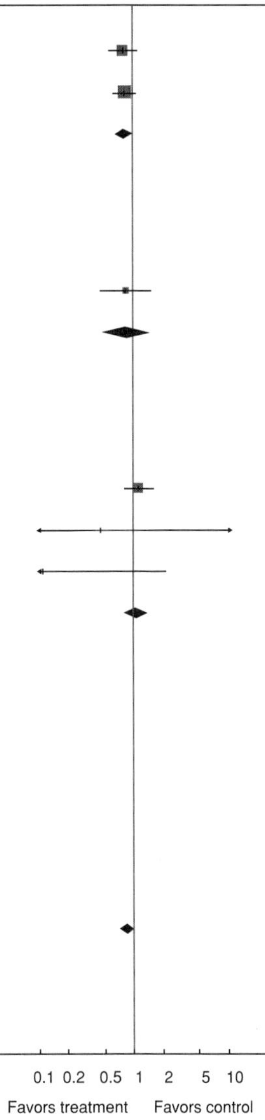

0.1 0.2 0.5 1 2 5 10

Favors treatment   Favors control

Figure 17.2 Low molecular weight heparins reduce the incidence of MI over all time periods. (Reproduced with permission from Magee et al. [47], © 2003 Cochrane Library.)

comparison of LMWHs included 438 patients with ACS who were randomized to receive open-label treatment with enoxaparin or tinzaparin [49]. The incidence of the composite endpoint of death, MI or recurrent angina was lower in the enoxaparin arm compared to the tinzaparin arm (12.3% vs 21.1%, $P = 0.015$). This result, however, was driven by the "softer" endpoint of recurrent angina. Additional work is needed to unequivocally recommend one particular LMWH over another. Moreover, as newer agents such as fundaparinox and oral thrombin inhibitors arrive on the market, these recommendations will likely need to be revised.

In summary, when given to patients with a history of typical angina accompanied by either a past medical history of coronary artery disease or ECG/cardiac enzyme change, LMWH is more efficacious in reducing MI and revascularization with fewer serious side-effects than UFH. Given the relative ease of use and predictable dose–response curve compared to UFH, LMWH is the unequivocal choice for the treatment of UA/NSTEMI.

There are limited data to recommend LMWH over UFH in the setting of PCI. Available evidence suggests that both therapies are safe and efficacious, although the two treatments have not been directly compared. One possible strategy is to substitute UFH for

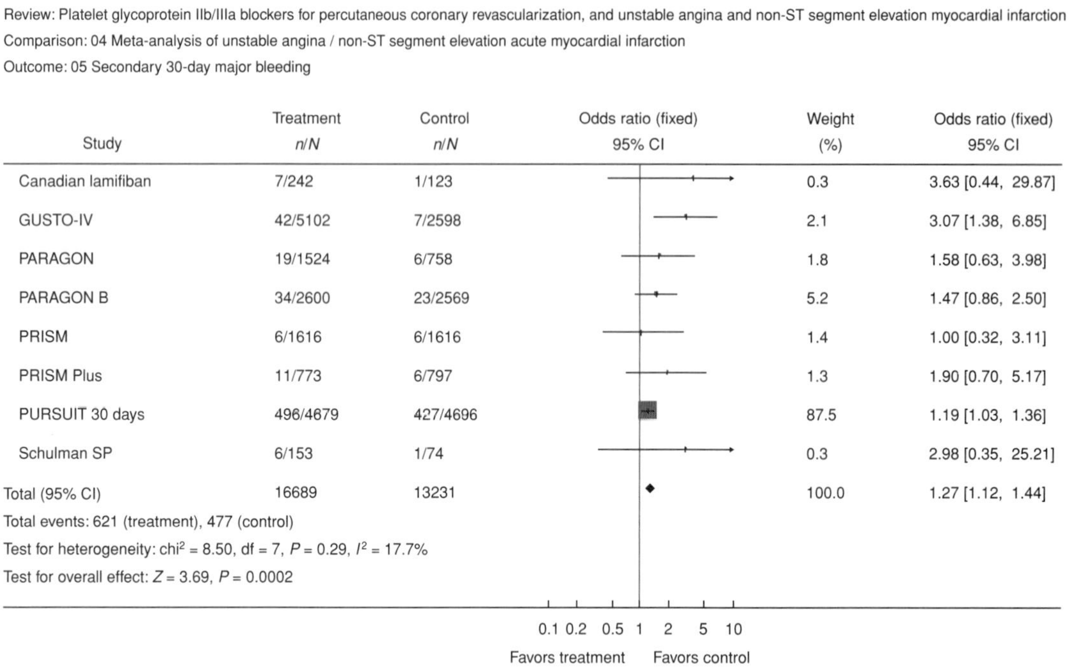

Review: Platelet glycoprotein IIb/IIIa blockers for percutaneous coronary revascularization, and unstable angina and non-ST segment elevation myocardial infarction

Comparison: 04 Meta-analysis of unstable angina / non-ST segment elevation acute myocardial infarction

Outcome: 05 Secondary 30-day major bleeding

Study	Treatment n/N	Control n/N	Odds ratio (fixed) 95% CI	Weight (%)	Odds ratio (fixed) 95% CI
Canadian lamifiban	7/242	1/123		0.3	3.63 [0.44, 29.87]
GUSTO-IV	42/5102	7/2598		2.1	3.07 [1.38, 6.85]
PARAGON	19/1524	6/758		1.8	1.58 [0.63, 3.98]
PARAGON B	34/2600	23/2569		5.2	1.47 [0.86, 2.50]
PRISM	6/1616	6/1616		1.4	1.00 [0.32, 3.11]
PRISM Plus	11/773	6/797		1.3	1.90 [0.70, 5.17]
PURSUIT 30 days	496/4679	427/4696		87.5	1.19 [1.03, 1.36]
Schulman SP	6/153	1/74		0.3	2.98 [0.35, 25.21]
Total (95% CI)	16689	13231		100.0	1.27 [1.12, 1.44]

Total events: 621 (treatment), 477 (control)

Test for heterogeneity: chi^2 = 8.50, df = 7, P = 0.29, I^2 = 17.7%

Test for overall effect: Z = 3.69, P = 0.0002

0.1 0.2 0.5 1 2 5 10

Favors treatment   Favors control

Figure 17.3 Platelet glycoprotein IIb/IIIa increases the incidence of major bleeding in patients with UA/NSTEMI. (Reproduced with permission from Bosch & Marrugat [52], © 2001 Cochrane Library.)

LMWH prior to PCI if the last LMWH dose was given more than 8–12 hours before the procedure [50].

Question 8: In patients with ACS (population), does the use of IIb/IIIa inhibitors in the ED setting (intervention) decrease mortality and morbidity (outcome) compared to routine care (control)?

Search strategy

- Cochrane Library: (unstable angina OR acute coronary syndrome) AND glycoprotein IIb/IIIa

The glycoprotein IIb/IIIa integrin present on platelets mediates the final common pathway in platelet aggregation [51]. Glycoprotein IIb/IIIa receptor antagonists induce profound platelet inhibition; however, this potential benefit in the treatment of ACS must be weighed against the potential for serious bleeding complications (Fig. 17.3). A Cochrane review identified eight trials involving 30,006 patients in which glycoprotein IIb/IIIa inhibitors were compared to standard care in patients with UA and NSTEMI [52]. Glycoprotein IIb/IIIa inhibitors were not associated with a decreased mortality at 20 days (OR = 0.90; 95% CI: 0.80 to 1.02) or 6 months (OR = 1.01; 95% CI: 0.88 to 0.95). Myocardial infarction (defined as an elevated troponin) was unfortunately not reported as a separate outcome. When death and MI were considered as a composite outcome, glycoprotein IIb/IIIa antagonists were superior to placebo at 30 days (OR = 0.91; 95% CI: 0.85 to 0.98; NNT =

100) and 6 months (OR = 0.88; 95% CI: 0.81 to 0.95; NNT = 77). Severe bleeding was described in all trials included in the analysis. Glycoprotein IIb/IIIa inhibitors significantly increased the rate of major bleeding (OR = 1.27; 95% CI: 1.12 to 1.44) with one additional severe bleed (e.g., intracranial or gastrointestinal bleeding) for every 1000 patients treated. Severe bleeding was defined as intracranial hemorrhage, cardiac tamponade or need for transfusion. Another meta-analysis with similar results advocated the use of glycoprotein IIb/IIIa inhibitors to reduce cardiac complications even in those patients with ACS not routinely scheduled for early revascularization [53].

From the same Cochrane review there is better evidence for the use of glycoprotein IIb/IIIa antagonists in patients with ACS undergoing percutaneous coronary revascularization where their use was associated with a significant reduction in mortality at 30 days (OR = 0.71; 95% CI: 0.52 to 0.97). Indeed, the authors of a third systematic review conducted a post hoc analysis that suggested that the reduction in mortality and MI observed in patients treated with glycoprotein IIb/IIIa inhibitors was restricted to those patients who received PCI (Fig. 17.4) [54].

The ACUITY Timing Trial (n = 9207) examined the routine upstream use of glycoprotein treatment strategy compared to deferred selective use in patients undergoing PCI [55]. Composite ischemic events at 30 days occurred in 7.9% of patients assigned to the deferred use compared with 7.1% of patients assigned to upstream administration (RR = 1.12; 95% CI: 0.97 to 1.29). Deferred use was associated with less frequent 30-day rates of major bleeding compared to routine upstream use (RR = 0.80; 95% CI: 0.67 to 0.95).

Review: Early invasive versus conservative strategies for unstable angina % non-ST elevation myocardial infarction in the stent era

Comparison: 01 All studies undertaken in the stent era regardless of glycoprotein IIb/IIIa receptor use

Outcome: 07 Intermediate myocardial infarction

Study	Invasive n/N	Conservative n/N	Relative risk (random) 95% CI	Weight (%)	Relative risk (random) 95% CI
01 Routine glycoprotein IIb/IIIa receptor antagonist use					
ICTUS	51/604	35/596		21.7	1.44 [0.95, 2.18]
TACTICS-TIMI 18	53/1114	76/1106		24.6	0.69 [0.49, 0.97]
Subtotal (95% CI)	1718	1702		46.3	0.99 [0.48, 2.02]
Total events: 104 (invasive), 111 (conservative)					
Test for heterogeneity: chi^2 = 7.11, df = 1, P = 0.008, I^2 = 85.9%					
Test for overall effect: Z = 0.03, P = 1					
02 No routine glycoprotein IIb/IIIa receptor antagonist use					
FRISC-II	105/1222	143/1235		28.6	0.74 [0.58, 0.94]
RITA-3	34/895	44/915		20.9	0.79 [0.51, 1.22]
VINO 2002	2/64	10/67		4.2	0.21 [0.05, 0.92]
Subtotal (95% CI)	2181	2217		53.7	0.72 [0.52, 0.98]
Total events: 141 (invasive), 197 (conservative)					
Test for heterogeneity: chi^2 = 2.89, df = 2, P = 0.24, I^2 = 30.8%					
Test for overall effect: Z = 2.07, P = 0.04					
Total (95% CI)	3899	3919		100.0	0.81 [0.59, 1.12]
Total events: 245 (invasive), 308 (conservative)					
Test for heterogeneity: chi^2 = 11.89, df = 4, P = 0.02, I^2 = 66.4%					
Test for overall effect: Z = 1.29, P = 0.2					

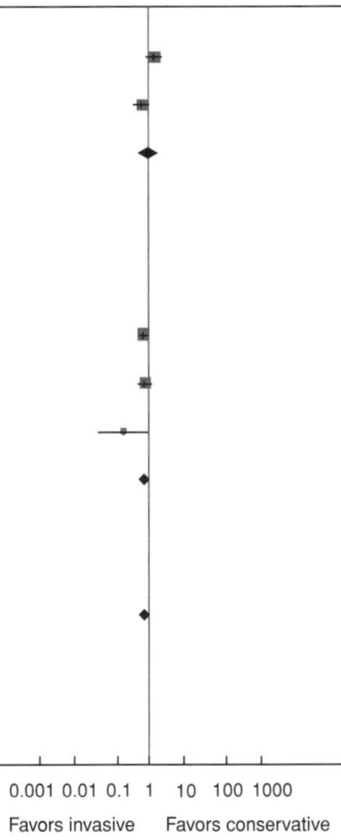

0.001 0.01 0.1 1 10 100 1000

Favors invasive   Favors conservative

Figure 17.4 Similar rates of intermediate MI were observed in the early invasive and conservative groups. (Reproduced with permission from Hoenig et al. [57], © 2006 Cochrane Library.)

In summary, the most current guidelines conclude that glycoprotein IIb/IIIa inhibitors offer benefit in patients with UA/NSTEMI who undergo PCI, particularly those who are high risk and troponin positive. In patients in whom an initial noninvasive conservative strategy is planned, the evidence for their benefit is less convincing [29].

Question 9: In patients with ACS (population), does immediate invasive strategy (intervention) improve mortality and morbidity (outcome) compared to a selective (conservative) strategy (control)?

Search strategy

- Cochrane Library: (unstable angina OR acute coronary syndrome) AND invasive strategy

There is clear evidence that patients with recurrent ischemia and coronary anatomy that is deemed appropriate have better outcomes if they undergo early PCI [56]. However, patients initially thought to have ACS are a heterogeneous group, and some will ultimately be diagnosed with a non-cardiac etiology for their chest pain. After the initial medical management of UA/NSTEMI, two different treatment strategies are possible. In an "early invasive" strategy, coronary angiography is routinely performed on all patients. In an "early conservative" strategy, only those patients who are considered at high risk with evidence of recurrent or provokable ischemia undergo coronary angiography. A Cochrane review that included five trials and 7818 patients offers the best evidence for choosing the most appropriate treatment strategy [57]. There was a trend towards increased mortality during the index hospitalization in the early invasive group (RR = 1.59; 95% CI: 0.96 to 2.64). However, in the two trials which followed subjects for at least 2 years, the mortality was significantly improved in patients who underwent early angiography (RR = 0.75; 95% CI: 0.62 to 0.92) with a NNT of 42 [58,59]. Early and intermediate MI was not reduced by an invasive strategy; however, late MI was significantly reduced (RR = 0.75; 95% CI: 0.61 to 0.91).

Two other systematic reviews also addressed this issue [60,61]. They did not include a more recent study that was identified in the Cochrane review [62] and included three additional trials from the pre-stent era [63–65]. All of the reviews consistently showed benefit in the early invasive group with respect to both refractory angina (RR = 0.67; 95% CI: 0.55 to 0.83) and re-hospitalization (RR = 0.67; 95% CI: 0.61 to 0.74). This must be weighed against the cost of more peri-procedural myocardial infarctions (RR = 2.05; 95% CI: 1.56 to 2.70) in the invasive group compared to the conservative group.

Clinically, the data suggest that an early invasive strategy is superior to a conservative approach. The trials have, however, enrolled a heterogeneous group of patients with varying levels of risk and event rates. In the future, the application of validated risk scores may allow clinicians to more accurately stratify those patients most likely to receive the maximum absolute benefit from an invasive strategy.

Conclusions

The patient's blood work returned and his cardiac markers were not elevated. He was given LMWH (100 mg enoxaparin subcutaneously), started on clopidogrel (300 mg loading dose orally) and admitted to the cardiac care unit. The next day, he had angiography, which demonstrated a significant narrowing of his left anterior descending coronary artery. He underwent successful angioplasty and stenting of the lesion with concurrent administration of a glycoprotein IIb/IIIa inhibitor. He recovered without incident and was discharged home, where he subsequently returned to his previous level of functioning.

Acute coronary syndromes are common presentations to the ED and require rapid diagnosis and treatment to prevent significant morbidity and mortality. The recommendations summarized here provide clinicians with the knowledge to appropriately risk-stratify patients with ACS so that they may receive maximal therapy to prevent platelet aggregation and thrombus formation, thereby limiting cardiac ischemia and ultimately myocardial infarction or death.

Acknowledgments

To my wife, Beth, and family – for your love, support and patience.

Conflicts of interest

None were reported.

References

1 Nourjah P. *National Hospital Ambulatory Medical Care Survey: 1997 emergency department summary*. National Center for Health Statistics, Hyattsville, MD, 1999 (data from *Vital Health Stat* 1999;**304**).

2 National Center for Health Statistics. *Detailed Diagnoses and Procedures: National Hospital Discharge Survey, 1996*. National Center for Health Statistics, Hyattsville, MD, 1998 (data from *Vital Health Stat* 1998;**138**).

3 Kong DF, Blazing MA, O'Connor CM. The health care burden of unstable angina. *Cardiol Clin* 1999;**17**:247–61.

4 Jackevicius CA, Tu K, Filate WA, et al. Trends in cardiovascular drug utilization and drug expenditures in Canada between 1996 and 2001. *Can J Cardiol* 2003;**19**:1366–9.

5 Topal EJ. Economics and quality of care for patients with acute coronary syndromes: the impending crisis. *Clin Cardiol* 2002;**25**(Suppl 1):9–15.

6 Braunwald E, Jones RH, Mark DB, et al. Diagnosing and managing unstable angina. *Circulation* 1994;**90**:613–22.

7 Antman EM, Cohen M, Bernink PJ, et al. The TIMI risk score for unstable angina/non-ST elevation MI. *JAMA* 2000;**284**:835–42.

8 Eagle KA, Lim MJ, Dabbous OH, et al. A validated prediction model for all forms of acute coronary syndrome estimating the risk of 6-month post-discharge death in an international registry. *JAMA* 2004;**291**:2727–33.

9 Boersma E, Pieper KS, Steyerber EW, et al. Predictors of outcome in patients with acute coronary syndromes without persistent ST-segment elevation. *Circulation* 2000;**101**:2557–67.

10 Yan AT, Jong P, Yan RT, et al. Clinical trial-derived risk model may not generalize to real-world patients with acute coronary syndrome. *Am Heart J* 2004;**148**:1020–27.

11 Harrell FE, Jr., Califf RM, Pryor DB, et al. Evaluating the yield of medical tests. *JAMA* 1982;**247**:2543–6.

12 Sabatine MS, McCabe CH, Morrow DA, et al. Identification of patients at high risk for death and a cardiac ischemic event after hospital discharge. *Am Heart J* 2002;**143**:966–70.

13 Cannon CP, Weintraub WS, Demopoulos LA, et al. Comparison of early invasive and conservative strategies in patients with unstable coronary syndromes treated with the glycoprotein IIb/IIIa inhibitor tirofiban. *N Engl J Med* 2001;**344**:1879–87.

14 Morrow DA, Antman EM, Snapinn S, et al. An integrated clinical approach to predicting the benefit of tirofiban in non-ST elevation acute coronary syndromes: application of the TIMI risk score for UA/NSTEMI in PRISM-PLUS. *Eur Heart J* 2002;**23**:223–9.

15 Scirica BM, Cannon CP, Antman EM, et al. Validation of the Thrombolysis In Myocardial Infarction (TIMI) risk score for unstable angina pectoris and non-ST-segment-elevation myocardial infarction in the TIMI III registry. *Am J Card* 2002;**90**:303–5.

16 Budaj A, Yusuf S, Mehta SR, et al. Benefit of clopidogrel in patients with acute coronary syndromes without ST-segment elevation in various risk groups. *Circulation* 2002;**106**:1622–6.

17 Pollack CV, Sites FD, Shofer FS, et al. Application of the TIMI risk score for unstable angina and non-ST elevation acute coronary syndrome to an unselected emergency department chest pain population. *Acad Emerg Med* 2006;**13**:13–18.

18 Chase M, Robey JL, Zogby KE, et al. Prospective validation of the thrombolysis in myocardial infarction risk score in the emergency department chest pain population. *Ann Emerg Med* 2006;**48**:252–9.

19 Araujo Goncalves P, Ferreira J, Aguiar C, Seabra-Gomes R. TIMI, PURSUIT, and GRACE risk scores: sustained prognostic value and interaction with revascularization in NSTE-ACS. *Eur Heart J* 2005;**26**:865–72.

20 Lyon R, Morris AC, Caesar D, Gray S, Gray A. Chest pain presenting to the Emergency Department – to stratify risk with GRACE or TIMI? *Resuscitation* 2007;**74**(1):90–93.

21 Antithrombotic Trialists' Collaboration. Collaborative meta-analysis of randomised trials of antiplatelet therapy for prevention of death, myocardial infarction, and stroke in high risk patients. *BMJ* 2002;**324**:71–86.

22 CAPRIE Steering Committee. A randomised, blinded trial of clopidogrel versus aspirin in patients at risk of ischaemic events (CAPRIE). *Lancet* 1996;**348**:1329–39.

23 Yusuf S, Shao F, Mehta S, et al. The clopidogrel in unstable angina to prevent recurrent events (CURE) trial. *N Engl J Med* 2001;**345**:494–502.

24 Mehta S, Yusuf S, Peters RJG, et al. Effects of pretreatment with clopidogrel and aspirin followed by long-term therapy in patients undergoing percutaneous coronary intervention: the PCI-CURE study. *Lancet* 2001;**358**:527–33.

25 Balsano F, Rizzon P, Violi F, et al. Antiplatelet treatment with ticlopidine in unstable angina. *Circulation* 1990;**82**:17–26.

26 McLean DS, Sabatine MS, Guo W, McCabe CH, Cannon CP. Benefits and risks of clopidogrel pretreatment before coronary artery bypass grafting in patients with ST-elevation myocardial infarction treated with fibrinolytics in CLARITY-TIMI 28. *J Thromb Thrombolysis* 2007;**24**(2):85–91.

27 Sabatine MS, Cannon CP, Gibson CM, et al. Addition of clopidogrel to aspirin and fibrinolytic therapy for myocardial infarction with ST-segment elevation. *N Engl J Med* 2005;**352**:1179–89.

28 Lange RA, Hillis LD. Concurrent antiplatelet and fibrinolytic therapy. *N Engl J Med* 2005;**352**:1248–50.

29 Anderson JL, Adams CD, Antman EM, et al. ACC/AHA 2007 guidelines for the management of patients with unstable angina/non-ST-elevation myocardial infarction. *J Am Coll Cardiol* 2007;**50**:1–157.

30 Yusuf S, Collins R, MacMahon S, Peto R. Effect of intravenous nitrates on mortality in acute myocardial infarction: an overview of the randomised trials. *Lancet* 1988;**1**:1088–92.

31 Gruppo Italiano per lo Studio della Sopravvivenza nell'infarto Miocardico. GISSI-3: effects of lisinopril and transdermal glyceryl trinitrate singly and together on 6-week mortality and ventricular function after acute myocardial infarction. *Lancet* 1994;**343**:1115–22.

32 ISIS-4 (Fourth International Study of Infarct Survival) Collaborative Group. ISIS-4: a randomised factorial trial assessing early oral captopril, oral mononitrate, and intravenous magnesium sulphate in 58,050 patients with suspected acute myocardial infarction. *Lancet* 1005;**345**:669–85.

33 Karlberg KE, Saldeen T, Wallin R, et al. Intravenous nitroglycerin reduces ischaemia in unstable angina pectoris: a double-blind placebo-controlled study. *J Intern Med* 1998;**243**:25–31.

34 Doucet S, Malekianpour M, Theroux P, et al. Randomized trial comparing intravenous nitroglycerin and heparin for treatment of unstable angina secondary to restenosis after coronary artery angioplasty. *Circulation* 2000;**101**:955–61.

35 HINT Research Group. Early treatment of unstable angina in the coronary care unit: a randomized, double blind, placebo controlled comparison of recurrent ischaemia in patients treated with nifedipine or metoprolol or both. *Br Heart J* 1986;**56**:400–413.

36 Gottlieb SO, Weisfeldt ML, Ouyang P, et al. Effect of the addition of propranolol to therapy with nifedipine for unstable angina pectoris: a randomized, double-blind, placebo-controlled trial. *Circulation* 1986;**73**:331–7.

37 Brunner M, Faber TS, Greve B, et al. Usefulness of carvediolol in unstable angina pectoris. *Am J Cardiol* 2000;**85**:1173–8.

38 Hohnloser SH, Meinertz T, Klingenheben T, et al. Usefulness of esmolol in unstable angina pectoris. *Am J Cardiol* 1991;**67**:1319–23.

39 COMMIT Collaborative Group. Addition of clopidogrel to aspirin in 45852 patients with acute myocardial infarction: randomized placebo-controlled trial. *Lancet* 2005;**366**:1607–21.

40 Task FM, Lopez-Sendo J, Swedberg K, et al. Expert consensus document on beta-adrenergic receptor blockers: the Task Force on Beta-Blockers of the European Society of Cardiology. *Eur Heart J* 2004;**25**:1341–62.

41 Magee K, Campbell SG, Moher D, Rowe BH. Heparins versus placebo for acute coronary syndromes. *Cochrane Database Syst Rev* 2008;**2**:CD003462 (doi: 10.1002/14651858.CD003462).

42 Eikelboom JW, Anand SS, Malmberg K, Weitz JI, Warkentin TE. Unfractionated heparin and low-molecular-weight-heparin in acute coronary syndrome without ST elevation: a meta-analysis. *Lancet* 2000;**355**:1936–42.

43 Gurfinkel EP, Manos EJ, Mejail RI, et al. Low molecular weight heparin versus regular heparin or aspirin in the treatment of unstable angina and silent ischemia. *J Am Coll Cardiol* 1995;**26**:313–18.

44 Fragmin during Instability in Coronary Artery Disease (FRISC) Study Group. Low-molecular-weight-heparin during instability in coronary artery disease. *Lancet* 1996;**347**:561–8.

45 Fareed J, Hoppensteadt D, Jeske W, et al. Low molecular weight heparins: are they different? *Can J Cardiol* 1988;**14**:28E–34E.

46 Warkentin TE, Levine MN, Hirsh J, et al. Heparin-induced thrombocytopenia in patients treated with low molecular weight heparin or unfractionated heparin. *N Engl J Med* 1995;**332**:1330–35.

47 Magee K, Sevcik W, Moher D, Rowe BH. Low molecular weight heparins versus unfractionated heparin for acute coronary syndromes. *Cochrane Database Syst Rev* 2003;**1**:CD002132 (doi: 10.1002/14651858).

48 Suvarna TT, Parikh JA, Keshave R, Pillai MG, Pahlanani DB, Gandhi MJ. Comparison of clinical outcome of fixed-dose subcutaneous low molecular weight heparin (tinzaprin) with conventional heparin in unstable angina: a pilot study. *Indian Heart J* 1997;**49**:159–62.

49 Michalis LK, Katsouras CS, Papamichael N, et al. Enoxaparin versus tinzaparin in non-ST-segment elevation acute coronary syndromes: the EVET trial. *Am Heart J* 2003;**146**:304–10.

50 Wong GC, Giugliano RP, Antman EM. Use of low molecular weight heparins in the management of acute coronary artery syndromes and percutaneous coronary intervention. *JAMA* 2003;**289**:331–42.

51 Phillips DR, Charo IF, Parise LV, Fitzgerald LA. The platelet membrane glycoprotein IIb-IIIa complex. *Blood* 1988;**71**:831–3.

52 Bosch X, Marrugat J. Platelet glycoprotein IIb/IIIa blockers for percutaneous coronary revascularization, and unstable angina and non-ST-segment elevation myocardial infarction. *Cochrane Database Syst Rev* 2001;**4**:CD002130 (doi: 10.1002/14651858).

53 Boersma E, Harrington RA, Moliterno DJ, et al. Review: glycoprotein IIb/IIIa inhibitors reduced death or MI in acute coronary syndromes not routinely scheduled for revascularization. *Lancet* 2002;**359**:189–98.

54 Roffi M, Chew DP, Mukherjee D, et al. Platelet glycoprotein IIb/IIIa inhibition in acute coronary syndromes. Gradient of benefit related to the revascularization strategy. *Eur Heart J* 2002;**23**:1441–8.

55 Stone GW, Bertrand ME, Moses JW, et al. Routine upstream initiation versus deferred selective use of glycoprotein IIb/IIIa inhibitors in acute coronary syndromes. *JAMA* 2007;**297**:591–602.

56 Michalis LK, Stroumbis CS, Pappas K, et al. Treatment of refractory unstable angina in geographically isolated areas without cardiac surgery. Invasive versus conservative strategy (TRUCS study). *Eur Heart J* 2000;**23**:1954–9.

57 Hoenig MR, Doust JA, Aroney CN, Scott IA. Early invasive versus conservative strategies for unstable angina and non-ST-elevation myocardial infarction in the stent era. *Cochrane Database Syst Rev* 2006;**3**:CD004815 (doi: 10.1002/14651858).

58 Lagerqvist B, Husted S, Kontny F, et al. A long-term perspective on the protective effects of an early invasive strategy in unstable coronary artery

disease: two-year follow-up of the FRISC-II invasive study. *J Am Coll Cardiol* 2002;**40**:1902–14.

59 Fox KA, Poole-Wilson PA, Henderson RA, et al. Interventional versus conservative treatment for patients with unstable angina or non-ST-elevation myocardial infarction: the British Heart Foundation RITA 3 randomised trial, Randomized Intervention Trial of unstable Angina. *Lancet* 2002;**360**:743–51.

60 Choudhry NK, Singh JM, Barolet A, Tomlinson GA, Detsky AS. How should patients with unstable angina and non-ST-segment elevation myocardial infarction be managed? A meta-analysis of randomized trials. *Am J Med* 2005;**118**:465–74.

61 Mehta S, Cannon CP, Wallentin L, et al. Routine vs selective invasive strategies in patients with acute coronary syndromes: a collaborative meta-analysis of randomized trials. *JAMA* 2005;**93**:2908–17.

62 de Winter RJ, Winhausen F, Cornel JH, et al. Early invasive versus selectively invasive management for acute coronary syndromes. *N Engl J Med* 2005;**353**:1095–104.

63 Anderson HV, Cannon CP, Stone PH, et al. A randomized comparison of tissue-type plasminogen activator versus placebo and early invasive versus early conservative strategies in unstable angina and non-W wave myocardial infarction. *J Am Coll Cardiol* 1995;**26**:1643–50.

64 Boden WE, O'Rourke RA, Crawford MS, et al. Outcomes in patients with acute non-Q-wave myocardial infarction randomly assigned to an invasive as compared with a conservative management strategy. Veterans Affairs Non-Q-Wave Infarction Strategies in Hospital (VANQWISH) Trial Investigators. *N Engl J Med* 1998;**338**:1785–92.

65 McCullough PA, O'Neil WW, Graham M, et al. A prospective randomized trial of triage angiography in acute coronary syndromes ineligible for thrombolytic therapy. Result of the Medicine versus Angiography in Thrombolytic Exclusion (MATE) trial. *J Am Coll Cardiol* 1998;**32**:596–605.

66 Yan AT, Yan RT, Tan M, et al. Risk scores for risk stratification in acute coronary syndromes: useful but simpler is not necessarily better. *Eur Heart J* 2007;**29**:1072–8.

18 Acute Myocardial Infarction

Bjug Borgundvaag

Schwartz/Reisman Emergency Centre, Mount Sinai Hospital, Toronto, Canada

Case scenario

A 52-year-old man presented to the emergency department (ED) at 8:15 p.m. with a 1-hour history of constant, mid-sternal chest pressure radiating to his left axilla, jaw and back. He reported having similar but less severe discomfort, primarily with exertion, in the previous 2 days. His previous episodes had resolved within a few minutes of resting, and never exceeded 20 minutes in duration. He reported a 35 pack/year history of smoking, and a family history of myocardial infarction (MI) (his father, at age 54); however, he had no other cardiac risk factors, and denied taking any medications.

The patient appeared uncomfortable and was diaphoretic. His vital signs were pulse 124 beat/min, blood pressure 147/101 mmHg, respiratory rate 68 beats/min and SO_2 (2 L O_2 by nasal prongs) of 96%. His weight was 88 kg. His jugular venous pressure (JVP) was 2 cm above the sternal angle, his heart sounds were normal, and no murmurs were present. His chest was clear, there were no signs of congestive heart failure, and the remainder of his physical exam was unremarkable.

The 12-lead electrocardiogram (ECG) is shown in Fig. 18.1 and the 15-lead ECG is shown in Fig. 18.2. A diagnosis of acute ST elevation myocardial infarction (STEMI) was made. Since this patient met generally accepted criteria for revascularization therapy, all treatment options were considered (e.g., primary angioplasty, fibrinolysis, a combination of the two, and no revascularization therapy). You discussed the options with your patient, who asked which option will result in the best outcome in his case.

Background

STEMI is a commonly encountered problem in the ED. The mortality associated with STEMI is front-end loaded, with the majority

Evidence-based Emergency Medicine. Edited by Brian H. Rowe
© 2009 Blackwell Publishing, ISBN: 978-1-4051-6143-5.

of adverse outcomes occurring in the first hours to days after the onset of the MI [1]. From the first studies comparing fibrinolysis with placebo treatment, it has been recognized that time to fibrinolysis is the critical determinant of outcome [2]. The relationship between time to treatment and outcomes also applies to patients undergoing mechanical revascularization [3], suggesting that every effort be made to reduce time to revascularization regardless of treatment modality.

Historically, the use of fibrinolytics in acute MI has been used as an example of the importance of evidence-based medicine in treatment decisions in health care. In 1992, a group of researchers led by Lau conducted a systematic review examining the role of fibrinolysis in the treatment of acute MI [4]. This cumulative analysis proved that conclusive evidence favoring the use of these agents existed long before the mega-trial era and even longer before the treatment was advised as "routine" treatment in standard text books. Knowing the delay is in knowledge translation, this likely prolonged the "care gap" in acute MI, a gap between what is known and what is practiced in medicine. The delay in translating this evidence meant that many hundreds of thousands of patients were denied the opportunity of effective care.

Traditionally, STEMI patients have been treated with fibrinolysis in the ED, and the emphasis has been on early identification and administration of lytic agents. It has long been recognized, however, that not all patients with STEMI are effectively treated with fibrinolysis. Angiographic studies have shown that 46% of STEMI patients treated with fibrinolysis continue to have an occluded infarct-related artery within 90 minutes of lytic administration [5]. While enormous effort has been devoted to improving the effectiveness and safety of fibrinolytic agents (increasing fibrin specificity, development of bolus agents) and improved adjuvant treatments (primarily antithrombin and antiplatelet therapy), improvements in outcomes using pharmacotherapy have been very modest. Frustration with the slow pace of improvement has resulted in renewed interest in mechanical reperfusion options. The most significant changes to the management of STEMI in the last 10 years have been the result of advances in primary angioplasty, also referred to as a percutaneous coronary

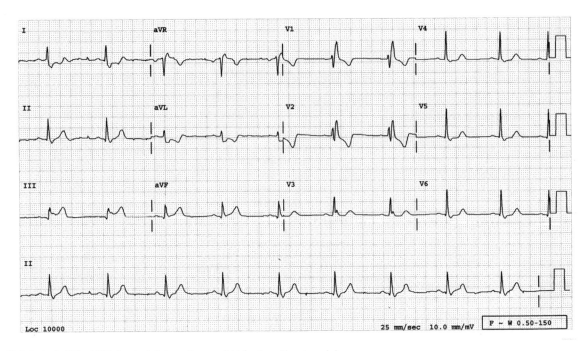

Figure 18.1 Patient's 12-lead ECG showing inferior wall myocardial infarction with reciprocal changes.

intervention (PCI). The mechanical approach has been widely accepted to be superior to the pharmacological one [6]; however, important limitations to this generalization exist, especially pertaining to timing and availability of the procedure. There are significant challenges to providing mechanical reperfusion in a timely fashion, and inclusion of PCI in the routine management of STEMI has greatly increased the complexity of care for STEMI patients, especially in facilities which do not have around-the-clock interventional cardiology availability. This chapter examines the role of fibrinolytics, PCI and other interventions in the

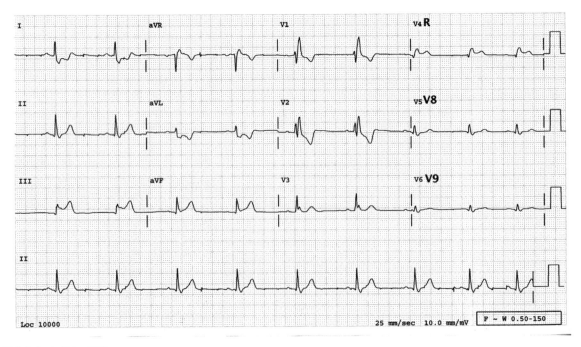

Figure 18.2 Patient's 15-lead ECG.

evidence-based treatment of patients presenting to the ED with a STEMI.

Clinical questions

In order to address the issues of greatest relevance to your patients and to help in searching the literature for the evidence regarding these issues, you should structure your clinical questions as recommended in Chapter 1.

1 In patients with suspected STEMI (population), does the use of prehospital 12-lead ECG (intervention) reduce time to ECG and reduce mortality (outcomes) compared to standard treatment (control)?

2 In patients with the confirmed diagnosis of STEMI (population), does the prehospital administration of fibrinolysis (intervention) reduce death, repeat chest pain or revascularization procedures (outcomes) compared to in-ED fibrinolytic administration (control)?

3 In patients with STEMI (population), does the administration of acetyl-salicylic acid (ASA) (intervention) reduce death, repeat chest pain or revascularization (outcomes) compared to non-ASA treatment (control)?

4 In patients with STEMI (population), does the administration of β-blockers (intervention) reduce death, repeat chest pain or revascularization (outcomes) compared to standard care (control)?

5 In patients with STEMI (population), does the administration of fibrinolysis (intervention) reduce death, repeat chest pain or revascularization (outcomes) compared to standard care (control)? If so, which patients should receive treatment?

6 In patients with the presumed diagnosis of STEMI (population), does primary angioplasty (intervention) reduce death, repeat chest pain or revascularization (outcomes) compared to patients administered with fibrinolysis (control)?

7 In patients with STEMI who receive fibrinolysis (population), does the administration of heparin as adjunctive therapy (intervention) reduce mortality, revascularization and complications (outcomes) compared to fibrinolysis alone (control)?

General search strategy

Cardiology is a unique field in which randomized controlled trials and systematic reviews are available for many of the key ED questions. In fact, one of the first systematic reviews published that identified a practice gap was published on the fibrinolytic treatment of acute MI [4]. Electronic databases such as the Cochrane Library, MEDLINE and EMBASE were searched first looking for systematic reviews and meta-analyses. Clinical trials, cohort studies, consensus statements and pertinent review articles were identified. The Clinical Guideline Clearinghouse (www.guideline.gov)

and American College of Emergency Physicians clinical policies were also searched.

Critical appraisal of the literature

Question 1: In patients with suspected STEMI (population), does the use of prehospital 12-lead ECG (intervention) reduce time to ECG and reduce mortality (outcomes) compared to standard treatment (control)?

Search strategy

- MEDLINE: (pre-hospital OR prehospital OR EMS OR emergency medical services) AND (12-lead ECG OR ECG OR EKG OR electrocardiography) AND (AMI OR MI OR myocardial infarction)

The axiom "time is muscle" has been shown to be true since the original studies investigating the use of systemic fibrinolysis for the treatment of STEMI [2]. Since STEMI remains a leading cause of death around the world, significant effort has been directed towards the rapid identification and treatment of patients suffering from this condition.

The World Health Organization (WHO) definition of acute MI includes a combination of at least two of the following three characteristic symptoms: (i) typical symptoms (e.g., chest discomfort); (ii) enzyme rise and fall over an expected time course; and (iii) typical ECG changes evolving into the development of Q waves. While these criteria have recently been amended to include the use of more cardiac specific markers (troponins [7]), and additional tools are available at some hospitals, the tools available to most emergency physicians have remained essentially constant. As such, the diagnosis of acute MI in the ED has remained heavily dependent on the evaluation of these three criteria.

Clearly, in STEMI, the key diagnostic tool is the ECG, and timeliness of this test is of critical importance. For example, the current American Heart Association quality standard for time to ECG evaluation in patients with suspected ischemic chest pain is 10 minutes [8].

There are several theoretical reasons to believe that a strategy which moves the actual diagnosis of STEMI to the prehospital setting may prove beneficial in the management of STEMI:

1 In many instances, the distance between a patient's location and the nearest treatment facility can be considerable. There is evidence that the diagnosis and treatment (with fibrinolytic therapy) of STEMI in the field results in better outcomes, especially if transport times are long

2 Advance notification of ED personnel that a STEMI patient is en route may allow a better level of preparedness at the receiving ED. Registry data have shown that such patients receive more aggressive treatment and have improved outcomes. Canto et al. [9] demonstrated that patients who received a prehospital 12-lead ECG were more likely to receive in-hospital fibrinolytic therapy, angiography and revascularization treatment. This approach translated into a significantly reduced in-hospital mortality from 12% to 8% (OR = 0.83; 95% CI: 0.71 to 0.96).

3 As medical systems develop, and primary angioplasty becomes increasingly available, the ability to make a diagnosis in the field will allow first responders to be able to direct patients to the best available resource for their treatment. For example, transportation of patients directly to the cardiac catheterization lab (bypassing the ED completely) will save time and improve outcomes [10–12].

For these reasons, consensus guidelines encourage the use of prehospital ECGs [8].

Two recent meta-analyses have been performed on the effectiveness of prehospital ECG, although each used slightly different selection criteria. These analyses, while both small, are consistent in their findings, with slightly different magnitudes of benefit. Brainard et al. [13] included four studies, with a total of only 99 patients, and demonstrated a reduction in time to reperfusion therapy of 22 minutes (95% CI: 20 to 24 minutes). Patients who had a prehospital ECG had a mean time to reperfusion of 36.5 minutes (95% CI: 32.4 to 40.6 minutes) compared to 58.5 minutes (95% CI: 56.1 to 60.9 minutes). Morrison et al. [14] included three of the same studies as Brainard with two more recent studies, with a total of 181 patients. They found a mean reduction in door-to-needle time of 36.1 minutes (95% CI: 9.3 to 63 minutes), with no significant increase in on-site time.

In summary, there are several theoretical reasons for believing that obtaining a prehospital ECG reduces time to treatment and may improve outcomes, and data from existing small studies demonstrate consistent benefit. Data from large-scale randomized controlled trials are lacking; however, it seems sensible for EDs and emergency medical services (EMS) programs to develop coordinated strategies for identifying patients in the prehospital setting using ECGs and transporting these patients rapidly. While this is an important strategy, it only applies to the perhaps one-quarter of STEMI patients who attend the ED via ambulance [15]. Consequently, EDs must develop strategies to identify patients who have STEMI through rapid ECG testing.

Question 2: In patients with the confirmed diagnosis of STEMI (population), does the prehospital administration of fibrinolysis (intervention) reduce death, repeat chest pain or revascularization procedures (outcomes) compared to in-ED fibrinolytic administration (control)?

Search strategy

- MEDLINE: (pre-hospital OR prehospital OR EMS OR emergency medical services OR transportation of patients) AND (thrombolysis OR revascularization OR primary angioplasty) AND (chest pain OR AMI OR MI OR myocardial infarction)

The primary goal in the treatment of STEMI is to deliver revascularization therapy as quickly as possible. The ultimate expression of this philosophy has been to try and initiate revascularization therapy at the earliest point of care.

In urban areas where ED services are minutes away, prehospital fibrinolysis may not make sense; however, there are many circumstances where it may be possible to considerably reduce time to fibrinolysis and improve outcomes by initiating therapy in the field. In their 1997 review, the United States National Heart Attack Alert Program concluded that prehospital fibrinolysis reduces mortality in the subgroup of patients with long (> 1 hour) transport times [16].

A meta-analysis of mortality and prehospital fibrinolysis, which included 6434 patients randomized in six clinical trials, was published in 2000 [17]. This analysis demonstrated a significantly reduced in-hospital mortality for patients treated with fibrinolysis in the prehospital phase compared to those treated in hospital (OR = 0.83; 95% CI: 0.70 to 0.98). These results were consistent regardless of the training and experience of the EMS provider. The evidence suggests that this reduction in mortality was largely due to a significant reduction in the time to initiation of fibrinolysis, from 162 to 104 minutes for patients treated in hospital and prehospital, respectively.

Though data from large-scale randomized controlled trials is not available, more recent data from smaller studies performed in a variety of settings (Europe, North America) and using EMS providers with varying degrees of training (paramedics, doctors) are consistent with the above findings. These studies have demonstrated that prehospital fibrinolysis is feasible, reduces time to treatment, and improves patient outcomes [18,19]. Data from the non-randomized Registry of Cardiac Intensive Care in Sweden [20] demonstrate a significant reduction in both time to fibrinolysis (113 vs 165 minutes, $P < 0.001$) and 1-year mortality (OR = 0.71; 95% CI: 0.55 to 0.92) for prehospital fibrinolysis compared to in-hospital treatment.

The optimal choice of antithrombin therapy for patients receiving prehospital fibrinolysis remains somewhat questionable, particularly in patients over the age of 75 years. In the relatively small ($n = 1639$) ASSENT-3 Plus trial [19], the prehospital use of full-dose enoxaparin (30 mg IV bolus immediately followed by the first 1 mg/kg SC dose) in this population was associated with a large, significant excess (6.7% vs 0.8%, $P = 0.01$) in intracranial hemorrhage compared to intravenous (IV) unfractionated heparin (UFH). No such increase in intracranial hemorrhage was observed in this population using the same dosing regimen in the ASSENT-3 trial, or the much larger ExTRACT-TIMI-25 trial [21] (which used a modified, lower dose of enoxaparin in patients over 75 years). This raises the possibility that the excess intracranial hemorrhage rate in the ASSENT-3 Plus trial was a spurious finding, or that factors related to transportation or administration of enoxaparin in the field may be associated with excessive hemorrhage, especially without dosing adjustment.

In summary, prehospital fibrinolysis has been shown to be feasible, to reduce time to revascularization treatment, and to improve

Hours from pain onset	Vascular deaths/patient Aspirin		(% dead) Placebo tablets		Odds ratio & 95% CI Aspirin better	Placebo better
0–1	34/356		43/358			
2	80/953		103/955			
3	109/1243		149/1243			
4	109/1181		138/1178			
Subtotal: 0–4	332/3733	(8.9%)	433/3734	(11.6%)		25% SD7
5–12	366/3633		451/3636			
13–24	106/1221		132/1230			
Subtotal: 5–24	472/4854	(9.7%)	583/4866	(12.0%)		21% SD6
Total: 0–24	804/8587	(9.4%)	1016/8600	(11.8%)		23% SD4 odds reduction

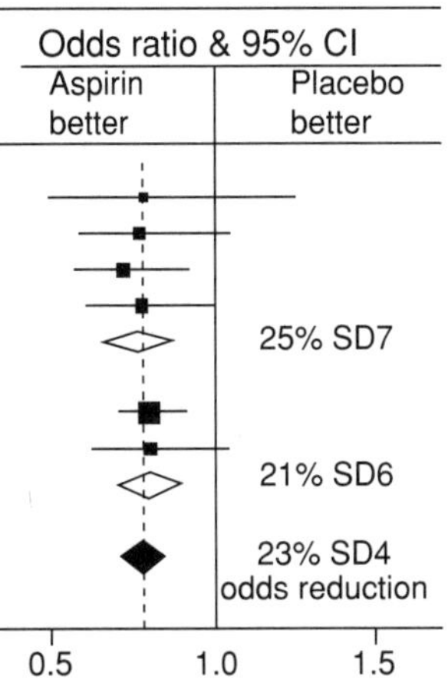

0.5   1.0   1.5

Figure 18.3 Reduction in odds of vascular death in days 0 to 35, subdivided by time from pain onset.

outcomes. While this approach has been integrated into health care systems in some areas, particularly in Europe, it has not been widely adopted in other parts of the world. Efforts should be made to increase the availability of this form of treatment delivery, especially in settings where transport times are long.

Question 3: In patients with STEMI (population), does the administration of acetyl-salicylic acid (ASA) (intervention) reduce death, repeat chest pain or revascularization (outcomes) compared to non-ASA treatment (control)?

Search strategy

- MEDLINE: (ASA OR acetylsalicylic acid) AND (AMI OR MI OR myocardial infarction)

The evidence for the benefit of antiplatelet therapy at reducing cardiovascular morbidity and mortality in patients at high risk of occlusive vascular events in general is excellent and consistent [22]. The evidence for the use of ASA in the setting of STEMI is derived from a single, large ($n = 17,187$) randomized controlled trial. The Second International Study of Infarct Survival (ISIS-2) [23] demonstrated that ASA alone (160 mg/day for 1 month following MI), or in combination with streptokinase (SK), produced a highly significant reduction in mortality (Fig. 18.3).

ASA alone was effective in reducing mortality over the first 35 days following STEMI, from 11.8% to 9.4% (OR = 0.77; 95% CI: 0.70 to 0.85). The magnitude of this effect was approximately equivalent to the effect of SK alone. The effects of ASA and SK were synergistic. The combined treatment reduced mortality from 13.2% to 8.0% (OR = 0.57; 95% CI: 0.50 to 66), and exceeded the benefit of either ASA or SK alone. Consistent with the Antithrombotic Trialists' Collaboration meta-analysis above [22], in ISIS-2, ASA was associated with significant reductions in reinfarction, cardiac arrest and stroke.

In ISIS-2 the times to both ASA and SK treatment were recorded. Unlike the effects observed with fibrinolysis, the effect of ASA was independent of the time of administration over the first 24 hours. There was no increase in major bleeds (requiring transfusion or intracranial hemorrhage), though there was a slight increase (1.9% to 2.5% (OR = 1.3, $P < 0.01$)) in minor bleeds.

In summary, ISIS-2 demonstrates that 1 month of ASA at a dose of 160 mg/day, started immediately in 1000 patients with STEMI, would result in 25 fewer deaths. While most patients with STEMI do currently receive ASA either by the EMS, or on arrival at hospital, efforts should be made to ensure that *all* eligible patients with suspected STEMI receive this treatment.

Question 4: In patients with STEMI (population), does the administration of β-blockers (intervention) reduce death, repeat chest pain or revascularization (outcomes) compared to standard care (control)?

Search strategy

- MEDLINE: (adrenergic beta antagonists OR propranolol OR beta blockers OR beta-blockade) AND (AMI OR MI OR myocardial infarction)

Prior to the fibrinolytic era, the use of β-blockers in the post-MI setting was well studied. In their comprehensive review of the subject at the time, Yusuf et al. [24] reached several important conclusions. Firstly, despite the large number of studies, they concluded that the effect of IV β-blockers (started immediately upon hospital admission) on short-term mortality was slight (3.4% vs 3.6% for treated and controls, respectively), and not statistically significant. Moreover, they deferred judgment until the publication of a soon to be published definitive study (ISIS-1), and conceded that the 95% confidence intervals around their estimates could allow for as much as a 20% reduction in mortality in an adequately powered study. Their analysis of the pooled long-term

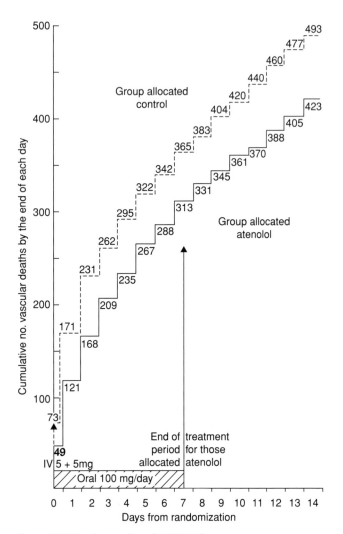

Figure 18.4 Vascular mortality in the ISIS-1 trial.

benefit of oral β-blockers (started within days of the onset of MI) in almost 20,000 patients demonstrated a significant reduction in deaths (RR = 0.77; 95% CI: 0.70 to 0.85).

The definitive trial of immediate IV β-blockade on hospital admission for STEMI was the First International Study of Infarct Survival (ISIS-1 [25]), in which patients (n = 16,027) were randomized to atenolol (5–10 mg IV immediately, followed by 100 mg/day orally for 7 days) or a placebo control. This study demonstrated a small, but significant, reduction in vascular mortality in patients in the β-blocker group at the end of the treatment period (3.89% vs 4.57%; OR = 0.85; 95% CI: 0.73 to 0.99). Interestingly, all of this benefit was observed in days 0 to 1 (Fig. 18.4).

ISIS-1 also demonstrated a slight (5% vs 3.4%, P < 0.0001) increase in the use of inotropic agents, which occurred chiefly during the first day of admission. There was no disproportionate excess of deaths for those patients receiving β-blockers and inotropic agents compared to control patients receiving inotropic agents. However, the excess use of inotropic agents in the atenolol group appeared greater in the small proportion of patients with

atrial fibrillation (1.6%) and the suggestion of cardiogenic shock (combination of systolic blood pressure < 120 mmHg and heart rate > 90 beats/min: 2% of patients).

The recently published, very large (n = 45,852) COMMIT trial has called the immediate use of IV β-blocker therapy in the setting of STEMI into question. In this trial, patients with suspected MI were randomized to metoprolol (up to 15 mg IV, then 200 mg oral daily for 4 weeks or until hospital discharge, mean 15 days) or matching placebo. The key findings of this study were that metoprolol had no effect on mortality (7.7% mortality in the metoprolol group vs 7.8% in the control group (OR = 0.99; 95% CI: 0.92 to 1.05)). Patients treated with metoprolol did have fewer reinfarctions and episodes of ventricular fibrillation; however, this was counterbalanced by a significant increase in cardiogenic shock (OR = 1.30; 95% CI: 1.19 to 1.41).

How can the negative findings of the COMMIT trial be reconciled with the beneficial effects of β-blockers observed in the earlier ISIS-1 study? The most likely explanation lies in the patient selection for each study. COMMIT enrolled a significant number of patients with evidence of significant heart failure (25% with Killip class II or III). While the ISIS-1 manuscript does not specify the number of patients in heart failure at enrollment, only 2% of patients had the combination of systolic blood pressure < 120 mmHg and a heart rate of > 90 beats/min. Additionally, only 10.8% of patients in ISIS-1 had a systolic blood pressure lower than 120 mmHg, compared to 33% of patients in COMMIT. It seems unlikely that the divergent results were caused by different medications. The previously mentioned meta-analysis by Yusuf included a variety of β-blockers, and, in the MIAMI study [26], metoprolol, at the same dose as that used in COMMIT, was shown to have a net beneficial effect on outcomes of similar magnitude to that observed with atenolol in ISIS-1. Finally, since all the studies of β-blockade in the setting of STEMI predating COMMIT were performed prior to the routine use of fibrinolysis for STEMI patients, it is possible that the there is an early hazard associated with the use of β-blockade which potentiates the clearly documented increase in mortality on the first day of treatment with fibrinolytic therapy.

In summary, meta-analysis of older studies indicates a significant and meaningful reduction in mortality associated with long-term β-blocker use in post-MI patients. The large ISIS-1 study found that immediate intravenous administration of atenolol in the setting of STEMI produced significant and meaningful reductions in mortality, and that this survival benefit was confined to the first 48 hours following the onset of MI. The more recent COMMIT study contradicts the findings of the earlier ISIS-1 study, and suggests that β-blocker use in the first hours to days following STEMI is associated with no net clinical benefit due to an increased incidence of cardiogenic shock associated with their use. While the immediate use of IV β-blockers in the setting of STEMI is still recommended, caution is required and these medications should not be given to patients with evidence of congestive heart failure, bradycardia or hypotension until their hemodynamic status is stable.

Question 5: In patients with STEMI (population), does the administration of fibrinolysis (intervention) reduce death, repeat chest pain or revascularization (outcomes) compared to standard care (control)? If so, which patients should receive treatment?

Search strategy

- MEDLINE: (thrombolysis OR fibrinolytic agents OR streptokinase OR thrombolytic therapy OR tissue plasminogen activator) AND (AMI OR MI OR myocardial infarction)

The effectiveness of fibrinolysis in the management of STEMI is one of the best-studied treatments in clinical medicine. Following initial studies demonstrating the effectiveness of streptokinase delivered via the intracoronary route, definitive studies showing both the effectiveness and safety of intravenous SK were undertaken. The first study to unequivocally show this effect was the landmark Effectiveness of Intravenous Fibrinolytic Treatment in Acute Myocardial Infarction (GISSI) study published in 1986 [2]. In this study, 11,806 patients presenting within the first 12 hours after the onset of symptoms were randomized to treatment with either 1.5 million units SK over 60 minutes or to the control group. The GISSI investigators drew several important conclusions from their study.

1 Treatment with intravenous SK significantly reduced mortality from 13% in controls to 10.7% in the SK treated group (RR = 0.81; 95% CI: 0.72 to 0.90).

2 Treatment with SK was associated with significantly better outcomes unless treatment was initiated more than 6 hours following the onset of symptoms.

3 The reduction in mortality associated with SK treatment was greatest when it was administered soon after the onset of symptoms. Patients treated with SK within 1 hour of the onset of symptoms had an approximately 50% reduction in mortality (RR = 0.49; 95% CI: 0.34 to 0.69), whereas patients treated within 3–6 hours after the onset of symptoms had a more modest benefit (RR = 0.80; 95% CI: 0.66 to 0.98).

A multitude of smaller studies investigating the effects of intravenous SK had been performed prior to GISSI, though none were adequately powered to demonstrate a mortality benefit. Following the publication of the GISSI study, a meta-analysis of these smaller studies was performed by Lau et al. [4]. The results of this meta-analysis were consistent with the findings of the GISSI study, and demonstrated a treatment benefit of the same magnitude (OR = 0.74; 95% CI: 0.59 to 0.92).

Following the demonstration of the effectiveness of SK for STEMI, additional studies have further refined this treatment strategy. The landmark GUSTO-1 trial [27], directly compared tissue plasminogen activator (t-PA), given at an accelerated rate, with SK. This very large ($n = 41,021$) study found a small (14% relative risk reduction, approximately 1% absolute reduction) but significant (95% CI: 5.9 to 21.3; $P = 0.001$) reduction in mortality associated with the use of t-PA compared to SK. Although mortality was reduced, there was an increase in the rate of hemorrhagic stroke rates in patients treated with t-PA compared to SK (0.72% vs 0.49%, equaling an excess of four hemorrhagic strokes per 1000 patients treated). On the basis of this trial, accelerated t-PA has been considered the gold standard of fibrinolytic therapy.

Despite the large size of the fibrinolysis studies, uncertainty remained over which patients would experience reduced mortality with this treatment. For example, there was uncertainty regarding the effectiveness of fibrinolysis in patients without ST elevation, those presenting more than 6 hours after the onset of symptoms, elderly patients and those in cardiogenic shock. These questions were addressed in a meta-analysis performed by the Fibrinolytic Therapy Trialists' (FTT) Collaborative Group, which included 58,600 patients who had been enrolled in studies comparing fibrinolysis with placebo treatment [28]. The key findings of this analysis were that patients with anterior STEMI and new left bundle branch block (LBBB) benefit the most from fibrinolysis, irrespective of other clinical factors, and that the benefit of treatment was greater the earlier it was initiated, especially in those treated within the first 6 hours after the onset of symptoms. The full results of the study are presented in Fig. 18.5.

In summary, there is overwhelming evidence regarding the effectiveness of fibrinolysis in the treatment of STEMI. This treatment is most effective when given early, and to patients with anterior STEMI or LBBB; however, it is also effective in patients with inferior STEMI. There is an increased risk of bleeding associated with the use of fibrinolysis, especially the risk of intracranial hemorrhage; however, the benefits of treatment for patients with ST elevation or LBBB on their presenting ECG significantly outweigh the risks of treatment.

Question 6: In patients with the presumed diagnosis of STEMI (population), does primary angioplasty (intervention) reduce death, repeat chest pain or revascularization (outcomes) compared to patients administered fibrinolysis (control)?

Search strategy

- MEDLINE: primary angioplasty AND (myocardial infarction OR MI OR AMI)

Coronary angiography performed on 2431 patients as part of the GUSTO study demonstrated that normal coronary blood flow in the infarct-related artery was present at 90 minutes following accelerated t-PA in only 54% of patients [5]. Despite enormous effort to improve the effectiveness of pharmacological treatment of STEMI, this result has remained largely unchanged over the last 15 years. Frustration with this lack of progress has led to increased interest and significant advances in mechanical reperfusion options (primary PCI) in recent years. Initial progress in this area was very slow, suffering from the same limitations as the original

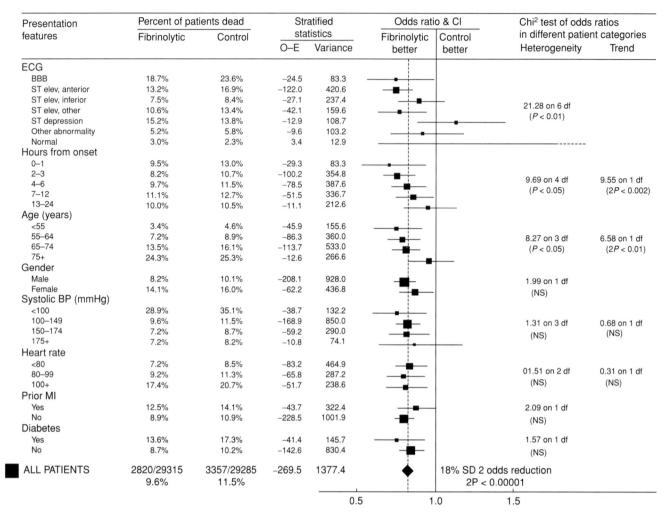

Presentation features	Percent of patients dead		Stratified statistics		Odds ratio & CI		Chi² test of odds ratios in different patient categories	
	Fibrinolytic	Control	O–E	Variance	Fibrinolytic better	Control better	Heterogeneity	Trend
ECG								
BBB	18.7%	23.6%	−24.5	83.3				
ST elev, anterior	13.2%	16.9%	−122.0	420.6				
ST elev, inferior	7.5%	8.4%	−27.1	237.4			21.28 on 6 df	
ST elev, other	10.6%	13.4%	−42.1	159.6			(P < 0.01)	
ST depression	15.2%	13.8%	−12.9	108.7				
Other abnormality	5.2%	5.8%	−9.6	103.2				
Normal	3.0%	2.3%	3.4	12.9				
Hours from onset								
0–1	9.5%	13.0%	−29.3	83.3				
2–3	8.2%	10.7%	−100.2	354.8			9.69 on 4 df	9.55 on 1 df
4–6	9.7%	11.5%	−78.5	387.6			(P < 0.05)	(2P < 0.002)
7–12	11.1%	12.7%	−51.5	336.7				
13–24	10.0%	10.5%	−11.1	212.6				
Age (years)								
<55	3.4%	4.6%	−45.9	155.6				
55–64	7.2%	8.9%	−86.3	360.0			8.27 on 3 df	6.58 on 1 df
65–74	13.5%	16.1%	−113.7	533.0			(P < 0.05)	(2P < 0.01)
75+	24.3%	25.3%	−12.6	266.6				
Gender								
Male	8.2%	10.1%	−208.1	928.0			1.99 on 1 df	
Female	14.1%	16.0%	−62.2	436.8			(NS)	
Systolic BP (mmHg)								
<100	28.9%	35.1%	−38.7	132.2				
100–149	9.6%	11.5%	−168.9	850.0			1.31 on 3 df	0.68 on 1 df
150–174	7.2%	8.7%	−59.2	290.0			(NS)	(NS)
175+	7.2%	8.2%	−10.8	74.1				
Heart rate								
<80	7.2%	8.5%	−83.2	464.9				
80–99	9.2%	11.3%	−65.8	287.2			01.51 on 2 df	0.31 on 1 df
100+	17.4%	20.7%	−51.7	238.6			(NS)	(NS)
Prior MI								
Yes	12.5%	14.1%	−43.7	322.4			2.09 on 1 df	
No	8.9%	10.9%	−228.5	1001.9			(NS)	
Diabetes								
Yes	13.6%	17.3%	−41.4	145.7			1.57 on 1 df	
No	8.7%	10.2%	−142.6	830.4			(NS)	
■ ALL PATIENTS	2820/29315 9.6%	3357/29285 11.5%	−269.5	1377.4	◆		18% SD 2 odds reduction 2P < 0.00001	

0.5   1.0   1.5

Figure 18.5 Proportional effects of fibrinolytic therapy on mortality during days 0 to 35, subdivided by presentation features. BP, blood pressure; BBB, branch bundle block; ECG, electrocardiogram; O-E, observed minus expected.

intra-coronary SK studies, namely that it is difficult to provide this service in a timely fashion.

Three separate meta-analyses of studies comparing primary PCI with fibrinolysis have been performed, starting in 1995 [6,29,30], and the most recent of these includes all studies. In aggregate, the data from the clinical trials comparing primary PCI with fibrinolysis demonstrate a significant reduction in short-term (defined as 4–6 weeks) mortality (OR = 0.73; 95% CI: 0.62 to 0.86), as well as other important endpoints. For example, the combined endpoint of death, reinfarction and stroke was reduced from 14% to 8% (OR = 0.53; 95% CI: 0.45 to 0.63).

The criticism of primary PCI has not been related to efficacy, but rather that it is very difficult to perform in a timely fashion. The relationship between increasing door to balloon time for primary PCI and increasing mortality has been convincingly demonstrated [3,31]. In a meta-analysis of outcomes for studies comparing primary PCI and fibrinolysis as a function of PCI-related delay (the time interval between when the patient could have had fibrinolysis

and when they did have balloon inflation during primary PCI), the authors demonstrated that if primary PCI-related time delay exceeded 62 minutes the mortality advantage gained by primary PCI over fibrinolysis was lost [32]. They also noted that the mean PCI-related time delay in the 21 studies they included in their analysis was only 39.5 minutes. This study has led to the general recommendation in the current American College of Cardiology/American Heart Association guidelines for the management of STEMI that routine primary PCI should be performed within 90 minutes of first medical contact [8].

The relative mortality benefit of primary PCI over fibrinolysis, as a function of PCI-related delay, has recently been better defined using data from the very large (n = 192,509) National Registry of MI (data from June 1994 through August 2003) [33]. This study demonstrated that the time at which the advantage of primary PCI over fibrinolysis is lost depends on a variety of patient factors including age, location of infarction and prehospital delay (Fig. 18.6).

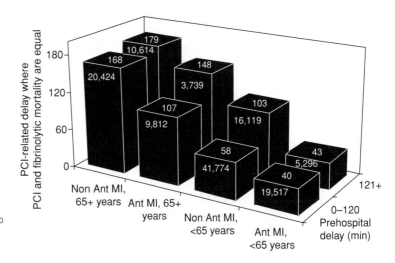

Figure 18.6 Effect of PCI-related time delay on mortality compared to fibrinolysis by clinical factors. Ant MI, anterior myocardial infarction; Non Ant MI, non-anterior myocardial infarction.

Data from the large ($n = 27{,}080$) Second National Registry of Myocardial Infarction in the USA demonstrated a median "door-to-balloon time" of 1 hour 56 minutes at participating US hospitals, with only 8% of patients having a door-to-balloon time of 60 minutes or less [34]. Time delays to primary PCI outside of the clinical trial setting may be one of the key factors explaining why outcomes in studies performed in clinical practice in community settings have reported no benefit of primary PCI over fibrinolysis [35].

In summary, primary PCI when performed in a timely fashion in the clinical trial setting provides superior outcomes compared to fibrinolysis. Most hospitals do not have interventional cardiology services, and even in those that do, obtaining a primary PCI for STEMI within the recommended time guidelines remains challenging. The time delay to PCI, beyond which the benefit of primary PCI over fibrinolysis is lost, is variable and depends on a variety of patient characteristics. Emergency physicians planning to refer STEMI patients for primary PCI should be aware of the typical delays to treatment in their institution, and treat patients accordingly.

Question 7: In patients with STEMI who receive fibrinolysis (population), does the administration of heparin as adjunctive therapy (intervention) reduce mortality, revascularization and complications (outcomes) compared to fibrinolysis alone (control)?

Search strategy

- MEDLINE: (heparin OR low molecular weight heparin OR enoxaparin) AND (MI OR myocardial infarction OR AMI)

The safety and efficacy of a variety of antithrombin therapies (agents and doses) in patients with STEMI has been studied intensively, yet until recently the role of anticoagulation in this setting has been unclear. Intravenous UFH has been a part of standard therapy for patients treated with fibrin-specific fibrinolytics since the original GUSTO-1 study [27], and has been recommended to prevent systemic emboli in patients with anterior STEMI. Recently, the low molecular weight heparins (LMWHs) have been introduced in the clinical setting of STEMI, increasing the therapeutic options. The role of either UFH or LMWH in conjunction with SK and other non-fibrin-specific agents was the subject of a meta-analysis of randomized trials evaluating the efficacy and safety of UFH and LMWH and designed to clarify this issue [36]. In this meta-analysis, the following combinations were considered: (i) UFH versus control (four trials; $n = 1239$); (ii) LMWH versus placebo (four trials; $n = 16{,}943$); and (iii) LMWH versus UFH (six trials; $n = 7098$).

From the included studies, compared to controls, UFH was not effective in reducing death or reinfarction. In contrast, LMWH for 4–8 days compared to placebo treatment reduced death by approximately 10%, and reinfarction by approximately 25%. When directly compared, LMWH reduced infarction by almost 50%, with no effect on mortality compared to UFH. Table 18.1 summarizes the results of these trials on benefits of treatment, as well as risk of stroke and minor and major bleeding.

Since the publication of the above meta-analysis, a very large randomized controlled double blind clinical trial of enoxaparin versus UFH has been completed. In the ExTRACT-TIMI 25 study [37], 20,506 patients with STEMI treated with fibrinolysis and ASA were randomized to receive enoxaparin or fully weight-adjusted UFH. The somewhat complex dosing of both agents was carefully considered in order to minimize bleeding complications.

Enoxaparin was administered as a 30 mg IV bolus followed in 15 minutes by 1.0 mg/kg SC every 12 hours for patients under 75, and 0.75 mg/kg SC every 12 hours without an IV bolus dose for patients over the age of 75. For the first two subcutaneous injections, the dose of 100 mg (patients under 75) or 75 mg (patients 75 and older) was not to be exceeded. For patients with a creatinine clearance of less than 30 ml/min, the dose of enoxaparin was reduced to 1.0 mg/kg every 24 hours. Enoxaparin was to be continued until hospital discharge or a maximum of 8 days.

Table 18.1 Summary of evidence table for the effect of heparin treatment on reinfarction, death, stroke and bleeding during hospitalization at 7 days.

Comparison	Reinfarction OR (95% CI)	Death OR (95% CI)	Stroke OR (95% CI)	Minor bleeding OR (95% CI)	Major bleeding OR (95% CI)	Intracranial bleeding OR (95% CI)
UFH vs control	1.08 (0.58 to 1.99)	1.04 (0.62 to 1.78)	2.55 (0.85 to 7.68)	1.72 (1.22 to 2.43)	1.21 (0.67 to 2.18)	2.30 (0.59 to 8.95)
LMWH vs placebo	0.72 (0.58 to 0.90)	0.90 (0.80 to 0.99)	1.19 (0.84 to 1.70)	3.24 (2.12 to 4.91)	2.70 (1.83 to 3.99)	2.18 (1.07 to 4.52)
LMWH vs UFH	0.57 (0.45 to 0.73)	0.92 (0.74 to 1.13)	1.38 (0.95 to 2.01)	1.26 (1.12 to 1.43)	1.30 (0.98 to 1.72)	1.18 (0.74 to 1.87)

CI, confidence interval; LMWH, low molecular weight heparin; OR, odds ratio; UFH, unfractionated heparin.

UFH was administered as a 60 U/kg (maximum 4000 U) bolus, and then a 12 U/kg/h infusion (to be started 15 minutes after the bolus dose, with an initial maximum of 1000 U/h). Anticoagulation was monitored to maintain an activated partial thromboplastin time of 1.5 to 2.0 times the control time. Intravenous UFH was to be continued for at least 48 hours, but could be continued for longer at the treating physician's discretion. For both enoxaparin and UFH, the IV bolus dose was to be omitted if patients had received open-label UFH (at least 4000 U) in the 3 hours prior to randomization.

The therapy received in ExTRACT-TIMI 25 was relevant to contemporary practice. Approximately 20% of patients were treated with SK, with the remainder treated with the fibrin-specific fibrinolytic agents tenecteplase (20%), alteplase (55%) and reteplase (5%). Approximately 85% received β-blockers, one-third received clopidogrel and 70% received a statin. The median duration of treatment for the enoxaparin and UFH treatments were 7 and 2 days, respectively; the mean duration of hospitalization was 10 days. Three-quarters of patients were treated with medical therapy alone, with 23% undergoing angioplasty (2.8% as rescue for failed fibrinolysis, and 20% as an urgent or elective procedure), and 2.8% undergoing a coronary bypass procedure.

The key findings of ExTRACT-TIMI 25 were consistent with the previously discussed meta-analysis. Enoxaparin therapy was not associated with a reduction in mortality but did result in a small, albeit significant, reduction in reinfarction and urgent revascularizations. Table 18.2 summarizes the various efficacy outcomes at 48 hours, 8 days and 30 days.

The slightly improved outcomes with enoxaparin came at the cost of additional bleeding complications. The rates of major

Table 18.2 Efficacy outcomes for UFH vs enoxaparin in acute myocardial infarction.

Outcome	Enoxaparin ($n = 10,220$) Number (%)	Unfractionated heparin ($n = 10,223$) Number (%)	Relative risk (95% CI)	P value
Outcome at 48 hours				
Death or non-fatal MI	478 (4.7)	531 (5.2)	0.90 (0.80 to 1.01)	0.08
Death	383 (3.7)	390 (3.8)	0.98 (0.85 to 1.12)	0.76
Non-fatal MI	95 (0.9)	141 (1.4)	0.67 (0.52 to 0.87)	0.002
Urgent revascularization	74 (0.7)	96 (0.9)	0.77 (0.57 to 1.04)	0.09
Death, non-fatal MI or urgent revascularization	548 (5.3)	622 (6.1)	0.88 (0.79 to 0.98)	0.02
Outcome at 8 days				
Death or non-fatal MI	740 (7.2)	954 (9.3)	0.77 (0.71 to 0.85)	<0.001
Death	559 (5.5)	605 (5.9)	0.92 (0.82 to 1.03)	0.15
Non-fatal MI	181 (1.8)	349 (3.4)	0.52 (0.43 to 0.62)	<0.001
Urgent revascularization	145 (1.4)	247 (2.4)	0.59 (0.48 to 0.72)	<0.001
Death, non-fatal MI or urgent revascularization	874 (8.5)	1181 (11.6)	0.74 (0.68 to 0.80)	<0.001
Outcome at 30 days				
Primary efficacy endpoint (death or non-fatal MI)	1017 (9.9)	1223 (12.0)	0.83 (0.77 to 0.90)	<0.001
Death	708 (6.9)	765 (7.5)	0.92 (0.84 to 1.02)	0.11
Non-fatal MI	309 (3.0)	458 (4.5)	0.67 (0.58 to 0.77)	<0.001
Urgent revascularization	213 (2.1)	286 (2.8)	0.74 (0.62 to 0.88)	<0.001
Death, non-fatal MI or urgent revascularization	1199 (11.7)	1479 (14.5)	0.81 (0.75 to 0.87)	<0.001

*Non-fatal myocardial infarction (MI) indicates that a patient had a recurrent MI and had not died by the time shown.

†Urgent revascularization denotes episodes of recurrent MI (without infarction) that drove the clinical decision to perform coronary revascularization during the same hospitalization.

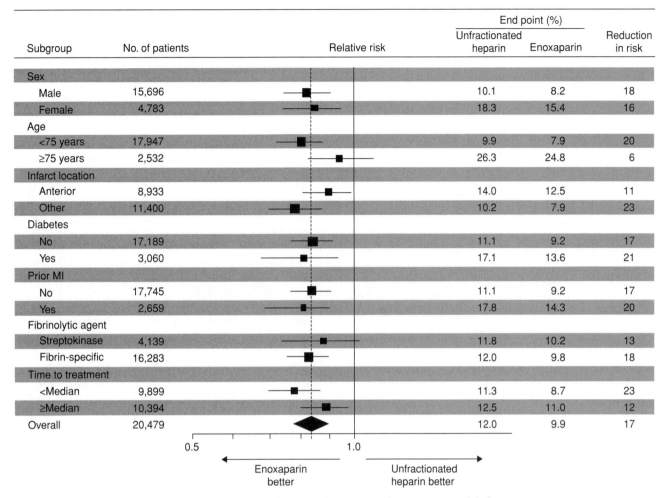

Subgroup	No. of patients	Relative risk	End point (%) Unfractionated heparin	Enoxaparin	Reduction in risk
Sex					
Male	15,696		10.1	8.2	18
Female	4,783		18.3	15.4	16
Age					
<75 years	17,947		9.9	7.9	20
≥75 years	2,532		26.3	24.8	6
Infarct location					
Anterior	8,933		14.0	12.5	11
Other	11,400		10.2	7.9	23
Diabetes					
No	17,189		11.1	9.2	17
Yes	3,060		17.1	13.6	21
Prior MI					
No	17,745		11.1	9.2	17
Yes	2,659		17.8	14.3	20
Fibrinolytic agent					
Streptokinase	4,139		11.8	10.2	13
Fibrin-specific	16,283		12.0	9.8	18
Time to treatment					
<Median	9,899		11.3	8.7	23
≥Median	10,394		12.5	11.0	12
Overall	20,479		12.0	9.9	17

0.5   1.0

Enoxaparin better   Unfractionated heparin better

Figure 18.7 Relative risks of absolute event rates for the primary endpoint at 30 days in various subgroups. MI, myocardial infarction.

bleeding – as defined by the severity scoring system devised by the TIMI group (which includes intracranial hemorrhage) – at 30 days were 1.4% in the UFH group and 2.1% in the enoxaparin group (absolute increase of 0.7%, 53% increase in relative risk, $P < 0.001$). The rate of intracranical hemorrhage specifically was not increased with enoxaparin treatment. The relative risks and absolute event rates for the primary endpoint (death or non-fatal recurrent MI through to 30 days) for the various subgroups are shown in Fig. 18.7.

In summary, STEMI patients treated with ASA do not appear to benefit from IV UFH therapy in combination with fibrinolytic therapy compared to controls. This conclusion should be tempered by the fact that limited data exist for this comparison (a total of only 1239 patients with 42 reinfarctions and 58 deaths). When such patients are treated with LMWH, they have a slight but significant reduction in death and reinfarction compared to placebo controls, and a slight but significant reduction in reinfarction compared to patients treated with IV UFH. Additionally, patients treated with enoxaparin are at a slight (0.7% absolute increase) but significantly higher risk of major bleeding, excluding intracranial hemorrhage.

Conclusions

Returning to the case scenario above, your patient was diagnosed with a STEMI. He was administered ASA, IV β-blockers (metoprolol 5 mg), oxygen and IV nitroglycerin. Cardiac labs and a chest radiograph were ordered while treatment was initiated. His pain and cardiogram remained unchanged, and his chest radiograph was normal, so 20 minutes from arrival he was deemed to be eligible for revascularization. Since your hospital does not maintain 24-hour availability of primary PCI, and because it was well after normal operating hours, you doubt the catheterization lab staff would be immediately available. There is an interventional site 10 blocks away that advertises 24/7 PCI capacity, and you attempt to contact the cardiologist on call regarding further treatment. The final choice is whether or not you should initiate fibrinolytic therapy at your own ED immediately. In this case, given the patient's early presentation, lack of contraindications/risk factors for intracranial hemorrhage, and the anticipated delay to primary PCI, you administered thrombolytics (t-PA) and arranged for transfer in the event of treatment failure. The patient revascularized in the ED within 90 minutes of receiving fibrinolysis, and received delayed angioplasty 12 hours later at the receiving hospital after being found to have a lesion correctable with coronary stenting. He recovered without incident, and was discharged home 3 days after hospitalization.

Overall, impressive strides have been made in the treatment of acute MI in developed countries in the last two decades and mortality from this disease has declined. Routine "wait and see" therapy for acute MI in the 1980s has evolved to include bolus thrombolytic therapy and now primary PCI. Recognition of acute MI remains a priority in all EMS and ED settings; prehospital ECG and thrombolysis are safe and effective interventions, and ED physicians with medical control of this service should make efforts to expand their application. ECGs should be obtained within 10 minutes of arrival in EDs and thrombolytics should be administered within 30 minutes of arrival or PCI should be initiated within 90 minutes of arrival. Additional treatments with ASA, β-blockers and oxygen are all important adjuncts to therapy. While UFH appears to add little to the treatment of STEMI patients, the use of LMWH does appear to result in slight improvement in outcomes at the cost of increased bleeding.

References

1 Kleiman NS, White HD, Ohman EM, et al. Mortality within 24 hours of thrombolysis for myocardial infarction. The importance of early reperfusion. The GUSTO Investigators, Global Utilization of Streptokinase and Tissue Plasminogen Activator for Occluded Coronary Arteries. *Circulation* 1994;**90**:2658–65.

2 Anonymous. Effectiveness of intravenous thrombolytic treatment in acute myocardial infarction. Gruppo Italiano per lo Studio della Streptochinasi nell'Infarto Miocardico (GISSI). *Lancet* 1986;**1**:397–402.

3 De Luca G, Suryapranata H, Ottervanger JP, Antman EM. Time delay to treatment and mortality in primary angioplasty for acute myocardial infarction: every minute of delay counts. *Circulation* 2004;**109**:1223–5.

4 Lau J, Antman EM, Jimenez-Silva J, Kupelnick B, Mosteller F, Chalmers TC. Cumulative meta-analysis of therapeutic trials for myocardial infarction. *N Engl J Med* 1992;**327**:248–54.

5 Anonymous. The effects of tissue plasminogen activator, streptokinase, or both on coronary-artery patency, ventricular function, and survival after acute myocardial infarction. The GUSTO Angiographic Investigators. *N Engl J Med* 1993;**329**:1615–22.

6 Keeley EC, Boura JA, Grines CL. Primary angioplasty versus intravenous thrombolytic therapy for acute myocardial infarction: a quantitative review of 23 randomised trials. *Lancet* 2003;**361**:13–20.

7 Anonymous. Myocardial infarction redefined – a consensus document of the Joint European Society of Cardiology/American College of Cardiology Committee for the redefinition of myocardial infarction. *Eur Heart J* 2000;**21**:1502–13.

8 Antman EM, Anbe DT, Armstrong PW, et al. ACC/AHA guidelines for the management of patients with ST-elevation myocardial infarction: a report of the American College of Cardiology/American Heart Association Task Force on Practice Guidelines (Committee to Revise the 1999 Guidelines for the Management of Patients with Acute Myocardial Infarction). *Circulation* 2004;**110**:e82–292.

9 Canto JG, Rogers WJ, Bowlby LJ, French WJ, Pearce DJ, Weaver WD. The prehospital electrocardiogram in acute myocardial infarction: is its full potential being realized? National Registry of Myocardial Infarction 2 Investigators. *J Am Coll Cardiol* 1997;**29**:498–505.

10 Andersen HR, Nielsen TT, Rasmussen K, et al. A comparison of coronary angioplasty with fibrinolytic therapy in acute myocardial infarction. *N Engl J Med* 2003;**349**:733–42.

11 Widimsky P, Budesinsky T, Vorac D, et al. Long distance transport for primary angioplasty vs immediate thrombolysis in acute myocardial infarction. Final results of the randomized national multicentre trial – PRAGUE-2. *Eur Heart J* 2003;**24**:94–104.

12 Steg PG, Bonnefoy E, Chabaud S, et al. Impact of time to treatment on mortality after prehospital fibrinolysis or primary angioplasty: data from the CAPTIM randomized clinical trial. *Circulation* 2003;**108**:2851–6.

13 Brainard AH, Raynovich W, Tandberg D, Bedrick EJ. The prehospital 12-lead electrocardiogram's effect on time to initiation of reperfusion therapy: a systematic review and meta-analysis of existing literature. *Am J Emerg Med* 2005;**23**:351–6.

14 Morrison LJ, Brooks S, Sawadsky B, McDonald A, Verbeek PR. Prehospital 12-lead electrocardiography impact on acute myocardial infarction treatment times and mortality: a systematic review. *Acad Emerg Med* 2006;**13**:84–9.

15 Hutchings CB, Mann NC, Daya M, et al. Patients with chest pain calling 9-1-1 or self-transporting to reach definitive care: which mode is quicker? *Am Heart J* 2004;**147**:35–41.

16 Selker HP, Zalenski RJ, Antman EM, et al. An evaluation of technologies for identifying acute cardiac ischemia in the emergency department: a report from a National Heart Attack Alert Program Working Group. *Ann Emerg Med* 1997;**29**:13–87.

17 Morrison LJ, Verbeek PR, McDonald AC, Sawadsky BV, Cook DJ. Mortality and prehospital thrombolysis for acute myocardial infarction: a meta-analysis. *JAMA* 2000;**283**:2686–92.

18 Steg PG, Bonnefoy E, Chabaud S, et al. Impact of time to treatment on mortality after prehospital fibrinolysis or primary angioplasty: data from the CAPTIM randomized clinical trial. *Circulation* 2003;**108**:2851–6.

19 Wallentin L, Goldstein P, Armstrong PW, et al. Efficacy and safety of tenecteplase in combination with the low-molecular-weight heparin enoxaparin or unfractionated heparin in the prehospital setting: the Assessment of the Safety and Efficacy of a New Thrombolytic Regimen (ASSENT)-3 PLUS randomized trial in acute myocardial infarction. *Circulation* 2003;**108**:135–42.

20 Bjorklund E, Stenestrand U, Lindback J, Svensson L, Wallentin L, Lindahl B. Pre-hospital thrombolysis delivered by paramedics is associated with reduced time delay and mortality in ambulance-transported real-life patients with ST-elevation myocardial infarction. *Eur Heart J* 2006;**27**:1146–52.

21 Antman EM, Morrow DA, McCabe CH, et al. Enoxaparin versus unfractionated heparin with fibrinolysis for ST-elevation myocardial infarction. *N Engl J Med* 2006;**354**:1477–88.

22 Antithrombotic Trialists' Collaboration. Meta-analysis of randomised trials of antiplatelet therapy for prevention of death, myocardial infarction, and stroke in high risk patients. *BMJ* 2002;**324**:71–86.

23 Anonymous. Randomised trial of intravenous streptokinase, oral aspirin, both, or neither among 17,187 cases of suspected acute myocardial infarction: ISIS-2. ISIS-2 (Second International Study of Infarct Survival) Collaborative Group. *Lancet* 1988;**2**:349–60.

24 Yusuf S, Peto R, Lewis J, Collins R, Sleight P. Beta blockade during and after myocardial infarction: an overview of the randomized trials. *Prog Cardiovasc Dis* 1985;**27**:335–71.

25 Anonymous. Randomised trial of intravenous atenolol among 16 027 cases of suspected acute myocardial infarction: ISIS-1. First International Study of Infarct Survival Collaborative Group. *Lancet* 1986;**2**: 57–66.

26 Anonymous. Metoprolol in acute myocardial infarction (MIAMI). A randomised placebo-controlled international trial. The MIAMI Trial Research Group. *Eur Heart J* 1985;**6**:199–226.

27 Anonymous. An international randomized trial comparing four thrombolytic strategies for acute myocardial infarction. The GUSTO Investigators. *N Engl J Med* 1993;**329**:673–82.

28 Anonymous. Indications for fibrinolytic therapy in suspected acute myocardial infarction: collaborative overview of early mortality and major morbidity results from all randomised trials of more than 1000 patients. Fibrinolytic Therapy Trialists' (FTT) Collaborative Group. *Lancet* 1994;**343**:311–22.

29 Weaver WD, Simes RJ, Betriu A, et al. Comparison of primary coronary angioplasty and intravenous thrombolytic therapy for acute myocardial infarction: a quantitative review. *JAMA* 1997;**278**:2093–8.

30 Michels KB, Yusuf S. Does PTCA in acute myocardial infarction affect mortality and reinfarction rates? A quantitative overview (meta-analysis) of the randomized clinical trials. *Circulation* 1995;**91**:476–85.

31 Cannon CP, Gibson CM, Lambrew CT, et al. Relationship of symptom-onset-to-balloon time and door-to-balloon time with mortality in patients undergoing angioplasty for acute myocardial infarction. *JAMA* 2000;**283**:2941–7.

32 Nallamothu BK, Bates ER. Percutaneous coronary intervention versus fibrinolytic therapy in acute myocardial infarction: is timing (almost) everything? *Am J Cardiol* 2003;**92**:824–6.

33 Pinto DS, Kirtane AJ, Nallamothu BK, et al. Hospital delays in reperfusion for ST-elevation myocardial infarction: implications when selecting a reperfusion strategy. *Circulation* 2006;**114**:2019–25.

34 Cannon CP, Gibson CM, Lambrew CT, et al. Relationship of symptom-onset-to-balloon time and door-to-balloon time with mortality in patients undergoing angioplasty for acute myocardial infarction. *JAMA* 2000;**283**:2941–7.

35 Every NR, Parsons LS, Hlatky M, Martin JS, Weaver WD. A comparison of thrombolytic therapy with primary coronary angioplasty for acute myocardial infarction. Myocardial Infarction Triage and Intervention Investigators. *N Engl J Med* 1996;**335**:1253–60.

36 Eikelboom JW, Quinlan DJ, Mehta SR, Turpie AG, Menown IB, Yusuf S. Unfractionated and low-molecular-weight heparin as adjuncts to thrombolysis in aspirin-treated patients with ST-elevation acute myocardial infarction: a meta-analysis of the randomized trials. *Circulation* 2005;**112**:3855–67.

37 Antman EM, Morrow DA, McCabe CH, et al. Enoxaparin versus unfractionated heparin with fibrinolysis for ST-elevation myocardial infarction. *N Engl J Med* 2006;**354**:1477–88.

19 Acute Decompensated Heart Failure

Brett Jones[2] & Sean P. Collins[1]

[1] Department of Emergency Medicine, University of Cincinnati, Cincinnati, USA
[2] Ya vapai Medical Center, Prescott, USA

Case scenario

A 68-year-old female presented to the emergency department (ED) with 4 days of increasing shortness of breath. She also stated she had experienced increasing dyspnea on exertion over the same time period, as well as three-pillow orthopnea. She had a past medical history significant for heart failure, coronary artery disease, hypertension and chronic obstructive pulmonary disease (COPD). She noted a dull pressure in her chest; however, she denied any radiation of the pain or associated symptoms such as nausea or dizziness. On physical examination she was in moderate respiratory distress with a blood pressure of 205/125 mmHg, a respiratory rate of 26 breaths/min, a heart rate of 95 beats/min and oxygen saturation (SaO_2) of 89% on a non-rebreather face mask providing 15 L/min of oxygen flow. Auscultation of her chest revealed bi-basilar rales with faint, diffuse expiratory wheezes. She was also noted to have bilateral lower extremity pitting edema. The chest radiograph was consistent with pulmonary edema, and her electrocardiogram (ECG) showed evidence of left ventricular hypertrophy; there were no acute changes when compared with prior ECGs. Her first set of cardiac markers were negative, her complete blood count was unremarkable, and her renal profile was within normal limits, with the exception of a creatinine of 1.6 mg/dl (baseline = 1.1 mg/dl). Her B-type natriuretic peptide (BNP) was 960 pg/ml. You administered repeated doses of sublingual nitroglycerin and a dose of intravenous diuretic (furosemide 80 mg). Her repeat blood pressure was 180/95 and she continued to exhibit increased work of breathing. Intubation was a consideration and your student questioned whether the benefit of non-invasive ventilation (NIV) as an adjunct outweighed the risk(s) in this patient.

Evidence-based Emergency Medicine. Edited by Brian H. Rowe
© 2009 Blackwell Publishing, ISBN: 978-1-4051-6143-5.

Background

As many as 5 million Americans have heart failure, with an additional 550,000 new cases diagnosed annually. Heart failure accounts for more than 1 million hospital admissions annually, which has risen 175% from 1979 to 2004. It is the leading discharge diagnosis for all patients >65 years of age, in whom the incidence approaches 10 per 1000 population. Annual death rate is approximately 20% and the estimated cost of heart failure in the United States for 2007 is nearly $33.2 billion [1].

In the USA, approximately 80% of all patients admitted with acute decompensated heart failure (ADHF) initially present to the ED [2]. Between 1992 and 2001, there were 10.5 million ED visits for ADHF, with an admission rate of 70–80% [3,4]. As heart failure is primarily a disease of the elderly, these numbers are projected to increase [3,5].

The cornerstone of treatment for ADHF has been vasodilators, diuretics and oxygen. The rationale for the above treatments is to decrease preload, afterload and pulmonary congestion. Developments in the diagnosis and treatment of ADHF in the past decade are discussed herein.

Clinical questions

1 In patients with ADHF (population), are there any features of the clinical assessment (intervention) that predict (diagnostic test characteristic) which patients are likely to have ADHF (outcome)?

2 In patients with undifferentiated acute dyspnea who present to the ED (population), does a natriuretic peptide measurement (intervention) improve the sensitivity or specificity (diagnostic test characteristics) compared to clinical assessment alone (control)?

3 In patients with ADHF (population), what is the efficacy and safety (outcomes) of initiating nitroglycerin treatment compared to oxygen and diuretic treatment?

4 In patients with ADHF (population), does non-invasive positive pressure ventilation (intervention) decrease intubation

rates and/or mortality (outcomes) compared to standard care (control)?

5 In patients with ADHF (population), does administration of nesiritide (i.e., recombinant BNP) affect renal function and/or mortality (outcomes) compared to standard care (control)?

6 In patients with ADHF (population), are there any clinical factors (intervention) that predict (objective test characteristic) which patients can be safely discharged home (outcome)?

7 In patients with ADHF felt to be non-high risk (population), does observation unit management (intervention) reduce ED relapse and conserve hospital resources (outcomes) compared to hospital admission (control)?

General search strategy

PubMed was searched in a systematic manner using a combination of search terms specific to each question. Preferences were given to studies that enrolled patients in the ED and studied acute heart failure. Specific inclusion and exclusion criteria are delineated under each question of interest.

Critical review of the literature

Question 1: In patients with ADHF (population), are there any features of the clinical assessment (intervention) that predict (diagnostic test characteristic) which patients are likely to have ADHF (outcome)?

Search strategy

- PubMed: (CHF OR congestive heart failure OR acute heart failure) AND diagnosis AND (ED OR emergency department) AND (physical examination OR clinical examination)

The history and physical examination have traditionally been a cornerstone in the diagnostic work-up of the dyspneic ED patient. With the recent introduction of natriuretic peptides, however, history and physical examination have been less emphasized. Are there history or physician examination findings that should lead the examining clinician to strongly consider ADHF as the leading diagnosis? The aforementioned search strategy sought to identify studies that utilized ED data to enroll patients with ADHF. Review articles were excluded. The search identified 13 studies that met these inclusion criteria [6–17]. A systematic review summarized the findings from 12 of these 13 studies.

The systematic review included 12 articles that evaluated history and physical examination findings in dyspneic ED patients to diagnose ADHF. Helpful findings in the clinical history include a history of heart failure (positive likelihood ratio, +LR = 5.8; 95% CI: 4.1 to 8.0). Other historical findings traditionally associated with ADHF were less helpful; paroxysmal nocturnal dyspnea (+LR = 2.6; 95% CI: 1.5 to 4.5), orthopnea (+LR = 2.2; 95% CI:

1.2 to 3.9) and complaints of edema (+LR = 2.1; 95% CI: 0.9 to 5.0) all had likelihood ratios that would not significantly impact decision making. Physical examination findings that were found to be helpful include the S3 gallop (+LR = 11; 95% CI: 4.9 to 25.0) and the abdomino-jugular reflex (+LR = 6.4; 95% CI: 0.8 to 51.0). Unfortunately the high likelihood ratios encountered with these examination findings were largely a result of their high specificities. Their low sensitivities (<25%) make them poor screening tools.

In summary, clinicians should seek out a previous history of heart failure to assist in confirming the diagnosis of heart failure. In addition to the classic findings associated with heart failure, clinicians should specifically listen for an S3 gallop and test for the abdomino-jugular reflex to aid in diagnostic certainty.

Question 2: In patients with undifferentiated acute dyspnea who present to the ED (population), does a natriuretic peptide measurement (intervention) improve the sensitivity or specificity (diagnostic test characteristics) for diagnosing acute heart failure compared to clinical assessment alone (control)?

Search strategy

- PubMed: (BNP OR natriuretic peptide) AND (CHF OR heart failure) AND (dyspnea OR emergency department). Studies were limited to those that were prospectively conducted in the ED, excluded patients with concurrent myocardial infarction, and had a criterion standard of acute heart failure

Dyspnea is a predominant feature of ADHF, as well as many other ED presentations such as asthma and COPD exacerbations. Wheezing can also be a significant feature in each of these disease processes. It is not uncommon for patients to suffer symptoms as a consequence of heart failure, COPD and/or asthma simultaneously, and thus it can be difficult to distinguish the primary cause of an acute respiratory distress presentation.

B-type natriuretic peptide (BNP) is secreted by the right and left ventricles as a pro-hormone in response to increased pressure. It is cleaved into BNP and NT-proBNP. BNP decreases preload and afterload, increases the glomerular filtration rate, and decreases sodium reabsorption [18]. Natriuretic peptides have been shown to be elevated in persons with ADHF. Therefore, the use of these peptides as markers of ADHF has been the subject of considerable research in the past decade.

The aforementioned search identified 17 original studies that have investigated the diagnostic utility and clinical impact of measuring BNP in patients with dyspnea. Further, three systematic reviews and one critical appraisal have also been published. The most comprehensive systematic review was performed by Wang et al. in 2005 and its findings are summarized in Table 19.1 [19]. This review focused only on BNP because there was limited information about NT-proBNP at the time of publication. Korenstein

BNP level	Sensitivity	Specificity	Positive LR (95% CI)	Negative LR (95% CI)
>50 pg/ml	0.97	0.44	1.7 (1.2 to 2.6)	0.06 (0.03 to 0.12)
>100 pg/ml	0.93	0.66	2.7 (2.0 to 3.9)	0.11 (0.07 to 0.16)
>250 pg/ml	0.89	0.81	4.6 (2.6 to 8.0)	0.14 (0.06 to 0.33)

Table 19.1 Systematic review of BNP use in dyspneic patients with possible acute heart failure.

CI, confidence interval; LR, likelihood ratio.

et al. performed a similar study [20]. The critical appraisal by Schwam in 2004 [21] provided excellent details about three individual studies, but did not attempt to pool data. The systematic review by Doust et al. in 2004 [22] did not specifically focus on ED patients and is thus the least relevant.

The largest study to date evaluating serum BNP levels in the diagnosis of heart failure was performed by Maisel et al. [23]. In this study, BNP levels were obtained from 1586 patients with a chief complaint of dyspnea. The gold standard diagnosis was determined by chart review performed by cardiologists who were blinded to BNP levels. When compared with history, physical examination and any other laboratory value, BNP levels were found to be the most significant predictor of ADHF. They noted a diagnostic accuracy of 83.4% when a cut-point of 100 pg/ml was utilized. Sensitivity and specificity were 90% and 76% (negative likelihood ratio, $-LR = 0.13$; 95% CI: 0.11 to 0.16), respectively.

In a European study, Mueller et al. evaluated BNP measurement in the ED with respect to length of hospital stay and total cost of treatment in the context of a randomized controlled trial [24]. Four hundred and fifty-two patients were enrolled; 225 had bedside point-of-care BNP determination as part of their emergency assessment, while 227 did not. The authors found the initial BNP determination reduced both hospital (75% vs 85%) and intensive care unit admissions (15% vs 14%). They also noted a decrease in median length of stay (LOS) (8 vs 11 days) as well as lower mean cost of treatment (US$5410 vs $7264). Mortality at 30 days was not significantly different between the two groups. While one would expect an earlier diagnosis of ADHF to affect hospital LOS and decrease further diagnostic testing and costs, many other factors likely contribute to total hospital LOS and cost. Furthermore, the median LOS in this study (8–11 days) was much higher than that encountered in US hospitals (median 4–5 days).

The Wang systematic review [19] suggests that BNP at low levels (<100 pg/ml) have a reasonable $-LR$ (0.11; 95% CI: 0.07 to 0.16) for excluding acute heart failure. The appraisal of the Maisel study by Schwam [21] revealed similar findings. A useful $-LR$ was felt to occur at levels <80 pg/ml ($-LR = 0.33$; 95% CI: 0.23 to 0.50). Further, Schwam's findings suggest that BNP levels needed to be over 400 pg/ml ($+LR = 5.0$; 95% CI: 3.3 to 7.9) or over 1000 pg/ml ($+LR = 16$; 95% CI: 10 to 26) to be useful in confirming acute heart failure as a diagnosis. Korenstein's systematic review [20] revealed similar results, with a $-LR$ of 0.14 at levels <100 pg/ml and a $+LR$ of 7.6 at levels >400 pg/ml.

Similar to the Maisel trial mentioned above, Januzzi et al. investigated NT-proBNP in the evaluation of dyspnea [15]. Six hundred patients were enrolled and the primary endpoint was a comparison of NT-proBNP versus clinical judgment in correctly diagnosing ADHF. Also similar to the Maisel trial, the authors found NT-proBNP to be the single most accurate predictor of ADHF (OR = 44; 95% CI: 21.0 to 91.0). At a cut-point of 900 pg/ml, sensitivity and specificity for the diagnosis of ADHF were 90% and 76% ($-LR = 0.13$; 95% CI: 0.9 to 0.20), respectively. The negative predictive value was 94% and diagnostic accuracy was 87%. Previous head-to-head comparisons have found similar test characteristics between NT-proBNP and BNP. Hence, it would be expected that NT-proBNP might be helpful in a similar manner: only very low (<300 pg/ml) and very high (>1000 pg/ml) values would be useful in excluding and diagnosing acute heart failure.

Overall, natriuretic peptides appear to be somewhat helpful in the diagnosis of ADHF; however, they are particularly helpful at very low (to exclude ADHF) or very high (to confirm ADHF) levels. The American College of Emergency Physicians issued a clinical policy statement regarding the evaluation and treatment of ADHF in October 2006 [25]. One of the main thrusts of the statement was serum BNP determination in the evaluation of dyspneic ED patients for whom decompensated heart failure should be a consideration. The authors assigned serum BNP determination a moderate clinical certainty recommendation and further recommended cut-off values (i.e., ruling out and ruling in) of 100 and 500 pg/ml, respectively. Serum NT-ProBNP also received a moderate clinical certainty recommendation with upper and lower limits of 300 and 1000 pg/ml, respectively.

Question 3: In patients with ADHF (population), what is the efficacy and safety (outcomes) of initiating nitroglycerin treatment compared to oxygen and diuretic treatment (control)?

Search strategy

- PubMed: nitroglycerin AND (acute heart failure OR congestive heart failure) AND furosemide. Limits: clinical trial, randomized clinical trial
- PubMed: further nitroglycerin AND emergency department AND heart failure

Nitroglycerin has been a cornerstone of therapy in ADHF. It has been used in several forms including sublingual, topical and intravenous. The use of nitroglycerin in the treatment of ADHF is recommended by the American College of Emergency Physicians, the Heart Failure Society of America and the European Society of Cardiology [25–27]. Registry data suggest it has a better safety profile than dobutamine or milrinone, and one similar to nesiritide [28].

The aforementioned search identified one original prospective investigation of ED patients with acute heart failure who were randomized to: (i) predominantly isosorbide dinitrate; or (ii) predominantly furosemide [29]. The authors randomized 110 patients to receive either: (i) 3 mg isosorbide dinitrate IV every 5 minutes plus furosemide 40 mg IV; or (ii) isosorbide dinitrate 1 mg/h (titrated 1 mg/h every 10 minutes) plus furosemide 80 mg IV every 15 minutes. This study found significant differences in oxygen saturation, subsequent intubation and myocardial infarction, all in favor of the high-dose isosorbide group (all $P < 0.05$). There was no significant difference in the in-hospital mortality ($P = 0.61$). Several other studies have investigated nitroglycerin against novel inotropes and vasodilators, but these studies are difficult to extrapolate to the ED setting [30–33].

A subset of ADHF patients may derive particular benefit from nitrate therapy. Approximately 50% of patients with acute heart failure will present with a systolic blood pressure over 140 mmHg [34–36]. These patients tend to be older, female, have a history of diastolic dysfunction, and often have acute symptoms that have been present for less than 24–48 hours. Because of the shorter symptom duration they are more likely to have acute pulmonary edema (both on physical examination and chest radiograph) rather than generalized edema (weight gain, leg edema). Symptoms are often the result of a significant increase in afterload and fluid misdistribution rather than total body fluid overload. This subset of patients is most likely to benefit from a predominant vasodilator strategy as discussed in the previous trial.

In summary, despite guideline recommendation to use nitroglycerin in ADHF, the evidence for doing so is relatively weak. The subset of patients most likely to benefit from a predominant vasodilator strategy are likely those with hypertension upon ED presentation.

Question 4: In patients with ADHF (population), does non-invasive positive pressure ventilation (intervention) decrease intubation rates and/or mortality (outcomes) compared to standard care (control)?

Search strategy

- PubMed: (pulmonary edema OR congestive heart failure OR heart failure) AND (positive pressure ventilation OR noninvasive ventilation OR noninvasive positive pressure ventilation OR NPPV OR BiPAP OR CPAP). Limits: randomized clinical trials and human studies in the English language

Non-invasive ventilation was introduced as a treatment modality for acute cardiogenic pulmonary edema in the mid-1990s based on observations that it was a useful adjunct for other forms of respiratory disorders such as COPD [37,38]. The two basic forms of NIV are continuous positive airway pressure (CPAP) and non-invasive positive pressure ventilation (NPPV, or BiPAP (bi-level positive airway pressure)). CPAP involves a constant level of positive pressure during both inhalation and exhalation, whereas BiPAP alternates between two levels of pressure – a higher inspiratory pressure and a lower expiratory pressure. In addition to decreasing the work of breathing, CPAP also decreases afterload without decreasing cardiac index, and it is thought BiPAP acts via the same mechanism.

The search identified 12 studies that met our criteria [39–50]. Several of these investigated CPAP and/or BiPAP versus standard oxygen treatment (typically a non-rebreather oxygen mask with 10 L/min flow), a few compared CPAP versus BiPAP alone, and three systematic reviews were also included. The identified studies encompassed a wide variety of study designs (different primary endpoints), as well as results. While some studies demonstrated significant differences in outcomes such as intubation or mortality rates, these differences were not always statistically significant. It is also unclear whether a true difference between CPAP and BiPAP exists. Consequently, meta-analyses have been performed in an effort to pool data and increase the statistical power to identify differences not apparent in individual trials (Table 19.2).

Pang et al. performed a meta-analysis of NIV versus standard oxygen therapy in 1998 [51]. Data were pooled from three studies that compared CPAP and/or BiPAP to standard medical therapy. The authors specifically investigated the effect(s) of NPPV on mortality and the need for intubation. They found that CPAP was associated with a reduced rate of intubation (RR $= -26\%$; 95% CI: -14% to -38%) and a trend toward decreased mortality (RR $= -6.6\%$; 95% CI: -16% to $+3\%$) when compared to standard oxygen therapy. The pooled analysis neither confirmed nor excluded the value of BiPAP compared to standard therapy alone.

Masip et al. performed a meta-analysis of trials comparing NIV (i.e., CPAP and BiPAP) to standard oxygen therapy in the treatment of acute cardiogenic pulmonary edema [52]. Fifteen trials were included and involved data from 727 patients. Primary endpoints were in-hospital mortality and intubation rate. The secondary endpoint was myocardial infarction. From this review, it was shown that NIV significantly decreased the relative mortality risk by 43% (CPAP 46%, BiPAP 37%). This was statistically significant for CPAP, but BiPAP results failed to reach statistical significance. It was also shown that NIV significantly reduced the relative intubation risk by 57% ($P < 0.001$), and the results were statistically significant for both CPAP and BiPAP ($P < 0.001$ and $P = 0.002$, respectively). Overall rates of myocardial infarction were not significantly different between standard oxygen therapy and either mode of non-invasive ventilation (RR $= 0.89$; 95% CI: 0.69 to 1.17).

Similarly, Collins et al. also performed a meta-analysis comparing NIV to standard oxygen therapy in the treatment of acute

Table 19.2 Systematic reviews evaluating non-invasive positive pressure ventilation in the treatment of acute decompensated heart failure.

	Type of study	Patients (n)	Treatments compared	Pooled RR intubation (95% CI)	Pooled RR mortality (95% CI)	Significant findings
Pang et al. [51]	Meta-analysis	3 trials (180 patients)	CPAP vs SOT	0.74 (0.62 to 0.86)	0.94 (0.84 to 1.03)	CPAP decreases intubation rate. Non-significant trend toward decreased mortality
Masip et al. [52]	Meta-analysis	15 trials (727 patients)	BiPAP vs CPAP vs SOT	0.43 (0.32 to 0.57)	0.55 (0.40 to 0.78)	NIV decreases intubation rate and mortality rate. No significant differences between CPAP and BiPAP
Collins et al. [53]	Meta-analysis	11 trials (494 patients)	BiPAP vs CPAP vs SOT	0.43 (0.21 to 0.87)	0.61 (0.41 to 0.91)	NIV decreases intubation rate and mortality rate. No significant differences between CPAP and BiPAP

BiPAP, bi-level positive airway pressure; CPAP, continuous positive airway pressure; LOS, length of stay; NIV, non-invasive ventilation; SOT, standard oxygen therapy.

cardiogenic pulmonary edema [53]. This systematic review focused on ED patients only, making it most applicable to this chapter. Data from 11 ED trials were evaluated. Primary endpoints were hospital mortality and intubation rates. Of these trials, three compared CPAP to standard oxygen therapy, two compared BiPAP to standard oxygen therapy, four compared CPAP to BiPAP alone, and two compared CPAP to BiPAP with a standard oxygen therapy control. Seven of the trials included mortality data when comparing NIV to standard oxygen therapy. The pooled analysis of 494 patients suggested that NIV, in addition to standard medical therapy, significantly reduced hospital mortality compared to standard medical therapy alone (RR = 0.61; 95% CI: 0.41 to 0.91). Similarly, a pooled analysis of six studies and 436 patients suggested that NIV was associated with a significant decrease in intubation rates (RR = 0.43; 95% CI: 0.21 to 0.87).

In summary, the above findings suggest that both CPAP and BiPAP are useful adjuncts in the ED treatment of ADHF. The American College of Emergency Physicians extended a moderate clinical certainty recommendation for the use of CPAP, while BiPAP was given a preliminary, inconclusive or conflicting evidence, or based on panel consensus recommendation due to the concern for potential myocardial ischemia and/or infarction [25].

Question 5: In patients with ADHF (population), does administration of nesiritide (i.e., recombinant BNP) affect renal function and/or mortality (outcomes) compared to standard care (control)?

Search strategy

- PubMed: nesiritide AND (congestive heart failure OR acute heart failure) AND (emergency department OR treatment). Limits: clinical trial, randomized controlled trial

Due to the neuro-hormonal effects, and the increased serum levels of BNP in the setting of heart failure, it has been speculated that recombinant BNP may be a therapeutic addition to the treatment of acute exacerbations of heart failure. The literature search above was performed seeking original trials and studies of patients with acute heart failures which were not the result of an acute coronary syndrome. The search identified 10 original articles and three systematic reviews that evaluated the use of nesiritide in acute heart failure patients (Table 19.3) [5,54–62].

In 2002, the VMAC Investigators published a report comparing nesiritide (recombinant BNP) to nitroglycerin in the treatment of decompensated heart failure [31]. They enrolled 489 patients; primary endpoints were changes in pulmonary capillary wedge pressures (PCWP) and subjective improvement in dyspnea. After 15 minutes, significant reductions in PCWP were noted in the nesiritide group when compared to either nitroglycerin or placebo ($P < 0.05$). These differences continued to be significant for 3 hours, at which time patients in the placebo group were randomized to cross over into either the nesiritide or nitroglycerin group. After 24 hours, the reduction in PCWP was still significantly greater in the nesiritide group when compared to the nitroglycerin group ($P = 0.04$). There was no difference, however, in resolution of dyspnea between the nitroglycerin and nesiritide groups, although both treatments were significantly more effective than placebo at 3 hours.

In 2005, Sackner-Bernstein published two meta-analyses investigating the development of acute renal insufficiency and death associated with nesiritide use [63,64]. For the effect on renal function, data from five randomized studies involving 1269 patients were analyzed. These pooled results suggested that nesiritide, either in low- or high-dose regimens, significantly increased the risk of worsening renal function (22% vs 15%), as defined by a rise in serum creatinine >0.5 mg/dl (RR = 1.52; 95% CI: 1.16 to 2.00). Although renal function was significantly reduced by nesiritide

Table 19.3 Systematic reviews evaluating nesiritide administration in the treatment of acute decompensated heart failure.

	Type of study	Patients (*n*)	Treatments compared	Pooled RR worsening renal function (95% CI)	Pooled RR 30-day mortality (95% CI)	Significant findings
Sackner-Bernstein [63]	Meta-analysis	1269 (pooled from 5 randomized trials)	Nesiritide vs non-inotrope controls	1.52 (1.16 to 2.00)		Nesiritide increases risk of worsening renal function. No difference in dialysis
Sackner-Bernstein [64]	Meta-analysis	862 (pooled from 3 randomized trials)	Nesiritide vs non-inotrope controls		1.74 (0.97 to 3.12)	Nesiritide associated with increased risk of death within 30 days
Arora [65]	Meta-analysis	1507 (pooled from 6 trials)	Nesiritide vs placebo or active comparator		1.33 (0.84 to 2.10)	

CI, confidence interval; RR, relative risk.

administration, there was no difference in hemodialysis between the two groups (RR = 1.18; 95% CI: 0.5 to 2.76).

The same group also pooled data from three randomized trials involving 862 patients, and determined the risk of 30-day mortality associated with nesiritide administration [64]. They found that the administration of nesiritide was associated with an increased risk of death (7.2% vs 4.0%) when compared to non-inotrope-based therapy (RR = 1.74; 95% CI: 0.97 to 3.12).

The third meta-analysis that was identified pooled data from seven trials involving 1717 patients [65]. All included trials were randomized, controlled with double-blind or open-label design. However, one of the trials enrolled outpatients, so a separate analysis was performed with the patients from this trial excluded [66]. The authors found a pooled RR of 30-day mortality of 1.33 (95% CI: 0.84 to 2.10) in favor of control therapy.

In summary, given the concern for a potential increase in the risk of death and worsening renal failure, nesiritide should not be considered a first-line agent for the treatment of ADHF in the ED. The American College of Emergency Physicians also recommended Nesiritide not be considered first-line therapy based on a Class C recommendation (based on preliminary, inconclusive, or conflicting evidence).

Question 6: In patients with ADHF (population), are there any clinical factors (intervention) that predict (objective test characteristic) which patients can be safely discharged home (outcome)?

Search strategy

- PubMed: (CHF OR congestive heart failure OR acute heart failure) AND (prognosis OR risk stratification) AND (ED OR emergency department)

Over 80% of ADHF admissions originate in an ED and account for a majority of expenditures, yet it has been suggested up to 50% could be discharged home after initial therapy [67–69]. However, patients with ADHF have an in-hospital mortality of 4–7%, and 60-day mortality and recidivism rates of 10% and 25%, respectively [31,33,34,37]. Further, current ADHF guidelines for ED and hospital disposition are based on little or no empirical evidence. This can result in an overestimation of risk leading to unnecessary admissions and prolonged hospital LOS [68,70–75]. Over the past two decades, studies have identified high-risk patients with ADHF based on specific physiological variables (e.g., vital signs, serum creatinine levels) [76–87]. Efforts to identify the features that characterize a low-risk patient, and possibly enable ED discharge, seem warranted.

The aforementioned search strategy sought to identify studies that utilized ED data to enroll patients with ADHF. Studies that enrolled heart failure patients as a result of acute myocardial infarction were excluded. The search identified seven studies that met these inclusion criteria [70,76,79,81,88–90]. There were no systematic reviews identified. The majority of these studies were based on retrospectively collected data, often from pre-existing registries using *International Classification of Diseases*, 9th revision (ICD-9) codes to identify ED patients with ADHF. One of the studies was a follow-up from the same cohort of patients presented previously [89,90]. Two of the studies focused on observation unit patients and their associated outcomes [88,91]; however, they did identify features associated with decreased adverse events and hospital LOS. Those patients with normal or high blood pressure, normal serum sodium and preserved renal function were less likely to have adverse events, but a true "low-risk" cohort has yet to be identified.

In summary, discharge decisions by emergency physicians for patients with ADHF are not evidence based. A prospectively derived, ED-based predictive instrument that stratifies patients into low-, intermediate- and high-risk of short-term (less than 2 weeks) outcomes has yet to be developed. An ongoing investigation led by emergency medicine investigators, supported by the National Heart, Lung and Blood Institute, aims to answer this question [92].

Question 7: In patients with ADHF felt to be non-high risk (population), does observation unit management (intervention) reduce ED relapse and conserve hospital resources (outcomes) compared to hospital admission (control)?

Search strategy

- PubMed: observation unit AND (acute heart failure OR heart failure OR CHF OR pulmonary edema) AND/OR emergency department

The growth of observation unit (OU) medicine under the direction of emergency physicians provides an ideal opportunity for further risk stratification after initial therapy, maximizing the clinical applicability of these questions to the emergency setting. The OU provides a safe, less costly alternative to hospitalization, where patients can receive up to 24 hours of care to further delineate the need for admission [93–95]. Characterizing patients with ADHF as being appropriate for the OU, and thus decreasing hospital admission rates, could result in significant cost savings.

Using the search strategy above and focusing on non-review articles and studies that took place in ED-based OU's, we identified four articles [88,91,96,97]. No prospective randomized trials or systematic reviews were identified. Another article was only presented in abstract format, and a final article was a prospective randomized trial of a therapeutic intervention (nesiritide) compared to standard OU care [5,98]. Two of the articles had similar criteria for selecting patients for OU management [96,97]. Their protocols suggested that afebrile patients with preserved renal function, no ECG or biomarker evidence of ischemia, and not needing a titratable intravenous medication for blood pressure control were reasonable candidates for OU management. Compared to hospital admission, both studies found OU management to be associated with a significant cost saving and no difference in 30-day event rates. The third article examined predictors of successful OU discharge after ADHF management [88]. An elevated blood urea nitrogen was found to be the only predictor of hospital admission after OU management in a multi-variate model. Unfortunately, the study did not consider recidivism or death after OU management (discharge or admission). As a consequence, its conclusions regarding the efficacy of OU management are limited. The final study suggested that patients with a preserved systolic blood pressure (>160 mmHg) and normal troponin levels were good candidates for safe OU management and discharge [91].

In summary, while awaiting validated predictive instruments to assist with ADHF risk stratification, OU management is a reasonable alternative to hospital admission in non-high-risk patients. Preliminary data suggest ADHF patients with preserved renal function, no evidence of ongoing cardiac ischemia and well-maintained

blood pressure are reasonable candidates for safe OU management and discharge.

Conclusions

The aforementioned patient was diagnosed with ADHF based on clinical examination findings and an elevated BNP value. She received several doses of sublingual nitroglycerin followed by nitroglycerin paste applied to her anterior chest wall. She responded well to the administration of furosemide and diuresed appropriately, with significant improvement of her symptoms. Her respirations became less labored with NPPV and she no longer required adjunctive therapy by the time she was transferred to the ward. She had no ECG changes and had negative cardiac biomarkers throughout her entire hospitalization. She was discharged on hospital day 3 with a final diagnosis of ADHF.

ADHF is a common and problematic condition in the ED from both diagnostic and management perspectives. Since dyspnea can be caused by a myriad of pathophysiological mechanisms, the diagnosis can be challenging. The available data suggest that either very high or very low natriuretic peptides values can be helpful in the diagnostic work-up of dyspneic ED patients. Two recent meta-analyses suggest that NIV, in addition to standard care, decreases intubation rates and mortality in ADHF. Use of other treatments, including diuretics, oxygen and inotropes, are less evidence based, yet still form part of the recommendations for treatment. While nesiritide appears to be as efficacious as nitroglycerin with respect to dyspnea improvement and PCWP reduction, safety concerns relegate it to second-line therapy in ED patients with ADHF. Finally, discharge decision making and risk stratification for patients with ADHF is problematic and has not been well delineated. This will be an important area of future research whose results will likely have a profound impact on health policy.

References

1 American Heart Association. *Heart Disease and Stroke Statistics – 2007 update.* American Heart Association, Dallas, 2006.

2 Adams KF, Jr., Fonarow CG, Emerman CL, et al. Characteristics and outcomes of patients hospitalized for heart failure in the United States: rationale, design, and preliminary observations from the first 100,000 cases in the Acute Decompensated Heart Failure National Registry (ADHERE). *Am Heart J* 1005;**149**(2):209–16.

3 Hugli O, Braun JE, Kim S, Pelletier AJ, Camargo CA, Jr. United States emergency department visits for acute decompensated heart failure, 1992 to 2001. *Am J Cardiol* 2005;**96**(11):1537–42.

4 Peacock W, Fonarow GC, Emerman CL, Mills RM, Wynne J. Impact of early initiation of intravenous therapy for acute decompensated heart failure on outcomes in ADHERE. *Cardiology* 2006;**107**(1):44–51.

5 Peacock WF, Holland R, Gyarmathy R, et al. Observation unit treatment of heart failure with nesiritide: results from the proaction trial. *J Emerg Med* 2005;**29**(3):243–52.

6 Springfield CL, Sebat F, Johnson D, Lengle S, Sebat C. Utility of impedance cardiography to determine cardiac vs. noncardiac cause of dyspnea in the emergency department. *Congest Heart Fail* 2004;**10**(2 Suppl 2):14–16.

7 Marantz PR, Kaplan MC, Alderman MH. Clinical diagnosis of congestive heart failure in patients with acute dyspnea. *Chest* 1990;**97**(4):776–81.

8 Morrison LK, Harrison A, Krishnaswamy P, Kazanegra R, Clopton P, Maisel A. Utility of a rapid B-natriuretic peptide assay in differentiating congestive heart failure from lung disease in patients presenting with dyspnea. *J Am Coll Cardiol* 2002;**39**(2):202–9.

9 McCullough PA, Nowak RM, McCord J, et al. B-type natriuretic peptide and clinical judgment in emergency diagnosis of heart failure: analysis from Breathing Not Properly (BNP) Multinational Study. *Circulation* 2002;**106**(4):416–22.

10 Knudsen CW, Omland T, Clopton P, et al. Diagnostic value of B-type natriuretic peptide and chest radiographic findings in patients with acute dyspnea. *Am J Med* 2004;**116**(6):363–8.

11 Logeart D, Saudubray C, Beyne P, et al. Comparative value of Doppler echocardiography and B-type natriuretic peptide assay in the etiologic diagnosis of acute dyspnea. *J Am Coll Cardiol* 2002;**40**(10):1794–800.

12 Knudsen CW, Riis JS, Finsen AV, et al. Diagnostic value of a rapid test for B-type natriuretic peptide in patients presenting with acute dyspnea effect of age and gender. *Eur J Heart Fail* 2004;**6**(1):55–62.

13 Bayes-Genis A, Santalo-Bel M, Zapico-Muniz E, et al. N-terminal pro-brain natriuretic peptide (NT-proBNP) in the emergency diagnosis and in-hospital monitoring of patients with dyspnoea and ventricular dysfunction. *Eur J Heart Fail* 2004;**6**(3):301–8.

14 Dao Q, Krishnaswamy P, Kazanegra R, et al. Utility of B-type natriuretic peptide in the diagnosis of congestive heart failure in an urgent-care setting. *J Am Coll Cardiol* 2001;**37**(2):379–85.

15 Januzzi JL, Jr., Camargo CA, Anwaruddin S, et al. The N-terminal Pro-BNP investigation of dyspnea in the emergency department (PRIDE) study. *Am J Cardiol* 2005;**95**(8):948–54.

16 Mueller T, Gegenhuber A, Poelz W, Haltmayer M. Diagnostic accuracy of B type natriuretic peptide and amino terminal proBNP in the emergency diagnosis of heart failure. *Heart* (British Cardiac Society) 2005;**91**(5):606–12.

17 Mueller C, Frana B, Rodriguez D, Laule-Kilian K, Perruchoud AP. Emergency diagnosis of congestive heart failure: impact of signs and symptoms. *Can J Cardiol* 2005;**21**(11):921–4.

18 Mayo DD, Colletti JE, Kuo DC. Brain natriuretic peptide (BNP) testing in the emergency department. *J Emerg Med* 2006;**31**(2):201–10.

19 Wang CS, FitzGerald JM, Schulzer M, Mak E, Ayas NT. Does this dyspneic patient in the emergency department have congestive heart failure? *JAMA* 2005;**294**(15):1944–56.

20 Korenstein D, Wisnivesky JP, Wyer P, Adler R, Ponieman D, McGinn T. The utility of B-type natriuretic peptide in the diagnosis of heart failure in the emergency department: a systematic review. *BMC Emerg Med* 2007;**7**:6.

21 Schwam E. B-type natriuretic peptide for diagnosis of heart failure in emergency department patients: a critical appraisal. *Acad Emerg Med* 2004;**11**(6):686–91.

22 Doust JA, Glasziou PP, Pietrzak E, Dobson AJ. A systematic review of the diagnostic accuracy of natriuretic peptides for heart failure. *Arch Intern Med* 2004;**164**(18):1978–84.

23 Maisel AS, Krishnaswamy P, Nowak RM, et al. Rapid measurement of B-type natriuretic peptide in the emergency diagnosis of heart failure. *N Engl J Med* 2002;**347**(3):161–7.

24 Mueller C, Laule-Kilian K, Schindler C, et al. Cost-effectiveness of B-type natriuretic peptide testing in patients with acute dyspnea. *Arch Intern Med* 2006;**166**(10):1081–7.

25 Silvers SM, Howell JM, Kosowsky JM, Rokos IC, Jagoda AS. Clinical policy: critical issues in the evaluation and management of adult patients presenting to the emergency department with acute heart failure syndromes. *Ann Emerg Med* 2007;**49**(5):627–69.

26 Heart Failure Society of America. HFSA 2006 comprehensive heart failure practice guideline. *J Card Fail* 2006;**12**(1):e1–2.

27 Nieminen MS, Bohm M, Cowie MR, et al. Executive summary of the guidelines on the diagnosis and treatment of acute heart failure: the Task Force on Acute Heart Failure of the European Society of Cardiology. *Eur Heart J* 2005;**26**(4):384–416.

28 Abraham WT, Adams KF, Fonarow GC, et al. In-hospital mortality in patients with acute decompensated heart failure requiring intravenous vasoactive medications: an analysis from the Acute Decompensated Heart Failure National Registry (ADHERE). *J Am Coll Cardiol* 2005;**46**(1):57–64.

29 Cotter G, Metzkor E, Kaluski E, et al. Randomised trial of high-dose isosorbide dinitrate plus low-dose furosemide versus high-dose furosemide plus low-dose isosorbide dinitrate in severe pulmonary oedema. *Lancet* 1998;**351**(9100):389–93.

30 Collins SP, Hinckley WR, Storrow AB. Critical review and recommendations for nesiritide use in the emergency department. *J Emerg Med* 2005;**29**(3):317–29.

31 VMAC Investigators. Intravenous nesiritide vs nitroglycerin for treatment of decompensated congestive heart failure: a randomized controlled trial. *JAMA* 2002;**287**(12):1531–40.

32 Gheorghiade M, Konstam MA, Burnett JC, Jr., et al. Short-term clinical effects of tolvaptan, an oral vasopressin antagonist, in patients hospitalized for heart failure: the EVEREST Clinical Status Trials. *JAMA* 2007;**297**(12):1332–43.

33 Cuffe MS, Califf RM, Adams KF, Jr., et al. Short-term intravenous milrinone for acute exacerbation of chronic heart failure: a randomized controlled trial. *JAMA* 2002;**287**(12):1541–7.

34 Adams KF, Jr., Fonarow GC, Emerman CL, et al. Characteristics and outcomes of patients hospitalized for heart failure in the United States: rationale, design, and preliminary observations from the first 100,000 cases in the Acute Decompensated Heart Failure National Registry (ADHERE). *Am Heart J* 2005;**149**(2):209–16.

35 Fonarow G, Abraham WT, Albert NM, et al. Characteristics, treatment and outcomes of patients hospitalized for heart failure with preserved systolic function: a report from OPTIMIZE-HF. *J Am Coll Cardiol* 2006;**47**(4 Suppl A):47A.

36 Cleland JG, Swedberg K, Follath F, et al. The EuroHeart Failure survey programme – a survey on the quality of care among patients with heart failure in Europe. Part 1: patient characteristics and diagnosis. *Eur Heart J* 2003;**24**(5):442–63.

37 Brochard L, Mancebo J, Wysocki M, et al. Noninvasive ventilation for acute exacerbations of chronic obstructive pulmonary disease. *N Engl J Med* 1995;**333**(13):817–22.

38 Plant PK, Owen JL, Elliott MW. Early use of non-invasive ventilation for acute exacerbations of chronic obstructive pulmonary disease on general respiratory wards: a multicentre randomised controlled trial. *Lancet* 2000;**355**(9219):1931–5.

39 Park M, Lorenzi-Filho G, Feltrim MI, et al. Oxygen therapy, continuous positive airway pressure, or noninvasive bilevel positive pressure

ventilation in the treatment of acute cardiogenic pulmonary edema. *Arq Bras Cardiol* 2001;**76**(3):221–30.

40 Mehta S, Jay GD, Woolard RH, et al. Randomized, prospective trial of bilevel versus continuous positive airway pressure in acute pulmonary edema. *Crit Care Med* 1997;**25**(4):620–28.

41 Bersten AD, Holt AW, Vedig AE, Skowronski GA, Baggoley CJ. Treatment of severe cardiogenic pulmonary edema with continuous positive airway pressure delivered by face mask. *N Engl J Med* 1991;**325**(26):1825–30.

42 Crane SD, Elliott MW, Gilligan P, Richards K, Gray AJ. Randomised controlled comparison of continuous positive airways pressure, bilevel non-invasive ventilation, and standard treatment in emergency department patients with acute cardiogenic pulmonary oedema. *Emerg Med J* 2004;**21**(2):155–61.

43 Kelly CA, Newby DE, McDonagh TA, et al. Randomised controlled trial of continuous positive airway pressure and standard oxygen therapy in acute pulmonary oedema; effects on plasma brain natriuretic peptide concentrations. *Eur Heart J* 2002;**23**(17):1379–86.

44 L'Her E, Duquesne F, Girou E, et al. Noninvasive continuous positive airway pressure in elderly cardiogenic pulmonary edema patients. *Intensive Care Med* 2004;**30**(5):882–8.

45 Levitt MA. A prospective, randomized trial of BiPAP in severe acute congestive heart failure. *J Emerg Med* 2001;**21**(4):363–9.

46 Nava S, Carbone G, DiBattista N, et al. Noninvasive ventilation in cardiogenic pulmonary edema: a multicenter randomized trial. *Am J Respir Crit Care Med* 2003;**168**(12):1432–7.

47 Park M, Sangean MC, Volpe M de S, et al. Randomized, prospective trial of oxygen, continuous positive airway pressure, and bilevel positive airway pressure by face mask in acute cardiogenic pulmonary edema. *Crit Care Med* 2004;**32**(12):2407–15.

48 Bellone A, Monari A, Cortellaro F, Vettorello M, Arlati S, Coen D. Myocardial infarction rate in acute pulmonary edema: noninvasive pressure support ventilation versus continuous positive airway pressure. *Crit Care Med* 2004;**32**(9):1860–65.

49 Bellone A, Vettorello M, Monari A, Cortellaro F, Coen D. Noninvasive pressure support ventilation vs. continuous positive airway pressure in acute hypercapnic pulmonary edema. *Intensive Care Med* 2005;**31**(6):807–11.

50 Cross AM, Cameron P, Kierce M, Ragg M, Kelly AM. Non-invasive ventilation in acute respiratory failure: a randomised comparison of continuous positive airway pressure and bi-level positive airway pressure. *Emerg Med J* 2003;**20**(6):531–4.

51 Pang D, Keenan SP, Cook DJ, Sibbald WJ. The effect of positive pressure airway support on mortality and the need for intubation in cardiogenic pulmonary edema: a systematic review. *Chest* 1998;**114**(4):1185–92.

52 Masip J, Roque M, Sanchez B, Fernandez R, Subirana M, Exposito JA. Noninvasive ventilation in acute cardiogenic pulmonary edema: systematic review and meta-analysis. *JAMA* 2005;**294**(24):3124–30.

53 Collins SP, Mielniczuk LM, Whittingham HA, Boseley ME, Schramm DR, Storrow AB. The use of noninvasive ventilation in emergency department patients with acute cardiogenic pulmonary edema: a systematic review. *Ann Emer Med* 2006;**48**(3):260–69, e1–4.

54 Burger AJ, Horton DP, LeJemtel T, et al. Effect of nesiritide (B-type natriuretic peptide) and dobutamine on ventricular arrhythmias in the treatment of patients with acutely decompensated congestive heart failure: the PRECEDENT study. *Am Heart J* 2002;**144**(6):1102–8.

55 Burger AJ, Elkayam U, Neibaur MT, et al. Comparison of the occurrence of ventricular arrhythmias in patients with acutely decompensated con-

gestive heart failure receiving dobutamine versus nesiritide therapy. *Am J Cardiol* 2001;**88**(1):35–9.

56 Hobbs RE, Miller LW, Bott-Silverman C, James KB, Rincon G, Grossbard EB. Hemodynamic effects of a single intravenous injection of synthetic human brain natriuretic peptide in patients with heart failure secondary to ischemic or idiopathic dilated cardiomyopathy. *Am J Cardiol* 1996;**78**(8):896–901.

57 Marcus LS, Hart D, Packer M, et al. Hemodynamic and renal excretory effects of human brain natriuretic peptide infusion in patients with congestive heart failure. A double-blind, placebo-controlled, randomized crossover trial. *Circulation* 1996;**94**(12):3184–9.

58 Clarkson PB, Wheeldon NM, MacFadyen RJ, Pringle SD, MacDonald TM. Effects of brain natriuretic peptide on exercise hemodynamics and neurohormones in isolated diastolic heart failure. *Circulation* 1996;**93**(11):2037–42.

59 Colucci WS, Elkayam U, Horton DP, et al. Intravenous nesiritide, a natriuretic peptide, in the treatment of decompensated congestive heart failure. Nesiritide Study Group. *N Engl J Med* 2000;**343**(4):246–53.

60 Lainchbury JG, Richards AM, Nicholls MG, et al. The effects of pathophysiological increments in brain natriuretic peptide in left ventricular systolic dysfunction. *Hypertension* 1997;**30**(3/1):398–404.

61 Mills RM, LeJemtel TH, Horton DP, et al. Sustained hemodynamic effects of an infusion of nesiritide (human b-type natriuretic peptide) in heart failure: a randomized, double-blind, placebo-controlled clinical trial. Natrecor Study Group. *J Am Coll Cardiol* 1999;**34**(1):155–62.

62 Wang DJ, Dowling TC, Meadows D, et al. Nesiritide does not improve renal function in patients with chronic heart failure and worsening serum creatinine. *Circulation* 2004;**110**(12):1620–25.

63 Sackner-Bernstein JD, Kowalski M, Fox M, Aaronson K. Short-term risk of death after treatment with nesiritide for decompensated heart failure: a pooled analysis of randomized controlled trials. *JAMA* 2005;**293**(15):1900–905.

64 Sackner-Bernstein JD, Skopicki HA, Aaronson KD. Risk of worsening renal function with nesiritide in patients with acutely decompensated heart failure. *Circulation* 2005;**111**(12):1487–91.

65 Arora RR, Venkatesh PK, Molnar J. Short and long-term mortality with nesiritide. *Am Heart J* 2006;**152**(6):1084–90.

66 Yancy CW, Saltzberg MT, Berkowitz RL, et al. Safety and feasibility of using serial infusions of nesiritide for heart failure in an outpatient setting (from the FUSION I trial). *Am J Cardiol* 2004;**94**(5):595–601.

67 Graff L, Orledge J, Radford MJ, Wang Y, Petrillo M, Maag R. Correlation of the Agency for Health Care Policy and Research congestive heart failure admission guideline with mortality: peer review organization voluntary hospital association initiative to decrease events (PROVIDE) for congestive heart failure. *Ann Emerg Med* 1999;**34**(4/1):429–37.

68 Smith WR, Poses RM, McClish DK, et al. Prognostic judgments and triage decisions for patients with acute congestive heart failure. *Chest* 2002;**121**(5):1610–17.

69 Polanczyk CA, Rohde LE, Philbin EA, Di Salvo TG. A new casemix adjustment index for hospital mortality among patients with congestive heart failure. *Med Care* 1998;**36**(10):1489–99.

70 Rame JE, Sheffield MA, Dries DL, et al. Outcomes after emergency department discharge with a primary diagnosis of heart failure. *Am Heart J* 2001;**142**(4):714–19.

71 Hunt SA, Abraham WT, Chin MH, et al. ACC/AHA 2005 Guideline update for the diagnosis and management of chronic heart failure in the adult – summary article, a report of the American College of Cardiology/American Heart Association Task Force on Practice Guidelines

(Writing Committee to update the 2001 guidelines for the evaluation and management of heart failure). *J Am Coll Cardiol* 2005;**46**(6):1116–43.

72 Hunt SA, Baker DW, Chin MH, et al. ACC/AHA guidelines for the evaluation and management of chronic heart failure in the adult: executive summary. *J Heart Lung Transplant* 2002;**21**(2):189–203.

73 HFSA. HFSA guidelines for the management of patients with heart failure due to left ventricular systolic dysfunction – pharmacological approaches. *Congest Heart Fail* 2000;**6**(1):11–39.

74 Hunt SA, Abraham WT, Shin MH, et al. Guidelines for the evaluation and management of heart failure. Report of the American College of Cardiology/American Heart Association Task Force on Practice Guidelines (Committee on Evaluation and Management of Heart Failure). *J Am Coll Cardiol* 1995;**26**(5):1376–98.

75 Konstam M, Dracup K, Baker D. *Heart Failure: Evaluation and care of patients with left-ventricular systolic dysfunction.* Clinical Practice Guidelines No. 11. Agency for Health Care Policy and Research, Rockville, MD, 1994:94.

76 Auble TE, Hsieh M, Gardner W, et al. A prediction rule to identify low-risk patients with heart failure. *Acad Emerg Med* 2005;**12**(6):514–21.

77 Harjai KJ, Thompson HW, Turgut T, Shah M. Simple clinical variables are markers of the propensity for readmission in patients hospitalized with heart failure. *Am J Cardiol* 2001;**87**(2):234–7, A9.

78 Chin MH, Goldman L. Correlates of early hospital readmission or death in patients with congestive heart failure. *Am J Cardiol* 1997;**79**(12):1640–44.

79 Katz MH, Nicholson BW, Singer DE, Kelleher PA, Mulley AG, Thibault GE. The triage decision in pulmonary edema. *J Gen Intern Med* 1988;**3**(6):533–9.

80 Esdaile JM, Horwitz RI, Levinton C, Clemens JD, Amatruda JG, Feinstein AR. Response to initial therapy and new onset as predictors of prognosis in patients hospitalized with congestive heart failure. *Clin Invest Med* 1992;**15**(2):122–31.

81 Villacorta H, Rocha N, Cardoso R, et al. Hospital outcome and short-term follow-up of elderly patients presenting to the emergency unit with congestive heart failure. *Arq Bras Cardiol* 1998;**70**(3):167–71.

82 Butler J, Hanumanthu S, Chomsky D, Wilson JR. Frequency of low-risk hospital admissions for heart failure. *Am J Cardiol* 1998;**81**(1):41–4.

83 Plotnick GD, Kelemen MH, Garrett RB, Randall W, Fisher ML. Acute cardiogenic pulmonary edema in the elderly: factors predicting in-hospital and one-year mortality. *South Med J* 1982;**75**(5):565–9.

84 Lee DS, Austin PC, Rouleau JL, Liu PP, Naimark D, Tu JV. Predicting mortality among patients hospitalized for heart failure: derivation and validation of a clinical model. *JAMA* 2003;**290**(19):2581–7.

85 Selker HP, Griffith JL, D'Agostino RB. A time-insensitive predictive instrument for acute hospital mortality due to congestive heart failure: development, testing, and use for comparing hospitals: a multicenter study. *Med Care* 1994;**32**(10):1040–52.

86 Chin MH, Goldman L. Correlates of major complications or death in patients admitted to the hospital with congestive heart failure. *Arch Intern Med* 1996;**156**(16):1814–20.

87 Fonarow GC, Adams KF, Jr., Abraham WT, Yancy CW, Boscardin WJ. Risk stratification for in-hospital mortality in acutely decompensated heart failure: classification and regression tree analysis. *JAMA* 2005;**293**(5):572–80.

88 Burkhardt J, Peacock WF, Emerman CL. Predictors of emergency department observation unit outcomes. *Acad Emerg Med* 2005;**12**(9):869–74.

89 Brophy JM, Deslauriers G, Boucher B, Rouleau JL. The hospital course and short term prognosis of patients presenting to the emergency room with decompensated congestive heart failure. *Can J Cardiol* 1993;**9**(3):219–24.

90 Brophy JM, Deslauriers G, Rouleau JL. Long-term prognosis of patients presenting to the emergency room with decompensated congestive heart failure. *Can J Cardiol* 1994;**10**(5):543–7.

91 Diercks DB, Peacock WF, Kirk JD, Weber JE. ED patients with heart failure: identification of an observational unit-appropriate cohort. *Am J Emerg Med* 2006;**24**(3):319–24.

92 Storrow AB, Collins S, Disalvo T, Han J. *Improving Heart Failure Risk Stratification in the ED: Stratify 1R01HL088459-01.* NHLBI, Vanderbilt University, Nashville, 2007.

93 Storrow AB, Collins SP, Lyons MS, Wagoner LE, Gibler WB, Lindsell CJ. Emergency department observation of heart failure: preliminary analysis of safety and cost. *Congest Heart Fail* 2005;**11**:68–72.

94 Peacock WFt, Albert NM. Observation unit management of heart failure. *Emerg Med Clin North Am* 2001;**19**(1):209–32.

95 Peacock W, Young J, Collins S, Diercks D, Emerman C. Heart failure observation units: optimizing care. *Ann Emerg Med* 2006;**47**(1):22–33.

96 Storrow AB, Collins SP, Lyons MS, Wagoner LE, Gibler WB, Lindsell CJ. Emergency department observation of heart failure: preliminary analysis of safety and cost. *Congest Heart Fail* 2005;**11**(2):68–72.

97 Peacock WF, Remer EE, Aponte J, Moffa DA, Emerman CE, Albert NM. Effective observation unit treatment of decompensated heart failure. *Congest Heart Fail* 2002;**8**(2):68–73.

98 Kosowsky JM, Gasaway MD, Hamilton CA, Storrow AB. Preliminary experience with an emergency department observation unit protocol for heart failure. *Acad Emerg Med* 2000;**7**(10):1171.

20 Atrial Fibrillation

Barry Diner

Department of Emergency Medicine, Emory University School of Medicine, Emory University, Atlanta, USA

Clinical scenario

A 78-year-old male presented to the emergency department (ED) at 8:00 a.m. complaining of palpitations that started at exactly 11:30 p.m. while watching television. The patient was alert and oriented with mild shortness of breath and an ongoing sensation of palpitations. His vital signs were respiratory rate 24 breaths/min, blood pressure 160/95 mmHg (right = left arm) and heart rate 160 beats/min; he was afebrile. This was the patient's fifth episode with palpitations over the past 18 months and all but this one had resolved spontaneously upon presentation to the ED. The only common mitigating factor that the patient could remember was that prior to three of these episodes the patient had a single glass of malt whisky.

Examination of his lungs revealed clear breath sounds. On auscultation of his heart he had a systolic ejection murmur graded 2/6 with an irregularly irregular pulse. His jugular veins were not distended and his lower extremities demonstrated no edema. The remainder of his clinical exam was within normal limits. An electrocardiogram (ECG) was performed that demonstrated atrial fibrillation (AF) with a ventricular rate of 160. One of the residents suggested that his rate be controlled and consideration given to cardioverting the patient in the ED.

After controlling the heart rate with intravenous diltiazem, the patient's pulse decreased to 105 beats/min with a BP of 140/80 mmHg. Although the patient continued to experience palpitations, he felt significantly better. The patient described completing a 24-hour Holter monitor recording several months ago, ordered by his family doctor in an attempt to investigate the cause of his palpitations; however, the results were unhelpful. The patient was not placed on any medications, except for a daily enteric-coated acetyl-salicylic acid (ASA).

The patient was eager to resolve his current medical problem, due to how symptomatic he felt. He wanted to know how to stop these episodes from happening in the future and was extremely concerned about this diagnosis since his older brother recently had a stroke that was related to this same condition.

Background

Atrial fibrillation (AF) is a condition where atrial rhythm irregularity creates asynchrony of ventricular firing. AF is the single most common and serious chronic cardiac rhythm disturbance, and it is also the most common form of cardiac arrhythmia managed in North American EDs [1]. An estimated 2.3 million people in North America and 4.5 million people in the European Union have paroxysmal or persistent AF [2]. In an unselected population, the prevalence of AF is approximately 2% [3]. The incidence of AF increases from less than 0.1% per year in people younger than 40 years of age to over 1.5% per year among women and 2% among men older than 80 years of age [4]. According to the National Hospital Ambulatory Medical Care Survey over a 10-year period from 1995 to 2004, the overall proportion of AF was 36.2 per 10,000 ED visits, which represented an annual increase of 5% from baseline (95% CI: 2% to 8%) [5]. Over the past 20 years the hospital admission for AF is on the rise by 66% due to the aging of the population, a rising prevalence of chronic heart disease, more frequent diagnosis through the use of ambulatory monitoring devices, and other factors [6].

Atrial fibrillation is responsible for substantial morbidity, disability and mortality in the general population. Deaths associated with AF have increased dramatically over the past two decades [7]. The most common complication of AF is an acute thromboembolic event to the brain causing transient (transient ischemic attacks, TIAs) or permanent (stroke or cerebrovascular accident) neurological impairment. The risk of other thromboembolic phenomena (e.g., ischemic limb, renal or bowel infarction, etc.) is increased in patients with AF. AF alone increases the risk of stroke 4–5-fold; approximately 15% of all ischemic strokes are attributable to AF [8].

Evidence-based Emergency Medicine. Edited by Brian H. Rowe
© 2009 Blackwell Publishing, ISBN: 978-1-4051-6143-5.

Atrial fibrillation is a common and challenging arrhythmia that presents to the ED on a regular basis. There are several specific evidence-based practice guidelines that can aid in diagnosis, treatment and prevention [9]. Unfortunately, the recommended algorithms are often not followed and impressive practice variation amongst emergency physicians has been observed. Specific examples lie in the difference of AF admission to hospital between the USA (64%) and Canada (40%) [10,11]. The American Heart Association recommends a three-pronged approach to the treatment of AF: control of the ventricular rate, restoration of sinus rhythm (where appropriate) and prevention of thromboembolism [12].

Given the fact that the rate of admission for AF continues to climb and untreated AF can lead to devastating sequelae, the need for a more evidence-based approach to this disease is clear [13]. A better understanding of the disease and its associated risks would encourage physicians to be more cognizant of the management and prevention of AF.

Clinical questions

1 In adults with acute atrial fibrillation of known duration (population), does cardioversion to normal sinus rhythm in less than 48 hours (intervention) result in different thromboembolic risks (outcome) compared to AF of >48 hours' duration (control)? Which patients with new-onset AF should receive attempts at cardioversion and which should receive only conservative treatment with rate control and thromboembolism prophylaxis?

2 In adults with acute atrial fibrillation (population), do β-blockers (intervention) control the ventricular rate (outcome) more effectively and safely compared to calcium channel blockers (control)?

3 In adults with acute atrial fibrillation (population), is pharmacological (chemical) cardioversion (intervention) as effective in conversion to sinus rhythm (outcome) compared to placebo (control)?

4 In adults with acute atrial fibrillation (population), what is the efficacy and safety (outcomes) of monophasic electrical cardioversion (intervention) compared to biphasic electrical cardioversion (control)?

5 In adults with acute non-valvular atrial fibrillation (population), do antiplatelets (ASA) (intervention) decrease the risk of thromboembolic complications (especially stroke) (outcome) compared to placebo (control)?

6 In adults with acute non-valvular atrial fibrillation (population), do oral anticoagulants (warfarin; intervention) decrease the risk of thromboembolic complications (especially stroke) (outcome) compared to placebo (control)?

7 In adults with acute non-valvular atrial fibrillation (population), is ASA (intervention) as effective in reducing the risk of thromboembolic complications (especially stroke) (outcome) compared to oral anticoagulants (control)?

8 In adults with atrial fibrillation (population), does electrical/pharmacological cardioversion (intervention) to sinus rhythm reduce the annual risk of stroke, peripheral embolism and mortality (outcomes) compared to rate control (control)?

General search strategy

A large number of studies have been published in the area of atrial fibrillation treatment, diagnosis, causation and prevention. Consequently, a clinician looking for evidence-based resources must be vigilant or he/she could easily become overwhelmed with the search results. The first approach when examining a topic area with a large number of published papers is to search for a systematic review. Searching the Cochrane Library identified a number of relevant reviews for this chapter. Next, MEDLINE and EMBASE searches using terms for population (AF) AND setting (terms for "emergency" or "acute"), and the exclusion of postoperative period identified the population. With each question in treatment, terms for the therapeutic intervention (e.g., electrical cardioversion OR anti-arrhythmia agents) were used. For adverse outcomes questions, "risks" or "adverse outcomes" (TIA, stroke, thromboembolism, etc.) were sought. Finally, a search filter limiting results to evidence-based medicine (EBM) reviews and English language was employed. Finally, wherever possible, recent and evidence-based clinical practice guidelines on AF or acute thromboembolic event were searched to identify consensus recommendations.

Critical review of the literature

Question 1: In adults with acute atrial fibrillation of known duration (population), does cardioversion to normal sinus rhythm in less than 48 hours (intervention) result in different thromboembolic risks (outcome) compared to AF of >48 hours' duration (control)? Which patients with new-onset AF should receive attempts at cardioversion and which should receive only conservative treatment with rate control and thromboembolism prophylaxis?

Search strategy

- Cochrane Library: atrial fibrillation AND cardioversion
- MEDLINE: atrial fibrillation AND cardioversion. Limited to EBM reviews

There are a number of ways in which AF is classified, and each is reflected in the treatment approach used for the disease. One commonly accepted approach is to refer to AF as chronic (recurrent, persistent) or acute. Within the acute AF classification, most guidelines refer to two distinct groups: those with AF for ≤48 hours and those with AF for >48 hours [14]. Recent AF is classified on the basis of history, and those who cannot determine the exact timing of AF symptoms are automatically classified as having AF of >48 hours' duration. The remainder of this discussion will focus on patients who present to the ED with recent-onset AF of ≤48 hours' duration, since the risk of thromboembolic phenomena associated with cardioverting AF of >48 hours' duration is unacceptably high [9].

The above search of the Cochrane Library did not identify any systematic reviews addressing cardioversion. The MEDLINE search revealed one relevant article which was not a systematic review [15]. The most recent guidelines set out by the American Heart Association (AHA) and the American College of Cardiology (ACC), published in 2006, allow for immediate cardioversion of patients with AF if the duration of symptoms is of less than 48 hours. Although clinical management is based on the presumption that atrial thrombus formation requires continued AF of approximately 48 hours' duration, thrombi have been identified by transesophageal electrocardiography (TEE) within shorter intervals [16,17]. Cardioversion carries a risk of thromboembolism unless anticoagulation prophylaxis is initiated well before the procedure, and this risk is greatest when the arrhythmia has been present for more than 48 hours [9]. In patients with atrial fibrillation that lasts for more than 48 hours, the immediate risk of experiencing a thromboembolic event is between 5% and 7% if not preceded by anticoagulation [9,18,19]. This risk decreases to 0–1.6% if 2–4 weeks of prophylactic anticoagulation and TEE are performed [20–22].

The AHA/ACC recommendation is generally accepted as the gold standard for selecting which patients are candidates for immediate cardioversion in the ED. The entire basis of this recommendation is founded on one prospective non-randomized study of 375 patients who had AF clinically estimated to be of less than 48 hours' duration. The rate of thromboembolic events in this cohort was 0.8% (95% CI: 0.2% to 2.4%). In addition, no significant difference was found in the incidence of thromboembolism after conversion between patients for whom anticoagulation therapy was initiated on presentation, 0.8% (95% CI: 0.02% to 4.1%), and those for whom it was not, 0.9% (95% CI: 0.1% to 3.1%) [15].

In summary, electrical cardioversion carries a risk of acute thromboembolic event complications, which clinical practice guidelines dichotomize as high (AF >48 hours) and low (AF <48 hours) risk. The evidence for this, although based on a single study, is consistent with consensus recommendations. The priority issues for emergency physicians are to obtain a clear history of the duration of AF, and make decisions on the risks associated with acute thromboembolic event complications.

Question 2: In adults with acute atrial fibrillation (population), do β-blockers (intervention) control the ventricular rate (outcome) more effectively and safely compared to calcium channel blockers (control)?

Search strategy

- Cochrane Library: atrial fibrillation AND treatment AND rate control
- MEDLINE: atrial fibrillation AND treatment AND rate control

The Cochrane Library search did not identify any systematic reviews that addressed the question outlined above. One systematic review was identified from the Agency for Healthcare Research and Quality (AHRQ) Evidence-Based Practice Centers guidelines on the management of acute AF, published in 2003. This AHRQ-funded evidence report found 48 trials assessing 17 different agents for rate control in AF [23]. Additional searches of both MEDLINE (1950 to the present) and the Cochrane central registry of controlled trials produced one additional study that was not included in the AHRQ report that compared β-blockers to calcium channel blockers [24].

In hemodynamically stable patients, controlling the ventricular rate with oral or intravenous medications is often the priority in the ED as a means of improving symptoms. It is the ventricular rate that not only determines the sensation of palpitations and racing heart beat, but may also determine the development of complications, especially in the elderly. Controlling the patient's ventricular rate can improve the patient's status by allowing for better ventricular filling, reduced myocardial oxygen demand, and improved cardiac output. According to the AHA guidelines, in the presence of rapid ventricular response, depression of the atrioventricular node is indicated as the initial treatment of AF, assuming that the underlying cause is not Wolf–Parkinson–White syndrome [9]. Beta-blockers and calcium channel blockers have not been proven to be effective as agents that convert AF to sinus rhythm; however, they are indicated for rate control [25].

Figure 20.1 summarizes the results of the AHRQ systematic review that show that intravenous and oral calcium channel blockers in the acute and outpatient setting were more effective than placebo or digoxin in reducing the ventricular rate both at rest and during exercise. The results for β-blockers were not as consistent (Fig. 20.2). Metoprolol and atenolol were found to improve heart rate both at rest and during exercise.

In a randomized, blinded controlled study that compared the effectiveness of IV diltiazem and metoprolol in 40 patients with AF, both were safe and effective for the management of rapid ventricular rate. However, rate control was achieved more quickly and the percentage decrease in ventricular rate was higher with diltiazem (0.25 mg/kg IV, maximum 25 mg) than with metoprolol (0.15 mg/kg, maximum 10 mg) [24].

In summary, both calcium channel blockers and β-blockers are effective in reducing the ventricular rate in response to AF; however, calcium channel blockers appear to act faster. After an examination of contraindications, emergency physicians can use either to rate control symptomatic patients in the ED.

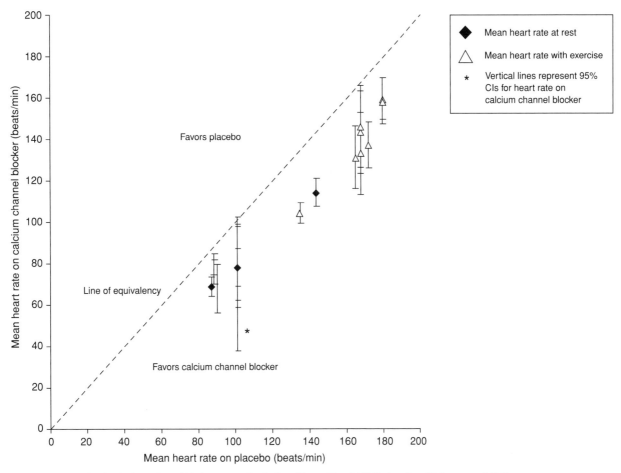

Figure 20.1 Rate control trials of calcium channel blockers versus placebo for subjects with atrial fibrillation. (From McNamara et al. [31]).

Question 3: In adults with acute atrial fibrillation (population), is pharmacological (chemical) cardioversion (intervention) as effective in conversion to sinus rhythm (outcome) compared to placebo (control)?

Search strategy

- Cochrane Library: atrial fibrillation AND treatment
- MEDLINE: atrial fibrillation AND treatment AND therapy AND drug therapy. Limited to English language and EBM review

The Cochrane Library search failed to identify any systematic reviews that addressed the question outlined above. The AHRQ Evidence-Based Practice Centers guidelines on the management of acute AF published in 2003 report synthesized data from 46 trials assessing several different classes of anti-arrhythmics compared to placebo. Additional searches of MEDLINE (1950 to the present) and the Cochrane central registry of controlled trials produced two additional systematic reviews that were published prior to this review (2001 and 2002) which reached similar overall conclusions [26,27].

There are two distinct options to achieve "rhythm control" in acute AF: chemical cardioversion and electrical cardioversion. Chemical cardioversion, which does not require sedation, has a lower success rate ranging from 30% to 70% depending on the choice of drug used (see Question 4 below for cardioversion rates with electrical therapy) [28]. The other main disadvantage of this strategy is related to the pro-arrhythmic potential and side-effect profile of the drugs used for rhythm control. Most medications currently used to prevent and/or treat atrial or ventricular arrhythmias have effects on the entire heart, including both healthy and damaged tissue. These drugs, which globally block ion channels in the heart, have long been associated with other forms of life-threatening arrhythmia such as torsades de pointes, vary with respect to time to conversion and the potential side-effects (i.e., hypotension, gastrointestinal upset), and could lead to increased rather than decreased mortality in selected patient population (e.g., congestive heart failure) [29]. In a consecutive cohort of AF patients that presented to the ED, the rate of chemical cardioversion was 62% compared to 89% with electrical cardioversion [30].

This review of the literature identified 46 randomized clinical trials on acute pharmacological conversion of AF that included the following anti-arrhythmics agents: quinidine and

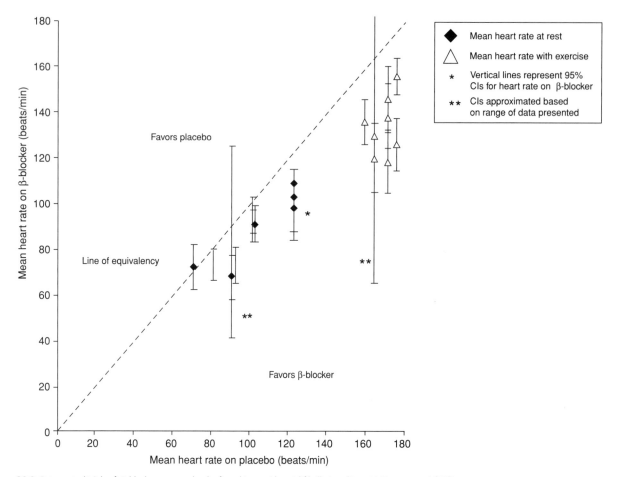

Figure 20.2 Rate control trials of β-blockers versus placebo for subjects with atrial fibrillation. (From McNamara et al. [31]).

procainamide (class Ia), flecainide and propafenone (class Ic), β-blockers (class II), amiodarone, sotalol, ibutilide and dofetilide (class III), verapamil, diltiazem (class IV), and digoxin (class V). Older agents such as β-blockers, calcium channel blockers (verapamil, diltiazem) and digoxin are currently viewed as relatively ineffective for the restoration of sinus rhythm [31]. The summary information on the efficacy of each drug is presented in Fig. 20.3.

There is *strong evidence* (defined in the AHRQ report as: OR > 1.0, 99% CI does not include 1.0 ($P < 0.01$)) of efficacy for the following agents compared with control treatment: flecainide, propafenone, and ibutilide/dofetilide. There is *moderate evidence* (defined in the AHRQ report as: OR >1.0, 95% CI does not include 1.0, but 99% CI does includes 1.0 ($0.01 < P < 0.05$)) of efficacy for propafenone and quinidine in regard to conversion of AF. Only about one-half of the included studies specifically mentioned ventricular fibrillation, polymorphic ventricular tachycardia and/or torsade de pointes as potential adverse effects of treatment. The rate of ventricular arrhythmia was as high as 12% with quinidine [32] and 9% using ibutilide [33].

In summary, chemical cardioversion is a viable option in the ED for patients with acute AF. The limitations include pro-arrhythmic effects of treatment, so patient selection is important (i.e., to be

avoided in the setting of underlying heart disease). In addition, the rate of success is much lower than with electrical cardioversion and the need for cardiac ED monitoring may be as long as 12 hours for the assessment of drug-induced dysrhythmia [29]. Recent success with a protocol approach consisting of attempts to chemically cardiovert (with IV procainamide) followed by electrical cardioversion has led to high success rates and infrequent complications [34].

Question 4: In adults with acute atrial fibrillation (population), what is the efficacy and safety (outcomes) of monophasic electrical cardioversion (intervention) compared to biphasic electrical cardioversion (control)?

Search strategy

- Cochrane Library: atrial fibrillation AND cardioversion AND electric countershock
- MEDLINE: atrial fibrillation AND (cardioversion OR electric countershock OR monophasic cardioversion). Limited to EBM reviews

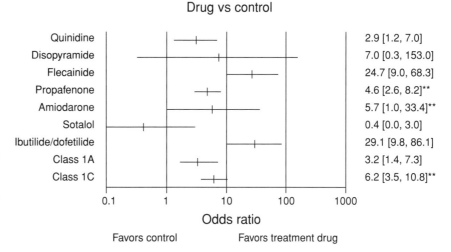

Drug vs control

	Odds ratio
Quinidine	2.9 [1.2, 7.0]
Disopyramide	7.0 [0.3, 153.0]
Flecainide	24.7 [9.0, 68.3]
Propafenone	4.6 [2.6, 8.2]**
Amiodarone	5.7 [1.0, 33.4]**
Sotalol	0.4 [0.0, 3.0]
Ibutilide/dofetilide	29.1 [9.8, 86.1]
Class 1A	3.2 [1.4, 7.3]
Class 1C	6.2 [3.5, 10.8]**

Favors control   Favors treatment drug

Figure 20.3 Comparison of drug classes compared to placebo in converting AF in the acute setting. Vertical bars are point estimates. Horizontal bars and numbers in brackets are 95% confidence intervals using a fixed-effects model unless otherwise indicated; **confidence interval using a random-effects model. The control treatment includes groups receiving placebo, verapamil, diltiazem or digoxin. (From McNamara et al. [31].)

Cardioversion of AF is one of the oldest therapies in cardiovascular medicine and in 1962 Lown et al. reported the efficacy of direct-current cardioversion of AF to sinus [35]. Cardioversion to sinus rhythm is performed in order to improve cardiac function, relieve symptoms and decrease the risk of thrombus formation [36]. There are two options for cardioversion, chemical and electrical, both with different rates of success. The reported rates of successful electrical cardioversion of acute AF to sinus rhythm vary from 70% to 99% in the literature [37–39]. The disadvantage of this procedure is that it requires procedural sedation, which carries its own potential risks. In addition, electrical cardioversion can cause pain, is more labor intensive and may require multiple attempts. Yet this treatment option has been shown to be safe in the ED [40]. It is the quickest way of establishing normal sinus rhythm and is the treatment of choice for patients that are in AF and considered to be hemodynamically unstable or who are experiencing myocardial ischemia or significant congestive heart failure. The evidence suggests that high initial energy is significantly more effective than low levels and that 200 J should be used for initial cardioversion regardless of whether a monophasic or biphasic waveform defibrillator is employed [41,42].

The above search of the Cochrane Library did not identify any systematic reviews addressing cardioversion. The MEDLINE search revealed four relevant articles which were not systematic reviews. Three of the four studies were randomized prospective trials that enrolled a total of 425 patients and the fourth was a prospective non-randomized cohort that enrolled 679 AF patients who were cardioverted. All four trials demonstrated that biphasic cardioversion is more successful than monophasic, with conversion rates ranging from 60% to 95% (compared to 22–79% for monophasic) [43–46]. All studies showed statistically significant differences. The patient population ranged from AF that was <48 hours in duration to patients who had AF for longer than a year. Importantly, these studies were not ED-initiated studies and no trials restricted to ED patients were found. One of the four studies with 203 patients demonstrated that biphasic cardioversion re-

quired fewer shocks (1.7 ± 1.0 vs 2.8 ± 1.2, $P < 0.0001$), lower total energy (217 ± 176 vs 548 ± 335 J, $P < 0.0001$), and was associated with a lower frequency of dermal injury (17% vs 41%, $P < 0.0001$) [43]. Finally, in another one of the studies, with 165 patients, the reported relative risk for successful cardioversion using biphasic technique was 4.2 (95% CI: 1.3 to 13.9) (Table 20.1) [46].

In summary, biphasic electrical cardioversion is more effective than monophasic when treating patients with AF. It is also requires fewer shocks, lower energy and results in less frequent side-effects.

Question 5: In adults with acute non-valvular atrial fibrillation (population), do antiplatelets (ASA) (intervention) decrease the risk of thromboembolic complications (especially stroke) (outcome) compared to placebo (control)?

Question 6: In adults with acute non-valvular atrial fibrillation (population), do oral anticoagulants (warfarin) (intervention) decrease the risk of thromboembolic complications (especially stroke) (outcome) compared to placebo (control)?

Question 7: In adults with acute atrial fibrillation (population), is ASA (intervention) as effective in reducing the risk of thromboembolic complications (especially stroke) (outcome) compared to oral anticoagulants (control)?

Search strategy

- Cochrane Library: atrial fibrillation AND treatment AND prevention AND anti-platelet AND thrombosis AND cerebrovascular accident
- MEDLINE: atrial fibrillation AND treatment AND prevention AND anti-platelet AND thrombosis AND cerebrovascular accident

Table 20.1 Summary of evidence from studies comparing biphasic to monophasic electrical cardioversion in patients with atrial fibrillation (AF).

Study	Design	*n*	Population	Biphasic (%)	Monophasic (%)	*P*-value	Odds ratio (95% CI)
Mittal et al. 2000 [46]	RCT	165	AF: elective cardioversion	94	79	0.005	0.23 (0.08 to 0.66)
Page et al. 2002 [43]	RCT	203	AF: elective cardioversion (<48 hours to >1 year)				
100 J				60	22	<0.0001	0.19 (0.10 to 0.35)
150 J				77	44	<0.0001	0.23 (0.13 to 0.43)
200 J				90	53	<0.0001	0.13 (0.06 to 0.28)
Gurevitz et al. 2005 [44]	Cohort	679	AF (>48 hours)	93	81	0.007	0.32 (0.20 to 0.51)
Ricard et al., 2001 [45]	RCT	57	Paroxysmal (>48 hours and <7 days) or chronic (>7 days)	86	51	0.02	0.22 (0.06 to 0.82)

RCT, randomized controlled trial.

Atrial fibrillation is responsible for substantial morbidity, disability and mortality in the general population. The most common complication of AF is an acute thromboembolic event to the brain (stroke or cerebrovascular accident) representing the most devastating outcome in AF. AF is associated with an increased long-term risk of stroke [47]. The rate of stroke in patients with non-valvular AF is about 5% per year which is about 2–7 times greater than patients without AF [48]. Approximately one out of six ischemic strokes are attributable to AF [49]. The annual rate of stroke attributed to AF increases with age from 1.5% at age 50–59 years to approximately 23.5% at age 80–89 years [48]. In the Framingham Heart Study the risk of stroke increased fivefold in patients with rheumatic heart disease compared to patients without the disease [50].

The need for anticoagulation or antiplatelet therapy is essential to AF treatment and the prevention of stroke. Prior thromboembolism, heart failure, hypertension, increasing age and diabetes mellitus have consistently emerged as independent risk factors

Table 20.2 Risk factors for ischemic stroke and systemic embolism in patients with non-valvular atrial fibrillation.* (Reproduced with permission from Fuster et al. [9], courtesy of the American Heart Association and the American College of Cardiology.)

Risk factors	Relative risk
Previous stroke or TIA	2.5
Diabetes mellitus	1.7
History of hypertension	1.6
Heart failure	1.4
Advanced age (continuous, per decade)	1.4

*Data derived from collaborative analysis of five untreated control groups in primary prevention trials. Relative risk refers to comparison of patients with AF to patients without these risk factors.
TIA, transient ischemic attack.

for ischemic stroke associated with non-valvular AF (Table 20.2). Embolic cerebrovascular events such as stroke or TIA are clearly the single largest complication in patients without valvular heart disease.

There are several approaches to risk stratifying patients in terms of the likelihood with which they can develop stroke related to AF. These include expert consensus and recursive partitioning that assist in selecting low-, intermediate- and high-risk patients. The CHADS$_2$ (Cardiac Failure, Hypertension, Age, Diabetes, Stroke (Doubled)) scoring system incorporates several approaches by developing a scoring system that ranks patients from 0 to 5, giving 2 points for TIA or stroke and 1 point for all other risk factors (Table 20.3) [51,52].

The expected stroke rate (95% CI) per 100 patient-years without antithrombotic therapy increases by a factor of 1.5 for each 1-point increase in the CHADS$_2$ score, with a c statistic (the c index is closely related to the area under the receiver operating curve (ROC) and provides a score from 0 to 1.0 (or 0–100%) with higher values indicating greater model fitting) of 0.82 (95% CI: 0.80 to 0.84). The CHADS$_2$ index was the most accurate predictor of stroke compared to the Atrial Fibrillation Investigators (AFI) and the Stroke Prevention in Atrial Fibrillation (SPAF) predictors [51].

The AHA 2006 AF guidelines have summarized stroke risks and roles of both anticoagulation and antiplatelet therapy for the prevention of thromboembolic events (Tables 20.4, 20.5) and defined these risk factors (Fig. 20.4).

Given the similarity and inter-connectivity of the three questions above, we have elected to produce a grouped response, based on the search strategy described above. The results of our search provided us with eight systematic reviews and one protocol from the Cochrane Collaboration that specifically dealt with therapy and AF. The eight trials were compared to a mega meta-analysis published by the authors of two of the Cochrane reviews. Included studies were compared and all relevant studies were incorporated in this most recent review, together with several additional studies not originally included [53].

Table 20.3 Stroke risk in patients with non-valvular AF not treated with anticoagulation according to the CHADS₂ index. (Reproduced with permission from Fuster et al. [9], courtesy of the American Heart Association and the American College of Cardiology.)

CHADS₂ risk criteria	Score
Prior stroke or TIA	2
Age >75 years	1
Hypertension	1
Diabetes mellitus	1
Heart failure	1

Patients (*n* = 1733)	Adjusted stroke rate %/year (95% CI)	CHADS₂ score
120	1.9 (1.2 to 3.0)	0
463	2.8 (2.0 to 3.8)	1
523	4.0 (3.1 to 5.1)	2
337	5.9 (4.6 to 7.3)	3
220	8.5 (6.3 to 11.1)	4
65	12.5 (8.2 to 17.5)	5
5	18.2 (10.5 to 27.4)	6

CI, confidence interval; TIA, transient ischemic attack.

Antiplatelet therapy

In seven trials involving almost 4000 patients, the relative risk reduction of stroke for those treated with aspirin compared to placebo or no therapy was 19% (95% CI: –1 to 35). The numbers needed to treat (NNT) in order to prevent one stroke were 125 and 40 for primary and secondary prevention, respectively [53]. In another similar Cochrane review, the risk of major hemorrhage (cerebral hemorrhage or a bleed requiring transfusion or hospitalization) from aspirin was not different to that of placebo or no therapy (OR = 0.81; 95% CI: 0.37 to 1.78) in two trials involving 1680 patients (AFASAK [54], SPAF-I [55]). In five trials involving 3762 patients, outcomes such as intracranial and extracranial hemorrhage and all-cause mortality were calculated. There was no statistical or clinically important difference when comparing aspirin to control or no treatment.

In summary, antiplatelet agents, such as ASA, are effective in preventing strokes in patients with AF compared to no treatment

Table 20.4 Thromboembolic risk factors for patients with atrial fibrillation. (Reproduced with permission from Fuster et al. [9], courtesy of the American Heart Association and the American College of Cardiology.)

Less validated or "weaker" risk factors	Moderate-risk factors	High-risk factors
Female gender	Age greater than or equal to 75 years	Previous stroke, TIA or embolism
Age 65 to 74 years	Hypertension	Mitral stenosis
Coronary artery disease	Heart failure	Prosthetic heart valve
Thyrotoxicosis	LV ejection fraction 35% or less	
	Diabetes mellitus	

LV, left ventricular; TIA, transient ischemic attack.

or control. The safety profile of ASA suggests this is an excellent agent for many patients with AF.

Anticoagulation therapy

In six trials involving 2900 patients and a mean of 1.6 years' follow-up per patient, adjusted dose warfarin relative risk reduction (RRR) for all strokes was 64% (95% CI: 49% to 74%) compared to control or placebo (Fig. 20.5). The absolute risk reductions (ARRs) were 2.7% (NNT = 37) and 8.4% (NNT = 12) per year for primary and secondary prevention, respectively. In a subgroup analysis involving only ischemic stroke, adjusted dose warfarin reduced events compared to control or placebo (RRR = 67%; 95% CI: 54% to 77%). For both primary and secondary prevention studies, adjusted dose warfarin demonstrated a non-statistical increase in major extracranial bleeding with a RRR of 66% (95% CI: –18% to 235%) and only six cases of intracranial bleeding in the treatment group compared to three in the control arm. Using a composite safety outcome (intracranial and extracranial hemorrhage and all-cause mortality), adjusted dose warfarin reduced all-cause mortality by 26% (95% CI: 3% to 43%) compared to control or placebo only. The rates of intracranial and extracranial hemorrhage were not statistically different in the intervention or control groups [53].

In summary, anticoagulation with warfarin is effective in preventing strokes in patients who suffer from chronic AF when compared to no treatment or control. The safety profile of warfarin demands a more cautious treatment approach and suggests that an individualized risk–benefit approach needs to be adopted for each patient in the use of these agents.

Anticoagulation versus antiplatelet therapy

Overall, eight trials involving 3647 patients compared adjusted-dose warfarin (with a target international normalized ratio (INR)

Risk category	Recommended therapy
No risk factors	ASA, 81–325 mg daily
One moderate-risk factor	ASA, 81–325 mg daily or warfarin (INR: 2.0 to 3.0, target 2.5)
Any high-risk factor or more than one moderate-risk factor	Warfarin (INR: 2.0 to 3.0, target 2.5)

Table 20.5 Antithrombotic therapy for patients with atrial fibrillation. (Reproduced with permission from Fuster et al. [9], courtesy of the American Heart Association and the American College of Cardiology.)

ASA, acetyl-salicylic acid; INR, international normalized ratio.

ranging from 2 to 4) to various dosages of aspirin. The summary analysis indicated that warfarin was more effective in reducing stroke (RRR = 38%; 95% CI: 18 to 52); and both primary (ARR = 0.7%/year) and secondary (ARR = 7.0%/year) prevention also demonstrated a benefit with warfarin compared to ASA (Fig. 20.6). The NNTs to prevent primary and secondary stroke are 143 and 14, respectively [53]. In a large study that included 6707 patients with 171 strokes comparing dose-adjusted warfarin with clopidogrel and ASA, anticoagulation was shown to be superior (RRR = 40%; 95% CI: 18% to 56%) [56]. In all eight of the trials the risk of intracranial hemorrhage increased by 128% compared to aspirin with a non-statistical increase in major extracranial hemorrhage and a statistical decrease in all-cause mortality.

In summary, warfarin was more effective than ASA and/or clopidogrel in preventing strokes in patients with AF. The safety profile of warfarin poses a risk for major bleeding, especially intracranial hemorrhage. The need to establish a risk–benefit profile for each patient is essential prior to commencing treatment.

Question 8: In adults with atrial fibrillation (population), does electrical/pharmacological cardioversion (intervention) to sinus rhythm reduce the annual risk of stroke, peripheral embolism and mortality (outcomes) compared to rate control (control)?

Search strategy

- Cochrane Library: atrial fibrillation AND treatment
- MEDLINE: atrial fibrillation AND treatment. Limited to English language and EBM review

The Cochrane Library search produced one protocol that included five trials: AFFIRM, HOTCAFE, PIAF, RACE, STAF [57–61]. The MEDLINE search revealed three systematic reviews relevant to this topic. All studies that were included in the Cochrane protocol were included in all three systematic reviews without exception.

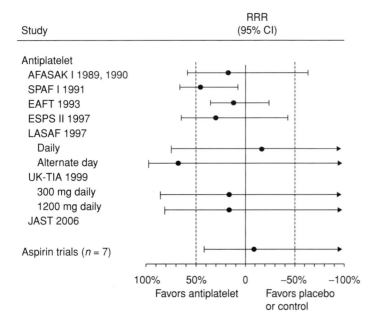

Figure 20.4 Antiplatelet agents compared with placebo or control. (Reproduced with permission from Hart et al. [53], courtesy of the American College of Physicians.)

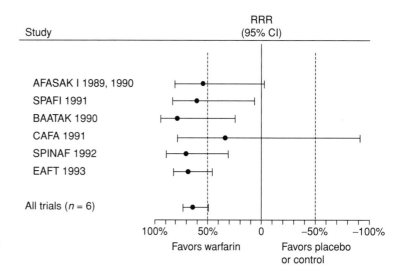

Figure 20.5 Adjusted dose warfarin compared with placebo or control. (Reproduced with permission from Hart et al. [53], courtesy of the American College of Physicians.)

There are two general therapeutic strategies used in treating patients with AF. First, in the management strategy referred to as "rate control", AF is permitted to continue and control of the ventricular response is achieved by suppressing the atrioventricular node using a variety of therapies (e.g., digoxin, calcium channel blockers, β-blockers). This strategy also generally requires chronic anticoagulation therapy with warfarin to prevent thromboembolic complications. The advantage to this approach is that it avoids the risks of conversion (e.g., thromboembolism, pain, pro-arrhythmias, other adverse effects of anti-arrhythmic therapy) and may be an efficient alternative resulting in lower costs to the health care system. Alternatively, in the management strategy referred to as "rhythm control", efforts are made to convert AF to normal sinus rhythm, which may be maintained with other pharmacological agents. The advantage of this approach is that it potentially avoids the need for anticoagulants, reduces patient symptoms and may improve quality of life.

Recent data suggest that providing rate control without cardioversion (pharmacological) may result in similar or better outcomes than converting the patient back into normal sinus rhythm [62]. The five trials include 5239 patients; however, none of these trials specifically included patients from the ED setting. Four of the trials dealt exclusively with persistent AF patients, and the largest of the five trails, the AFFIRM trial (4060 patients), enrolled patients with first or recurrent, paroxysmal or persistent AF at high risk for stroke who had a history of AF for at least 6 hours in the past 6 months. Only 1778 of the patients were actually in AF at the time of randomization [57]. Unfortunately, since the majority of these patients were not enrolled from the ED with acute AF, the generalizability of these results to the ED setting may be problematic.

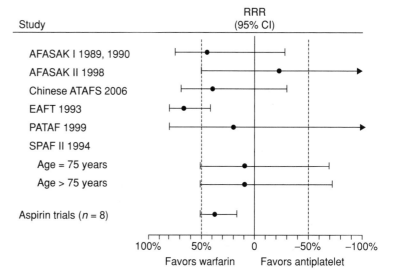

Figure 20.6 Adjusted dose warfarin compared with antiplatelet agents. (Reproduced with permission from Hart et al. [53], courtesy of the American College of Physicians.)

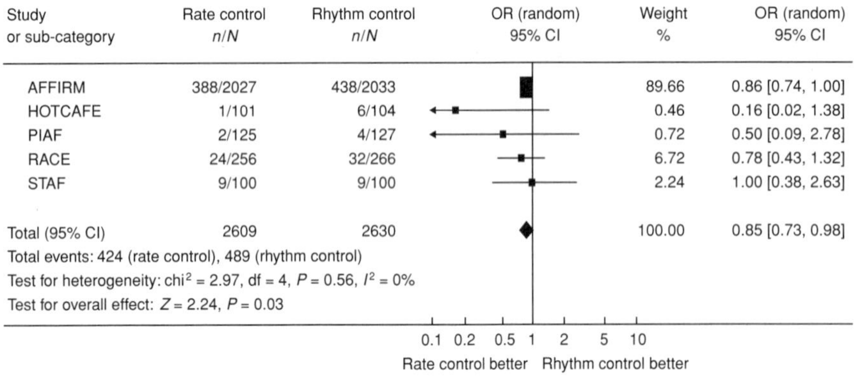

Study or sub-category	Rate control n/N	Rhythm control n/N	OR (random) 95% CI	Weight %	OR (random) 95% CI
AFFIRM	388/2027	438/2033		89.66	0.86 [0.74, 1.00]
HOTCAFE	1/101	6/104		0.46	0.16 [0.02, 1.38]
PIAF	2/125	4/127		0.72	0.50 [0.09, 2.78]
RACE	24/256	32/266		6.72	0.78 [0.43, 1.32]
STAF	9/100	9/100		2.24	1.00 [0.38, 2.63]
Total (95% CI)	2609	2630		100.00	0.85 [0.73, 0.98]

Total events: 424 (rate control), 489 (rhythm control)
Test for heterogeneity: chi² = 2.97, df = 4, P = 0.56, I² = 0%
Test for overall effect: Z = 2.24, P = 0.03

0.1 0.2 0.5 1 2 5 10
Rate control better   Rhythm control better

Figure 20.7 Summary of all-cause mortality and thromboembolic stroke outcomes in studies of rate versus rhythm control in atrial fibrillation. (Reproduced with permission from Testa et al. [63], courtesy of Oxford University Press.)

Overall, the rate control strategy had a significantly lower risk of all-cause death and thromboembolic stroke (OR = 0.85; 95% CI: 0.73 to 0.98) (Fig. 20.7) [63]. When events are evaluated separately there was a non-significant trend towards reduced risk of death (OR = 0.87; 95% CI: 0.74 to 1.02) and thromboembolic stroke (OR = 0.8; 95% CI: 0.6 to 1.07), respectively. Therefore, the NNT to avoid one death and one thromboembolic stroke was 50 and 100, respectively [63].

The rate of major bleeding (intracranial and extracranial) was similar between the rate and rhythm control strategies (OR = 1.12; 95% CI: 0.82 to 1.53) (Fig. 20.8) [63].

The results of these five trials contradict the commonly held perception that maintaining sinus rhythm is superior to rate control. The evidence identifies a reduction in the combined endpoint (death and thromboembolic stroke) for rate control compared to rhythm control. Furthermore, this is accomplished without any increase in bleeding, which could be anticipated with chronic anticoagulation. The AFFIRM trial demonstrated that there was a trend towards increased mortality in the rhythm control arm of the study (hazard ratio = 1.15; 95% CI: 0.99 to 1.34). The rate of the composite endpoint of death, disabling stroke, disabling anoxic encephalopathy, major bleeding or cardiac arrest was also similar in both groups (P = 0.33) [57].

In summary, although much of this evidence is not specific to ED practice, the importance of this body of work in the general treatment of AF patients is clear. Overall, current evidence cannot precisely guide emergency physicians in the management of acute AF; symptomatic patients would probably benefit from rate control efforts over rhythm control. Given that "AF begets AF", emergency physicians may wish to consider rate control and anticoagulation for patients who have had multiple episodes or who are asymptomatic.

Conclusions

The 78-year-old patient was diagnosed with AF based on history, clinical findings and an ECG, which is the gold standard for confirming this arrhythmia. He received a single 20 mg dose of intravenous diltiazem for rate control, which slowed his heart rate down to 105 beats/min. Following normal laboratory work-up, and several hours of observation, the patient remained in AF and was still complaining of mild palpitations. The patient was presented with two options for cardioversion, electrical or chemical. The patient selected electrical and was successfully cardioverted with 100 J (biphasic). The patient was observed for 2 hours in the ED where he remained in sinus rhythm and was asymptomatic.

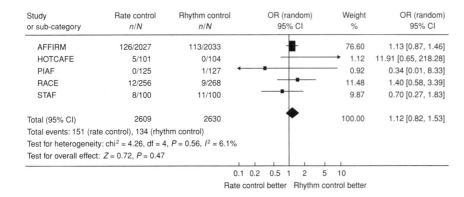

Study or sub-category	Rate control n/N	Rhythm control n/N	OR (random) 95% CI	Weight %	OR (random) 95% CI
AFFIRM	126/2027	113/2033		76.60	1.13 [0.87, 1.46]
HOTCAFE	5/101	0/104		1.12	11.91 [0.65, 218.28]
PIAF	0/125	1/127		0.92	0.34 [0.01, 8.33]
RACE	12/256	9/268		11.48	1.40 [0.58, 3.39]
STAF	8/100	11/100		9.87	0.70 [0.27, 1.83]
Total (95% CI)	2609	2630		100.00	1.12 [0.82, 1.53]

Total events: 151 (rate control), 134 (rhythm control)
Test for heterogeneity: chi² = 4.26, df = 4, P = 0.56, I² = 6.1%
Test for overall effect: Z = 0.72, P = 0.47

0.1 0.2 0.5 1 2 5 10
Rate control better   Rhythm control better

Figure 20.8 Summary of major bleeding complications in studies of rate versus rhythm control in atrial fibrillation. (Reproduced with permission from Testa et al. [63], courtesy of Oxford University Press.)

He was discharged home on warfarin because of his age and underlying hypertensive disease.

Acute AF is the most common arrhythmia seen in the ED. Management, stroke prevention and disposition are the three issues that emergency physicians must consider when treating patients with AF. The available data suggest that calcium channel blockers are more effective than β-blockers for achieving rate control, which is the primary therapeutic intervention recommended for rapid AF. The current recommendations suggest that cardioverting AF patients who have had less than 48 hours of symptoms is safe; however, there is only one non-randomized study that supports this practice. Over the last several years there has been increasing evidence to support rate over rhythm control when dealing with AF patients. Most guidelines support rate control over rhythm control due to the lower incidence of long-term side-effects; however, unfortunately none of the studies included patients in the ED. Systematic review evidence suggests that both ASA and warfarin (but not the combination) are more effective in preventing stroke in patients with AF than placebo. In addition, warfarin was found to be superior to ASA, although in association with a small increased risk of intracranial bleeding. Final disposition of patients who present with acute AF has not been well studied and the variability for disposition decisions among ED physicians has been documented. Currently, there are no practice guidelines that deal specifically with risk stratification and outpatient treatment of patients with AF who present to the ED for acute exacerbations of chronic AF or new-onset AF. With the rising cost of health care this is an important area of future research that will have an impact on how we treat and seek appropriate disposition for patients with AF.

Acknowledgments

Thanks to the Robert W. Woodruff Foundation with collaboration from the CDC Foundation, and scientific and technical assistance from the Centers for Disease Control and Prevention.

Conflicts of interest

Dr. Diner has received study funding from Astellas Pharmaceutical for participation in a multi-centered trial of atrial fibrillation management.

References

1 Martinez JA. Management of Acute Atrial Fibrillation, Scientific assembly of the American College of Emergency Physicians, October 13, 1999. Las Vegas, Nevada, 1999.

2 Go AS, Hylek EM, Phillips KA, et al. Prevalence of diagnosed atrial fibrillation in adults: national implications for rhythm management and stroke prevention: the Anticoagulation and Risk Factors in Atrial Fibrillation (ATRIA) Study. *JAMA* 2001;**285**:2370–75.

3 Ukami AZ, Ezekowitz MD. Contemporary management of atrial fibrillation. *Med Clin North Am* 1995;**79**;1135–52.

4 Friberg J, Scharling H, Gadsboll N, et al. Sex-specific increase in the prevalence of atrial fibrillation (the Copenhagen City Heart Study). *Am J Cardiol* 2003;**92**:1419–23.

5 Diner BM, Ratcliff JJ, Pitts SR, Rowe BH. Emergency department presentations of atrial fibrillation (AF) in the United States. *Can J Emerg Med* 2004;**6**:202.

6 Friberg J, Buch P, Scharling H, et al. Rising rates of hospital admissions for atrial fibrillation. *Epidemiology* 2003;**14**:666–72.

7 Wattigney WA, Mensah GA, Croft JB. Increased atrial fibrillation mortality: United States, 1980–1998. *Am J Epidemiol* 2002;**155**:819–26.

8 Masoudi FA, Goldschlager N. The medical management of atrial fibrillation. *Cardiol Clin* 1997;**15**(4):689–719.

9 Fuster V, Ryden LE, Cannom DS, et al. ACC/AHA/ESC 2006 guidelines for the management of patients with atrial fibrillation – executive summary: a report of the American College of Cardiology/American Heart Association Task Force on Practice Guidelines and the European Society of Cardiology Committee for Practice Guidelines (Writing Committee to Revise the 2001 Guidelines for the Management of Patients with Atrial Fibrillation). *Circulation* 2006;**114**:700–752.

10 Diner BM, Ratcliff JJ, Pitts SR, Rowe BH. Emergency department presentations of atrial fibrillation (AF) in the United States. *Can J Emerg Med* 2004;**6**:202.

11 Diner BM, Yiannakoulis N, Holroyd BR, et al. Emergency department presentations of atrial fibrillation (AF) in Alberta, Canada. *Can J Emerg Med* 2003;**5**(3):179–209.

12 Prystowsky EN, Benson DW, Fuster V, et al. Management of patients with atrial fibrillation. *Circulation* 1996;**93**:1262–77.

13 Wattigney WA, Mensah GA, Croft JB. Increasing trends in hospitalization of older Americans for cardiac conduction disorder or arrhythmias, 1991–1998. *J Am Geriatr Soc* 2001;**49**:763–70.

14 Li H, Easley A, Barrington W, et al. Evaluation and management of atrial fibrillation in the emergency department. *Emerg Med Clinic North Am* 1998;**16**:389–403.

15 Wegner MJ, Caulfield TA, Danias PG, et al. Risk for clinical thromboembolism associated with conversion to sinus rhythm in patients with atrial fibrillation lasting less than 48 hours. *Ann Intern Med* 1997;**126**(8):615–20.

16 Stoddard MF, Dawkins PR, Prince CR, et al. Left atrial appendage thrombus is not uncommon in patients with acute atrial fibrillation and a recent embolic event: a transesophageal echocardiographic study. *J Am Coll Cardiol* 1995;**25**:452–9.

17 Manning WJ, Silverman DI, Waksmonski CA, et al. Prevalence of residual left atrial thrombi among patients with acute thromboembolism and newly recognized atrial fibrillation. *Arch Intern Med* 1995;**155**:2193–8.

18 Bjerkelund CJ, Orning OM. The efficacy of anticoagulant therapy in preventing embolism related to D.C. electrical cardioversion of atrial fibrillation. *Am J Cardiol* 1969;**23**:208–15.

19 Peterson P, Godtfredsen J. Embolic complications in paroxysmal atrial fibrillation. *Stroke* 1986;**17**:622–6.

20 Arnold AZ, Mick MJ, Mazurek RP, Loop FD, Trohman RG. Role of prophylactic anticoagulation for direct current cardioversion in patients with atrial fibrillation or atrial flutter. *J Am Coll Cardiol* 1992;**19**(4):851–5.

21 Manning WJ, Silverman DI, Keighley CS, Oettgen P, Douglas PS. Transesophageal echocardiographically facilitated early cardioversion from atrial fibrillation using short-term anticoagulation: final results of a prospective 4.5 year study. *J Am Coll Cardiol* 1995;**25**:1354–61.

22 Manning WJ, Silverman DI, Gordon SP, Krumholz HM, Douglas PS. Cardioversion from atrial fibrillation without prolonged anticoagulation with use of transesophageal echocardiography to exclude the presence of atrial thrombi. *N Engl J Med* 1993;**328**:750–55.

23 McNamara RL, Tamariz LJ, Segal JS, Bass EB. Management of atrial fibrillation: review of the evidence for the role of pharmacologic therapy, electrical cardioversion, and echocardiography. *Ann Intern Med* 2003;**139**:1018–33.

24 Demircan C, Cikriklar HI, Engindeniz Z, et al. Comparison of the effectiveness of intravenous diltiazem and metoprolol in the management of rapid ventricular rate in atrial fibrillation. *Emerg Med J* 2005;**2**(6):411–14.

25 Raghaven AR, Decker WW, Melo TD. Management of atrial fibrillation in the emergency department. *Emerg Med Clin North Am* 2005;**23**:1127–39.

26 Nichol G, McAlister F, Pham B, et al. Meta-analysis of randomised controlled trials of the effectiveness of antiarrhythmic agents at promoting sinus rhythm in patients with atrial fibrillation. *Heart* 2002;**87**(6):535–43.

27 Slavik RS, Tisdale JE, Borzak S. Pharmacologic conversion of atrial fibrillation: a systematic review of available evidence. *Prog Cardiovasc Dis* 2001;**44**(2):121–52.

28 Fuster V, Ryden LE, Asinger RW, et al. ACC/AHA/ESC guidelines for the management of patients with atrial fibrillation: a report of the American College of Cardiology/American Heart Association Task Force on Practice Guidelines and the European Society of Cardiology Committee for Practice Guidelines and policy conferences (Committee to Develop Guidelines for the Management of Patients with Atrial Fibrillation). *J Am Coll Cardiol* 2001;**38**:1231–65.

29 Flaker GC, Blackshear JL, McBride R, Kronmal RA, Halperin JL, Hart RG. Antiarrhythmic drug therapy and cardiac mortality in atrial fibrillation. The Stroke Prevention in Atrial Fibrillation Investigators. *J Am Coll Cardiol* 1992;**20**(3):527–32.

30 Michael JA, Stiell IG, Agarwal S, et al. Cardioversion of paroxysmal atrial fibrillation in the emergency department. *Ann Emerg Med* 1999;**33**(4):379–87.

31 McNamara RL, Bass EB, Miller MR, et al. *Management of New Onset Atrial Fibrillation*. Evidence Report/Technology Assessment No. 12 (prepared by the Johns Hopkins University Evidence-based Practice Center in Baltimore, MD under Contract No. 290-97-0006). AHRQ Publication Number 01-E026. Agency for Healthcare Research and Quality, Rockville, MD, 2001.

32 Hohnloser SH, van de Loo A, Baedeker F. Efficacy and proarrhythmic hazards of pharmacologic cardioversion of atrial fibrillation: prospective comparison of sotalol versus quinidine. *J Am Coll Cardiol* 1995;**26**(4):852–8.

33 Ellenbogen KA, Stambler BS, Wood MA, et al. Efficacy of intravenous ibutilide for rapid termination of atrial fibrillation and atrial flutter: a dose–response study. *J Am Coll Cardiol* 1996;**28**(1):130–36.

34 Stiell IG, Clement CM, Symington C, Dickinson G, Perry J, Vaillancourt C. The Ottawa aggressive protocol for ED management of acute atrial fibrillation. *Acad Emerg Med* 2007;**14**(5):S9.

35 Lown B, Amarasingham R, Neuman J. New method for terminating cardiac arrhythmias: use of synchronized capacitor discharge. *JAMA* 1962;**182**:548–55.

36 Pritchett EL. Management of atrial fibrillation. *N Engl J Med* 1992;**326**:1264–71.

37 Van Gelder IC, Crijns HJ, van Gilst WH, et al. Prediction of uneventful cardioversion and maintenance of sinus rhythm from direct-current electrical cardioversion of chronic atrial fibrillation and flutter. *Am J Cardiol* 1991;**68**:41–6.

38 Lundstrom T, Ryden L. Chronic atrial fibrillation. Long-term results of direct current conversion. *Acta Med Scand* 1988;**223**:53–9.

39 Niebauer MJ, Brewer JE, Chung MK, et al. Comparison of the rectilinear biphasic waveform with the monophasic damped sine waveform for external cardioversion of atrial fibrillation and flutter. *Am J Cardiol* 2004;**93**:1495–9.

40 Michael JA, Stiell IG, Argwal S, et al. Cardioversion of paroxysmal atrial fibrillation in the emergency department. *Ann Emerg Med* 1999;**33**:379–87.

41 Joglar JA, Hamdan MH, Ramaswamy K, et al. Initial energy for elective external cardioversion of persistent atrial fibrillation. *Am J Cardiol* 2000;**86**:348–50.

42 Wozakowska-Kaplon B, Janion M, Sielski J, et al. Efficacy of biphasic shock for transthoracic cardioversion of persistent atrial fibrillation: can we predict energy requirements? *Pacing Clin Electrophysiol* 2004;**27**:764–8.

43 Page RL, Kerber RE, Russell JK, et al. Biphasic versus monophasic shock waveform for conversion of atrial fibrillation: the results of an international randomized, double-blind multicenter trial. *J Am Coll Cardiol* 2002;**39**:1956–63.

44 Gurewitz OT, Ammash NM, Malouf JF, et al. Comparative efficacy of monophasic and biphasic waveforms for transthoracic cardioversion of atrial fibrillation and atrial flutter. *Am Heart J* 2005;**149**:316–21.

45 Ricard P, Levy S, Boccara G. External cardioversion of atrial fibrillation: comparison of biphasic vs monophasic waveform shocks. *Europace* 2001;**3**:96–9.

46 Mittal S, Ayati S, Stein KM, et al. Transthoracic cardioversion of atrial fibrillation: comparison of rectilinear biphasic versus damped sine wave monophasic shocks. *Circulation* 2000;**101**:1282–7.

47 Atrial Fibrillation Investigators. Risk factors for stroke and efficacy of antithrombotic therapy in atrial fibrillation. Analysis of pooled data from five randomized controlled trials. *Arch Intern Med* 1994;**154**:1449–57.

48 Wolf PA, Abbott RD, Kannel WB. Atrial fibrillation as an independent risk factor for stroke: the Framingham Study. *Stroke* 1991;**22**:983–8.

49 Hart RG, Halperin JL. Atrial fibrillation and thromboembolism: a decade of progress in stroke prevention. *Ann Intern Med* 1999;**131**:688–95.

50 Wolf PA, Dawber TR, Thomas HE, Jr., et al. Epidemiologic assessment of chronic atrial fibrillation and risk of stroke: the Framingham study. *Neurology* 1978;**28**:973–7.

51 Gage BF, Waterman AD, Shannon W, et al. Validation of clinical classification schemes for predicting stroke: results from the National Registry of Atrial Fibrillation. *JAMA* 2001;**285**:2864–70.

52 van Walraven WC, Hart RG, Wells GA, et al. A clinical prediction rule to identify patients with atrial fibrillation and a low risk for stroke while taking aspirin. *Arch Intern Med* 2003;**163**:936–43.

53 Hart RG, Pearce LA, Aguilar MI. Meta-analysis: antithrombotic therapy to prevent stroke in patients who have nonvalvular atrial fibrillation. *Ann Intern Med* 2007;**146**:857–67.

54 Petersen P, Boysen G, Godtfredsen J, Andersen ED, Andersen B. Placebo-controlled, randomised trial of warfarin and aspirin for prevention of thromboembolic complications in chronic atrial fibrillation. The Copenhagen AFASAK study. *Lancet* 1989;**1**:175–9.

55 Stroke Prevention in Atrial Fibrillation Study. Final results. *Circulation* 1991;**84**:527–39.

56 ACTIVE Writing Group on behalf of the ACTIVE Investigators. Clopidogrel plus aspirin versus oral anticoagulation for atrial fibrillation in the Atrial fibrillation Clopidogrel Trial with Irbesartan for prevention of Vascular Events (ACTIVE W): a randomised controlled trial. *Lancet* 2006;**367**:1903–12.

57 Wyse DG, Waldo AL, DiMarco JP, et al., Atrial Fibrillation Follow-up Investigation of Rhythm Management (AFFIRM) Investigators. A comparison of rate control and rhythm control in patients with atrial fibrillation. *N Engl J Med* 2002;**347**:1825–33.

58 Opolski G, Torbicki A, Kosior D, et al. Rhythm control versus rate control in patients with persistent atrial fibrillation. Results of the HOT CAFE Polish Study. *Kardiol Pol* 2003;**59**:1–16.

59 Hohnloser SH, Kuck KH, Lilienthal J. Rhythm or rate control in atrial fibrillation. Pharmacological intervention in atrial fibrillation (PIAF): a randomized trial. *Lancet* 2000;**356**:1789–94.

60 Van Gelder IC, Hagens VE, Bosker HA, et al., Rate Control versus Electrical Cardioversion for Persistent Atrial Fibrillation Study Group. A comparison of rate control and rhythm control in patients with recurrent persistent atrial fibrillation. *N Engl J Med* 2002;**347**:1834–40.

61 Carlsson J, Miketic S, Windeler J, et al., STAF Investigators. Randomized trial of rate-control versus rhythm-control in persistent atrial fibrillation: the Strategies of Treatment of Atrial Fibrillation (STAF) study. *J Am Coll Cardiol* 2003;**41**:1690–96.

62 Wyse DG, Waldo AL, DiMarco JP, et al., Atrial Fibrillation Follow-up Investigation of Rhythm Management (AFFIRM) Investigators. A comparison of rate control and rhythm control in patients with atrial fibrillation. *N Engl J Med* 2002;**347**:1825–33.

63 Testa L, Biondi-Zoccai GG, Dello Russo A, Bellocci F, Andreotti F, Crea F. Rate-control vs. rhythm-control in patients with atrial fibrillation: a meta-analysis. *Eur Heart J* 2005;**26**(19):2000–2006.

21 Ventricular and Supraventricular Arrhythmias

Eddy S. Lang & Eli Segal

Department of Family Medicine, McGill University, Montreal *and* Department of Emergency Medicine,
SMBD Jewish General Hospital, Montreal, Canada

Case scenario

A 62-year-old male presented to the emergency department (ED) for epigastric discomfort, dyspepsia and diaphoresis that began 2 hours before presentation. Upon arrival, the triage nurse identified a rapid pulse and a blood pressure of 110/70 mmHg (right arm). An electrocardiogram (ECG) was performed revealing a wide complex tachycardia of approximately170 beats/min.

The patient was known to have cardiovascular risk factors including hyperlipidemia and a strong family history for premature coronary artery disease. His medications included a lipid-lowering agent (atorvastatin 20 mg) as well as a preventive dose of 80 mg of aspirin as advised by his family physician. He denied, however, any past personal history of atherosclerotic heart disease and did not report exertional chest or respiratory symptoms. According to the patient he had successfully completed a cardiac stress test 7 years earlier.

The patient denied ongoing chest pain or syncope although he did admit to having been somewhat lightheaded when the symptoms started and felt somewhat short of breath in the ED. He denied a history of palpitations or arrhythmia and at his annual physical examination 1 year previously was told that his ECG was normal.

Physical examination revealed a moderately obese and anxious gentleman with a respiratory rate of 22 breaths/min and a heart rate persisting at 170 beats/min. There was no evidence of jugular venous distension, peripheral edema or rales, and heart sounds were inaudible. The nurses wondered if you wanted them to prepare this patient for electrical cardioversion.

Background

Ventricular tachycardia (VT) is defined as abnormal and rapid patterns of electrical activity originating within myocardial tissue

and manifesting as a wide complex arrhythmia. VT is further classified as monomorphic when occurring at a consistent rate and amplitude and polymorphic when waveforms are more variable and chaotic. Torsades de pointes is a specific kind of polymorphic VT associated with a prolonged QT interval and a characteristic twisting pattern to the wave signal. It is often associated with drug toxicity and electrolyte disturbances.

Ventricular fibrillation (VF) is characterized by irregular and chaotic electrical activity and ventricular contraction in which the heart immediately loses its ability to function as a pump. Pulseless VT and VF are the primary causes of sudden cardiac death. VF and VT associated with cardiovascular collapse, cardiac arrest and sudden cardiac death are abrupt pulseless arrhythmias. The annual incidence of sudden cardiac death is believed to approach 2 per 1000 population; however, this can vary depending on the prevalence of cardiovascular disease in the population [1]. It is estimated that 300,000 sudden cardiac deaths are recorded annually in the USA, representing 50% of all cardiovascular mortality in that country [2]. Data from Holter monitor studies suggest that about 85% of sudden cardiac deaths are the result of VT/VF [3].

Ventricular tachycardia is diagnosed by a QRS width complex of >120 ms and an electrical rhythm of >130 beats/min. Non-pulseless (stable) VT has the same electrical characteristics as VT but without hemodynamic compromise. In this chapter we will focus on the diagnosis and treatments of ventricular and supraventricular tachyarrhythmias (SVTs). Atrial fibrillation (AF) has been assigned a specific chapter in this text (see Chapter 20) and other specific therapies for VT- and VF-associated cardiac arrest in the prehospital setting are covered in Chapter 22.

Ventricular arrhythmias occur as a result of structural heart disease arising primarily from myocardial ischemia or cardiomyopathies. In developed nations, VT is believed to occur most typically in the context of myocardial ischemia. As a result, major risk factors for VT reflect those that lead to progressive coronary artery disease. Specific additional risk factors attributed to VT and sudden cardiac death include dilated cardiomyopathy (especially with ejection fractions of <30%), age (peak incidence 45–75 years) and male sex [1]. VF and VT associated with cardiac arrest results in a

Evidence-based Emergency Medicine. Edited by Brian H. Rowe
© 2009 Blackwell Publishing, ISBN: 978-1-4051-6143-5.

lack of oxygen delivery and major ischemic injury to vital organs. If untreated this condition is uniformly fatal within minutes.

Supraventricular tachycardias are rapid and abnormal heart rhythms in which the origin of the electrical signal is either the atria or the atrioventricular (AV) node. These rhythms require the atria or the AV node for either initiation or maintenance. This is in contrast to VTs, which are tachycardias that are independent of the atria or AV node. SVT is a general term that describes a number of different arrhythmias of the heart, each with a different mechanism of impulse maintenance. AF is the most commonly encountered SVT, but paroxysmal SVT, multifocal atrial tachycardia and Wolff–Parkinson–White constitute other entities that often present to the ED. In the absence of conduction abnormalities, SVT is diagnosed as the presence of a rapid narrow complex tachycardia noted on either the ECG or rhythm strip. Also characteristic is the frequent absence of atrial activity in the form of a P-wave. Many SVTs are self-limited entities, while others can be associated with serious hemodynamic manifestations when heart rates exceed 150/min.

Clinical questions

1 In clinically stable patients with a wide complex tachy-dysrhythmia (population), are there valid and reliable clinical and electrocardiographic criteria (diagnostic test characteristics) that can discriminate between VT and SVT with aberrant conduction (outcome)?

2 In patients with SVT (patients), does adenosine (intervention) effectively convert patients to normal sinus rhythm (outcome) compared with calcium channel blockers (control)?

3 In patients with cardiac arrest associated with shock resistant VT or VF (population), does anti-arrhythmic therapy with amiodarone (intervention) result in normal neurological outcome (outcome) more often than standard care with or without lidocaine?

4 In patients with cardiac arrest associated with shock resistant VT or VF (population), does anti-arrhythmic therapy with lidocaine (intervention) result in normal neurological outcome (outcome) more often than standard care with or without lidocaine?

5 In patients with cardiac arrest associated with shock resistant VT or VF (population), does anti-arrhythmic therapy (e.g., bretylium, procainamide) (intervention) provide a more favorable neurological outcome (outcome) than standard care and defibrillation (control)?

6 In patients with *stable* VT (population), does anti-arrhythmic therapy (e.g., lidocaine, amiodarone, sotalol, procainamide) (intervention) convert patients to normal sinus rhythm more frequently (outcome) than standard care and synchronized cardioversion (control)?

7 In patients with torsades de pointes (polymorphic VT) (population), does magnesium sulfate (intervention) convert patients to normal sinus rhythm more frequently (outcome) than standard care and cardioversion (control)?

General search strategy

You begin to address these questions by searching for evidence in the common electronic databases such as the Cochrane Library, MEDLINE and EMBASE looking specifically for systematic reviews and meta-analyses. The Cochrane Database of Systematic Reviews includes high-quality systematic review evidence on therapy for ventricular tachycardia and supraventricular tachycardia and the Database of Abstracts of Reviews of Effects (DARE) includes systematic review evidence on the diagnosis of VT and VF. You also search the Cochrane Central Register of Controlled Trials (CENTRAL), MEDLINE and EMBASE to identify randomized controlled trials (RCTs) that became available after the publication date of the systematic review or, if no systematic reviews were identified, to locate high-quality RCTs that directly address the clinical question. In addition, updated, evidence-based clinical practice guidelines (CPGs) on advanced cardiac life support are accessed to determine the consensus rating of topics lacking more robust support.

Critical review of the literature

Question 1: In clinically stable patients with a wide complex tachy-dysrhythmia (population), are there valid and reliable clinical and electrocardiographic criteria (diagnostic test characteristics) that can discriminate between VT and SVT with aberrant conduction (outcome)?

Search strategy

- MEDLINE: ventricular tachycardia OR supraventricular tachycardia OR wide complex tachycardia OR electrocardiogram

Wide complex tachycardia (WCT) frequently presents a diagnostic dilemma for clinicians. Although several causes exist, the main priority in the clinical setting is to distinguish VT from other arrhythmias. VT carries a significantly worse prognosis and failure to recognize it and initiate appropriate treatment can lead to dire consequences for the patient [4]. Misdiagnosing a WCT as VT when it is truly another arrhythmia (most commonly supraventricular tachycardia with aberrancy (SVTwA)), while potentially exposing the patient to unnecessary testing in the electrophysiology laboratory, carries a much lower risk to the patient. Therefore, a diagnostic method is required that has a high sensitivity, while a lower specificity can be tolerated (i.e., SnOut – a sensitive strategy, which if yielding a negative result, rules out the condition in question).

While it is widely accepted that older patients with a history of heart disease are at greater risk for VT, clinical criteria are not sufficiently reliable to distinguish between VT and non-VT causes

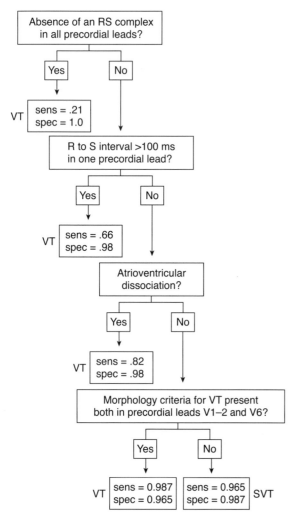

Figure 21.1 Brugada algorithm for distinguishing ventricular tachycardia (VT) from supraventricular tachycardia (SVT). sens, sensitivity; spec, specificity. (Reprinted with permission from Brugada et al. [6], courtesy of Lippincott Williams & Wilkins.)

of WCT. A common misconception is that VT is unlikely in the absence of hemodynamic instability. Misdiagnosis of VT as SVTwA based upon hemodynamic stability can lead to inappropriate and potentially dangerous therapy [4,5].

Several algorithms have been developed to distinguish VT from non-VT rhythms based upon ECG criteria. The Brugada algorithm, building upon earlier studies that examined the frequency of specific ECG morphology in VT and non-VT rhythms, uses a sequential four-step process (Fig. 21.1) [6]. Griffith et al. developed a simplified process, examining for two criteria – the presence of ECG findings typical of bundle branch block and independent P-waves (AV dissociation) – in an effort to maximize the sensitivity for the detection of VT (Fig. 21.2) [7]. Both algorithms had high sensitivities and specificities in their original validation set; however, when re-tested (by non-expert ECG readers), the sensitivities and specificities were not as high as their derivation set (Table 21.1) [8,9].

Another method, using a Bayesian approach, identified six clinical criteria based upon data from previous studies and calculated the likelihood ratios for predicting VT or SVTwA (Fig. 21.3) [10]. To calculate the probability of VT, a pre-test odds of 4 (i.e., 4:1) is used, based upon a relative VT prevalence of 80% versus 20% for SVTwA. The pre-test odds are then multiplied by the likelihood ratio for each of the six criteria that are interpretable to generate the post-test odds of VT. One advantage of this approach is that criteria that are uninterpretable do not prevent determination of the probability of a diagnosis, a potential drawback in the sequential approach of other algorithms. However, due to the greater number of criteria involved, the Bayesian method is more complicated to apply than the other two methods. An on-line calculator would facilitate its implementation. In the face of the complexity of the Bayesian method, despite the increased accuracy in validation trials, the Griffith algorithm is likely to be the most sensible method to implement in practice [8].

In summary, determining the specific cause of a WCT remains a challenge to the clinician. The ideal tool, combining a high sensitivity for VT with ease of use, has yet to be validated for the non-expert. Future computer decision aids may facilitate the process. In the meantime, it is important to remember that the safest course of action is to assume that the cause of the WCT is VT. When in doubt, treat for VT [11].

Question 2: In patients with SVT (population), does adenosine (intervention) effectively convert patients to normal sinus rhythm (outcome) compared with calcium channel blockers (control)?

Search strategy

- MEDLINE: narrow complex tachycardia OR supraventricular tachycardia OR adenosine OR calcium channel blocker

Supraventricular tachycardia is a regular tachycardia that is caused by re-entry, an abnormal circuit either within the AV node or via an accessory pathway that allows for a continuous wave of depolarization. Patients with SVT most commonly present to the ED with palpitations (including increased or irregular heart beat) and chest pain [12]. In the hemodynamically stable patient with SVT, prior to initiation of drug therapy, a trial of vagal maneuvers may convert up to 28% of SVT in the ED setting [13]. Hemodynamically unstable patients should receive immediate synchronized cardioversion [14]. For SVT resistant to vagal maneuvers, the most commonly recommended medications are adenosine and calcium channel blockers. Both act by inhibiting conduction through the AV node, thereby terminating the re-entrant rhythm at the root of most SVTs.

A Cochrane review including eight RCTs involving 577 participants compared adenosine to calcium channel blockers for the treatment of SVT [15]. In the pooled analysis, successful conversion to normal sinus rhythm occurred in 92% of the adenosine

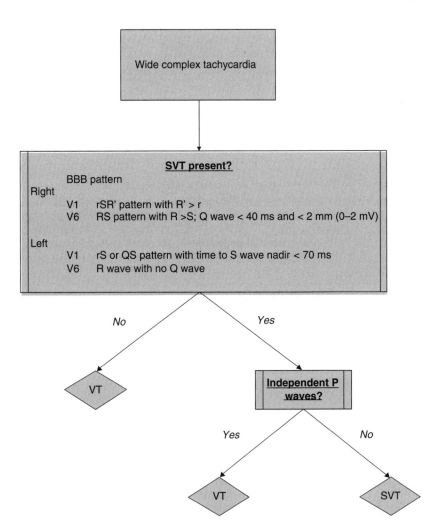

Figure 21.2 Griffith algorithm for the diagnosis of wide complex tachycardia. BBB, branch bundle block; SVT, supraventricular tachycardia; VT, ventricular tachycardia. (Adapted with permission from Griffith et al. [7], courtesy of Elsevier.)

group compared with 89% of the verapamil group (OR = 0.67; 95% CI: 0.38 to 1.16) (Fig. 21.4). In the four studies that reported time to normal sinus rhythm, adenosine demonstrated a significantly shorter time; however, the times to reversion could not be combined due to significant heterogeneity. There was an insignificant difference in relapse rate between the two drugs (OR = 0.27; 95% CI: 0.06 to 1.23) in favor of verapamil. Aside from the conversion rate, other factors, such as cost and side-effect profile, may be a factor in which medication is selected. In Canada, adenosine is nearly 10 times as expensive as verapamil (approximately $20 vs $2, respectively); however, adenosine has a slightly quicker onset

of action, which may translate into decreased monitoring time and therefore the use of fewer resources.

The frequency of side-effects may also play an important role in choosing one drug over the other. Minor adverse events, including chest tightness, nausea, shortness of breath, headache and flushing, occurred more commonly with adenosine than with verapamil (OR = 0.13; 95% CI: 0.05 to 0.29) (Fig. 21.5). One major side-effect, hypotension, was documented more often with verapamil than adenosine (OR = 8.6; 95% CI: 0.88 to 83.86) (Fig. 21.6).

In summary, adenosine is as effective as the calcium channel blocker verapamil; however, short-term side-effects are more

Table 21.1 Test characteristics of the diagnostic criteria for the diagnosis of wide complex tachycardia.

| Algorithm | Original derivation study | | Validation set | | | |
| | | | Lau & Ng [8] | | Isenhour et al. [9] | |
	Sensitivity	Specificity	Sensitivity	Specificity	Sensitivity	Specificity
Brugada [6]	98.7	96.5	92	44	79–91	43–70
Griffith [7]	96	64	92	44		
Bayesian [10]	95	52	97	56		

ECG features	LR
ORS width	
≤ 0.14 second	0.31
> 0.14 and ≤ 0.16 second	0.46
> 0.16 second	22.86
ORS axis	
Right superior (–90° to ± 180°)	7.86
Left (–80° to – 90°) (RBBB type)	8.21
Right (+120° to ± 180°) (LBBB type)	3.93
None of the above	0.47
V morphology in RBBB pattern	
Taller left peak	50
Biphasic Rs or qR	4.03
Triphasic rsR or rR'	0.21
None of the above	1.41
V or V morphology in LBBB pattern	
(a) r ≥ 0.04 second, or (b) Notched S downstroke, or (c) Delayed S nadir > 0.06 second	50
None of the above	0.13
Interval to intrinsicoid deflection in V_6	
≥ 0.06 second	19.30
< 0.08 second	0.46
V_6 morphology	
Monophasic QS	50
Biphasic rS (r:S < 1) (RBBB type)	50
Triphasic qRs (R:S < 1) (RBBB type)	0.13
None of the above	0.57

The LRs quoted relate to the factor by which the odds of ventricular tachycarida (VT) to supraventricular tachycardia with aberrant conduction (SVTAC) need to be multiplied when the associated ECG features is present. Thus if the LR is > 1, the presence of that particular features should be regarded as a positive test, as it favors the diagnosis of VT over SVTAC, while if the LR is < 1, the presence of that particular feature should be regarded as a negative test, as if favors the diagnosis of SVTAC over VT.

Figure 21.3 Diagnostic criteria included in the Bayesian diagnostic algorithm for wide complex tachycardia (WCT) and their likelihood ratios (LRs) due to test results. ECG, electrocardiogram; LBBB, left branch bundle block; RBBB, right branch bundle block. (Reprinted with permission from Lau et al. [10], courtesy of Wiley-Blackwell Publishing.)

frequent and the costs are higher. One approach may be to inquire whether a patient would prefer a slightly faster medication that is likely to cause minor side-effects versus one that is overall better tolerated but more likely to cause a major side-effect (hypotension). Diltiazem, a calcium channel blocker with less negative effects on myocardial contractility than verapamil in vitro (approximately $3 per treatment), has not been studied in comparison to adenosine for the management of SVT. However, it appears to have efficacy similar to verapamil in terminating SVT [16].

Question 3: In patients with cardiac arrest associated with shock resistant VT or VF (population) does anti-arrhythmic therapy with amiodarone (intervention) result in normal neurological outcome (outcome) more often than standard care with or without lidocaine?

Search strategy

- MEDLINE: ventricular tachycardia OR ventricular fibrillation OR cardiac arrest OR lidocaine OR amiodarone OR return of spontaneous circulation

Ventricular arrhythmias occur primarily in the setting of myocardial ischemia or cardiomyopathies. Pulseless VT and VF are the main causes of sudden cardiac death, but other ventricular tachyarrhythmias can occur without hemodynamic compromise. Cardiac arrest associated with ventricular tachyarrhythmias is managed with cardiopulmonary resuscitation and electrical defibrillation. Pharmacotherapy, an adjunct to those fundamental interventions, has been the subject of a number of trials conducted in the context of prehospital cardiac arrest.

Two major trials, the ARREST (Amiodarone in the Out-of-hospital Resuscitation of Refractory Sustained Ventricular Tachyarrhythmia) and ALIVE (Amiodarone versus Lidocaine in Prehospital Ventricular Fibrillation Evaluation) trials conducted in the early 1990s examined the role of amiodarone in comparison to either placebo or lidocaine, respectively, in a population of cardiac arrest patients with shock resistant VT or VF [17,18]. The ARREST population (504 people with cardiac arrest and shock resistant VF or pulseless VF developing at some point during resuscitation) revealed that there were significantly more people who survived to admission to hospital when amiodarone was administered (44%) compared to placebo (34%) (OR = 0.66; 95% CI: 0.46 to 0.94) [17]. However, no significant difference in survival to hospital discharge (a proxy for reasonable neurological recovery) was observed between amiodarone- and placebo-treated patients (OR = 0.98; 95% CI: 0.59 to 1.64). This RCT also found similar results between amiodarone and placebo in the number of the people who survived to discharge from hospital who returned to independent living or work (OR = 0.81; 95% CI: 0.31 to 2.14).

In the comparison of amiodarone with lidocaine, the ALIVE trial (347 people with cardiac arrest and shock resistant VT or VF developing at some point during their resuscitation) found that

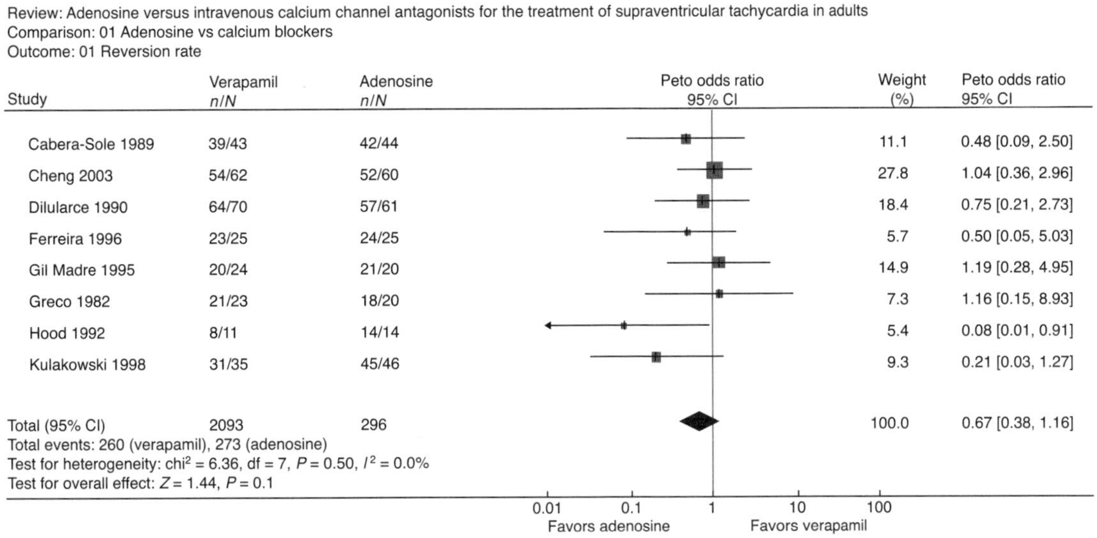

Review: Adenosine versus intravenous calcium channel antagonists for the treatment of supraventricular tachycardia in adults
Comparison: 01 Adenosine vs calcium blockers
Outcome: 01 Reversion rate

Study	Verapamil n/N	Adenosine n/N	Peto odds ratio 95% CI	Weight (%)	Peto odds ratio 95% CI
Cabera-Sole 1989	39/43	42/44		11.1	0.48 [0.09, 2.50]
Cheng 2003	54/62	52/60		27.8	1.04 [0.36, 2.96]
Dilularce 1990	64/70	57/61		18.4	0.75 [0.21, 2.73]
Ferreira 1996	23/25	24/25		5.7	0.50 [0.05, 5.03]
Gil Madre 1995	20/24	21/20		14.9	1.19 [0.28, 4.95]
Greco 1982	21/23	18/20		7.3	1.16 [0.15, 8.93]
Hood 1992	8/11	14/14		5.4	0.08 [0.01, 0.91]
Kulakowski 1998	31/35	45/46		9.3	0.21 [0.03, 1.27]
Total (95% CI)	2093	296		100.0	0.67 [0.38, 1.16]

Total events: 260 (verapamil), 273 (adenosine)
Test for heterogeneity: chi^2 = 6.36, df = 7, P = 0.50, I^2 = 0.0%
Test for overall effect: Z = 1.44, P = 0.1

0.01   0.1   1   10   100
Favors adenosine   Favors verapamil

Figure 21.4 Reversion rate of adenosine versus calcium channel blockers for the treatment of supraventricular tachycardia. (Reproduced with permission from Holdgate & Foo [15], © Cochrane Library.)

a significantly larger proportion of people survived to hospital admission with amiodarone compared with lidocaine (OR = 0.46; 95% CI: 0.26 to 0.82). However, it found no significant difference in survival to discharge from hospital between amiodarone and lidocaine (OR = 0.6; 95% CI: 0.19 to 1.77).

Both the ARREST and ALIVE trials reported data on the potential harms associated with these interventions. The ARREST trial found that there was significantly more hypotension (59% with amiodarone vs 48% with placebo; P = 0.04) and bradycardia (41% with amiodarone vs 25% with placebo; P = 0.004) in people who took amiodarone compared with placebo and who had either a transient or a sustained return of spontaneous circulation. The ALIVE trial reported that pressor drugs were needed both for people who took amiodarone and people who took lidocaine (OR = 1.8; 95% CI: 0.7 to 4.69) [18]. The RCT also reported that treatment for bradycardia was required in both groups (OR = 1.06; 95% CI: 0.64 to 1.74).

In the ALIVE trial, the median interval from dispatch to drug administration was 24 minutes; 22.8% of amiodarone-treated patients survived to hospital admission compared to 12.0% of lidocaine-treated patients (P = 0.009) [18]. If the study drug was given within 24 minutes after dispatch, 27.7% of amiodarone patients and 15.3% of lidocaine patients survived to hospital admission (P = 0.05).

It is worth noting that neither the ARREST nor the ALIVE trials were powered to detect a difference in hospital discharge rate/meaningful neurological survival. As neither study found an advantage with regard to either of these outcomes it is conceivable that amiodarone use might simply lead to increased consumption of hospital intensive care unit (ICU) resources without patient benefit. Although methodologically sound, the selection of admission to hospital ICU as these studies' primary outcome is problematic though possibly unavoidable given the cost and logistical issues as-

sociated with a significantly larger trial. However, important developments in post-resuscitative care (i.e., therapeutic hypothermia) might actually allow the increased ICU admission rate associated with amiodarone to translate into a clinical benefit as it relates to neurological recovery from cardiac arrest.

There is no evidence that giving any anti-arrhythmic drug routinely during human cardiac arrest increases rate of survival to hospital discharge. In comparison with placebo and lidocaine, the use of amiodarone in shock refractory VF improves the short-term outcome of survival to hospital admission. Despite the lack of human long-term outcome data, it is reasonable to continue to use anti-arrhythmic drugs on a routine basis.

In summary, one high-quality RCT found that more people survived to hospital admission with amiodarone compared with placebo [17]. However, it found no significant difference in survival to hospital discharge. Another RCT found that more people survived to hospital admission with amiodarone compared with lidocaine [18]. However, it also found no significant difference in survival to hospital discharge. Amiodarone was associated with more hypotension and bradycardia than placebo.

Question 4: In patients with cardiac arrest associated with shock resistant VT or VF (population), does anti-arrhythmic therapy with lidocaine (intervention) result in normal neurological outcome (outcome) more often than standard care and placebo?

Search strategy

- MEDLINE: ventricular tachycardia OR ventricular fibrillation OR cardiac arrest OR lidocaine OR return of spontaneous circulation

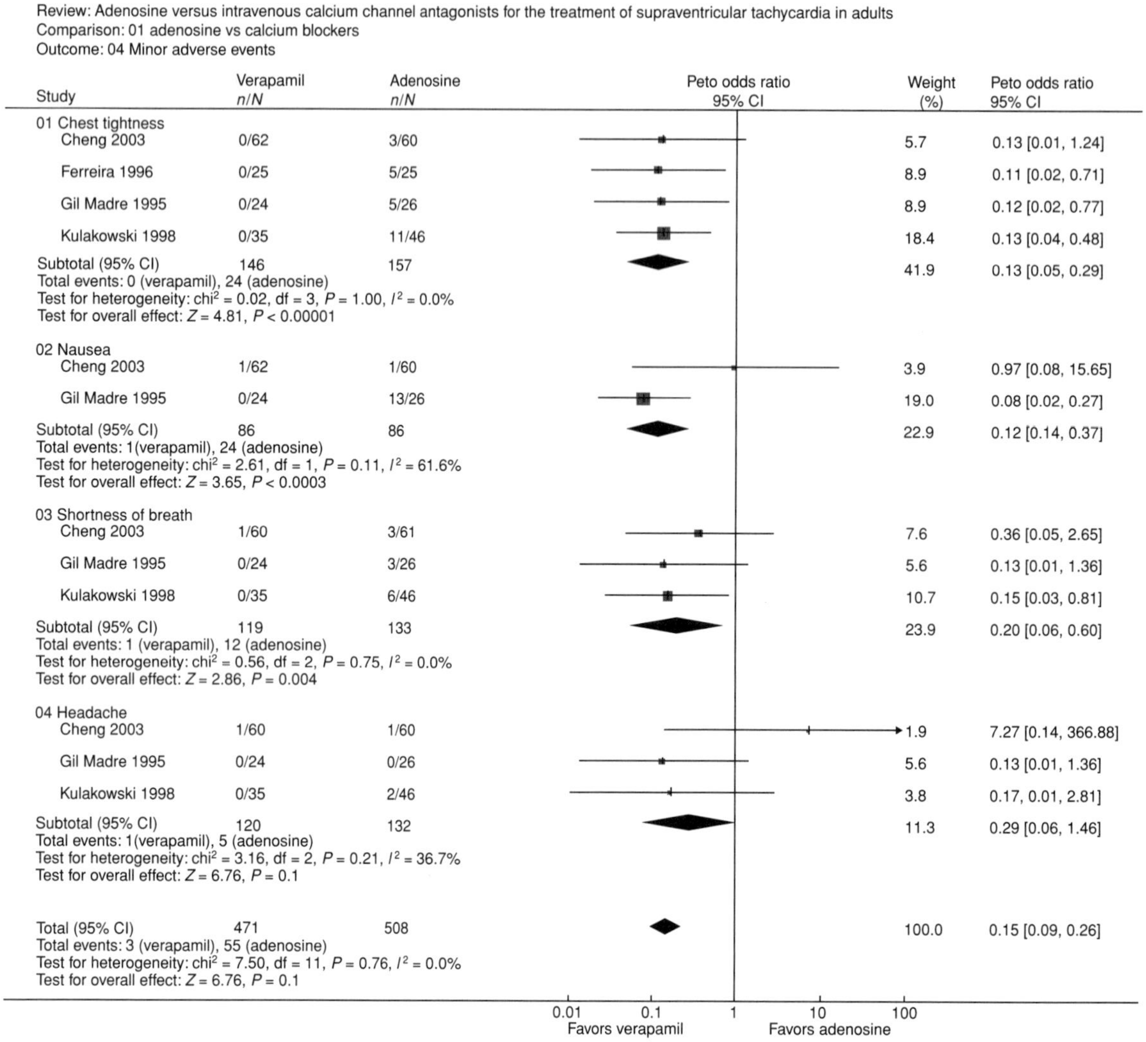

Review: Adenosine versus intravenous calcium channel antagonists for the treatment of supraventricular tachycardia in adults
Comparison: 01 adenosine vs calcium blockers
Outcome: 04 Minor adverse events

Study	Verapamil n/N	Adenosine n/N	Peto odds ratio 95% CI	Weight (%)	Peto odds ratio 95% CI
01 Chest tightness					
Cheng 2003	0/62	3/60		5.7	0.13 [0.01, 1.24]
Ferreira 1996	0/25	5/25		8.9	0.11 [0.02, 0.71]
Gil Madre 1995	0/24	5/26		8.9	0.12 [0.02, 0.77]
Kulakowski 1998	0/35	11/46		18.4	0.13 [0.04, 0.48]
Subtotal (95% CI)	146	157		41.9	0.13 [0.05, 0.29]

Total events: 0 (verapamil), 24 (adenosine)
Test for heterogeneity: chi^2 = 0.02, df = 3, P = 1.00, I^2 = 0.0%
Test for overall effect: Z = 4.81, P < 0.00001

02 Nausea					
Cheng 2003	1/62	1/60		3.9	0.97 [0.08, 15.65]
Gil Madre 1995	0/24	13/26		19.0	0.08 [0.02, 0.27]
Subtotal (95% CI)	86	86		22.9	0.12 [0.14, 0.37]

Total events: 1(verapamil), 24 (adenosine)
Test for heterogeneity: chi^2 = 2.61, df = 1, P = 0.11, I^2 = 61.6%
Test for overall effect: Z = 3.65, P < 0.0003

03 Shortness of breath					
Cheng 2003	1/60	3/61		7.6	0.36 [0.05, 2.65]
Gil Madre 1995	0/24	3/26		5.6	0.13 [0.01, 1.36]
Kulakowski 1998	0/35	6/46		10.7	0.15 [0.03, 0.81]
Subtotal (95% CI)	119	133		23.9	0.20 [0.06, 0.60]

Total events: 1 (verapamil), 12 (adenosine)
Test for heterogeneity: chi^2 = 0.56, df = 2, P = 0.75, I^2 = 0.0%
Test for overall effect: Z = 2.86, P = 0.004

04 Headache					
Cheng 2003	1/60	1/60		1.9	7.27 [0.14, 366.88]
Gil Madre 1995	0/24	0/26		5.6	0.13 [0.01, 1.36]
Kulakowski 1998	0/35	2/46		3.8	0.17 [0.01, 2.81]
Subtotal (95% CI)	120	132		11.3	0.29 [0.06, 1.46]

Total events: 1(verapamil), 5 (adenosine)
Test for heterogeneity: chi^2 = 3.16, df = 2, P = 0.21, I^2 = 36.7%
Test for overall effect: Z = 6.76, P = 0.1

Total (95% CI)	471	508		100.0	0.15 [0.09, 0.26]

Total events: 3 (verapamil), 55 (adenosine)
Test for heterogeneity: chi^2 = 7.50, df = 11, P = 0.76, I^2 = 0.0%
Test for overall effect: Z = 6.76, P = 0.1

```
0.01    0.1      1      10    100
   Favors verapamil   Favors adenosine
```

Figure 21.5 Minor adverse event rate during treatment of supraventricular tachycardia with adenosine compared to intravenous calcium channel blockers. (Reproduced with permission from Holdgate & Foo [15], © Cochrane Library.)

Review: Adenosine versus intravenous calcium channel antagonists for the treatment of supraventricular tachycardia in adults
Comparison: 01 Adenosine vs calcium blockers
Outcome: 05 Hypotension

Study	Verapamil n/N	Adenosine n/N	Peto odds ratio 95% CI	Weight (%)	Peto odds ratio 95% CI
Cabera-Sole 1989	0/25	0/25		0.0	Not estimable
Dilularce 1990	1/70	0/61		33.6	6.50 [0.13, 330.51]
Ferreira 1996	0/25	0/25		0.0	Not estimable
Hood 1992	1/11	0/14		33.3	9.71 [0.19, 503.30]
Kulakowski 1998	1/35	0/46		33.1	10.12 [0.19, 528.94]
Total (95% CI)	166	171		100.0	8.60 [0.88, 83.86]

Total events: 3 (verapamil), 0 (adenosine)
Test for heterogeneity: chi^2 = 0.03, df = 2, P = 0.99, I^2 = 0.0%
Test for overall effect: Z = 1.85, P = 0.06

```
0.001  0.01   0.1     1     10   100  1000
      Favors verapamil   Favors adenosine
```

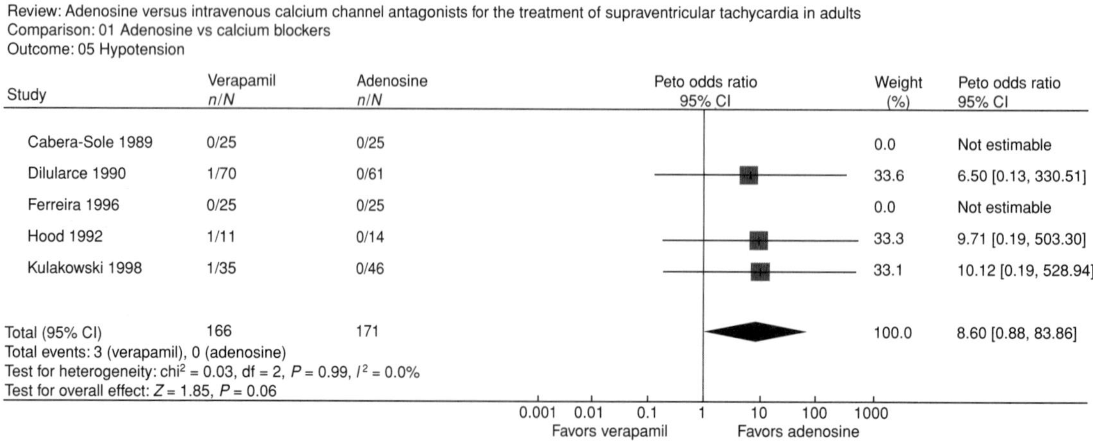

Figure 21.6 Rate of hypotension during treatment of supraventricular tachycardia with adenosine compared to intravenous calcium channel blockers. (Reproduced with permission from Holdgate & Foo [15], © Cochrane Library.)

Supported by evidence-based guidelines issued by the American Heart Association (AHA), lidocaine, until recently, was an established agent for the treatment of cardiac arrest-associated arrhythmias [19]. In previous versions of these guidelines, lidocaine retained its status as an acceptable anti-arrhythmic for use in the treatment of shock refractory VF and pulseless VT, even though the evidence supporting its efficacy was noted to be extremely poor and methodologically weak. Specifically there are no RCTs comparing lidocaine to placebo in an out-of-hospital or in-hospital cardiac arrest context. The AHA 2000 conference experts concluded that lidocaine could continue to be used for VF/VT but that, given the antiquated evidence, it merits a lower evidence grading (class indeterminate). Lidocaine has also not been recommended for routine prophylaxis of ventricular arrhythmias in the setting of acute myocardial infarction since 1992 [19]. Conference experts in 2000 also concluded that the data did not justify changing the classification of lidocaine to an *evidence-of-harm* agent [20]. In the 2005 update of the guidelines, lidocaine as an anti-arrhythmic option in shock resistant cardiac arrest due to VT/VF was dropped as a consideration [21]. As noted in Question 3 above, one high-quality RCT (ALIVE trial) suggests that lidocaine is inferior to amiodarone for the outcome of admission to the hospital ICU [19].

In summary, there is no sound scientific basis to support the use of lidocaine as a primary treatment in shock resistant VT or VF in the setting of cardiac arrest.

Question 5: In patients with cardiac arrest associated with shock resistant VT or VF (population), does anti-arrhythmic therapy (e.g., bretylium, procainamide) (intervention) provide a more favorable neurological outcome (outcome) than standard care and defibrillation (control)?

Search strategy

- MEDLINE: ventricular tachycardia OR ventricular fibrillation OR cardiac arrest OR lidocaine OR amiodarone OR bretylium OR procainamide OR return of spontaneous circulation

Bretylium was first thought to have a promising role in the resuscitation of cardiac arrest patients with either VF or asystole. A small emergency-based study reported a nearly 30% difference in return of spontaneous circulation among 59 patients (35% vs 6%) [22]. However, two smaller RCTs conducted in the prehospital setting found no difference in clinical outcomes between bretylium and lidocaine [23,24]. The first of these latter prehospital RCTs (100 people with out-of-hospital and persistent VF after initial shock) found no significant difference between lidocaine and bretylium given after the first shock in terms of discharge from hospital (23% with lidocaine vs 21% with bretylium; $P > 0.1$) [23]. This study also reported that pressor drugs were needed in both arms (33% with lidocaine vs 37% with bretylium; $P = $ NS). The second RCT

(91 people with refractory VT) found no significant difference between lidocaine and bretylium in the proportion of people who survived to hospital discharge (10% with lidocaine vs 5% with bretylium; $P = $ NS) [24]. However, in this RCT, people were given the alternative drug if they did not respond to the first drug.

There are no RCTs comparing procainamide or bretylium versus placebo for the clinical outcomes of interest; however, the Cardiac Arrest in Seattle: Conventional versus Amiodarone Drug Evaluation (CASCADE) trial demonstrated better results for amiodarone in comparison with procainamide for the secondary prevention of cardiac arrest among survivors [25]. From a practical perspective, the time required to infuse procainamide is usually long (generally recommended as a slow infusion over several minutes) and this would make it a less favorable choice in acute or unstable conditions as a preferred drug. It might, however, be considered an option for recurrent VT/VF.

Question 6: In patients with *stable* VT (population), does anti-arrhythmic therapy (e.g., lidocaine, amiodarone, sotalol, procainamide) (intervention) convert patients to normal sinus rhythm more frequently (outcome) than standard care and synchronized cardioversion (control).

Search strategy

- MEDLINE: ventricular tachycardia OR lidocaine OR sotalol OR procainamide OR amiodarone OR cardioversion

Stable VT is an infrequent, yet potentially life-threatening, condition encountered in the ED setting. A patient with stable VT, akin to the patient described in the clinical scenario, is characterized by a WCT presumed to be ventricular in origin and not associated with either hypotension or other signs of cardiovascular decompensation such as congestive heart failure or chest pain. In the literature review conducted for the November 2005 update of the AHA/American College of Cardiology (ACC) clinical practice guidelines on advanced cardiac life support, Domanovits noted the paucity of relevant research in patients requiring acute management of stable VT [26]. Instead most of the literature on this question draws upon conclusions from electrophysiological laboratory studies and animal research. In this section we will briefly review the literature as it pertains to each of the four anti-arrhythmic medications noted in the question.

There are no prospective trials of patients with stable VT treated with lidocaine. There is only one prospective randomized trial that examined the benefit of lidocaine in the setting of stable VT and then ostensibly as a prophylactic agent. In this prehospital trial of lidocaine (400 mg) administered intramuscularly in over 6000 patients suspected of suffering a myocardial infarction, lidocaine-treated patients were less likely to develop VF within 15 minutes of randomization than control patients (OR = 0.17; 95% CI: 0.04 to 0.74) [27]. Other than that study, all of the evidence for lidocaine in stable VT is drawn from case series literature, which in general suggests a very low level of termination for stable VT, generally in the range of 20% [28,29]. Therefore, the benefit of administration of intravenous lidocaine for patients with acute myocardial infarction or in patients with or without a history of coronary artery disease for the treatment of stable VT in the hospital setting is questionable.

The evidence base for the treatment of stable VT with amiodarone is somewhat more robust. Somberg randomized 29 patients with shock resistant VT to either up to two 150 mg boluses of amiodarone or two 100 mg boluses of lidocaine [30]. Immediate VT termination was achieved in 14 patients (78%) with amiodarone versus three patients (27%) on lidocaine ($P < 0.05$). After 1 hour, 67% of those on amiodarone and 9% on lidocaine were alive and free of VT ($P < 0.01$). Amiodarone had a 33% drug failure rate, whereas there was a 91% drug failure rate for lidocaine. The 24-hour survival was 39% on amiodarone and 9% on lidocaine (OR = 0.16, $P < 0.01$). Although much of the evidence in support of amiodarone comes from case series literature there appears to be a promising role for amiodarone in the setting of ischemic heart disease or depressed left ventricular function.

Both Helmy and Shutzenberger reported the effective termination of VT in a majority of their case series of patients with significantly impaired ejection fractions and failure to respond to other treatments [31,32]. Of note, a multi-center comparison of high-dose amiodarone (1.8 g/day) and low-dose amiodarone (0.2 g/day) versus a third arm consisting of bretylium revealed similar survival rates, though they showed an advantage of the higher-dose amiodarone over the lower-dose amiodarone, the former being equivalent to the effect of bretylium [33]. Therefore, administration of amiodarone for patients with preserved or depressed left ventricular function, for the treatment of spontaneous sustained monomorphic VT and recurrent VT as well as for shock resistant and/or drug refractory VT (electrical storm) in the hospital setting can be recommended.

Procainamide is another valid option in patients with stable VT. In an RCT of 29 patients with VT, procainamide was superior to lidocaine in terminating spontaneously occurring VT (OR = 15; 95% CI: 2.5 to 91.5) [34]. Of a total of 41 VT episodes, four of 15 responded to lidocaine and 20 of 26 could be terminated with procainamide ($P < 0.01$). Administration of procainamide for patients with spontaneously occurring monomorphic VT is thus preferred over lidocaine. The 2006 AHA/ACC guidelines on the management of ventricular arrhythmias established procainamide as the only agent with a weight of *evidence favors use* (single RCT or non-randomized studies) designation [11]. Amiodarone is also designated as *evidence favors use* but with lower levels of evidence [11].

Finally, in a RCT of 33 patients with VT but not in cardiac arrest, intravenous sotalol resulted in a superior rate of VT termination compared to lidocaine [35]. Sotalol was significantly more effective than lidocaine in an intention-to-treat basis (OR = 10.1; 95% CI: 2.0 to 52.2). Although concerns about the safety of IV sotalol have been raised, a meta-analysis showed that the overall risk of torsades de pointes in patients treated with a single infusion of IV

sotalol is approximately 0.1% [29]. Therefore, administration of sotalol to adult patients with spontaneous sustained stable VT is recommended and should be preferred over lidocaine.

In summary, the most promising agents for use in the termination of VT in a hemodynamically stable patient include amiodarone, procainamide and sotalol, all administered as intravenous therapies. Additional research with head-to-head comparisons among these agents would be useful.

Question 7: In patients with torsades de pointes (polymorphic VT) (population), does magnesium sulfate (intervention) convert patients to normal sinus rhythm more frequently (outcome) than standard care and cardioversion?

Search strategy

- MEDLINE: ventricular tachycardia OR torsades de pointes OR cardiac arrest OR magnesium sulfate OR cardioversion OR QT interval

Torsades de pointes (TdP) is a polymorphic VT that has a characteristic alternating electric polarity and amplitude, such that the rhythm appears to twist about its axis. Patients may present with palpitations, seizures, syncope or in cardiac arrest. In one series of patients with sudden cardiac death while undergoing Holter monitoring, 12.7% had TdP [36]. TdP most commonly occurs in patients with a long QT interval, which may be congenital or more commonly acquired through disease or drugs (especially anti-arrhythmics). Patients with TdP who are hemodynamically unstable require immediate high-dose unsynchronized defibrillation [37].

Medical treatment of TdP is appropriate when a patient is hemodynamically stable. Several treatments have been described, including withdrawal of any offending drugs (e.g., dialysis or bicarbonate therapy in certain tricyclic antidepressant overdoses), correction of electrolyte abnormalities, isoproterenol, overdrive pacing and magnesium [38].

Magnesium has been cited as a first-line agent to use in the treatment of TdP (AHA 2005 guidelines); however, no clinical trials have directly compared magnesium to cardioversion or other interventions [37]. Only two observational studies report the use of magnesium for TdP. In one case series 17 patients with polymorphic VT were treated with IV magnesium [39]. Twelve had a prolonged QT interval as measured from the sinus beat immediately preceding the VT, while five patients had a normal QT interval. Of the 12 patients with prolonged QT intervals, nine were on anti-arrhythmics prior to the onset of TdP. Four patients received other interventions prior to magnesium (two with lidocaine, one with isoproterenol and one with cardiac pacing), however these were either ineffective or were discontinued secondary to patient discomfort. All 12 cases converted to sinus rhythm after either one bolus (9/12) or two boluses (3/12) of MgSO$_4$. The magnesium was given as an intravenous bolus of 2 g within 1–2 minutes and in most patients this was followed by a continuous infusion (3–20 mg/min). In the same series, five other patients with normal QT interval polymorphic VT received 2–6 g of magnesium with no effect. The VT in these five patients responded to IV lidocaine (3/5) or procainamide (2/5). No adverse effects of magnesium administration were reported. In another case series, 25 patients with monomorphic VT and four patients with TdP were treated with 2 g of magnesium glutamate [40]. Magnesium effectively interrupted all four cases of TdP but only in eight of 25 patients with monomorphic VT.

Although the evidence is scanty, magnesium has a large therapeutic index with few adverse reactions in the usual doses and when administered slowly [41]. In the limited published experience with TdP there were no reported adverse outcomes from its administration.

In summary, magnesium appears effective in terminating polymorphic VT associated with a long QT interval (the most common cause of TdP); however, it is unclear if it has efficacy in polymorphic VT with a normal QT interval or monomorphic VT. While it may be difficult or impossible to determine if a patient with polymorphic VT had a long QT interval prior to the onset of the arrhythmia, magnesium treatment is safe and potentially effective, and should be considered as a first-line agent in hemodynamically stable patients.

Conclusions

You suspect that the patient has either VT or a SVT with aberrancy, but you are unsure of the diagnosis and how to proceed with treatment. As the patient is hemodynamically stable, you step to the computer situated in your resuscitation room and do a quick search. Using PubMed clinical queries, you select "narrow, specific search" for diagnosis and enter ventricular tachycardia. Unfortunately, this yields far too many hits, and a quick scan of the first few do not reveal any that look applicable to your situation. You decide to refine your search, using the following search items: "ventricular tachycardia supraventricular tachycardia electrocardiogram not ICD". The fourth citation appears to directly address your question [8]. Using the algorithm presented in the article, you decide that your patient's rhythm is indeed VT. You then proceed to consult the Cochrane Library for recommendations on treatment of the VT. Unfortunately, there do not appear to be any helpful documents in the Cochrane reviews. You then turn to the TRIP (Turning Research Into Practice) database, available freely to all on the web. Searching using the term "stable ventricular tachycardia", the results under the "Guidelines" menu yield a promising hit. The fourth citation listed, the AHA 2006 guidelines for the management of patients with ventricular arrhythmias, recommend starting the patient on procainamide. As your patient has no contraindications to procainamide, you order the infusion. Twenty minutes later the patient successfully converts into a sinus rhythm.

Ventricular and supraventricular arrhythmias constitute both common and potentially life-threatening presentations to the ED. Perhaps more than any other domain of emergency care, their management often requires quick action and a consistent and reliable approach. The decision algorithms and treatment recommendations summarized here present a rational method of managing these conditions.

Acknowledgments

The author wishes to thank Dr. Marwan Al Raisi for his contribution to this chapter.

References

1 Engelstein ED, Zipes DP. Sudden cardiac death. In: Alexander RW, Schlant RC, Fuster V, eds. *The Heart, Arteries and Veins.* McGraw-Hill, New York, 1998:1081–112.

2 Myerburg RJ, Castellanos A. Cardiac arrest and sudden cardiac death. In: Braunwald E, ed. *Heart Disease: A textbook of cardiovascular medicine.* WB Saunders, Philadelphia, 1997:742–79.

3 de Vreede-Swagemakers JJ, Gorgels AP, Dubois-Arbouw WI, et al. Out-of-hospital cardiac arrest in the 1990s: a population-based study in the Maastricht area on incidence, characteristics and survival. *J Am Coll Cardiol* 1997;**30**:1500–505.

4 Stewart RB. Wide complex tachycardia: misdiagnosis and outcome after emergent therapy. *Ann Intern Med* 1986;**104**:766–71.

5 Dancy M, Camm AJ, Ward D. Misdiagnosis of chronic recurrent ventricular tachycardia. *Lancet* 1985;**2**:320–23.

6 Brugada P, Brugada J, Mont L, Smeets J, Andries EW. A new approach to the differential diagnosis of a regular tachycardia with a wide QRS complex. *Circulation* 1991;**83**:1649–59.

7 Griffith MJ, Garratt CJ, Mounsey P, Camm AJ. Ventricular tachycardia as default diagnosis in broad complex tachycardia. *Lancet* 1994;**343**:386–8.

8 Lau EW, Ng GA. Comparison of the performance of three diagnostic algorithms for regular broad complex tachycardia in practical application. *Pacing Clin Electrophysiol* 2002;**25**:822–7.

9 Isenhour JL, Craig S, Gibbs M, Littmann L, Rose G, Risch R. Wide-complex tachycardia: continued evaluation of diagnostic criteria. *Acad Emerg Med* 2000;**7**:769–73.

10 Lau EW, Pathamanathan RK, Ng GA, Cooper J, Skehan JD, Griffith MJ. The Bayesian approach improves the electrocardiographic diagnosis of broad complex tachycardia. *Pacing Clin Electrophysiol* 2000;**23**:1519–26.

11 Zipes, DP, Camm, AJ, Borggrefe, M, et al. ACC/AHA/ESC 2006 guidelines for management of patients with ventricular arrhythmias and the prevention of sudden cardiac death – executive summary. A report of the American College of Cardiology/American Heart Association Task Force and the European Society of Cardiology Committee for Practice Guidelines (Writing Committee to Develop Guidelines for Management of Patients with Ventricular Arrhythmias and the Prevention of Sudden Cardiac Death). *J Am Coll Cardiol* 2006;**48**:1064.

12 Murman DH, McFonald AJ, Pelletier AJ, Camargo CA. US emergency department visits for supraventricular tachycardia, 1993–2003. *Acad Emerg Med* 2007;**14**:578–81.

13 AHA/ECC. Management of symptomatic bradycardia and tachycardia. *Circulation* 2005;**112**:IV67–77.

14 Lim SH, Anantharaman V, Teo WS, Goh PP, Tan AT. Comparison of treatment of supraventricular tachycardia by Valsalva maneuver and carotid sinus massage. *Ann Emerg Med* 1998;**31**:30–35.

15 Holdgate A, Foo A. Adenosine versus intravenous calcium channel antagonists for the treatment of supraventricular tachycardia in adults. *Cochrane Database Syst Rev* 2006;**4**:CD005154.

16 Lim SH, Anantharaman V, Teo WS. Slow-infusion of calcium channel blockers in the emergency management of supraventricular tachycardia. *Resuscitation* 2002;**52**:167–74.

17 Kudenchuk PJ, Cobb LA, Copass MK, et al. Amiodarone for resuscitation after out-of-hospital cardiac arrest due to ventricular fibrillation. *N Engl J Med* 1999;**341**:871–8.

18 Dorian P, Cass D, Schwartz B, et al. Amiodarone as compared with lidocaine for shock-resistant ventricular fibrillation. *N Engl J Med* 2002;**346**:884–90.

19 American Heart Association. Guidelines for cardiopulmonary resuscitation emergency cardiac care. *JAMA* 1992;**268**:2212–302.

20 American Heart Association in collaboration with the International Liaison Committee on Resuscitation. Guidelines 2000 for cardiopulmonary resuscitation and emergency cardiovascular care. Part 6: Advanced cardiovascular life support. Section 5: Pharmacology I: agents for arrhythmias. *Circulation* 2000;**102**:I112–28.

21 ECC Committee, Subcommittees and Task Forces of the American Heart Association. Part 7.2: Management of cardiac arrest 2005 American Heart Association guidelines for cardiopulmonary resuscitation and emergency cardiovascular care. *Circulation* 2005;**112**: IV58–66.

22 Nowak RM, Bodnar TJ, Dronen S, et al. Bretylium tosylate as initial treatment for cardiopulmonary arrest: randomized comparison with placebo. *Ann Emerg Med* 1981;**10**:404–7.

23 Haynes RE, Chinn TL, Copass MK, et al. Comparison of bretylium tosylate and lidocaine in management of out of hospital ventricular fibrillation: a randomized clinical trial. *Am J Cardiol* 1981;**48**: 353–6.

24 Olson DW, Thompson BM, Darin JC, et al. A randomized comparison study of bretylium tosylate and lidocaine in resuscitation of patients from out-of-hospital ventricular fibrillation in a paramedic system. *Ann Emerg Med* 1984;**13**:807–10.

25 Greene HL. The CASCADE study: randomized antiarrhythmic drug therapy in survivors of cardiac arrest in Seattle. CASCADE Investigators. *Am J Cardiol* 1993;**72**:70F–74F.

26 American Heart Association Guidelines for Cardiopulmonary Resuscitation and Emergency Cardiovascular Care. Adult Basic Life Support. Part 7.3: Management of Symptomatic Bradycardia and Tachycardia Part 7.3: Circulation. 2005;**112**: IV-67-IV-77.

27 Koster RW, Dunning AJ. Intramuscular lidocaine for prevention of lethal arrhythmias in the prehospitalization phase of acute myocardial infarction. *N Engl J Med* 1985;**313**:1105–10.

28 Armengol RE, Graff J, Baerman JM, Swiryn S. Lack of effectiveness of lidocaine for sustained, wide QRS complex tachycardia. *Ann Emerg Med* 1989;**18**:254–7.

29 Marill KA, Greenberg GM, Kay D, Nelson BK. Analysis of the treatment of spontaneous sustained stable ventricular tachycardia. *Acad Emerg Med* 1997;**4**:1122–8.

30 Somberg JC, Bailin SJ, Haffajee CI, et al., Amio-Aqueous Investigators. Intravenous lidocaine versus intravenous amiodarone (in a new aqueous formulation) for incessant ventricular tachycardia. *Am J Cardiol* 2002;**90**:853–9.

31 Schutzenberger W, Leisch F, Kerschner K, Harringer W, Herbinger W. Clinical efficacy of intravenous amiodarone in the short term treatment of recurrent sustained ventricular tachycardia and ventricular fibrillation. *Br Heart J* 1989;**62**:367–71.

32 Helmy I, Herre JM, Gee G, et al. Use of intravenous amiodarone for emergency treatment of life-threatening ventricular arrhythmias. *J Am Coll Cardiol* 1988;**12**:1015–22.

33 Kowey PR, Levine JH, Herre JM, et al. Randomized, double-blind comparison of intravenous amiodarone and bretylium in the treatment of patients with recurrent, hemodynamically destabilizing ventricular tachycardia or fibrillation. The Intravenous Amiodarone Multicenter Investigators Group. *Circulation* 1995;**92**:3255–63.

34 Gorgels AP, van den Dool A, Hofs A, et al. Comparison of procainamide and lidocaine in terminating sustained monomorphic ventricular tachycardia. *Am J Cardiol* 1996;**78**:43–6.

35 Ho DS, Zecchin RP, Richards DAB, Uther JB, Ross DL. Double-blind trial of lignocaine versus sotalol for acute termination of spontaneous sustained ventricular tachycardia. *Lancet* 1994;**344**:18–23.

36 Bayes de Luna A, Coumel P, Leclercq JF. Ambulatory sudden cardiac death: mechanisms of production of fatal arrhythmia on the basis of data from 157 cases. *Am Heart J* 1989;**117**:151–9.

37 AHA/ECC. Management of symptomatic bradycardia and tachycardia. *Circulation* 2005;**112**:IV67–77.

38 Keren A, Tzivoni D, Gavish D, Levi J, Gottlieb S, Benhorin J, Stern S. Etiology, warning signs and therapy of torsade de pointes. A study of 10 patients. *Circulation* 1981;**64**:1167–74.

39 Tzivoni D, Banai S, Schuger C, et al. Treatment of torsade de pointes with magnesium sulfate. *Circulation* 1988;**77**:392–7.

40 Manz M, Pfeiffer D, Jung W, Lueritz B. Intravenous treatment with magnesium in recurrent persistent ventricular tachycardia. *New Trends Arrhythmias* 1991;**7**:437–42.

41 Kaye P, O'Sullivan I. The role of magnesium in the emergency department. *Emerg Med J* 2002;**19**:288–91.

22 Cardiac Arrest

Riyad B. Abu-Laban[1] & Michael Shuster[2]

[1]Division of Emergency Medicine, University of British Columbia, Vancouver, *and* Department of Emergency Medicine, Vancouver General Hospital, Vancouver, Canada
[2]Department of Emergency Medicine, Mineral Springs Hospital, Banff, Canada

Case scenario

A 52-year-old man is transported to the emergency department (ED) by emergency medical services (EMS) after resuscitation from an out-of-hospital cardiac arrest. The paramedics report he had complained of chest heaviness, and subsequently collapsed. His wife, who witnessed the event, immediately called 911 and followed dispatcher instructions to perform chest compressions until EMS arrived.

After noting ventricular fibrillation (VF) on the cardiac monitor, the paramedics continued chest compressions to minimize time without cardiopulmonary resuscitation (CPR) and charged a biphasic defibrillator to 150 J. Following defibrillation, they immediately recommended CPR and established an intravenous line. Intubation was not performed since bag mask ventilation was deemed to be effective. A rhythm and pulse check 2 minutes later identified pulseless VF, which the paramedics shocked at 150 J, restarting CPR immediately after defibrillation. With CPR ongoing, they administered 1 mg of epinephrine IV. Two minutes later they identified a junctional rhythm at 80/min and palpable pulses. The paramedics stopped CPR and inserted a laryngeal mask airway (LMA) prior to transport.

Upon ED arrival, the patient was unresponsive and was being ventilated through the LMA. End tidal CO_2 was 29 mmHg and there was good air entry bilaterally. The pulse was 92 beats/min and the blood pressure was 115/70 mmHg. An electrocardiogram (ECG) showed no evidence of acute ischemia. While the patient was being readied for cardiac care unit transfer, the emergency nurse asked if therapeutic hypothermia should be initiated.

Evidence-based Emergency Medicine. Edited by Brian H. Rowe
© 2009 Blackwell Publishing, ISBN: 978-1-4051-6143-5.

Background

Out-of-hospital cardiac arrest treated by the EMS has an annual incidence of approximately 155,000 episodes in the USA. Successful management of cardiac arrest involves the application, coordination and interaction of many interventions. Outcome is influenced by numerous factors including cardiac arrest etiology, witnessed arrest, early bystander CPR, initial cardiac rhythm, early defibrillation and patient co-morbidities. Moreover, even when a cardiac arrest victim survives to hospital admission, subsequent care-giver decisions and post-resuscitation care may have a profound effect on survival.

In most communities, the rate of survival to hospital discharge is less than 5%; however, far higher rates occur in specific patient subgroups and optimized systems. CPR, new technologies, drug interventions and post-resuscitation care have all received significant research attention in recent years and are discussed in the 2005 cardiac arrest guidelines [1].

Clinical questions

1 In adults in cardiac arrest (population), does the addition of ventilations (intervention) to chest compressions (control) during bystander CPR improve the rate of return of spontaneous circulation or survival to hospital discharge (outcomes)?

2 In adults who have an out-of-hospital cardiac arrest (population), does public access to automated defibrillators (intervention) increase the rate of survival to hospital discharge (outcome) compared to routine emergency medical services response (control)?

3 In adults in ventricular fibrillation or pulseless ventricular tachycardia (population), does biphasic defibrillation (intervention) increase the rate of rhythm conversion (outcome) compared to monophasic defibrillation (control)?

4 In adults in cardiac arrest (population), does establishing an airway with endotracheal intubation, a laryngeal mask airway or a

combitube (intervention) improve survival (outcome) compared to bag mask ventilation (intervention)?

5 In adults in cardiac arrest (population), does the administration of pharmacotherapy (specifically vasopressors, atropine, antiarrhythmics, thrombolytics, aminophylline, sodium bicarbonate) (intervention) increase the rate of survival to hospital discharge or return of spontaneous circulation (outcomes) compared to CPR and defibrillation alone (control)?

6 In adults who achieve return of spontaneous circulation following cardiac arrest (population), does the administration of therapeutic hypothermia (intervention) increase the rate of survival to hospital discharge (outcome) compared to supportive care (control)?

7 In adults who have an out-of-hospital cardiac arrest (population), are there evidence-based guidelines (intervention) that accurately identify a subset of patients for whom resuscitation efforts are futile and should not be commenced or should be discontinued (outcome)?

General search strategy

The topic of cardiac arrest can be first addressed by searching for systematic reviews and randomized controlled trials in common electronic databases such as MEDLINE and EMBASE. A large body of evidence exists on this topic; however, despite this, few meta-analyses have been published in cardiac arrest, and no Cochrane reviews were identified for the questions above. Finally, relevant, regularly updated, evidence-based clinical practice guidelines (CPGs) on cardiac arrest are accessed and reviewed to determine the consensus recommendations in areas lacking high-level evidence.

Critical review of the literature

Question 1: In adults in cardiac arrest (population), does the addition of ventilations (intervention) to chest compressions (control) during bystander CPR improve the rate of return of spontaneous circulation or of survival to hospital discharge (outcomes)?

Search strategy

- MEDLINE and EMBASE: chest compression alone CPR OR continuous compressions OR continuous chest compressions OR cardiocerebral resuscitation OR chest compression only CPR OR (CPR AND without AND ventilations)

Although the necessity of ventilations during CPR has historically been taken for granted, recent studies have challenged this assumption. Because of the proven benefit of early CPR, the frequent

reluctance of bystanders to provide mouth-to-mouth ventilation to strangers, and the relative difficulty of providing effective ventilations, the notion of endorsing compression-only CPR for the public has captured attention.

In 1993, Berg and colleagues found that 16 swine who received chest compressions without ventilation for 12 minutes during cardiac arrest were resuscitated neurologically intact [2]. The results of this landmark study were subsequently replicated in a number of swine and canine models. In a model analogous to an out-of-hospital cardiac arrest, 30 swine who underwent 3 minutes of untreated VF were randomized to receive 12 minutes of either CPR with a 15:2 compression:ventilation ratio or continuous chest compression CPR followed by defibrillation. Neurologically normal 24-hour survival was significantly higher in the group receiving continuous chest compression CPR (12 vs two of 15 cases, $P < 0.0001$) [3]. A follow-up study added two additional groups: (i) CPR with a 50:5 compression:ventilation ratio; and (ii) 4 minutes of continuous chest compressions, followed by 8 minutes of 100:2 ratio CPR [4]. Collectively, these animal studies suggest that two factors favor the effectiveness of continuous chest compression CPR: passive air exchange caused by chest compressions and increased efficiency of uninterrupted chest compressions.

Three human studies of compression-only CPR have been published to date. In a before/after study, a rural EMS service implemented a new CPR protocol whereby unstacked defibrillations were preceded by 200 uninterrupted chest compressions and initial airway management with an oral pharyngeal device and supplemental oxygen [5]. In the 3 years prior to implementation of the new protocol 14 of 92 patients (15%) survived neurologically intact compared with 16 of 33 patients (48%) after implementation of the new protocol ($P < 0.001$).

A non-significant but favorable trend was found when 520 callers to 911 were randomized to phone instruction on compression-only CPR or compressions with mouth-to-mouth ventilations [6]. Survival to hospital discharge was 14.6% in the compression-only group and 10.4% in the compression plus ventilation group ($P = 0.18$). The variable length of time to complete the training in each group, interruptions in compressions in order to ventilate, and possibility of an increased regurgitation rate in patients who received mouth-to-mouth ventilation [7] may have affected the results of this study. A prospective observational study found an increased likelihood of favorable neurological outcome in 439 patients with compression-only CPR compared to 712 patients who received standard CPR (OR = 1.5; 95% CI: 0.9 to 2.5) [8].

In summary, although the evidence is limited and further studies are needed, it is conceivable that bystander compression-only CPR is as effective as, and possibly more effective than, CPR with mouth-to-mouth ventilations. The 2005 guidelines recommend that lay persons do chest compression-only CPR when they are unable or unwilling to perform rescue breaths, and that EMS dispatchers consider such an approach when providing telephone instruction in CPR [1].

Question 2: In adults who have an out-of-hospital cardiac arrest (population), does public access to automated defibrillators (intervention) increase the rate of survival to hospital discharge (outcome) compared to routine emergency medical services response (control)?

Search strategy

- MEDLINE and EMBASE: (public OR layperson) AND (electric countershock OR defibrillation)

Automated external defibrillators (AEDs) can be used by individuals with minimal or no training to rapidly analyze the cardiac rhythm and deliver an electric countershock when indicated. As studies emerged describing the successful use of AEDs by personnel with limited medical knowledge, the notion of what constitutes "advanced" cardiac arrest care has blurred. Given the simplicity of use of modern AEDs, our increased awareness that early defibrillation increases survival, and the fact that few EMS systems achieve ideal response times, the expansion of AED availability beyond the boundaries of standard EMS systems has received attention.

Public access defibrillation (PAD) is a commonly used term, although the word "public" is variably defined and ranges from family members or other true lay-people, with no duty to provide care, to "non-traditional responders" with a duty to respond in medical emergencies but who traditionally have not provided medical interventions. PAD is a generic term for the use of AEDs by any such individuals, either within or outside a structured EMS system, and either with or without specific training. A number of papers have described hypothetical outcome benefits and cost-effectiveness of PAD in different settings.

A 3-year prospective observational study of AEDs use by trained security officers in 32 casinos examined 148 cardiac arrests, of which 90 (61%) were witnessed and involved an initial rhythm of VF [9]. The survival to discharge rate was 38% (56 patients) overall and 59% (53 patients) within the witnessed VF group. Most arrests were witnessed, the rate of CPR prior to defibrillation was high, and the mean interval from collapse to first defibrillation in the witnessed VF group was 4.4 minutes. A second study described the results of the deployment of AEDs on selected American Airlines aircraft for use by trained flight attendants or at the request of bystander physicians [10]. Over a 2-year period, AEDs were used on 200 occasions, 191 in the aircraft and nine in the terminal. There were 15 patients defibrillated, of whom six (40%) survived to hospital discharge with complete neurological recovery. Similar results were obtained in a 2-year study of AED deployment in public areas in Chicago airports [11]. Eighteen of 21 cardiac arrest victims had VF and 11 survived to hospital discharge (61%), all with good neurological outcomes. With two exceptions, AED operators were airline passengers (often with a medical background) or airport employees with no duty to respond. Positive results have also been reported using trained layperson volunteers responding with AEDs within an existing EMS system in Italy [12], and in community-based models of PAD using trained responders in Helsinki [13] and Seattle [14].

The largest and most rigorous study of PAD to date was a prospective randomized trial conducted between 2000 and 2003 in 993 "community units" across 24 North American regions [15]. Over 19,000 volunteer layperson responders whose primary job description did not include the responsibility to provide medical assistance during emergencies, were trained in AED use. There were more survivors to hospital discharge in the units assigned to volunteers trained in CPR plus the use of AEDs than in the units assigned to volunteers trained only in CPR (RR = 2.0; 95% CI: 1.1 to 3.8). Small studies have also been published on the favorable use of PAD in high school [16] and in non-inpatient hospital areas [17].

In summary, it is clear that PAD can improve cardiac arrest survival in selected situations involving trained, and possibly untrained, non-traditional providers functioning as part of a larger EMS system. Local factors including estimated cardiac arrest frequency, witnessed arrest and bystander CPR rates, and EMS response times must be carefully considered for informed decision making. The outcome benefit and/or cost-effectiveness of widespread deployment of AEDs for use by the general public has not been established [18], and the 2005 guidelines state lay rescuer AED programs will have the greatest potential impact if they are established in selected locations with a high likelihood of cardiac arrests [1].

Question 3: In adults in ventricular fibrillation or pulseless ventricular tachycardia (population), does biphasic defibrillation (intervention) increase the rate of rhythm conversion (outcome) compared to monophasic defibrillation (control)?

Search strategy

- MEDLINE and EMBASE: biphasic AND defibrillation AND human

Until recently, defibrillation waveform was not a consideration since all defibrillators were monophasic. New defibrillators use a biphasic waveform, but many monophasic defibrillators remain in use. Biphasic defibrillation has replaced monophasic in implantable defibrillators for a number of reasons including lower energy requirements, lower defibrillation threshold, reduced post-shock ECG abnormality, and smaller device size. A meta-analysis of seven studies involving a total of 1129 patients in electrophysiology labs or during implantable defibrillator testing found that defibrillation with a 200 J biphasic waveform was more efficacious than 200 J monophasic shocks (RR of post-shock VF or asystole = 0.19; 95% CI: 0.06 to 0.60) and equally efficacious at biphasic energies of 115–130 J compared to standard 200 J monophasic shocks (RR of post-shock VF or asystole = 1.07; 95% CI: 0.66 to 1.74) [19].

Four prospective randomized controlled trials have compared monophasic and biphasic defibrillation in cardiac arrest, although shock success was defined differently in each study. When shock success was defined as any non-VF rhythm for > 5 seconds, the first-shock success rate was 66% (44/67) for monophasic and 92% (44/48) for biphasic defibrillation ($P < 0.001$) [20]. When shock success was defined as any organized rhythm within 1 minute of defibrillation, success was 45% (31/69) for monophasic and 69% (35/51) biphasic defibrillation ($P < 0.01$) [21]. When shock success was defined as an organized rhythm within 5 seconds following one to three shocks, success was 33.7% (28/83) for monophasic and 52.3% (45/86) for biphasic defibrillation ($P < 0.01$) [22]. And when shock success was defined as termination of VF (to either asystole or an organized rhythm $\leq$ 120 beats/min) at 5, 10 and 20 seconds, first-shock success rate was 82% (75/91) for monophasic and 88% (65/74) for biphasic defibrillation ($P = 0.33$) [23]. Based on the definitions of each study, biphasic defibrillation was judged more effective than monophasic defibrillation in three of the four studies and equivalent in the fourth study.

Interpreting the above studies is problematic, since converting VF to another non-perfusing rhythm is not necessarily a desirable outcome. Moreover, the outcome of rhythm conversion is not as clinically relevant as survival to hospital admission or neurologically intact survival to hospital discharge. None of the four randomized controlled trials found a significant difference in survival to hospital admission or to hospital discharge; however, all were underpowered to detect such a difference.

In summary, there is sufficient evidence to conclude that biphasic defibrillation is as effective as, or more effective than, monophasic defibrillation for rhythm conversion, and the 2005 guidelines endorse biphasic defibrillation for this reason [1]. The effect, if any, of defibrillation waveform on survival is unknown.

Question 4: In adults in cardiac arrest (population), does establishing an airway with endotracheal intubation, a laryngeal mask airway or a combitube (intervention) improve survival (outcome) compared to bag mask ventilation (intervention)?

Search strategy

- MEDLINE and EMBASE: (LMA OR combitube OR endotracheal intubation OR tracheal intubation) AND resuscitation AND clinical trial

Endotracheal intubation has long been considered the gold standard technique of airway management; however, recent studies showing high rates of complications – some lethal – have led experts to question whether endotracheal intubation is the best method of airway management during resuscitation.

The only controlled clinical trial comparing bag mask airway management to endotracheal intubation (ETI) was conducted in pediatric out-of-hospital patients using even/odd day treatment allocation. There was no significant difference between the bag mask group and the ETI group in survival (OR = 0.82; 95% CI: 0.61 to 1.11) or good neurological outcome (OR = 0.87; 95% CI: 0.62 to 1.22). Although the complication rates in both groups were similar, the rates in the ETI group of failure and of esophageal displacement were high (and all of the patients with the latter complication died), and on-scene times were significantly longer in the ETI group [24].

The only adult clinical trial involved an indirect assessment of different airway management strategies in cardiac arrest victims treated by basic and advanced paramedics. The "bundle" of advanced skills studied in this large trial, which included ETI and drug administration, was not found to affect survival rates [25].

The LMA and combitube have been recommended as airway management alternatives to the endotracheal tube or bag mask ventilation. The ease of learning to insert these devices has been assessed in manikin and operating room studies, which found insertion rates faster than ETI and ventilation volumes equivalent to ETI and equivalent to or better than bag mask ventilation. A clinical trial found that when patients were ventilated with the bag mask alone or bag mask followed by ETI, the incidence of gastric regurgitation during CPR was 12.4%. When patients were ventilated with the LMA alone or LMA followed by ETI, the incidence of regurgitation was 3.5% [26]. Other clinical trials, comparing the advanced airways to one another or to bag masks, have evaluated speed of insertion, ability to ventilate, volume of ventilation, oxygenation levels and failure rates, but to date no clinical trials have studied survival rates.

In summary, it is apparent that any of the standard airway devices can ventilate, and that each has advantages and disadvantages. There is insufficient evidence to conclude that any device is superior for patient-oriented outcomes. It is possible that the best method of airway management may depend on individual care giver ability and expertise, rather than on an inherent superiority of any specific device. The 2005 guidelines consider the endotracheal tube, LMA and combitube to be acceptable alternatives to bag mask ventilation, but caution that there is no evidence that advanced airway interventions improve outcome from cardiac arrest so interruption of CPR to perform endotracheal intubation may not be justified [1].

Question 5: In adults in cardiac arrest (population), does the administration of pharmacotherapy (specifically vasopressors, atropine, anti-arrhythmics, thrombolytics, aminophylline, sodium bicarbonate) (intervention) increase the rate of survival to hospital discharge or return of spontaneous circulation (outcomes) compared to CPR and defibrillation alone (control)?

Search strategy

- MEDLINE and EMBASE: (heart arrest OR cardiopulmonary resuscitation) AND (epinephrine OR vasopressin OR atropine OR lidocaine OR admiodarone OR procainamide OR bretylium OR

thrombolytic therapy OR fibrinolytic agents OR tissue plasminogen
activator OR streptokinase OR urokinase OR aminophylline OR
sodium bicarbonate) AND clinical trial

Vasopressors

Epinephrine has consistently been recommended by cardiac arrest
guidelines, largely because of dog studies performed by Pearson
and Redding in the early 1960s [27]. In the late 1980s and early
1990s a number of case reports and methodologically weak studies suggested a benefit from "high-dose epinephrine". A meta-
analysis described five randomized double-blind trials comparing epinephrine dosing strategies and concluded that there is
no evidence of a benefit from high and/or escalating doses of
epinephrine, and that the trend favors standard dosing [28]. More
recently there has been interest in vasopressin in cardiac arrest.
A meta-analysis described five trials comparing vasopressin and
epinephrine and concluded there is no clear evidence of an advantage of one agent over the other [29]. No human clinical trials
were identified that compared any vasopressor to placebo. The
2005 guidelines recommend that a vasopressor be given in asystole or pulseless electrical activity, or if ventricular fibrillation or
ventricular tachycardia (VT) persists after administration of one
or two shocks and CPR [1].

Atropine

Although there are theoretical reasons why atropine may be beneficial in bradyasystolic cardiac arrest, no human clinical trials of
this intervention were identified. The 2005 guidelines are based on
consensus only, and recommend that 1 mg of atropine be administered every 3–5 minutes to a total of 3 mg [1].

Anti-arrhythmics

The use of anti-arrhythmics in cardiac arrest during or following ventricular rhythms has historically been commonplace. A
few small trials have compared an anti-arrhythmic to placebo in
such situations. A randomized, double-blind, placebo-controlled
study of 504 patients given amiodarone or lidocaine during out-of-
hospital cardiac arrest found those in the amiodarone group were
more likely to be admitted to hospital alive (44% vs 33%; OR =
1.6; 95% CI: 1.1 to 2.4) [30]. A small crossover study of 29 patients
also concluded amiodarone was more effective than lidocaine
in shock resistant VT [31]. Finally, a randomized, double-blind,
placebo-controlled study of 347 out-of-hospital cardiac patients
given amiodarone or lidocaine found 22.8% of patients treated
with amiodarone, compared to 12.0% of patients treated with lidocaine, survived to hospital admission (OR = 2.2; 95% CI: 1.2 to
3.8) [32]. Neither this study, nor the first trial, found a difference
in survival to hospital discharge between the two groups; however, neither study was powered to detect such a difference. The
2005 guidelines advise the administration of amiodarone (or lidocaine, if amiodarone is unavailable) be considered if VF or pulseless VT persists after two or three shocks, CPR and vasopressor

administration. A more in-depth discussion on the issue of anti-
arrhythmics in cardiac arrest can be found in Chapter 21.

Thrombolytics

A number of case reports and small case series published over the
last two decades have suggested a benefit from thrombolysis in cardiac arrest, particularly in the setting of pulmonary embolism. Two
methodologically weak studies of tissue plasminogen activator
(t-PA) have suggested a benefit of thrombolysis in a general cardiac
arrest population [33,34], as did a small study of tenecteplase [35].
However, a randomized double-blind trial of placebo versus t-PA
in 233 undifferentiated cardiac arrest patients with pulseless electrical activity was negative, and excluded a t-PA-related increase in
survival-to-hospital discharge rate of over 4.8% [36]. A 2006 meta-
analysis of CPR with and without thrombolytic agents concluded
that thrombolysis can improve neurological function and survival to discharge; however, the conclusions of this meta-analysis
are questionable as it involved low-quality heterogeneous studies and inexplicably excluded the negative, double-blind, placebo-
controlled trial [37]. The negative results of a large European trial
of thrombolysis in cardiac arrest were published in narrative form
in 2006, refuting the conclusions of this meta-analysis and supporting the conclusions of the prior randomized trial [38]. The
2005 guidelines endorse the consideration of thrombolytics on a
"case by case" basis when pulmonary embolism is suspected as the
cause of a cardiac arrest, primarily because of numerous dramatic
case reports and case series suggesting the possibility of a benefit
in such a population.

Aminophylline

Several case reports and three small clinical trials have suggested
a possible benefit from aminophylline in bradyasystolic cardiac
arrest. However, a randomized, double-blind, placebo-controlled
trial of 971 patients found that although there was a higher incidence of non-sinus tachyarrhythmias with aminophylline (34.6%
vs 24.5%, $P = 0.004$), there was no difference in return of spontaneous circulation (ROSC) (24.5% vs 23.7%, $P = 0.778$) and
no evidence of a subgroup or interactive effect from aminophylline on multivariate analysis [39]. A recently published meta-
analysis identified the four aforementioned trials, and concluded
that aminophylline has no impact on clinically relevant outcomes
in cardiac arrest [40]. Aminophylline is not endorsed in the 2005
guidelines [1].

Sodium bicarbonate

In recent years there have been recommendations against the use
of sodium bicarbonate in cardiac arrest. The only identified randomized trial of bicarbonate enrolled 792 patients over a 4-year
period and found no difference in survival in those who received
bicarbonate versus placebo (7.4% vs 6.7%, $P = 0.88$). However,
in a controversial and unplanned subgroup analysis, a trend towards improved survival with bicarbonate in prolonged arrest
(>15 minutes) was reported [41]. The 2005 guidelines do not endorse sodium bicarbonate as a first-line or routine agent in cardiac

Study	Treatment n/N	Control n/N	RR (95% CI fixed)	Weight %	RR (95% CI fixed)
Bernard	22/43	23/24		23.7	0.76 [0.52, 1.10]
HACA	50/136	69/137		63.5	0.73 [0.55, 0.96]
Hachimi-Idrissi	13/16	13/14		12.8	0.87 [0.66, 1.15]
Total (95% CI)	85/195	105/185		100.0	0.75 [0.62, 0.92]

Test for heterogeneity: chi² = 1.15, df = 2, P = 0.56
Test for overall effect: Z = 2.79, P = 0.005

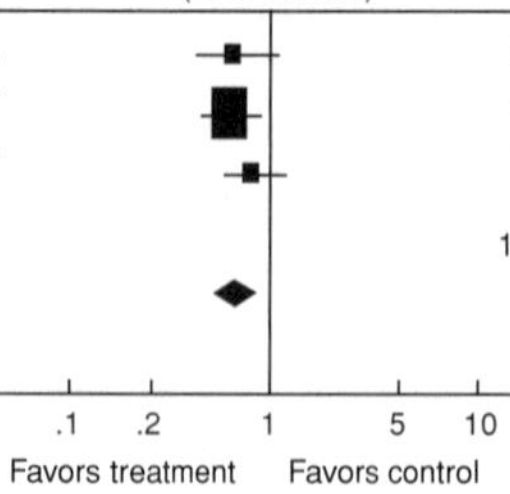

.1 .2 1 5 10
Favors treatment   Favors control

Figure 22.1 Comparison of in-hospital mortality between patients treated with mild hypothermia and control groups in three clinical trials. (Reproduced with permission from the Canadian Journal of Emergency Medicine [46]).

arrest, except in special circumstances such as hyperkalemia or cyclic antidepressant overdose [1].

Summary

The benefit, if any, from pharmacotherapy in cardiac arrest remains unproven, largely because very few placebo-controlled trials have been performed. There is compelling evidence that amiodarone is superior to lidocaine in improving short-term survival; however, no drug intervention has been convincingly demonstrated to increase survival to hospital discharge. It remains unclear whether the use of thrombolytics in highly selected cardiac arrest patients may be beneficial.

Question 6: In adults who achieve return of spontaneous circulation following cardiac arrest (population), does the administration of therapeutic hypothermia (intervention) increase the rate of survival to hospital discharge (outcome) compared to supportive care (control).

Search strategy

- MEDLINE and EMBASE: (heart arrest OR cardiopulmonary resuscitation) AND (hypothermia, induced OR circulatory arrest, deep hypothermia induced)

Cerebral ischemia may persist for many hours following ROSC, and it has been hypothesized that therapeutic hypothermia may, through various mechanisms, reduce anoxic brain injury and improve outcomes.

A feasibility study on hypothermia induced by a helmet device in 30 patients demonstrated encouraging results [42], and in 2002 two large and rigorous studies on this topic were published. The first was a multi-centre randomized trial with blinded outcome assessment that enrolled 273 patients with ROSC following VF or pulseless VT in nine centres across five European countries [43]. Cooling was commenced prehospital and continued for 24 hours before passive rewarming. Mortality at 6 months was 41% in the hypothermia group and 55% in the normothermia group (RR = 0.74; 95% CI: 0.58 to 0.95). Cerebral outcomes were also improved in the hypothermia group. The second study was an Australian clinical trial of 77 patients with ROSC following VF, and involved

alternate day treatment allocation [44]. Of 43 patients treated with hypothermia for 12 hours followed by active rewarming, 21 (49%) survived to hospital discharge with good neurological outcome compared to nine of 34 patients (26%) in the normothermia group ($P = 0.046$).

Two meta-analyses have been published on this topic [45,46], both of which identified the aforementioned trials and concluded that hypothermia was beneficial. Figure 22.1, adapted from the more rigorous of the two meta-analyses, shows a Forrest plot illustrating the overall benefit from hypothermia on risk of death (RR = 0.75; 95% CI: 0.62 to 0.92). This meta-analysis concluded that seven patients would require treatment with hypothermia to prevent one in-hospital death (95% CI: 4 to 25) [46].

Although the number of trials and patients studied is small, there is compelling evidence that mild (32–34°C) therapeutic hypothermia reduces mortality and improves neurological outcomes in patients with ROSC and coma after VF or pulseless VT cardiac arrest, and the 2005 guidelines endorse such an approach. Recent papers have suggested the early cooling of such patients is feasible in the non-study setting. The potential benefit, if any, of hypothermia in patients with ROSC after asystole or pulseless electrical activity remains undetermined and thus only a minority of cardiac arrest patients would qualify for this therapy.

Question 7: In adults who have an out-of-hospital cardiac arrest (population), are there evidence-based guidelines (intervention) that accurately identify a subset of patients for whom resuscitation efforts are futile and should not be commenced or should be discontinued (outcome)?

Search strategy

- MEDLINE and EMBASE: (heart arrest OR cardiopulmonary resuscitation) AND (termination OR medical futility)

Since most cardiac arrest resuscitations fail to achieve sustained ROSC, care givers regularly face the difficult task of deciding when resuscitation efforts are futile. Irrefutable evidence of death or the presence of an advanced directive are clear indications that it is inappropriate to commence CPR, but such criteria are uncommon. Thus, EMS providers routinely begin CPR while simultaneously gathering information and determining whether a shockable rhythm exists. As a result, the questions of when and on whom to terminate resuscitative efforts have received increasing attention. Many EMS systems and organizations have developed guidelines for advanced care providers to terminate resuscitative efforts; however, such guidelines have not been extensively studied and there is significant variability in their application [47]. Only recently have researchers begun to address the question of termination guidelines for basic life support paramedics using AEDs.

A retrospective case series of 1068 cardiac arrests found that transport of patients who did not achieve ROSC resulted in a 0.4% survival to discharge rate and poor neurological outcomes among the few survivors [48]. A similar study of 1461 cardiac arrests found that in patients who did not achieve ROSC within 25 minutes, only 0.6% survived to discharge (all with persistent VF) [49]. Another study of 414 cardiac arrests found no survivors among patients with a non-shockable rhythm, no bystander CPR and more than 15 minutes from collapse to EMS arrival [50]. In 1999, the National Association of EMS Physicians published a position paper recommending that termination of resuscitation be considered in patients who receive at least 20 minutes of advanced care resuscitative efforts and who remain in pulseless electrical activity or asystole with no ROSC. This approach was evaluated in 366 prospective and 135 retrospective cases of cardiac arrest and found to be 100% specific for non-survival to hospital discharge [51].

A prospective cohort study of 3888 cardiac arrests with an initial rhythm of asystole managed by basic life support paramedics using AEDs identified nine patients who survived to hospital discharge, three of whom had an unwitnessed arrest without bystander CPR [52]. There were no survivors in cases with a call-to-response interval of over 8 minutes. Recently, the Termination of Resuscitation Trial (TOR), involving 24 Ontario EMS systems, was published [53]. This was a prospective validation of a previously derived clinical prediction rule for basic life support paramedics using AEDs. The rule recommends termination of resuscitation when there is no ROSC, no shocks administered, and the arrest is not witnessed by EMS personnel. In 1240 patients, the rule recommended termination in 776 cases, four (0.5%) of whom survived. Implementation of the rule would have reduced transports from 100% to 37.4% of cases. Inclusion of post hoc additional factors (a response interval over 8 minutes as suggested by the OPALS study or unwitnessed cardiac arrest) was found to improve the correct identification of survivors at the expense of transporting a larger proportion of patients.

Finally, another prospective cohort study was published by the OPALS group [54] comparing the performance of three aforementioned termination guidelines [50,52,53]. Although all three guidelines were touted to have 100% sensitivity for predicting survivors when derived, when evaluated using a dataset of 13,684 cardiac arrest cases, all recommended termination for at least one patient who survived. The TOR rule had the best overall diagnostic performance (sensitivity 99.5%, specificity 52.9%, positive predictive value 9.3%, negative predictive value 100%); however, this approach would have advised termination of resuscitation in three patients who survived.

In summary, although guidelines exist that alone or in combination can facilitate the decision to terminate resuscitation efforts, perfect decision rules have not been identified and the 2005 guidelines provide no specific recommendations in this regard [1]. Given the challenges in defining futility and the boundaries of "appropriate care", it would seem prudent to consult widely when determining whether and how to adopt termination guidelines in a particular jurisdiction. The TOR authors aptly stated "prediction rules for the termination of resuscitation efforts should remain advisory and ... should be tempered by the full clinical picture, taking into account the very small possibility of successful resuscitation when the prediction rules suggest termination" [53].

Conclusions

The patient in the scenario above was transferred to the cardiac care unit after therapeutic hypothermia was initiated in the ED. He went on to survive to hospital discharge with no adverse neurological sequelae.

Given the myriad of factors influencing cardiac arrest outcomes, a low baseline survival rate and the notorious difficulty of carrying out high-quality resuscitation research, it is perhaps not surprising that it is difficult (and perhaps often impossible) to demonstrate that the addition of a single intervention to the sequence of cardiac arrest treatment influences survival to hospital discharge. It is for this reason that surrogate outcomes like defibrillation success, ROSC and short-term survival are often employed. For some interventions the use of such outcomes may be the most feasible evidence of effectiveness.

Cardiac arrest guidelines have existed since the 1960s to address the stressful nature of cardiac arrest resuscitations and the fact that care givers must make rapid decisions based, as much as possible, on correct interpretation of a huge volume of literature [55]. In 1993 the International Liaison Committee on Resuscitation (ILCOR) was established to coordinate the efforts of resuscitation organizations throughout the world. The ILCOR recommendations provide evidence for best practice based on a rigorous and transparent approach to literature evaluation and expert consensus [56]. The 2005 guidelines [1] were noteworthy for their emphasis on the importance of minimizing "hands off time" through a new 30:2 compression:ventilation ratio and the elimination of post-shock rhythm analysis and pulse checks. Readers with an interest in delving further into the evidence on a particular cardiac arrest topic are encouraged to review the 2005 guidelines and the publicly available evidence evaluation worksheets upon which they were based (see www.c2005.org). Revised guidelines are scheduled to be released in 2010.

Future cardiac arrest research is likely to involve collaborations and consortiums for the purposes of conducting megatrials. "Bundled" therapies, rather than single interventions, may be the subject of research attention. Knowledge translation (see Chapter 2), CPR optimization, new technologies, cardiocerebral resuscitation and post-resuscitation care are likely to receive increased research attention in the years to come.

References

1 ECC Committee, Subcommittees and Task Forces of the American Heart Association. 2005 American Heart Association guidelines for cardiopulmonary resuscitation and emergency cardiovascular care. *Circulation* 2005;**112**(24 Suppl):IV1–203.

2 Berg RA, Kern KB, Sanders AB, Otto CW, Hilwig RW, Ewy GA. Bystander cardiopulmonary resuscitation. Is ventilation necessary? *Circulation* 1993;**88**(4/1):1907–15.

3 Kern KB, Hilwig RW, Berg RA, Sanders AB, Ewy GA. Importance of continuous chest compressions during cardiopulmonary resuscitation: improved outcome during a simulated single lay-rescuer scenario. *Circulation* 2002;**105**(5):645–9.

4 Sanders AB, Kern KB, Berg RA, Hilwig RW, Heidenrich J, Ewy GA. Survival and neurologic outcome after cardiopulmonary resuscitation with four different chest compression-ventilation ratios. *Ann Emerg Med* 2002;**40**(6):553–62.

5 Kellum MJ, Kennedy KW, Ewy GA. Cardiocerebral resuscitation improves survival of patients with out-of-hospital cardiac arrest. *Am J Med* 2006;**119**(4):335–40.

6 Hallstrom A, Cobb L, Johnson E, Copass M. Cardiopulmonary resuscitation by chest compression alone or with mouth-to-mouth ventilation. *N Engl J Med* 2000;**342**(21):1546–53.

7 Virkkunen I, Kujala S, Ryynanen S, et al. Bystander mouth-to-mouth ventilation and regurgitation during cardiopulmonary resuscitation. *J Intern Med* 2006;**260**(1):39–42.

8 SOS-KANTO Study Group. Cardiopulmonary resuscitation by bystanders with chest compression only (SOS-KANTO): an observational study. *Lancet* 2007;**369**:920–26.

9 Valenzuela TD, Roe DJ, Nichol G, Clark LL, Spaite DW, Hardman RG. Outcomes of rapid defibrillation by security officers after cardiac arrest in casinos. *N Engl J Med* 2000;**343**(17):1206–9.

10 Page RL, Joglar JA, Kowal RC, et al. Use of automated external defibrillators by a U.S. airline. *N Engl J Med* 2000;**343**(17):1210–16.

11 Caffrey SL, Willoughby PJ, Pepe PE, Becker LB. Public use of automated external defibrillators. *N Engl J Med* 2002;**347**(16):1242–7.

12 Capucci A, Aschieri D, Piepoli MF, Bardy GH, Iconomu E, Arvedi M. Tripling survival from sudden cardiac arrest via early defibrillation without traditional education in cardiopulmonary resuscitation. *Circulation* 2002;**106**:1065–70.

13 Kuisma M, Castren M, Nurminen K. Public access defibrillation in Helsinki – costs and potential benefits from a community-based pilot study. *Resuscitation* 2003;**56**:149–52.

14 Culley LL, Rea TD, Murray JA, et al. Public access defibrillation in out-of-hospital cardiac arrest. A community based study. *Circulation* 2004;**109**:1859–63.

15 Hallstrom AP, Ornato JP, Weisfeldt M, et al. Public-access defibrillation and survival after out-of-hospital cardiac arrest. *N Engl J Med* 2004;**351**(7):637–46.

16 England HE, Hoffman C, Hodgman T, et al. Effectiveness of automated external defibrillators in high schools in greater Boston. *Am J Cardiol* 2005;**95**:1484–6.

17 Friedman FD, Dowler K, Link MS. A public-access defibrillation programme in non-inpatient hospital areas. *Resuscitation* 2005;**69**:407–11.

18 Nichol G, Valenzuela T, Roe D, Clark L, Huszti E, Wells GA. Cost effectiveness of defibrillation by targeted responders in public settings. *Circulation* 2003;**108**(6):697–703.

19 Faddy SC, Powell J, Craig JC. Biphasic and monophasic shocks for transthoracic defibrillation: a meta analysis of randomised controlled trials. *Resuscitation* 2003;**58**(1):9–16.

20 Schneider T, Martens PR, Paschen H, et al. Multicenter, randomized, controlled trial of 150-J biphasic shocks compared with 200- to 360-J monophasic shocks in the resuscitation of out-of-hospital cardiac arrest victims. Optimized Response to Cardiac Arrest (ORCA) Investigators. *Circulation* 2000;**102**(15):1780–87.

21 van Alem AP, Chapman FW, Lank P, Hart AA, Koster RW. A prospective, randomised and blinded comparison of first shock success of monophasic and biphasic waveforms in out-of-hospital cardiac arrest. *Resuscitation* 2003;**58**(1):17–24.

22 Morrison LJ, Dorian P, Long J, et al. Out-of-hospital cardiac arrest rectilinear biphasic to monophasic damped sine defibrillation waveforms with advanced life support intervention trial (ORBIT). *Resuscitation* 2005;**66**(2):149–57.

23 Kudenchuk PJ, Cobb LA, Copass MK, Olsufka M, Maynard C, Nichol G. Transthoracic incremental monophasic versus biphasic defibrillation by emergency responders (TIMBER): a randomized comparison of monophasic with biphasic waveform ascending energy defibrillation for the resuscitation of out-of-hospital cardiac arrest due to ventricular fibrillation. *Circulation* 2006;**114**(19):2010–18.

24 Gausche M, Lewis RJ, Stratton SJ, et al. Effect of out-of-hospital pediatric endotracheal intubation on survival and neurological outcome: a controlled clinical trial. *JAMA* 2000;**283**(6):783–90.

25 Stiell IG, Wells GA, Field B, et al. Advanced cardiac life support in out-of-hospital cardiac arrest. *N Engl J Med* 2004;**351**(7):647–56.

26 Stone BJ, Chantler PJ, Baskett PJ. The incidence of regurgitation during cardiopulmonary resuscitation: a comparison between the bag valve mask and laryngeal mask airway. *Resuscitation* 1998;**38**(1):3–6.

27 Pearson JW, Redding JS. The role of epinephrine in cardiac resuscitation. *Anesth Analg* 1963;**42**(5):599–606.

28 Vandycke C, Martens P. High dose versus standard dose epinephrine in cardiac arrest – a meta-analysis. *Resuscitation* 2000;**45**:161–6.

29 Aung K, Htay T. Vasopressin for cardiac arrest. A systematic review and meta-analysis. *Arch Intern Med* 2005;**165**:17–24.

30 Kudenchuk PJ, Cobb LA, Copass MK, et al. Amiodarone for resuscitation after out-of-hospital cardiac arrest due to ventricular fibrillation. *N Engl J Med* 1999;**341**(12):871–8.

31 Somberg JC, Bailin SJ, Haffajee CI, et al. Intravenous lidocaine versus intravenous amiodarone (in a new aqueous formulation) for incessant ventricular tachycardia. *Am J Cardiol* 2002;**90**:853–9.

32 Dorian P, Cass D, Schwartz B, Cooper R, Gelaznikas R, Barr A. Amiodarone as compared with lidocaine for shock-resistant ventricular fibrillation. *N Engl J Med* 2002;**346**(12):884–90.

33 Bottiger BW, Bode C, Kern S, et al. Efficacy and safety of thrombolytic therapy after initially unsuccessful cardiopulmonary resuscitation: a prospective clinical trial. *Lancet* 2001;**357**:1583–5.

34 Lederer W, Lichtenberger C, Pechlaner C, Kroesen G, Baubin M. Recombinant tissue plasminogen activator during cardiopulmonary resuscitation in 108 patients with out-of-hospital cardiac arrest. *Resuscitation* 2001;**50**:71–6.

35 Bozeman WP, Kleiner DM, Ferguson LK. Empiric tenecteplase is associated with increased return of spontaneous circulation and short term

survival in cardiac arrest patients unresponsive to standard interventions. *Resuscitation* 2006;**69**:399–406.

36 Abu-Laban RB, Christenson JM, Innes GD, van Beek CA, Wagner KP, McKnight RD. Tissue plasminogen activator in cardiac arrest with PEA. *N Engl J Med* 2002;**346**(20):1522–8.

37 Li X, Fu Q, Jing X, et al. A meta–analysis of cardiopulmonary resuscitation with and without the administration of thrombolytic agents. *Resuscitation* 2006;**70**:31–6.

38 Clappers N, Verheugt FWA. Hotlines sessions of the 28th European Congress of Cardiology/World Congress of Cardiology 2006. *Eur Heart J* 2006;**27**:2896–9.

39 Abu-Laban RB, McIntyre CM, Christenson JM, et al. Aminophylline in bradyasystolic cardiac arrest: a randomized placebo-controlled trial. *Lancet* 2006;**367**:1577–84.

40 Hurley KF. Does the administration of intravenous aminophylline improve survival in adults with bradysystolic cardiac arrest? *Can J Emerg Med* 2007;**9**(1):26–9.

41 Vukmir RB, Katz L, Sodium Bicarbonate Study Group. Sodium bicarbonate improves outcome in prolonged cardiac arrest. *Am J Emerg Med* 2006;**24**:156–61.

42 Hachimi-Idrissi S, Corne L, Ebinger G, Michotte Y, Huyghens L. Mild hypothermia induced by a helmet device: a clinical feasibility study. *Resuscitation* 2001;**51**:275–81.

43 Hypothermia after Cardiac Arrest Study Group. Mild therapeutic hypothermia to improve the neurologic outcome after cardiac arrest. *N Engl J Med* 2002;**346**(8):549–56.

44 Bernard SA, Gray TW, Buist MD, et al. Treatment of comatose survivors of out-of-hospital cardiac arrest with induced hypothermia. *N Engl J Med* 2002;**346**(8):557–63.

45 Holzer M, Bernard SA, Hachimi-Idrissi S, Roine RO, Sterz F, Mullner M. Hypothermia for neuroprotection after cardiac arrest: systematic review and individual patient data meta-analysis. *Crit Care Med* 2005;**33**(2):414–18.

46 Cheung KW, Green RS, Magee KD. Systematic review of randomized controlled trials of therapeutic hypothermia as a neuroprotectant in post cardiac arrest patients. *Can J Emerg Med* 2006;**8**(5):329–37.

47 Eckstein M, Stratton SJ, Chan LS. Termination of resuscitative efforts for out-of-hospital cardiac arrests. *Acad Emerg Med* 2005;**12**(1):65–70.

48 Kellerman AL, Hackman BB, Somes G. Predicting the outcome of unsuccessful prehospital advanced cardiac life support. *JAMA* 1993;**270**(12):1433–6.

49 Bonnin MJ, Pepe PE, Kimball KT, Clark PS. Distinct criteria for termination of resuscitation in the out-of-hospital setting. *JAMA* 1993;**270**(12):1457–62.

50 Marsden AK, Ng GA, Dalziel K, Cobbe SM. When is it futile for ambulance personnel to initiate cardiopulmonary resuscitation? *BMJ* 1995;**311**:49–51.

51 Cone DC, Bailey ED, Spackman AB. The safety of a field termination-of-resuscitation protocol. *Prehosp Emerg Care* 2005;**9**(3):276–81.

52 Petrie DA, De Maio V, Stiell IG, Dreyer J, Martin M, O'Brien J. Factors affecting survival after prehospital asystolic cardiac arrest in a basic life support-defibrillation system. *Can J Emerg Med* 2001;**3**(3):186–92.

53 Morrison LJ, Visentin LM, Kiss A, et al. Validation of a rule for termination of resuscitation in out-of-hospital cardiac arrest. *N Engl J Med* 2006;**355**(5):478–87.

54 Ong ME, Jaffey J, Stiell I, Nesbitt L. Comparison of termination-of-resuscitation guidelines for basic life support-defibrillator providers in out-of-hospital cardiac arrest. *Ann Emerg Med* 2006;**47**(4):337–43.

55 Abu-Laban RB. Reflections on ACLS. *Can J Emerg Med* 2005;**7**(6):415–16.

56 Shuster M. 2005 emergency cardiovascular care guidelines. *Can J Emerg Med* 2006;**8**(1):37–42.

4 General Medical Conditions

23 Severe Sepsis and Septic Shock

Peter W. Greenwald[1], Scott Weingart[2] & H. Bryant Nguyen[3]

[1]Division of Emergency Medicine, New York–Presbyterian Hospital,
Weill Medical College of Cornell University, New York, USA
[2]Division of Emergency Critical Care, Department of Emergency Medicine,
Mount Sinai School of Medicine, New York, USA
[3]Departments of Emergency Medicine and Medicine, Division of Pulmonary and Critical Care Medicine,
Loma Linda University, Loma Linda, USA

Case scenario

A 66-year-old woman presented to the emergency department (ED) with a history of recurrent urinary tract infections and several admissions to the hospital for pyelonephritis. On presentation to the ED, she reported a 4-day history of dysuria. On the morning prior to coming to the ED she had developed a subjective fever, vomited three times, and felt very weak, sweaty and dizzy, so she asked her daughter to accompany her to the ED.

On arrival at the ED, she had the following vital signs: heart rate of 96 beats/min, respiratory rate of 28 breaths/min, blood pressure of 82/40 mmHg (left arm) and oxygen saturation of 94% (on room air). Her physical exam was remarkable for diaphoresis, costovertebral angle tenderness on the left, and suprapubic tenderness. The remainder of her physical exam was normal.

Laboratory results were remarkable for: leukocytosis (white blood cells (WBCs) = 23,000/mm^3), an anion gap of 20, a creatinine of 3.0 mg/dl (229 μmol/L) from baseline 1.5 mg/dl (114 μmol/L), venous lactate of 6.2 mmol/L, hemoglobin of 8 g/dL (80 g/L) and a platelet count of 122,000/μl. Urine microscopy demonstrated >100 WBCs per high power field with many bacteria and few red blood cells. You concluded that the patient was suffering from a serious urinary tract infection that had ascended to her kidneys. Chest radiograph and computer tomography of the abdomen failed to identify an alternate source of infection.

You immediately established intravenous lines and started fluid resuscitation (20 ml/kg bolus), placed her on oxygen and initiated antibiotic therapy. The patient's daughter asked you to help her understand what was happening to her mother and what her prognosis was.

Background

This patient is suffering from a life-threatening infection. Although she has pyelonephritis, her condition can best be described as *septic shock*. The terminology we use to describe systemic infection was established by a consensus conference in 1992 and revised in 2002 [1,2]. Four terms are used to describe the systemic response to infection:
1 Systemic inflammatory response syndrome (SIRS).
2 Sepsis.
3 Severe sepsis.
4 Septic shock.

The systemic inflammatory response syndrome is the systemic response to a variety of severe clinical insults. The response is manifested by two or more of the following:
1 Temperature >38°C or <36°C (>100.4°F or <96.8° F).
2 Heart rate >90 beats/min.
3 Respiratory rate >20 breaths/min or $PaCO_2$ <32 mmHg.
4 White blood cell count >12,000/mm^3 or <4000 per mm^3, or >10% bands.

These physiological changes should represent an acute alteration from baseline in the absence of another known cause for such abnormalities, such as chemotherapy inducing leukopenia. SIRS is seen in association with a large number of clinical conditions. Non-infectious pathological causes may include pancreatitis, ischemia, multiple trauma, tissue injury, hemorrhagic shock, immune-mediated organ injury and the exogenous administration of such putative mediators of the inflammatory process as tumor necrosis factor and other cytokines.

Sepsis is the presence of SIRS with confirmation of infection. Infection is defined as either:
• the microbial phenomenon mediated by inflammatory response to the presence of microorganism; *or*
• the invasion of normally sterile tissue by those organisms. Early in the course of sepsis, infection is more often suspected than proven.

Severe sepsis is sepsis associated with organ dysfunction, hypoperfusion or sepsis-induced hypotension. Hypoperfusion abnormalities include, but are not limited to, lactic acidosis, oliguria or an acute alteration in mental status. Sepsis-induced hypotension is a systolic blood pressure <90 mmHg or a reduction >40 mmHg from baseline in the absence of other causes of hypotension.

Septic shock is severe sepsis that continues despite adequate fluid resuscitation along with the persistence of hypoperfusion abnormalities (see above). Patients who are receiving inotropic or vasopressor agents may not be hypotensive at the time perfusion abnormalities are measured, but they still have septic shock because vasopressors are needed to support their blood pressure.

Mortality from septic shock has traditionally been thought to be approximately 50% [3]. Recent prospective observational cohort studies have suggested that mortality rates as low as 20–30% may be obtainable using modern therapies [4–9]. There is a growing appreciation that care delivered early in the disease course may affect mortality in ways that are not possible later in the disease process. Active areas of research and discussion in the care of severe sepsis and septic shock patients include mortality prediction, timing of antibiotic administration, protocol-driven hemodynamic optimization (early goal-directed therapy), recombinant human activated protein C (rhAPC) administration, glycemic control, physiological dose steroid repletion, and low tidal volume mechanical ventilation (lung protective strategy). We will focus here on the evidence underlying early interventions applicable in the ED.

Clinical questions

In order to address the issues of greatest relevance to your patients and to help in searching the literature for the evidence regarding these issues, you structure your clinical questions as recommended in Chapter 1.

1 For adult patients in the first 24 hours of severe sepsis or septic shock (population), are there validated criteria (prognostic indicators) for assigning mortality risk (outcome)?

2 For adult patients in the first 24 hours of severe sepsis or septic shock (population), does timing and choice of antibiotics (intervention and comparison) lower mortality (outcome) compared to delayed delivery and/or broad spectrum therapy (control)?

3 For adult patients in the first 24 hours of severe sepsis or septic shock (population), does the institution of bundled therapy/early hemodynamic optimization (intervention) lower mortality (outcome) compared to standard therapy (control)?

4 For adult patients in the first 24 hours of severe sepsis or septic shock (population), does colloid resuscitation (intervention) lower mortality (outcome) compared to standard crystalloid resuscitation (control)?

5 For adult patients in the first 24 hours of severe sepsis or septic shock (population), do other vasopressors (intervention) lower mortality (outcome) compared to dopamine (control)?

6 For adult patients in the first 24 hours of severe sepsis or septic shock (population), do patients receiving a specific transfusion threshold (intervention) have lower mortality (outcome) than patients who either do not receive transfusion or transfusion to the same threshold (control)?

7 For adult patients in the first 24 hours of severe sepsis or septic shock (population), does administration of rhAPC (intervention) improve mortality (outcome) compared to patients who do not receive this therapy (control)?

8 For adult patients in the first 24 hours of severe sepsis or septic shock (population), do patients receiving tight glycemic control (intervention) have lower mortality (outcome) than patients receiving standard therapy (control)?

9 For adult patients in the first 24 hours of severe sepsis or septic shock (population), do patients receiving corticosteroids (intervention) have lower mortality (outcome) than patients who do not receive corticosteroids (control)?

10 For adult patients in the first 24 hours of severe sepsis or septic shock who are mechanically ventilated (population), do patients receiving low tidal volume ventilation (intervention) have lower mortality (outcome) than patients who receive high tidal volume ventilation (control)?

General search strategy

You perform a search using the electronic databases MEDLINE and EMBASE and also the Database of Abstracts of Reviews of Effects (DARE), ACP Journal Club and the Cochrane Library looking particularly for systematic reviews and individual randomized controlled trials pertinent to the ED management of severe sepsis or septic shock. For the purposes of this chapter studies that enrolled patients within the first 24 hours of severe sepsis or septic shock were targeted. Articles that enrolled intensive care unit (ICU) patients were included if there was particular relevance, if they explicitly reported data from patients early in the course of severe sepsis or septic shock, or if they were the highest grade evidence available. Animal studies were excluded, as were studies that reported physiological outcomes rather than outcomes like mortality and disability that are of direct importance to patients.

Critical review of the literature

Question 1: For adult patients in the first 24 hours of severe sepsis or septic shock (population), are there validated criteria (prognostic indicators) for assigning mortality risk (outcome)?

Search strategy

- MEDLINE, EMBASE, Cochrane, DARE, ACP Journal Club and CENTRAL: (severe sepsis OR septic shock) AND (hypotension OR outcome assessment) AND (severity of illness index OR mortality OR survival rate OR prognosis)

Overall, 274 studies were screened, of which 82 articles that reviewed clinical rules and biochemical markers were considered relevant. Of the markers evaluated, lactate has been studied more extensively than the others. There are prospectively validated mortality prediction rules that have been applied to patients with sepsis. Most of them have not enrolled patients while in the ED. These rules include the following:

• Multiple Organ Dysfunction Score (MODS) [10].
• Acute Physiology and Chronic Health Evaluation (APACHE) II, III and IV [11–13].
• Sepsis-related Organ Failure Assessment (SOFA) [14].
• Mortality probability models (MPM) II and III [15,16].
• Mortality in Emergency Department Sepsis (MEDS) score [16,17].
• Simplified and complete septic shock scoring system [18].
• Rapid Emergency Medicine Score (REMS) [19].

Of these, the MEDS system may be the most appropriate for risk stratification in the ED. Unlike the other tools, MEDS was developed from an ED population of patients who presented with infection (infection defined as the need for blood cultures) and is readily calculated from clinical criteria and basic laboratory results available to the ED practitioner. Our search recovered five studies pertaining to the MEDS scoring system, the initial derivation study, three validation studies, and one study expanding the use of the MEDS prediction tool to risk of death within 1 year of the index hospital visit [17,20–22]. One of the validation studies is internal (performed at the same center on a different group of patients) [22] and two are external validations [21,23]. One external validation study applies the MEDS rule specifically to patients with severe sepsis, and in this validation the MEDS rule outperforms APACHE II. The other validation study examined sepsis patients in the ED. The MEDS score had discriminatory capability similar to its derivation set, and better than the biochemical markers it was tested against [23]. APACHE II, MEDS and studies validating MEDS are summarized in Table 23.1. The MEDS score criteria and associated risk predictions are shown in Tables 23.2 and 23.3.

The APACHE II score is the most widely used mortality prediction tool for critically ill patients. APACHE II uses physiological and laboratory values to predict mortality in the critically ill [17,18,24–26]. Although its accuracy in septic ICU patients has been demonstrated, in one multi-centered study of ED patients the APACHE II score was only a moderate predictor of 14-day mortality, and in a second study of adult severe sepsis patients in the ED, the MEDS score outperformed the APACHE II score. [21,27]. Part of this lack of accuracy in the ED may be the result of the ED population behaving differently than the ICU patients from whom APACHE II was derived; by the time patients arrive in the ICU, their condition may be significantly stabilized. It has been shown that the hourly rates of change of severity scoring systems (APACHE II, SAPS II and MODS) are greater in the ED than any other time in the first 72 hours of hospitalization [24]. Another factor to be aware of in the APACHE II scoring system is that clinicians need to calculate an APACHE II score *prior* to the use of rhAPC (see Question 7 below). Only high-risk patients without

contraindication to rhAPC whose APACHE II score is greater than or equal to 25 should receive rhAPC.

Lactate levels are included elements required for entry into bundled therapy protocols for patients with severe sepsis or septic shock (see Question 3 below). When obtained, the results can also help with predicting prognosis. In one prospective cohort study of ED patients, higher lactate levels were associated with increased mortality [28]. At a level of ≥ 4.0 mmol/L the odds ratio of death within 72 hours was 4.9 (95% CI: 3.1 to 7.9). The ability to decrease an elevated lactate in ED patients has been associated with survival using logistic regression modeling on an ED data set; in this data set there was an approximately 11% decrease in the likelihood of mortality for each 10% increase in lactate clearance [29].

Dozens of other biochemical markers have been evaluated as markers of severity in severe sepsis and septic shock. With the exception of lactate, there is not sufficient evidence to recommend the routine use of these markers in the ED to aid decision making.

In summary, clinicians should calculate the MEDS score, obtain serial lactate levels and monitor the change in lactate (lactate clearance rate) to help assess prognosis. In severe sepsis patients, the APACHE II score should be calculated to guide the use of rhAPC (see Question 7 below). Emergency physicians should be cautious when these tools are used in the early onset of severe sepsis and septic shock when patient status is subject to rapid change.

Question 2: For adult patients in the first 24 hours of severe sepsis or septic shock (population), does timing and choice of antibiotics (intervention and comparison) lower mortality (outcome) compared to delayed delivery and/or broad spectrum therapy (control)?

Search strategy

• MEDLINE, EMBASE, Cochrane, DARE, ACP Journal Club and CENTRAL: (severe sepsis OR septic shock OR sepsis) AND (antibiotic timing OR antibiotic choice OR emergency department OR antibacterial agent) AND (time factors OR hospital mortality OR treatment outcome)

From nearly 500 articles identified, 32 were considered relevant. Prospective animal studies have demonstrated increased survival with antibiotic administration in the setting of laboratory models of septic shock. No prospective human studies were identified evaluating the timing or appropriateness of antibiotics on patient survival. The human studies that were identified were primarily retrospective cohort analyses. Several trials using this design suggest early antibiotic administration is associated with increased survival, and that the initial use of antibiotics that are effective against pathogens eventually cultured is associated with higher survival [30–40].

Kumar et al. retrospectively evaluated 2731 patients in the early phase of septic shock and found a 7.6% (95% CI: 3.6% to 9.9%) reduction in survival associated with each additional hour's delay

Table 23.1 Clinical prediction rules for severe sepsis and septic shock relevant to emergency medicine.

Rule	Physiological variables	Population	Performance
Mortality in Emergency Department Sepsis (MEDS) score [17]	Yes/no to the following (with a weighted point scale): Terminal illness <30 days Tachypnea or hypoxia Septic shock Platelets <150,000 Bands >5% Age >65 years Lower respiratory infection Nursing home resident Altered mental status	Single center adults in the ED at risk for infection (as indicated by the physician ordering a blood culture); $N = 3179$	Mortality: 0–4 points, 1.1% 5–7 points, 4.4% 8–12 points, 9.3% >13 points, 39%
Acute Physiology and Chronic Health Evaluation (APACHE II) [11]	Temperature Mean arterial pressure Heart rate Respiratory rate $(A-a)PO_2$ or PAO_2 Arterial pH Bicarbonate (if no arterial blood gas) Sodium Potassium Creatinine Hematocrit White blood cell count Glasgow Coma Score Age Chronic health	Intensive care admissions from 13 hospitals; $N = 5815$	APACHE II performs less well in the ED than in its original derivation set. The predictive accuracy of the APACHE II score gradually increases over the first 24 hours of hospitalization [18,24] ICU mortality: 0–4 points, 4% 5–9 points, 8% 10–14 points, 15% 15–19 points, 25% 20–24 points, 40% 25–29 points, 55% 30–34 points, 75% >34 points, 85%
Howell et al. [22]	Internal validation of MEDS score	Single center adults in the ED at risk for infection (as indicated by the physician ordering a blood culture); $N = 2132$	Mortality: 0–4 points, 0.4% 5–7 points, 3.3% 8–12 points, 6.6% >13 points, 31.6%
Chen et al. [21]	External validation of MEDS score	ED patients being admitted to non-surgical ICUs with severe sepsis or septic shock; $N = 302$	Patients with a MEDS score >12 had a significantly higher 28-day mortality rate (48.9% vs 17.5%). The MEDS score out-performed APACHE II in this validation set
Lee et al. [23]	External validation of MEDS score	ED patients with sepsis; $N = 525$ (399 with sepsis, 102 with severe sepsis, 24 with septic shock)	MEDS had a better discriminative power than procalcitonin or C-reactive protein levels. The MEDS score performed better in this validation set than in the original derivation study

ED, emergency department; ICU, intensive care unit.

in initiation of antibiotic therapy during the first 6 hours following the onset of hypotension [32]. In multivariate analysis of the same data set, time to initial antibiotic was more closely associated with survival than appropriateness of antibiotic, time to vasopressor administration, choice of vasopressor or volume of fluid resuscitation. The association between early antibiotic and survival persisted after adjustment for site of infection, APACHE II score and number of organ failures. Observational studies are ultimately only able to assess association, so despite this strong association between early antibiotic and survival, a causal relationship is not proven.

Overall, the association between early antibiotic administration and increased survival is clinically and physiologically plausible based on evidence from the observational studies. Practitioners should attempt to give appropriate antibiotics as soon as possible for patients with severe sepsis or septic shock.

Table 23.2 MEDS score predictors of mortality [17].

	Odds ratio mortality (95% CI)	Point score
Terminal illness <30 days	6.1 (3.6 to 10.2)	6
Tachypnea or hypoxia	2.7 (1.6 to 4.3)	3
Septic shock	2.7 (1.2 to 5.7)	3
Platelets <150,000	2.5 (1.5 to 4.3)	3
Bands >5%	2.3 (1.5 to 3.5)	3
Age >65 years	2.2 (1.3 to 3.6)	3
Lower respiratory infection	1.9 (1.2 to 3.0)	2
Nursing home resident	1.9 (1.2 to 3.0)	2
Altered mental status	1.6 (1.0 to 2.6)	2

Question 3: For adult patients in the first 24 hours of severe sepsis or septic shock (population), does the institution of bundled therapy/early hemodynamic optimization (intervention) lower mortality (outcome) compared to standard therapy (control)?

Search strategy

- MEDLINE, EMBASE, Cochrane, DARE, ACP Journal Club and CENTRAL: (severe sepsis OR septic shock OR sepsis) AND (hypotension OR outcome assessment) AND (severity of illness index OR mortality OR survival rate OR prognosis)

We designed Question 3 to evaluate the overall effect of bundle implementation. Search Questions 4 to 6 were designed to evaluate the data supporting each of the components of bundle implementation. We also evaluated questions pertaining to inotrope use, central venous pressure (CVP) monitoring/targeting and central venous oxygen saturation ($ScvO_2$) monitoring/targeting. We did not find high-grade evidence pertaining to these bundle elements as isolated therapies.

Overall, from 30 papers that were considered relevant, the highest grade evidence resulting from our search included two randomized controlled trials, five before/after studies of bundle implementation, and one before/after analysis of a different type of bundle implementation. Results are summarized in Table 23.4.

Bundled therapies of hemodynamic optimization combine a number of interventions into a treatment protocol for the care of

Table 23.3 MEDS score tabulation [17].

Point range	MEDS risk group	28-day mortality
0–4	Very low	1.1%
5–7	Low	4.4%
8–12	Moderate	9.3%
13–15	High	16.1%
>15	Very high	39%

patients with severe sepsis or septic shock. The best-known example of this type of therapy is early goal-directed therapy (EGDT) [41]. This bundle includes the following components:

- Volume resuscitation of CVP as a reflection of preload.
- Vasoactive agent optimization of mean arterial pressure as a reflection of afterload.
- Blood transfusion and/or inotrope optimization of $ScvO_2$ as a reflection of oxygen content and contractility as the final goal in optimizing oxygen delivery.

The highest level of evidence available arises from two prospective controlled trials. The initial EGDT study was a prospective, partially blinded, randomized controlled trial that demonstrated an absolute reduction in mortality from 46.5% to 30.5% with the application of bundled therapy in ED patients with severe sepsis or septic shock [41]. A second prospective randomized trial used a similar bundle for ICU patients within 4 hours of the onset of septic shock. This study likewise demonstrated a reduction in mortality, from 73.2% to 53.7% [42]. Six additional studies of the implementation of an EGDT protocol were also identified [4–7,9,43]. Four of these studies used a before/after comparison design, and reported mortality in cohorts before implementation of the EGDT group as compared to cohorts after implementation [5–7,9]. Each of these four reported decreased mortality in the post-implementation cohorts; in two studies the improvement reached statistical significance. Two studies evaluated the association of successful completion of bundle elements with mortality, finding increased mortality in the group that did not receive all the elements of the bundle [4,8]. Interestingly, one before/after study was identified that predated the others by over 20 years. In 1978, a before/after mortality comparison was performed for patients with septic shock; this study demonstrated a statistically significant fall in mortality from 71% in the before bundle group to 47% after the bundle was implemented [44].

The treatment algorithm employed in the EGDT bundle, from the randomized trial mentioned above, consists of an initial fluid administration of 20 ml/kg to patients who have severe sepsis with lactate >4 mmol/L or septic shock criteria. For patients meeting these criteria, CVP monitoring is established with a central line with the tip in the superior vena cava (SVC). Preload is optimized by bringing the CVP to 8 mmHg (12 mmHg if intubated) by the administration of additional fluids. Once the CVP is optimized, if the mean arterial pressure has not improved to greater than 65 mmHg, vasopressors are started, and titrated to a mean arterial pressure of >65 mmHg. $ScvO_2$ is also monitored; in the original study this was obtained through the use of a continuous reading fiberoptic catheter placed in the SVC (the same catheter that is used to measure the CVP). Transfusion was also performed to reach a hematocrit of 30%, and an inotrope (dobutamine) was started as needed to achieve a $ScvO_2$ of >70%. This therapy is shown in Fig. 23.1.

Early goal-directed therapy constitutes an advance in the treatment of severe sepsis and septic shock. Rivers et al. found a reduction in mortality using bundled care that, if applied to six patients

Table 23.4 Summary of evidence for bundled therapy in severe sepsis and septic shock.

Study	Population	Design	Outcome
Rivers et al. [41]	ED patients with severe sepsis or septic shock; $N = 263$	Prospective, randomized, partially blinded EGDT compared to standard care over 6 hours	Mortality in EGDT group: 38/130 (29.2%)* Mortality in control: 59/133 (44.3%)* RRR = 0.34 (95% CI: 0.09 to 0.53) NNT = 6.6 (95% CI: 3.8 to 28.7)

Lin et al. [42]	Patients within 4 hours of onset of septic shock ($N = 224$); patients were admitted from the ED ($N = 86$) and from medical wards ($N = 138$)	Prospective, randomized, unblinded study with bundle similar to EGDT, $ScvO_2$ not monitored, and urine output goals targeted	In-hospital mortality:
			    In bundle group: 58/108
			    In control group: 85/116
			    RRR = 0.27 (95% CI: 0.104 to 0.397)
			    NNT = 5.1 (95% CI: 3.2 to 14.3)
			ED subset ICU mortality:
			    In bundle group: 13/27
			    In control group: 25/46
			RRR = 0.40 (95% CI: 0.018 to 0.644)
			NNT = 4.57 (95% CI: 2.5 to 123.7)

Jones et al. [6]	ED patients with severe sepsis or septic shock; $N = 156$	Before/after clinical intervention of EGDT	Mortality in EGDT group: 14/77 (18%) Mortality in control group: 21/79 (27%) RRR = 0.32 (95% CI: 0.23 to 0.625)
Shapiro et al. [5]	ED patients with severe sepsis or septic shock; $N = 167$	Before/after clinical intervention with EGDT	Mortality in EGDT group: 16/79 (20.3%) Mortality in control group: 15/51 (29.4%) RRR = 0.31 (95% CI: 0.27 to 0.62)
Micek et al. [7]	ED patients with septic shock; $N = 120$	Before/after clinical intervention with EGDT	Mortality in EGDT group: 18/60 (30%) Mortality in control group: 29/60 (48.3%) RRR = 0.38 (95% CI: 0.22 to 0.61) NNT = 5.5 (95% CI: 2.9 to 115.3)
Kortgen et al. [9]	ICU patients; $N = 60$	Before/after clinical intervention with EGDT	Mortality in EGDT group: 8/30 (27%) Mortality in control group: 16/30 (53%) RRR = 0.50 (95% CI: 0.05 to 0.75) NNT = 3.8 (95% CI: 2.1 to 53.2)
Gao et al. [4]	Adult patients with severe sepsis or septic shock on medical or surgical wards or ED; $N = 101$	Observational cohort. Comparison of mortality when care was compliant with a completed bundle vs when care was not compliant (groups were similar in severity of illness)	Mortality in compliant group: 12/52 (23%) Mortality in control group: 24/49 (49%) RRR = 0.53 (95% CI: 0.18 to 0.73) NNT = 3.9 (95% CI: 2.4 to 13.8)
Nguyen et al. [8]	Patients presenting to the ED who met criteria for severe sepsis or septic shock; $N = 330$	Observational cohort. Comparison of mortality when care was compliant with a completed bundle vs when care was not compliant (groups were similar in severity of illness)	Mortality in compliant group: 16/77 (20.8%) Mortality in control group: 100/253 (39.5%) RRR = 0.47((95% CI: 0.19 to 0.67) NNT = 5.3 (95% CI: 3.6 to 14.4)
Ledingham & McArdle [44]	Patients with shock on admission to an ICU by a shock response team; $N = 113$	Before/after implementation study	Mortality in bundle group: 39/78 (50%) Mortality in control group: 25/35 (71%) RRR = 0.30 (95% CI: 0.03 to 0.45) NNT = 4.7 (95% CI: 2.7 to 58.6)

*Rivers et al. used the Kaplan–Meier product-limit method – percentages here are calculated directly from observed data.

CI, confidence interval; ED, emergency department; EGDT, early goal-directed therapy; ICU, intensive care unit; NNT, number needed to treat; RRR, relative risk reduction; $ScvO_2$, central venous oxygen saturation.

with septic shock, will save one patient who otherwise would have died [41]. Although the two prospective trials and the before/after studies are reassuring regarding validating the efficacy of bundled therapy, validation in a prospective multi-center trial is needed. A

federally funded multi-centered randomized trial to perform this validation is in its beginning stages [45].

In summary, bundled therapy for severe sepsis or septic shock is supported by high-quality evidence, and has the potential to have

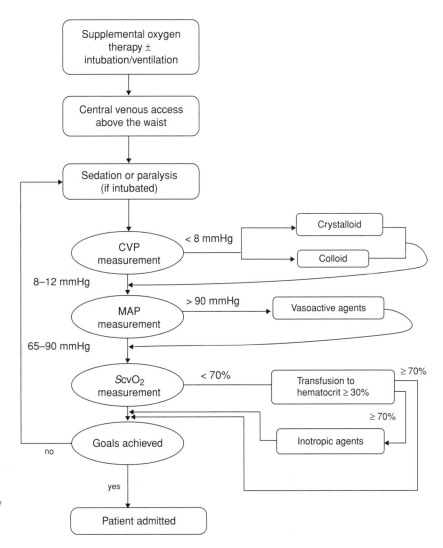

Figure 23.1 Flow diagram for early goal-directed therapy (EGDT) [41]. CVP, central venous pressure; MAP, mean arterial pressure; ScvO₂, central venous oxygen saturation.

an impressive impact on patient mortality. The evidence suggests that the application of this therapy to six patients will result in the survival of one patient who otherwise would have died. The application of bundled therapy is strongly encouraged for patients with severe sepsis or septic shock.

Question 4: For adult patients in the first 24 hours of severe sepsis or septic shock (population), does colloid resuscitation (intervention) lower mortality (outcome) compared to standard crystalloid resuscitation (control)?

Search strategy

- MEDLINE, EMBASE, Cochrane, DARE, ACP Journal Club and CENTRAL: (severe sepsis OR septic shock OR sepsis) AND colloid AND crystalloid

Overall, the above search identified 61 relevant citations for inclusion. There were no human studies specifically studying the effect of fluid administration on septic shock mortality in the first 24 hours of care. Two randomized human trials investigated colloid versus crystalloid administration in the ICU setting [46,47].

The Safe Study Investigators (SSI group) evaluated the administration of albumin as compared to saline for the resuscitation of critically ill ICU patients. Enrollment was not limited by duration of symptoms, and not limited to septic shock, but over 25% of patients were admitted from the ED, and 18% of patients enrolled had severe sepsis. Pre-planned subgroup analysis was performed for patients who had severe sepsis. In this subset analysis 30.7% died in the albumin group, as compared to 35.3% in the saline group (RR of death in albumin treatment = 0.87, 95% CI: 0.74 to 1.02) [46].

Upadhyay et al. performed an open-label randomized study comparing saline to colloid in the resuscitation of pediatric septic shock, targeting CVP as an endpoint. Thirty-day mortality was 29% in the saline group and 31% in the colloid group, a difference that did not reach statistical significance. Groups also did not differ in hemodynamic stability at 6 or 12 hours, nor did they differ in the number of organ systems that failed [47].

In summary, the administration of fluids to help maintain blood pressure in the setting of severe sepsis and septic shock is widely accepted. Fluid resuscitation is recommended as standard therapy; however, there is little research evidence to support this component of therapy, and no evidence favoring the use colloid over crystalloid. The use of early fluid resuscitations is strongly recommended as part of a sepsis care bundle.

Question 5: For adult patients in the first 24 hours of severe sepsis or septic shock (population), do other vasopressors (intervention) lower mortality (outcome) compared to dopamine (control)?

Search strategy

- MEDLINE, EMBASE, Cochrane, DARE, ACP Journal Club and CENTRAL: (severe sepsis OR septic shock OR sepsis) AND (dopamine OR norepinephrine OR vasopress* OR hypertensive factor OR vasoconstrictor agent OR noradrenaline)

This search identified 31 relevant citations. The highest graded evidence identified was two human prospective randomized trials [48,49] and 11 human observational cohort studies [50–60]. The

Cochrane Collaboration also reviewed the topic for all literature up to 2003 [61]. The most pertinent studies are summarized in Table 23.5.

There is no definitive evidence to support the specific choice of vasopressor. One of the cohort studies [59], two prospective randomized trials [48,49] and preliminary data from a prospective randomized controlled trial (the Vasopressin in Septic Shock Trial, VASST) [62] warrant further discussion:

1 The SOAP study was a multi-centered, retrospective, observational cohort of patients with shock. One-third of the patients in the cohort had septic shock [59]. Logistic regression was used to look for factors associated with mortality. Of the parameters tested, SOFA score, age, cancer, medical illness (as opposed to surgical illness), higher fluid balance and dopamine and epinephrine administration were independently associated with 30-day mortality.

2 Lauzier et al. prospectively evaluated norepinephrine as compared to vasopressin in early septic shock in a randomized open-label trial. There were no significant differences noted in mortality between the two groups, although the study was underpowered to detect anything but large differences in mortality (total $n = 23$) [49]. Annane et al. performed a prospective, randomized, double-blinded multi-centered trial on patients with septic shock during the first 24 hours following becoming vasopressor dependent. They compared dobutamine and norepinephrine to epinephrine alone, and found no significant difference in mortality between groups at 28 days [48].

3 VASST was a prospective, multi-centered, randomized trial that included patients in the first 24 hours of septic shock [62]. The

Table 23.5 Summary of evidence for vasopressor use in severe sepsis and septic shock.

Study	Population	Design	Outcome
Annane et al. [48]	Patients with septic shock admitted to one of 19 participating ICUs in France; $N = 330$	Prospective, randomized, double-blinded, multi-centered trial on patients with septic shock during the first 24 hours following becoming vasopressor dependent, comparing dobutamine and norepinephrine to epinephrine alone	Mortality in epinepherine group: 64/161 (40%) Mortality in norepinepherine plus dobutamine: 58/169 (34%) RRR = −0.16 (95% CI: −0.54 to 0.05)
Sakr et al. [59]	ICU patients ($N = 3147$); some with shock ($N = 1058$)	Multi-centered, retrospective, observational cohort in 198 European ICUs	Mortality with dopamine: 187/135 (49.9%) Mortality without dopamine: 285/683 (41.7%) RRR of dopamine = 1.69 (95% CI: 1.47 to 1.94) NNH = 4.9 (95% CI: 3.82 to 6.84)

Russell [62]	Patients with septic shock requiring vasopressors for >6 hours and one additional organ failure present for <24 hours; $N = 779$	Prospective randomized trial evaluating 30-day mortality using low-dose vasopressin compared to norepinephrine	For less severe septic shock:
			  Mortality with norepinephrine: 35.7%
			  Mortality with vasopressin: 26.5%
			  NNT = 10.9*
			This was a pre-planned sub-group analysis. No statistical significance was found between treatment arms overall, and no significant difference was found for more severe sepsis

*At time of press these data were not yet published.

CI, confidence interval; ICU, intensive care unit; NNH, number needed to harm; NNT, number needed to treat; RRR, relative risk reduction.

trial was designed to demonstrate a difference in 30-day mortality using low-dose vasopressin (defined as 0.03 U/min) compared to norepinephrine. Results were stratified by severity of septic shock in a pre-planned subset analysis (less severe septic shock was defined as patients requiring norepinephrine 5–14 μg/min to maintain their blood pressure at time of enrollment). For these less severely ill patients, vasopressin administration reportedly provided a significant survival advantage. Preliminary results are listed in Table 23.5.

In summary, early evidence suggests that vasopressin administration confers survival advantage in less severe septic shock; however, this evidence is preliminary and caution is advised prior to widespread practice change. The use of dopamine may be associated with increased mortality in shock, but a causal relationship has not been proven. The use of vasopressors in septic shock to maintain blood pressure at a level that supports blood flow to vital organs is widely accepted. The use of dobutamine is supported as a component of bundled therapy.

Question 6: For adult patients in the first 24 hours of severe sepsis or septic shock (population), do patients receiving a specific transfusion threshold (intervention) have lower mortality (outcome) than patients who either do not receive transfusion or transfusion to the same threshold (control)?

Search strategy

- MEDLINE, EMBASE, Cochrane, DARE, ACP Journal Club and CENTRAL: (severe sepsis OR septic shock OR sepsis) AND (blood transfusion OR transfusion OR exchange transfusion OR whole blood)

Although several studies have demonstrated increased delivery of oxygen to the tissues after transfusion in patients with severe sepsis or septic shock, the effect of transfusion of packed red blood cells isolated from other therapies on the mortality of patients with severe sepsis or septic shock has not been studied [63–65].

Hebert et al. evaluated transfusion thresholds in ICU patients (not specifically severe sepsis or septic shock). This multi-center prospective randomized trial compared ICU patients who were maintained at a hemoglobin of 10–12 g/dl to patients maintained at a hemoglobin of 7–9 g/dl [66]. Overall, 30-day mortality was similar in the two groups (23.3% vs 18.7%); however, among patients with APACHE II score <20 and in patients <55 years of age, the lower transfusion threshold was associated with significantly lower mortality (16.1% vs 8.7% mortality, number needed to treat (NNT) = 13.5, and 13.0% vs 5.7% mortality, NNT = 13.7, respectively). In no group analyzed was the higher transfusion level beneficial.

In summary, although severe sepsis or septic shock patients have not been studied specifically, a transfusion target of 7–9 g/dl (70–80 g/L) is appropriate, with the exception of patients with evidence of hypoperfusion being transfused to meet the $ScvO_2$ goal of greater than 70% in EGDT (see Question 3 above).

Question 7: For adult patients in the first 24 hours of severe sepsis or septic shock (population), does administration of rhAPC (intervention) improve mortality (outcome) compared to patients who do not receive this therapy (control)?

Search strategy

- MEDLINE, EMBASE, Cochrane, DARE, ACP Journal Club and CENTRAL: (severe sepsis OR septic shock OR sepsis) AND (anticoagulants OR protein c OR recombinant protein OR blood coagulation factor inhibitor OR disseminated intravascular coagulation OR drotrecogin alpha OR rhAPC OR rh APC OR recombinant activated protein c)

The Cochrane Collaboration reviewed activated human recombinant protein C (rhAPC) use in severe sepsis in 2007. They found, using pooled data analysis, that for 28-day mortality, rhAPC did not reduce the risk of death at 28 days in adult participants with severe sepsis or septic shock (pooled RR reduction = 0.08; 95% CI: –0.18 to 0.28). The findings were similar when data were pooled for patients with APACHE II score ≥25 (RR reduction = 0.10; 95% CI: –0.49 to 0.46) [67].

In a multi-centered, prospective, randomized controlled study, rhAPC was demonstrated to reduce mortality in patients with severe sepsis from 30.8% in the placebo group to 24.7% in the rhAPC group (RR reduction = 0.20; 95% CI: 0.065 to 0.31; NNT = 17, 95% CI: 10 to 54). A pre defined analysis showed that rhAPC conferred greatest benefit in patients with APACHE II scores ≥25 [68]. Benefit may also be greater when rhAPC is initiated within the first 24 hours of severe sepsis [69]. In patients with single organ dysfunction or an APACHE II score <25 there was no survival benefit from rhAPC administration [70].

The administration of rhAPC is not without cost and side-effect concerns. The administration of rhAPC was associated with a 3.5% incidence of serious bleeding (defined as intracranial bleeding, bleeding requiring more than 3 U of blood in 48 hours, or bleeding that was considered life-threatening) compared to 2.0% in the placebo group ($P = 0.06$). Intracranial hemorrhage occurred in 0.2% compared to 0.1%, respectively [69]. Risk of serious bleeding in pooled analysis of adult patients from a Cochrane review was 1.68 (95% CI: 1.19 to 2.38) [67].

In conclusion, for patients with no contraindication to rhAPC who have severe sepsis with multiple organ dysfunction and an APACHE II score ≥25, rhAPC may be administered after careful consideration.

Question 8: For adult patients in the first 24 hours of severe sepsis or septic shock (population), do patients receiving tight glycemic control (intervention) have lower mortality (outcome) than patients receiving standard therapy (control)?

Search strategy

• MEDLINE, EMBASE, Cochrane, DARE, ACP Journal Club and CENTRAL: (severe sepsis OR septic shock OR sepsis) AND (insulin OR blood glucose OR glycemic control OR hypoglycemic agents OR hypoglycemia OR antidiabetic agent OR tight glycemic control) AND (critical illness)

The above search identified 171 citations, of which 21 were relevant to this question. Although tight glycemic control appears to provide a survival benefit to surgical ICU patients [71], and reduced morbidity (but not mortality) to medical ICU patients [72], there has been no study to evaluate the effectiveness of this therapy in the setting of severe sepsis or septic shock patients in the ED [71–76].

In summary, while perhaps appealing, tight glycemic control in the ED for severe sepsis or septic shock remains an untested and unproven therapy. Emergency physicians should focus initially on other issues such as fluid therapy, antibiotics and hemodynamic optimization before addressing tight glycemic control.

Question 9: For adult patients in the first 24 hours of severe sepsis or septic shock (population), do patients receiving corticosteroids (intervention) have lower mortality (outcome) than patients who do not receive corticosteroids (control)?

Search strategy

• MEDLINE, EMBASE, Cochrane, DARE, ACP Journal Club and CENTRAL: (severe sepsis OR septic shock OR sepsis) AND (steroid OR corticosteroid OR adrenal cortex hormone OR glucocorticoid)

The search identified 40 potentially relevant studies, of which the important ones are summarized in Table 23.6. Several studies were identified that suggested a trend to increased survival or more rapid improvement of septic shock for patients who received physiological dose steroid repletion [77–82]. This finding, however, is not supported by the results of a recent prospective, multi-centered trial [83].

One multi-centered, prospective, randomized trial enrolled mechanically ventilated patients with persistent hypotension and septic shock (all patients were still hypotensive after fluids and vasopressor therapy) comparing administration of low-dose hydrocortisone and fludrocortisone to patients who did not receive steroids [79]. This study demonstrated a reduction in mortality for patients receiving corticosteroids who were non-responders to the adrenocorticotrophic hormone (ACTH) stimulation test (relatively adrenal insufficient). This result was significant only after

Table 23.6 Summary of evidence for corticosteroid administration in severe sepsis and septic shock.

Study	Population	Design	Outcome
CORTICUS (in progress) [83]	Septic shock patients in the first 72 hours of illness; $N = 500$	Prospective, randomized controlled trial on septic shock patients in the first 72 hours of illness randomized to hydrocortisone or placebo	Full data set not yet published 28-day mortality rate, hydrocortisone group: 33% 28-day mortality rate, placebo group: 31% This difference is not significant
Annane et al. [79]	ICU mechanically ventilated patients with persistent hypotension and early in course of septic shock; $N = 300$	Prospective, randomized controlled trial on patients receiving either hydrocortisone (50 mg intravenous bolus every 6 hours) and fludrocortisone (50 μg tablet once daily) or matching placebo	For adrenally insufficient patients Corticosteroid treatment group mortality: 60/113 (53%) Placebo group mortality: 73/116 (63%) RRR = 0.16 (95% CI: −0.05 to 0.32) These results only became statistically significant after adjustment for severity
Oppert et al. [78]	ICU patients early in the course of septic shock; $N = 41$	Prospective, randomized controlled trial All patients received an adrenocorticotropic hormone test, then were randomized to receive either low-dose hydrocortisone (50 mg bolus followed by a continuous infusion of 0.18 mg/kg/h) or matching placebo	Time to cessation of vasopressor support (primary endpoint) was significantly shorter in hydrocortisone-treated patients compared with placebo (53 hours vs 120 hours, $P < 0.02$)

CI, confidence interval; ICU, intensive care unit; RRR, relative risk reduction.

statistically adjusting for differences in severity between groups. Of note, there was no a non-significant trend in the direction of increased mortality among patients with normal adrenal function patients who received steroids.

A recent prospective, multi-centered, randomized, placebo-controlled trial, the Corticosteroid Therapy of Septic Shock (CORTICUS) trial, has been completed and awaits publication [83]. The CORTICUS trial enrolled septic shock patients in the first 72 hours of illness and compared treatment with hydrocortisone to care without steroids. The patients in this study could not be hypotensive at the time of enrollment. Slightly over half the patients in each group had relative adrenal insufficiency (did not respond to the ACTH stimulation test). The trial was terminated early because interim analysis suggested no difference between the corticosteroid and control treatment arms. There was also no difference between groups when results were stratified between ACTH responders and non-responders. The difference between the results obtained in the CORTICUS trial and the Annane study may be the result of differences in the severity of illness for patients in each trial. Patients in the Annane study were more ill than those enrolled in CORTICUS.

Overall, there appears to be no role for routine corticosteroid administration for patients with severe sepsis. For patients with septic shock, based on the preliminary data from the CORTICUS trial, there is no benefit from corticosteroid therapy. The Annane trial, which enrolled patients with more severe sepsis, reported improved survival with corticosteroids after statistical adjustment for severity. It may be appropriate to navigate these disparate results by only using corticosteroids in septic shock patients who are adrenal insufficient and who remain hypotensive despite vasopressor administration.

Question 10: For adult patients in the first 24 hours of severe sepsis or septic shock who are mechanically ventilated (population), do patients receiving low tidal volume ventilation (intervention) have lower mortality (outcome) than patients who receive high tidal volume ventilation (control)?

Search strategy

- MEDLINE, EMBASE, Cochrane, DARE, ACP Journal Club and CENTRAL: (severe sepsis OR septic shock OR sepsis) AND (ventilator OR artificial ventilator OR tidal volume OR low volume ventilator) AND (survival analysis OR hospital mortality)

There have been several prospective randomized trials comparing low tidal volume mechanical ventilation (defined as 6 ml/kg) to historically conventional tidal volume ventilation targeted at 12 ml/kg in intensive care patients with acute lung injury (ALI) or acute respiratory distress syndrome (ARDS) [84–89]. These trials have included a large number of septic shock patients. Most of these trials show a mortality benefit to low tidal volume ven-

tilation. None of the trials demonstrate harm caused by low tidal volumes. No studies of lung volume have been performed in the ED setting, and no studies have been done specifically on patients with severe sepsis or septic shock. For the heterogeneous group of critically ill patients who have been studied, the use of low tidal volume ventilation significantly reduces mortality.

In summary, although low tidal volume ventilation has not been studied specifically in the ED or specifically in septic shock patients, it has become an accepted practice in patients with ALI or ARDS and is recommended for severe sepsis and septic shock patients who require mechanical ventilation.

Conclusions

Returning to your patient in the clinical scenario, her blood pressure remained unchanged after a 20 ml/kg fluid bolus and intravenous antibiotics. Several hours into her course of treatment the patient became confused, her respiratory rate increased to 36 breaths/min, and blood gas analysis demonstrated a metabolic acidosis and respiratory alkalosis with a pH of 7.06. The patient was intubated for airway protection and imminent respiratory failure, and placed on low tidal volume (6 ml/kg) mechanical ventilation.

A central line with a distal fiberoptic port allowing continuous $ScvO_2$ measurement was placed in her subclavian vein. Her initial CVP was 2 mmHg and $ScvO_2$ was 52%. She required a total of 6 L of normal saline before her CVP reached 12 mmHg. She received piperacillin/tazobactam, a fluoroquinolone and vancomycin within her first 2 hours in the ED. Despite her CVP reaching 12 mmHg, her blood pressure remained low, so she was started on a norepinephrine drip and her blood pressure increased to 110/50 mmHg (mean arterial pressure = 70 mmHg). The patient's $ScvO_2$ was still 61% after the above measures, and she was transfused 2 U of packed red blood cells, which raised her hemoglobin to 10.5 g/dl and $ScvO_2$ to 72%. Her APACHE II score was calculated to be 29, and she was administered rhAPC after screening for contraindications. After an initially rocky course, the patient stabilized, was discharged from the ICU after 7 days and from the hospital after a further 10 days.

It is now clear that early aggressive care in the treatment of severe sepsis and septic shock saves lives, placing sepsis care alongside myocardial infarction, trauma and stroke in its need for appropriate, timely intervention. The literature on the diagnosis, prognostication and treatment of severe sepsis and septic shock in the ED setting is limited. The use of lactate and a physiological scoring system such as MEDS and APACHE II will facilitate identification of high-risk patients. Early antibiotic administration together with a bundled approach to hemodynamic optimization improves survival. Consideration should be given to the administration of rhAPC for patients with severe sepsis, multiple organ dysfunction and APACHE II scores >25 if they do not have contraindications to the medication. More studies are needed to further evaluate individual components of these therapies.

Acknowledgments

The authors would like to thank Martha Prescott, MLS Director Berkshire Health Sciences Library for her research assistance and organizational support in the development of this chapter.

References

1 Bone RC, Balk RA, Cerra FB, et al. Definitions for sepsis and organ failure and guidelines for the use of innovative therapies in sepsis. The ACCP/SCCM Consensus Conference Committee. American College of Chest Physicians/Society of Critical Care Medicine. *Chest* 1992;**101**(6):1644–55.

2 Levy MM, Fink MP, Marshall JC, et al. 2001 SCCM/ESICM/ACCP/ATS/SIS International Sepsis Definitions Conference. *Crit Care Med* 2003;**31**(4):1250–56.

3 Angus DC, Linde-Zwirble WT, Lidicker J, Clermont G, Carcillo J, Pinsky MR. Epidemiology of severe sepsis in the United States: analysis of incidence, outcome, and associated costs of care. *Crit Care Med* 2001;**29**(7):1303–10.

4 Gao F, Melody T, Daniels DF, Giles S, Fox S. The impact of compliance with 6-hour and 24-hour sepsis bundles on hospital mortality in patients with severe sepsis: a prospective observational study. *Crit Care* (London) 2005;**9**(6):R764–70.

5 Shapiro NI, Howell MD, Talmor D, et al. Implementation and outcomes of the Multiple Urgent Sepsis Therapies (MUST) protocol. *Crit Care Med* 2006;**34**(4):1025–32.

6 Jones AE, Focht A, Horton JM, Kline JA. Prospective external validation of the clinical effectiveness of an emergency department-based early goal-directed therapy protocol for severe sepsis and septic shock. *Chest* 2007;**132**(2):425–32.

7 Micek ST, Roubinian N, Heuring T, et al. Before–after study of a standardized hospital order set for the management of septic shock. *Crit Care Med* 2006;**34**(11):2707–13.

8 Nguyen HB, Corbett SW, Steele R, et al. Implementation of a bundle of quality indicators for the early management of severe sepsis and septic shock is associated with decreased mortality. *Crit Care Med* 2007;**35**(4):1105–12.

9 Kortgen A, Niederprum P, Bauer M. Implementation of an evidence-based "standard operating procedure" and outcome in septic shock. *Crit Care Med* 2006;**34**(4):943–9.

10 Marshall JC, Cook DJ, Christou NV, Bernard GR, Sprung CL, Sibbald WJ. Multiple organ dysfunction score: a reliable descriptor of a complex clinical outcome. *Crit Care Med* 1995;**23**(10):1638–52.

11 Knaus WA, Draper EA, Wagner DP, Zimmerman JE. APACHE II: a severity of disease classification system. *Crit Care Med* 1985;**13**(10):818–29.

12 Knaus W, Wagner D, Draper E. APACHE III study design: analytic plan for evaluation of severity and outcome in intensive care unit patients. Development of APACHE. *Crit Care Med* 1989;**17**(12/2):S181–5.

13 Zimmerman JE, Kramer AA, McNair DS, Malila FM. Acute Physiology and Chronic Health Evaluation (APACHE) IV: hospital mortality assessment for today's critically ill patients. *Crit Care Med* 2006;**34**(5):1297–310.

14 Vincent JL, Moreno R, Takala J, et al. The SOFA (Sepsis-related Organ Failure Assessment) score to describe organ dysfunction/failure. On behalf of the Working Group on Sepsis-Related Problems of the European Society of Intensive Care Medicine. *Intensive Care Med* 1996;**22**(7):707–10.

15 Lemeshow S, Teres D, Klar J, Avrunin JS, Gehlbach SH, Rapoport J. Mortality Probability Models (MPM II) based on an international cohort of intensive care unit patients. *JAMA* 1993;**270**(20):2478–86.

16 Higgins TL, Teres D, Copes WS, Nathanson BH, Stark M, Kramer AA. Assessing contemporary intensive care unit outcome: an updated Mortality Probability Admission Model (MPM0-III). *Crit Care Med* 2007;**35**(3):827–35.

17 Shapiro NI, Wolfe RE, Moore RB, Smith E, Burdick E, Bates DW. Mortality in Emergency Department Sepsis (MEDS) score: a prospectively derived and validated clinical prediction rule. *Crit Care Med* 2003;**31**(3):670–75.

18 Baumgartner JD, Bula C, Vaney C, Wu MM, Eggimann P, Perret C. A novel score for predicting the mortality of septic shock patients. *Crit Care Med* 1992;**20**(7):953–60.

19 Olsson T, Lind L. Comparison of the Rapid Emergency Medicine Score and APACHE II in nonsurgical emergency department patients. *Acad Emerg Med* 2003;**10**(10):1040–48.

20 Shapiro NI, Howell MD, Talmor D, Donnino M, Ngo L, Bates DW. Mortality in Emergency Department Sepsis (MEDS) score predicts 1-year mortality. *Crit Care Med* 2007;**35**(1):192–8.

21 Chen CC, Chong CF, Liu YL, Chen KC, Wang TL. Risk stratification of severe sepsis patients in the emergency department. *Emerg Med J* 2006;**23**(4):281–5.

22 Howell MD, Donnino MW, Talmor D, Clardy P, Ngo L, Shapiro NI. Performance of severity of illness scoring systems in emergency department patients with infection. *Acad Emerg Med* 2007;**14**(8):709–14.

23 Lee CC, Chen SY, Tsai CL, et al. Prognostic value of mortality in emergency department sepsis score, procalcitonin, and c-reactive protein in patients with sepsis at the emergency department. *Shock* 2007;**29**(30):322–7.

24 Nguyen HB, Rivers EP, Havstad S, et al. Critical care in the emergency department: a physiologic assessment and outcome evaluation. *Acad Emerg Med* 2000;**7**(12):1354–61.

25 Jacobs S, Zuleika M, Mphansa T. The Multiple Organ Dysfunction Score as a descriptor of patient outcome in septic shock compared with two other scoring systems. *Crit Care Med* 1999;**27**(4):741–4.

26 Arabi Y, Al Shirawi N, Memish Z, Venkatesh S, Al-Shimemeri A. Assessment of six mortality prediction models in patients admitted with severe sepsis and septic shock to the intensive care unit: a prospective cohort study. *Crit Care* (London) 2003;**7**(5):R116–22.

27 Man SY, Chan KM, Wong FY, et al. Evaluation of the performance of a modified Acute Physiology and Chronic Health Evaluation (APACHE II) scoring system for critically ill patients in emergency departments in Hong Kong. *Resuscitation* 2007;**74**(2):259–65.

28 Shapiro NI, Howell MD, Talmor D, et al. Serum lactate as a predictor of mortality in emergency department patients with infection. *Ann Emerg Med* 2005;**45**(5):524–8.

29 Nguyen HB, Rivers EP, Knoblich BP, et al. Early lactate clearance is associated with improved outcome in severe sepsis and septic shock. *Crit Care Med* 2004;**32**(8):1637–42.

30 Harbarth S, Garbino J, Pugin J, Romand JA, Lew D, Pittet D. Inappropriate initial antimicrobial therapy and its effect on survival in a clinical trial of immunomodulating therapy for severe sepsis. *Am J Med* 2003;**115**(7):529–35.

31 Harbarth S, Garbino J, Pugin J, Romand JA, Pittet D. Lack of effect of combination antibiotic therapy on mortality in patients with pneumococcal sepsis. *Eur J Clin Microbiol Infect Dis* 2005;**24**(10):688–90.

32 Kumar A, Roberts D, Wood KE, et al. Duration of hypotension before initiation of effective antimicrobial therapy is the critical determinant of survival in human septic shock. *Crit Care Med* 2006;**34**(6):1589–96.

33 Larche J, Azoulay E, Fieux F, et al. Improved survival of critically ill cancer patients with septic shock. *Intensive Care Med* 2003;**29**(10):1688–95.

34 Leibovici L, Pitlik SD, Konisberger H, Drucker M. Bloodstream infections in patients older than eighty years. *Age Ageing* 1993;**22**(6):431–42.

35 Leone M, Bourgoin A, Cambon S, Dubuc M, Albanese J, Martin C. Empirical antimicrobial therapy of septic shock patients: adequacy and impact on the outcome. *Crit Care Med* 2003;**31**(2):462–7.

36 Leroy O, Santre C, Beuscart C, et al. A five-year study of severe community-acquired pneumonia with emphasis on prognosis in patients admitted to an intensive care unit. *Intensive Care Med* 1995;**21**(1):24–31.

37 Rodriguez A, Rello J, Neira J, et al. Effects of high-dose of intravenous immunoglobulin and antibiotics on survival for severe sepsis undergoing surgery. *Shock* 2005;**23**(4):298–304.

38 Sainio V, Kemppainen E, Puolakkainen P, et al. Early antibiotic treatment in acute necrotising pancreatitis. *Lancet* 1995;**346**(8976):663–7.

39 Falagas ME, Siempos, II, Bliziotis IA, Panos GZ. Impact of initial discordant treatment with beta-lactam antibiotics on clinical outcomes in adults with pneumococcal pneumonia: a systematic review. *Mayo Clin Proc* 2006;**81**(12):1567–74.

40 Garnacho-Montero J, Garcia-Garmendia JL, Barrero-Almodovar A, Jimenez-Jimenez FJ, Perez-Paredes C, Ortiz-Leyba C. Impact of adequate empirical antibiotic therapy on the outcome of patients admitted to the intensive care unit with sepsis. *Crit Care Med* 2003;**31**(12):2742–51.

41 Rivers EP, Nguyen HB, Havstad S, et al. Early goal-directed therapy in the treatment of severe sepsis and septic shock. *N Engl J Med* 2001;**345**(19):1368–77.

42 Lin SM, Huang CD, Lin HC, Liu CY, Wang CH, Kuo HP. A modified goal-directed protocol improves clinical outcomes in intensive care unit patients with septic shock: a randomized controlled trial. *Shock* 2006;**26**(6):551–7.

43 Nguyen HB, Corbett SW, Menes K, et al. Early goal-directed therapy, corticosteroid, and recombinant human activated protein C for the treatment of severe sepsis and septic shock in the emergency department. *Acad Emerg Med* 2006;**13**(1):109–13.

44 Ledingham IM, McArdle CS. Prospective study of the treatment of septic shock. *Lancet* 1978;**1**(8075):1194–7.

45 Anon. Protocolized Care for Early Septic Shock (ProCESS). Available at http://www.clinicaltrials.gov/ct/show/NCT00510835;jsessionid=7391ED783DF2B751930230235AE530EE?order=15.

46 The SSI. A comparison of albumin and saline for fluid resuscitation in the intensive care unit. *N Engl J Med* 2004;**350**(22):2247–56.

47 Upadhyay M, Singhi S, Murlidharan J, et al. Randomized evaluation of fluid resuscitation with crystalloid (saline) and colloid (polymer from degraded gelatin in saline) in pediatric septic shock. *Indian Pediatr* 2005;**42**(3):223–31.

48 Annane D, Vignon P, Renault A, et al. Norepinephrine plus dobutamine versus epinephrine alone for management of septic shock: a randomised trial. *Lancet* 2007;**370**(9588):676–84.

49 Lauzier F, Levy B, Lamarre P, Lesur O. Vasopressin or norepinephrine in early hyperdynamic septic shock: a randomized clinical trial. *Intensive Care Med* 2006;**32**(11):1782–9.

50 Hall LG, Oyen LJ, Taner CB, et al. Fixed-dose vasopressin compared with titrated dopamine and norepinephrine as initial vasopressor therapy for septic shock. *Pharmacotherapy* 2004;**24**(8):1002–12.

51 Malay MB, Ashton RC, Jr., Landry DW, et al. Low-dose vasopressin in the treatment of vasodilatory septic shock. *J Trauma-Injury Infect Crit Care* 1999;**47**(4):699–705.

52 Dunser MW, Mayr AJ, Ulmer H, et al. Arginine vasopressin in advanced vasodilatory shock: a prospective, randomized, controlled study. *Circulation* 2003;**107**(18):2313–19.

53 Boccara G, Ouattara A, Godet G, et al. Terlipressin versus norepinephrine to correct refractory arterial hypotension after general anesthesia in patients chronically treated with renin-angiotensin system inhibitors. *Anesthesiology* 2003;**98**(6):1338–44.

54 Martin C, Papazian L, Perrin G, Saux P, Gouin F. Norepinephrine or dopamine for the treatment of hyperdynamic septic shock? *Chest* 1993;**103**(6):1826–31.

55 Marik PE, Mohedin M. The contrasting effects of dopamine and norepinephrine on systemic and splanchnic oxygen utilization in hyperdynamic sepsis. *JAMA* 1994;**272**(17):1354–7.

56 Ruokonen E, Takala J, Kari A, Saxen H, Mertsola J, Hansen EJ. Regional blood flow and oxygen transport in septic shock. *Crit Care Med* 1993;**21**(9):1296–303.

57 Levy B, Bollaert PE, Charpentier C, et al. Comparison of norepinephrine and dobutamine to epinephrine for hemodynamics, lactate metabolism, and gastric tonometric variables in septic shock: a prospective, randomized study. *Intensive Care Med* 1997;**23**(3):282–7.

58 Seguin P, Bellissant E, Le Tulzo Y, et al. Effects of epinephrine compared with the combination of dobutamine and norepinephrine on gastric perfusion in septic shock. *Clin Pharmacol Ther* 2002;**71**(5):381–8.

59 Sakr Y, Reinhart K, Vincent JL, et al. Does dopamine administration in shock influence outcome? Results of the Sepsis Occurrence in Acutely Ill Patients (SOAP) study. *Crit Care Med* 2006;**34**(3):589–97.

60 Obritsch MD, Jung R, Fish DN, MacLaren R. Effects of continuous vasopressin infusion in patients with septic shock. *Ann Pharmacother* 2004;**38**(7/8):1117–22.

61 Mullner M, Urbanek B, Havel C, Losert H, Waechter F, Gamper G. Vasopressors for shock. *Cochrane Database Syst Rev* 2004;**3**:CD003709.

62 Russell JA, Walley KR, Singer J, et al., for the VASST Investigators. Hemodynamic support of sepsis. Vasopressin versus norepinephrine infusion in patients with septic shock. *N Engl J Med* 2008; **358**(9):877–87.

63 Lorente JA, Landin L, De Pablo R, Renes E, Rodriguez-Diaz R, Liste D. Effects of blood transfusion on oxygen transport variables in severe sepsis. *Crit Care Med* 1993;**21**(9):1312–18.

64 Conrad SA, Dietrich KA, Hebert CA, Romero MD. Effect of red cell transfusion on oxygen consumption following fluid resuscitation in septic shock. *Circ Shock* 1990;**31**(4):419–29.

65 Yu M, Levy MM, Smith P, Takiguchi SA, Miyasaki A, Myers SA. Effect of maximizing oxygen delivery on morbidity and mortality rates in critically ill patients: a prospective, randomized, controlled study. *Crit Care Med* 1993;**21**(6):830–38.

66 Hebert PC, Wells G, Blajchman MA, et al. A multicenter, randomized, controlled clinical trial of transfusion requirements in critical care. Transfusion Requirements in Critical Care Investigators, Canadian Critical Care Trials Group. *N Engl J Med* 1999;**340**(6):409–17.

67 Marti-Carvajal A, Salanti G, Cardona AF. Human recombinant activated protein C for severe sepsis. *Cochrane Database Syst Rev* 2007;**3**:CD004388.

68 Bernard GR, Vincent JL, Laterre PF, et al. Efficacy and safety of recombinant human activated protein C for severe sepsis. *N Engl J Med* 2001;**344**(10):699–709.

69 Vincent JL. Drotrecogin alfa (activated) in the treatment of severe sepsis. *Expert Rev Antiinfective Ther* 2006;**4**(4):537–47.

70 Abraham E, Laterre PF, Garg R, et al. Drotrecogin alfa (activated) for adults with severe sepsis and a low risk of death. *N Engl J Med* 2005;**353**(13):1332–41.

71 van den Berghe G, Wouters P, Weekers F, et al. Intensive insulin therapy in the critically ill patient. *N Engl J Med* 2001;**345**(19):1359–67.

72 van den Berghe G, Wilmer A, Hermans G, et al. Intensive insulin therapy in the medical ICU. *N Engl J Med* 2006;**354**(5):449–61.

73 Turina M, Christ-Crain M, Polk HC, Jr. Diabetes and hyperglycemia: strict glycemic control. *Crit Care Med* 2006;**34**(9 Suppl):S291–300.

74 van den Berghe G, Wouters PJ, Bouillon R, et al. Outcome benefit of intensive insulin therapy in the critically ill: insulin dose versus glycemic control. *Crit Care Med* 2003;**31**(2):359–66.

75 Pittas AG, Siegel RD, Lau J. Insulin therapy for critically ill hospitalized patients: a meta-analysis of randomized controlled trials. *Arch Intern Med* 2004;**164**(18):2005–11.

76 Pittas AG, Siegel RD, Lau J. Insulin therapy and in-hospital mortality in critically ill patients: systematic review and meta-analysis of randomized controlled trials. *J Parenteral Enteral Nutr* 2006;**30**(2):164–72.

77 Yildiz O, Doganay M, Aygen B, Guven M, Kelestimur F, Tutuu A. Physiological-dose steroid therapy in sepsis (ISRCTN36253388). *Crit Care* (London) 2002;**6**(3):251–9.

78 Oppert M, Schindler R, Husung C, et al. Low-dose hydrocortisone improves shock reversal and reduces cytokine levels in early hyperdynamic septic shock. *Crit Care Med* 2005;**33**(11):2457–64.

79 Annane D, Sebille V, Charpentier C, et al. Effect of treatment with low doses of hydrocortisone and fludrocortisone on mortality in patients with septic shock. *JAMA* 2002;**288**(7):862–71.

80 Fernandez J, Escorsell A, Zabalza M, et al. Adrenal insufficiency in patients with cirrhosis and septic shock: effect of treatment with hydrocortisone on survival. *Hepatology* 2006;**44**(5):1288–95.

81 Briegel J, Forst H, Haller M, et al. Stress doses of hydrocortisone reverse hyperdynamic septic shock: a prospective, randomized, double-blind, single-center study. *Crit Care Med* 1999;**27**(4):723–32.

82 Bollaert PE, Charpentier C, Levy B, Debouverie M, Audibert G, Larcan A. Reversal of late septic shock with supraphysiologic doses of hydrocortisone. *Crit Care Med* 1998;**26**(4):645–50.

83 Sprung CL. Corticosteroid Therapy of Septic Shock – Corticus. A multi-national, prospective, double-blind, randomized, placebo-controlled study. clinical trails number NCT00147004. Available at http://clinicaltrials.gov/ ct/show/NCT00147004.

84 Brower RG, Shanholtz CB, Fessler HE, et al. Prospective, randomized, controlled clinical trial comparing traditional versus reduced tidal volume ventilation in acute respiratory distress syndrome patients. *Crit Care Med* 1999;**27**(8):1492–8.

85 Stewart TE, Meade MO, Cook DJ, et al. Evaluation of a ventilation strategy to prevent barotrauma in patients at high risk for acute respiratory distress syndrome. Pressure- and Volume-Limited Ventilation Strategy Group. *N Engl J Med* 1998;**338**(6):355–61.

86 Amato MB, Barbas CS, Medeiros DM, et al. Effect of a protective-ventilation strategy on mortality in the acute respiratory distress syndrome. *N Engl J Med* 1998;**338**(6):347–54.

87 Sakr Y, Vincent JL, Reinhart K, et al. High tidal volume and positive fluid balance are associated with worse outcome in acute lung injury. *Chest* 2005;**128**(5):3098–108.

88 Villar J, Kacmarek RM, Perez-Mendez L, Aguirre-Jaime A. A high positive end-expiratory pressure, low tidal volume ventilatory strategy improves outcome in persistent acute respiratory distress syndrome: a randomized, controlled trial. *Crit Care Med* 2006;**34**(5):1311–18.

89 Hickling KG, Walsh J, Henderson S, Jackson R. Low mortality rate in adult respiratory distress syndrome using low-volume, pressure-limited ventilation with permissive hypercapnia: a prospective study. *Crit Care Med* 1994;**22**(10):1568–78.

24 Delirium

Denise Nassisi & Andy Jagoda

Department of Emergency Medicine, Mount Sinai School of Medicine, New York, USA

Clinical scenario

An 82-year-old male was brought to the emergency department (ED) by his home care worker because he was confused and not himself on the day of presentation. He lived alone and the home care worker stated that the patient initially would not let her in the house; however, he eventually relented. He refused to eat breakfast or take his medication, and his conversation had not been making sense. His past history was significant for mild dementia, coronary artery disease, hypertension and prostate disease. He was on several unknown medications, although the health care aide volunteered to retrieve them, if needed.

At triage, the nurse evaluation revealed: an irregular and rapid pulse of 128 beats/min, temperature of 38.5°C (oral), respiratory rate of 20 breaths/min, blood pressure of 150/90 mmHg (left arm) and pulse oximetry of 95% on room air. The patient was escorted to the ED treatment area where he became agitated when the staff tried to have him undress. He refused to allow the nurse to draw blood samples or establish an intravenous line; he started shouting at the staff to stop harming him and he attempted to leave the ED and return home.

You diagnose acute delirium; however, the cause is as yet unknown. The resident working with you asked whether phenothiazines would be safe in elderly agitated patients like yours. The nurses requested four-point restraints as well as a catheter be placed in his bladder because they did not feel they would have the time to deal with his behavior in the overcrowded ED. Once again, the resident wondered about the effectiveness of this intervention for patients with delirium. Finally, the family arrived and wondered what the cause of their father's confusion was. They had never seen him act this way.

Background

Delirium poses a particularly challenging clinical scenario to practitioners in the ED. Managing the delirious agitated patient requires a coordinated approach that gains control of the situation while facilitating the diagnostic work-up. Patients presenting to the ED with altered mental status should be assumed to be delirious until proven otherwise. Altered mental status is a common ED presentation accounting for 5–10% of all ED visits.

Delirium is an organic mental syndrome defined by a global disturbance in consciousness and cognition. It is characterized by a disturbance in attention and memory impairment. Hallmarks of delirium include global cognitive impairment, relatively rapid onset of symptoms and a fluctuating clinical course (Box 24.1). Delirium is caused by a medical condition, substance intoxication or withdrawal or medication side-effects. The underlying mechanism of delirium is poorly understood and its pathophysiology has not been well elucidated.

Delirium is a medical emergency requiring prompt evaluation and treatment. The treatment of delirium is two fold: the behavioral symptoms of the delirium need to be controlled in order to facilitate patient assessment and management, and the underlying cause of the delirium must be addressed and treated. In patients with delirium, a potentially life-threatening etiology may exist and prompt intervention may be life saving. Therapeutic interventions may be required even before a specific underlying etiology is identified. Immediately life-threatening etiologies (e.g., hypoxia, hypoglycemia, hypotension) must be rapidly identified, with medical evaluation and stabilization occurring in parallel. The presence of delirium requires a thorough evaluation for a serious and potentially life-threatening etiology. Since delirium is a multi-factorial disorder, the differential diagnosis of delirium is extensive. Common causes of delirium include infections, insufficiency of any major organ, medication or substance use or withdrawal, electrolyte disturbances and dehydration (Box 24.2). Elderly and medically compromised individuals are particularly susceptible to its development.

Evidence-based Emergency Medicine. Edited by Brian H. Rowe
© 2009 Blackwell Publishing, ISBN: 978-1-4051-6143-5.

Box 24.1 Key features of delirium.

- Altered level of consciousness ranging from stupor to agitation
- Inattention, decreased ability to focus
- Fluctuating course over hours or days
- Disturbance in sleep/wake cycle
- Precipitated by medical illness, substance intoxication/withdrawal or medication effect

---

Delirium is a syndrome and not a specific disease, thus identifying the underlying etiology requires a comprehensive approach that includes a history and physical and diagnostic testing (Box 24.3). The clinical manifestations of delirium are highly variable. Patients may present hyperactively with agitation or hypoactively with a depressed sensorium. Delirium may be misdiagnosed and incorrectly assumed to be a manifestation of a psychiatric disturbance or of dementia. Subtle cases of delirium may not be recognized without a thorough evaluation of the patient's mental status. In one prospective study of 229 hospitalized elderly patients with delirium, agitation was present in less than one-third of cases [1]. The evaluation of a combative and agitated delirious patient is an especially problematic clinical situation. Pharmacological agents should be considered when the patient has the potential to harm themselves or others, or is impeding medical evaluation and treatment.

The study of delirium is challenging due to the heterogeneity of patient characteristics and plethora of underlying etiologies, as well as its characteristic fluctuating clinical course. In reviewing available pharmacological agents for the treatment of agitated patients, this chapter focuses on the non-psychiatric patient population. We avoided studies of decompensated psychiatric patients with acute psychosis (see Part 7).

Box 24.2 Differential diagnosis of etiologies of delirium.

- Hypoxemia/hypercarbia
- Hypoglycemia/hyperglycemia
- Hypotension and hypoperfusion
- Dehydration
- Electrolyte disturbance (sodium, calcium, magnesium, phosphorus)
- Infection/sepsis (pneumonia, urinary tract infection)
- Alcohol and drug toxicity or withdrawal
- Medication/vitamin deficiencies (Wernicke's)
- Central nervous system lesion, injury, infection (cerebrovascular accident, subdural hematoma, meningitis, encephalitis)
- Endocrinopathies (thyroid, adrenal)
- Cardiac disease (myocardial infarction, congestive heart failure, arrhythmia)
- Hyperthermia or hypothermia

Box 24.3 Physical assessment of the patient with delirium.

- Vital signs including accurate temperature measurement
- Physical examination with thorough neurological exam
- Oxygen saturation
- Rapid glucose determination
- Chemistry including electrolytes, renal function and liver function panels
- Urinalysis
- Chest X-ray
- Electrocardiogram
- Dependent upon the clinical scenario consider: computerized tomography scan of the head, lumbar puncture, blood cultures, toxicology screening, thyroid function

---

Clinical questions

In order to address the issues of greatest relevance to your patients and to help in searching the literature for the evidence regarding these issues, you should structure your clinical questions as recommended in Chapter 1.

1 Among elderly patients presenting to the ED with an acute medical complaint (population), what is the sensitivity and specificity (diagnostic test characteristics) of the Confusion Assessment Method (CAM) (test) in diagnosing delirium (outcome) compared with routine clinical diagnosis using history and physical exam (criterion standard)?

2 In patients presenting to the ED with a diagnosis of delirium (population), what is the in-hospital, 6-month mortality rate and morbidity (increased length of hospitalization, reduced functional ability, need for long-term placement) (outcomes) for patients who receive appropriate medical care?

3 In ED patients with undifferentiated acute agitation (population), does the use of benzodiazepines or antipsychotics (intervention) reduce agitation and/or adverse effects (outcomes) compared to no treatment (comparison)?

4 In ED patients with undifferentiated acute agitation (population), does the combined use of benzodiazepines with antipsychotics (intervention) reduce agitation and/or adverse effects (outcomes) compared to either a benzodiazepine or antipsychotic alone (comparison)?

5 In ED patients with undifferentiated acute agitation (population), does the use of atypical antipsychotic agents (intervention) reduce agitation and/or adverse effects (outcomes) compared to typical antipsychotic agents alone (comparison)?

6 In patients presenting to the ED with a diagnosis of delirium (population), does the use of droperidol (intervention) increase the risk of cardiac dysrhythmias (outcome) compared to the use of other antipsychotic drugs (comparison)?

7 In elderly patients hospitalized from the ED (population), are there strategies (intervention) that emergency physicians can employ to reduce the risk of delirium developing (outcome) compared to standard care (comparison)?

General search strategy

Electronic databases such as the Cochrane Library, MEDLINE and EMBASE were searched, first looking for systematic reviews and meta-analyses. Clinical trials, cohort studies, consensus statements and pertinent review articles were identified. The Clinical Guideline Clearinghouse (www.guideline.gov) and American College of Emergency Physicians (ACEP) clinical policies were also searched.

Critical review of the literature

Question 1: Among elderly patients presenting to the ED with an acute medical complaint (population), what is the sensitivity and specificity (diagnostic test characteristics) of the Confusion Assessment Method (CAM) (test) in diagnosing delirium (outcome) compared with routine clinical diagnosis using history and physical exam (criterion standard)?

> #### Search strategy
>
> • Cochrane Library, MEDLINE and EMBASE: confusion assessment method AND (sensitiv* [title/abstract] OR sensitivity and specificity [MeSH] OR diagnos* [title/abstract] OR diagnosis [MeSH:noexp] OR diagnostic* [MeSH:noexp] OR diagnosis, differential [MeSH:noexp] OR diagnosis [subheading:noexp])
>
> • Cochrane Library, MEDLINE and EMBASE: delirium AND (systematic [sb] OR specificity and sensitivity)

The diagnosis of delirium requires an assessment of mental status. There are a variety of mental status tests that can be used in the ED to assess mental status including the Mini Mental Status Examination (MMSE). The MMSE is used to test for cognition, which includes orientation, registration, attention and calculation, recall, visual–spatial ability and language. A low score is nonspecific and not diagnostic of a specific disorder. The MMSE must be interpreted with caution in patients with delirium because the delirious patient has impairment with attention, which interferes with exam performance [2,3]. The Confusion Assessment Method (CAM) has been proposed as an easy-to-use, sensitive and specific diagnostic tool to screen for delirium in patients. The CAM is based upon the criteria of the DSM-IV (*Diagnostic and Statistical Manual of Mental Disorders*, 4th edn) for the diagnosis of delirium [4]. The CAM instrument is outlined in Box 24.4. Briefly, this tool has four key features: (i) acute onset and fluctuating course; (ii) inattention; (iii) disorganized thinking; and (iv) altered level

> #### Box 24.4 Confusion Assessment Method (CAM) diagnostic algorithm.
>
> 1 Acute onset and fluctuating course
> 2 Inattention, distractibility
> 3 Disorganized thinking, illogical or unclear ideas
> 4 Alteration in consciousness
> The diagnosis of delirium requires the presence of both features 1 *and* 2, plus *either* feature 3 or 4

of consciousness. The first two features and one of the last two must be present to make the diagnosis of delirium.

The CAM is an instrument that can distinguish between delirium and other types of cognitive impairment. It has a sensitivity of 93–100% and a specificity of 90–95% for the diagnosis of delirium when compared with the diagnosis according to trained psychiatrists [5]. Studies of the use of the CAM in the ED are limited. One study utilized the CAM to evaluate elderly ED patients and found a prevalence of delirium of 10% [6]. A prospective study of 110 patients compared the CAM administered by geriatricians with administration by trained lay interviewers, and demonstrated that the CAM can be used successfully by trained lay interviewers in the ED [7]. A cohort study demonstrated that utilization of the CAM in ED patients aged 65 years and older found a prevalence of delirium of 10%; however only 17% of these cases were clinically recognized and charted by ED physicians as having delirium [8].

A study by Elie et al. of 477 patients aged 65 and older in the ED (excluding critically ill patients) compared the sensitivity of the clinical diagnosis of delirium of ED physicians with that of trained research psychiatrists administering both the CAM and MMSE [9]. The prevalence of delirium was found to be 9.6%; the sensitivity of the ED physician diagnosis was only 35.3% with a specificity of 98.5%.

In China, a study of 87 patients aged 65 and over consecutively admitted from the ED to medical wards compared a psychiatrist's diagnosis, the CAM and a consensus diagnosis and concluded that a consensus diagnosis by a trained rater (using the CAM and multiple observation points) may be a more sensitive approach to diagnosis [10]. While this mode of consensus diagnosis is impractical in the ED setting, this study does have implications for the design of future delirium studies and in the determination of what is the gold standard for the diagnosis of delirium.

Many would argue against the use of the CAM test in the busy setting of the ED, citing that the addition of a bedside screening test is both impractical and time consuming. When taking into consideration the mortality associated with delirium, however, the CAM test may be the first step in a valuable risk management strategy. A prospective observational convenience sample of 297 patients aged 70 and older was screened with the CAM for delirium and it was reported that 37% (11 of 30) of patients who met the criteria of delirium were discharged home [11,12].

Unfortunately, one study found that even when the results of the CAM test were provided to emergency physicians who missed the diagnosis of delirium (five patients), management was unchanged, and patients were still sent home [13]. The author of this article suggested it may be a quality-of-care issue, and ED physicians may need further education regarding the significance of delirium. Of the five patients with delirium who were discharged home, four had poor outcomes at follow-up.

In summary, because patients with delirium represent a high-risk population in both mortality and morbidity, the high prevalence of mental status impairment in the elderly population, and the increasing number of elderly patients presenting to the ED, due diligence is needed in addressing this at risk population. The CAM test appears to be a useful test in the screening of patients with delirium in the ED setting though further studies are needed to assess whether it alters management and ultimately patient care.

Question 2: In patients presenting to the ED with a diagnosis of delirium (population), what is the in-hospital, 6-month mortality rate and morbidity (increased length of hospitalization, reduced functional ability, need for long-term placement) (outcomes) for patients who receive appropriate medical care?

Search strategy

- MEDLINE, EMBASE and Cochrane Library: delirium AND (prognos* [title/abstract] OR (first [title/abstract] AND episode [title/abstract]) OR cohort [title/abstract])

Most published studies of the rates of delirium are based on hospitalized patients; however, some of these include patients who were admitted through the ED. Studies of hospital mortality rates in patients with delirium range from 22% to 76% [14–16]. Hospital mortality rates in patients who develop delirium have been reported to be as high as the mortality rate associated with acute myocardial infarction or sepsis.

Delirium is a marker for serious underlying medical illness. The presence of delirium is an important prognostic determinant associated with an increase in morbidity and mortality. However, published studies have not always adequately evaluated delirium as an independent predictor of increased adverse outcome and have failed to adjust for severity of illness and co-morbidities. More recent studies have attempted to address this issue.

In a prospective study of 727 patients conducted at three sites reported by Inouye et al. [17], the relationship of delirium at admission to death alone (35 events at discharge and 98 at 3-months' follow-up), and to length of hospital stay, were not statistically significant. The relatively small number of in-hospital deaths in the combined sample, with a limited power of 32% to detect a significant association, precluded drawing any definitive conclusions about the effect of delirium on hospital mortality. By the 3-month follow-up, the number of deaths in the combined sample increased, yielding a statistically significant association of delirium and mortality in the crude analysis. However, after multivariate adjustment, the effect was diminished (adjusted OR = 1.6; 95% CI: 0.8 to 3.2) and no longer achieved statistical significance.

A follow-up study of hospitalized delirious patients demonstrated a 62% increase in mortality at 1 year [18]. One prospective, consecutive series study of 238 critical care patients in Tokyo demonstrated that the patients who developed delirium (16%) had a longer length of hospital stay but did not have a higher rate of mortality [19].

Delirium was found to be an independent predictor of mortality at 6 months in a study of patients evaluated in two Montreal EDs who were discharged without hospital admission [20]. A study of patients in England admitted to an acute geriatric service screened 225 patients for delirium using DSM-III criteria with outcome measures of mortality, length of stay, complications and institutional placement [21]. While adjusting for age, co-morbidity, prior cognitive impairment and disability, delirium was independently associated with prolonged hospital stay, functional decline during hospitalization, increased risk of developing a hospital-acquired complication, and with increased admission to long-term care.

In summary, the majority of research efforts in this field arise from the identification of delirium in hospitalized patients; however, these data are likely generalizable to the ED population. Overall, delirium is common and outcome is poor. Further studies with sufficient numbers of patients are needed to evaluate delirium as an independent predictor of adverse outcomes. The identification and appropriate treatment of this condition early in the ED is an important issue and will likely have an impact on patient outcomes.

Question 3: In ED patients with undifferentiated acute agitation (population), does the use of benzodiazepines or antipsychotics (intervention) reduce agitation and/or adverse effects (outcomes) compared to no treatment (comparison)?

Search strategy

- MEDLINE and Cochrane Library: emergency service, hospital [Majr] AND (benzodiazepines [MeSH] OR antipsychotic agents [MeSH]) AND (psychomotor agitation [MeSH] OR delirium [MeSH])

Pharmacological therapy is necessary in delirious patients who are agitated and are a danger to themselves or others, or are impeding medical evaluation and care. To date there are no randomized, placebo-controlled trials to establish the efficacy or safety of any medication in the management of delirium. Unfortunately, there is little evidence in the literature to guide the pharmacological treatment of acute agitation in the elderly population. Most studies of the emergent sedation of acutely agitated patients are in a younger patient population and typically include substance abusers and patients with underlying psychiatric disturbances (e.g., psychotic or mood disorders), often without other concomitant medical problems. There are several studies that evaluate the long-term management of chronic agitation but not acute agitation in the demented elderly.

Pharmacological options include the benzodiazepines and the typical and atypical antipsychotic agents. For rapid sedation of an acutely agitated patient the intravenous (IV) route is preferred. In situations where establishing an IV route is difficult or hazardous because of the patient's agitation, the intramuscular route may be necessary. In general, oral sedation has little role in the uncooperative, acutely agitated patient in an emergency setting. However, an oral agent may be considered if symptoms of agitation are not severe and may be considered prior to the escalation of symptoms:

1 *Haloperidol*: this is commonly used for the treatment of agitation because its use is rarely associated with respiratory depression, hypotension or anticholinergic side-effects. Numerous studies have demonstrated its efficacy in treating aggression, however most of these studies were of younger patients with a known psychiatric disorder [22]. Haloperidol was recommended as a drug of choice for managing the patient with delirium by the American Psychiatric Association in their 1999 practice guideline [23]. In one retrospective case series of 136 disruptive ED patients (mean age 33 years), haloperidol was demonstrated to be safe and effective [24]. In a randomized double-blind study of hospitalized AIDS (acquired immune deficiency syndrome) patients with delirium, haloperidol or chlorpromazine were found superior to lorazepam in controlling symptoms [25].

2 *Midazolam*: this is the benzodiazepine that has the fastest onset of action and the shortest duration of effect. In a study by Nobay et al. in younger patients (mean age 41 years) IM midazolam had a significantly shorter onset of action and shorter duration of effect than both IM haloperidol and IM lorazepam [26]. In a study comparing IM midazolam, IM ziprasidone and IM droperidol [27], respiratory depression requiring supplemental oxygen administration (but no intubation or bag mask ventilation) was a frequent adverse effect in the midazolam group. Additionally, patients who received midazolam were more likely to require subsequent rescue medication to maintain sedation. An Australian study of patients, primarily with psychiatric disturbances and abusing substances, compared IV midazolam with IV droperidol. Both agents achieved rapid adequate sedation; however, patients receiving midazolam were more likely to need airway management (including one patient who required intubation) and to require further sedation at 60 minutes [28].

3 *Lorazepam*: numerous studies have demonstrated the efficacy of IM lorazepam for the sedation of the agitated young patient in the ED [26,29,30]. Only one randomized controlled trial investigated its use in the delirious elderly patient [31]. In this study, lorazepam was more ef-

fective than placebo in reducing agitation and was well tolerated; however, the risk of respiratory depression was not specifically assessed.

In several clinical scenarios, such as alcohol withdrawal, benzodiazepines are the preferred sedative agent [23,32]. Benzodiazepines are particularly effective in agitated patients with sympathomimetic toxidromes, such as in cocaine and phencyclidine intoxication [33]. In patients with Parkinson's disease, benzodiazepines should be considered because they are not associated with extrapyramidal symptoms, as the antipsychotics drugs are. Benzodiazepines should also be considered when prevention of seizures is important.

The evidence to guide the evaluation and pharmacological management of delirium and acute agitation is limited. A search of the Cochrane Database of Systematic Reviews yielded a review of haloperidol in chronic agitation in elderly demented patients [34]. The Clinical Guideline Clearinghouse (www.guideline.gov) and ACEP clinical policies were also searched.

There is limited evidence from uncontrolled studies to guide current management. Available pharmacological options include antipsychotics and benzodiazepines. The ideal agent for treating undifferentiated acutely agitated patients would be one that is effective with a rapid onset of action and minimal or no side-effects. Patients often require emergent sedation before full knowledge of their medical history and presenting illness is known. Pharmacological therapy in the medically ill and elderly is complicated by their underlying disease process as well as altered pharmacokinetics and pharmacodynamics. The elderly are particularly susceptible to drug side-effects due to decreased renal and hepatic function, as well as confounding polypharmacy. In general, drugs should be administered at the lowest effective dose.

In 1999 the ACEP published a "Clinical policy for the initial approach to patients presenting with altered mental status" which critically reviewed the literature and provided an evaluation framework; it did not address specific pharmacological interventions [35]. In January 2006 the ACEP published the clinical policy: "Critical issues in the diagnosis and management of the psychiatric patient in the emergency department" [22]. This policy focused primarily on medically stable patients with acute psychiatric disturbances; however, the pharmacological management section addresses undifferentiated agitation including delirium. The review found no level A (high degree of clinical certainty) evidence, although it provided a level B recommendation (moderate clinical certainty) for a benzodiazepine or conventional antipsychotic as monotherapy in the acutely agitated undifferentiated patient in the ED.

The American Psychiatric Association published in 1999 the "Practice guideline for the treatment of patients with delirium" [23]. This document reviewed the literature and made graded recommendations based on the strength of evidence regarding psychiatric management, environmental and supportive interventions, and pharmacological interventions. It provided a comprehensive analysis of delirium and emphasized the need for a multidisciplinary approach. Overall, this group recommended haloperidol as the drug of choice for patients with delirium. One systematic review was identified that evaluated the pharmacological management of agitation in emergency settings [36]. However, this study evaluated agitation in a psychiatric ED population and not in a medically ill, delirious population.

In summary, pharmacologic management is necessary in more severe cases of agitation in which patients are a danger to themselves or others, or are impeding medical evaluation and care. Good evidence from well designed studies to guide pharmacologic treatment is limited. At the present time, the best available evidence supports the use of either typical antipsychotics (e.g., haloperidol or droperidol) or a benzodiazepine (e.g. lorazepam or midazolam). The benzodiazepines are preferred in patient with drug related agitation or in patients with Parkinsonism or at risk of anti-cholinergic complications.

Question 4: In ED patients with undifferentiated acute agitation (population), does the combined use of benzodiazepines with antipsychotic agents (intervention) reduce agitation and/or adverse effects (outcomes) compared to either a benzodiazepine or antipsychotic alone (comparison)?

Search strategy

- MEDLINE and Cochrane Library: emergency service, hospital [Majr] AND (benzodiazepines [MeSH] OR antipsychotic agents [MeSH]) AND (psychomotor agitation [MeSH] OR delirium [MeSH])

The combination of an antipsychotic and a benzodiazepine is often used for the rapid tranquilization of acutely agitated, violent, younger patients. A study of haldoperidol and lorazepam, in patients with an average age of only 34.2 years, demonstrated that the combination of the two was more effective than either drug alone [30]. In studies of agitated psychiatric patients by Garza-Trevino et al. [37] and Bieniek et al. [38], the combination of IM lorazepam and IM haloperidol resulted in more rapid onset of sedation than monotherapy. A systematic review by Yildiz et al., of previously published studies of primarily psychiatric ED patients, concluded that a combination of haloperidol and lorazepam was an effective rapid tranquilization method [36]. The treatment of elderly agitated patients with a combination drug therapy has not been studied and in general it is thought best to minimize the number of medications when treating elderly patients. However, the American Psychiatric Association's practice guideline for the treatment of delirium cited combination therapy with a typical antipsychotic and a benzodiazepine as potentially beneficial in that it allows for the use of a lower dose of each medication and thus lower the risks of each drug's side-effects [23].

In summary, once again, high-quality evidence from well-designed studies to guide pharmacological treatment is limited. At the present time, the best available evidence supports the use of monotherapy with either typical antipsychotics (e.g., haloperidol

or droperidol) or a benzodiazepine (e.g., lorazepam or midazolam). Combination treatments are poorly studied and likely too risky in this population of patients.

Question 5: In ED patients with undifferentiated acute agitation (population), does the use of atypical antipsychotic agents (intervention) reduce agitation and/or adverse effects (outcomes) compared to typical antipsychotic agents alone (comparison)?

Search strategy

- Cochrane Library: delirium AND antipsychotics

A Cochrane systematic review identified three studies that compared the efficacy and safety of haloperidol with risperidone, olanzapine and quetiapine in the treatment of delirium [39]. The authors found no evidence that low-dosage haloperidol was more efficacious compared with the atypical antipsychotics in the management of delirium or has a greater frequency of adverse drug effects than atypical antipsychotics. High-dose haloperidol was associated with a greater incidence of side-effects, mainly Parkinsonism, than the atypical antipsychotic agents. These are cautious conclusions based on small studies of limited scope.

In summary, low-dose haloperidol and the agents in the atypical antipsychotic class appear effective in the treatment of delirium. The choice may depend on the availability and physician preference. The side-effects associated with high-dose haloperidol are sufficiently frequent and severe to suggest that this approach should be avoided.

Question 6: In patients presenting to the ED with a diagnosis of delirium (population), does the use of droperidol (intervention) increase the risk of cardiac dysrhythmias (outcomes) compared to the use of other antipsychotic drugs (comparison), in emergency department patients with undifferentiated acute agitation (population)?

Search strategy

- MEDLINE and Cochrane Library: emergency service, hospital [Majr] AND (droperidol OR antipsychotic agents [MeSH]) AND cardiac arrhythmia [MeSH]

Droperidol has been used effectively for the rapid tranquilization of acutely agitated and violent patients in the ED [33]. Droperidol is more potent, more sedating, has a more rapid onset and has a shorter half-life than haloperidol. Intramuscular droperidol has been demonstrated to have more rapid onset and greater efficacy than IM haloperidol alone for patients with acute psychosis [40,41]. In 2001, the Food and Drug Administration (FDA) placed a "black box" warning for droperidol because of reports of death

Table 24.1 Summary of droperidol studies.

Study	*N* Setting/population	Design	Study
Chase & Biros [43]	2468 ED setting/undifferentiated	Retrospective review	Chart review of patients who received droperidol
Richards et al. [33]	202 ED setting/undifferentiated with a majority of substance abusers	Randomized, un-blinded	Droperidol vs lorazepam
Thomas et al. [40]	68 ED setting/undifferentiated	Prospective randomized double-blinded	Droperidol vs haloperidol
Martel et al. [27]	144 ED setting/undifferentiated	Prospective randomized double-blinded	Droperidol vs midazolam vs ziprasidone
Knott et al. [28]	153 ED setting/primarily psychiatric and substance abusers	Randomized double-blinded	Droperidol vs midazolam
Resnick & Burton [41]	27 ED and acute psychiatric ward/acute psychosis	Randomized	Droperidol vs haloperidol

associated with QTc prolongation and the development of torsades de pointes. Some controversy exists in the literature regarding the boxed warning issued to droperidol given the decades of successful clinical use [42].

Using the search above, a total of six studies were identified (Table 24.1). A retrospective review of its use and safety in 2500 ED patients, including 141 patients over the age of 66, found that complications were negligible [43]. In a review of 12,000 patients treated with droperidol for agitation, no dysrhythmic events were observed [44]. There is evidence to suggest that haloperidol, as well as all of the other antipsychotics, is also associated with QTc prolongation and torsades de pointes [45–47].

A study by Martel et al. of acute undifferentiated agitation in patients with a mean age of 37 years (range 19 to 68 years) compared 5 mg of IM midazolam with 5 mg of IM droperidol and 20 mg of IM ziprasidone [27]. All three agents were found to be effective sedative agents, however the ziprasidone group was more likely to remain agitated at 15 minutes. No cardiac dysrhythmias were noted. Respiratory depression requiring supplemental oxygen was more likely with midazolam.

An Australian study of patients primarily with psychiatric disturbances and abusing substances, compared IV midazolam with IV droperidol. Both agents achieved rapid adequate sedation; however, patients receiving midazolam were more likely to need airway management (including one patient who required intubation) and to require further sedation at 60 minutes [28].

There are two small studies that examine the use of droperidol in the prehospital setting. Rosen et al. compared 5 mg of droperidol IV to placebo in 46 patients. There was significantly greater sedation at 5 and 10 minutes, and no significant side-effects except one occurrence of akathisia that had no associated morbidity

[48]. Another study of 53 patients showed a reduction in agitation using IM droperidol without significant adverse events [49].

In summary, droperidol in the hospital and prehospital setting appears safe.

Question 7: In elderly patients hospitalized from the ED (population), are there strategies (intervention) that emergency physicians can employ to reduce the risk of delirium developing (outcome) compared to standard care (comparison)?

Search strategy

- Cochrane Library: delirium AND prevention

There are a number of interventions that have been studied to prevent delirium in hospitalized patients. This issue is an important one for emergency physicians, since the development of delirium in hospitalized patients will increase their length of stay and exacerbate already impressive problems with overcrowding that exist in EDs in developed countries. A variety of issues may contribute to delirium, such as the development of an intercurrent infection, electrolyte abnormalities, and so forth. Interventions may be system-wide or relate to a specific intervention. They include programs of education for ward nursing staff [50], non-pharmacological intervention protocols targeting specific risk factors and implemented by a trained interdisciplinary team [51], and a specialist nursing intervention to educate nursing staff, assess and change medication, encourage mobilization and improve the environment of the patient [52].

A Cochrane review on this topic identified six such trials, involving over 800 patients [53]. To date, the trials have been limited; in fact, no completed studies in hospitalized medical care of the elderly, general surgery, cancer or intensive care patients were identified. In one trial, 126 hip fracture patients were randomized to a multidisciplinary team, and this reduced the development of severe delirium in the post-operative period. In another trial of low-dose haloperidol prophylaxis, there was no difference in delirium incidence but the severity and duration of a delirium episode and length of hospital stay were all reduced. Trials of education were not identified.

In summary, there are some interventions currently in practice that show promise to reduce delirium in hospitalized patients and emergency physicians can likely contribute to this goal by following a few simple steps. Further research should enlighten this field in the coming years.

Conclusions

Returning to the original patient scenario, the staff attempted to verbally calm and reassure the patient; however, he became even more agitated. He was given a dose of haloperidol (5 mg intramuscularly) to calm him down to allow for a thorough medical assessment. Once sedated, examination failed to reveal any abnormalities apart from his altered mental status. His chest radiograph was normal, his electrolytes were all normal, his blood glucose was 10.2 mmol/L and his hemoglobin was 132 g/L. He had no evidence of abnormal leukocytes and his white blood cell count was 11.2. His urinalysis demonstrated 50 white blood cells per high powered field (hpf), 10–20 red blood cells/hpf, some casts and "many" bacteria. A urinary tract infection was diagnosed, antibiotic treatment was initiated and he was admitted to the inpatient general internal medical service. He required further treatment with haloperidol for agitation during his inpatient hospital stay. Although his confusion improved when the infection cleared his mental status did not return to baseline and he was placed in a nursing home upon hospital discharge.

Delirium is a common presenting problem in the ED and may develop in patients following the decision to hospitalize. Emergency physicians may require specialized tools (e.g., CAM) to improve diagnostic sensitivity and should attempt to identify the causes of delirium. The differential diagnosis is wide and investigations must be wide ranging. In many cases, the patient requires chemical restraints to protect themselves and others from injury and to facilitate the completion of the investigation. The typical antipsychotics (e.g., haloperidol and droperidol) remain effective sedative agents for the management of acutely agitated patients. There is evidence that both haloperidol and droperidol, as well as the new generation atypical antipsychotics, are relatively safe although all have been associated with QTc interval prolongation. The Federal Drug Agency's warning for droperidol introduced concerns regarding usage of this agent though subsequent analyses question the validity of the warning. Indeed, the 2006 ACEP clinical policy recommends that droperidol be considered when rapid sedation is required. Finally, efforts to avoid the development of delirium in elderly hospitalized patients while in the ED remain unclear at this time.

References

1 Francis J, Martin D, Kapoor WN. A prospective study of delirium in hospitalized elderly. *JAMA* 1990;**263**:1097–101.

2 Nelson A, Fogel BS, Faust D. Bedside cognitive screening instruments: a critical assessment. *J Nerv Ment Dis* 1986;**174**(2):73–83.

3 Folstein MF, Folstein SE, McHugh PR. Mini-mental state. A practical method for grading the cognitive state of patients for the clinician. *J Psychiatr Res* 1975;**12**(13):189–98.

4 American Psychiatric Association. *Diagnostic and Statistical Manual of Mental Disorders*, 4th edn. American Psychiatric Association, Washington, 1994:124–33.

5 Inouye S, van Dyck C, Alessi C, et al. Clarifying confusion: the confusion assessment method. *Ann Intern Med* 1990;**113**:941–8.

6 Naughton B, Moran M, Kadah H, et al. Delirium and other cognitive impairment in older adults in an emergency department. *Ann Emerg Med* 1995;**25**(6):751–5.

7 Monette J, Galbaud du Fort G, Fung S, et al. Evaluation of the confusion assessment method (CAM) as a screening tool for delirium in the emergency room. *Gen Hosp Psychiatry* 2001;**23**:20–25.

8 Lewis L, Miller K, Morley J, et al. Unrecognized delirium in ED geriatric patients. *Am J Emerg Med* 1995;**13**(2):142–5.

9 Elie M, Rousseau F, Cole M, et al. Prevalence and detection of delirium in elderly emergency department patients. *Can Med Am J* 2000;**163**(8): 977–81.

10 Zou Y, Cole M, Premeau F, et al. Detection and diagnosis of delirium in the elderly: psychiatrist diagnosis, confusion assessment method, or consensus diagnosis? *Int Psycho Geriatr* 1998;**10**(3):303–8.

11 Hustey F, Meldon S, Palmer R. Prevalence and documentation of impaired mental status in elderly emergency department patients. *Acad Emerg Med* 2000;**7**(10):1166.

12 Hustey F, Meldon S. The prevalence and documentation of impaired mental status in elderly emergency department patients. *Ann Emerg Med* 2002;**39**(3):248–53.

13 Hustey F, Meldon S, Smith M, Lex C. The effect of mental status screening on the care of elderly emergency department patients. *Ann Emerg Med* 2003;**41**(5):678–84.

14 Pompei P, Foreman M, Rudberg M, et al. Delirium in hospitalized older persons: outcome and predictors. *J Am Geriatr Soc* 1994;**42**:809–15.

15 Dolan M, Hawkes W, Zimmerman S, et al. Delirium on hospital admission in aged hip fracture patients: prediction of mortality and 2-year functional outcomes. *J Gerontol A Biol Sci Med Sci* 2000;**58**:M527–34.

16 Levkoff SE, Besdine RW, Wetle T. Acute confusional states (delirium) in the hospitalized elderly. *Annu Rev Gerontol Geriatr* 1986;**6**:1–26.

17 Inouye S, Rushing J, Foreman M, et al. Does delirium contribute to poor hospital outcomes? A three-site epidemiologic study. *J Gen Intern Med* 1998;**13**:234–42.

18 Leslie D, Zhang Y, Holford T, et al. Premature death associated with delirium at 1-year follow-up. *Arch Intern Med* 2005;**165**(14):1657–62.

19 Kishi Y, Iwasaki Y, Takezawa K, et al. Delirium in critical care unit patients admitted through an emergency room. *Gen Hosp Psychiatry* 1995;**1**(5):371–9.

20 Kakuma R, du Fort G, Arsenault L, et al. Delirium in older emergency department patients discharged home; effect on survival. *J Am Geriatr Soc* 2003;**5**:443–50.

21 O'Keefe S, Lavan J. The prognostic significance of delirium in older hospital patients. *J Am Geriatr Soc* 1997;**45**(2):247–8.

22 American College of Emergency Physicians. Critical issues in the diagnosis and management of the psychiatric patient in the emergency department. *Ann Emerg Med* 2006;**47**:79–99.

23 American Psychiatric Association. Practice guideline for the treatment of patients with delirium. *Am J Psych* 1999;**156**(Suppl 5):1–20.

24 Clinton JE, Sterner S, Stelmachera Z, Ruiz E. Haloperidol for sedation of disruptive emergency patients. *Ann Emerg Med* 1987;**16**:319–22.

25 Breitbart W, Marotta R, Platt M, et al. A double blind trial of haloperidol, chlorpromazine, and lorazepam in the treatment of delirium in hospitalized AIDS patients. *Am J Psychiatry* 1996;**153**:231–7.

26 Nobay F, Simon B, Levitt M, Dresden G. A prospective, double-blind, randomized trial of midazolam versus haloperidol versus lorazepam in the chemical restraint of violent and severely agitated patients. *Acad Emerg Med* 2004;**11**:744–9.

27 Martel M, Serzinger A, Miner J, et al. Management of acute undifferentiated agitation in the emergency department: a randomized double-blind trial of droperidol, ziprasidone, and midazolam. *Acad Emerg Med* 2005;**12**:1167–72.

28 Knott J, Taylor D, Castle D. Randomized clinical trial comparing intravenous midazolam and droperidol for sedation of the acutely agitated patient in the emergency department. *Ann Emerg Med* 2006;**47**:61–7.

29 Salzman C, Solomon D, Miyawaki E, et al. Parenteral lorazepam versus parenteral haloperidol for the control of psychotic disruptive behavior. *J Clin Psychiatry* 1991;**52**:177–80.

30 Battaglia J, Moss S, Rush J, et al. Haloperidol, lorazepam, or both for psychotic agitation? A multicenter, prospective, double-blind, emergency department study. *Am J Emerg Med* 1997;**15**:335–40.

31 Meehan KM, Wang H, David SR, et al. Comparison of rapidly acting intramuscular olanzapine, lorazepam and placebo: a double-blind, randomized study in acutely agitated patients with dementia. *Neuropsychopharmacology* 2002;**26**:494–504.

32 Mayo-Smith M, Beecher L, Fischer T, et al. Management of alcohol withdrawal delirium. An evidence-based practice guideline. *Arch Intern Med* 2004;**164**:1405–12.

33 Richards JR, Derlet RW, Duncan DR. Chemical restraint for the agitated patient in the emergency department: lorazepam versus droperidol. *J Emerg Med* 1998;**16**:567–73.

34 Lonegran E, Luxenberg J, Colford J. Haloperidol for agitation in dementia. *Cochrane Database Syst Rev* 2002;**2**:CD002852 (doi: 10.1002/14651858.CD002852).

35 American College of Emergency Physicians. Clinical policy for the initial approach to patients presenting with altered mental status. *Ann Emerg Med* 1999;**33**:251–81.

36 Yildiz A, Sachs G, Turgay A. Pharmacologic management of agitation in emergency settings. *Emerg Med J* 2003;**20**:339–46.

37 Garza-Trevino E, Hollister L, Overall J, et al. Efficacy of combinations of intramuscular antipsychotics and sedative-hypnotics for control of psychotic agitation. *Am J Psychiatry* 1989;**146**:1598–601.

38 Bieniek S, Wonby R, Penalver A, et al. A double-blind study of lorazepam versus the combination of haloperidol and lorazepam in managing agitation. *Pharmacotherapy* 1998;**18**:57–62.

39 Lonergan E, Britton AM, Luxenberg J, Wyller T. Antipsychotics for delirium. *Cochrane Database Syst Rev* 2007;**2**:CD005594 (doi: 10.1002/14651858.CD005594.pub2).

40 Thomas H, Schwartz E, Petrilli R. Droperidol versus haloperidol for chemical restraint of agitated and combative patients. *Ann Emerg Med* 1992;**21**:407–13.

41 Resnick M, Burton B. Droperidol versus haloperidol in the initial management of agitated patients. *J Clin Psychiatry* 1984;**45**:298–9.

42 Horowitz B, Bizovi K, Morena R. Droperidol – behind the black box warning. *Acad Emerg Med* 2002;**9**:615–18.

43 Chase PB, Biros MH. A retrospective review of the use and safety of droperidol in a large, high-risk, inner-city emergency department patient population. *Acad Emerg Med* 2002;**9**:1402–10.

44 Shale J, Shale C, Mastin W. A review of the safety and efficacy of droperidol for the rapid sedation of severely agitated and violent patients. *J Clin Psychiatry* 2003;**64**:500–505.

45 Wilt J, Minnema A, Johnson R, Rosenblum A. Torsades de pointes associated with the use of intravenous haloperidol. *Ann Intern Med* 1993;**119**:391–4.

46 Sharma N, Rosman H, Padhi D, Tisdale J. Torsades de pointes associated with intravenous haloperidol in critically ill patients. *Am J Cardiol* 1998;**81**:238–40.

47 Jackson T, Ditmanson L, Phibba B. Torsades de pointes and low-dose oral haloperidol. *Arch Intern Med* 1997;**157**:2013–15.

48 Rosen C, Ratliff A, Wolfe R, et al. The efficacy of intravenous droperidol in the prehospital setting. *J Emerg Med* 1997;**15**:13–17.

49 Hick J, Mahoney B, Lappe M. Prehospital sedation with intramuscular droperidol: a one-year pilot. *Prehosp Emerg Care* 2001;**5**:391–4.

50 Rockwood K. Educational interventions in delirium. *Dement Geriatr Cogn Disord* 1999;**10**:426–9.

51 Inouye S, Bogardus S, Charpentier PA. A multicomponent intervention to prevent delirium in hospitalized older patients. *N Engl J Med* 1999;**340**:669–76.

52 Wanich C, Sullivan-Marx E, Gottlieb G, Johnson J. Functional status outcomes of a nursing intervention in hospitalized elderly. *Image J Nurs Sch* 1992;**24**(3):201–7.

53 Siddiqi N, Stockdale R, Britton AM, Holmes J. Interventions for preventing delirium in hospitalised patients. *Cochrane Database Syst Rev* 2007;**2**:CD005563 (doi: 10.1002/14651858.CD005563.pub2).

25 Caring for the Elderly

Christopher R. Carpenter[1], Michael Stern[2] & Arthur B. Sanders[3]

[1] Division of Emergency Medicine, St. Louis School of Medicine, Washington University, St. Louis, USA
[2] Department of Medicine, Division of Emergency Medicine, Weill Cornell Medical Center, New York, USA
[3] Department of Emergency Medicine, University of Arizona College of Medicine, Tucson, USA

Case scenario

An 80-year-old male came to the emergency department (ED) after a fall, which occurred in the course of getting up at night to urinate. His daughter brought him to the ED out of concern that he might have broken his right hip in the fall. He was able to walk but complained of pain in the right hip area. He had no loss of consciousness with the fall, did not hit his head, and denied chest pain or shortness of breath. He stated he had been feeling poorly for a week and his daughter confirmed that he had "not been himself". The patient lived independently and his daughter checked in on him each weekend. Past medical history included: myocardial infarction with angioplasty 10 years previously, stable congestive heart failure, diabetes mellitus, hypertension, hypothyroidism, dyslipidemia, seasonal allergies, depression and osteoarthritis. There was no history of dementia. Medications included: metoprolol, lisinopril, furosemide, digoxin, levothyroxine, atorvastatin, niaspan, rosiglitazone, glyburide, aspirin, mirtazapine, diazepam, naproxen and diphenhydramine.

On physical exam, vital signs were: BP 160/90; pulse 90 beats/min, respirations 18 breaths/min, temperature 38°C (oral) and oxygen saturation 95% on room air. Chest and abdominal exam were unremarkable; mental status exam showed the patient to be oriented but unable to recall three items. The neurological exam was otherwise non-focal. There was mild tenderness in the right greater trochanteric area but full range of motion of the hip.

The physician on duty noted no radiographic evidence of a hip fracture, but the family was more interested in understanding why the patient fell. His daughter was concerned by his apparent cognitive deficit on mental status testing. The emergency physician identified the patient's low grade fever and polypharmacy as potential clues to the etiology of the fall. The differential diagnosis included infection, adverse drug reaction or drug interaction,

acute coronary syndrome with exacerbation of congestive heart, a metabolic abnormality, or a combination of these. In addition to hip X-rays, the ED work-up included chest radiograph, electrocardiogram (ECG) and laboratory blood work. The only positive findings were an elevated blood glucose (10 mmol/L) and a urine analysis showing 50 white blood cells per high powered field. The patient was started on antibiotics and admitted to the hospital with plans to re-evaluate his medications and mental status after his urinary tract infection cleared.

Background

According to the most recent US Census Bureau data, there are currently more than 35 million people aged 65 years and over – that is, 13% of the population – living in the United States. Similar statistics can be found in other parts of the developed world. By 2030, this percentage will increase to approximately 21% of the US population, or 76 million people. Moreover, the fastest growing segment of the population is the age group 85 and older [1]. Compared with previous generations, older people today are living longer and healthier lives, remaining independent and highly functional well past retirement. At the same time, many still suffer from profound functional impairment and disabling disease. Acute exacerbations of chronic illness and severe decompensation from a debilitated baseline cause elderly patients to seek emergency care in ever increasing numbers. This in turn places a premium on a number of issues of assessment and management of this population in the ED, some of which have been specially targeted for focused consideration in this chapter.

The complexity of elderly patients' clinical presentations and subsequent management, their consumption of ED resources, and their length of stay in the ED are all significantly higher than for younger patients [2,3]. The most recent United States ambulatory care ED data noted over 50 visits per 100 persons age 65 or older, with 70 ED visits per 100 persons over age 75 [4]. The trend of increased ED usage among older patients for both their acute and sub-acute health care needs is projected to continue in Canada

Evidence-based Emergency Medicine. Edited by Brian H. Rowe
© 2009 Blackwell Publishing, ISBN: 978-1-4051-6143-5.

[5], Australia [6], the United Kingdom [7] and the United States [8], further exacerbating ED overcrowding and substantial delays awaiting inpatient bed availability for all patients. In addition, traditional hospitalization is not without risk, including nosocomial infections, delirium and iatrogenic injuries [9]. One novel solution is the hospital in home (HIH) care model, which brings health care professionals to the patient's home to provide active treatment for a condition that would otherwise mandate traditional hospital inpatient management.

The elderly represent a population of ED patients with unique characteristics that differ significantly compared with younger patients. Emergency physicians must incorporate many of the following considerations into their clinical practice in order to provide what the Society for Academic Emergency Medicine Geriatric Task Force recommended as a more comprehensive model of care [10]. One such model, comprehensive geriatric assessment (CGA), is a multidisciplinary, interdisciplinary diagnostic evaluation to both coordinate and integrate treatment plans [11]. CGA can be applied to either inpatients or outpatients. Inpatient models can be geographically localized to one area of an institution or a multidisciplinary team assessing patients to deliver recommendations to the physicians caring for the patients. The effects of the physiology of aging (i.e., loss of physiological reserve, diminished hemostatic mechanisms, altered metabolism) produce atypical disease presentations, as well as important differences in how patients evolve clinically while in the emergency setting. The particular pathophysiology of older patients is manifested by disproportionately represented geriatric syndromes, such as falls, polypharmacy and delirium, which almost never follow the tenet of Ocham's razor.

Dementia is highly prevalent in the elderly population and represents the majority of mental status impairment. Alzheimer's disease and cerebrovascular ischemia (vascular dementia) are irreversible and represent the two most common causes of dementia. Age is the strongest risk factor for dementia affecting approximately 3–11% of people aged 65 years and older and 25–47% of those older than 85 in the United States, with an annual economic cost estimated to be $100 billion [12–14]. In Beijing, the prevalence of dementia is 2.5% over age 60, while England [15], Europe [16] and Australia [17] report prevalence rates similar to the USA, and all are increasing [17–19]. Among the patients over age 65 who present to an ED, cognitive dysfunction is even more common, with an estimated prevalence rate ranging from 16% to 22% [20,21], yet clinicians often do not recognize dementia on routine history and physical examination [22–24].

Among community-dwelling older adults, 30–60% fall each year and approximately half of them experience multiple falls [25]. Ten percent of falls result in significant injury, and up to 50% of older people requiring hospitalization for injuries from a fall die within 1 year [26]. Fall incidence rises with increasing age and is highest among individuals > 80 years old [25,27,28]. In the USA, 18% of ED visits are by people over age 65, and falls account for approximately 10% of their visits to EDs and 6% of urgent hospitalizations, most of which are due to hip fractures [29]. Between 25% and 75% of community-dwelling individuals with

fall-related hip fractures do not recover their pre-fracture level of function in ambulation or activities of daily living (ADLs) [30].

Disproportionate co-morbidity coupled with diminished physiological reserve, increased cognitive dysfunction and atypical presentations all result in increased disease-specific mortality for older adults. One quantitative measure of treatment effect is the number needed to treat (NNT), the inverse of the absolute risk reduction (see Chapter 1) [31,32]. If treatment effects remain constant over age groups, then increases in age-related mortality will result in a lower NNT [31]. For example, assume a hypothetical therapy reduces mortality risk by 10% (relative risk reduction) in a study including both younger and older patients and that the mortality risk in patients younger than 50 years is 10% without treatment and 20% in patients older than 50 years without treatment. The drug will reduce the 10% mortality risk in the younger patients by 10%, yielding an absolute risk reduction of 1% and a NNT of 100. The same drug will reduce the 20% risk in the older patients by the same 10%, yielding an absolute risk reduction of 2% and a NNT of 50. Hence only half as many older patients as younger patients will need to be treated with the drug over the time period in question to save one life. Failing to recognize this principle, clinicians sometimes express reluctance about recommending well-established interventions to older adults due to concerns about increased risk of adverse effects. In withholding such recommendations, they frequently overlook the fact that the increased therapeutic impact of the intervention in the higher risk older patient tends to far outweigh the increased risk of adverse effects. In other words, the decrease in NNT is clinically much more significant than is the corresponding decrease in number needed to harm. In deciding whether to apply the results of effective interventional trials to older adults, therefore, one should not use age alone as a contraindication to extrapolating similar or better results to geriatric patients [33].

Clinical questions

In order to address the issues of most relevance to geriatrics and to help in searching the literature for the evidence regarding these issues, you structure your clinical questions as recommended in Chapter 1.

1 In older ED patients with possible dementia (population), what are the sensitivity and specificity (diagnostic test characteristics) of dementia screening tools (tests) to diagnose dementia (outcome)?

2 In older ED patients at high risk for falls (population), do fall prevention tools (intervention) reduce the number of falls, the risk of recurrent falls or fall-related injuries (outcomes) compared with no application of fall prevention tools (control)?

3 In older community-dwelling adults presenting to the ED with uncomplicated, non-critical medical conditions (e.g., isolated cellulitis or pneumonia) (population), does admission to "hospital in home" (intervention) reduce mortality, re-hospitalization rates, hospital length of stay or patient or care-giver satisfaction scores (outcomes) compared with those managed in traditional inpatient hospitals (control)?

4 Do older adults in the ED (population) who undergo polypharmacy screening prior to ED discharge (intervention), have lower 6-month adverse drug-related events (outcomes) compared with those older ED adults who do not (control)?

5 Do older adult ED patients (population) who undergo comprehensive geriatric assessment (CGA) prior to ED discharge (intervention) have lower hospitalization rates (outcomes) at 1 year compared with those older ED adults not receiving CGA (control)?

6 In older adult ED patients being discharged to home (population), does the use of prognostic screening tools such as the Triage Risk Screening Tool or the Identification of Seniors at Risk tool (prognostic indicators) identify a subset of patients at high risk for death or decline (outcomes) calling for admission or close outpatient follow-up instead of standard medical management?

General search strategy

Searching for systematic reviews, meta-analyses and high-quality randomized controlled trials (RCTs), the initial search strategy for questions related to therapy included the Cochrane Library, MEDLINE and EMBASE. Because diagnostic and prognostic questions are not often readily identified in the Cochrane Library, MEDLINE clinical queries (sensitive) were also used for such questions.

Critical appraisal of the literature

Question 1: In older ED patients with possible dementia (population), what are the sensitivity and specificity (diagnostic test characteristics) of dementia screening tools (tests) to diagnose dementia (outcome)?

Search strategy

- MEDLINE and EMBASE: dementia AND (sensitiv*[title/abstract] OR sensitivity and specificity[MeSH terms] OR diagnos*[title/abstract] OR diagnosis[MeSH:noexp] OR diagnostic*[MeSH:noexp] OR diagnosis, differential[MeSH:noexp] OR diagnosis[subheading:noexp])

The search strategy for the Cochrane Library identified no systematic reviews addressing this question. The MEDLINE and EMBASE searches identified several articles relevant to this question including one systematic review [34–36].

Twenty-five different screening instruments have been described [34], such as the Short Portable Mental Status Questionnaire, Clock Drawing Test, Modified Mini Mental Status Examination (MMSE), Mini-Cog, Six-Item Screener (SIS), Hopkins' Verbal Learning Test and the 7-minute screen. None of these have been adequately evaluated in primary care settings or the ED [13].

The MMSE consists of 19 questions and tasks, each scored by an observer to a total of 30 possible points, with a higher score designating a higher level of cognitive function [37]. Among other factors affecting "normal values", the median MMSE varies by age, gender, race and educational level [34,38]. The standard MMSE cut-off score is defined as abnormal if it is equal to or below 24, yielding a median positive likelihood ratio (+LR) of 6.3 and a median negative likelihood ratio (−LR) of 0.19 for cognitive dysfunction on a general population of adults aged 60–100 [34,39]. All studies reviewed used the DSM-IV (or similar criteria) as the reference standard. Eight studies evaluating the MMSE were examined and found to have similar findings to the 1996 Agency for Health Care Research and Quality narrative review and guidelines [40]. The MMSE provides the best dementia screening tool for primary care populations, but generally requires 7–10 minutes to administer. It may therefore be less ideal for ED settings. Furthermore, the MMSE suffers from false positives in less educated populations [41], false negatives in those with higher education [42], and diminished ability to identify mild impairment [43]. Another feature limiting the practicality of the MMSE as an ED screening tool is a renewed interest in copyright issues [44] aimed at restricting the use of the MMSE except from authorized reproductions [37,38] or the Psychological Assessment Resources, Inc. website [45].

The Hopkins' Verbal Learning Test may be preferred for mild impairment or in highly educated patients [43]. In comparing a cross-section of geriatric psychiatry patients with mild dementia and those with no dementia using DSM-IV as the criterion standard, the Hopkins' Verbal Learning Test demonstrated a +LR of 4.8 and −LR of 0.05 without diminished discriminatory ability based upon education compared with the MMSE, which demonstrated a +LR of 12.6 and a −LR of 0.13 [43]. The studies that have evaluated elderly patients in the ED have been small, cross-sectional and have predominantly focused on the shorter cognitive function tests [20,46]. One single-center, prospective, cross-sectional study compared the test characteristics and accuracy of the SIS and Mini-Cog in 149 older ED patients by randomizing subjects to have either the SIS or the Mini-Cog. The study used the MMSE as the criterion standard and found the SIS to be superior, with a +LR of 6.6 (95% CI: 3.5 to 13) and a −LR of 0.06 (95% CI: 0.01 to 0.44) [36].

Finally, several screening tests employing informant-based functional questionnaires, such as the Functional Activities Questionnaire (FAQ) [40] and the Informant Questionnaire on Cognitive Decline in the Elderly (IQCODE), have been studied. A meta-analysis summarized 10 studies (involving subjects from hospital, clinic and community settings) directly comparing an informant questionnaire with brief cognitive tests (MMSE) as the criterion standard; the informant questionnaire was found to have a summary +LR and −LR of 4.3 and 0.18, respectively [35]. Although the author concluded that informant questionnaires are as effective as brief cognitive tests at screening for dementia, the meta-analysis did not provide any subject inclusion criteria or reference the accepted criterion standard DSM-IV.

In summary, the evidence supports the ED use of the MMSE to test for dementia in older adults recognizing that alternative screening tests more accurately identify early-stage cognitive dysfunction and dementia in highly educated populations.

Question 2: In older ED patients at high risk for falls (population), do fall prevention tools (intervention) reduce the number of falls, the risk of recurrent falls or fall-related injuries (outcomes) compared with no application of fall prevention tools (control)?

Search strategy

- Cochrane, MEDLINE and EMBASE: falls AND prevention AND MEDLINE AND (systematic review OR meta-analysis OR metaanalysis) AND elderly

Our search yielded three systematic reviews related to our question [47–49] and one individual trial of direct relevance to an ED-based falls prevention program [50]. The only randomized controlled study based in the ED, the Prevention of Falls in the Elderly Trial (PROFET), was an intervention to decrease the risk of recurrent falls in community-dwelling patients over the age of 65 who presented to the ED having fallen. It involved a structured interdisciplinary approach that resulted in a significant reduction in the number of falls [50]. Participants randomized to the intervention group underwent a detailed medical and occupational therapy assessment by unspecified medical personnel with referral to relevant services if indicated, versus no such assessment in the control group. The risk of falling was significantly reduced in the intervention group (OR = 0.39; 95% CI: 0.23 to 0.66), as was the risk of recurrent falls (OR = 0.33; 95% CI: 0.16 to 0.68) at 12-month follow-up with a NNT of 5 (95% CI: 3.4 to 9.6) to prevent one fall. In addition, the odds of hospital admission were lower in the intervention group and the decline in the Barthel ADL scores with time was greater in the control group ($P < 0.00001$).

Gillespie et al.'s Cochrane review assessed the effects of primary and secondary prevention interventions designed to reduce the incidence of falls in elderly people living in the community and in institutional or hospital care [47]. Unfortunately, none of these interventions were based specifically in the ED setting, although many minor and injurious falls result in ED presentation. Trials that evaluated multidisciplinary, multi-factorial, health/environment risk factor screening / intervention programs in the community appeared most likely to be beneficial. Programs involving muscle strengthening, balance retraining, home hazard assessment and modification, withdrawal of psychotropic medication and Tai Chi group exercise were also likely to be beneficial in the prevention of falls. McClure et al. conducted a Cochrane review to assess the effectiveness of population-based interventions, defined as coordinated, community-wide, multi-strategy initiatives, for reducing fall-related injuries among older people [48]. All five included studies showed downward trends in fall-related injuries.

An important limitation of available evidence is the paucity of trials of ED-based interventions. A systematic review to determine whether EDs should institute a falls prevention program for older patients was conducted as part of a project to evaluate prevention and screening interventions in the ED [49]. Of 26 unreferenced articles that were reviewed, none investigated the primary or secondary prevention of falls in older ED patients. Further research is needed to determine both the diagnostic test characteristics of ED-based falls prevention screening tools and the efficacy of those prevention tools in reducing both the number of falls and the morbidity and mortality associated with fall-related injuries [51].

In summary, one RCT of a structured ED-based secondary falls prevention program reduced falls and hospital admissions while preventing functional decline among older adults. Community-based primary and secondary fall prevention programs have proven successful at reducing fall-related injury, but none have been initiated from the ED.

Question 3: In older community-dwelling adults presenting to the ED with uncomplicated, non-critical medical conditions (e.g., isolated cellulitis or pneumonia) (population), does admission to "hospital in home" (intervention) reduce mortality, re-hospitalization rates, hospital length of stay or patient or care-giver satisfaction scores (outcomes) compared with those managed in traditional inpatient hospitals (control)?

Search strategy

- MEDLINE and EMBASE: hospital at home AND ((clinical[title/abstract] AND trial[title/abstract]) OR clinical trials[MeSH terms] OR clinical trial[publication type] OR random*[title/abstract] OR random allocation[MeSH terms] OR therapeutic use[MeSH subheading])) AND elderly AND home care services, hospital-based/standards

Our search yielded one Cochrane review [52] related to our question and two relevant clinical trials [53,54]. The Cochrane review included 22 trials, of which 13 evaluated predominantly elderly medical inpatients, although only five of these included schemes operating from an ED [55–59]. Two additional studies have been published since the Cochrane review [53,54]. These two trials and the five emergency medicine pertinent trials in the Cochrane review are summarized in Table 25.1. Overall, these studies lend support to the evidence base on HIH and suggest mortality is unaffected by an HIH option. Moreover, this option unblocks ED and inpatient beds, results in few readmissions, and improves patient and provider satisfaction.

There remain several issues associated with this approach. First, patient selection is complex and safety is a major concern. In all of

Table 25.1 Summary of evidence table for hospital in the home compared to traditional inpatient care.

Study	Sample	Intervention/outcome	Effect size	Conclusion
Davies et al. [56]	ED-based RCT of 150 patients with COPD	HIH versus inpatient care. Outcomes included 2-week and 3-month mortality and admission	M: ND (9% vs 8%) A: 9% HIH admission	ND
Caplan et al. [55]	ED-based RCT of 100 patients with GM problems	HIH (within 24 hours of admission) Outcomes included ED LOS, complications, patient and care-giver satisfaction and mortality	ED LOS: 4.4-hour reduction M: ND (3 vs 4) PS: 78% vs 40%, $P < 0.0001$ CS: 55% vs 27%, $P > 0.0001$ C: reduced in HIH	HIH reduces ED LOS and hospital-related complications while improving patient and care-giver satisfaction without increasing mortality
Leff et al. [54]	ED-based cohort study of 454 patients with selected GM problems	HIH Outcomes included home arrival of nurse, physician and medical supplies, ED LOS, complications, patient satisfaction and cost of care	Nurse: 20 minutes Physician: 1.8 hours Supplies: 2.2 hours ED LOS: favored control (5.5 vs 6.4 hours, $P < 0.001$) Delirium: OR 0.26 (95% CI: 0.12 to 0.57) Critical C: 0% HIH vs 6%, $P < 0.001$) PS: 7 vs 6 ($P < 0.001$) favoring HIH Cost: HIH saved US$2398 (95% CI: $1376 to $3631)	HIH increased ED LOS by 1 hour, but reduced geriatric complication rates and patient/care giver satisfaction without increasing mortality
Gonzalez-Barcala et al. [53]	ED-based cohort study of patients with acute respiratory conditions (pneumonia or COPD exacerbations)	HIH compared to sex-matched controls who met the HIH-entry criteria but were instead admitted to hospital Outcomes included 3-month mortality, LOS and readmission	LOS: 7 vs 12 days, $P = 0.001$) 3-month A: ND (14% vs 24%) M: ND (16% vs 10%, $P = 0.451$).	HIH decreased LOS without increasing 3-month mortality or readmission rates
Ricauda et al. [57]	ED-based cohort of geriatric patients within 24 hours of first acute ischemic stroke symptom onset	HIH compared to GMW Outcomes included 6-month mortality, functional impairment, depression and admission to rehabilitation and long-term facilities	M: ND (23% vs 21%) FI: ND D: favors HIH (GMW 17 vs HIH 10, $P < 0.001$) Disposition home: favors HIH (GMW 46% vs HIH 98%, $P < 0.001$)	ND in mortality HIH reduces patient depression and nursing home admissions
Shepperd et al. [58]	Hospital-based RCT of 538 patients aged > 60 years with ED discharge home or early hospital discharge for orthopedic surgery or medical admission	HIH compared to GMW Outcomes included 3-month general health status, physical limitations, admission, mortality and patient and care-giver satisfaction	Elderly medical patients A: GMW 11% vs HIH 26% M: 9% GMW vs HIH 18% PS favored HIH: GMW 20% vs HIH 62% CS: ND COPD A: GMW 35% vs HIH 53% M: ND (18% vs 20%) CS: ND	ND in mortality, readmission rates, or care-giver satisfaction Medical patients prefer HIH care, COPD patients prefer GMW care
Wilson et al. [59]	Office-based RCT of 199 patients (median age 84 years) referred for hospitalization	HIH compared to GMW. Outcomes included LOS, 2-week and 3-month functional impairment, mortality and admission	FI: ND 3-month M: GMW 31% vs HIH 26% Initial hospital LOS: GMW 14.5 days vs HIH 8 days, $P = 0.026$; Total care LOS: GMW 16 days vs HIH 9 days, $P = 0.031$	ND in FI, mortality or readmission rates, but significantly reduced LOS favoring HIH model

A, admission; C, complications; CI, confidence interval; COPD, chronic obstructive pulmonary disease; CS, care-giver satisfaction; D, depression; ED, emergency department; FI, functional impairment; GM, general medicine; GMW, general medical ward; HIH, hospital in home; LOS, length of stay; M, mortality; ND, no difference; OR, odds ratio; PS, patient satisfaction; RCT, randomized controlled trial.

the studies, patients were carefully selected for this option. For example, because of the extensive criteria used by Leff et al. [54], 78% of all potentially eligible subjects were removed from eligibility. Reassuringly, 60% of eligible subjects who were approached did consent to the HIH model of care. Second, while the overall costs associated with an HIH eventually appear less expensive than the inpatient admission, a coordinated and dedicated team appears to be necessary to manage the patients and administrative issues associated with a problem of this nature. Finally, as emergency patients increase in complexity and acuity, the viability of a program of this nature may be reduced. For example, as fewer of these sick elderly ED patients qualify for discharge, application of the HIH may be restricted to fewer patients or only in EDs seeing less acute patients.

In summary, current evidence suggests that compared with traditional hospital admissions, HIH care for selected geriatric populations with stroke, chronic obstructive pulmonary disease or uncomplicated infections may lower costs without influencing 6-month mortality. Moreover, HIH appears to reduce iatrogenic complications and enhance patient and care-giver satisfaction. Evolving therapeutic options and local resource availability will likely impact settings and situations where HIH is most beneficial to individuals and communities, but widespread application of an out-of-hospital care model will require effectiveness trials to verify acceptability and patient safety in environments where alternatives to inpatient care are not already established [51]. The expense of designing and implementing HIH models among heterogeneous communities are potential obstacles to large studies.

Question 4: Do older adults in the ED (population) who undergo polypharmacy screening prior to ED discharge (intervention), have lower 6-month adverse drug-related events (outcomes) compared with those older ED adults who do not (control)?

Search strategy

- MEDLINE and EMBASE: polypharmacy AND ((clinical[title/abstract] AND trial[title/abstract]) OR clinical trials[MeSH terms] OR clinical trial[publication type] OR random*[title/abstract] OR random allocation[MeSH terms] OR therapeutic use[MeSH subheading])

Our search yielded no relevant systematic reviews evaluating the assessment or treatment of geriatric polypharmacy in the ED. Our MEDLINE review revealed several non-ED-based RCTs of older adults of limited relevance to emergency medicine and two trials of pharmacist interventions during or following an ED evaluation [60,61]. A British RCT of home-based pharmacist intervention on patients over the age of 80 within 8 weeks of ED discharge demonstrated a higher subsequent readmission rate in the intervention group compared to the control group (RR 1.3, 95% CI1.07-1.68) with no difference in mortality or quality of life measures [60].

A subsequent economic analysis of these results did not find home-based medication review by a pharmacist in those over the age of 80 to be cost-effective [62]. An uncontrolled, single-center, ED-based pharmacist intervention demonstrated over US$1 million savings over 3 months; however, this study did not specifically assess the recognition of over-prescribing or adverse drug-related events involving geriatric patients. Pharmacist interventions included dosing recommendations, allergy and drug duplication notification, drug compatibility issues, and alternative drug options [61]. Other non-ED-based RCTs have also demonstrated no effect of home-based medication reviews by a pharmacist on hospital admissions, mortality or death, although some demonstrate a reduction in overall prescribing.

In summary, geriatric polypharmacy is an expensive, prevalent problem resulting in iatrogenic adverse drug reactions and medication non-compliance. Effective ED-based interventions to identify or reduce polypharmacy are yet to be reported or validated.

Question 5: Do older adult ED patients (population) who undergo comprehensive geriatric assessment (CGA) prior to ED discharge (intervention), have lower subsequent hospitalization rates (outcome) at 1 year compared to those older ED adults not receiving CGA (control)?

Search strategy

- MEDLINE, EMBASE and Cochrane: comprehensive geriatric assessment AND ((clinical[title/abstract] AND trial[title/abstract]) OR clinical trials[MeSH terms] OR clinical trial[publication type] OR random*[title/abstract] OR random allocation[MeSH terms] OR therapeutic use[MeSH subheading])

Our search identified one Cochrane review protocol [63], two meta-analyses [64,65] and one relevant clinical trial [66]. One Australian randomized controlled ED-based outpatient model of CGA, the Discharge of Elderly from the ED (DEED II) study, was not included in either meta-analysis and consisted of a geriatric nurse's intake evaluation of subjects' functional status and presenting illness, which occurred after the decision to discharge home had been made. For the next month, each subject's case was individually discussed at weekly multidisciplinary care meetings including a geriatrician, physiotherapist and geriatric nurse with recommendations forwarded to the respective patient's primary care provider. The primary outcome measure was all hospital admissions within 30 days and 18 months of the index ED evaluation. Subjects, physicians and researchers were not blinded to the allocation arm and researchers did not ascertain whether recommended interventions actually occurred. CGA patients demonstrated reductions in hospitalization at 30 days (16.5% vs 22.2%, $P = 0.048$) and 18 months (44.4% vs 54.3%, $P = 0.007$). The DEED II research team had a pre-existing framework upon which to build their CGA outpatient model limiting the external validity of their study [66].

Stuck's meta-analysis of 28 inpatient studies, involving over 9000 randomized subjects, demonstrated a 35% 6-month mortality reduction and a 12% reduction in readmission rates while preserving physical and cognitive functioning with CGA [65]. One subsequent meta-analysis of outpatient CGA for the frail elderly found no mortality benefit [64]. However, another meta-analysis of home visits to prevent nursing home admission and functional decline observed a reduction in functional decline among trials using multi-dimensional assessments [67].

In summary, the current evidence on effectiveness of CGA involves a complex series of interdependent interventions on a heterogeneous group of patients. The challenge is to identify the effective components, in addition to those populations most likely to benefit from ED-initiated interventions. Future research should delineate the impact of inpatient and outpatient CGA teams upon primary outcomes of independent survival and death, along with secondary outcome measures of functional status, resource use, most effective models (ward vs team), optimal team compositions, admission criteria (age vs diagnosis) and regional sustainability [51].

Question 6: In older adult ED patients being discharged to home (population), does the use of prognostic screening tools such as the Triage Risk Screening Tool or the Identification of Seniors at Risk tool (prognostic indicators) identify a subset of patients at high risk for death or decline (outcomes) calling for admission or close outpatient follow-up instead of standard medical management?

Search strategy

- MEDLINE, EMBASE and Cochrane: geriatric screening emergency AND (incidence[MeSH:noexp] OR mortality[MeSH terms] OR follow up studies[MeSH:noexp] OR prognos*[text word] OR predict*[text word] OR course*[text word])

Our search identified one systematic review [68] and two relevant trials [69,70]. The systematic review identified 26 relevant articles addressing elderly adults discharged home from the ED. Some of the research they identified included observational studies or retrospective reviews of interventions such as telephone follow-up, pre-discharge physical therapy, functional assessment, case coordinator directed interventions, staff educational models, rapid placement services, and home health visitors following ED discharge. The systematic review also identified six ED-based RCTs, including one pre-discharge screening tool. The three most important studies are summarized in Table 25.2.

McCusker et al. developed and validated the Identification of Seniors at Risk (ISAR; Box 25.1) tool, a six-item questionnaire completed by patients in the ED to identify those at increased post-discharge risk of death, nursing home admission or clinically significant functional decline within 6 months [69]. Functional

decline was assessed using the Older American Resources and Services Activities of Daily Living Scale during enrollment and via telephone follow-up at 6 months. Two or more affirmative responses on ISAR identified a high-risk older adult characterized by 10% 6-month mortality, 2.9% increased risk of institutionalization and 16% increased risk of diminished functional independence. A subsequent RCT used a research associate to administer the ISAR to eligible patients. The ISAR is limited by the patient's ability to understand and complete the survey and has only been validated in Montreal.

Meldon et al. prospectively evaluated a different six-item questionnaire, the Triage Risk Screening Tool (TRST; Box 25.2), administered by nursing staff at two urban academic EDs. Two or more affirmative responses on the TRST were considered high risk [70]. An additional single-center evaluation of the TRST has noted prognostic accuracy in identifying older adults at increased risk of 30- and 120-day functional decline [71].

In summary, two older adult prognostic screening tools have been developed to identify the subset at risk for increased mortality and functional decline in the months following ED discharge: ISAR and TRST. Acting upon the ISAR results reduced functional decline, but increased health care resource utilization and returns to the ED.

Conclusions

The elderly gentleman with the fall and fever would benefit from a review of indications and age appropriateness for his multiple medications. Furthermore, age- and education-appropriate screening for cognitive dysfunction could accurately identify dementia while still in the ED. If the decision to discharge home had been made, prognostic screening tools would have identified whether he was at high risk for short-term functional decline or ED recidivism to guide the emergency medicine clinicians in arranging close primary physician follow-up and family monitoring. Future alternatives to traditional hospitalization models may permit this patient the opportunity to safely recover from his infection-related fall in the comfort of his own home while outpatient fall prevention initiatives launched from the ED might prevent recurrent accidental injury.

Aging adults represent an unprecedented demographic tsunami for 21st century medicine. High-quality, age-specific evidence is lacking for the large majority of presenting ED complaints and geriatric syndromes. Among the few instances where sufficient evidence exists to report, the impact of screening diagnostic tests and preventive interventions for dementia, falls and polypharmacy have failed to improve mortality or quality of life and none have been demonstrated to be cost-effective. Alternative models of multidisciplinary care such as the HIH and CGA must be explored to help alleviate the inevitably worsening ED overcrowding while improving patient- and care-giver-important outcomes. Geriatric patients' diminished physiological reserve, co-morbidity burden

Table 25.2 Summary of evidence for geriatric prognostic screening tools in the ED.

Study	Sample	Intervention/outcome	ES	Conclusion
McCusker et al. [72]	ED-based RCT of 388 community-dwelling discharged adults over the age of 65 with an ISAR score of 2–6	Brief, standardized geriatric nursing assessment intervention group compared with usual care control group Outcomes included change in patient and care-giver functional status and mental health status at 4 months	Intervention increased primary care physician and home care services referral rates Intervention reduced 4-month functional decline (adjusted OR = 0.53; 95% CI: 0.31 to 0.91), but had no effect on patient depressive symptoms, care-giver outcomes or satisfaction with care	Brief standardized nursing assessment and referral to primary and home care services among high-risk ISAR patients reduces 4-month functional decline
McCusker et al. [73]	ED-based RCT of 345 community-dwelling discharged adults over the age of 65 with an ISAR score of 2–6	Brief, standardized geriatric nursing assessment intervention group compared with usual care control group Outcomes included referrals and visits to the primary physician and clinics, home care services and return ED visits at 1 month	Intervention increased referral to clinics (OR = 4.0; 95% CI: 1.7 to 9.5) or primary physician (OR = 1.9; 95% CI: 1.0 to 3.4), but patient adherence to primary physician follow-up was low Intervention increased receipt of home care services at 1 month (OR = 2.3; 95% CI: 1.1 to 5.1) and return ED visits (OR = 1.6; 95% CI: 1.0 to 2.6)	Brief standardized nursing assessment increases one-month referral to home care services, but not primary physician follow-up among high-risk ISAR patients
Meldon et al. [70]	ED-based prospective observational study of 650 community-dwelling adults over the age of 65	Composite of ED recidivism, hospital admission or nursing home admission at 30 and 120 days	High-risk TRST vs low-risk TRST: Composite 30-day risk: RR = 2.2 (95% CI: 1.7 to 2.9) Composite 120-day risk: RR = 1.5 (95% CI: 1.3 to 1.8) ED use at 30 days: RR = 1.7 (95% CI: 1.2 to 2.3) ED use at 120 days: RR = 1.5 (95% CI: 1.2 to 1.8) Hospital admission at 30 days: RR = 3.3 (95% CI: 2.2 to 5.1) Hospital admission at 120 days: RR = 2.1 (95% CI: 1.6 to 2.7) Nursing home admission at 120 days: RR = 6.2 (95% CI: 1.8 to 21.5)	High-risk TRST score associated with increased risk for ED recidivism, hospital admission, and nursing home placement 30 and 120 days after ED screening

CI, confidence interval; ED, emergency department; ISAR, Identification of Seniors at Risk Tool; OR, odds ratio; RCT, randomized controlled trial; RR, relative risk; TRST, Triage Risk Screening Tool.

Box 25.1 Triage Risk Screening Tool (TRST).

- History or evidence of cognitive impairment (poor recall or not oriented)
- Difficulty walking/transferring or recent falls
- Five or more medications
- ED use in previous 30 days or hospitalization in previous 90 days
- ED registered nurse concern for elder abuse/neglect, substance abuse, medication non-compliance, activities of daily living problems or other issues

and atypical presentations offer emergency medicine professionals a novel opportunity: if we can compassionately and effectively care for them, we will have improved the care for all age groups.

Box 25.2 Identification of Seniors at Risk (ISAR).

- Before the illness or injury that brought you to the emergency department, did you need someone to help you on a regular basis?
- Since the illness or injury brought you to the emergency department, have you needed more help than usual to care for yourself?
- Have you been hospitalized for one or more nights during the past 6 months?
- In general, do you see well?
- In general, do you have serious problems with your memory?
- Do you take more than three different medications every day?

Acknowledgments

The authors would like to acknowledge the assistance of Lowell Gerson in organizing the content and themes of this chapter.

Conflicts of interest

Dr. Carpenter is supported by a Jahnigen Career Development Grant from the John Hartford Foundation and the American Geriatrics' Society. Dr. Sanders and Dr. Stern have no conflicts of interest to declare.

References

1 He W, Sengupta M, Velkoff VA, De Barros KA. 65+ in the United States: 2005. US Census Bureau Current Population Reports No. P23-209. US Government Printing Office, Washington, 2005.

2 McNamara RM, Rousseau E, Sanders AB. Geriatric emergency medicine: a survey of practicing emergency physicians. *Ann Emerg Med* 1992;**21**(7):796–801.

3 Singal BM, Hedges JR, Rousseau EW, et al. Geriatric patient emergency visits. Part I: Comparison of visits by geriatric and younger patients. *Ann Emerg Med* 1992;**21**(7):802–7.

4 Nawar EW, Niska RW, Xu J. National Hospital Ambulatory Medical Care Survey: 2005 Emergency Department Summary. Advance Data from Vital and Health Statistics No. 386. National Center for Health Statistics, Hyattsville, 2007.

5 Eagle J, Rideout E, Price P, et al. Misuse of the emergency department by the elderly patient: myth or reality. *J Emerg Nurs* 1993;**19**:212–18.

6 Chu K, Brown A, Pillay R. Older patients' utilisation of emergency department resources: a cross-sectional study. *Aust Health Rev* 2001;**24**(3):44–52.

7 Downing A, Wilson R. Older people's use of accident and emergency services. *Age Ageing* 2005;**34**(1):24–30.

8 Aminzadeh F, Dalziel WB. Older adults in the emergency department: a systematic review of patterns of use, adverse outcomes, and effectiveness of interventions. *Ann Emerg Med* 2002;**39**(3):238–47.

9 Creditor MC. Hazards of hospitalization of the elderly. *Ann Intern Med* 1993;**118**(3):219–23.

10 Sanders AB, Witzke DB, Jones JS, et al. Principle of care and application of the geriatric emergency care model. In: Sanders AB, ed. *Emergency Care of the Elder Person.* Beverly Cracom Publications, St. Louis, 1996:59–93.

11 Rubenstein LZ, Stuck AE, Siu AL, et al. Impact of geriatric evaluation and management programs on defined outcomes: overview of the evidence. *J Am Geriatr Soc* 1991;**39**(9/2):8S–16S.

12 Amo PS, Levine C, Memmott MM. The economic value of informal caregiving. *Health Affairs* 1999;**18**(2):182–8.

13 Boustani M, Peterson B, Hanson L, et al. Screening for dementia in primary care: a summary of the evidence for the U.S. Preventive Services Task Force. *Ann Intern Med* 2003;**138**(11):927–37.

14 Ernst RL, Hay JW. The US economic and social costs of Alzheimer's disease revisited. *Am J Public Health* 1994;**84**(8):1261–4.

15 Brayne C. Incidence of dementia in England and Wales: The MRC Cognitive Function and Ageing Study. *Alzheimer Dis Assoc Disord* 2006;**20**(Suppl 2):S47–51.

16 Lobo A, Launer LJ, Fratiglioni L, et al. Prevalence of dementia and major subtypes in Europe: a collaborative study of population-based cohorts. *Neurology* 2000;**54**(11 Suppl 5):S4–9.

17 Jorm AF, Dear KBG, Burgess NM. Projections of future numbers of dementia cases in Australia with and without prevention. *Aust NZJ Psychiatry* 2005;**39**(11–12):959–63.

18 Li S, Yan F, Li G, et al. Is the dementia rate increasing in Beijing? Prevalence and incidence of dementia 10 years later in an urban elderly population. *Acta Psychiatr Scand* 2006;**115**(1):73–9.

19 Wancata J, Musalek M, Alexandrowicz R, et al. Number of dementia sufferers in Europe between the years 2000 and 2050. *Eur Psychiatry* 2003;**18**(6):303–13.

20 Hustey FM, Meldon SW. The prevalence and documentation of impaired mental status in elderly emergency department patients. *Ann Emerg Med* 2002;**39**(3):248–53.

21 Naughton BJ, Moran MB, Kadah H. Delirium and other cognitive impairment in older adults in an emergency department. *Ann Emerg Med* 1995;**25**:751–5.

22 Cooper B, Bickel H, Schaufele M. Early development and progression of dementing illness in the elderly: a general-practice based study. *Psychol Med* 1996;**26**(2):411–19.

23 O'Connor DW, Pollitt PA, Hyde JB, et al. Do general practitioners miss dementia in elderly patients? *BMJ* 1988;**297**(6656):1107–10.

24 Valcour VG, Masaki KH, Curb D, et al. The detection of dementia in the primary care setting. *Arch Intern Med* 2000;**160**:2964–8.

25 Rubenstein LZ, Josephson KR. The epidemiology of falls and syncope. *Clin Geriatr Med* 2002;**18**(2):141–58.

26 Evans R. Trauma and falls. In: Sanders AB, ed. *Emergency Care of the Elder Person.* Beverly Cracom Publications, St. Louis, 1996: 153–70.

27 Kingma J, Ten Duis HJ. Severity of injuries due to accidental fall across the life span: a retrospective hospital-based study. *Percept Mot Skills* 2000;**90**(1):62–72.

28 Scott VJ, Gallagher EM. Mortality and morbidity related to injuries from falls in British Columbia. *Can J Public Health* 1999;**90**(5):343–7.

29 Tinetti ME. Clinical practice: preventing falls in elderly persons. *N Engl J Med* 2003;**348**(1):42–9.

30 Magaziner J, Simonsick EM, Kashner TM, et al. Predictors of functional recovery one year following hospital discharge for hip fracture: a prospective study. *J Gerontol* 1990;**45**(3):M101–7.

31 Barratt A, Wyer PC, Hatala R, et al. Tips for learners of evidence-based medicine: 1. Relative risk reduction, absolute risk reduction, and number needed to treat. *Can Med Assoc J* 2004;**171**(4):353–8.

32 Cordell WH. Number needed to treat (NNT). *Ann Emerg Med* 1999;**33**(4):433–6.

33 Alter DA, Manuel DG, Gunraj N, et al. Age, risk–benefit trade-offs, and the projected effects of evidence-based therapies. *Am J Med* 2004;**116**:540–45.

34 Holsinger T, Deveau J, Boustani M, et al. Does this patient have dementia? *JAMA* 2007;**297**(21):2391–404.

35 Jorm AF. Methods of screening for dementia: a meta-analysis of studies comparing an informant questionnaire with a brief cognitive test. *Alzheimer Dis Assoc Disord* 1997;**11**(3):158–62.

36 Wilber ST, Lofgren SD, Mager TG, et al. An evaluation of two screening tools for cognitive impairment in older emergency department patients. *Acad Emerg Med* 2005;**12**(7):612–16.

37 Folstein MF, Folstein SE, McHugh PR. Mini-mental state: a practical method for grading the cognitive state of patients for the clinician. *J Psychiatr Res* 1975;**12**(3):189–98.

38 Crum RM, Anthony JC, Bassett SS, et al. Population-based norms for the Mini-Mental State Examination by age and educational level. *JAMA* 1993;**269**(18):2386–91.

39 Heun R, Papassotiropoulos A, Jennssen F. The validity of psychometric instruments for detection of dementia in the elderly general population. *Int J Geriatr Psychiatry* 1998;**13**:368–80.

40 Costa PT, Williams TF, Sommerfield M, et al. Early identification of Alzheimer's disease and related dementias. Clinical Practice Guideline No. 19 (AHCPR Publication No. 97-703). US Department of Health and Human Services, Agency for Health Care Policy and Research, Rockville, 1996.

41 Anthony JC, LeResche L, Niaz U, et al. Limits of the 'Mini-Mental State' as a screening test for dementia and delirium among hospital patients. *Psychol Med* 1982;**12**:397–408.

42 Ihl R, Frolich L, Dierks T, et al. Differential validity of psychometric tests in dementia of the Alzheimer type. *Psychiatry Res* 1992;**44**(4):93–106.

43 Frank RM, Byrne GJ. The clinical utility of the Hopkins Verbal Learning Test as a screening test for mild dementia. *Int J Geriatr Psychiatry* 2000;**15**(4):317–24.

44 Powsner S, Powsner D. Cognition, copyright, and the classroom. *Am J Psychiatry* 2005;**162**(3):627–8.

45 Mini Mental Status Exam. Psychological Assessment Resources, Inc., 2005. Available at http://www.minimental.com (accessed May 26, 2008).

46 Gerson LW, Counsell SR, Fontanarosa PB, et al. Case finding for cognitive impairment in elderly emergency department patients. *Ann Emerg Med* 1994;**23**(4):813–17.

47 Gillespie LD, Gillespie WJ, Robertson MC, et al. Interventions for preventing falls in elderly people. *Cochrane Database Syst Rev* 2003;**4**:CD000340 (doi: 10.1002/14651858.CD000340).

48 McClure R, Turner C, Peel N, et al. Population-based interventions for the prevention of fall-related injuries in older people. *Cochrane Database Syst Rev* 2005;**1**:CD004441 (doi: 10.1002/14651858.CD004441.pub2).

49 Weigand JV, Gerson LW. Preventive care in the emergency department: should emergency departments institute a falls prevention program for elder patients? A systematic review. *Acad Emerg Med* 2001;**8**(8):823–6.

50 Close JCT, Ellis M, Hooper R, et al. Prevention of Falls in the Elderly Trial (PROFET): a randomised controlled trial. *Lancet* 1999;**353**:93–7.

51 Carpenter CR, Gerson LW. Geriatric emergency medicine. In: LoCicero J, Rosenthal RA, Katic M, et al., eds. *New Frontiers in Geriatrics Research: An agenda for surgical and related medical specialties*, 2nd edn. American Geriatrics Society, New York, 2008:45–71. Available at http://www.americangeriatrics.org/specialists/NewFrontiers.

52 Shepperd S, Iliffe S. Hospital at home versus in-patient hospital care. *Cochrane Database Syst Rev* 2005;**3**:CD000356 (doi: 10.1002/14651858.CD14000356.pub14651852).

53 Gonzalez-Barcala FJ, Reino AP, Paz-Esquete JJ, et al. Hospital at home for acute respiratory patients. *Eur J Internal Med* 2006;**17**:402–7.

54 Leff B, Burton L, Mader SL, et al. Hospital at home: feasibility and outcomes of a program to provide hospital-level care at home for acutely ill older patients. *Ann Intern Med* 2005;**143**:798–808.

55 Caplan GA, Ward JA, Brennan NJ, et al. Hospital in the home: a randomised controlled trial. *Med J Aust* 1999;**170**:156–60.

56 Davies L, Wilkinson M, Bonner S, et al. Hospital at home versus hospital care in patients with exacerbations of chronic obstructive pulmonary disease: prospective randomised controlled trial. *BMJ* 2000;**321**(7271):1265–8.

57 Ricauda NA, Bo M, Molaschi M, et al. Home hospitalization service for acute uncomplicated first ischemic stroke in elderly patients: a randomized trial. *J Am Geriatr Soc* 2004;**52**:278–83.

58 Shepperd S, Harwood D, Jenkinson C, et al. Randomised controlled trial comparing hospital at home care with inpatient hospital care. I: Three month follow up of health outcomes. *BMJ* 1998;**316**:1786–91.

59 Wilson A, Parker H, Wynn A, et al. Randomised controlled trial of effectiveness of Leicester hospital at home scheme compared with hospital care. *BMJ* 1999;**319**(7224):1542–6.

60 Holland R, Lenaghan E, Harvey I, et al. Does home based medication review keep older people out of hospital? The HOMER randomised controlled trial. *BMJ* 2005;**330**(7486):293–7.

61 Lada P, Delgado G. Documentation of pharmacists' interventions in an emergency department and associated cost avoidance. *Am J Health-System Pharmacy* 2007;**64**(1):63–8.

62 Pacini M, Smith RD, Wilson EC, et al. Home-based medication review in older people: is it cost effective? *Pharmacoeconomics* 2007;**25**(2):171–80.

63 Ellis G, Whitehead M, Robinson D, et al. Comprehensive geriatric assessment for older adults admitted to hospital: a systematic review (Protocol). *Cochrane Database Syst Rev* 2006;**4**:CD006211 (doi: 10.1002/14651858.CD006211).

64 Kuo HK, Scandrett KG, Dave J, et al. The influence of outpatient comprehensive geriatric assessment on survival: a meta-analysis. *Arch Gerontol Geriatric* 2004;**39**:245–54.

65 Stuck AE, Siu AL, Wieland GD, et al. Comprehensive geriatric assessment: a meta-analysis of controlled trials. *Lancet* 1993;**342**(8878): 1032–6.

66 Caplan GA, Williams AJ, Daly B, et al. A randomized, controlled trial of comprehensive geriatric assessment and multidisciplinary intervention

after discharge of elderly from the emergency department – The DEED II study. *J Am Geriatr Soc* 2004;**52**(9):1417–23.

67 Stuck AE, Egger M, Hammer A, et al. Home visits to prevent nursing home admission and functional decline in elderly people: systematic review and meta-regression analysis. *JAMA* 2002;**287**(8):1022–8.

68 Hastings SN, Heflin MT. A systematic review of interventions to improve outcomes for elders discharged from the emergency department. *Acad Emerg Med* 2005;**12**(10):978–86.

69 McCusker J, Bellavance F, Cardin S, et al. Detection of older people at increased risk of adverse health outcomes after an emergency visit: the ISAR screening tool. *J Am Geriatr Soc* 1999;**47**(10):1229–37.

70 Meldon SW, Mion LC, Palmer RM, et al. A brief risk-stratification tool to predict repeat emergency department visits and hospitalizations in older patients discharged from the emergency department. *Acad Emerg Med* 2003;**10**:224–32.

71 Hustey FM, Mion LC, Connor JT, et al. A brief risk stratification tool to predict functional decline in older adults discharged from emergency department. *J Am Geriatr Soc* 2007;**55**(8):1269–74.

72 McCusker J, Verdon J, Tousignant P, et al. Rapid emergency department intervention for older people reduces risk of functional decline: results of a multicenter randomized trial. *J Am Geriatr Soc* 2001;**49**(10):1272–81.

73 McCusker J, Dendukuri N, Tousignant P, et al. Rapid two-stage emergency department intervention for seniors: impact on continuity of care. *Acad Emerg Med* 2003;**10**(3):233–43.

26 Syncope

Richard Lappin[1] & James Quinn[2]

[1]Department of Emergency Medicine, New York–Presbyterian Hospital, Weill Cornell Medical Center, New York, USA
[2]Division of Emergency Medicine, Stanford University, Stanford, USA

Clinical scenario

An 85-year-old woman was brought to the emergency department (ED) by ambulance for evaluation of a syncopal episode. She was sitting in church with her friend on a warm summer morning when she said she did not feel well. A few seconds later she turned "as white as a ghost" and slumped forward as several people nearby lowered her gently to the floor. Her friend reported that she began to wake up about a minute later and vomited once. By the time the ambulance arrived several minutes later she was fully awake. The paramedics found normal vital signs.

In the ED she had no complaints. She recalled being momentarily dizzy before she fainted, but denied other associated symptoms. She reported a history of mild hypertension well controlled with a diuretic and that she took an aspirin daily, but had no history of heart disease. She had had no recent illnesses or changes in her medications. Although she denied previous syncope, her friend recalled an episode at dinner in a restaurant several years earlier when she became diaphoretic and briefly unresponsive at the end of the meal. Her doctor told her she had had a transient ischemic attack (TIA).

On examination she appeared well with the following vitals: pulse rate 67 beats/min, respiration rate 14 breaths/min, blood pressure 162/58 mmHg bilaterally, temperature 37.3°C (oral) and SaO_2 97% (on room air). Her general physical and neurological examinations were normal. The stool occult blood test was negative. There were no orthostatic changes in heart rate or blood pressure. Her electrocardiogram (ECG) showed only non-specific T-wave flattening, unchanged from a prior tracing. A complete blood count and electrolytes were normal.

The patient insisted that she felt fine, and wanted to go home. Her friend, however, was terrified by this episode and thought that the patient should be admitted to the hospital. Your resident

agreed and argued that syncope without a prolonged prodrome is highly suspicious for an arrhythmia. She pointed out that the patient's age, abnormal ECG and history of hypertension were all risk factors for heart disease and life-threatening arrhythmias and suggested that, because syncope is sometimes the only symptom of a myocardial infarction in the elderly, the patient needed to be admitted for serial cardiac enzymes.

Background

Syncope is a common symptom with a broad differential diagnosis. The overall incidence of self-reported syncope among participants in the Framingham Heart Study was 6.2 per 1000 person-years, with a sharp increase in incidence above the age of 70 [1]. The lifetime cumulative incidence of syncope in a general population aged 35–60 years was reported as 35% in one Dutch study [2]. Approximately 1–1.5% of all ED visits are syncope related [3,4], and the annual cost of syncope-related hospitalizations in the USA has been estimated at over $2.4 billion [5].

The etiology of syncope ranges from harmless cardiovascular reflexes to life-threatening conditions such as myocardial infarction (MI) and ventricular arrhythmias. The most common causes by far are the various forms of benign, neurally mediated syncope often referred to as "vasovagal" or "situational". The possibility that a syncopal episode was caused by a ventricular tachyarrhythmia generates considerable anxiety among clinicians, though in unselected ED populations less than 2% of syncope is ultimately attributed to such an arrhythmia. Unless syncope occurs in a monitored setting, the cause of a particular syncopal episode is usually a matter of conjecture based on circumstantial evidence.

Patients with immediately life-threatening conditions are usually identified in the ED because of abnormal vital signs, ongoing complaints or ECG abnormalities. By the time they are evaluated by an ED physician, however, most patients with uncomplicated

Evidence-based Emergency Medicine. Edited by Brian H. Rowe
© 2009 Blackwell Publishing, ISBN: 978-1-4051-6143-5.

syncope have normal vital signs, no symptoms and a normal or non-diagnostic ECG. Some will have a history consistent with some form of benign, situationally triggered syncope. Others, though, have neither an ongoing acute condition nor a diagnostic history. Evaluation of these patients involves searching for evidence of a medical condition that would put the patient at risk for an adverse outcome. Several large prospective cohort studies have identified risk factors for long-term (1–5-year) mortality and morbidity in patients with syncope; these include older age, abnormal ECG, history of cardiovascular disease (especially congestive heart failure) and history of ventricular arrhythmia. The emergency physician, however, is primarily concerned with short-term outcome over the days or weeks following a visit to the ED, rather than long-term outcome, which may have little or no causal connection to the index syncopal event. Evidence regarding the short-term outcomes of syncope patients has become available only in the past few years. This chapter examines the diagnostic evaluation of syncope, the ability of clinicians and prediction rules to predict adverse outcomes, and the challenges of deciding ED disposition for these patients.

Clinical questions

In order to address the issues of greatest relevance to your patients and to help in searching the literature for the evidence regarding syncope, a series of questions regarding diagnosis, prognosis and treatment should be structured as recommended in Chapter 1.

1 In stable patients presenting to the ED with syncope (population), how often does a structured diagnostic work-up done in the ED (tests) identify a likely cause of syncope (outcome)?

2 In stable adult patients presenting to the ED with syncope and without ischemic symptoms or ECG changes (population), what proportion are ruled in for myocardial infarction (target disease) when subjected to a defined protocol for detection of myocardial infarction (tests)?

3 In stable patients presenting to the ED with syncope (population), what are the sensitivity and specificity (diagnostic test characteristics) of prediction rules based on initial ED evaluation (test) for diagnosing adverse outcomes within a 1-week and 4-week period (outcomes)?

4 In stable patients presenting to the ED with syncope (population), what are the sensitivity and specificity (diagnostic test characteristics) of physician clinical judgment (test) for diagnosing adverse outcomes within a 1-week and 4-week period (outcomes)?

5 In stable patients with syncope for whom evaluation in the ED provides no diagnosis (population), does hospitalization (intervention) decrease short-term adverse outcomes (outcome) compared to standard ED evaluation and discharge (comparison)?

6 In stable patients presenting to the ED with syncope (population), does a designated syncope unit or protocol (intervention) improve the rate of diagnosis or decrease hospital admission (outcomes) compared to standard ED evaluation by individual practitioner discretion (comparison)?

General search strategy

You turn first to the Cochrane Library, but your search reveals no systematic reviews pertaining to outcome or management of ED patients with syncope. You turn to MEDLINE, but because syncope as a symptom can be associated with myriad disease processes, searches using the term "syncope" yield vast numbers of studies in which syncope is not the major concern. A search of the MEDLINE database using the controlled vocabulary of the medical subject headings (MeSH) allows you to specify syncope as the major subject of the study.

Question 1: In stable patients presenting to the ED with syncope (population), how often does a structured diagnostic work-up done in the ED (tests) identify a likely cause of syncope (outcome)?

Search strategy

- MEDLINE: (syncope/diagnosis [MeSH] OR syncope/etiology [MeSH]) AND prospective studies [MeSH]

Your MEDLINE search yields four prospective studies [6–9] available in English in which a defined diagnostic protocol and diagnostic criteria were applied to an unselected group of adult patients presenting to the ED with syncope (Table 26.1). Other studies enrolled only a selected subgroup of patients (e.g., those hospitalized for evaluation), addressed only the yield of a specific diagnostic test (e.g., cardiac telemetry), followed adverse outcomes rather than diagnoses, or provided insufficient data to assess the contribution of ED evaluation to final diagnostic yield.

Kapoor et al. [10] was the first of a series of highly influential papers that investigated the diagnosis and outcome of patients with syncope [6,11,12]. These studies were notable for their prospective cohort design, rigorous diagnostic criteria and longitudinal follow-up, and their results are often cited in discussions of the diagnostic yield of the ED evaluation for syncope. However, the Kapoor studies recruited a mixed population of patients, not only from the ED but also from inpatient floors and outpatient clinics. They reported the diagnostic yield of each step of a standardized syncope evaluation, but not the yield of an actual ED evaluation. A 1990 summary paper reported data from a cohort of 433 patients; in this group, the elements of a basic ED evaluation (history, physical exam and ECG) assigned a diagnosis to 37% of patients, which represented 63% of all diagnoses made [6].

The Osservatorio Epidemiologico della Sincope nel Lazio 2 (OESIL 2) study reported markedly lower rates of ED diagnosis. They looked at the implementation of a simplified diagnostic algorithm in a prospective cohort of 195 patients presenting to the ED with syncope at nine community hospitals; results were compared with a historical control group [7]. Only 22% of patients

Table 26.1 Diagnostic yield of emergency department evaluation for syncope.

Study	Population	Definition of syncope	Elements of ED evaluation	Classification of ED diagnoses	Diagnostic criteria for benign syncope	Further testing	Cumulative diagnostic yield	ED diagnostic yield	Proportion of all diagnoses made in ED
Kapoor [6]	433 patients (mixed ED, inpatients, outpatients); age criteria not stated	Sudden transient loss of consciousness and postural tone (coma, shock, dizziness, seizure, cardioversion excluded)	Hx, exam, ECG, lab tests (initial evaluation, not all in ED)	Cause assigned by initial evaluation, suggestive findings requiring confirmation, or unknown	"Vasodepressor" required precip event (fear, pain, etc); "situational" syndromes were cough, micturition and defecation	As per clinician judgment	59%	37%	63%
OESIL 2: Ammirati et al. [7]	195 ED patients over age 12	Sudden transient loss of consciousness and postural tone with spontaneous recovery	Hx, exam, ECG, hemoglobin, glucose	Conclusive or hypothesized	Not described	Predetermined protocol; HUT to confirm suspected NMS or diagnosed undetermined cases	83%	22%	27%
Sarasin et al. [8]	650 ED patients over age 18	Sudden transient loss of consciousness and postural tone with spontaneous recovery (coma, shock, dizziness, seizure excluded)	Hx, exam, ECG, orthostatics, bilat carotid massage	Strongly suspected, suspected or undetermined	"Vasodepressor" required precip event (fear, pain, etc); "situational" syndromes were cough, micturition and defecation	Predetermined protocol: HUT to diagnose vasovagal disorders	81%	69%	85%
EGSYS-2: Brignole et al. [9]	541 ED patients over age 18 seen within 24 hrs of syncope	Not explicitly defined	Hx, exam, ECG, orthostatics	Certain, suspected or unexplained	Situational syndromes also included postprandial syncope	Predetermined protocol: HUT to diagnose "non-classical" vasovagal syncope: CSM for older healthy patients with recurrent syncope or syncope with neck turning	98%	50%	51%

CSM, carotid sinus massage; ECG, electrocardiogram; ED, emergency department; HUT, head-up tilt test; Hx, history; NMS, neurally mediated syncope.

were assigned a diagnosis after the first step assessment; this group represented 27% of all diagnoses made. Other studies, by contrast, have reported significantly higher rates of initial ED diagnosis. Sarasin et al. [8] conducted a prospective cohort study of 650 patients presenting with syncope to the ED of a single, large, tertiary care hospital. For 69% of patients a cause of syncope was "strongly suspected" after the initial ED evaluation; this represented 85% of all diagnoses made. The Evaluation of Guidelines in Syncope Study 2 (EGSYS-2) [9] prospectively assessed the performance of the European Society of Cardiology guidelines [13,14] for the management of syncope in a cohort of 541 patients who presented to the ED at 11 general hospitals. The initial evaluation – history, physical exam and ECG – was considered diagnostic in 50% of cases, and a final diagnosis was assigned in a remarkable 98% of cases.

Across studies, the reported diagnostic yield of a typical ED evaluation has varied from 20% to 70%, and the ED evaluation has provided anywhere from 27% to 85% of final diagnoses. In addition to the absence of a diagnostic gold standard for syncope, several factors might contribute to the high variability in these observations. First, although definitions of syncope were consistent between studies, patient population and the timing of evaluation were not. Kapoor [6] recruited a mixed population of patients from the ED, inpatient floors and outpatient clinics, many enrolled days after their syncopal episode when physical findings might have resolved and historical details might be forgotten. This may have reduced the diagnostic yield of the initial evaluation. Most subsequent studies have recruited patients at the time of presentation to the ED, and EGSYS-2 [9] specifically excluded patients seen more than 24 hours after syncope. A second likely factor is the definition of the standard ED evaluation itself. Routine measurement of orthostatic vital signs in the ED, for example, appeared to markedly increase diagnostic yield, and Sarasin et al. [8] reported that fully 24% of their syncope patients had orthostatic hypotension. Thirdly, diagnostic criteria are variable. Recognition of situational syndromes (such as postprandial syncope) that were not well known 25 years ago may have increased diagnostic yield in later studies. Lastly, the level of diagnostic certainty required to assign a diagnosis may be a source of variation: some studies required ED diagnoses to be "definitive" or "certain", while others referred to a "strongly suspected" cause. This variation in terminology might reflect real differences in willingness to assign a clinical diagnosis in the ED without further testing. Head-up tilt testing, not used by Kapoor, was used extensively in later studies to diagnose neurally mediated syncope, although there is no way of verifying the accuracy of the tilt test when used for this purpose [15]. The use of a test to diagnose or confirm neurally mediated syncope might have made some clinicians reluctant to assign this diagnosis in the ED on clinical grounds.

In summary, a thorough ED evaluation will identify a likely cause of syncope in more than 50% of cases. Awareness of situational syndromes and routine measurement of orthostatic vital signs may significantly increase diagnostic yield.

Question 2: In stable adult patients presenting to the ED with syncope and without ischemic symptoms or ECG changes (population), what proportion are ruled in for myocardial infarction (target disease) when subjected to a defined protocol for detection of myocardial infarction (tests)?

Search strategy

• MEDLINE: syncope [Majr] AND myocardial infarction

Your MEDLINE search yields many studies of the mechanisms of syncope in patients who have had MI, and of the incidence of MI as a long-term adverse outcome in patients who have had syncope. You find only three studies that focused on the incidence of MI diagnosed soon after syncope in patients presenting to the ED [16–18]. All three, however, examined selected subgroups of patients with syncope (Table 26.2). Grossman et al. retrospectively studied patients over age 65 who were inconsistently investigated for acute coronary syndrome (ACS), even when they had complained of ischemic symptoms; 2% of these patients were diagnosed with MI [16]. Georgeson et al. studied a subgroup of 251 patients with syncope and no chest pain within a cohort of 5762 patients who presented to the ED with symptoms of possible cardiac ischemia (chest pain, dyspnea, nausea and vomiting, dizziness, syncope) [17]. Eighteen (7%) were diagnosed with ACS; all had ischemic abnormalities on their initial ECG, and most had ST segment elevations. At least some also had ischemic symptoms other than chest pain, such as arm, neck, shoulder or throat pain or dyspnea, but the proportion was not specified. Link et al. retrospectively studied patients admitted through the ED for syncope or near-syncope over a 1-year period [18]. Of 104 admitted patients, 80 underwent a full 'rule-out MI' protocol of serial ECGs and cardiac enzymes. One patient ruled in for MI, and one was diagnosed with unstable angina; both patients presented with a clinical history of unstable angina.

The diagnostic studies identified as relevant to Question 1 were not concerned specifically with myocardial infarction; however, they did report the number of patients who were assigned a final diagnosis of MI. Some also detailed the proportion of patients who were diagnosed in the ED and provided limited information about the clinical presentation of these patients. The same search also identifies several studies of adverse short-term outcomes after syncope that reported specific data on MI. All of these studies enrolled unselected patients with syncope, but investigation for ACS was applied to a subset of patients according to the judgment of their physicians, leaving open the possibility that some patients with ACS were missed.

Kapoor reported very low rates of MI (approximately 1%) in patients with syncope [6,10]. Patients with MI were apparently identified by their initial ECG; their clinical history was not described, and no patient was diagnosed by cardiac enzymes. More recent cohort studies have also found very low rates of ACS. Sarasin

Table 26.2 Proportion of syncope patients diagnosed with cardiac ischemia.

Study	Population	Proportion evaluated with cardiac enzymes	Definition of cardiac ischemia	Proportion diagnosed with cardiac ischemia	Proportion of patients with cardiac ischemia diagnosed by initial ECG	Prop of patients with cardiac ischemia reporting ischemic symptoms
Georgeson et al. [17]	250 ED patients with syncope and no chest pain	All (initial and 48 hours)	WHO criteria for MI*; ischemic symptoms with compatible ECG/ETT/catheter for non-infarct ischemia	4% with MI 3% with non-infarct ischemia	All	Not specified
Link et al. [18]	104 admitted patients with syncope or near-syncope (retrospective)	80 (77%)	Elevated cardiac enzymes (MI); UAP not defined	1% with MI 1% with UAP	Not specified	2 of 2 with unstable angina sx
Grossman et al. [16]	319 ED patients over 65 years with syncope (retrospective)	45% (62% of the 72% that were admitted)	Elevated CPK-MB or troponin	2% with MI	All	2 of 3 with chest discomfort (third with dementia)
Kapoor [6]	433 patients with syncope: ED, inpatients, clinics	Not specified	Evolutionary ECG changes or elevated cardiac enzymes	1% with MI	Not specified	Not specified
Sarasin et al. [8]	650 ED patients with syncope	All with initial CPK, otherwise not specified	WHO criteria for MI*	1.4% with MI	All	Not specified
EGSYS-2: Brignole et al. [9]	541 ED patients with syncope	Not specified	Ischemic symptoms with ECG ischemia	2% with ischemia	Not specified	All
SFSR: Quinn et al. [4]	684 ED patients with syncope or near-syncope	Not specified	Troponin elevation or ECG change with discharge diagnosis of MI	3.1% with MI	Not specified	Not specified
SFSR: Sun et al. [21]	477 ED patients with syncope or near-syncope	Not specified	Troponin elevation or ECG change with cardiologist diagnosis of MI	0.2% with MI	Not specified	Not specified

*World Health Organization (WHO) criteria combine symptoms, ECG changes and cardiac enzyme elevations [34]. CPK, creatine phosphokinase; CPK-MB, creatine phosphokinase, MB isoenzyme; ECG, electrocardiogram; ETT, exercise tolerance test; MI, myocardial infarction; UAP, unstable angina pectoris.

et al. reported that only 9 of 650 patients (1.4%) were diagnosed with an ACS [8]. The authors stated that all patients with an ACS were identified on presentation by initial ECG, but it is unclear whether any patients with a normal ECG underwent further evaluation for ischemia. In EGSYS-2, 11 of 541 patients (2%) were considered to have syncope secondary to myocardial ischemia. Again, it is unclear whether patients without ischemic symptoms or ECG features were investigated for ischemia, and how many patients, if any, underwent serial cardiac enzyme testing [9].

The derivation study for the San Francisco Syncope Rule (SFSR; designed to predict short-term adverse outcomes) reported numbers of patients diagnosed with MI, defined as any troponin elevation or ECG change associated with a discharge diagnosis of MI [4]. Using this standard, 3.1% of all syncope patients in the derivation study were considered to have had an MI within 7 days of presentation. As the authors pointed out, the significance of small troponin elevations is unclear, as they are seen in many clinical settings other than acute coronary syndromes [19,20]. In the independent SFSR validation study of Sun et al., in which diagnosis of MI required not only an ECG change or increase in troponin but also documentation that a cardiology consultant agreed with the diagnosis, only one of 477 patients was diagnosed with MI on presentation to the ED and no patient received the diagnosis over the subsequent 7 days [21].

In summary, the available data suggest that acute coronary syndromes are quite unusual in patients who present to the ED with a primary complaint of syncope. Patients whose syncope is associated with other ischemic symptoms or ischemic ECG features merit investigation for ACS. Whether patients who present with syncope in the absence of these ischemic indicators have any significant incidence of ACS remains unclear. There are no convincing data to support the routine investigation of otherwise asymptomatic syncope patients for ACS.

Question 3: In stable patients presenting to the ED with syncope (population), what are the sensitivity and specificity (diagnostic test characteristics) of prediction rules based on initial ED evaluation (test) for diagnosing adverse outcomes within a 1-week and 4-week period (outcomes)?

Search strategy

- MEDLINE: syncope [Majr] AND (risk assessment [MeSH] OR risk factors [MeSH]) AND predictive value of tests [MeSH]

Almost all of the literature concerning the risk stratification of patients with syncope published over the past 25 years has looked at long-term outcomes, from 1 to 5 years after an index syncopal event. Your MEDLINE search identifies five prospective studies of rules based on initial ED evaluation that were designed to predict adverse short-term outcomes among unselected adult patients with syncope (Table 26.3) [4,21–24].

The SFSR was the first clinical prediction rule designed to identify patients at risk for serious short-term outcomes [4]. The derivation study was a prospective cohort study of adult patients presenting with syncope or near-syncope at a single large university teaching hospital. Serious outcomes were defined broadly to include not only acute clinical events and diagnoses (such as MI or hemorrhage), but also inpatient medical interventions related to the syncope (such as pacemaker insertion or surgery for abdominal aortic aneurysm) or any condition related to the syncope that caused or was likely to cause a return to the hospital and subsequent admission. Patients were followed to see if they had suffered a serious outcome within 7 days of their ED visit.

Of 684 patients who entered the study, 79 (11.5%) had serious outcomes by day 7, including five (0.7%) who died. As might be expected from the brief follow-up horizon, the serious outcomes included a large proportion of acute processes such as MI and gastrointestinal hemorrhage. A decision rule was derived that considered five factors: abnormal ECG (defined as non-sinus rhythm or new changes compared with previous ECG), a complaint of shortness of breath, hematocrit less than 30%, a triage systolic blood pressure less than 90 mmHg, and a history of congestive heart failure. The presence of one or more of these factors identified the patient as being at high risk for a serious outcome. Application of the rule classified 45% of the patients as "high risk". The prediction rule had a sensitivity of 96% (95% CI: 92% to 100%) and a specificity of 62% (95% CI: 58% to 66%), correctly identifying 76 of 79 serious outcomes. The authors questioned the clinical significance of the three patients missed by the rule – two patients with small troponin elevations of unclear significance (one of whom had a normal cardiac catheterization) and one patient readmitted for recurrent syncope for which no cause was found. Older age, a powerful predictor of adverse long-term outcomes [12], predicted serious short-term outcomes as well, but with a specificity too poor to be useful in the predictive model.

The validation study applied the prediction rule to a second patient cohort at the same medical center, with two important differences. First, this study followed patients and ascertained outcomes at 30 days, compared to the previous study which obtained 7-day outcomes. Second, the study analyzed the performance of the prediction rule only for the subset of patients who did not have a serious outcome diagnosed at the time of their ED evaluation [22]. Both changes, arguably, apply the prediction rule in a manner closer to the actual concerns and practice of ED physicians. Of 760 patients in the validation cohort (791 ED visits) there were 108 serious outcomes at 30 days (13.7%); of these, 6.8% were present and diagnosed in the ED, and the remaining 6.8% were diagnosed after the initial ED evaluation. The prediction rule identified 52 of the 53 patients who had serious outcomes diagnosed after ED evaluation, with a sensitivity of 98% (95% CI: 89% to 100%) and specificity of 56% (95% CI: 52% to 60%).

To date, one large independent validation study of the prediction rule has been published by Sun et al., evaluating the accuracy of the SFSR at another large, tertiary care academic center [21]. This study followed outcomes at 7 days (the time used by the

Table 26.3 Performance of the San Francisco Syncope Rule (SFSR).

Study	Outcome period	Symptoms	Definition of syncope	Sensitivity	Specificity	Comments
SFSR derivation: Quinn et al. [4]	7 days	Syncope or near-syncope	Transient LOC with return to baseline neurological status; near-syncope not defined	96%	62%	All serious outcomes
SFSR validation: Quinn et al. [22]	30 days	Syncope or near-syncope	Transient LOC with return to baseline neurological status; near-syncope not defined	98%	56%	Serious outcomes not apparent in ED
SFSR independent validation: Sun et al. [21]	7 days	Syncope or near-syncope	Transient LOC; near-syncope defined as imminent LOC	89% / 69%	42% / 42%	All serious outcomes / Serious outcomes not apparent in ED
ROSE pilot study: Reed et al. [23]	3 months	Syncope	Transient LOC	100%	46%	All serious outcomes
SFSR independent validation: Cosgriff et al. [24]	7 days	Syncope or near-syncope	Transient LOC with return to baseline neurological function; near-syncope defined as near LOC	90%	57%	All serious outcomes

ED, emergency department; LOC, loss of consciousness; ROSE, Risk Stratification Of Syncope in the Emergency Department; SFSR, San Francisco Syncope Rule.

SFSR derivation study) rather than at 30 days (as in the original validation study). The definition of an abnormal ECG, based on specific predefined features without reference to prior tracings, was different from that of Quinn et al. [4]. Of 477 patients, 11.7% had a serious outcome at 7 days, 8.4% diagnosed in the ED and 3.4% diagnosed after the index ED visit. When used to predict all serious outcomes, the SFSR had a sensitivity of 89% (95% CI: 81% to 97%) and specificity of 42% (95% CI: 37% to 48%); when used to predict outcomes not apparent in the ED, the sensitivity was only 69% (95% CI: 46% to 92%) and specificity was 42% (95% CI: 37% to 48%).

Other tests of the SFSR are still in preliminary stages. A small pilot study for the UK-based Risk Stratification Of Syncope in the Emergency Department (ROSE) project assessed the performance of the SFSR for adverse outcomes at 1 week, 1 month and 3 months [23]. For 3-month outcomes, the SFSR had a sensitivity of 100% and specificity of 46%. A small validation study from Australia found a sensitivity of 90% (95% CI: 60% to 99%) and specificity of 57% (95% CI: 46% to 67%) for 7-day outcomes [24]. Another prediction rule, based on Boston syncope criteria, has recently been published in abstract form [25].

Several factors may have contributed to variations in the performance of the prediction rule between these studies (see Table 26.3). Most of the studies included an unspecified proportion of patients with near-syncope, a group that can include patients with dizziness of neurological rather than hemodynamic cause. Some studies did not require a return to baseline neurological status after syncope, leaving the possibility that patients with hemodynamic instability or stroke might have been included. The definition of abnormal ECG in the original SFSR studies (non-sinus rhythm or new changes) did not specify which new changes were considered significant, nor which ECG features were considered abnormal for patients with no prior tracing on record [4,22].

It is important to realize that the "serious outcomes" of the SFSR did not consist of only adverse clinical events. The authors of the SFSR deliberately used a combined outcome measure that included not only clinical events (e.g., cardiac arrest), but also diagnostic test results (e.g., troponin elevation) and procedural outcomes (e.g., blood transfusion for anemia). In effect, this results in different definitions of serious outcome for admitted and discharged patients. Some diagnostic results that were defined as serious outcomes – for example, asymptomatic troponin elevation – will only be detected if the patient is hospitalized, and some medical procedures that were defined as serious outcomes – such as the elective insertion of a pacemaker – are more likely to occur in the first few weeks after syncope if the patient is hospitalized. This disparity between outcomes criteria for admitted and discharged patients might have caused the prediction rule to be fitted more closely to the outcomes of admitted patients, and might have made clinical variables that predict admission look like predictors of adverse outcome. Defining interventions that can be elective (such as blood transfusion) as serious outcomes introduces another possible distortion. It is possible, for example, that a hematocrit below 30 emerged as a predictor of serious outcomes not because it predicted adverse clinical events, but simply because physicians are inclined to transfuse patients with a hematocrit below this threshold. Unfortunately, the published studies do not report the extent to which each of the five components of the rule predicted specific serious outcomes.

Despite these limitations, prediction rules based on short-term adverse outcomes – exemplified by the SFSR – could be a valuable adjunct to a physician's clinical judgment in deciding the disposition of ED patients with syncope of unclear cause. However, physicians are unlikely to adopt any absolute prediction rule for syncope unless its sensitivity for adverse outcomes approaches 100%. The subjective nature of the definition of syncope and the application of the predictor and outcome variables suggest that an absolute prediction rule in the true sense is likely not possible. Because the numbers of patients with serious short-term outcomes not apparent in the ED are very small, the confidence intervals around estimates of sensitivity and specificity for this group in the SFSR are still quite broad. Larger studies, enrolling thousands of patients, may be necessary to define the accuracy of the prediction rule, and even then it will likely not be sensitive enough to be the determining factor for disposition.

Question 4: In stable patients presenting to the ED with syncope (population), what are the sensitivity and specificity (diagnostic test characteristics) of physician clinical judgment (test) for diagnosing adverse outcomes within a 1-week and 4-week period (outcomes)?

Search strategy

- MEDLINE: syncope [Majr] AND (risk assessment [MeSH] OR risk factors [MeSH]) AND predictive value of tests [MeSH]

Although physicians decide the disposition of thousands of syncope patients each day, there have been, until recently, remarkably few data concerning the performance of physician judgment in predicting the short-term outcomes of their patients. Your MEDLINE search identifies only one study that assessed the sensitivity and specificity of physician judgment in predicting adverse short-term outcomes (Table 26.4) [26].

Quinn et al. compared of the accuracy of the SFSR to physician judgment in predicting short-term serious outcomes [26]. The study utilized the same patient cohort as the original SFSR derivation paper. After evaluating each patient, ED physicians were asked to estimate prospectively the probability of a serious outcome within 7 days, and their decision to admit or discharge the patient was recorded. Physician judgment that a patient had a 2% or less chance of a serious outcome was defined as "low risk" for the purpose of comparison with the SFSR. Physicians classified 54% of patients as low risk; this group had 1.4% serious outcomes and no deaths. The SFSR classified 55% of patients as low risk; this group had 0.8% serious outcomes. Physician judgment had a sensitivity of 94% and specificity of 52%, compared with 96% and 62%, respectively, for the SFSR. The SFSR had an accuracy of 66%, compared with 57% for physician judgment.

Other studies comparing physician judgment to prediction rules have actually used physician decision to admit as a surrogate for physician prediction of adverse outcome. The validation study of the SFSR reported that the prediction rule identified 52 of the 53 patients who had serious 30-day outcomes and complete prediction rule data available (98% sensitivity), while physicians admitted 51 of the 54 patients with serious outcomes (96% sensitivity) [22]. The independent validation study of the SFSR performed by Sun et al. reported that the prediction rule identified 89% of all serious 7-day outcomes, and 69% of those not apparent at initial ED evaluation, while physicians decided to admit 100% of patients who went on to have a serious 7-day outcome [21]. It is possible that – since the definition of syncope in this study did not include a return to baseline neurological function – the poor performance of the prediction rule reflected the inclusion of unstable patients. In the ROSE pilot study, physicians admitted all patients who had serious outcomes at 3 months [23].

In summary, the limited data available suggest that physicians are able to identify almost all of the 10–15% of syncope patients who will have adverse short-term outcomes, but do so by admitting up to two-thirds of their patients with syncope. These studies do not tell us, however, whether physician judgment could be improved through the use of risk stratification to achieve a lower admission rate.

Question 5: In stable patients with syncope for whom evaluation in the ED provides no diagnosis (population), does hospitalization (intervention) decrease short-term adverse outcomes (outcome) compared to standard ED evaluation and discharge (comparison)?

Search strategy

- MEDLINE: syncope [Majr] AND hospitalization [MeSH]

Hospitalization for patients with syncope is appropriate if it can prevent or treat an adverse short-term outcome. While clearly indicated for those diagnosed at presentation with a serious acute condition such as MI, its benefit for patients with syncope of unknown cause is considerably less obvious because the rate of short-term adverse events among these patients is so low – approximately 7% over the 30 days following presentation [21,22]. Nevertheless, hospitalization for this group might be justified if those at risk cannot be reliably identified in advance. Your MEDLINE search finds

Table 26.4 Test characteristics of physician clinical judgment compared to the San Francisco Syncope Rule (SFSR) for predicting adverse short-term outcomes. (From Quinn et al. [26].)

	Proportion classified as low risk	Serious outcomes in low-risk group	Sensitivity	Specificity	Accuracy
Physician judgment	54%	1.4%	94%	52%	66%
SFSR	55%	0.8%	96%	62%	57%

no studies that compared the outcomes of patients with a negative ED evaluation who were randomized to either hospitalization or outpatient evaluation.

In summary, given the lack of evidence regarding the benefits of hospitalization, it appears reasonable and prudent to recommend hospitalization primarily for patients at risk for short-term (7–30-day) adverse events. More accurate identification of this small group, perhaps by refinement of prediction rules for short-term outcomes, might allow a significant decrease in hospitalization.

Question 6: In stable patients presenting to the ED with syncope (population), does a designated syncope unit or protocol (intervention) improve the rate of diagnosis or decrease hospital admission (outcomes) compared to standard ED evaluation by individual practitioner discretion (comparison)?

Search strategy

- MEDLINE: syncope [Majr] AND (hospitalization [MeSH] OR practice guidelines [MeSH])

Numerous commentators have argued that the evaluation of patients with syncope is inadequate, with unnecessarily high rates of hospital admission, long hospital stays, high costs, underutilization of appropriate diagnostic tests and a low overall rate of diagnosis. Although a number of practice recommendations have been published, it is unclear to what extent these have changed practitioner's behavior [13,14,27,28]. This situation has led to the suggestion that implementing syncope diagnostic protocols or establishing dedicated syncope units might improve diagnostic yield and efficiency.

Your MEDLINE search reveals two studies that tried to estimate the potential effect of practice guidelines on hospital admission. Elesber et al. retrospectively examined the potential impact of application of the American College of Emergency Physicians (ACEP) level B recommendations for admission of patients with syncope (admit patients with structural heart disease, coronary artery disease, evidence of heart failure, older age, abnormal ECG or hematocrit < 30) using the diagnosis of a cardiac cause of syncope as a surrogate for appropriateness of admission [29]. Of 200 ED patients included in the study, 58% were admitted, including 23 of the 24 who ultimately received a cardiac diagnosis. Fifty-seven patients (29%) met the ACEP level B recommendations for admission, including all of those assigned a cardiac diagnosis. Application of the ACEP recommendations would have been 100% sensitive and 81% specific for cardiac diagnosis, and would have reduced the admission rate by half. Bartoletti et al. prospectively compared hospital admissions with recommendations of the European Society of Cardiology (ESC) guidelines for the management of syncope. Of 566 patients with syncope, 50.1% were admitted, while 39.1% had one or more criteria for admission according to the guidelines [30].

Two studies reported the actual results of implementing a syncope protocol. In OESIL 2, investigators prospectively implemented a diagnostic algorithm for syncope and compared diagnostic yield with a historical control from an earlier observational study [7]. Overall, 83% of patients evaluated according to the standardized algorithm were assigned a diagnosis, compared with only 46% of historical controls. The investigators did not provide data regarding objective outcomes such as admission rates, length of stay, morbidity and mortality. EGSYS 2 was a multi-center, prospective study that compared the outcomes of 745 patients with syncope managed according to a standardized protocol based on the ESC guidelines with those of a similar group of 929 patients managed according to usual practice 3 years earlier [31]. The standardized-care group had a lower rate of hospitalization (39% vs 47%), shorter hospital stay (7.2 vs 8.1 days) and lower rate of unexplained syncope (5% vs 20%) than the usual-care group.

Two studies examined the performance of specialized syncope units. EGSYS compared syncope evaluation at six hospitals that had specialized syncope units to evaluation at six matched hospitals without such units [32]. Unfortunately, the total number of patients (30) referred to these units was very small, and represented only 11% of all syncope patients evaluated at these hospitals. Syncope unit hospitals had a slightly lower rate of admission (43% vs 49%), with the same diagnostic yield and in-hospital mortality rate. The Syncope Evaluation in the Emergency Department Study (SEEDS) was a small, single-center, prospective, randomized trial that compared standard ED care with admission to a designated ED syncope unit for the subset of patients whose cause of syncope was not identified in an initial ED evaluation and who were deemed to be at "intermediate risk" according to criteria modified from the ACEP policy statement on syncope [33]. Of the 262 patients with syncope of unclear cause who consented to the study, 39% were classified as intermediate risk. Patients in the designated syncope unit received continuous cardiac telemetry for up to 6 hours and vital sign measurements (including orthostatics) every hour. Additional investigations such as echocardiography, tilt-table testing, carotid sinus massage and electrophysiology consultation could be obtained while patients were in the syncope unit, or within 72 hours at an outpatient heart rhythm center.

Shifting inpatient testing to the ED caused diagnostic yield to increase from 10% in the standard-care group (patients who had recurrent symptoms during their ED stay) to 67% in the syncope-unit group. However, by the end of the follow-up period, the overall (accumulative) rate of diagnosis for patients in the syncope unit (82%) was nearly identical to those who received standard care (81%). The difference in admission rate was substantial: only 43% of patients in the syncope unit were recommended for admission, compared with 98% of those randomized to standard care. Because of the lower admission rate, total inpatient time was much lower in the syncope-unit group than the standard-care group (140 vs 64 patient-days); the effect of the syncope unit on length of stay in the ED itself was not reported. There was no significant difference in survival at 2 years between the standard-care group (90%) and the syncope-unit group (97%).

The success of the syncope unit depended crucially on the ready availability of specialized diagnostic tests such as echocardiography and tilt-table testing, either in the ED or on an outpatient basis within days of discharge. Elaborate inpatient testing and prompt specialist follow-up might not be possible for smaller hospitals. Even for larger centers with greater resources, the establishment of a syncope unit would require considerable effort and expense. Standardized syncope protocols may offer a modest decrease in admission rates and higher ED diagnostic yield without demanding the same resources.

Conclusions

Your assessment of your patient's history – syncope during prolonged upright posture in a warm environment – leads you to suspect that this was a benign, neurally mediated event. Although she has several risk factors associated with long-term mortality, such as her age and abnormal ECGs, she does not have any of the predictors of adverse short-term outcome specified by the SFSR. In addition, she has neither ischemic symptoms nor ECG evidence of ischemia. You know that there are few data to suggest that she would benefit from hospitalization. You combine your clinical judgment with the known risk factors and decide to let her go home and follow up with her physician.

Syncope is an extremely common presenting problem in the ED, with the potential for adverse outcomes. Emergency physicians need to combine clinical judgment with known risk factors prior to making decisions about disposition. Many of the risk factors associated with poor outcomes can be identified by using a decision rule (especially the SFSR).

Acknowledgments

The authors would like to thank Dr. Peter Wyer for his generous and thoughtful advice throughout the preparation of this chapter.

Conflicts of interest

The authors have no financial conflicts of interest to declare; Dr. Quinn is the lead author on the derivation of the San Francisco Syncope Rule.

References

1 Soteriades ES, Evans JC, Larson MG, et al. Incidence and prognosis of syncope. *N Engl J Med* 2002;**347**:878–85.

2 Ganzeboom KS, Mairuhu G, Reitsma JB, et al. Lifetime cumulative incidence of syncope in the general population: a study of 549 Dutch subjects aged 35–60 years. *J Cardiovasc Electrophysiol* 2006;**17**:1172–6.

3 Sun BC, Emond JA, Camargo CA. Characteristics and admission patterns of patients presenting with syncope to U.S. emergency departments, 1992–2000. *Acad Emerg Med* 2004;**11**:1029–34.

4 Quinn JV, Stiell IG, McDermott DA, et al. Derivation of the San Francisco Syncope Rule to predict patients with short-term serious outcomes. *Ann Emerg Med* 2004;**43**:224–32.

5 Sun BC, Emond JA, Camargo CA. Direct medical costs of syncope-related hospitalizations in the United States. *Am J Cardiol* 2005;**95**:668–71.

6 Kapoor WN. Evaluation and outcome of patients with syncope. *Medicine* 1990;**69**:160–75.

7 Ammirati F, Colivicchi F, Santini M. Diagnosing syncope in clinical practice. Implementation of a simplified diagnostic algorithm in a multicentre prospective trial – the OESIL 2 study (Osservatorio Epidemiologico della Sincope nel Lazio). *Eur Heart J* 2000;**21**:935–40.

8 Sarasin FP, Louis-Simonet M, Carballo D, et al. Prospective evaluation of patients with syncope: a population-based study. *Am J Med* 2001;**111**:177–84.

9 Brignole M, Menozzi C, Bartoletti A, et al. A new management of syncope: prospective systematic guideline-based evaluation of patients referred urgently to general hospitals. *Eur Heart J* 2006;**27**:76–82.

10 Kapoor WN, Karpf M, Wieand S, et al. A prospective evaluation and follow-up of patients with syncope. *N Engl J Med* 1983;**309**:197–204.

11 Kapoor WN, Hanusa BH. Is syncope a risk factor for poor outcomes? Comparison of patients with and without syncope. *Am J Med* 1996;**100**:646–55.

12 Martin TP, Hanusa BH, Kapoor WN. Risk stratification of patients with syncope. *Ann Emerg Med* 1997;**29**:459–66.

13 Brignole M, Alboni P, Benditt D, et al. Task force on syncope, European Society of Cardiology. Part 1. The initial evaluation of patients with syncope. *Europace* 2001;**3**:253–60.

14 Brignole M, Alboni P, Benditt D, et al. Guidelines on management (diagnosis and treatment) of syncope – update 2004. *Eur Heart J* 2004;**25**:2054–72.

15 Sheldon R. Tilt testing for syncope: a reappraisal. *Curr Opin Cardiol* 2005;**20**:38–41.

16 Grossman SA, Van Epp S, Arnold R, et al. The value of cardiac enzymes in elderly patients presenting to the emergency department with syncope. *J Gerontol A Biol Sci Med Sci* 2003;**58A**:1055–8.

17 Georgeson S, Linzer M, Griffith JL, et al. Acute cardiac ischemia in patients with syncope. *J Gen Intern Med* 1992;**7**:379–86.

18 Link MS, Lauer EP, Homoud MK, et al. Low yield of rule-out myocardial infarction protocol in patients presenting with syncope. *Am J Cardiol* 2001;**88**:706–7.

19 Hamm CW, Giannitsis E, Katus HA. Cardiac troponin elevations in patients without acute coronary syndrome (Editorial). *Circulation* 2002;**106**:2871–2.

20 Jeremias A, Gibson CM. Narrative review: alternate causes for elevated cardiac troponins when acute coronary syndromes are excluded. *Ann Internal Med* 2005;**142**:786–91.

21 Sun BC, Mangione CM, Merchant G, et al. External validation of the San Francisco Syncope Rule. *Ann Emerg Med* 2007;**49**:420–27.

22 Quinn JV, McDermott DA, Stiell IG, et al. Prospective validation of the San Francisco Syncope Rule to predict patients with serious outcomes. *Ann Emerg Med* 2006;**47**:448–54.

23 Reed MJ, Newby DE, Coull AJ, et al. The Risk Stratification Of Syncope in the Emergency Department (ROSE) pilot study: a comparison of existing syncope guidelines. *Emerg Med J* 2007;**24**:270–75.

24 Cosgriff TM, Kelly AM, Kerr D. External validation of the San Francisco Syncope Rule in the Australian context. *Can J Emerg Med* 2007;**9**: 157–61.

25 Grossman S, Lieberman R, Bar J, et al. Reducing admissions utilizing the Boston Syncope Criteria (Abstract). *Acad Emerg Med* 2007;**14**:S47.

26 Quinn JV, Stiell IG, McDermott DA, et al. The San Francisco Syncope Rule vs physician judgment and decision making. *Am J Emerg Med* 2005;**23**:782–6.

27 American College of Emergency Physicians. Clinical policy: critical issues in the evaluation and management of patients with syncope. *Ann Emerg Med* 2001;**37**:771–6.

28 Strickberger SA, Benson W, Biaggioni I, et al. AHA/ACCF scientific statement on the evaluation of syncope. *J Am Coll Cardiol* 2006;**47**:473–84.

29 Elesber AA, Decker WW, Smars PA, et al. Impact of the application of the American College of Emergency Physicians recommendations for the admission of patients with syncope on a retrospectively studied population presenting to the emergency department. *Am Heart J* 2005;**149**:826–31.

30 Bartoletti A, Fabiani P, Adriani P, et al. Hospital admission of patients referred to the emergency department for syncope: a single-hospital prospective study based on the application of the European Society of Cardiology Guidelines on syncope. *Eur Heart J* 2006;**27**:83–8.

31 Brignole M, Ungar A, Bartoletti A, et al. Standardized-care pathway vs. usual management of syncope patients presenting as emergencies at general hospitals. *Europace* 2006;**8**:644–50.

32 Brignole M, Disertori M, Menozzi C, et al. Management of syncope referred urgently to general hospitals with and without syncope units. *Europace* 2003;**5**:293–8.

33 Shen WK, Decker WW, Smars PA, et al. Syncope evaluation in the emergency department (SEEDS). A multidisciplinary approach to syncope management. *Circulation* 2004;**110**:3636–45.

34 World Health Organization. *Multinational Monitoring of Trends and Determinants in Cardiovascular Disease (MONICA Projects)*. Manual of Operations No. WHO/MNC/82.2. World Health Organization, Geneva, 1983:248.

27 General Toxicology

Luke Yip,[1] Nicole Bouchard[2] & Marco L. A. Sivilotti[3]

[1] Department of Emergency, The Prince Charles Hospital, Chermside, Queensland, Australia *and* Rocky Mountain Poison and Drug Center, Denver *and* Department of Medicine, Division of Medical Toxicology, Denver Health Medical Center, Denver *and* School of Pharmacy, University of Colorado Health Sciences Center, Denver, USA

[2] Emergency Medicine Department, New York–Presbyterian Hospital, Columbia University Medical Center, New York *and* New York City Poison Control Center, New York, USA

[3] Departments of Emergency Medicine *and* Pharmacology and Toxicology, Queen's University, Kingston *and* Ontario Poison Centre, Toronto, Canada

SCENARIO 1

Clinical scenario

A 19-year-old female arrived in the emergency department (ED) after she had ingested two packets of oral contraceptive pills over 1 hour following an argument with her boyfriend. She was crying and upset. Her vital signs were normal, except for a heart rate of 110 beats/min. Physical examination was unremarkable.

A 47-year-old female presented to the ED 3–4 hours after overdosing on an extended-release formulation of verapamil and rapidly lost consciousness while being assessed by the nursing staff. Her vital signs were: heart rate 60 beats/min, blood pressure 80/40 mmHg and respiratory rate 10 breaths/min. Physical examination was remarkable for the absence of a gag reflex and coma. The electrocardiogram (ECG) demonstrated a sinus bradycardia and a first-degree heart block. Laboratory data were normal except for a serum bicarbonate of 20 mmol/L and a glucose of 18.1 mmol/L (325 mg/dl).

Background

It has been estimated 1% of ED visits in the United States are poisoning related [1]. Patient presentation is diverse and spans a clinical spectrum from inconsequential to immediately life-threatening overdoses. Among the time-honoured and accepted medical treatments is the use of gastrointestinal decontamination (GID) for ingested poisons. "Gastrointestinal" refers to both gastric and intestinal components of this procedure. Gastric decontamination can be achieved by either administration of ipecac syrup or gastric lavage. Intestinal decontamination can be effective by either the administration of activated charcoal or whole bowel irrigation, which

may have the additional benefit of gastric decontamination. GID may also be accomplished by surgical or manual interventions. Physicians have routinely used gastric decontamination followed by activated charcoal with or without a cathartic. Over the past 20 years routine GID for all overdose patients has been questioned and scrutinized. Clinical studies have provided an opportunity to evaluate GID strategies for the poisoned patient. GID strategies continue to evolve and their refinement in patient selection, ingestant, technique and timing considerations are targets of thoughtful analysis and future research.

The art of medical toxicology encompasses intuition, common sense, logic, rational thought and clinical experience. These concepts gave rise to the principles of minimizing systemic absorption and decreasing gastrointestinal transit time of an ingestant. In contrast, the science of medical toxicology provided increasing evidence towards a less aggressive approach in GID for the heterogeneous population of unselected overdose patients. The apparent contradictions between the art and the science have generated significant controversies and debates in clinical toxicology. This has been reflected in wide variations between treatment recommendations, which may be inconsistent with position statements and conclusions from published studies, and different opinions among toxicologists who made substantial contributions to the development of these statements [2–4].

An evidence-based approach to clinical practice is only as good as the evidence. Position statements on GID have provided an extraordinary review of the literature [5–10]. However, the vast majority of available data for analysis were derived from models that do not necessarily reflect clinical reality.

Clinical questions

In order to address the issues of greatest relevance to your patients and to help in searching the literature for the evidence regarding toxicology issues, each scenario will be followed by a series of questions structured as recommended in Chapter 1.

Evidence-based Emergency Medicine. Edited by Brian H. Rowe
© 2009 Blackwell Publishing, ISBN: 978-1-4051-6143-5.

1 In adult patients with an acute drug overdose (population), does gastric emptying (ipecac syrup, gastric lavage) compared to activated charcoal (comparison) as initial treatment (intervention) prevent clinical deterioration or improve clinical outcome (outcomes)?

2 In adult patients with an acute overdose (population), does activated charcoal compared with observation (comparison) as initial treatment (intervention) prevent clinical deterioration or improve clinical outcome (outcomes)?

General search strategy

The search included efforts to identify controlled clinical trials (CCTs), randomized clinical trials (RCTs), systematic reviews from evidence-based medicine reviews (Cochrane Library, ACP Journal Club) and traditional electronic searching (e.g., MEDLINE) using the following search terms: gastrointestinal decontamination, decontamination, gastric emptying, gastric lavage, emptying, lavage, ipecac and charcoal. When no trials were identified, position papers were searched for consensus recommendations.

Question 1: In adult patients with an acute drug overdose (population), does gastric emptying (ipecac syrup, gastric lavage) compared to activated charcoal (comparison) as initial treatment (intervention) prevent clinical deterioration or improve clinical outcome (outcomes)?

> **Search strategy**
>
> • Cochrane and MEDLINE: (gastrointestinal decontamination OR decontamination, gastric emptying OR gastric lavage OR emptying, lavage OR ipecac) AND (RCTs OR systematic reviews)

There were four studies involving some form of gastric emptying technique followed by administration of activated charcoal compared to administration of activated charcoal alone (Table 27.1) [11–14]. These CCTs included a total of 2025 predominately adults representing a heterogeneous group of unselected patients with an acute drug overdose. Seriously sick patients and individual toxins of clinical consequence comprised a small subgroup. Patients were usually excluded from the study if there was ingestion of hydrocarbons, corrosives, iron, strychnine, camphor, heavy metals, monoamine oxidase inhibitors, digoxin, formaldehyde, mushrooms, modified-release products, lithium, acetaminophen (paracetamol), alcohol or other substances not absorbed to activated charcoal. Gastric emptying was accomplished by either ipecac syrup or gastric lavage. Activated charcoal was administered either alone or in combination with a cathartic. The outcomes included clinical deterioration or improvement, length of stay, hospital admission and complications (e.g., aspiration pneumonia, artificial ventilation). Outcome assessment occurred at least

4–6 hours after treatment. In spite of these similarities, significant differences between studies made pooling of results inappropriate.

The methodology of these studies limits generalizations. However, it does permit some conclusions to be made regarding the initial GID of a *heterogeneous* adult population presenting to an ED following an acute oral drug overdose. Gastric emptying does not appear to improve clinical outcomes, except perhaps in patients who were obtunded and presented to the ED within 1 hour of their overdose, and omission of gastric lavage may not be associated with clinical deterioration [11]. The data were insufficient to preclude benefit in severely sick patients presenting beyond 1 hour from their overdose and were limited by low power, selection bias, lack of objective confirmation of overdose and limited adjustment for severity. Since timing of overdoses is often unreliable and arrival to an ED within 1 hour of an overdose is unusual, this finding may not provide much guidance to clinicians. Adverse events (e.g., aspiration, intubation, ventilator use, intensive care unit admission, esophageal perforation) were more common in the gastric emptying group.

In summary, gastric emptying should not be routinely performed on all drug overdose patients. In most cases the administration of activated charcoal with a cathartic and supportive care are sufficient treatment to achieve a satisfactory clinical outcome. Whether gastric emptying can be omitted from the treatment protocol for every overdose patient remains to be determined. There are insufficient data to preclude benefit from gastric lavage followed by activated charcoal in severely sick patients presenting more than 1 hour from their overdose.

Question 2: In adult patients with an acute overdose (population), does activated charcoal compared with observation (comparison) as initial treatment (intervention) prevent clinical deterioration or improve clinical outcome (outcomes)?

> **Search strategy**
>
> • Cochrane and MEDLINE: charcoal AND overdose AND (RCTs OR systematic reviews)

There were three studies involving GID with activated charcoal compared to observation and supportive care (Table 27.2) [13,15,16]. Two CCTs included a total of 1930 adult patients and one RCT included 327 patients aged 16 years or older. The time between ingestion and treatment was reported only in the RCT, which included only patients presenting within 12 hours of their overdose; approximately 60% of these patients presented within 2 hours. The study population was a heterogeneous group of unselected patients with an acute drug overdose, and seriously sick patients and individual toxins of clinical consequence comprised a small subgroup. Exclusion criteria were similar to the Question 1 studies above. Activated charcoal was administered without a cathartic. The outcomes included clinical deterioration or

Table 27.1 Summary of evidence table for gastrointestinal decontamination with gastric emptying and activated charcoal.

Study	Population	Intervention	Control	Outcomes	Design	Effect measure	Summary
Kulig et al. [11]	592 patients with acute oral drug overdose; 5 patients < 5 years of age	GL (30–40 French tube) or IS followed by AC 30–50 g (20 g or 250 mg/kg for a child) plus $MgSO_4$ ($N = 286$)	AC 30–50 g (20 g or 250 mg/kg for a child) plus $MgSO_4$ ($N = 306$)	Clinical deterioration or improvement; observed $\geq$ 6 hours (except those admitted to the ICU)	CCT; consecutive patients; investigator could exclude patients	Clinical improvement ($P < 0.05$) in obtunded patients following GL (< 1 hour of OD); more aspiration and esophageal tear	GL (< 1 h of OD) may have a positive contribution in obtunded patients
Albertson et al. [12]	200 adult (> 18 years) patients with acute oral drug overdose (awake, cooperative with gag reflex)	IS 30 ml (repeated in 30 minutes if no response) followed by AC-S solution 1 g/kg ($N = 93$)	AC-S (1 g/kg) solution ($N = 107$)	Treatment-related complication rate; ED, hospital and ICU LOS; ICU/hospital admission	CCT; convenience sample and at discretion of investigator	Intervention group had more complications and ED LOS ($P < 0.05$); no difference in clinical outcomes	IS has an apparent negative contribution when administered prior to AC-S
Merigian et al. [13]	357 adult patients with symptomatic acute oral drug overdose	GL ("large bore Ewald tube") or IS followed by AC 50 g ($N = 163$)	AC 50 g (obtunded patients had limited gastric aspiration by nasogastric tube prior to AC) ($N = 194$)	Clinical deterioration or improvement; observed 4 hours	CCT; consecutive patients; investigator could exclude patients	Intervention group had more aspiration pneumonia and ventilator use ($P = 0.0001$) and ICU admission; control group had increased non-ICU admission	Gastric emptying has no apparent positive contribution and may be associated with increased complications and ICU admission
Pond et al. [14]	876 patients (> 13 years) with acute oral drug overdose	GL (36 French tube) or IS (30–50 ml; repeated if no response) followed by AC 50 g with sorbitol ($N = 459$)	AC 50 g slurry with sorbitol (200 ml) ($N = 417$)	Clinical deterioration or improvement; observed 6 hours; LOS	CCT; consecutive patients	No difference in clinical outcome between groups; control got AC-S sooner	Gastric emptying has no apparent positive contribution and delays AC-S administration

AC, activated charcoal; AC-S, activated charcoal with sorbitol; CCT, controlled clinical trial; ED, emergency department; GL, gastric lavage; ICU, intensive care unit; IS, ipecac syrup; LOS, length of stay; $MgSO_4$, magnesium sulfate; OD, overdose.

Table 27.2 Summary of evidence table for gastrointestinal decontamination without gastric emptying.

Study	Population	Intervention	Control	Outcomes	Design	Effect measure	Summary
Merigian et al. [13]	451 adult patients with asymptomatic acute oral drug overdose	AC 50 g ($N = 220$)	Observation ($N = 231$)	Clinical deterioration or improvement; observed 4 hours	CCT; consecutive patients; investigator could exclude patients	No difference in clinical outcome between groups	AC has no apparent positive contribution
Merigian & Blaho [15]	1479 adult patients with acute oral drug overdose	AC 50 g ($N = 399$)	Observation ($N = 1080$)	Clinical deterioration or improvement: observed ≥ 4 hours; incidence of vomiting, complications associated with overdose or treatment, and LOS	CCT; consecutive patients	Intervention group had increased ED LOS, incidence of vomiting ($P < 0.01$) and number of intubated ICU patients ($P = 0.01$); no increased ICU LOS; decreased non-ICU LOS	AC may have a positive contribution in decreasing non-ICU LOS but may be associated with increased complications, ICU admission and ED LOS
Cooper et al. [16]	327 patients (≥ 16 years) with acute drug overdose	AC 50 g slurry with water (200 ml) ($N = 166$)	Observation ($N = 161$)	LOS; requirement for ventilation, vomiting, incidence of aspiration and death	RCT; consecutive patients; investigator could exclude patients	No difference in clinical outcome between groups	AC has no apparent positive contribution

AC, activated charcoal; CCT, controlled clinical trial; ED, emergency department; ICU, intensive care unit; LOS, length of stay; RCT, randomized clinical trial.

improvement, length of stay, hospital admission and complications (e.g., vomiting, aspiration pneumonia, ventilator use, death). Outcome assessment occurred at least 4 hours after treatment. In spite of these similarities, significant differences between studies made pooling of results inappropriate.

The methodology of these studies limits generalizations. However, it does permit some general conclusions to be made regarding the initial GID of a *heterogeneous* adult population presenting to an ED following an acute oral drug overdose. A satisfactory clinical outcome may be achieved in most asymptomatic patients with a history of *trivial* overdose without GID. However, this result was tainted by the lack of objective confirmation that asymptomatic patients had ingested a toxic substance or a toxic (potentially lethal) dose of a substance.

In summary, activated charcoal does not appear to improve clinical outcomes in *generic* overdose patients, challenging the routine use of activated charcoal. Whether activated charcoal can be omitted from the treatment protocol for *every* adult overdose patient remains to be determined. There are insufficient data to preclude benefits from activated charcoal for selected overdose patients including the severely sick or most likely to deteriorate.

Conclusions

The first patient presented with a clinically inconsequential overdose (i.e., oral contraceptive pills) and is expected to have a satisfactory clinical outcome without GID. In contrast, the other patient in coma and shock following an overdose of a modified-release verapamil product may die in spite of maximal therapy. Since it has been 3–4 hours after ingestion and the patient is unconscious, ipecac-induced emesis would be contraindicated [8]. It is unknown if a 3–4-hour interval post-ingestion would preclude benefit from gastric lavage [7]. Additional methods of GID include a single dose of activated charcoal, multiple-dose activated charcoal, and whole bowel irrigation [5,9,10]. A straightforward rigorous scientific management guideline for this patient is not possible because the patient presented here was never the focus of any published RCT and was never adequately studied.

The results reported in clinical trials should be appreciated with an understanding that all studies to date are limited by (i) an under-representation of seriously sick patients; (ii) the heterogeneity of drug doses and formulations studied; (iii) a lack of objective quantifiable confirmation that patients had ingested a toxic substance or a toxic (potentially lethal) dose of a substance; and (iv) the lack of data for rigorous comparison of outcomes by patient presentation at hourly intervals [11–16]. The inability to confirm a patient had taken an overdose, much less a consequential overdose, may obscure any benefit GID may have on clinical outcome. The time dependency of GID has not been well characterized based on comparing patients presenting within 1 or 2 hours of their ingestion, and does not preclude GID considerations beyond 1 hour of an overdose [11,14,16]. Limited data are available to guide decisions on the small subset of patients with life-threatening ingestions.

The apparent lack of benefit from GID in general should not be construed to imply a benefit does not exist, and should not be justification to abandon therapies based on intuition, common sense, logic, rational thought and clinical experience.

The result of clinical research on GID appears to reflect the fact that most overdose patients presenting to an ED have clinically mild to moderate intoxications, are likely to have a satisfactory clinical outcome with mostly supportive care, and that routine gastrointestinal procedures do not improve clinical outcome. Obtunded patients who present within 1 hour of their overdose may benefit from gastric lavage.

Existing clinical evidence is entirely consistent with the premise that GID will have benefit in some clinical situations with minimal or proportionate risk to the patient. Patients with serious or life-threatening overdoses may benefit from gastric lavage followed by administration of activated charcoal, and it should be seriously considered and undertaken even when patients present more than 1 hour from their overdose. Activated charcoal should be considered in potentially serious overdose and when it appears likely that a significant amount of poison is present in the gastrointestinal tract.

SCENARIO 2

Clinical scenario

A 48-year-old undomiciled man presented to the ED with ethanol intoxication. He was diagnosed with left foot cellulitis, and admitted for IV antibiotics. While awaiting an inpatient bed, he awoke and complained of "the shakes" and malaise. He subsequently experienced two brief generalized seizures with a short post-ictal period. He was tremulous, anxious and restless, but oriented to person, place and time. The remainder of his physical and neurological examination was unremarkable.

His vital signs were: temperature 37.3°C (oral), heart rate 100 beats/min, blood pressure 130/90 mmHg, respiratory rate 18 breaths/min and pulse oximetry reading of 96% on room air. Finger stick capillary glucose was 105 mg/dl (5.8 mmol/L). The serum ethanol concentration at the time of the seizure was 57 mg/d (12 mmol/L). Other lab studies showed a white blood cell count of 13,000/ml; electrolytes, blood urea nitrogen (BUN), creatinine and hepatic profile were within normal limits. A chest X-ray and ECG were non-diagnostic.

Background

The care and disposition of patients with alcohol-related seizures (ARSs) is particularly relevant to emergency physicians since ARSs are a common occurrence in the ED, particularly in urban settings [17–19]. Seizures are the first manifestation of alcohol withdrawal syndrome in heavy drinkers and occur in 10% of patients during alcohol withdrawal. Seizures occur 7–48 hours after the last drink in 90% of patients. Most untreated patients will experience one to three generalized tonic-clonic, brief, self-limited seizures in rapid succession with a small percentage of patients progressing to status epilepticus and roughly one-third of patients will progress to delirium tremens [20–22]. The interval between the first to the last seizure is 6 hours or less in 85% of the patients.

Many patients with ARS exhibit no other signs or symptoms of withdrawal (e.g., tremor, diaphoresis, anxiety, tachycardia) despite relatively low or absent serum ethanol levels, although such signs do eventually become manifest in some cases [23,24]. Clinicians should not assume that ARSs are simply due to alcohol withdrawal. In one ED-based study, 26% of ARSs were attributed to head trauma, 16% to idiopathic seizure disorder, 6% to cerebrovascular accidents and 3% to toxic or metabolic abnormalities [20]. For this reason, the term ARS (rather than alcohol withdrawal seizure) is preferred (or "is used") to describe generalized tonic-clonic seizures that occur in the setting of chronic alcohol dependence [25].

Alcohol-related seizures are a manifestation of a diverse and interrelated array of pathological processes [17,20,23,25–28]:

• *Alcohol withdrawal*: abstinence or decreasing alcohol intake, especially rapid declines in serum ethanol precipitate ARS. A long history of heavy drinking (c. 300 g/day) is a strong risk factor, but not a prerequisite.

• *Epilepsy*: alcohol abuse exacerbates underlying epilepsy. The prevalence of epilepsy in alcoholics is triple that of the general population and is one of the most common causes of new-onset seizures in adults.

• *Structural brain lesions*: cerebrovascular accidents, head trauma, atrophy or tumors may cause seizures.

• *Co-ingestants*: an ARS may occur in association with the use of illicit drugs or medications. Rarely, severe intoxication with alcohol alone can precipitate ARSs.

Chronic alcohol consumption produces cerebral neurochemical alterations. Ethanol is a γ-aminobutyric acid (GABA) receptor-chloride channel agonist and an N-methy-D-aspartate receptor (NMDA) antagonist. With chronic exposure to ethanol the inhibitory GABA channel is down-regulated and the excitatory NMDA receptor is up-regulated [29–36]. Alcohol withdrawal seizures are thought to occur from rapid changes in this unbalanced state of receptor stimulation. Traditional anticonvulsants (e.g., phenytoin, carbamazepine) and medications that increase GABA tone (e.g., benzodiazepines, barbiturates) have both been proposed for the treatment of ARS [37]. Since there are no pure NMDA agonists currently available, there are no human studies to address their role in the treatment of ARS.

Clinical questions

3 In patients with alcohol-related seizures (population), does anticonvulsant therapy with phenytoin or carbamazepine (intervention) prevent recurrent seizures (outcome) compared to supportive care (comparison)?

4 In patients with alcohol-related seizures (population), do GABA agonists such as benzodiazepines or barbiturates (intervention) prevent recurrent seizures (outcome) compared to supportive care (comparison)?

General search strategy

The search for systematic reviews started with the Cochrane Library using search terms such as: alcohol-related seizures OR alcohol withdrawal AND (anticonvulsant; GABA agonists). The search for RCTs and systematic reviews was expanded to traditional electronic databases such as MEDLINE and EMBASE using search terms such as: (alcoholism OR alcohol-related seizures OR alcohol withdrawal OR alcohol withdrawal seizures OR alcohol OR seizures) AND (anticonvulsant; GABA agonists). The studies were restricted to human systematic reviews or RCTs and treatment.

Critical review of the literature

Question 3: In patients with alcohol-related seizures (population), does anticonvulsant therapy with phenytoin or carbamazepine (intervention) prevent recurrent seizures (outcome) compared to supportive care (comparison)?

Search strategy

• Cochrane Library: (alcohol-related seizures OR alcohol withdrawal) AND anticonvulsants

• MEDLINE and EMBASE: (alcoholism OR alcohol-related seizures OR alcohol withdrawal OR alcohol withdrawal seizures OR alcohol OR seizures) AND anticonvulsants

Rapid control of seizures is an undisputed goal in emergency medicine to reduce aspiration, and to prevent recurrent seizures and secondary trauma. Objectives differ between the management of acute ARSs in the ED, the prevention of alcohol withdrawal seizures in hospitalized inpatients, and the treatment of primary or secondary epilepsy with or without concurrent alcoholism. A Cochrane review updated in 2005 concluded that some anticonvulsants, particularly carbamazepine, are potentially beneficial in the treatment and prevention of alcohol withdrawal seizures in patients undergoing alcohol detoxification [38]. Studies involving patients in detoxification units undergoing treatment for alcohol withdrawal demonstrate conflicting findings regarding a role for phenytoin in preventing seizures [38]. Phenytoin is established therapy for seizures originating from a structural focus.

Overall, the search identified three RCTs that examined patients at high risk of alcohol-related seizures. They all compared phenytoin to placebo and measured recurrent witnessed seizures at least 6 hours after presentation. The results suggest phenytoin has no significant benefit when administered to non-epileptic patients with acute, undifferentiated ARSs (presumed to be from withdrawal) for secondary seizure prevention (Table 27.3, Fig. 27.1) [39–41]. While there are limitations to this body of research, these data generate a pooled result (Fig. 27.1) indicating phenytoin's ineffectiveness at preventing second seizures (pooled RR = 0.95; 95% CI: 0.56 to 1.61; I^2 index for heterogeneity = 0% [18]). It is important to note that patients with metabolic disorders, co-ingested drugs, severe withdrawal and recent trauma were excluded from these studies.

In summary, the use of IV phenytoin for the prevention of recurrent seizures in patients with ARSs secondary to alcohol withdrawal seizures cannot be supported. This conclusion should not be extrapolated to patients with severe head trauma, epilepsy or structural brain lesions.

Question 4: In patients with alcohol-related seizures (population), do GABA agonists such as benzodiazepines or barbiturates (intervention) prevent recurrent seizures (outcome) compared to supportive care (comparison)?

Search strategy

- Cochrane Library: (alcohol-related seizures OR alcohol withdrawal) AND GABA agonist drugs (i.e., benzodiazepine, barbiturates)

- MEDLINE and EMBASE: (alcoholism OR alcohol-related seizures OR alcohol withdrawal OR alcohol withdrawal seizures OR alcohol OR seizures) AND GABA agonists (i.e., benzodiazepine, barbiturates)

Only one prospective RCT has addressed benzodiazepine therapy in acute ARS in ED patients [37]. A Cochrane review updated in 2005 concluded that benzodiazepines were superior to other forms of therapy when seizures were examined as a subset of the more comprehensive clinical picture of the alcohol withdrawal syndrome [42].

In 1999, D'Onofrio and colleagues published their prospective, randomized, placebo-controlled, double-blind trial of 229 consecutive patients presenting with ARS in two US city hospital EDs [37]. Over a 21-month period, IV lorazepam (2 mg) or placebo were administered to 186 adult patients with a history of recent and chronic alcohol abuse and a witnessed generalized seizure not attributable to another cause (Table 27.4). The primary outcome was a second witnessed generalized seizure up to 6 hours after drug or placebo administration. Both seizures (RR = 0.13; 95% CI: 0.04 to 0.37) and hospitalizations (RR = 0.61; 95% CI: 0.42 to 0.90) were less frequent in the lorazepam group. After discharge, seven patients from the placebo group were transported by ambulance to another ED for recurrent seizures within 48 hours versus one in the lorazepam group.

In summary, IV lorazepam is effective at preventing multiple seizures and hospitalization for patients with uncomplicated ARSs. Emergency physicians should remain vigilant to exclude secondary causes of seizures and to detect patients at risk for major alcohol withdrawal.

Conclusions

The patient described above was given 2 mg of IV lorazepam immediately following the seizure. A computerized tomography scan of the head showed diffuse atrophy and no other abnormalities. He reported no history of epilepsy; however, he had experienced an ARS twice in the past. He had no history of hospitalization for major withdrawal. He was admitted to the medical service for continued treatment of cellulitis and alcohol withdrawal. During hospitalization, benzodiazepines were titrated according to a symptom-triggered structured assessment scale, and he remained seizure free.

Alcohol withdrawal and its consequences are important ED problems. Phenytoin does not appear to be of benefit in the treatment of acute ARS in the absence of structural lesions, severe head trauma or underlying epilepsy. Lorazepam appears to be effective treatment in preventing secondary ARSs. The management of patients with structural brain abnormality, severe head trauma or moderate to severe alcohol withdrawal should be individualized according to accepted guidelines and patient-specific situations.

SCENARIO 3

Clinical scenario

A 38-year-old cement worker arrived by ambulance to the ED for syncope and confusion. He was operating a gas-powered cutting tool for approximately 2 hours in the basement of a house when he became acutely unwell, exited the building and had a brief, witnessed loss of consciousness. His co-workers activated the emergency response system, and paramedics applied high-flow oxygen via a non-rebreather mask during transport to hospital. Upon ED arrival, the patient was awake and alert, complaining only of a mild headache.

Vital signs were unremarkable including a pulse oximetry reading of 100% on oxygen. Careful neurological examination failed to demonstrate deficits other than some hesitation and two instances of uncorrected digit reversal when he was asked to provide his 10-digit phone number backwards. A carboxyhemoglobin fraction of 0.27 (27%) was measured from a venous blood gas sample obtained about 30 minutes after oxygen was first applied, and about 45 minutes following the patient's exit from the building. The other co-workers were not affected. The nearest hyperbaric facility to this ED is approximately 250 km away.

Background

Carbon monoxide (CO) is a colorless, odorless, non-irritating gas generated by the incomplete combustion of hydrocarbon fuels. It is

Table 27.3 Summary of evidence for the effectiveness of phenytoin in treating alcohol-related seizures.

Study	Population	Intervention	Control	Outcomes	Design	Effect measure RR (95% CI)	Summary
Rathlev et al. [41]	100 consecutive adult patients with chronic alcohol abuse presenting with a seizure	IV phenytoin 15 mg/kg over 20 minutes	IV normal saline	Development of a second generalized seizure up to 6 hours after drug or placebo administration	Prospective, randomized, double-blind, placebo-controlled trial	RR = 1.1 (0.38 to 3.06)	Phenytoin has no apparent benefit in preventing recurrent ARS
Chance [40]	55 patients presenting with alcohol withdrawal seizures	IV phenytoin 15 mg/kg (max. 1000 mg)	IV normal saline	Development of a second generalized seizure up to 6 hours after drug or placebo administration	Prospective, randomized, double-blind, placebo-controlled trial	RR = 0.87 (0.41 to 1.8)	Phenytoin has no apparent benefit in preventing recurrent ARS
Alldredge et al. [39]	90 patients enrolled within 6 hours of a presumed alcohol-related seizure	IV phenytoin 1000 mg	IV normal saline	Development of a second generalized seizure up to 12 hours after drug or placebo administration	Prospective, randomized, double-blind, placebo-controlled trial	RR = 1.0 (0.35 to 2.8)	Phenytoin has no apparent benefit in preventing recurrent seizures in non-epileptic patients with ARS
Pooled data	245 patients	IV phenytoin 15 mg/kg	IV placebo	Witnessed seizure > 6 hours	3 prospective, randomized, double-blind, placebo-controlled trials	RR = 0.95 (0.56 to 1.61)	Phenytoin has no significant benefit in preventing recurrent ARS

ARS, alcohol-related seizure; CI, confidence interval; RR, relative risk.

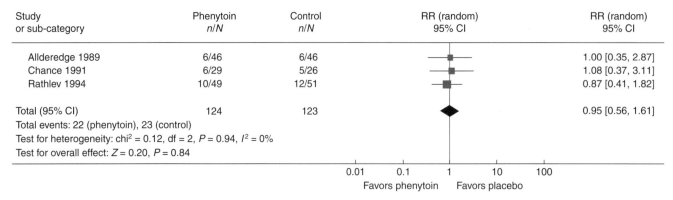

Study or sub-category	Phenytoin n/N	Control n/N	RR (random) 95% CI	RR (random) 95% CI
Allderedge 1989	6/46	6/46		1.00 [0.35, 2.87]
Chance 1991	6/29	5/26		1.08 [0.37, 3.11]
Rathlev 1994	10/49	12/51		0.87 [0.41, 1.82]
Total (95% CI)	124	123		0.95 [0.56, 1.61]

Total events: 22 (phenytoin), 23 (control)
Test for heterogeneity: chi^2 = 0.12, df = 2, P = 0.94, I^2 = 0%
Test for overall effect: Z = 0.20, P = 0.84

Figure 27.1 Phenytoin compared to placebo to prevent alcohol-related seizures.

estimated to be responsible for at least half of all poisoning fatalities worldwide. Small amounts are produced endogenously by heme metabolism, but toxicity results following inhalation of air containing more than 50 ppm of CO. Atmospheric CO concentrations are usually less than 10 ppm, but are higher in urban areas and congested motorways. Non-smokers have carboxyhemoglobin fractions of < 2%. Inhaled cigarette smoke contains 50–1000 ppm. Gasoline engines may produce up to 70,000 ppm CO and improper ventilation of this exhaust can cause death within minutes. Following emission control legislation, motor vehicles with catalytic converters typically exhaust CO at below 1000 ppm and the incidence of suicide following car exhaust collection has fallen dramatically [43]. Carbon monoxide detectors typically alarm after 15 minutes of 400 ppm exposure, or 180 minutes of 70 ppm exposure, which can result in a carboxyhemoglobin concentration of 10% with moderate exertion.

Moderately severe exposures present with a variety of non-specific symptoms such as headache, nausea, vomiting, blurred vision, chest pain, syncope, neurological deficits and transient confusion. Emergency physicians should remain vigilant for such cases to avoid discharging the patient back to the source of the exposure and missing multiple undiagnosed victims. The presence of seizures, coma, dysrhythmia, hypotension or myocardial ischemia denotes a severe exposure, which can culminate in cardiopulmonary arrest. Chronic moderate exposures can result in

apathy, insomnia, personality disturbances, cardiomegaly and cardiomyopathy. The diagnosis is easy to confirm by co-oximetry of a venous blood sample, but it must be entertained in the first place. There is mixed evidence regarding screening ED patients during the winter heating season for occult CO toxicity with pulse co-oximetry [44,45].

Carbon monoxide toxicity was once attributed to hemoglobin binding and interference with oxygen transport and delivery. However, it is now understood to be far more complex. Carbon monoxide itself has a myriad of direct effects on the microcirculation, binds to heme proteins and interferes with cellular respiration. At low physiological concentrations, it may play a beneficial role in signal transduction analogous to nitric oxide. At higher, toxic doses, tissue hypoxia despite circulatory perfusion, increased nitric oxide activity and free radical formation converge to cause end-organ toxicity. The prime target of CO toxicity is the nervous system, although the circulatory system is also affected [46,47]. The measured carboxyhemoglobin fraction should be interpreted to be a measure of exposure, and not of toxicity. Similarly, serial changes in carboxyhemoglobin fraction after removal from the source exposure represent simple competition with molecular oxygen, and do not necessarily correlate with the patient's clinical status or provide direct information on the clinical course. Pulse oximetry cannot distinguish between oxyhemoglobin and carboxyhemoglobin, and is falsely elevated in the presence of the latter.

Table 27.4 Randomized controlled trial for alcohol-related seizure treatment with benzodiazepines.

Study	Population	Intervention	Control	Outcomes	Design	Effect measure RR (95% CI)	Summary
D'Onofrio et al. [37]	186 adult patients with chronic alcohol abuse with a witnessed generalized seizure and a history of 1 + drinks in the previous 72 hours	IV lorazepam 2 mg	IV normal saline	Development of a second generalized seizure up to 6 hours after drug or placebo administration	Prospective, randomized, double-blind, placebo-controlled trial	RR (seizure) = 0.13 (0.04 to 0.37); RR (hospitalizations) = 0.61 (0.42 to 0.90)	Lorazepam reduces the risk of recurrent ARS in the emergency department and of hospitalization

ARS, alcohol-related seizure; CI, confidence interval; RR, relative risk.

Delayed neurological sequelae (DNS) may develop in a subset of patients usually 2–3 weeks following an acute exposure. A broad range of neuropsychiatric symptoms including disorientation, memory loss, hallucinations, motor disturbances, ataxia, impaired concentration, emotional lability, dementia, psychosis, Parkinsonism and incontinence have been described and are termed the *DNS syndrome*. Unfortunately, there are inconsistent definitions of DNS, which include patient self-reported symptoms and overt neurological deficits as well as subclinical findings on detailed neuropsychometric testing. It appears that more severely exposed patients are at greater risk of developing DNS, although it remains difficult to predict the likelihood of developing DNS in any given patient. Coma at presentation, increasing age and increased duration of exposure appear to be risk factors for developing DNS [48,49]. Most patients will recover within 1 year.

Treatment of CO toxicity begins with removal from the source, identification of other victims and empirical administration of high-flow oxygen. The possibilities of co-inhalants including cyanide following smoke inhalation and of co-ingestants following deliberate self-harm should be considered. High-flow oxygen competes with CO for binding to heme proteins including hemoglobin, and the carboxyhemoglobin fraction falls with a half-life of about 1 hour at an FiO_2 near 100% at sea level. The decision whether to provide higher doses of oxygen in a hyperbaric chamber remains highly controversial. Historically, it was assumed that the faster fall in carboxyhemoglobin with hyperbaric oxygen must be beneficial. Advocates of hyperbaric therapy now propose other benefits, including effects on free radical injury, neutrophil adhesion, alterations in myelin basic protein, nitric oxide synthetase activity and modulation of excitatory amino acid effects. An individualized decision for a given patient should be informed by the available and conflicting evidence.

General search strategy

The search included efforts to identify CCTs, RCTs, systematic reviews from evidence-based medicine reviews (Cochrane Library, ACP Journal Club) and traditional electronic searching (e.g., MEDLINE) using the following search terms: carbon monoxide and hyperbaric oxygen.

Clinical question

5 In patients with acute, unintentional exposure to carbon monoxide with syncope, elevated carboxyhemoglobin fraction and minor deficits of concentration (population), does the early administration of hyperbaric oxygen therapy (intervention) reduce the incidence of delayed neurological sequelae (outcome) compared to normobaric oxygen (control)?

Critical review of the literature

Question 5: In patients with acute, unintentional exposure to carbon monoxide with syncope, elevated carboxyhemoglobin fraction and minor deficits of concentration (population), does the early administration of hyperbaric oxygen therapy (intervention) reduce the incidence of delayed neurological sequelae (outcome) compared to normobaric oxygen (control)?

Search strategy

- Cochrane Library: carbon monoxide AND hyperbaric oxygen
- MEDLINE (1950 to August week 1, 2007): carbon monoxide. Limited to clinical trials (all phases) or RCTs
- Forward citation search and consultation with experts in the field

A total of seven prospective RCTs are available, of which only three report a benefit to hyperbaric oxygen [50–56]. A Cochrane review updated in 2004 concluded that the existing evidence did not establish whether hyperbaric oxygen reduced the incidence of adverse neurological outcomes [57]. Considerable heterogeneity exists between the studies with regard to design, population studied, hyperbaric and normobaric oxygen protocols, and outcomes measured. It is therefore informative to consider the two most recently published trials individually, especially since they are the only studies of high quality (Jadad score 5/5) and since they came to opposing conclusions (Table 27.5).

A randomized, double-blinded trial of 191 sequential patients referred to a single centre in Australia for CO poisoning was published in 1999 [54]. Multiple victims from the same exposure were assigned to the same intervention, resulting in a numerical imbalance between arms. At hospital discharge there was no difference in what appears to have been the primary outcome of persistent neurological sequelae (74% hyperbaric vs 68% control; adjusted OR = 1.7; 95% CI: 0.8 to 4.0). However, in the severely poisoned subgroup, the rate of persistent neurological sequelae was higher in the intervention group (85% hyperbaric vs 65% control; adjusted OR = 3.6 95% CI: 1.1 to 11.9). Substantially more subjects in the hyperbaric group (28% vs 15%; adjusted OR = 2.8; 95% CI: 1.3 to 6.2) were deemed clinically unwell after the third treatment and were re-treated, and this difference was particularly apparent in the large subgroup of severely poisoned patients (35% vs 13%; adjusted OR = 5.4; 95% CI: 2.0 to 14.8). Only half of the patients returned for the planned 1-month follow-up, but all five cases of new symptoms or deterioration on neuropsychological subtest scores by more than one standard deviation (the operational definition of DNS) occurred in the hyperbaric group. There were seven cases of ear barotraumas, and one seizure during hyperbaric oxygen therapy. Stratifying by delay to treatment, carboxyhemoglobin fraction, self-harm intent or endotracheal

Table 27.5 Summary of evidence for hyperbaric versus normobaric oxygen treatment of carbon monoxide poisoning.

Study	Population	Intervention	Control	Outcomes	Design	Effect measure; RR (95%CI)	Summary
Scheinkestel et al. [54]	191 sequential CO poisoned patients referred to a single facility; children, pregnant women and burn victims excluded; 69% intentional self-harm, 19% ventilated; 51% coma; average delay to treatment 7 hours	100-minute hyperbaric session (100% oxygen at 2.8 ATA for 60 minutes) daily for 3 days with high-flow (or 100%) oxygen between hyperbaric sessions; extended to 6 days if impaired after third treatment (N = 104)	Sham chamber session (1 ATA) daily with high-flow (or 100%) oxygen continuously for 3 days; extended to 6 days if impaired after third session (N = 87)	Persistent neurological sequelae = 2 of 7 neuropsychiatric subtest scores > 1 SD below the age- and education-adjusted norm at discharge	Randomized, double-blind trial; stratified by accidental vs intentional breathing, and by ventilated vs spontaneous breathing	74% hyperbaric vs 68% control (adjusted OR 1.7; 95% CI: 0.8 to 4.0)	Hyperbaric therapy does not appear to improve persistent neurologic sequelae at discharge
Weaver et al. [55]	152 patients with symptomatic CO exposure referred to a single facility; children, pregnant women and treatment delay > 24 hours excluded; 31% intentional, 8% ventilated; 49% loss of consciousness; average delay to treatment 6 hours	3 hyperbaric chamber sessions within a 24-hour interval: 100% oxygen at 3 ATA for 1 hour then 2 ATA for another hour (session 1), and at 2 ATA for 100 minutes (sessions 2 and 3) (N = 76)	3 sham chamber sessions pressurized to sea level (1 ATA) with 100% oxygen for the first session and air for the subsequent sessions (N = 76)	Cognitive sequelae at 6 weeks = 1 of 6 neuropsychological subtest scores > 2 SD below the demographically corrected norm, or 2 subtest scores > 1 SD, or self-reported difficulties with memory, attention or concentration and 1 subtest score > 1 SD (imputed to be present for patients with missing data)	Randomized, double-blind trial; stratified by loss of consciousness, delay to treatment < 6 or ≥ 6 hours, and by age < 40 or ≥ 40 years	25% hyperbaric vs 46% control (adjusted OR = 0.45; 95% CI: 0.22 to 0.92)	Hyperbaric therapy appears to reduce the frequency of cognitive sequelae at 6 weeks

ATA, atmospheres absolute; CI, confidence interval; CO, carbon monoxide; SD, standard deviation.

intubation did not demonstrate any benefit to hyperbaric oxygen by subgroup.

The main criticism of this study is the intensive oxygen therapy (continuous high-flow oxygen at 14 L/min via non-occlusive face mask or 100% O_2 via endotracheal tube) over several days in the control group, which does not reflect current practice. The high loss to follow-up also severely limits the ability to estimate the effect of hyperbaric oxygen on DNS. Finally, it is unclear whether explicit criteria were used to determine which subjects required re-treatment after 3 days, which generated the biggest signal of difference between groups.

The primary analysis of a randomized, double-blind trial of 152 patients referred to a single facility in Utah from 1992 to 1999 with symptomatic CO poisoning was reported in 2002 [55]. Subjects in either arm were only administered supplemental oxygen to maintain arterial oxygen saturation above 90%. Subjects randomized to the control arm received on average 6.9 ± 2.2 hours of oxygen in total. The trial was stopped at the third planned interim analysis for efficacy after 76 subjects had been randomized to each arm. The frequency of cognitive sequelae at 6 weeks was more common in the control group (25% hyperbaric vs 46% control; adjusted OR = 0.45; 95% CI: 0.22 to 0.92), primarily due to greater patient self-reports of memory difficulties (28% vs 51%; unadjusted OR = 0.37; 95% CI: 0.19 to 0.73). After adjustment for a baseline imbalance in cerebellar signs and for stratification variables, this difference no longer met the pre-specified criterion for early study termination. Fourteen subjects in the hyperbaric arm did not complete all three chamber sessions, mostly due to anxiety and ear barotrauma.

This study also has limitations. The primary outcome reported in the final manuscript is complicated and incorporates subjective patient complaints into objective neuropsychiatric testing, making it difficult to interpret the clinical significance of the observed difference. Critics have also suggested that this primary outcome may have changed during the course of the trial [58]. There was a large imbalance between groups at baseline for cerebellar dysfunction, the one factor predictive of neurological sequelae, and duration of exposure, both in favor of the hyperbaric group. Most of neuropsychological subtest scores were essentially normal at 6 weeks in both groups. Finally, due to the elevation of the treatment center (Salt Lake City elevation 1500 m, ambient pressure 0.85 atmospheres absolute) and a threshold for oxygen therapy of 90% saturation, a sub-optimal oxygen dose may have been used in the control group.

In summary, there is limited and conflicting evidence for hyperbaric oxygen administration to prevent DNS following carbon monoxide poisoning. It is unclear what subgroup of moderately to severely poisoned patients might benefit from this therapy, what treatment protocol to use and what treatment delay is permissible. The Cochrane review and others have concluded that the available evidence does not provide convincing support for hyperbaric oxygen treatment [57–61]. It is not possible to combine specific subgroups (e.g., severe poisoning, accidental exposure, treatment within 6 hours) from the various trials due to methodological heterogeneity. Any benefit would appear to be relatively modest at best, and must be contrasted with the limited access to hyperbaric facilities, the logistics and expense involved in transfer to a hyperbaric facility, and the morbidity of barotrauma, patient sequestration and hyperoxic seizures.

Conclusions

Any benefits of hyperbaric oxygen therapy appear to be small in unselected patients with CO poisoning, and need to be weighed against the risks and costs of hyperbaric treatment, including patient transfer. There are also no clinical trials comparing normobaric oxygen therapy at different dose intensities. In the absence of this evidence, most practitioners would recommend at least 6 hours of high-flow oxygen via a non-rebreather mask, and expect that the patient be neurologically and hemodynamically intact at the conclusion of this therapy. The patient should be advised regarding proper ventilation of exhaust and counseled about the possibility of developing delayed neurologic sequelae, as well as the natural history of these sequelae.

Acknowledgments

The authors would like to thank Ms. Diane Milette, Department of Emergency Medicine, University of Alberta, for her assistance with the formatting and referencing of this chapter.

Conflicts of interest

None were declared by any authors.

References

1 McCaig LF, Burt CW. Poisoning-related to emergency departments in the United States, 1993–1996. *J Toxicol Clin Toxicol* 1999;**37**(7):817–26.

2 Buckley N, Eddleston M. Paracetamol (acetaminophen) poisoning. *Clin Evid* 2006;**15**:1–9.

3 Buckley NA, Whyte IM, O'Connell DL, et al. Activated charcoal reduces the need for N-acetylcysteine treatment after acetaminophen (paracetamol) overdose. *J Toxicol Clin Toxicol* 1999;**37**:753–7.

4 Juurlink DN, McGuigan MA. Gastrointestinal decontamination for enteric-coated aspirin overdose: what to do depends on who you ask. *J Toxicol Clin Toxicol* 2000;**38**:465–70.

5 American Academy of Clinical Toxicology; European Association of Poisons Centres and Clinical Toxicologists. Position statement: single-dose activated charcoal. *Clin Toxicol* 2005;**43**:61–87.

6 American Academy of Clinical Toxicology; European Association of Poisons Centres and Clinical Toxicologists. Position statement: cathartics. *J Toxicol Clin Toxicol* 2004;**42**:243–53.

7 American Academy of Clinical Toxicology; European Association of Poisons Centres and Clinical Toxicologists. Position statement: gastric lavage. *J Toxicol Clin Toxicol* 2004;**42**:933–43.

8 American Academy of Clinical Toxicology; European Association of Poisons Centres and Clinical Toxicologists. *Position statement: ipecac syrup. J Toxicol Clin Toxicol* 2004;**42**:133–43.

9 American Academy of Clinical Toxicology; European Association of Poisons Centres and Clinical Toxicologists. Position statement: whole bowel irrigation. *J Toxicol Clin Toxicol* 2004;**42**:843–54.

10 American Academy of Clinical Toxicology; European Association of Poisons Centres and Clinical Toxicologists. Position statement and practice guidelines on the use of multi-dose activated charcoal in the treatment of acute poisoning. *J Toxicol Clin Toxicol* 1999;**37**:731–51.

11 Kulig K, Bar-Or D, Cantrill SV, Rosen P, Rumack BH. Management of acutely poisoned patient without gastric emptying. *Ann Emerg Med* 1985;**14**:562–7.

12 Albertson TE, Derlet RW, Foulke GE, Minguillon MC, Tharratt SR. Superiority of activated charcoal alone compared with ipecac and activated charcoal in the treatment of acute toxic ingestions. *Ann Emerg Med* 1989;**18**:56–9.

13 Merigian KS, Woodard M, Hedges JR, Roberts JR, Stuebing R, Rashkin MC. Prospective evaluation of gastric emptying in the self-poisoned patient. *Am J Emerg Med* 1990;**8**:479–83.

14 Pond SM, Lewis-Driver DJ, Williams GM, Green AC, Stevenson NW. Gastric emptying in acute overdose: a prospective randomised controlled trial. *Med J Aust* 1995;**163**:345–9.

15 Merigian KS, Blaho KE. Single-dose oral activated charcoal in the treatment of the self-poisoned patient: a prospective, randomized controlled trial. *Am J Ther* 2002;**9**:301–8.

16 Cooper GM, Le Couteur DG, Richardson D, Buckley NA. A randomized clinical trial of activated charcoal for the routine management of oral drug overdose. *Q J Med* 2005;**98**:655–60.

17 Earnest MP, Yarnell PR. Seizure admissions to a city hospital: the role of alcohol. *Epilepsia* 1976;**17**:387–93.

18 Hillborn ME. Occurrence of cerebral seizures provoked by alcohol abuse. *Epilepsia* 1980;**21**:459–66.

19 Isbell H, Fraser HF, Wilker A. An experimental study of the etiology of "run fits" and delirium tremens. *Q J Stud Alcohol* 1955;**16**:1–33.

20 Rathlev NK, Ulrish A, Shieh TC, et al. Etiology and weekly occurrence of alcohol-related seizures. *Acad Emerg Med* 2002;**9**:824–8.

21 Victor M, Adams RD. The effect of alcohol on the nervous system. *Res Publ Assoc Res Nerv Ment Dis* 1953;**32**:526–76.

22 Victor M, Braush C. The role of abstinence in the genesis of alcoholic epilepsy. *Epilepsia* 1966;**8**:1–20.

23 Ng SKC, Hauster WA, Brust JC, et al. Alcohol consumption and withdrawal in new-onset seizures. *N Engl J Med* 1988;**319**:666–73.

24 Morton AW, Laird LK, Crane FD, et al. A prediction model for identifying alcohol withdrawal seizures. *Am J Drug Alcohol Abuse* 1994;**20**:75–86.

25 Rathlev NK, Ulrich AS, Delanty N, D'Onofrio G. Alcohol-related seizures. *J Emerg Med* 2006;**31**:157–63.

26 Chan AW. Alcoholism and epilepsy. *Epilepsia* 1985;**26**:323–33.

27 Feussner JR, Linfors EW, Blesing CL, et al. Computed tomography brain scanning in alcohol withdrawal seizures. *Ann Int Med* 1981;**94**:519–22.

28 Rathlev NK, Urlich AS, Fish SS, D'Onofrio G. Clinical characteristics as predictors of recurrent alcohol-related seizures. *Acad Emerg Med* 2000;**7**:886–91.

29 Buck KJ, Eubanks JD, Hahner K, Sikela J, Harris H. Chronic ethanol treatment alters brain levels of gamma-aminobutyric acid receptor subunit mRNA. *J Neurochem* 1991;**57**:1452–5.

30 Keir WJ, Morrow AL. Differential expression of the GABAA receptor subunit MRNAs in ethanol-naïve withdrawal seizure resistant (WSR) vs. withdrawal seizure prone (WSP) mouse brain. *Brain Res Mol Brain Res* 1994;**25**:200–208.

31 Diamond I, Gordon AS. Cellular and molecular neuroscience of alcoholism. *Physiol Rev* 1997;**77**:1–20.

32 Cagetti E, Liang J, Spigelman I, Olsen RW. Withdrawal from chronic intermittent ethanol treatment changes subunit composition, reduces synaptic function, and decreases behavioral responses to positive allosteric modulators of GABAA receptors. *Mol Pharmacol* 2003;**63**:53–64.

33 Kumar S, Fleming RL, Morrow AL. Ethanol regulation of gamma-aminobutyric acid A receptors: genomic and nongenomic mechanisms. *Pharmacol Ther* 2004;**101**:211–26.

34 Grant KA, Valverius P, Hudspith M, Tabakoff B. Ethanol withdrawal seizures and the NMDA complex. *Eur J Pharm* 1990;**179**:289–96.

35 Hoffman PL, Grant KA, Snell LD, et al. NMDA receptor: role in ethanol withdrawal seizures. *Ann N Y Acad Sci* 1992;**654**:52–60.

36 Danysz W, Jankowska E, Galzewski S, Kostpwski W. The involvment of NMDA receptors in acute and chronic effects of alcohol. *Alcohol Clin Exp Res* 1992;**16**:499–504.

37 D'Onofrio G, Rathlev NK, Urlich AS, et al. Lorazepam for the prevention of recurrent seizures related to alcohol. *N Engl J Med* 1999;**340**:915–19.

38 Polycarpou A, Papanikolaou P, Ioannidis JPA, Contopoulos-Ioannidis DG. Anticonvulsants for alcohol withdrawal (Review). *Cochrane Database Syst Rev* 2005;**3**:CD005064 (doi:10.1002/14651858.CD005064.pub2).

39 Alldredge BK, Lowenstein DH, Simon RP. Placebo-controlled train of intravenous diphenlhydantoin for short-term treatment of alcohol withdrawal. *Am J Med* 1989;**87**:645–8.

40 Chance JF. Emergency department treatment of alcohol withdrawal seizures with phenytoin. *Ann Emerg Med* 1991;**20**:520–52.

41 Rathlev NK, D'Onofrio G, Fish SS, et al. The lack of efficacy of phenytoin in the prevention of recurrent alcohol-related seizures. *Ann Emerg Med* 1994;**23**:513–18.

42 Nyais C, Pakos E, Kyzas P, Ioannidis JPA. Benodiazepines for alcohol withdrawal (Review). *Cochrane Database Syst Rev* 2005;**3**:CD005063 (doi:10.1002/14651858.CD005063.pub2).

43 Mott JA, Wolfe MI, Alverson CJ, et al. National vehicle emissions policies and practices and declining US carbon monoxide-related mortality. *JAMA* 2002;**8**:988–95.

44 Suner S, Partridge R, Sucov A, Chee K, Valente J, Jay G. Non-invasive screening for carbon monoxide toxicity in the emergency department is valuable. *Ann Emerg Med* 2007;**49**(5):718–19.

45 O'Malley GF. Non-invasive carbon monoxide measurement is not accurate. *Ann Emerg Med* 2006;**48**(4):477–8.

46 Kalay N, Ozdogru I, Cetinkaya Y, et al. Cardiovascular effects of carbon monoxide poisoning. *Am J Cardiol* 2007;**99**(3):322–4.

47 Henry CR, Satran D, Lindgren B, Adkinson C, Nicholson CI, Henry TD. Myocardial injury and long-term mortality following moderate to severe carbon monoxide poisoning. *JAMA* 2006;**295**(4):398–402.

48 Choi IS. Delayed neurologic sequelae in carbon monoxide intoxication. *Arch Neurol* 1983;**40**(7):433–5.

49 Min SK. A brain syndrome associated with delayed neuropsychiatric sequelae following acute carbon monoxide intoxication. *Acta Psychiatr Scand* 1986;**73**(1):80–86.

50 Raphael JC, Elkharrat D, Jars-Guincestre MC, et al. Trial of normobaric and hyperbaric oxygen for acute carbon monoxide intoxication. *Lancet* 1989;**334**:414–19.

51 Ducasse JL, Celsis P, Marc-Vergnes JP. Non-comatose patients with acute carbon monoxide poisoning: hyperbaric or normobaric oxygenation? *Undersea Hyperb Med* 1995;**22**:9–15.

52 Thom SR, Taber RL, Mendiguren II, Clark JM, Hardy KR, Fisher AB. Delayed neuropsychologic sequelae after carbon monoxide poisoning: prevention by treatment with hyperbaric oxygen. *Ann Emerg Med* 1995;**25**(4):474–80.

53 Mathieu D, Wattel F, Mathieu-Nolf M, Durak C, Tempe JP, Bouachour G. Randomized prospective study comparing the effect of HBO versus 12 hours NBO in non comatose CO poisoned patients: results of the interim analysis. *Undersea Hyperb Med* 1996;**23**:7–8.

54 Scheinkestel CD, Bailey M, Myles PS, et al. Hyperbaric or normobaric oxygen for acute carbon monoxide poisoning: a randomised controlled clinical trial. *Med J Aust* 1999;**170**(5):203–10.

55 Weaver LK, Hopkins RO, Chan KJ, et al. Hyperbaric oxygen for acute carbon monoxide poisoning. *N Engl J Med* 2002;**347**:1057–67.

56 Raphael JC, Chevret S, Driheme A, Annane D. Managing carbon monoxide poisoning with hyperbaric oxygen (Abstract). *J Toxicol Clin Toxicol* 2004;**42**:455–6.

57 Juurlink DN, Buckley NA, Stanbrook MB, Isbister GK, Bennett M, McGuigan MA. Hyperbaric oxygen for carbon monoxide poisoning. *Cochrane Database Syst Rev* 2005;**1**:CD002041.

58 Buckley NA, Isbister GK, Stokes B, Juurlink DN. Hyperbaric oxygen for carbon monoxide poisoning: a systematic review and critical analysis of the evidence. *Toxicol Rev* 2005;**24**:75–92.

59 Silver S, Smith C, Worster A. The BEEM (Best Evidence in Emergency Medicine) Team. Should hyperbaric oxygen be used for carbon monoxide poisoning? *Can J Emerg Med* 2006;**8**:43–6.

60 Phin N. Carbon monoxide poisoning (acute). *Clin Evid* 2005;**13**:1732–43.

61 Gorman D, Drewry A, Huang YL, Sames C. The clinical toxicology of carbon monoxide. *Toxicology* 2003;**187**:25–38.

28 Toxicology: Acetaminophen and Salicylate Poisoning

Mark Yarema[1] & Richard Dart[2]

[1]Department of Emergency Medicine, Calgary Health Region, Calgary, Canada
[2]Rocky Mountain Poison and Drug Center, Denver, USA

Case scenario

A 42-year-old female was brought in by ambulance to the emergency department (ED) from home with depression, suicidal ideation and suspicion of an overdose. Her husband stated she had been depressed for approximately 3 months and he had been unable to get her to see a doctor. She had been drinking alcohol on the day of presentation and he believed she may have taken a combination of acetaminophen (APAP) and acetyl-salicylic acid (ASA) from the medicine cabinet. She had no other medical history apart from arthritis. She was alert and oriented, tearful, and cooperative. Her Glasgow Coma Score (GCS) was 15 and she had the following vital signs: pulse 120/min, respirations 24 breaths/min (shallow), SaO_2 94% on room air, temperature 37.5°C (oral) and blood pressure 120/60 mmHg (right arm = left arm). She complained of ringing in her ears and feeling nauseated. There was no sign of trauma. The medical student working with you wondered if this patient should undergo gastric lavage, receive charcoal and/or be administered an antidote?

Background

Acetaminophen ingestion is one of the leading causes of morbidity and mortality due to poisonings. The widespread availability of the drug and ease of access make it a popular choice for intentional poisonings and a common cause of unintentional poisonings. In North America, there are over 138,000 exposures and 300 deaths reported annually [1]. The principal mechanism of toxicity is hepatocellular injury. Under therapeutic conditions, sufficient reduced glutathione is available to detoxify the toxic intermediate of acetaminophen, N-acetyl-p-benzoquinonimine (NAPQI). In the overdose setting, the amount of glutathione available is inad-

Evidence-based Emergency Medicine. Edited by Brian H. Rowe
© 2009 Blackwell Publishing, ISBN: 978-1-4051-6143-5.

equate for NAPQI detoxification. NAPQI then binds to hepatic macromolecules and hepatic damage occurs, manifested as centrilobular necrosis [2–6].

For patients with potentially toxic APAP concentrations based upon the APAP treatment nomogram (the Rumack–Matthew nomogram, Fig. 28.1) [7], the current antidote of choice for APAP poisoning is N-acetylcysteine (NAC), which acts as a glutathione precursor and replacement. NAC has benefits in patients who present both before and after hepatic injury has developed [8–12].

Salicylates remain an important cause of poisonings and visits to EDs. In 2005 there were over 17,000 salicylate exposures reported to poison centers in North America [1]. Because of the difficulty in recognizing salicylate poisoning, it is likely under-reported in poison center data.

Salicylates cause toxicity by uncoupling oxidative phosphorylation. This produces an increase in anaerobic metabolism, resulting in acid–base disturbances, electrolyte and fluid imbalance, increased heat production, renal failure, altered glucose metabolism and bleeding disorders. Treatment of salicylate poisoning begins with early recognition of the poisoning and aggressive management, including steps to prevent absorption and enhance elimination.

This chapter will review the evidence-based approach to acetaminophen and salicylate poisonings.

Clinical questions

In order to address the issues of most relevance to your patient and to help in searching the literature for the evidence regarding these issues, you structure your clinical questions as recommended in Chapter 1.

1 In patients with intentional ingestion of acetaminophen (population), does gastric lavage (intervention) improve outcomes (e.g., decrease death, intubations, symptoms) (outcome) compared to conservative treatment (control)?

2 In patients with intentional ingestion of acetaminophen (population), does administration of activated charcoal (intervention)

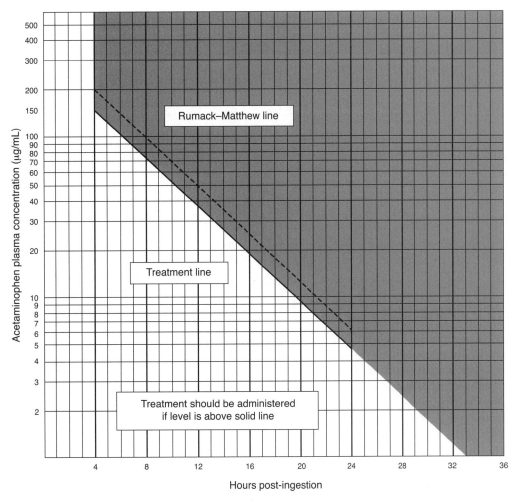

Figure 28.1 Acetaminophen treatment nomogram. Acetaminophen concentrations between 4 and 24 hours post-ingestion after an acute, single overdose may be plotted on the nomogram to estimate whether hepatotoxicity will result and whether *N*-acetylcysteine should be administered. To convert to SI units (μmol/L) multiply the concentration in μg/ml by 6.62. (Courtesy of E. Kuffner, McNeil Consumer and Specialty Pharmaceuticals, Fort Washington, PA, with permission.)

improve outcomes (e.g., decrease death, intubations, symptoms) (outcome) compared to conservative treatment (control)?

3 In patients with intentional ingestion of acetaminophen in the potentially toxic range on the treatment nomogram (population), does IV *N*-acetylcysteine (intervention) improve outcomes (e.g., decrease hepatotoxicity, mortality, symptoms) (outcome) compared to oral *N*-acetylcysteine treatment (control)?

4 In patients with intentional ingestion of acetaminophen who present in hepatic failure (population), does treatment with IV *N*-acetylcysteine (intervention) improve outcomes (e.g. decrease mortality, liver transplant) (outcome) compared to conservative treatment (control)?

5 In patients with intentional ingestion of salicylate compounds (population), does gastric lavage (intervention) improve outcomes (e.g., decrease death, intubations, symptoms) (outcome) compared to conservative treatment (control)? Are there groups of patients where the therapy may be more effective?

6 In patients with intentional ingestion of salicylate compounds (population), does administration of charcoal (intervention) improve out-

comes (e.g., decrease death, intubations, symptoms; outcome) compared to conservative treatment (control)?

7 In patients with intentional ingestion of salicylate compounds (population), does IV bicarbonate (intervention) improve outcomes (e.g., decrease death, intubations, symptoms) (outcome) compared to conservative treatment (control)?

8 In patients with an intentional ingestion of salicylate compounds (population), does dialysis (intervention) improve outcomes (e.g., decrease death, intubations, symptoms) (outcome) compared to conservative treatment (control)?

General search strategy

You begin to address these questions by searching for evidence in the common electronic databases such as the Cochrane Library, MEDLINE and EMBASE looking specifically for systematic reviews and meta-analyses. When a systematic review is identified, you also search for recent updates in the Cochrane Library and also search MEDLINE and EMBASE to identify randomized controlled trials (RCTs) that became available after the publication date of the systematic review.

Critical review of the literature: acetaminophen

Question 1: In patients with intentional ingestion of acetaminophen (population), does gastric lavage (intervention) improve outcomes (e.g., decrease death, intubations, symptoms) (outcome) compared to conservative treatment (control)?

Search strategy

- MEDLINE, Cochrane and EMBASE: (exp acetaminophen OR paracetamol) AND exp poisoning AND exp gastric lavage

Most reports studying the effectiveness of gastric lavage are randomized, controlled, crossover human volunteer studies that did not use a dose of APAP near the 150 mg/kg or 10 g dose thought necessary to increase risk of hepatotoxicity [13–15]. When compared to no treatment, gastric lavage was successful in reducing the bioavailability of APAP, as evidenced by decreased serum concentrations. It is not clear if gastric lavage reduces the incidence of hepatocellular injury when compared to no treatment.

A randomized trial of 60 patients who acutely ingested more than 5 g of APAP and were assigned to receive gastric lavage, activated charcoal, syrup of ipecac or no gastrointestinal decontamination found that gastric lavage was less effective than activated charcoal in reducing APAP absorption, as evidenced by decreasing serum APAP concentrations [14]. Similarly, an observational study of 162 patients admitted with potentially toxic APAP concentrations from 1987 to 1996 compared patients who were treated with gastric lavage plus activated charcoal to those treated with only activated charcoal [16]. The authors determined that the addition of gastric lavage did not significantly reduce the bioavailability of APAP compared to the use of activated charcoal alone. A Best Evidence Topic (BestBETs) review from the Manchester Royal Infirmary also concluded that gastric lavage was less effective than activated charcoal in reducing APAP concentrations in human volunteers [17].

In summary, the routine use of gastric lavage in acetaminophen poisoning is not indicated. Gastric lavage is an invasive procedure with the potential to result in complications. In the setting of a patient with a decreased level of consciousness, the patient requires airway protection before proceeding with treatment. The availability of other less invasive alternatives, such as activated charcoal, has also limited its utility.

Question 2: In patients with intentional ingestion of acetaminophen (population), does administration of activated charcoal (intervention) improve outcomes (e.g., decrease death, intubations, symptoms) (outcome) compared to conservative treatment (control)?

Search strategy

- MEDLINE, Cochrane and EMBASE: (exp acetaminophen OR paracetamol) AND exp poisoning AND (exp activated charcoal OR charcoal)

Most studies investigating the effectiveness of activated charcoal on APAP concentrations are randomized, controlled, crossover human volunteer studies in which the dose ingested is substantially lower than that thought to produce toxicity [13,18–22]. The summary of studies suggests that activated charcoal, given no later than 1–2 hours after an acetaminophen ingestion, reduces serum APAP concentrations. Because of their design, these studies are not able to assess whether administration of charcoal reduces the incidence of hepatocellular injury or improves outcome.

An observational study of 162 patients admitted with potentially toxic APAP concentrations after an overdose, from 1987 to 1996, compared patients who were treated with gastric lavage plus activated charcoal to those treated with only activated charcoal [16]. Treatment with activated charcoal within 2 hours post-ingestion resulted in fewer patients having potentially toxic APAP concentrations. Similar results were also found in a study involving children aged 6 years and younger, where activated charcoal administered within 2 hours of a potentially toxic ingestion resulted in significantly lower concentrations compared with untreated controls [23]. In a separate study investigating the routine use of activated charcoal for all patients presenting to an ED with an oral overdose, the use of activated charcoal did not reduce mortality, length of stay, vomiting or need for intensive care unit admission [24]. The most common medications ingested in that study included benzodiazepines, acetaminophen and selective serotonin re-uptake inhibitors. No comment was made on whether the addition of charcoal resulted in fewer patients requiring treatment with NAC. A BestBETs review from the Manchester Royal Infirmary concluded that activated charcoal should be given to all poisoned patients with a significant APAP poisoning who present acutely; however, no definition of what constituted a "significant poisoning" was provided [25].

In summary, the available evidence suggests that the routine use of activated charcoal for all patients presenting after APAP ingestion is unlikely to confer any outcome benefit. Patients treated with activated charcoal within 2 hours of their ingestion may have a reduction in subsequent serum APAP levels; however, it is unclear whether this translates into fewer patients treated with an antidote, or improved clinical outcomes. The use of charcoal, especially in patients with altered mental status, may result in complications such as aspiration, and therefore must be used cautiously. The effectiveness of NAC, especially in patients who are treated early (within 8 hours) after ingestion, also limits its necessity. In the absence of other clinical trial evidence, clinicians should consider charcoal for patients with recent (within 2 hours) APAP ingestion.

Question 3: In patients with intentional ingestion of acetaminophen in the potentially toxic range on the treatment nomogram (population), does IV N-acetylcysteine (intervention) improve outcomes (decrease hepatotoxicity, mortality, symptoms) (outcome) compared to oral N-acetylcysteine treatment (control)?

Search strategy

- MEDLINE, Cochrane and EMBASE – search: (exp acetaminophen OR paracetamol) AND exp poisoning AND exp acetylcysteine

The antidote of choice for APAP poisoning is NAC; however, considerable controversy exists regarding the route of delivery and duration of treatment. A 20-hour intravenous protocol has been used for several years in Canada, the United Kingdom, Australia, and other countries. In January 2004, the 20-hour IV NAC protocol was approved by the Food and Drug Administration (FDA) for use in the United States. The 20-hour protocol consists of a 150 mg/kg loading dose, followed by 50 mg/kg over 4 hours, and 100 mg/kg over 16 hours. A 72-hour oral protocol is also approved by the FDA for use, and consists of a 140 mg/kg loading dose followed by 70 mg/kg every 4 hours for 17 doses.

A Cochrane Library review, updated in 2006, summarized six studies involving 637 patients who were treated with IV NAC and 1634 patients from three studies who were treated with oral (PO) NAC from 0 to 24 hours post-ingestion [26]. There were no significant differences between the groups in terms of the incidence of hepatotoxicity, defined as a serum aspartate aminotransferase (AST) or alanine aminotransferase (ALT) greater than 1000 IU/L (IV vs PO: 13% vs 19%) or mortality (IV vs PO: 0.9% vs 0.6%), regardless of the time to treatment post-ingestion. No randomized controlled trials comparing the efficacy of IV and PO NAC exist.

Side-effects with both IV and PO NAC include nausea, vomiting and anaphylactoid reactions. Symptoms of anaphylactoid reactions include urticaria, facial flushing, pruritis, wheezing, dyspnea, edema and, in severe cases, cardiorespiratory collapse. The incidence of anaphylactoid reactions from IV NAC ranges from 6% to 48%. Most reactions occur within the first 2 hours of IV NAC therapy, leading to controversy over the duration of delivery for the initial dose (15 vs 60 minutes). A randomized controlled trial that compared 109 and 71 patients treated with the 15- and 60-minute loading doses, respectively, found no significant differences between the groups in terms of the incidence of anaphylactoid reac-

tions (18% vs 14%) [11]. In contrast, the Cochrane Hepato-Biliary Group found that the odds ratio was 1.98 (95% CI: 1.04 to 3.77) for an adverse event when treated with the 15-minute infusion [26]. No study has compared the incidence of adverse events or anaphylactoid reactions between IV and PO NAC.

In summary, given the approval of IV NAC in the United States, it seems unlikely that a prospective RCT comparing the effectiveness of IV versus PO NAC will ever be performed. Length of treatment, rather than route, is likely the more important determinant of a successful outcome. Treatment should be continued until serum transaminases and coagulation parameters are normal (or normalizing) and the serum acetaminophen concentration is undetectable [27]. Future research in this area should be directed at determining the optimal dose of IV NAC, especially for those patients treated early post-ingestion who may be at lower risk and may not require 20 hours of therapy.

Question 4: In patients with intentional ingestion of acetaminophen who present in hepatic failure (population), does treatment with IV N-acetylcysteine (intervention) improve outcomes (e.g. decrease mortality, liver transplant) (outcome) compared to conservative treatment (control)?

Search strategy

- MEDLINE, Cochrane and EMBASE – search: (exp acetaminophen OR paracetamol) AND exp poisoning AND exp acetylcysteine AND exp death AND exp liver failure

Hyperacute liver failure (onset of encephalopathy 0–7 days after the onset of jaundice) and acute liver failure (onset of encephalopathy 8–28 days after the onset of jaundice) after APAP poisoning are major risk factors associated with liver transplant and/or mortality, especially if the patient is not treated with IV NAC [28]. Harrison et al. [29] performed a retrospective analysis of 100 patients who developed acetaminophen-induced hepatic failure. Patients were divided into three groups according to the time that had elapsed between the overdose and the administration of IV NAC (received NAC within 10 hours, received NAC at 10 or more hours, or did not receive any antidote). Not receiving NAC was associated with a significantly higher incidence of encephalopathy (75% vs 51%, $P < 0.05$) and death (58% vs 37%, $P < 0.05$) compared to patients who received NAC 10 or more hours after their overdose. An RCT of patients presenting in APAP-induced fulminant hepatic failure compared continuous IV NAC (the 20-hour protocol continued indefinitely until recovery from encephalopathy or death) with standard liver care (intubation, sedation, insertion of pulmonary artery catheter) and demonstrated an absolute risk reduction of 28% (95% CI: 3% to 53%) in the IV NAC group [30]. The Peto odds ratio for death when treated with a continuous IV NAC infusion was 0.29 (95% CI: 0.09 to 0.94) [26].

In summary, patients who present in hepatic failure after either an acute supra-therapeutic or chronic acetaminophen ingestion should be provided treatment with IV NAC as part of their care. In this case, NAC should be continued beyond the initial 20-hour protocol. The third infusion (100 mg/kg in 1 L 5% dextrose in water (D5W) over 16 hours) should be repeated indefinitely until the international normalized ratio (INR) is less than 2, encephalopathy improves or the patient expires.

Critical review of the literature: salicylate

Question 5: In patients with intentional ingestion of salicylate compounds (population), does gastric lavage (intervention) improve outcomes (e.g., decrease death, intubations, symptoms) (outcome) compared to conservative treatment (control)? Are there groups of patients where the therapy may be more effective?

Search strategy

- MEDLINE, Cochrane and EMBASE: exp salicylate AND exp poisoning AND exp gastric lavage

The use of gastric lavage following ingestion of salicylate compounds has been the subject of considerable debate; however, evidence for or against this approach is extremely limited. One randomized trial was identified of 20 pediatric patients (12 years of age and younger) who had presented to the ED after ingesting an unknown amount of salicylate. The trial compared syrup of ipecac followed by gastric lavage with the same two therapies in reverse order [31]. Syrup of ipecac was more effective in removing salicylate from the stomach than gastric lavage, as demonstrated by greater amounts of salicylate measured in gastric contents. The symptoms experienced by the children and peak salicylate concentrations were not mentioned.

In general, the routine use of gastric lavage in salicylate poisoning is not indicated. Gastric lavage is an invasive procedure with the potential to result in complications. Its ability to improve patient outcomes has never been proven, including those who present to the ED within 60 minutes post-ingestion [32]. Moreover, in the setting of a patient with a decreased level of consciousness it requires airway protection before proceeding. The availability of other less invasive alternatives, such as activated charcoal, has also limited its utility.

In summary, unless the ingestion consists of large quantities likely to produce toxicity (>150 mg/kg) and is recent (within 1 hour post-ingestion), emergency physicians should not consider gastric lavage as an intervention for salicylate poisonings. Focus should be placed on alternative interventions for which evidence suggests a benefit.

Question 6: In patients with intentional ingestion of salicylate compounds (population), does administration of charcoal (intervention) improve outcomes (e.g., decrease death, intubations, symptoms) (outcome) compared to conservative treatment (control)?

Search strategy

- MEDLINE, Cochrane and EMBASE: exp salicylate AND exp poisoning AND (exp charcoal OR activated charcoal)

Most of the studies involving activated charcoal and salicylate are randomized human crossover volunteer studies designed to investigate whether repeat-dose activated charcoal improves elimination of salicylate [33–35]. None of these studies found that salicylate concentrations were significantly decreased by the use of repeated doses of activated charcoal. It must be emphasized that these trials used salicylate doses far below the 150 mg/kg thought to be the minimal amount required to cause toxicity. In addition, because these studies were designed to study the effect of charcoal on elimination, charcoal was usually given after absorption was thought to be complete, usually at least 4 hours post-ingestion.

Olsen et al. [36] performed a randomized, two-phase crossover study involving six volunteers who ingested 3.25 g aspirin followed by either low-volume whole bowel irrigation (3 L) or a combination of ipecac and single-dose activated charcoal. Both treatments were initiated 30 minutes post-ingestion. They determined that ipecac and charcoal produced significantly lower salicylate absorption than low-volume whole bowel irrigation, as evidenced by lower peak concentrations and area under the curve.

Hillman and Prescott [37] reported on the use of repeat-dose activated charcoal on five adults with salicylate poisoning. Prior to charcoal administration, all patients had received gastric lavage, and two had received forced alkaline diuresis. Charcoal was administered because of an unsatisfactory response to prior therapy. They compared salicylate concentrations to six control patients with salicylate poisoning who were treated with oral fluids alone. In the five poisoned patients, salicylate concentrations were lower than the controls. No clinical information was available on either group of patients, and therefore no comments about reductions in morbidity or mortality can be made.

In summary, the use of activated charcoal in the treatment of salicylate poisoning is warranted. The greatest benefit is likely to be achieved early (less than 1 hour) after ingestion. Whether single or repeat dosing is indicated is controversial [38,39]. In the absence of other clinical trial evidence, clinicians should consider the use of at least a single dose of activated charcoal for acute salicylate poisoning. Those receiving repeat dosing should receive 1 g/kg either orally or via a nasogastric tube as soon as salicylate poisoning is suspected (either by history or by a detectable serum level), followed by 0.25 g/kg 2 hours later. Care must be taken to ensure the patient does not develop any contraindications to its administration, such as a bowel obstruction or ileus. Salicylate concentrations and serum electrolytes should be followed every 2 hours during the patient's stay in the ED until there is evidence of a plateau or decline in the salicylate level accompanied by an improvement in clinical features and no development of an anion gap. Co-administration of ipecac is not recommended.

Question 7: In patients with intentional ingestion of salicylate compounds (population), does IV bicarbonate (intervention) improve outcomes (e.g., decrease death, intubations, symptoms) (outcome) compared to conservative treatment (control)?

Search strategy

- MEDLINE, Cochrane and EMBASE: exp salicylate AND exp poisoning AND (exp sodium bicarbonate OR bicarbonate)

When making a decision on the use of bicarbonate, clinicians must be aware of the restrictions of the Done nomogram for salicylate poisoning [40]. This treatment nomogram, developed in 1960, has several limitations that preclude its use for most salicylate poisonings. First, it was developed in pediatric patients and has been shown not to be as predictive of toxicity for adult salicylate ingestions [41]. Second, the nomogram assumes that salicylate elimination follows first-order elimination kinetics, rather than the more appropriate saturable (Michaelis–Menten) kinetics. Finally, and most importantly, the nomogram was intended to be applied only 6 hours or more after an acute ingestion. Treatment decisions must be made earlier than 6 hours post-ingestion in order to minimize absorption of salicylate from the gastrointestinal tract and to enhance elimination.

The use of a sodium bicarbonate solution for clinically important salicylate poisoning has been proposed to enhance elimination of salicylate from the urine. In a randomized crossover study, Vree et al. [42] studied the effect of urine alkalinization or acidification on elimination half-life in six human volunteers who ingested 1.5 g salicylate. They determined that under alkaline urine conditions (urine pH > 8.0) the elimination half-life was significantly lower than if the urine was kept acidic. Prescott et al. [43] studied 44 adults with salicylate poisoning who were allocated to receive oral fluids ($n = 16$), forced alkaline diuresis ($n = 16$), forced diuresis without sodium bicarbonate ($n = 6$) and sodium bicarbonate infusions without diuresis ($n = 6$) depending on the severity of their poisoning. Those patients with concentrations above 70 mg/dl (4.7 mmol/L) were excluded because the safety and efficacy of the therapies had not been established. All patients received gastric lavage prior to one of the above treatments. Decreased plasma salicylate concentrations and urinary recovery of salicylate was highest with those treated with sodium bicarbonate infusion alone, without the consequences of positive fluid balance, weight gain, hyponatremia and hypokalemia in those who received forced diuresis. No comments were made on relief of clinical symptoms or patient outcomes.

One option for preparing a bicarbonate infusion is to add 150 cm³ of 8.4% bicarbonate to 850 cm³ D5W and 40 meq KCl and infuse this solution at 250 cm³/h. Patients may require a second intravenous line for hydration purposes. Treatment should be continued until there is evidence of a decline in the salicylate level accompanied by an improvement in clinical features and no development of an anion gap. Arterial blood gases should be obtained as clinically indicated to ensure the serum pH is not above 7.55, at which point the infusion should be discontinued. Urine pH should be followed every hour with the goal of achieving a pH of 7.5–8.0. Proudfoot et al. [44] outline a comprehensive approach to urinary alkalinization for salicylate poisoning.

In summary, there are theoretical reasons and clinical evidence to support the use of a sodium bicarbonate solution for clinically important salicylate poisonings to enhance elimination of salicylate from the urine. The Done nomogram should not be used to assist the clinician in making decisions about the use of urinary alkalinization.

Question 8: In patients with intentional ingestion of salicylate compounds (population), does dialysis (intervention) improve outcomes (e.g., decrease death, intubations, symptoms) (outcome) compared to conservative treatment (control)?

Search strategy

- MEDLINE, Cochrane and EMBASE: exp salicylate AND exp poisoning AND (exp dialysis OR hemodialysis)

The literature supporting the use of hemodialysis for salicylate poisoning consists of case series and case reports. Higgins et al. [45] reported two cases of salicylate poisoning with tachypnea and tinnitus, and generalized tonic-clonic seizures with a salicylate concentration of 5 mmol/L. Hemodialysis was instituted for 4 hours, following which the salicylate concentrations decreased and clinical symptoms improved. A full recovery was made. Lund et al. [46] described a 24-year-old male who presented with tachypnea, tachycardia, diaphoresis, tremors and renal failure after ingesting 32,500 mg salicylate. Charcoal and sodium bicarbonate infusions were initiated. The initial salicylate concentration was 110 mg/dl (7.3 mmol/L). Hemodialysis was initiated for 4 hours and subsequently changed to sustained low-efficiency dialysis (SLED) for a further 12 hours. Salicylate levels decreased to 15 mg/dl (1 mmol/L) 4 hours after SLED was discontinued. No comment was made about improvements in the patient's clinical condition. While the reasons for the change to SLED from hemodialysis were not explicitly mentioned, SLED is reported to have advantages over hemodialysis in terms of greater hemodynamic stability. No trials exist that compare hemodialysis and SLED for the treatment of salicylate poisoning.

In summary, dialysis is effective in decreasing salicylate concentrations after acute poisoning. While the evidence is weak, the clinical use of hemodialysis for severe salicylate poisoning occurs regularly in most intensive care settings. No trials exist that compare dialysis with other decontamination or elimination methods such as sodium bicarbonate infusions. While no consensus statement exists, generally accepted recommendations for hemodialysis in salicylate-poisoned patients include pulmonary edema, seizures, coagulopathy, renal or hepatic failure, coma, a salicylate concentration above 100 mg/dl (7.2 mmol/L) or a rising salicylate concentration despite other therapies.

Conclusions

The patient was placed in a medical bed with cardiorespiratory monitoring. Blood was drawn for a complete blood count, electrolytes, acetaminophen, salicylate and ethanol concentration. Because of the possibility of multiple drug ingestion, the patient received 50 g of activated charcoal orally with no complications. A 4-hour post-ingestion acetaminophen concentration was 1200 μmol/L (181 μg/ml). Plotting this on the acetaminophen treatment nomogram (see Fig. 28.1) revealed a potentially toxic level. Her salicylate concentration was 3.5 mmol/L (48 mg/dl).

The patient was started on the 20-hour IV NAC protocol for her potentially toxic acetaminophen level and a bicarbonate infusion for both her elevated salicylate level and clinical features suggestive of salicylate poisoning.

The patient's liver chemistry and coagulation profile remained normal and the NAC was discontinued after the 20-hour infusion ended. Repeat salicylate concentrations and electrolytes were performed every 2 hours. After 12 hours of the bicarbonate infusion, her salicylate level had decreased to 1.5 mmol/L (20 mg/dl) with a normal anion gap; therefore the infusion was discontinued. She was cleared medically and transferred to psychiatry for further management.

Acetaminophen and salicylate are common poisons which, when unrecognized by the clinician, may result in significant morbidity and mortality. Prompt recognition, appropriate diagnostic testing, judicious use of gastrointestinal decontamination and timely use of antidotes such as *N*-acetylcysteine and sodium bicarbonate are the principles of treatment of toxicity from these agents.

Conflicts of interest

Dr. Yarema is the recipient of an unrestricted grant in aid from Cumberland Pharmaceuticals, which holds the NDA for Acetadote (acetylcysteine) Injection in the United States. Dr. Dart has received research funding and acted as a consultant for McNeil Consumer Products, the manufacturer of Tylenol. By the policy of Denver Health and Hospitals, all revenue is retained by Denver Health and Hospitals. Dr. Dart receives no salary, bonuses or incentives that are directly or indirectly related to fees paid to Denver Health by McNeil Consumer Products.

References

1 Lai MW, Klein-Schwartz W, Rodgers GC, et al. 2005 Annual report of the American Association of Poison Control Centers' National Poisoning and Exposure Database. *Clin Toxicol* (Phila) 2006;**44**(6–7):803–932.

2 Mitchell JR, Jollow DJ, Potter WZ. Acetaminophen-induced hepatic necrosis. IV. Protective role of glutathione. *J Pharmacol Exp Ther* 1973;**187**:211–17.

3 Mitchell JR, Jollow DJ, Potter WZ. Acetaminophen-induced hepatic necrosis. I. Role of drug metabolism. *J Pharmacol Exp Ther* 1973;**187**:185–94.

4 Mitchell JR, Thorgeirsson SS, Potter WZ, Jollow DJ, Keiser H. Acetaminophen-induced hepatic injury: protective role of glutathione in man and rationale for therapy. *Clin Pharmacol Ther* 1974;**16**(4):676–84.

5 Jollow DJ, Mitchell JR, Potter WZ. Acetaminophen-induced hepatic necrosis. II. Role of covalent binding in vivo. *J Pharmacol Exp Ther* 1973;**187**:195–202.

6 Jollow DJ, Thorgeirsson SS, Potter WZ, Hashimoto M, Mitchell JR. Acetaminophen-induced hepatic necrosis. VI. Metabolic disposition of toxic and nontoxic doses of acetaminophen. *Pharmacology* 1974;**12**(4–5):251–71.

7 Rumack BH, Peterson RG. Acetaminophen poisoning and toxicity. *Pediatrics* 1975;**55**(871):876.

8 Smilkstein MJ, Knapp GL, Kulig KW, Rumack BH. Efficacy of oral N-acetylcysteine in the treatment of acetaminophen overdose. Analysis of the national multicenter study (1976 to 1985). *N Engl J Med* 1988;**319**(24):1557–62.

9 Prescott LF, Illingworth RN, Critchley JA, Stewart MJ, Adam RD, Proudfoot AT. Intravenous N-acetylcysteine: the treatment of choice for paracetamol poisoning. *BMJ* 1979;**2**:1097–100.

10 Buckley NA, Whyte IM, O'Connell DL, Dawson AH. Oral or intravenous N-acetylcysteine. Which is the treatment of choice for acetaminophen (paracetamol) poisoning? *J Toxicol Clin Toxicol* 1999;**37**:759–67.

11 Kerr F, Dawson A, Whyte IM, et al. The Australasian Clinical Toxicology Investigators Collaboration randomized trial of different loading infusion rates of N-acetylcysteine. *Ann Emerg Med* 2005;**45**(4):402–8.

12 Harrison PM, Wendon JA, Gimson AE, Alexander GJ, Williams R. Improvement by acetylcysteine of hemodynamics and oxygen transport in fulminant hepatic failure. *N Engl J Med* 1991;**324**:1852–7.

13 Christophersen AB, Levin D, Hoegberg LC, Angelo HR, Kampmann JP. Activated charcoal alone or after gastric lavage: a simulated large paracetamol intoxication. *Br J Clin Pharmacol* 2002;**53**(3):312–17.

14 Underhill TJ, Greene MK, Dove AF. A comparison of the efficacy of gastric lavage, ipecacuanha and activated charcoal in the emergency management of paracetamol overdose. *Arch Emerg Med* 1990;**7**(3):148–54.

15 Grierson R, Green R, Sitar DS, Tenenbein M. Gastric lavage for liquid poisons. *Ann Emerg Med* 2000;**35**(5):435–9.

16 Buckley NA, Whyte IM, O'Connell DL, Dawson AH. Activated charcoal reduces the need for N-acetylcysteine treatment after acetaminophen (paracetamol) overdose. *J Toxicol Clin Toxicol* 1999;**37**(6):753–7.

17 Teece S, Hogg K. Gastric lavage in paracetamol poisoning. *Emerg Med J* 2004;**21**(1):75–6.

18 Rose SR, Gorman RL, Oderda GM, Klein-Schwartz W, Watson WA. Simulated acetaminophen overdose: pharmacokinetics and effectiveness of activated charcoal. *Ann Emerg Med* 1991;**20**(10):1064–8.

19 Yeates PJ, Thomas SH. Effectiveness of delayed activated charcoal administration in simulated paracetamol (acetaminophen) overdose. *Br J Clin Pharmacol* 2000;**49**(1):11–14.

20 Dordoni B, Willson R, Thompson R, Williams R. Reduction of absorption of paracetamol by activated charcoal and cholestyramine: a possible therapeutic measure. *BMJ* 1973;**3**:86–7.

21 Roberts JR, Gracely EJ, Schoffstall JM. Advantage of high-surface-area charcoal for gastrointestinal decontamination in a human acetaminophen ingestion model. *Acad Emerg Med* 1997;**4**(3):167–74.

22 Green R, Grierson R, Sitar DS, Tenenbein M. How long after drug ingestion is activated charcoal still effective? *J Toxicol Clin Toxicol* 2001;**39**(6):601–5.

23 Kirk MA, Peterson J, Kulig K, Lowenstein S, Rumack BH. Acetaminophen overdose in children: a comparison of ipecac versus activated charcoal versus no gastrointestinal decontamination (Abstract). *Ann Emerg Med* 1991;**20**(4):472–3.

24 Cooper GM, Le Couteur DG, Richardson D, Buckley NA. A randomized clinical trial of activated charcoal for the routine management of oral drug overdose. *Q J Med* 2005;**98**(9):655–60.

25 Richell-Herren K, Harrison M. Activated charcoal in paracetamol overdose. *J Accid Emerg Med* 2000;**17**:284.

26 Brok J, Buckley N, Gluud C. Interventions for paracetamol (acetaminophen) overdose (Review). *Cochrane Database Syst Rev* 2006;**2**: CD003328 (update of *Cochrane Database Syst Rev* 2002;3:CD003328; PMID: 12137690).

27 Betten D, Cantrell F, Thomas S, Williams S, Clark RF. A prospective evaluation of shortened course oral N-acetylcysteine for the treatment of acute acetaminophen poisoning. *Ann Emerg Med* 2007;**50**:272–9.

28 O'Grady JG, Schalm SW, Williams R. Acute liver failure: redefining the syndromes. *Lancet* 1993;**342**:273–5.

29 Harrison PM, Keays R, Bray GP, Alexander GJ, Williams R. Improved outcome of paracetamol-induced fulminant hepatic failure by late administration of acetylcysteine. *Lancet* 1990;**335**(8705):1572–3.

30 Keays R, Harrison PM, Wendon JA, et al. Intravenous acetylcysteine in paracetamol induced fulminant hepatic failure: a prospective controlled trial. *BMJ* 1991;**303**(6809):1026–9.

31 Boxer L, Anderson FP, Rowe DS. Comparison of ipecac-induced emesis with gastric lavage in the treatment of acute salicylate ingestion. *J Pediatr* 1969;**74**(5):800–803.

32 Vale JA. Position statement: gastric lavage. American Academy of Clinical Toxicology; European Association of Poisons Centres and Clinical Toxicologists (Review). *J Toxicol Clin Toxicol* 1997;**35**(7): 711–19.

33 Mayer AL, Sitar DS, Tenenbein M. Multiple-dose charcoal and whole-bowel irrigation do not increase clearance of absorbed salicylate. *Arch Intern Med* 1992;**152**(2):393–6.

34 Kirshenbaum LA, Mathews SC, Sitar DS, Tenenbein M. Does multiple-dose charcoal therapy enhance salicylate excretion? *Arch Intern Med* 1990;**150**:1281–3.

35 Ho JL, Tierney MG, Dickinson G. An evaluation of the effect of repeated doses of oral activated charcoal on salicylate elimination. *J Clin Pharmacol* 1989;**29**:366–9.

36 Olsen KM, Ma FH, Ackerman BH, Stull RE. Low-volume whole bowel irrigation and salicylate absorption: a comparison with ipecac-charcoal. *Pharmacotherapy* 1993;**13**(3):229–32.

37 Hillman RJ, Prescott LF. Treatment of salicylate poisoning with repeated oral charcoal. *BMJ* 1985;**291**(6507):1472.

38 Vale JA, Krenzelok EP, Proudfoot AT. Position statement and practice guidelines on the use of multi-dose activated charcoal in the treatment of acute poisoning. *J Toxicol Clin Toxicol* 1999;**37**(6):731–51.

39 Chyka PA, Seger D. Position statement: single-dose activated charcoal. *J Toxicol Clin Toxicol* 1997;**35**(7):721–41.

40 Done AK. Salicylate intoxication significance of measurements of salicylate in blood in cases of acute ingestion. *Pediatrics* 1960;**26**:800–807.

41 Dugandzic RM, Tierney MG, Dickinson GE, Dolan MC, McKnight DR. Evaluation of the validity of the Done nomogram in the management of acute salicylate intoxication. *Ann Emerg Med* 1989;**18**(11):1186–90.

42 Vree TB, Van Ewuk-Beneken Kolmer EWJ, Verwey-Van Wissen CPWGM, Hekster YA. Effect of urinary pH on the pharmacokinetics of salicylic acid, with its glycine and glucuronide conjugates in humans. *Int J Pharmacol Ther* 1994;**32**(10):550–58.

43 Prescott LF, Balali-Mood MI, Critchley JAJH. Diuresis or urinary alkalinisation for salicylate poisoning? *BMJ* 1982;**285**(6352):1383–6.

44 Proudfoot AT, Krenzelok EP, Vale JA. Position paper on urine alkalinization. *J Toxicol Clin Toxicol* 2004;**42**(1):1–26.

45 Higgins RM, Connolly JO, Hendry BM. Alkalinization and hemodialysis in severe salicylate poisoning: comparison of elimination techniques in the same patient. *Clin Nephrol* 1998;**50**(3):178–83.

46 Lund B, Seifert S, Mayersohn M. Efficacy of sustained low-efficiency dialysis in the treatment of salicylate toxicity. *Nephrol Dial Transplant* 2005;**20**:1483–4.

5 Injury

29 Mild Traumatic Brain Injury

Jeffrey J. Bazarian[1] & Will Townend[2]

[1]Departments of Emergency Medicine *and* Neurology, University of Rochester School of Medicine and Dentistry, Rochester, USA
[2]Department of Emergency Medicine, Hull Royal Infirmary, Hull, UK

Clinical scenario

A 42-year-old businessman had been attending a social club, where he had consumed around six glasses of wine over the preceding 3 hours. He lost his footing on a small run of stairs and fell down around four steps and landed on his head. He lost consciousness and has little recollection of falling, although he does remember the ambulance ride to the emergency department (ED). He has not vomited. He had some bleeding from his ear after the fall but this has now stopped.

On examination he is neurologically intact and fully conscious. He has no bruising or laceration to his head. He has some dried blood around the left external auditory meatus, but no ongoing blood or cerebrospinal fluid loss. He has a headache but no neck pain or tenderness. You wonder what the chances are that these findings indicate basal skull fracture.

You are aware that there is a risk of intracranial haematoma, despite his return to full consciousness. You decide to perform a computerized tomography (CT) scan of the brain. This shows no signs of intracranial bleeding. You consider the risk of subsequent neurological deterioration or prolonged post-concussive symptoms, and wonder if further hospital admission is necessary. The patient is requesting medication for relief of his headache, wants to know if he will develop post-concussive symptoms and asks when he can resume normal activities/work.

Background

Mild traumatic brain injury (TBI) is an important public health problem, affecting over 1.2 million Americans annually [1]. Despite the designation "mild", the adverse outcomes from this injury can be significant. Cognitive difficulties and post-concussive

Evidence-based Emergency Medicine. Edited by Brian H. Rowe
© 2009 Blackwell Publishing, ISBN: 978-1-4051-6143-5.

symptoms are well known sequelae and include headache, dizziness, difficulty concentrating, reduced short-term memory, inability to multi-task and problems with arithmetic computation. Less well known are motoric deficits, which include balance difficulties, dynamic gait instability and slowed simple reaction time. The long-term consequences of mild TBI are also significant. Approximately 30–50% of mild TBI patients are impaired 3 months after their injury, with 25% impaired at 1 year. A substantial number of patients become unemployed after suffering mild TBI. In addition, mild TBI has recently been recognized as a possible risk factor for both Alzheimer's disease and Parkinson's disease. Thus, there is significant impetus for clinicians to be able to recognize and treat mild TBI.

The most widely accepted definition of mild TBI involves a blow to the head (or rapid deceleration) with witnessed or self-reported loss of consciousness of less than 30 minutes, or amnesia of less than 24 hours, or any alteration in mental state at the time of the injury. In addition, patients must present with a Glasgow Coma Scale (GCS) score of 13–15 30 minutes or more after the injury [1,2]. This chapter searches for evidence for the important questions related to mild TBI in the emergency setting.

Clinical questions

1 In adult patients with mild TBI (population), do clinical signs and symptoms (measures) have sufficient sensitivity and specificity (diagnostic test characteristics) to safely rule out intracranial abnormalities on CT requiring surgical intervention?
2 In adult patients with mild TBI (population), do clinical signs and symptoms (measures) have sufficient reliability (diagnostic test characteristics) to safely be used in clinical decision rules (outcome)?
3 In adult patients with mild TBI (population), do CT scan abnormalities (measures) have sufficient sensitivity and specificity (diagnostic test characteristics) to safely discharge and rule out disabling symptoms beyond 3 months of injury (outcome)?

4 In adult patients with mild TBI (population), does admission to hospital for a period of observation compared to immediate discharge reduce the incidence of neurological deterioration or improve cognitive outcome/post-concussive symptoms (outcome)?

5 In adult patients with headache after mild TBI (population), does administration of analgesics compared to no analgesics reduce the duration of headache or other post-concussive symptoms (outcomes)?

6 In adult patients with mild TBI (population), does a period of refraining from physical exertion (intervention) compared to unrestricted physical activity (control) reduce the incidence of second impact syndrome, or improve cognitive outcome/post-concussive symptoms (outcomes)?

7 In adult patients with mild TBI (population), what signs and symptoms or biomarkers present immediately after the injury (risk factors) predict the development of post-concussive symptoms lasting 1 month or more (outcome)?

General search strategy

You begin to address these questions by searching for evidence in the common electronic databases such as MEDLINE, the Cochrane Library and EMBASE, looking specifically for systematic reviews and meta-analyses. In addition, you access relevant, updated and evidence-based clinical practice guidelines (CPGs) on mild TBI diagnosis and management in areas lacking evidence. A search of the Cochrane Library, MEDLINE and EMBASE databases found no systematic reviews of meta-analyses of diagnostic studies in mild TBI.

Critical review of the literature

Question 1: In adult patients with mild TBI (population), do clinical signs and symptoms (measures) have sufficient sensitivity and specificity (diagnostic test characteristics) to safely rule out intracranial abnormalities on CT requiring surgical intervention?

Search strategy

- MEDLINE: brain concussion AND X-ray computed tomography. Limited to diagnosis (sensitivity and specificity)

The initial clinical imperative in assessing a head-injured patient is to identify potentially life-threatening intracranial bleeding in a timely fashion, despite the rarity of such complications (0.4–1.0%) [3–6]. Diagnostic protocols must identify all such patients at risk. One approach is to perform a CT scan on all patients presenting to the ED following a blow to the head. Although safe in terms of detecting significant injury, this approach will be costly and expose many patients without intracranial injury (likely 92–94%)

to ionizing radiation [3,6], potentially on a number of occasions in their lifetime. In a number of health care settings this may be unaffordable, or indeed impractical.

A number of authors have sought to identify clinical indicators for risk stratification. A specific search was made for studies in which decision support guidelines, derived by recursive partitioning of prospectively recorded clinical data from mild TBI (initial GCS of 13–15) patients, were used. This highlighted four studies (Table 29.1) [3–6]. A search for external validation of these rules revealed a further four studies (Table 29.2) [7–10]. Variables vary from rule to rule; however, most include advanced age, seizures, vomiting and amnesia. Sensitivity for traumatic intracranial injuries on CT ranged from 95.2 to 100%, while specificity ranges were much lower at 17.3–49.6%. Thus, in general, these rules are better at correctly predicting normal CT scans than at identifying abnormal scans. Variation in estimates of sensitivity and specificity vary due to slightly different definitions of mild TBI and abnormal CT scans.

These decision rules were often validated in other settings to obtain a true reflection of their likely clinical worth (Table 29.2) [7,8]. Smits and co-workers evaluated the Canadian CT Head Rule (CCHR; Fig. 29.1) and the New Orleans Criteria (NOC; Fig. 29.2) in 3181 adults (GCS 13–15) and found both rules to be 100% sensitive for the detection of intracranial injury requiring surgical intervention (17 patients (0.5%)). The CCHR required 63% of patients to be scanned, and the NOC 94%. This reflects the design of each instrument, and the cost of the scan reduction when following the CCHR in this study is loss of sensitivity for any CT abnormality (83.4% vs 97.7% for the NOC).

Stiell and colleagues also performed a validation study of the CCHR and the NOC in 2707 patients (GCS 13–15). Forty-one patients (1.5%) required neurosurgical intervention. They reported 100% sensitivity for both rules (95% CI: 96% to 100%) for neurosurgical intervention and clinically significant CT abnormality (a composite endpoint including a clinical evaluation for 19.2% who did not undergo imaging in the ED). The CT rate for the CCHR was 52% and for the NOC was 88% in their patients.

Ibanez and colleagues used the NOC and the CCHR in a cohort of 1101 Spanish head-injured patients (age over 14 years, GCS 14–15, 1% undergoing surgery). They did not describe the prediction of the need for neurosurgical intervention, but the sensitivity for relevant scan findings were 85.5% (95% CI: 78% to 98%) for the CCHR and 95.2% (95% CI: 90.6% to 99.8%) for the NOC.

The CCHR has been adapted to develop UK National Institute for Health and Clinical Excellence (NICE) guidelines [9], with the addition of post-traumatic seizure, focal neurological deficits and coagulopathy as predictors. These were validated in a prospective series of 7955 Italian patients (age 10 years or more, GCS 14–15, neurosurgical intervention in 1.3%) by Fabbri and co-workers. The NICE guidelines showed a sensitivity of 94.4% (95% CI: 87.8% to 97.1%) for neurosurgical intervention and 93.5% sensitivity (95% CI: 91% to 95.2%) for intracranial lesions. They did not describe the neurosurgical procedure for the six NICE guideline-negative

Table 29.1 CT decision rule derivation studies for use of head CT after mild traumatic brain injury.

Study	Number of subjects	Indications for CT scanning	Sensitivity for intracranial traumatic CT findings (95% CI)	Specificity (95% CI)	Comments
New Orleans Criteria [3]	520 (validated in a further 909)	Vomiting, age >60 years, drug or alcohol intoxication, persistent anterograde amnesia, visible trauma above the clavicles, seizure	100% (95 to 100)	25% (22 to 28)	Mild TBI defined as GCS 15
Canadian CT Head Rule [4]	3121	GCS <15 at 2 hours after injury, suspected open or depressed skull fracture, any sign of basal skull fracture, two or more vomiting episodes, age >65 years, amnesia before impact of 30+ minutes, dangerous mechanism (e.g., pedestrian struck by a motor vehicle, occupant ejected from a motor vehicle, fall from height >1 m or five stairs)	98.4% (96 to 99)	49.6% (48 to 51)	Mild TBI defined as GCS 13–14 or GCS 15 with LOC/amnesia. Rule predicts clinically important CT abnormalities only (contusions <5 mm, SDH <4 mm, SAH 1 mm, isolated pneumocephaly, closed depressed skull fracture of outer table i.e., not contusions <5mm)
NEXUS II [6]	13,326	Evidence of skull fracture, scalp hematoma, neurological deficit, altered alertness, abnormal behavior, coagulopathy, persistent vomiting, age >65 years	95.2% (92.2 to 97.2)	17.3% (16.5 to 18.0)	Minor head injury not defined
CT in head injury patients [5]	3181	Presence of one or more of the following major criteria: Pedestrian/cyclist struck by vehicle, ejected from vehicle, vomiting, post-traumatic amnesia, clinical sign of skull fracture, GCS <15, GCS deterioration by ≥ 2 (1 hour after presentation), anticoagulant use, post-traumatic seizure, age ≥ 60 years *Or* Presence of more than one of the following minor criteria: Fall from any elevation, persistent anterograde amnesia, contusion of the skull, GCS deterioration by ≥ 2 (1 hour after presentation), neurological deficit, loss of consciousness, age 40–60 years	97.5%	22% (1 to 24)	Mild TBI defined as GCS 13–14 or GCS 15 and one risk factor

CI, confidence interval; CT, computerized tomography; GCS, Glasgow Coma Score; LOC, loss of consciousness; SAH, subarachnoid hemorrhage; SDH, subdural hemorrhage; TBI, traumatic brain injury.

patients. This underlines the possible confounding of this endpoint by variation in practice internationally.

The use of clinical data for decision support will depend on what the clinician aims to achieve. It appears that none of the decision instruments will enable detection of every lesion. Each of the rules described appears suitable to identify those at risk of death or disability from time-critical, surgically redeemable pathology. The trade-off is the miss rate for CT scan abnormality. Stiell and colleagues gained a consensus nationally for what a significant lesion might be, and consequently their reported sensitivity for its detection is higher in their validation study. The further question is whether it is vital to identify all lesions, as the consequences for the patient of non-surgical lesions is largely unknown, and the

outcome for those with normal scans is not uniformly favorable with regard to symptoms and function.

In summary, the approach where a CT scan is obtained for every head-injured patient is not practical or efficient. The alternative, where clinicians select a rule with a scan rate or sensitivity that suits the setting in which the patient is seen, seems reasonable and far more evidence based than clinical impression alone.

Question 2: In adult patients with mild TBI (population), do clinical signs and symptoms (measures) have sufficient reliability (diagnostic test characteristics) to safely be used in clinical decision rules (outcome)?

Study	Number of patients	Neurosurgical lesion sensitivity% (95% CI)	CT abnormality sensitivity% (95% CI)	Scan rate (%)
Smits et al. [7]	3181		"Important CT findings"	
NOC		100 (81.6 to 100)	99.2 (97.1 to 99.8)	97
CCHR		100 (81.6 to 100)	87.2 (82.6 to 90.9)	62.7
Stiell et al. [8]	2707		"Clinically important"	
NOC		100 (63 to 100)	100 (96 to 100)	88.0
CCHR		100 (91 to 100)	100 (96 to 100)	52.1
Ibanez et al. [9]	1101		"Relevant finding"	
NOC		–	95.2 (90.6 to 99.8)	83.6
CCHR		–	85.5 (78.0 to 98.0)	52.3
Fabbri et al. [10]	7995		Intracranial lesion	
NICE		94.4 (87.8 to 97.1)	93.5 (91 to 95.2)	34.4
Pooled	6989			
NOC		100 (99.93 to 100)	99.3 (99.0 to 99.4)	91.5
CCHR		100 (99.94 to 100)	97.0 (96.6 to 97.4)	57.0

Table 29.2 CT decision rule validation studies for the use of head CT after mild traumatic brain injury.

CCHR, Canadian CT Head Rule; CI, confidence interval; NOC, New Orleans Criteria.

Search strategy

• MEDLINE: brain concussion AND physical examination

The value of decision rules depends not only on their sensitivity and specificity, but also on the reliability of the variables employed in the rule. If one clinician's notion of amnesia, for example, differs significantly from another clinician's, then the validity and utility of the rule is diminished. Two of the four decision rule groups attempted to determine the reliability of variables used in their rules. The NEXUS II group [11] assessed the agreement between two emergency physicians in the determination of 19 variables in 3951 patients. They later used these variables in their derivation study [4]. They rated a kappa (κ) value of 0.50 to denote substantial agreement. All the values in their final model rated higher than 0.6. Stiell and co-workers, in their derivation of the CCHR, found high inter-rater reliability for possible open and basal skull fractures (κ = 0.85 and 0.76, respectively) [4]. There was more variability in the assessment of amnesia (κ = 0.52). In addition, the agreement between raters on some NOC variables, such as injury above the clavicles, was insufficient to be considered reliable (κ = 0.42) [4]. Variability in assessment of amnesia has been found in other studies of mild head injury [12]. Consequently, the current decision rules contain reliable historical and physical findings that can be safely used by most ED clinicians. It is the responsibility of those using the rules to understand the inclusion criteria, know how to reliably measure the included factors, and finally apply the rule.

Question 3: In adult patients with mild TBI (population), do CT scan abnormalities (measures) have sufficient sensitivity and specificity (diagnostic test characteristics) to safely discharge and rule out disabling symptoms beyond 3 months of injury (outcome)?

Search strategy

• MEDLINE: (brain concussion AND x-ray computed tomography AND neurologic deterioration) OR (brain concussion AND x-ray computed tomography AND post concussive syndrome/symptoms)

Having followed a decision rule, or indeed having simply ordered a scan, the clinician is faced with the decision of what to do next. Does the absence of an intracranial injury exclude the risk of neurological deterioration from the accumulation of extra-axial hematoma to the extent that patients can be immediately discharged from the ED?

Many emergency providers are not reassured by a normal head CT scan and believe that the chances of delayed intracranial bleeding and neurological deterioration are sufficient enough to warrant hospital observation [13]. These practices may have been born out of several case reports from the late 1980s and early 1990s describing the appearance of delayed epidural and subdural hematomas after an initially normal head CT scan. Since that time, however, several large prospective studies have demonstrated that the risk of delayed neurological deterioration or need for neurosurgical intervention is actually quite low in the setting of mild TBI and an initially normal head CT. In two prospective studies of 3322 mild

Canadian CT Head Rule

CT Head is only required for minor head injury patients with any one of the following findings. Minor head injury patients present with a GCS score of 13 to 15 after witnessed loss of consciousness, amnesia, or confusion.

High risk (for Neurological Intervention)

1. GCS score < 15 at 2 hours after injury
2. Suspected open or depressed skull fracture
3. Any sign of basal skull fracture *
4. Vomiting ≥ 2 episodes
5. Age ≥ 65 years

Medium-risk (for Brain Injury on CT)

6. Amnesia before impact = 30 minutes
7. Dangerous mechanism **

* Signs of Basal Skull Fracture:
- hemotympanum, 'racoon' eyes, CSF otorrhea / rhinorrhea, Battle's sign

** Dangerous Mechanism:
- pedestrian struck by motor vehicle
- occupant ejected from motor vehicle
- fall from elevation ≥ 3 feet or 5 stairs

Rule not applicable if:
- non-trauma case
- gCS < 13
- age < 16 years
- oral anticoagulant medication use or bleeding disorder
- obvious open skull fracture

Figure 29.1 Canadian CT Head Rule.

TBI patients observed for 24 hours, only one patient in whom the initial CT scan was negative needed urgent surgery (to remove facial fracture fragments that had intruded into the calvarium) [14,15]. Moreover, in a published review of 52 studies containing over 62,000 mild TBI patients, only three patients deteriorated following an initially normal CT scan [16]. Taken together, these studies would suggest that the risk of delayed neurological deterioration or need for neurosurgery after mild TBI given an initially normal head CT is in the order of 0.3–4 per 100,000.

Given the weight of the evidence, several consensus guidelines have recommended routine CT scanning for patients with mild TBI and hospital discharge for those without traumatic abnormality on the initial CT scan. These include the Eastern Association for the Surgery of Trauma [17] and the American College

New Orleans Criteria

CT Head is only required for minor head injury patients with any one of the following findings. Only applies to head injury patients with a GCS Score of 15.

1. **Headache**

2. **Vomiting**

3. **Age > 60 years**

4. **Drug or alcohol intoxication**

5. **Persistent anterograde amnesia**

6. **Trauma above the clavicle**

7. **Seizure**

Figure 29.2 New Orleans Criteria.

of Emergency Physicians [18]. An alternative approach would be to apply a clinical decision rule (CCHR or NOC) and discharge all those who are "rule negative" or "rule positive" with a negative image. This approach would be safe, reduce resource use and reduce ionizing radiation exposure.

Although the risk of neurological deterioration after a normal head CT is low, the risk of developing disabling post-concussive symptoms is not. Most studies reporting the incidence of post-concussive symptoms exclude those with traumatic abnormalities on head CT scan. Thus the 30–50% incidence of post-concussive symptoms quoted earlier in this chapter refers primarily to those with a normal initial CT scan. (It is unclear if traumatic abnormalities on head CT scan after mild TBI are associated with higher post-concussive syndrome risk [19,20].) Neuroimaging modalities such as diffusion-weighted magnetic resonance imaging (MRI) and single photon emission computed tomography (SPECT) frequently reveal evidence of brain injury after a concussion in the setting of a normal CT scan, underscoring the organic underpinnings of these symptoms [21]. In most patients, these symptoms resolve by 1–3 months; however, these symptoms persist beyond 1 year in approximately 25% of patients [1].

In summary, a normal head CT scan essentially rules out neurological deterioration but not the development of post-concussive symptoms. Practitioners should bear this in mind when informing patients what to expect after ED discharge for mild TBI.

Question 4: In adult patients with mild TBI (population), does admission to hospital for a period of observation compared to immediate discharge reduce the incidence of neurological deterioration or improved cognitive outcome/post-concussive symptoms (outcome)?

Search strategy

• MEDLINE: brain concussion AND observation

Even if the risk of neurological deterioration is low after a normal head CT scan, is there any value to observing patients in the hospital? This issue has been addressed in one controlled trial where immediate discharge after normal head CT was compared to in-hospital observation. Among the 2602 mild TBI patients included in the trial, mortality, need for neurosurgical intervention and the Extended Glasgow Outcome scale were similar in both groups [22]. Among those admitted for observation, overall costs were higher and time to neurosurgery was longer compared to those who received immediate CT scans.

For mild TBI patients who have an initially abnormal CT scan, hospitalization for neurosurgery or observation remains the standard of care. The need for neurosurgical intervention in such patients varies between 0.4% and 3% [23,24]. Among those who do not need neurosurgery, the rate of neurological deterioration, and thus the value of in-hospital observation, is less clear. Additionally,

the outcome for mild TBI patients neither scanned nor observed is also not known.

In summary, there appears to be no advantage to in-hospital observation for mild TBI patients with a normal head CT scan in terms of short-term outcome. However, the effect of observation on longer-term post-concussive symptoms remains unstudied.

Question 5: In adult patients with headache after mild TBI (population), does administration of analgesics compared to no analgesics reduce the duration of headache or other post-concussive symptoms (outcome)?

Search strategy

• MEDLINE: (brain concussion AND headache) OR posttraumatic headache. Limited to clinical trial

Headache is one of the most common symptoms after a concussion and often is the symptom that limits a patient's ability to return to normal daily activities [25]. Clinicians may be inclined not to treat headache after concussions for fear that analgesics will mask the symptoms of rising intracranial pressure, or interfere with platelet function and precipitate intracranial bleeding. As discussed in Question 3 above, however, the chances of bleeding or neurological deterioration are exceedingly rare in patients who have had a normal CT of the head. The evidence that analgesics may be of some benefit, however, is less clear. This issue had been examined in several, mostly uncontrolled studies (Table 29.3) [26–32]. The two drugs subjected to a controlled trial (piracetem and CDP-choline) had modest beneficial effects on headache. These trials were small and to date have not been followed up by more definitive trials.

In US emergency departments, the most common analgesics given acutely after mild TBI are acetaminophen and non-steroidal anti-inflammatory drugs [33]. However, the effectiveness of these medications for relieving headache after mild TBI has not been studied. In summary, symptomatic treatment with analgesics seems reasonable and safe; however, the preferred agent has yet to be identified.

Question 6: In adult patients with mild TBI (population), does a period of refraining from physical exertion (intervention) compared to unrestricted physical activity (control) reduce the incidence of second impact syndrome, or improve cognitive outcome/post-concussive symptoms (outcomes)?

Search strategy

• MEDLINE: brain concussion AND rest

Table 29.3 Pharmacological treatments for headache (HA) after mild traumatic brain injury (TBI).

Treatment	Timing of treatment after mild TBI	Study type	Number of patients	Outcome	Study
Piracetam	2–12 months	Double-blind, placebo-controlled trial	60	Significant reduction in mean HA scores among treated group	Hakkarainen & Hakamies [26]
Naltrexone	4 months to 6 years	Case report	2	Both patients had reduction in HA	Tennant et al. [27]
Dihydroergotoamine and metoclopramide	1 day to 3 years	Case series	34	85% had good to excellent HA relief	McBeath & Nanda [28]
CDP-choline	Unclear (during acute hospitalization)	Double-blind, placebo-controlled trial	14	HA relieved in 86% treated patients vs 57% placebo	Levin [29]
Divalproex sodium	More than 2 months	Case series	100	44% had 25–50% improvement in HA; 16% had >50% improvement	Packard [30]
Sumtriptan	Months-years	Case series	7	Reduction in HA in all patients	Gawel et al. [31]
Propranolol or amitryptiline or both or verapamil	1–30 months	Case series	35	70% had reduction in frequency and severity of HA	Weiss et al. [32]

Rest is commonly prescribed after mild TBI although its effectiveness remains unclear. A period of rest is generally thought to hasten recovery and lessen the severity of post-concussive symptoms, which affect 25–50% of mild TBI patients and contribute to long-term disability and unemployment [1]. Rest is also prescribed in the setting of sports-related mild TBI where the goal is to prevent a second fatal head blow during the period of neurological recovery (the so-called second impact syndrome) [34].

The effect of rest on the development of post-concussive symptoms was tested in a single randomized trial of 107 mild TBI patients. Compared to those who resumed activity immediately, those randomized to full bed rest for 6 days had similar post-concussive symptom scores at 2 weeks, 3 months and 6 months after injury [35]. The effect of rest on the development of second impact syndrome has not been subject to any controlled trial. Nevertheless, multiple consensus guidelines recommend a graded return to activities after sports-related mild TBI. These include the American Academy of Neurology, the Colorado Medical Society, the American College of Sports Medicine, and others [36].

In both sports and non-sports settings, the period of rest is typically guided by the patient's symptoms. However, some experts recommend that the duration of rest be guided by the return of normal cognitive performance, especially when there is suspicion that the patient might be minimizing symptoms [37]. Cognitive testing typically requires the involvement of a neuropsychologist or rehabilitation specialist, with attendant increased health care costs. The superiority of a cognitive-based guide to rest over a symptom-based guide has not been examined.

In summary, a period of rest seems to be a prudent and safe strategy to promote recovery after mild TBI and is recommended by several sports organizations. However, the superiority of this strategy over one where activity is not restricted has not been demonstrated.

Question 7: In adult patients with mild TBI (population), what signs and symptoms or biomarkers present immediately after the injury (risk factors) predict the development of post-concussive symptoms lasting 1 month or more (outcome)?

Search strategy

- MEDLINE: brain concussion AND observation

Not all patients who suffer a mild TBI will develop post-concussive symptoms. It is generally believed that both the severity of brain injury and the patient's psychological response to injury contribute to the development of post-concussive symptoms [38,39]. Several studies have examined the relationship between specific factors present immediately after injury to the development of post-concussive symptoms (Table 29.4) [40–43]. Female gender, serum S100 calcium binding protein B (S-100B) level >0.5 µg/L, presence of a skull fracture, headache and dizziness are all associated with an increased risk of post-concussive symptoms. Others have found female gender to be associated with poor outcome after mild TBI, the reasons for which are not entirely clear [44]. S-100B is a protein released from brain cells (astrocytes) when they are damaged after mild TBI. Although not currently available in North America, serum assays for S-100B are currently used clinically in Europe.

Clinicians could use these factors to decide which mild TBI patients should be targeted for early follow-up. Several studies have revealed that early follow-up for unselected mild TBI patients

Factor	Predicts PCS at what time interval?	OR or LR (95% CI)	Study
Female gender	1 month	7.8 (1.9 to 41.6)	Bazarian et al. [40]
Amnesia, both retrograde and anterograde	1 month	0.055 (0.002 to 0.47)	
Amnesia, both retrograde and anterograde	3 months	0.13 (0.0 to 0.93)	
Skull fracture	1 month	8.0 (2.6 to 24.6)	Savola & Hillbom [41]
Serum S-100B >0.5 μg/L	1 month	5.5 (1.6 to 18.6)	
Dizziness	1 month	3.1 (1.2 to 8.0)	
Headache	1 month	2.6 (1.0 to 6.5)	
Serum S-100B > 0.5 ug/L	9 months	2.67 (0.7 to 9.3)	Ingebrigtsen et al. [42]
Serum S-100B >0.48 ug/L	1 month	5.4 (3.3 to 8.7)	Townend et al. [43]

Table 29.4 Factors that predict post-concussive syndrome (PCS) after mild traumatic brain injury.

reduces long-term disability [45,46]. Such follow-up usually consists of education and/or cognitive rehabilitation. High-risk patients would be most likely to benefit from the effect of any intervention on follow-up.

Conclusions

The patient mentioned above underwent CT scanning, which revealed a basilar skull fracture but no traumatic abnormality to the brain. He was observed in the hospital for 24 hours and did not exhibit any worsening of his mental status. He received several doses of acetaminophen for headache with minimal relief and was released the following day. The patient was prescribed 1 week of rest at home but 3 weeks after hospital discharge he continued to have frequent daily headaches and dizziness, as well as difficulty concentrating. He has been unable to work since his head injury.

The management of mild traumatic brain injury is evolving. Efforts to understand the impact of hospitalization, rest and drugs on recovery depend on our ability to accurately identify patients with true neurological injury after a blow to the head. Improved diagnosis will facilitate future controlled trials of early pharmacological intervention. In the meantime, clinicians need to actively elicit the symptoms of mild TBI and judiciously order CT imaging. A normal CT scan does not exclude the risk of development of disabling post-concussive symptoms, although patients are safe to be discharged from the ED. Follow-up with experts may help; however, effective pharmacological interventions have yet to be identified.

Conflicts of interest

None were declared.

References

1 Centers for Disease Control and Prevention, National Center for Injury Prevention and Control. *Report to Congress. Mild Traumatic Brain Injury in the United States: Steps to prevent a serious public health problem.* Centers for Disease Control and Prevention, Atlanta, 2003.

2 Kay T, Harrington DE, Adams R, et al. Definition of mild traumatic brain injury. *J Head Trauma Rehab* 1993;8(3):86–7.

3 Haydel MJ, Preston CA, Mills TJ, Luber S, Blaudeau E, DeBlieux PMC. Indications for computed tomography in patients with minor head injury (Comment). *N Engl J Med* 2000;343(2):100–105.

4 Stiell IG, Wells GA, Vandemheen K, et al. The Canadian CT Head Rule for patients with minor head injury (Comment). *Lancet* 2001;357(9266):1391–6.

5 Smiths M, Dippel DWJ, Steyerberg EW, et al. Predicting intracranial traumatic findings on computed tomography in patients with minor head injury: the CHIP prediction rule. *Ann Intern Med* 2007;146(6):397–405.

6 Mower WRHJ, Herbert M, Wolfson AB, Pollack CV, Jr., Zucker MI, and NI Investigators. Developing a decision instrument to guide computed tomographic imaging of blunt head injury patients. *J Trauma Injury Infect Crit Care* 2005;59(4):954–9.

7 Smits M, Dippel DWJ, de Haan GG, et al. External validation of the Canadian CT Head Rule and the New Orleans Criteria in patients with minor head injury. *JAMA* 2005;294(12):1519–25.

8 Stiell IG, Clement CM, Rowe BH, et al. Comparison of the Canadian CT Head Rule and the New Orleans Criteria for CT scanning in patients with minor head injury. *JAMA* 2005;294(12):1511–18.

9 Ibanez, J, Arikan F, Pedraza S, et al. Reliability of clinical guidelines in the detection of patients at risk following mild head injury: results of a prospective study. *J Neurosurg* 2004;100(5):825–34.

10 Fabbri A, Servadei F, Marchesini G, et al. Clinical performance of NICE recommendations versus NCWFNS proposal in patients with mild head injury. *J Neurotrauma* 2005;22(12):1419–27.

11 Hollander JE, Lowery DW, Wolfson AS, et al. Interrater reliability of criteria used in assessing blunt head injury patients for intracranial injuries. *Acad Emerg Med* 2003;**10**(8):830–35.

12 King NS, Crawford S, Wenden FJ, Moss NE, Wade DT, Caldwell FE. Measurement of post-traumatic amnesia: how reliable is it? *J Neurol Neurosurg Psychiatry* 1997;**62**(1):38–42.

13 Harad FT, Kerstein MD. Inadequacy of bedside clinical indicators in identifying significant intracranial injury in trauma patients. *J Trauma Injury Infect Crit Care* 1992;**32**(3):359–63.

14 Livingston DH, Lavery RF, Passannante MR, et al. Emergency department discharge of patients with a negative cranial computed tomography scan after minimal head injury. *Ann Surg* 2000;**232**(1):126–32.

15 Nagy KK, Joseph KT, Krosner SM, et al. The utility of head computed tomography after minimal head injury. *J Trauma Injury Infect Crit Care* 1999;**46**(2):268–70.

16 Geijerstam J-L, Britton M. Mild head injury: reliability of early computed tomographic findings in triage for admission. *Emerg Med J* 2005;**22**(2):103–7.

17 Cushman JG, Agarwal N, Fabian TC, et al. Practice management guidelines for the management of mild traumatic brain injury: the EAST practice management guidelines work group. *J Trauma Injury Infect Crit Care* 2001;**51**(5):1016–26.

18 Jagoda AS, Cantrill SV, Wears RL, et al. Clinical policy: neuroimaging and decisionmaking in adult mild traumatic brain injury in the acute setting. *Ann Emerg Med* 2002;**40**(2):231–49.

19 Wallesch CW, Curio N, Kutz S, Jost S, Bartels C, Synowitz H. Outcome after mild-to-moderate blunt head injury: effects of focal lesions and diffuse axonal injury. *Brain Injury* 2001;**15**(5):401–12.

20 Williams DH, Levin HS, Eisenberg HM. Mild head injury classification. *Neurosurgery* 1990;**27**(3):422–8.

21 Bazarian JJ, Blyth B, Cimpello L. Bench to bedside: evidence for brain injury after concussion – looking beyond the computed tomography scan. *Acad Emerg Med* 2006;**13**(2):199–214.

22 Geijerstam J-L, Oredsson S, Britton M. Medical outcome after immediate computed tomography or admission for observation in patients with mild head injury: randomised controlled trial. *BMJ* 2006;**333**(7566):465.

23 Culotta VP, Sementilli M, Gerold K, Watts C. Clinicopathological heterogeneity in the classification of mild head injury. *Neurosurgery* 1996;**38**(2):245–50.

24 Stein SC, Ross SE. The value of computed tomographic scans in patients with low-risk head injuries. *Neurosurgery* 1990;**26**(4):638–40.

25 Alves W, Macciocchi SN, Barth JT. Postconcussive symptoms after uncomplicated mild head injury. *J Head Trauma Rehab* 1993;**8**(3):48–59.

26 Hakkarainen H, Hakamies L. Piracetam in the treatment of postconcussional syndrome. A double-blind study. *Eur Neurol* 1978;**17**(1):50–55.

27 Tennant FS, Wild J. Naltrexone treatment for postconcussional syndrome. *Am J Psychiatry* 1987;**144**(6):813–14.

28 McBeath J, Nanda A. Use of dihydroergotamine in patients with postconcussion syndrome. *Headache* 1994;**34**:148–51.

29 Levin HS. Treatment of postconcussional symptoms with CDP-choline. *J Neurol Sci* 1991;**103**(Suppl):S39–42.

30 Packard RC. Treatment of chronic daily posttraumatic headache with divalproex sodium. *Headache* 2000;**40**(9):736–9.

31 Gawel MJ, Rothbart P, Jacobs H. Subcutaneous sumatriptan in the treatment of acute episodes of posttraumatic headache. *Headache* 1993;**33**(2):96–7.

32 Weiss HD, Stern BJ, Goldberg J. Post-traumatic migraine: chronic migraine precipitated by minor head or neck trauma. *Headache* 1991;**31**(7):451–6.

33 Bazarian JJ, McClung J, Cheng Y, Flesher W, Schneider SM. Emergency department management of mild traumatic brain injury in the USA. *Emerg Med J* 2005;**22**(7):473–7.

34 Cantu RC. Second-impact syndrome. *Clin Sports Med* 1998;**17**(1):37–44.

35 de Kruijk JR, Leffers P, Meerhoff S, Rutten J, Twijnstra A. Effectiveness of bed rest after mild traumatic brain injury: a randomised trial of no versus six days of bed rest. *J Neurol Neurosurg Psychiatry* 2002;**73**(2):167–72.

36 McCrory P, Johnston K, Meeuwisse W, et al. Summary and agreement statement of the 2nd International Conference on Concussion in Sport, Prague 2004. *Br J Sports Med* 2005;**39**(4):196–204.

37 Van Kampen DA, Lovell MR, Pardini JE, Collins MW, Fu FH. The "value added" of neurocognitive testing after sports-related concussion. *Am J Sports Med* 2006;**34**(10):1630–35.

38 Ponsford J, Willmott C, Rothwell A, et al. Factors influencing outcome following mild traumatic brain injury in adults. *J Int Neuropsychol Soc* 2000;**6**(5):568–79.

39 Meares S, Shores EA, Batchelor J, et al. The relationship of psychological and cognitive factors and opioids in the development of the postconcussion syndrome in general trauma patients with mild traumatic brain injury. *J Int Neuropsychol Soc* 2006;**12**(6):792–801.

40 Bazarian JJ, Wong T, Harris M, Leahey N, Mookerjee S, Dombovy M. Epidemiology and predictors of post-concussive syndrome after minor head injury in an emergency population. *Brain Injury* 1999;**13**(3):173–89.

41 Savola O, Hillbom M. Early predictors of post-concussion symptoms in patients with mild head injury. *Eur J Neurol* 2003;**10**(2):175–81.

42 Ingebrigtsen T, Romner B, Kongstad P, Langbakk B. Increased serum concentrations of protein S-100 after minor head injury: a biochemical serum marker with prognostic value? *J Neurol Neurosurg Psychiatry* 1995;**59**(1):103–4.

43 Townend WJ, Guy M, Pani M, Martin B, Yates D. Head injury outcome prediction in the emergency department: a role for protein S-100B? *J Neurol Neurosurg Psychiatry* 2002;**73**(5):542–6.

44 Farace E, Alves WM. Do women fare worse: a metaanalysis of gender differences in traumatic brain injury outcome. *J Neurosurg* 2000;**93**:539–45.

45 Ponsford J, Willmott C, Rothwell A, et al. Impact of early intervention on outcome after mild traumatic brain injury in children. *Pediatrics* 2001;**108**(6):1297–303.

46 Wade DT, King NS, Wenden FJ, Crawford S, Caldwell FE. Routine follow up after head injury: a second randomised controlled trial. *J Neurol Neurosurg Psychiatry* 1998;**65**(2):177–83.

30 Neck Injuries

Marcia L. Edmonds[1] & Robert Brison[2]

[1] Division of Emergency Medicine, University of Western Ontario, London, Canada
[2] Departments of Emergency Medicine *and* Community Health and Epidemiology, Queen's University, Kingston, Canada

Clinical scenario

A 45-year-old male is brought to the emergency department (ED) by ambulance following involvement in a motor vehicle crash. He had lost control of his vehicle when swerving to miss a deer. He went into a ditch and did not roll over; however, he crashed into a fence post which deployed the driver side air-bag. He was transferred by ambulance with full spinal precautions on a spine board with rigid cervical immobilization. He was fully alert and oriented, recalled all events and complained only of neck pain and discomfort from lying on the backboard. His vital signs were normal with a Glasgow Coma Score (GCS) of 15 and normal sensation and movement of all limbs.

The patient requested that the restraints holding him on the board and the cervical collar be removed. He was confident that he was fine. At the scene he had extricated himself from his seatbelt and was standing at the roadside at the time of police and emergency services' arrival.

Prior to removing cervical spine precautions, a portable lateral cervical spine radiograph was obtained. This showed no suggestion of fracture, edema or instability down to the C7/T1 juncture. Anterior and odontoid views were subsequently performed in the ED radiology suite. These were also normal. One hour after the patient's arrival in the ED he complained of increasing discomfort from the backboard. No significant injuries were detected on chest, abdominal or pelvic exam, and a screening neurological exam was also normal. All restraints and the collar were removed and a full physical examination conducted. The patient had tenderness and stiffness across both trapezius muscles and cervical paraspinal muscles but scant midline tenderness. Despite this, he was able to actively rotate his head 60° in each direction. Moreover, there was no significant tenderness on palpation of the thoracic and lumbar spine regions. He was much more comfortable once he could sit up and move around.

Evidence-based Emergency Medicine. Edited by Brian H. Rowe
© 2009 Blackwell Publishing, ISBN: 978-1-4051-6143-5.

Your resident asks whether the patient's spine could have been cleared clinically, saving the patient time and discomfort and saving hospital radiology and nursing costs. She also wonders what the expected progression of his neck symptoms will be and what arrangements should be made for follow-up.

Background

Managing patients with trauma to the neck and cervical spine (C-spine) is an important and frequent component of emergency medicine practice. More than 1 million cases of suspected neck injury are seen in US ED's annually, most of which are diagnosed as soft tissue injuries [1]. A small proportion of these patients have clear risks for serious C-spine injury associated with neurological deficit or as a component of multiple traumas. Most patients seen in the ED for potential C-spine injury are alert, hemodynamically stable and are at low risk for fracture or ligamentous instability. Only 1–3% of these latter patients will be diagnosed with an unstable cervical injury or fracture [1,2]. Despite this, they are often brought to the ED in full spinal immobilization, often complaining of varying degrees of neck pain as well as discomfort from the spinal immobilization. A large proportion will undergo C-spine radiography as fears of missing a potentially devastating injury has lead to high use of radiography in these patients. Increasingly, special imaging has become the standard in many trauma centers, even for the most minor injury cases. Liberal use of radiographs and special imaging adds to health care costs and to the time that patients remain in the ED and restrained with C-spine precautions. Alert, stable trauma patients represent the majority of patients assessed for potential C-spine injury in the ED setting. It is also the group for which there is the greatest variation in patterns of ED practice to which current evidence can be applied. As such, this patient population will be the focus of this chapter. We will examine evidence for: (i) methods of clinical and radiological assessment for C-spine fracture and instability; and (ii) the management of stable soft tissue injuries of the neck and C-spine.

Clinical questions

1 In alert, stable patients presenting to the ED with possible cervical spine injury (population), what are the common mechanisms of injury (risk factors)? Is an understanding of the mechanism of injury (risk factors) helpful in predicting the risk of cervical spine fracture or instability (outcome)?

2 In alert, stable trauma patients (population), what is the sensitivity and specificity (diagnostic test characteristics) of the clinical examination (test) in detecting significant neck injuries (outcome)?

3 In alert, stable trauma patients (population), are there clinical decision rules (tests) that are adequately sensitive and specific (diagnostic test characteristics) to aid our decision making?

4 In alert, stable trauma patients (population), what plain film imaging tests (diagnostic tests) have sufficient sensitivity and specificity (diagnostic test characteristics) to detect the presence of clinically important cervical spine injury (outcome)?

5 In patients with no fracture identified on routine neck X-rays (population), are there clinical factors (historical features, symptoms, findings on physical exam) (tests) that are sufficiently sensitive and specific (diagnostic test characteristics) to indicate a need for further tests to exclude significant injuries (outcome)?

6 In trauma patients presenting to the ED with acute soft tissue injuries of the neck (population), what is the likelihood (prognosis) of developing a long-term pain syndrome of greater than 6 months (whiplash-associated disorder) (outcome)?

7 In ED patients presenting with acute soft tissue injuries of the neck (population), are there interventions (interventions) to prevent the development of long-term pain syndromes (outcomes) compared to routine follow-up in primary care (control)?

8 In patients with soft tissue injuries of the neck (population), what ED-based educational treatments (interventions) can reduce pain and improve quality of life (outcomes) compared to standard care (control)?

General search strategy

You begin to address these questions by searching for evidence in the common electronic databases such as the Cochrane Library, MEDLINE and EMBASE looking specifically for studies involving the diagnostic test characteristics of various imaging modalities for neck injuries or systematic reviews of those studies, as well as clinical prediction rules for patients with possible neck injuries. The Cochrane Library is a useful resource for questions regarding therapy of whiplash-associated disorder. When a systematic review is identified, we also searched for recent updates on the Cochrane Library and also searched MEDLINE and EMBASE to identify randomized controlled trials (RCTs) that became available after the publication date of the systematic review.

Searching for evidence synthesis: primary search strategy

- Cochrane Library: cervical spine fracture OR whiplash OR neck injury OR mechanical neck disorder
- MEDLINE and EMBASE: cervical vertebrae/injuries, radiography AND decision support technique AND spinal fractures (for decision rule questions)
- MEDLINE and EMBASE: cervical vertebrae/injuries, radiography AND sensitivity AND specificity (for diagnosis questions)
- MEDLINE and EMBASE: mechanical neck disorder AND review
- MEDLINE and EMBASE: whiplash AND (systematic review OR meta-analysis OR metaanalysis)
- MEDLINE and EMBASE: whiplash associated disorder AND prognosis

Question 1: In alert, stable patients presenting to the ED with possible cervical spine injury (population), what are the common mechanisms of injury (risk factors)? Is an understanding of the mechanism of injury (risk factors) helpful in predicting the risk of cervical spine fracture or instability (outcome)?

Search strategy

- MEDLINE and EMBASE: cervical vertebrae/injuries AND epidemiology AND risk factors

In the United States, more than 1.3 million cases of neck injury are seen in EDs every year. The prevalence of fracture or spinal cord injury in these patients is quite low (less than 3% in most series). In one study involving stable, alert trauma patients the proportion of fracture or spinal cord injury was 0.9% [1]. The most common mechanism of injury was motor vehicle crashes (70%). The range of collision forces described varied from those seen with simple rear-end collisions to those in a high-speed rollover. Other types of injuries included falls (approximately 10%), bicycle collisions (5%), assaults (5%) and collisions involving other motorized vehicles such as motorcycles (2%).

Certain injury patterns have been associated with specific mechanisms. For example, Jefferson's fracture (a burst fracture of C1) has been associated with an axial load to the head (such as occurs with a heavy load falling on the top of the head), and a Hangman's fracture (a bilateral pedicle fracture of C2) has been associated with forced hyper-extension of the head (such as the when the face forcibly strikes the dashboard) [3].

It has been previously noted that there is a higher incidence of C-spine fracture in association with severe head injury (about 10%) or severe facial injury [4]. Other significant predictors of spinal injury include increasing age, high energy cause (high speed car crash, fall) and the presence of focal neurological deficits [5]. A recent, large study further delineated factors associated with increased risk of fracture. Persons injured in a motor vehicle crash were at increased risk for fracture where there was a higher posted speed limit, vehicle rollover and failure to wear a seatbelt. Falls greater than 1 m were also associated with a higher risk of injury, with this risk increasing directly with the height of the fall. Simple rear-end crashes are associated with a very low risk for C-spine fracture [6].

In summary, patients with potential C-spine injury present commonly to the ED. However, fracture or ligamentous instability is uncommon. The most common mechanism of injury appears to be motor vehicle crashes (70%) followed remotely by falls. Knowledge of the injury mechanisms (and the fractures associated with some of these mechanisms) is an important consideration in the evaluation of these patients in the ED.

Question 2: In alert, stable trauma patients (population), what is the sensitivity and specificity (diagnostic test characteristics) of the clinical examination (test) in detecting significant neck injuries (outcome)?

Search strategy

- MEDLINE and EMBASE: cervical vertebrae/injuries, diagnosis AND clinical examination

Although the prevalence of C-spine fracture is low in alert, stable trauma patients, the consequences of missing an unstable spinal injury are potentially devastating. For this reason, any test used to rule out C-spine injury must have near 100% sensitivity to detect injuries to be a useful test in the ED [2].

The clinical examination has been studied for its ability to detect C-spine injury. In one study, the clinical examination (including a history of neck pain or neurological abnormality, GCS, presence of neurological deficits, presence of neck tenderness and range of motion of the neck) was found to have 91% sensitivity to detect C-spine injury with a specificity of 82.4% [7]. Another study found a similar specificity of 92.2% for unstructured physician judgment, although a lower specificity of 53.9% [8].

In the derivation of the Canadian C-spine Rule (CCR), the authors examined the inter-rater reliability of potential predictors of C-spine fracture in the clinical examination. The inter-rater reliability of several predictors was found to be quite variable ($\kappa > 0.6$ is considered good agreement, $\kappa = 0.4$–0.6 is moderate agreement) (Table 30.1).

In summary, physical examination is an important contributor to decisions. Although evidence demonstrates that some of the features of the clinical examination are reliably collected and sensitive in detecting significant injuries, none alone provides the high sensitivity (i.e., approximating 100%) needed to confidently rule out a C-spine injury. Question 3 examines the potential for combining this information to improve the sensitivity and specificity of diagnosis.

Table 30.1 Inter-rater reliability for predictors from the clinical examination [9].

Predictors	κ
Information from history	
Ambulatory at any time after injury	0.87
Midline posterior neck pain	0.69
Weakness in extremities	0.54
Posterolateral neck pain	0.45
Findings from physical examination	
Sitting position during examination	0.74
Distracting painful injuries	0.41
Unreliable finding due to drugs or alcohol	0.22
Neck tenderness midline	0.78
Able to actively flex neck	0.63

Question 3: In alert, stable trauma patients (population), are there clinical decision rules (tests) that are adequately sensitive and specific (diagnostic test characteristics) to aid our decision making?

Search strategy

- MEDLINE and EMBASE: cervical vertebrae/injuries AND decision support technique AND spinal fractures

A clinical decision rule is a decision-making tool that incorporates three or more variables from the history, clinical examination or simple tests that may be used to guide care of patients. A rule to aid assessment of low-risk trauma patients for potential C-spine injury would be useful as this is a common ED problem for which there is a wide variation in X-ray utilization rates between physicians and hospitals [1]. Most clinicians would consider a sensitivity approaching 100% to be of utmost importance in any rule evaluating patients with a potential C-spine injury, because of the risk of missing important injuries that may cause further morbidity if undetected. The specificity of a rule is also important, as a rule with near 100% sensitivity but low specificity (or a likelihood ratio (LR) approaching 1.0) would be expected to increase baseline radiography use with little opportunity to affect clinical decision making.

Two major decision rules for the detection of C-spine fracture in the ED have been developed and validated. The National Emergency X-ray Utilization Study (NEXUS) low-risk criteria were first described in 1992 and later validated in a large study of over 34,000 patients [2]. This study showed that patients presenting with potential C-spine injury, with a GCS of 13 or greater, did not need an X-ray if they met all of the five NEXUS criteria (Box 30.1).

In the initial validation study performed on the NEXUS low-risk criteria, which included 34,069 patients, 818 (2.4%) of whom had a C-spine injury, the sensitivity was found to be 99.0% (95% CI: 98.0% to 99.6%) and the specificity was 12.9% (95% CI: 12.8% to 13.0%) providing a positive LR of 1.14. Injuries were missed in only eight of 818 patients, and only two of these met the pre-set

---

Box 30.1. The NEXUS low-risk criteria.

- No posterior midline tenderness
- No evidence of intoxication
- A normal level of alertness
- No focal neurological deficit
- No painful distracting injuries

---

definition of a clinically significant injury (sensitivity for clinically significant injury = 99.6%; 95% CI: 98.6% to 100%) [2].

A second decision rule, the CCR, was subsequently developed and validated in a series of large Canadian cohort studies. Application of this rule involves three steps, as illustrated in Fig. 30.1). First, patients with three specified high-risk criteria are identified as requiring radiography. Second, patients with any of five low-risk criteria for injury are identified. Any patient not having at least one of these low-risk factors undergoes radiography. Third, patients with one of these five low-risk criteria are asked to actively rotate their neck. Those able to rotate 45° or more to both sides are cleared clinically, without the use of radiography [9].

In the study deriving the CCR, 8294 patients were assessed, of whom 151 (1.8%) had a clinically significant C-spine injury. The rule had 100% sensitivity (95% CI: 98% to 100%) and 42.5% specificity to identify these injuries [9]. In a subsequent validation study involving 8283 new patients, 169 (2.0%) of whom had a C-spine injury, the rule had 99.4% sensitivity and 40.4% specificity [10], providing a positive LR of 1.67. Combining these two studies, for a total of 16,363 patients, resulted in an overall sensitivity of 99.7% (95% CI: 98% to 100%) for the CCR.

The CCR and NEXUS were compared in a large validation study for the CCR by the study group that developed the CCR [10]. In this lower risk population (including stable, alert patients >16 years of age with acute trauma to the head or neck), the CCR performed better than NEXUS. This study included 8283 patients, 169 (2%) of whom had a clinically important injury; the CCR was both more sensitive (99.4% vs 90.7%, $P < 0.001$) and more specific than the NEXUS (45.1% vs 36.8%, $P < 0.001$). Positive LRs from this study were 1.81 and 1.44 for the CCR and NEXUS, respectively. This is an improved though still lower LR for the NEXUS rule in this lower risk population. Further, there was higher inter-observer agreement between clinicians applying the rules on the interpretation of both the individual components and the overall rule for the CCR than for the NEXUS. There were more cases where the CCR was indeterminate, however, due to physician reluctance to evaluate the range of motion of the neck in patients with low-risk criteria.

In summary, useful tools are available to assist clinicians in decisions on the need for radiology in patients with potential cervical spine injury. Overall, the CCR was superior to the NEXUS in most diagnostic test characteristics reported, and would lead to a lower proportion of patients requiring radiography with fewer missed injuries. The NEXUS may be useful to aid imaging decisions

in certain populations, including pediatric patients and more seriously injured patients both of whom were excluded from the CCR.

Question 4: In alert, stable trauma patients (population), what plain film imaging tests (diagnostic tests) have sufficient sensitivity and specificity (diagnostic test characteristics) to detect the presence of clinically important cervical spine injury (outcome)?

Search strategy

- MEDLINE and EMBASE: cervical vertebrae/injuries, radiography AND sensitivity and specificity

---

Traditional teaching and the current advanced trauma life support (ATLS) guidelines [11], recommend that the initial investigation for trauma patients should be a cross-table lateral view of the C-spine in the trauma room. If the patient is stable, this should be later supplemented with an anteroposterior (AP) and open-mouth odontoid view. It is frequently difficult to visualize the lower C-spine on the lateral view; a swimmer's view may be preformed to better visualize the lower C-spine in these patients. Early studies showed that these three views of the C-spine had >80% sensitivity and 97% specificity to detect fractures [12]. Adding extra views of the C-spine has been suggested to improve the ability to detect fractures; however, the results have been disappointing. The use of oblique views, which were proposed to help improve visualization of the lower C-spine and posterior elements, did not improve fracture detection, and in one study there was a suggestion of more X-ray interpretation errors with oblique films [13,14]. Similarly, the addition of flexion/extension views, proposed to increase detection of fractures or ligamentous instability, did not show any added benefit when three views of the C-spine were normal, did not detect important injuries that were missed on plain films, and did not provide further information that was not seen on helical computerized tomography (CT) [15–17].

Recent studies of patients at high risk for C-spine injury have suggested that the sensitivity of plain films to detect fracture is inadequate. Two studies demonstrate sensitivity as low as 32% to detect fractures [18,19]. A recent meta-analysis found a pooled sensitivity of only 52% for plain X-rays versus 98% for CT [20]; however, there appeared to be heterogeneity between the studies for the accuracy of plain X-rays ($P = 0.07$). The high-risk patients included in many of the studies in this meta-analysis were quite different from the low-risk, alert, stable trauma patient of prime interest to this discussion. In the more difficult trauma scenario studies, plain X-rays were often technically inadequate. Also, some of the fractures detected by CT would be considered clinically insignificant (it cannot be ascertained what the sensitivity for clinically significant fractures would be). Despite these reservations with the meta-analysis, this low sensitivity is concerning and has led several recent authors to suggest that CT should be the

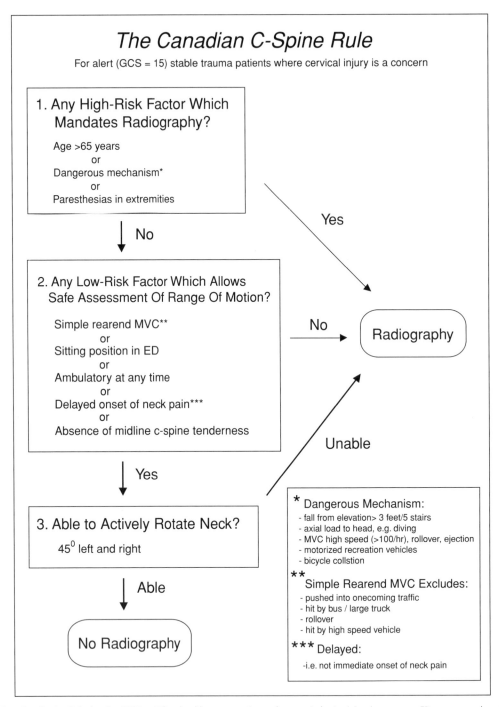

Figure 30.1 The Canadian C-spine Rule, for alert (GCS = 15) and stable trauma patients where cervical spine injury is a concern. ED, emergency department; MVC, motor vehicle collision. (Reproduced with permission, © 2001 *Journal of the American Medical Association.*)

initial imaging test for high-risk patients. Issues with CT including availability, cost and increased radiation exposure may limit its usefulness in low-risk patients [21].

Overall, these recent studies of high-risk populations provide little direction on how to best image a patient with a low risk of injury such as the one in the initial case. In an analysis of the patients included in the NEXUS study, when adequate three-view plain film X-rays were performed, the sensitivity of plain films was 89.4% and, more importantly, the negative predictive value was 99.9% in this relatively low-risk population [22]. Further studies to delineate the most appropriate imaging test in low-risk patients requiring imaging are needed.

Question 5: In patients with no fracture identified on routine neck X-rays (population), are there clinical factors (historical features, symptoms, findings on physical exam) (tests) that are sufficiently sensitive and specific (diagnostic test characteristics) to indicate a need for further tests to exclude significant injuries (outcome)?

Search strategy

- MEDLINE and EMBASE: cervical vertebrae/injuries AND radiography AND tomography, x-ray computed

Although the negative predictive value of a normal three-view C-spine series was 99.9% in the low-risk population included in the NEXUS study, there is some risk of missing significant neck fractures with the low sensitivity of plain X-rays. In the meta-analysis comparing CT and plain X-rays, CT was shown to be clearly superior to X-rays with a sensitivity of 98% [20]. However, using a CT scan as the initial investigation in all trauma patients undergoing cervical spine radiography is not a practical option; not only is there limited availability and a higher cost than with plain X-rays, but it exposes patients to a significantly higher dose of radiation [23].

There have been several retrospective studies to examine which patients are at higher risk of fracture and should undergo initial imaging with CT instead of or in addition to plain films. The presence of severe head injury, a high energy mechanism and focal neurological deficits, as well as being older than 50 years, are all potential useful predictors of the presence of C-spine fracture. No prospective studies or large validation studies, however, are available to guide our initial choice of imaging. Moreover, these studies have not specifically examined a low-risk population to determine if there are certain features in otherwise low-risk patients that would indicate a need for CT [5,24]. One cost-effectiveness study showed that screening with CT as the initial test for high- and moderate-risk trauma patients was cost-effective; however, more evidence is needed to clearly define the appropriate population for this strategy [25].

Even with a CT scan that is negative for fracture, there is a potential risk of missing ligamentous injury that could still lead to instability of the C-spine and the potential for delayed injury. Magnetic resonance imaging (MRI) has been shown to be more sensitive for detecting soft tissue injury than CT scans, and some have proposed that it may be needed in addition to CT in some patients. However, in one large, prospective study, it was found that even in severely injured patients with a low GCS, MRI did not diagnose any significant, unstable injuries in patients with normal CT results and a normal motor examination [26].

In summary, until new research is published, the current ED approach of using plain films followed by judicious use of CT or MRI to diagnose cervical pathology is the approach of choice in low-risk patients when images of the cervical spine are required.

Question 6: In trauma patients presenting to the ED with acute soft tissue injuries of the neck (population), what is the likelihood (prognosis) of developing a long-term pain syndrome of greater than 6 months (whiplash-associated disorder) (outcome)?

Search strategy

- Cochrane Library: Cervical Overview Group reviews
- MEDLINE and EMBASE: (mechanical neck disorder OR whiplash injuries OR whiplash associated disorder) AND prognosis

What happens to that vast majority of ED patients with cervical injury where a fracture is ruled out? Do they get better? How long does it take? A Cochrane review [27] suggests that that most estimates of the incidence of long-term pain syndromes lie between 20% and 40%. One ED-based study that enrolled all patients involved in rear-end motor vehicle crashes showed that 60% of patients developed moderate or severe pain in the first week post injury with this decreasing to approximately 50% and 40% at 1 and 2 months, respectively [28]. Overall, 37% of all patients continued to have moderate or severe pain at 3 months, with this proportion changing little at 6, 12 and 24 months.

In summary, even when patients do not suffer a clinically important fracture or dislocation, they may remain symptomatic for many weeks and months following injury.

Question 7: In ED patients presenting with acute soft tissue injuries of the neck (population), are there interventions (interventions) to prevent the development of long-term pain syndromes (outcomes) compared to routine follow-up in primary care (control)?

Search strategy

- Cochrane Library: Cervical Overview Group reviews
- MEDLINE and EMBASE: (mechanical neck disorder OR whiplash OR whiplash associated disorder) AND randomized controlled trial

Given that such a high proportion of patients with these injuries have short-term and long-term pain syndromes, provision of effective treatments in the acute care setting to reduce the symptoms and improve quality of life are important. While there are many studies assessing treatment of chronic neck pain, there are few that assess the utility of interventions provided to patients at or near the time of injury.

Evidence based on RCTs, and reported in two systematic reviews [29,30], exists to support the use of a multi-modal physical therapy approach for the early active mobilization of the neck to reduce pain in the short term as well as reducing the likelihood of developing long-term whiplash-associated disorders. These include use of postural, mobilization, stretching and strengthening exercises.

Gross et al. [30] report strong evidence of benefit for sustained reduction of pain and improvement in function for exercise plus mobilization/manipulation versus control in subjects with sub-acute/chronic mechanical neck disorders. Moderate benefit was found for neck stretching and strengthening exercises for chronic mechanical neck disorders. These are interventions that can be provided in the ED setting or through physical therapy follow-up.

The Cochrane Cervical Overview Group's systematic reviews found limited evidence to support the use of massage therapy [31] and no trials of the use of acupuncture [32] in the acute care of these patients. There was also no evidence to support the use of non-steroidal anti-inflammatory drugs (NSAIDs) over alternate analgesics in either the management of acute pain or the prevention of chronic pain [33]. While the recommendation of cryotherapy in the acute phase of any soft tissue injury is common practice, there is no RCT assessing for this benefit in patients with soft tissue injury to the neck. It does seem logical to use ice and avoid heat in the initial 2–3 days of wound healing.

In summary, many treatment options exist for emergency physicians when dealing with patients who have non-fracture, soft tissue injuries of the neck. It would appear that physical therapy is most effective; however, how this should be delivered and by whom remains unclear.

Question 8: In patients with soft tissue injuries of the neck (population), what ED-based educational treatments (interventions) can reduce pain and improve quality of life (outcomes) compared to standard care (control)?

Search strategy

- Cochrane Library: Cervical Overview Group reviews
- MEDLINE and EMBASE: (mechanical neck disorder OR whiplash OR whiplash associated disorder) AND patient education AND RCTs

Emergency department physicians and staff have limited time to teach patients exercises and explain the likely prognosis for their recovery in this or any other condition. Consequently, the possibility of having this provided by alternative methods has been the subject of clinical research. From the above search, three published RCTs were found and another is in progress [34–37].

There are two single-site RCTs where ED patients were asked to view educational videos that provided information describing the soft tissue injury pattern, the expected progression of symptoms and techniques for management of pain. Pain management included advice on the appropriate progression in use of cryotherapy, heat, analgesics, activity, specific postural, mobilization and strengthening exercises, and relaxation techniques. Each showed evidence of benefit in terms of decrease in pain and improved function [34,35]. Oliveira et al. demonstrated markedly reduced use of physician, physiotherapy and chiropractic services by patients who were provided with the educational video compared

with those receiving usual care [35]. This effect persisted for the 6-month follow-up period of that study.

In another study comparing different educational methods (generic vs specific evidence-based neck pamphlet) for patients with neck pain following injury, researchers were unable to demonstrate similar benefits [36]. For example, the rate of whiplash-associated disorder symptoms was no different between the two groups; however, the opening of a litigation claim was higher in the patient group receiving the specific evidence-based neck pamphlet. Overall, the authors concluded that written educational material provided to patients has yet to be proven effective in this setting. Finally, a large, cluster RCT is currently underway in the UK, where multiple interventions are being tested, including the *Back Book* [37,38].

In summary, there is clear evidence that early and active mobilization of the neck is useful in controlling short- and long-term symptoms in mechanical neck disorders and that there is a role for providing this information in the ED setting. Emergency physicians should either provide patients with some instruction on exercise therapies for management of these disorders or make referral for early follow-up with a physical therapist.

Conclusions

On reflection, we had to admit to our resident that the evidence would support an initial examination of our patient that would have negated the need for radiographs. Using our preferred decision rule, the CCR, there was no defined dangerous mechanism or clinical symptom that would indicate a need for radiography. Furthermore, the patient was ambulatory at the scene thus meeting a low-risk criterion, and able to rotate his neck 45° or more in each direction. If we had applied the CCR, we would have had the opportunity to remove restraints at the time of assessment, and saved our patient the discomfort of prolonged confinement and our department, the costs of radiography, and staff time in caring for this patient. Moreover, his contribution to our ED's overcrowding would have been reduced. Time saved would have been better spent discussing with this patient the nature of his soft tissue injury, including the importance of early and active range-of-motion and postural exercises in limiting the severity and duration of his pain. We also recognized that if we used this rule more often we might argue more effectively for the purchase of a DVD player for patient viewing of an educational video that would more efficiently provide the patient with information that would further support his or her efforts in recovery.

In summary, potential cervical spine injury is a common presentation to the ED setting. The use of clinical decision rules such as the CCR would safely reduce practice variation in the ED, reduce radiography ordering, reduce time to C-spine clearance and be cost-effective. In the setting of confirmed fracture or ligamentous instability, referral to the local spine service and/or admission is appropriate. In the absence of fracture or ligamentous injury, patients should be offered analgesia (physician preference), encouraged to mobilize the neck (and not wear a brace) and either be provided with patient education on how to manage their injury and avoid whiplash-associated disorder or be sent to a professional who can do this for them.

Acknowledgments

The authors would like to thank Shauna-Lee Konrad BA, BEd, MLIS, for her assistance with literature searching.

References

1 Stiell IG, Wells GA, Vandemheen K, et al. Variation in emergency department use of cervical spine radiography for alert, stable trauma patients. *Can Med Assoc J* 1997;**156**:1537–44.

2 Hoffman JR, Mower WR, Wolfson AB, Todd KH, Zucker MI. Validity of a set of clinical criteria to rule out injury to the cervical spine in patients with blunt trauma. *N Engl J Med* 2000;**343**:94–9.

3 Mirvis SE, Young JW, Lim C, Greenberg J. Hangman's fracture: radiologic assessment in 27 cases. *Radiology* 1987;**163**(3):713–17.

4 Crim JR, Moore K, Brodke D. Clearance of the cervical spine in multitrauma patients: the role of advanced imaging. *Semin Ultrasound CT MR* 2001;**22**(4):283–305.

5 Blackmore CC, Emerson SS, Mann FA, Koepsell RD. Cervical spine imaging in patients with trauma: determination of fracture risk to optimize use. *Radiology* 1999;**211**:759–65.

6 Thompson WL, Stiell IG, Clement C, Wells G, Brison RJ, for the Canadian C-Spine Rule Study Group. Association of injury mechanism with the risk of cervical spine fractures. *Can J Emerg Med* 2007 (submitted).

7 Gonzalez RP, Fried PO, Bukhalo M, Holevar MR, Falimirski ME. Role of clinical examination in screening for blunt cervical spine injury. *J Am Coll Surg* 1999;**189**:152–7.

8 Bandiera G, Stiell IG, Wells GA, et al., Canadian C-Spine and CT Head Study Group. The Canadian C-spine rule performs better than unstructured physician judgment. *Ann Emerg Med* 2003;**42**(3):395–402.

9 Stiell IG, Wells GA, Vandemheen KL, et al. The Canadian c-spine rule for radiography in alert and stable trauma patients. *JAMA* 2001;**286**:1841–8.

10 Stiell IG, Clement CM, McKnight RD, et al. The Canadian c-spine rule versus the NEXUS low-risk criteria in patients with trauma. *N Engl J Med* 2003;**349**:2510–18.

11 American College of Surgeons. *Advanced Trauma Life Support Manual*, 7th edn. American College of Surgeons, Chicago, 2005.

12 Macdonald RL, Schwartz ML, Mirich D, Sharkey PW, Nelson WR. Diagnosis of cervical spine injury in motor vehicle crash victims; how many x-rays are enough? *J Trauma* 1990;**30**:392–7.

13 Offerman SR, Holmes JF, Katzberg RX, Richards JR. Utility of supine oblique radiographs in detecting cervical spine injury. *J Emerg Med* 2006;**30**:189–95.

14 Ralston ME, Ecklund K, Emans JV, Torrey SB, Bailey MC, Schutzman SA. Role of oblique radiographs in blunt pediatric cervical spine injury. *Pediatr Emerg Care* 2003;**19**:68–72.

15 Brady WJ, Moghtader J, Cutcher D, Exline C, Young J. ED use of flexion-extension radiography in the evaluation of blunt trauma. *Am J Emerg Med* 1999;**17**:504–8.

16 Pollack CV, Henday GW, Martin DR, Hoffman JR, Mower WR. Use of flexion-extension radiographs of the cervical spine in blunt trauma. *Ann Emerg Med* 2001;**38**:8–11.

17 Spiteri V, Kotnis R, Singh P, et al. Cervical dynamic screening in spinal clearance; now redundant. *J Trauma* 2006;**61**:1171–7.

18 Gale S, Gracias VH, Reilly PM, Schwab CW. The inefficiency of plain radiography to evaluate the cervical spine after blunt trauma. *J Trauma* 2005;**59**:1121–5.

19 McCulloch PT, France J, Jones DL, et al. Helical computed tomography alone compared with plain radiographs with adjunct computer tomography to evaluate the cervical spine after high-energy trauma. *J Bone Joint Surg Am* 2005;**84**:2388–94.

20 Holmes JF, Akkinepalli R. Computed tomography versus plain radiography to screen for cervical spine injury; a meta-analysis. *J Trauma* 2005;**58**:901–5.

21 Nunez DB, Quencer RM. The role of helical CT in the assessment of cervical spine injuries. *Am J Radiol* 1998;**171**:951–7.

22 Mower WR, Hoffman JR, Pollack CV, Zucker MI, Browne BJ, Wolfson AB. Use of plain radiography to screen for cervical spine injuries. *Ann Emerg Med* 2001;**38**:1–7.

23 Rybicki F, Nawfel RD, Judy PF, et al. Skin and thyroid dosimetry in cervical spine screening: two methods for evaluation and a comparison between a helical CT and radiographic trauma series. *Am J Radiol* 2002;**179**:933–7.

24 Hanson JA, Blackmore CC, Mann FA, Wilson AJ. Cervical spine injury: a clinical decision rule to identify high-risk patients for helical CT screening. *Am J Radiol* 2000;**174**:713–17.

25 Blackmore CC, Ramsey SD, Mann FA, Deyo RA. Cervical spine screening with CT in trauma patients: a cost-effectiveness analysis. *Radiology* 1999;**212**:117–25.

26 Schuster R, Waxman K, Sanchez B, et al. Magnetic resonance imaging is not needed to clear cervical spines in blunt trauma patients with normal computed tomographic results and no motor deficits. *Arch Surg* 2005;**140**:762–6.

27 Verhagen AP, Scholten-Peeters GGM, de Bie RA, Bierma-Zeinstra SMA. Conservative treatments for whiplash. *Cochrane Database Syst Rev* 2004;**1**:CD003338 (doi: 10.1002/14651858.CD003338.pub2).

28 Brison RJ, Hartling L, Pickett W. Prospective study of neck injuries following rear-end motor vehicle collisions. *J Musculoskeletal Pain* 2000;**8**(1–2):97–113.

29 Kay TM, Gross A, Goldsmith C, Santaguida PL, Hoving J, Bronfort G, Cervical Overview Group. Exercises for mechanical neck disorders. *Cochrane Database Syst Rev* 2005;**3**:CD004250 (doi: 10.1002/14651858.CD004250.pub3).

30 Gross AR, Goldsmith C, Hoving JL, et al., Cervical Overview Group. Conservative management of mechanical neck disorders: a systematic review. *J Rheumatol* 2007;**34**(5):1083–102.

31 Haraldsson BG, Gross AR, Myers CD, et al., Cervical Overview Group. Massage for mechanical neck disorders. *Cochrane Database Syst Rev* 2006;**3**:CD004871 (doi: 10.1002/14651858.CD004871.pub3).

32 Trinh KV, Graham N, Gross AR, et al., Cervical Overview Group. Acupuncture for neck disorders. *Cochrane Database Syst Rev* 2006;**3**:CD004870 (doi: 10.1002/14651858.CD004870.pub3).

33 Peloso P, Gross A, Haines T, Trinh K, Goldsmith CH, Aker P, Cervical Overview Group. Medicinal and injection therapies for mechanical neck disorders. *Cochrane Database Syst Rev* 2004;**2**:CD000319 (doi: 10.1002/14651858.CD000319.pub3).

34 Brison RJ, Hartling L, Dostaler S, et al. A randomized controlled trial of an educational intervention to prevent the chronic pain of whiplash

associated disorders following rear-end motor vehicle collisions. *Spine* 2005;**30**(16):1799–807.

35 Oliveira A, Gevirtz R, Hubbard D. A psycho-educational video used in the emergency department provides effective treatment for whiplash injuries. *Spine* 2006;**31**(15):1652–7.

36 Ferrari R, Rowe BH, Majumdar SR, et al. Simple educational intervention to improve the recovery from acute whiplash: results of a randomized, controlled trial. *Acad Emerg Med* 2005:**12**(8):699–706.

37 Lamb SE, Gates S, Underwood MR, et al., MINT Study Team. Managing Injuries of the Neck Trial (MINT): design of a randomised controlled trial of treatments for whiplash associated disorders. *BMC Musculoskeletal Disord* 2007;**8**(7):12.

38 Royal College of General Practitioners, NHS Executive. *The Back Book: The best way to deal with back pain; get back active*, 2nd edn. HMSO, London, 2002.

31 Ankle Injuries

Jerome Fan

Department of Emergency Medicine, McMaster University, Hamilton, Canada

Clinical scenario

A 23-year-old male university student with a previous history of several "ankle sprains" suffered an inversion injury while playing basketball on an indoor surface. He was unable to immediately weight bear and presents 2 hours later to the emergency department (ED) with a grossly swollen right ankle; however, he could place weight on his heel if pushed. He requested an "X-ray" of his ankle to make sure he hadn't broken it and a cast to protect his joint in the icy weather. He also wanted to know if there was anything else he should be doing to improve his healing from this injury and whether there was something that can be done for his pain and swelling. Finally, before he left, he wanted to know if there was any way he could prevent this from happening in the future.

Background

Ankle injuries are one of the most common musculoskeletal complaints that EDs in developed countries treat on an annual basis. It is estimated that 5–10 million ankle injuries occur in the United States per year [1]. The estimated annual cost of managing ankle injuries is in the range of $2 billion [1]. Similar statistics can be found in the United Kingdom where it is estimated that one ankle injury occurs per 10,000 population per day; costing 40 million Euro annually per 1 million population [2,3]. The prevalence of fractures in patients presenting to an ED with a traumatic ankle complaint is less than 15%, suggesting that the large majority of these injuries are sprains [4–8]. Given medico-legal concerns, missing an ankle fracture may result in significant morbidity for patients as well as medico-legal ramifications for physicians.

For a clinician practicing emergency medicine, missing a fracture is not an acceptable option. Consequently, most patients receive an ankle and/or foot radiograph when presenting with this complaint. There are a number of reasons why this may be

problematic. First, using the numbers cited above, the majority of patients are subjected to needless radiation from this practice. Second, radiographs delay departure and contribute to ED overcrowding and patient dissatisfaction. Finally, the cost of frequent use of low-cost investigation can be enormous. For example, the cost of ankle radiography per year to the US and Canadian health care systems may be as much as $500 million [9]. Therefore, despite the lackluster interest in this topic, it actually has an enormous impact on health care economics and judicious use of radiography is important.

In addition to ruling out fractures, emergency medicine consultants must also be knowledgeable in the management of the more prevalent injury, the ankle sprain. This injury accounts for 2–6% of all those seeking treatment in an ED [10]. These sprains are most commonly isolated over the lateral ligamentous complex and rarely involve only the medial deltoid ligament. The Leach classification (Table 31.1) is commonly used to grade the severity of lateral ankle sprains [11]. Despite the number of these injuries, there is impressive practice variation with respect to the management of this problem, suggesting a lack of evidence-based guidelines. Clinicians have prescribed anti-inflammatory drugs, cryotherapy, ultrasound, functional treatments, physiotherapy, cast immobilization and even surgery for ankle sprains [12–14].

The purpose of this chapter is twofold. First, it will provide readers with evidence-based guidelines to help decide when to order X-rays in ankle-injured patients in a manner that is clinically safe and cost-effective. Second, it will provide the latest evidence-based methods of treating acute ankle sprains and chronic ankle instability and ways to prevent future re-injury.

Clinical questions

1 In patients with ankle injuries seen in the ED (population), are there clinical criteria (measurements) that can define a patient's probability of sustaining a fracture (outcome)?

2 In patients with ankle injuries seen in the ED (population), are there valid and reliable clinical tools (clinical prediction guides)

Evidence-based Emergency Medicine. Edited by Brian H. Rowe
© 2009 Blackwell Publishing, ISBN: 978-1-4051-6143-5.

Table 31.1 Leach classification of lateral ankle sprains. (Reproduced with permission from Dalton & Schweinle [11].)

Injury grade	Functional grade	Anatomic injury	Laxity tests	Recovery (weeks)
I	Stable	Partial tear ATF, intact CFL	−ADT −TTT	1–3
II	Stable	Complete tear ATF, ± partial tear CFL	+ADT −TTT	2–6
III	Unstable	Complete tear ATF, complete tear CFL	+ADT +TTT	4–30

ADT, anterior drawer test; ATF, anterior talofibular; CFL, calcaneofibular ligament; TTT, telar tilt test.

that are sufficiently powerful to assist in the diagnosis of an ankle fracture (outcome)?

3 In patients with ankle injuries seen in the ED (population), does the decision to order an X-ray (intervention) improve patient satisfaction (outcome) compared to not having a radiograph ordered (control)?

4 In patients with ankle injuries seen in the ED (population), is the clinical decision rule (intervention) cost-effective (outcome) compared to physicians' experience (control)?

5 In ED patients with a negative radiograph or decision rule (population), does cast immobilization (intervention) shorten time to return to work/sport, reduce pain and reduce instability (outcomes) compared to functional care (control)?

6 In ED patients with a negative radiograph or decision rule (population), does any specific functional ankle support (intervention) shorten time to return to work/sport, reduce pain and reduce instability (outcomes) compared to other alternative functional ankle support strategies (control)?

7 In ED patients with a negative radiograph or decision rule (population), does physiotherapy (intervention) improve healing, reduce pain and stiffness and prevent further sprains (outcomes) compared to no physiotherapy (control)?

8 For ED patients with an ankle sprain (population), does external ankle support (intervention) prevent further sprains (outcome) compared to no support (control)?

9 In patients with chronic ankle instability who present to the ED with further ankle sprains (population), does surgery (intervention) prevent further injuries (outcome) compared to routine care (control)?

Critical review of the literature

Question 1: In patients with ankle injuries seen in the ED (population), are there clinical criteria (measurements) that can define a patient's probability of sustaining a fracture (outcome)?

Search strategy

- OVID MEDLINE: (reproducibility of results/ OR reliability.mp) AND (ankle.mp OR ankle injuries/ OR ankle/) AND (physical exam$.mp OR physical examination/)

The reliability of the physical exam for ankle-injured patients has been studied in three papers. The first paper described a prospective cohort study using a convenience sample of patients with an acute blunt injury to the ankle [15]. This study measured the inter-observer physician reliability of 22 physical findings using a standardized data collection form. The physicians came from a pool of 21 individuals, where each patient was examined by a single random pair of physicians, each blinded to the other's assessment [15]. The second and third papers were clinical studies employed in the derivation and validation of the Ottawa Ankle Rules. Both these studies used similar methods to the first in determining the inter-observer reliability of the clinical findings [16–18].

From these studies, the only findings that were reliable (kappa, $\kappa \geq 0.6$) and were significantly associated with ankle fractures were the following: inability to bear weight both immediately and in the ED (OR = 9.3; 95% CI: 5.1 to 17.1), swelling of the lateral malleolus within the first 6 hours (OR = 8.3; 95% CI: 4.2 to 16.5), bone tenderness of the inferior tip (OR = 2.5; 95% CI: 1.5 to 4.2) or posterior edge of the lateral malleolus (OR = 6.2; 95% CI: 3.6 to 10.6), and bone tenderness of the inferior tip (OR = 4.2; 95% CI: 2.5 to 7.2) or posterior edge of the medial malleolus (OR = 9.9; 95% CI: 5.4 to 18.2). For the foot, findings that were reliable ($\kappa \geq 0.5$) and were significantly associated with foot fractures were the following: bony tenderness at the base of the fifth metatarsal (OR = 29.3; 95% CI: 6.8 to 126.5) or any bony tenderness at the base of the fifth metatarsal, cuboid or navicular (OR = 21.8; 95% CI: 1.3 to 362.8).

In summary, the evidence suggests there are certain clinical findings that are both reliable and predictive for ankle and/or foot fractures for patients presenting with blunt ankle/foot injuries. We shall see in the next section how these findings can be combined in an effective manner to produce a guideline that best rules out the need for radiography.

Question 2: In patients with ankle injuries seen in the ED (population), are there valid and reliable clinical tools (clinical prediction guides) that are sufficiently powerful to assist in the diagnosis of an ankle fracture (outcome)?

Search strategy

- OVID: (exp decision support techniques/ OR exp decision support systems, clinical/ OR exp decision making/ OR decision support.mp OR clinical decision rule$.mp OR clinical decision support.mp OR decision rule$.mp) AND (ankle injuries/ OR ankle/ OR foot/ OR foot injuries/ OR ankle.mp OR foot.mp)

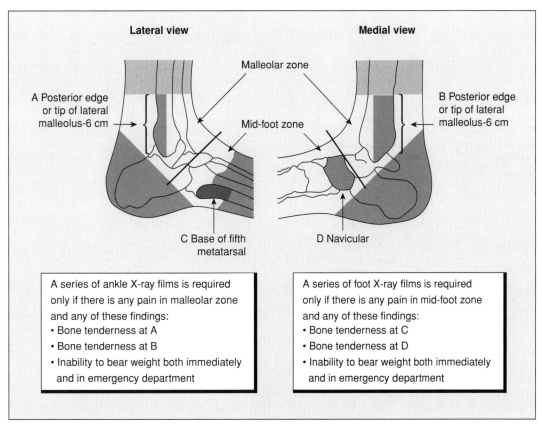

Figure 31.1 Ottawa Ankle Rule. (Reproduced with permission from Stiell et al. [33], courtesy of the *Journal of the American Medical Association.*)

Prior to 1992, there was a paucity of guidelines to assist physicians on when to order X-rays for patients with acute ankle injuries. Since then, rigorous methods for creating clinical decision rules have been developed. They include determining the reliability of clinical findings (developing factors), deriving a rule to maximize the fracture detection rate (derivation phase), prospectively testing the rule to ensure validity (validation phase) and implementing the rule in a setting outside the immediate development sites (implementation phase). Using these methods in multi-center fashion, the Ottawa Ankle Rule (OAR) (Fig. 31.1) was developed [16–18]. Subsequent to this, numerous validation and implementation trials have been performed independently by researchers around the globe. A systematic review of these studies was performed to summarize the diagnostic test characteristics of the OAR [19]. The sensitivity, specificity and negative likelihood ratios were 97.6% (95% CI: 96.4% to 98.9%), 31.5% (inter-quartile range (IQR): 23.8% to 44.4%) and 0.10 (95% CI: 0.06 to 0.16), respectively. These characteristics were consistent across site of injury (ankle vs foot), children versus adults, and ≤ 48 hours versus >48 hrs at initial assessment. There was some evidence that suggested that if the prevalence of fractures was >3.74% (IQR: 1.73% to 8.26%), the ability of this clinical decision rule to rule out fractures was slightly poorer, as shown by a negative likelihood ratio of 0.22 (95% CI: 0.10 to 0.51). The study also concluded that despite its

working well in children, there were only seven studies and the OAR accuracies must be viewed with caution [19].

Subsequent to the publication of this systematic review, a Netherland study compared the diagnostic accuracy between the OAR and two other locally derived clinical decision rules (named the Utrecht and Leiden rules) for detecting fractures. The authors found that the OAR had the greatest sensitivity (98%; 95% CI: 87% to 100%) compared to the Utrecht (59%; 95% CI: 42% to 74%) and Leiden (88%; 95% CI: 74% to 96%) rules. However, the area under the receiver operating curve (ROC) (area under curve, AUC) for the OAR (0.76; 95% CI: 0.69 to 0.84) was significantly less than for the two local rules: Utrecht, 0.83 (95% CI: 0.76 to 0.89) and Leiden, 0.84 (95% CI: 0.78 to 0.90). Overall, this study demonstrates that the OAR has the best ability to detect all clinically significant fractures; however, its ability to discriminate between those with and without fractures is less than these two other clinically decision rules. Since the identification of a fracture is more important (sensitivity) than reducing radiographic utilization (specificity), the OAR appears more clinically useful [20].

Interestingly, the same authors, using the same data from the above study, compared the performance of the OAR with physician judgment after using a structured data collection form (Fig. 31.2). They found that the sensitivity of detecting *all* fractures (including clinically insignificant ones) with physician judgment (82%;

Ankle Injury Data Collection Form

Patient information, such as ID number, sex and age

Inspection

	Yes	No
Unable to bear weight (4 steps)	☐	☐
Deformity	☐	☐
Hematoma	☐	☐
Pallor	☐	☐
Swollen medial or lateral metatarsal	☐	☐
Swollen fifth metatarsal	☐	☐
Swollen Achilles tendon	☐	☐
Traffic accident	☐	☐

Examination

	Yes	No
Pain on palpation lateral malleolus	☐	☐
Pain on palpation medial malleolus	☐	☐
Pain on palpation base/fifth metatarsal	☐	☐
Pain on palpation navicular bone	☐	☐
Pain on palpation Achilles tendon	☐	☐
Pulseless posterior tibal artery	☐	☐
Instability	☐	☐
Crepitation	☐	☐
Pain on axial compression	☐	☐

What do you think is the probability of ankle fracture in this patient after considering the information from the history and physical examination

☐ 0 1 5 10 20 30 40 50 60 70 80 90 95 99 100 ☐

Do you want to send this patient for radiographic examination? Yes ☐ No ☐

Name of physician: ____________________

Function: ____________________

Figure 31.2 Structured data collection form. (From Glas et al. [21].)

95% CI: 72% to 90%) versus the OAR (89%; 95% CI: 80% to 95%) was comparable. Furthermore, they found that physician pre-test probability estimates for fractures were accurate when the prevalence of fracture was <10%; however, physicians overestimated probability when the prevalence of fracture was >10%. The overall discriminative ability was greater for physician judgment compared to the OAR as shown by the AUC: 0.80 (95% CI: 0.74 to 0.87) versus 0.69 (95% CI: 0.62 to 0.76), respectively [21].

In summary, it can be concluded that there is clinical utility for using both the OAR and physician judgment together for patients with ankle injuries. When the pre-test probability of a fracture is less than 10% after a systematic evaluation with a proper history and physical exam (on a structured data collection form), radiography is not required and the OAR will not help with the decision-making process. However, when the probability is greater than 10%, the OAR can help physicians determine if X-rays are necessary. Using this combination approach, the number of unnecessary X-rays may be further reduced without increasing the number of missed fractures as occurs in using either the OAR or physician judgment alone.

Question 3: In patients with ankle injuries seen in the ED (population), does the decision to order an X-ray (intervention) improve patient satisfaction (outcome) compared to not having a radiograph ordered (control)?

Search strategy

- OVID: (exp patient satisfaction/ OR patient satisfaction.mp OR satisfaction) AND Ottawa ankle rule$.mp

One major concern for physicians treating ankle-injured patients is their dissatisfaction with not having an X-ray taken. This concern is driven by the fear of missing a fracture and subsequent litigation as well as believing that X-rays are necessary to meet patient expectations. With the development of the OAR, physicians now have a guideline to rule out fractures with excellent sensitivity without the need for radiography, which addresses the first reason for concern. The second reason has been less well studied. There was only one moderate-quality, prospective, cross-sectional survey identified investigating patient satisfaction with respect to receiving and not receiving an X-ray for ankle injuries [22]. Patients who had no X-rays and those with negative radiographs were interviewed 2 weeks after ED discharge with a structured telephone interview. Information on their radiographic utilization and outpatient and hospital visits was collected. This survey achieved an acceptable response rate of 69–77%.

In this study, physicians used the OAR as a guide to determine those who did not require an X-ray. Despite the majority of physicians (76%) reporting support for the clinical practice guidelines (CPGs), many (64%) felt patient expectations negatively influence their use of the OAR CPG. The patient satisfaction outcomes in this study, however, show that these assumptions are unfounded. The results showed that the patients who did not receive X-rays were equally satisfied with the ED physician care compared to patients who had X-rays (89% vs 90%, $P = 0.16$). Moreover, 80% of patients not receiving X-rays were satisfied with the decision not to perform radiography. The proportions of patients rating ED care as excellent, very good, good, fair or poor were similar between the two groups ($P = 0.12$).

In summary, with the limited evidence available, it does not appear that the decision to order or not to order radiographs for ankle injuries impacts on patient satisfaction. Patients appear to be equally satisfied with either approach. From a practical standpoint, when X-rays are not ordered, it is important to explain to patients how we arrive at this decision to ensure patients receive the health information that they expect from a medical encounter.

Question 4: In patients with ankle injuries seen in the ED (population), is the clinical decision rule (intervention) cost-effective (outcome) compared to physicians' experience (control)?

Search strategy

- OVID: (exp economics, medical/ OR exp costs and cost analysis/ OR exp cost-benefit analysis/ OR exp economics/ OR economic evaluation.mp OR exp models, economic/) AND (Ottawa Ankle rule$ OR Leiden.mp OR Utrecht.mp)

Economic evaluations of new health technologies (e.g., drugs, diagnostic equipment, decision rules, program interventions, etc.) are important in estimating the wider impact on the health care system and assist in deciding where to allocate resources. Among the clinical decision rules described above, only the OAR has undergone formal economic evaluation. We identified a single deterministic cost-effectiveness decision analysis using 1995 data from a before/after implementation trial of the OAR into Canadian emergency departments. This evaluation compared the use of the OAR

versus no OAR in evaluating ankle-injured patients from a societal perspective. Several deterministic sensitivity analyses were performed that included lowering the OAR negative predictive value from 100% to 98.5%, the incorporation of lawsuit probabilities and varying levels of litigation settlement amounts, as well as increasing and decreasing the cost of radiography by 50%. Medical and non-medical costs associated with a missed fracture were added to the cost calculations.

The baseline analysis results demonstrated an estimated cost saving per patient of $8.89 in 1995 Canadian dollars. The cost savings per patient if the negative predictive value of the OAR was lowered to 98.5% and the probability of a lawsuit was 1%, was $7.16. The threshold value for a probability of a lawsuit at which the cost-effectiveness of the OAR was reduced to $0 was 50%. Extrapolating to a population of 100,000 patients with ankle injuries seen in the ED annually, the cost savings to society would be $730,145 [23].

Unfortunately, this study has two major methodological limitations. First, the authors do not incorporate any uncertainty into their cost and outcome calculations. Second, they use a high diagnostic sensitivity in their worse-case scenario analysis, whereas the literature now would suggest that the OAR sensitivity may be as low as 96%. The inclusion of uncertainty and a more realistic OAR sensitivity may have significantly altered the results of this study. Furthermore, in order to evaluate whether a diagnostic strategy or intervention is worth investing in, information about its cost–utility and cost–benefit are also important. However, no published studies have investigated this issue. Therefore, as the current literature stands, while promising, the economic value of using the OAR requires further testing.

Question 5: In ED patients with a negative radiograph or decision rule (population), does cast immobilization (intervention) shorten time to return to work/sport, reduce pain and reduce instability (outcomes) compared to functional care (control)?

Search strategy

- Cochrane: acute ankle AND immobilization

The amount of pain and gait disability from an ankle sprain depends on the severity of the ligament damage as well as patient perception of the injury. Although most patients will require crutch-assisted ambulation initially, it is unclear whether complete immobilization with a rigid cast will improve clinical outcomes compared to functional treatments (e.g., rest, tensor, ice, early ambulation, etc.) alone. A Cochrane system review of 21 randomized controlled trials (RCTs) involving 2184 participants demonstrated a significant decrease in time to return to work for functionally treated patients (weighted mean difference, WMD = 8.23 days; 95% CI: 6.31 to 10.16) compared to those who received a cast. This decrease in time to return to work persisted even when only high-quality studies were pooled (WMD = 12.89 days; 95% CI: 7.10 to 18.67) [24].

This review also showed that there was a decrease in time to return to sport (WMD = 4.88 days; 95% CI: 1.50 to 8.25) and an increase in number of patients returning to sports activities at long-term follow-up (RR = 1.86; 95% CI: 1.22 to 2.86). Similarly, there was a decrease in short-term swelling (RR = 1.74; 95% CI: 1.17 to 2.59) and an increase in patient satisfaction (RR = 1.83; 95% CI: 1.09 to 3.07) with the functional treatment. Interestingly, objective instability as assessed by the talar tilt test was greater in patients with rigid immobilization (WMD = 2.60; 95% CI: 1.24 to 3.34). All these effects disappeared after pooling only high-quality studies; however, none of these outcomes reversed in direction to favor rigid immobilization. There were no significant differences between treatment arms for pain, recurrent sprain or range of motion [24].

In summary, the best evidence suggests that functional treatment is clinically superior to rigid cast immobilization for ankle-injured patients without a fracture. Although this Cochrane review only studied patients with lateral ligament complex injuries, it is unlikely that the patho-physiology is significantly different for medial complex injuries to which the evidence does not apply. A comparison of functional treatments for ankle sprains is described in the next section of this chapter.

Question 6: In ED patients with a negative radiograph or decision rule (population), does any specific functional ankle support (intervention) shorten time to return to work/sport, reduce pain and reduce instability (outcomes) compared to other alternative functional ankle support strategies (control)?

Search strategy

- Cochrane: acute ankle AND functional support

As shown above, functional treatments of acute ankle sprains have superior clinical outcomes compared to rigid immobilization [24]. However, there are a myriad of functional treatments, each for a different financial cost, available for an emergency physician to choose from. A Cochrane systematic review of nine trials, involving 892 patients, grouped these treatments into four types: elastic bandage/stockings, tape (adhesive or elastic athletic tape), canvas-like or nylon lace-up ankle support, and semi-rigid ankle support with a stirrup [25]. Meta-analytical comparisons between each pair of functional treatments were performed to provide evidence-based recommendations.

The pooling of four studies showed that use of semi-rigid ankle supports compared to elastic bandages resulted in a shorter time period to return to work (WMD = 4.24 days; 95% CI: 2.42 to 6.06) (Fig. 31.3). One RCT found that semi-rigid ankle supports had a faster return to sport compared to elastic bandages (WMD = 9.60 days; 95% CI: 6.34 to 12.86). The use of elastic bandages compared to tape resulted in fewer skin and other complications (RR = 0.11; 95% CI: 0.01 to 0.86). Lace-up ankle support had better results for persistent swelling at short-term follow-up when compared with semi-rigid ankle support (RR = 4.19; 95% CI: 1.26 to 13.98), elastic bandage (RR = 5.48; 95% CI: 1.69 to 17.76) and tape (RR = 4.07; 95% CI: 1.21 to 13.68). None of the comparisons revealed any superior treatment in the reduction of pain, instability or recurrent injury. Unfortunately, because of the heterogeneity of outcome reporting in the primary studies, proper comparisons between each of the functional treatments could not be adequately made. An RCT protocol has been published, in which its objective is to compare different methods of mechanical support and to examine the cost-effectiveness of each strategy [26]. Results of this study will provide more definite conclusions.

A search of RCTs after this published systematic review in 2004 found a rigorous RCT that compared air casting with elastic bandages versus each alone, and casting, in grade 2 and 3 sprains in ED patients with first time ankle injuries. This study found that the group with a combined air casting–elastic bandage returned to pre-injury walking and stair climbing earlier than either modality alone in grade 1 tears ($P < 0.01$). Functional treatments outperformed casting in grade 2 tears ($P = 0.0001$) and no difference was found between an air cast versus fiberglass cast in grade 3 tears ($P > 0.8$) (Table 31.2) [27].

In summary, there is sufficient evidence demonstrating that a removable semi-rigid ankle support (i.e., an air cast) is the best single functional treatment of ankle sprains, although combining it with an elastic bandage may be the ideal treatment.

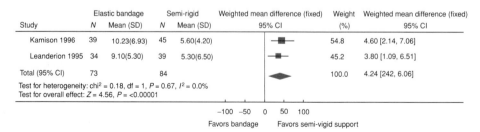

Figure 31.3 Elastic bandage versus semi-rigid support: return to work (days). (Reproduced with permission from Kerkhoff et al. [25], © Wiley, Cochrane Library Database.)

Table 31.2 Different functional supports. (Reproduced with permission from Beynnon et al. [27].)

Primary outcome	Grade I			Grade II			Grade III		
	Plastic warp	Air-stirrup ankle brace	Air-stirrup ankle brace with warp	Plastic warp	Air-stirrup ankle warp	Air-stirrup ankle brace with warp	Cast	Air-stirrup ankle brase	Cast
Number of days required to return to:									
Normal (pre-injury) walking	11.16	10.22	4.62	11.67	12.28	10.10	24.12	18.56	19
Normal (pre-injury) stair climbing	13.05	11.42	5.46	12.28	10.28	11.72	17.94	15.21	21.05

Plaster or fiberglass lower-leg casts are generally not helpful and impose greater restrictions on activities of daily living (e.g., bathing, wearing shoes). Moreover, casting poses the increased disadvantage of increased risk venous thromboembolism. For patients who have to pay for their own commercial ankle support, their immediate cost is in the range of 80 to 100 Canadian dollars, which can be prohibitive for some consumers. However, the higher upfront cost may be balanced by the earlier return to income-generating activities. Thus, the overall economic impact of these various therapeutic options requires further study.

Question 7: In ED patients with a negative radiograph or decision rule (population), does physiotherapy (intervention) shorten time to return to work/sport, reduce pain and stiffness and prevent further sprains (outcomes) compared to no physiotherapy (control)?

Search strategy

- Cochrane: acute ankle AND rehabilitation

Physiotherapy is an oft prescribed intervention for both acute ankle sprains as well as chronic ankle instability. The goals of physiotherapy after an acute ankle sprain are to improve return to baseline function and provide secondary prevention of injury recurrence. Several systematic reviews have addressed this topic to varying degrees. All these reviews were unfortunately plagued with small trial numbers/samples, poor quality studies with heterogeneous populations and incomplete outcome reporting. Interpretation of any of the pooled outcomes must be viewed with caution. Furthermore, no high-quality review or RCT was found studying clinical outcomes such as return to work/sport, and pain or stiffness reduction. Fortunately, "recurrent sprains" was a frequent cited outcome.

Of these systematic reviews, the highest quality review was located in the Cochrane Library. This review examined both rehabilitative and prevention strategies [28]. For patients with acute ankle sprains, an ankle disk (wobble board) exercise program showed a trend in reducing the number of recurrent ankle sprains compared to controls (RR = 0.46; 95% CI: 0.21 to 1.01) in a single study. In a worse case scenario analysis that included data for 13 missing and excluded patients, however, the trend disappeared (RR = 0.97; 95% CI: 0.54 to 1.73). Similarly, a single study evaluating a supervised program emphasizing balance exercises (including the use of an ankle disk) compared to controls found a trend in reduction of ankle re-injuries at 1-year follow-up (RR = 0.24; 95% CI: 0.06 to 0.99). This result reversed in direction in a worse case scenario accounting for the 25% loss to follow-up in the original study (RR = 1.73; 95% CI: 0.93 to 3.21).

In terms of prevention strategies, this same review failed to find evidence to suggest that there is any injury reduction for ankle disk training, warm-up exercises for specific muscle groups, leg muscle stretching, injury awareness and instruction for exercises, or multi-component tailored prophylactic programs in reducing the number of ankle sprains [28].

In summary, there is insufficient evidence to demonstrate that physiotherapy is useful in helping patients with acute ankle sprains return to work/sport earlier, reduce pain or stiffness, or prevent future ankle injuries. As one qualitative study reported, however, "All patients that received physiotherapy were impressed with their treatment" [29]. Further studies are required to determine the value of physiotherapy in patients with ankle sprains. In the mean time, it may be prudent to propose that referral to physiotherapy be performed by the primary care provider at the follow-up visit.

Question 8: For ED patients with an ankle sprain (population), does external ankle support (intervention) prevent further sprains (outcomes) compared to no support (control)?

Search strategy

- Cochrane: acute ankle AND external ankle support

After sustaining a painful ankle injury, most if not all patients are concerned with what they can personally do to prevent the same injury in the future. As shown in the above section, there is insufficient evidence to definitively suggest physiotherapy as a modality of prevention. Sports medicine experts have also suggested the use of external ankle supports to provide additional stability in order to prevent ankle sprains.

We identified a high-quality Cochrane systematic review of interventions used to prevent ankle sprains. This review showed that external ankle supports compared to controls were beneficial. Statistical pooling of five trials involving 3682 participants showed that the use of direct external ankle support reduced the number of future ankle sprains (RR = 0.53; 95% CI: 0.40 to 0.69) (Fig. 31.4) [28]. Isolating only patients with a previous history of ankle sprains, the use of external supports reduced the number of future sprains (RR = 0.33; 95% CI: 0.20 to 0.53). Interestingly, those who did not have a prior history did not benefit (RR = 0.73; 95% CI: 0.52 to 1.03). The types of supports evaluated in these studies included semi-rigid ankle orthoses (e.g., air casts) and ankle braces.

In summary, there is excellent evidence demonstrating that external ankle supports such as air casts and ankle braces help prevent ankle sprains. This particular finding is especially strong for those with previous histories of ankle sprains. Unfortunately, the participants involved in these trials were primarily young, active adult males playing sports. Caution is warranted when generalizing these findings to children, females and older adults. Overall, any persons involved in high-risk activities or who have medical or social conditions that predispose them to recurrent ankle injuries are advised to utilize external ankle support as a useful preventive strategy.

Question 9: In patients with chronic ankle instability who present to the ED with further ankle sprains (population), does surgery (intervention) prevent further injuries (outcomes) compared to routine care (control)?

Search strategy

• Cochrane: chronic ankle instability AND surgery

Approximately 10–20% of patients after an acute ankle ligament injury will develop a chronically unstable ankle. This condition is defined by a feeling of giving away that persists for more than 6 months [30]. This instability is caused by a disturbed proprioception of the joint and its surrounding muscles [31]. It is this group of individuals that present to EDs with recurrent ankle sprains. The advice to these patients is usually conservative management with physiotherapy and some form of external ankle support; however, if symptoms persist, surgical treatments are sometimes tried.

A high-quality Cochrane review of surgical and conservative management of chronic ankle instability found insufficient evidence to recommend any particular management strategy for this population [32]. This result was due to the poor methodological quality of all primary studies available in the literature. Studies examining different types of surgical repairs either did not evaluate any functional outcomes, such as return to work or sport or prevention of recurrent ankle sprains, or the outcome effects were lost when study heterogeneity was accounted for by a random effects model. This problem was similar for the authors' evaluation of studies comparing different conservative ankle training methods. Unfortunately, there was no high-quality RCT found that directly compared surgical with conservative treatment for patients with chronic ankle instability. Nor were there any RCTs identified that evaluated orthotics or external ankle supports for this patient population [32].

As emergency physicians, the best current advice for patients with chronic instability that present with a new ankle sprain would be the use of a functional external rigid ankle support immediately for the treatment of the acute injury. After the acute injury period, patients should use such external supports in the long term for

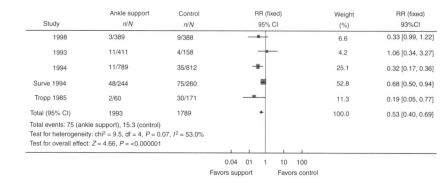

Figure 31.4 External ankle support versus control: ankle sprains outcome. (Reproduced with permission from Handoll et al. [28], © Wiley, Cochrane Library Database.)

any high-risk physical activity and for persistent symptoms until better evidence is available.

Conclusions

Using the Ottawa Ankle Rule, it was determined that the above mentioned university student did not require an X-ray. The patient was provided with crutches to weight bear as tolerated and advised to purchase an air cast for external ankle support during his recovery and for future sporting activities. Non-steroidal anti-inflammatory drugs NSAIDS were prescribed as well as the RICE (rest, ice, compression, elevation) regimen.

Ankle injuries are common problems faced by emergency physicians. This chapter outlines the most reliable predictors of ankle fractures and a well-validated clinical decision rule (Ottawa Ankle Rule) to assist in the ordering of ankle radiography to rule out fractures in a cost-effective manner. After ruling out a fracture and diagnosing a sprain, the use of external ankle supportive devices provides the best clinical recovery for the acute event and prevention of future injuries.

Acknowledgments

The author would like to thank Dr. Andrew Worster for his ongoing support with the research activities by associate staff physicians at McMaster University in the Department of Emergency Medicine.

Conflicts of interests

None were reported.

References

1 Garrick JG, Requa RK. The epidemiology of foot and ankle injuries in sports. *Clin Sports Med* 1988;**7**:29–36.

2 Katcherian DA. Soft-tissue injuries of the ankle. In: Dutter LD, Mizel MS, Pfeffer GB, eds. *Orthopaedic Knowledge Update: Foot and ankle.* American Academy of Orthopaedic Surgeons, Rosemont, IL, 1994:241–53.

3 Zeegers AVCM. *Het supinatieletsel van de enkel.* University of Utrecht, Utrecht, 1995.

4 Lloyd S. Selective radiographic assessment of acute ankle injuries in the emergency department: barriers to implementation. *Can Med Assoc J* 1986;**135**:973–4.

5 Brooks SC, Potter BT, Rainey JB. Inversion injuries of the ankle: clinical assessment and radiographic review. *BMJ* 1981;**282**:607–8.

6 Vargish T, Clarke WR, Young RA, et al. The ankle injury: indications for the selective use of x-rays. *Injury* 1983;**14**:507–12.

7 Montague AP, McQuillan RF. Clinical assessment of apparently sprained ankle and detection of fracture. *Injury* 1985;**16**:545–6.

8 Sujitkumar P, Hadfield JM, Yates DW. Sprain or fracture? An analysis of 2000 ankle injuries. *Arch Emerg Med* 1986;**3**:101–6.

9 Stiell IG, Greenberg GH, McKnight RD, et al. Decision rules for the use of radiography in acute ankle injuries: refinement and prospective validation. *JAMA* 1993;**269**:1127–32.

10 Stephensen N. *Ankle Sprain.* Rene Vejlsgaard Medical Yearbook, Copenhagen, 1981.

11 Dalton JD, Schweinle JE. Randomized controlled non-inferiority trial to compare extended release acetaminophen and ibuprofen for the treatment of ankle sprains. *Ann Emerg Med* 2006;**48**(5):615–23.

12 Cooke MW, Lamb SE, Marsh J, Dale J. A survey of current consultant practice of treatment of severe ankle sprains in emergency departments in the United Kingdom. *Emerg Med J* 2003;**20**:505–7.

13 Birrer RB, Fani-Salek MH, Totten VY, Herman LM, Politi V. Managing ankle injuries in the emergency department. *J Emerg Med* 1999;**17**(4): 651–60.

14 Van der Windt D, Van der Heijden G, Van den Berg S, Ter Riet G, de Winter AF, Bouter LM. Therapeutic ultrasound for acute ankle sprains. *Cochrane Database Syst Rev* 2002;**1**:CD001250 (doi: 10.1002/14651858. CD001250).

15 Stiell IG, McKnight RD, Greenberg GH, Nair RC, McDowell I, Wallace GJ. Interobserver agreement in the examination of acute ankle injury patients. *Am J Emerg Med* 1992;**10**:14–17.

16 Landis JR, Koch GG. The measurement of observer agreement for categorical data. *Biometrics* 1977;**33**:159–74.

17 Stiell IG, Greenberg GH, McKnight RD, Nair RC, McDowell I, Worthington JR. A study to develop clinical decision rules for the use of radiography in acute ankle injuries. *Ann Emerg Med* 1992;**21**:384–90.

18 Stiell IG, Greenberg GH, McKnight RD, et al. Decision rules for the use of radiography in acute ankle injuries. Refinement and prospective validation. *JAMA* 1993;**269**(9):1127–32.

19 Bachmann LM, Kolb E, Koller MT, Steurer J, ter Riet G. Accuracy of Ottawa ankle rules to exclude fractures of the ankle and mid-foot: systematic review. *BMJ* 2003;**326**:417–24.

20 Pijnenburg, ACM, Glas AS, de Roos MAJ, et al. Radiography in acute ankle injuries: the Ottawa Ankle Rules versus local diagnostic decision rules. *Ann Emerg Med* 2002;**39**:599–604.

21 Glas AS, Pijnenburg ACM, Lijmer JG, et al. Comparison of diagnostic decision rules and structured data collection in assessment of acute ankle injury. *Can Med Assoc J* 2002;**166**(6):727–33.

22 Wilson DE, Noseworthy TW, Rowe BH, Holroyd BR. Evaluation of patient satisfaction and outcomes after assessment for acute ankle injuries. *Am J Emerg Med* 2002;**20**:18–22.

23 Anis AH, Stiell IG, Stewart DG, Laupacis A. Cost-effectiveness analysis of the Ottawa Ankle Rules. *Ann Emerg Med* 1995;**26**(4):422–8.

24 Kerkhoffs GMMJ, Rowe BH, Assendelft WJJ, Kelly K, Struijs PAA, van Dijk CN. Immobilization and functional treatment for acute lateral ankle ligament injuries in adults. *Cochrane Database Syst Rev* 2002;**3**:CD003762 (doi: 10.1002/14651858.CD003762).

25 Kerkhoff GMMJ, Struijs PAA, Marti RK, Assendelft WJJ, Blankevoort L, van Dijk CN. Different functional treatment strategies for acute lateral ankle ligament injuries in adults. *Cochrane Database Syst Rev* 2002;**3**:CD002938 (doi:10.1002/14651858.CD002938).

26 Lamb SE, Nakash RA, Withers EJ, et al. Clinical and cost effectiveness of mechanical support for severe ankle sprains: design of a randomized controlled trial in the emergency department (ISRCTN 37807450).

BMC Musculoskeletal Disord 2005;**6**(1):1–8. Available at http://www.biomedcentral.com/1471-2474/6/1.

27 Beynnon BD, Renstrom PA, Haugh L, Uh BS, Barker H. A prospective, randomized clinical investigation of the treatment of first-time ankle sprains. *Am J Sports Med* 2006;**34**(9):1401–12.

28 Handoll HHG, Rowe BH, Quinn KM, de Bie R. Interventions for preventing ankle ligament injuries. *Cochrane Database Syst Rev* 2001;**3**: CD000018 (doi 10.1002/14651858.CD000018).

29 Brooks SC, Potter BT, Rainey JB. Treatment for partial tears of the lateral ligament of the ankle: a prospective trial. *BMJ* 1981;**282**:606–7.

30 Karlsson J, Eriksson BI, Sward L. Early functional treatment for acute ligament injuries of the ankle joint. *Scand J Med Sci Sports* 1996;**6**(6):341–5.

31 Matsusaka N, Yokoyama S, Tsurusaki T, Inokuchi S, Okita M. Effect of ankle disk training combined with tactile stimulation to the leg and foot on functional instability of the ankle. *Am J Sports Med* 2001;**29**(1):25–30.

32 De Vries JS, Krips R, Sierevelt IN, Blankevoort L, van Dijk CN. Interventions for treating chronic ankle instability. *Cochrane Database Syst Rev* 2006;**4**:CD004124 (doi 10.1002/14651858.CD004124.pub2).

33 Stiell IG, McKnight RD, Greenberg GH, et al. Implementation of the Ottawa Ankle Rule. *JAMA* 1994;**271**(11):827–32.

32 Knee Injuries

Anita Pozgay & Elisabeth Hobden

Department of Emergency Medicine, The Ottawa Hospital, Ottawa, Canada

Case scenario

A 30-year-old female comes to your emergency department (ED) unable to weight bear and complaining of knee swelling and pain after she collided with another alpine skier at the local ski resort. She had to be escorted down the ski hill via sled by the ski patrol. Further history reveals the swelling was immediate and there was no "popping" sound. You examine her and find a 3+ effusion and a knee locked in 20° of flexion. The skin and neurovascular status of the leg are intact. Further attempts to examine her menisci, ligaments and patella result in her guarding due to severe pain. You decide to send her for a knee radiograph (anteroposterior and lateral views), which demonstrate soft tissue swelling consistent with the clinical examination and no obvious fracture. You wonder whether magnetic resonance imaging (MRI) would be better than the radiograph?

You decide to place her leg in a straight leg splint and give her crutches instructing her not to walk on the affected leg until seen by an orthopedic surgeon the following week. She asks why she needs to see an orthopedic surgeon; does she require surgery? A friend of hers had a knee injury that resolved after several physiotherapy sessions. Should she seek the services of a physiotherapist instead? In the meantime, what about the pain and swelling? You explain the RICE (rest, ice, compression, elevation) concept to her. How many times a day should she ice her knee? You recall a colleague telling a patient, 3–4 times a day for 3 days, and recite the same instructions to your patient. You give her a prescription for acetaminophen with codeine, but she wonders if plain ibuprofen or acetaminophen is sufficient? Finally, she wonders when she could return to work and her regular activities?

Evidence-based Emergency Medicine. Edited by Brian H. Rowe
© 2009 Blackwell Publishing, ISBN: 978-1-4051-6143-5.

Background

Sports-related injuries are an increasingly common cause of presentation to the ED. These injuries are more frequent as the population ages, and more people are participating in physical activity. In the USA, the Centers for Disease Control and Prevention (CDC) report that one in five visits to EDs are for injuries sustained during sports and recreation [1]. In young adults, injuries are the highest cause of mortality. The population of older adults is increasing as is their participation in sports and recreation; however, little is known about their risk of injury. In 1996, US emergency department statistics showed a 54% increase in sports and recreational injuries in persons older than 65 years compared to 1990.

A 10-year epidemiological study of knee injuries at a sports clinic in Switzerland [1,2] showed a 45% prevalence of internal derangement. Most of these internal injuries were anterior cruciate ligament (ACL) ruptures (22.3%) with or without medial meniscus (10.8%) and medial cruciate ligament (MCL) (7.9%) lesions. Injury to the posterolateral stabilizers was uncommon. The most common sports activities resulting in knee injuries were alpine skiing and soccer; however, clearly this varies based on location. A study by Burt and Overspeck [3] in the USA concluded that cycling and basketball were the most common sports causing knee injuries. This likely reflects a greater proportion of people participating in these sports rather than the assumption they are more dangerous than others.

Motor vehicle collisions are another frequent cause of knee injuries. Knee injuries were the third leading cause of bodily injury after the head and neck in the US National Accident Sampling System (NASS) database from 1975 to 1995 [4]. These resulted in estimated health care expenditures of $425–740 million.

A community-based study [5] of acute knee injuries (less than 1 month after injury) showed the annual incidence rate as 278 per 100,000 overall. The most common causes were sports injuries (36%) followed by non-sports-related twists or bends (26.5%), falls (21.1%) and other trauma (8.6%). Overall, 71% of patients were referred to an orthopedic surgeon if they had a presumed internal knee derangement (e.g., meniscal tear/injuries, cruciate ligament ruptures). Most patients were treated with the following conservative therapies: analgesics (81%), ice (70%), crutches/cast/cane/tensor (65%) and rest (63%). Physiotherapy was recommended in approximately half of the patients.

Despite the high prevalence and cost of knee injuries in many parts of the world, education of medical students and residents is lacking [6]. For example, Canadian data demonstrate that only 51% of family medicine teaching programs require musculoskeletal training. Moreover, therapeutic strategies are based on emulation and tradition more than evidence. This chapter aims to identify and summarize all pertinent evidence on knee injuries by addressing the following questions.

Clinical questions

1 In adults with acute knee injuries (population), are the sensitivities and specificities of various physical examination techniques (diagnostic test characteristics) sufficient to predict further management (intervention) without imaging modalities?
2 In adults with acute knee injuries (population), are there valid and reliable clinical criteria (clinical prediction guides) that can direct radiography to rule out a fracture (outcome)?
3 In adults with an acute knee injury (population), does MRI (intervention) identify injuries and predict the need for subsequent treatment/arthroscopy (outcome) better than history and directed physical examination (control)?
4 In adults with acute knee injuries and negative radiographs (population), does ice (intervention) allow earlier return to work/play (outcome) compared to treatment without ice (control)?
5 In adults with acute knee injuries and negative radiographs (population), does treatment with non-steroidal anti-inflammatory drugs (NSAIDs) (intervention) reduce pain and swelling (outcome) faster and more completely compared to acetaminophen with or without a narcotic (control)?
6 In adults with acute knee injuries and negative radiographs (population), does physiotherapy (intervention) allow earlier return to work/play (outcome) compared to a period of immobilization or no treatment (control)?
7 In adults with knee injuries (population), does early referral to an orthopedic surgeon or musculoskeletal specialist (intervention) reduce morbidity and complications (outcomes) compared to usual care (control)?

General search strategy

Knee injuries are poorly coded in most electronic search engines. For example, knee injuries may be classified as meniscal, ligamentous, soft tissue and fracture injuries. Consequently, the following databases were searched looking for knee injuries limited to adults, human, English language, clinical trials and systematic reviews (therapy), and sensitivity and specificity (diagnosis):

MEDLINE (PubMed), EMBASE, the Cochrane Library and Sport Discus. Sport Discus is a sports medicine database encompassing coaching, athletic and physiotherapy information from the athlete's point of view and includes not only journal format, but textbooks and other publication types.

Question 1: In adults with acute knee injuries (population), are the sensitivities and specificities of various physical examination techniques (diagnostic test characteristics) sufficient to predict further management (intervention) without imaging modalities?

Search strategy

- MEDLINE, EMBASE, Cochrane Library and Sport Discus: (knee injuries [MeSH] OR knee injury [text word]) AND specificity

The physical examination in acute knee injuries is complex and involves inspection, palpation and range of motion, as well as maneuvers to assess ligamentous instability (medial and lateral collateral ligaments, anterior and posterior cruciate ligaments), presence of effusion and meniscal injury. The examination of the knee has been criticized as being inaccurate, making the diagnosis elusive [7–10]. Moreover, the examination often leads to referral for diagnostic imaging or directly to an orthopedic surgeon.

An acute knee injury may result in a tense hemarthrosis and/or a joint locked in flexion, making the exam difficult. Most studies on the clinical examination of the knee have been performed by orthopedic surgeons at least a week post injury when the effusion has improved or resolved. This overestimates the sensitivity and specificity of the knee examination, especially since the prevalence of serious ligamentous or meniscal injuries are much higher in these settings. Also, orthopedic surgeons usually have more experience examining knees, further inflating the sensitivity and specificity of the examination. Finally, lack of blinding may have introduced verification bias since the orthopedic surgeons knew the clinical diagnosis at arthroscopy.

The most cited meta-analysis on the accuracy of the physical examination of the knee is one such review plagued by the heterogeneity of its individual studies, most of which were composed of patients referred to orthopedic surgeons, and thus invoke spectrum bias [11]. Despite these limitations, the study provided sensitivity and specificity data from individual studies and calculated the pooled likelihood ratios (LRs) for specific examination maneuvers, thereby overcoming the dependency on the prevalence of the condition. For predicting ACL injury, the anterior drawer test had a positive LR (+LR) of 3.8 (95% CI: 0.7 to 0.22) and a negative LR (−LR) of 0.30 (95% CI: 0.05 to 1.50), meaning that a patient with an ACL tear was 3.8 times more likely to have a positive anterior drawer test than one without such a lesion (Table 32.1). The Lachman test showed a +LR of 42 (95% CI: 2.7

Table 32.1 Summary likelihood ratios of meta-analyses on the diagnostic evaluation of ligamentous and meniscal injuries to the knee.

	Solomon et al. [11,37]		Scholten et al. [8–10]		Jackson et al. [12,38]	
	29 studies (15 ACL/5 PCL/9 meniscus)		17 studies for ACL		35 studies (11 ACL/4 meniscus/2 PCL)	
	$N = 2691$		13 for meniscus		Primary Care physician or orthopedic surgeon	
	Patients referred to orthopedic surgeon		Patients referred to orthopedic surgeon		Reference standard: arthrotomy or arthroscopy	
	Reference standard: arthroscopy		Reference standard: arthrotomy, arthroscopy or MRI			
Diagnostic test	+LR (95% CI)	−LR (95% CI)	+LR	−LR	+LR (95% CI)	−LR (95% CI)
ACL						
Composite exam*	25 (2.1 to 306)	0.04 (0.01 to 0.48)	N/A	N/A	15 (5.1 to 23)	0.27 (0.1 to 0.4)
Anterior drawer	3.8 (0.7 to 0.22)	0.3 (0.05 to 1.5)	5.4–87.9	0.1–0.8	N/A	N/A
Lachman	42† (2.7 to 651)	0.1 (0 to 0.4)	2.0–102	0.1–0.4	N/A	N/A
Pivot shift	N/A	N/A	8.2–26.9	0.5–0.8	N/A	N/A
PCL						
Composite exam*	21 (2.1 to 205)	0.05 (0.01 to 0.5)	N/A	N/A	16.2 (5.2 to 25)	0.2 (0.13 to 0.49)
Meniscus						
Joint line tenderness	0.9 (0.8 to 1.0)	1.1 (1.0 to 1.3)	0.8–14.9	0.2–2.1	1.1 (0.7 to 1.6)	0.8 (0.3 to 3.5)
McMurray	1.3 (0.9 to 1.7)	0.8 (0.6 to 1.1)	1.5–9.5	0.4–0.9	17.3 (2.7 to 68)	0.5 (0.3 to 0.8)

*All ACL or PCL tests combined.

†Data based on only one study.

ACL, anterior cruciate ligament; LR, likelihood ratio; MRI, magnetic resonance imaging; N/A, not applicable; PCL, posterior cruciate ligament.

to 651.0) and a −LR of 0.1 (95% CI: 0 to 0.4); however, this was only based on one study for which sensitivity and specificity data could be extrapolated and thus produced wide confidence intervals. LR data for the pivot shift test could not be derived since there were no specificities reported. There were only five studies involving diagnostic tests for the posterior cruciate ligament (PCL), of which three permitted calculation of LRs. However, two of these based their PCL testing on the "general examination" (they did not specify if this meant the general knee exam or general tests for the PCL). No conclusions could be made on the accuracy of these tests.

Nine studies evaluated diagnostic tests for meniscal lesions including most commonly joint line tenderness and the McMurray test. Five studies based their results on a composite examination rather than the specific tests. Only two studies provided LRs for joint line tenderness, and three studies provided LRs for the McMurray test (Table 32.1). Since the positive and negative LRs overlap unity neither of these tests have any predictive power in isolation.

Two meta-analyses by Scholten et al. on the accuracy of meniscal and ACL diagnostic tests used meta-regression to address the heterogeneity amongst the 13 and 17 studies included, respectively [8,10]. The resulting summary receiver operating curves (ROCs) were used to estimate positive and negative predictive values based on previous prevalences of meniscal or ACL lesions. Ranges of LRs

are reported for the individual studies but no summary LRs could be derived due to the wide heterogeneity of the studies (Table 32.1). Although the results of these meta-analyses must be taken as preliminary at best, the conclusions reached were: (i) for diagnosing meniscal pathology, only the McMurray test had a good positive predictive value (PPV); and (ii) for diagnosing an ACL lesion, the pivot shift test has a high PPV and the Lachman has a high negative predictive value (a negative test rules it out). The anterior drawer test was not shown to be helpful diagnostically.

Jackson and colleagues [12] reviewed 35 studies of the physical examination of the knee in acute (<1 week) injuries for patients seen by primary care physicians (internists, family practitioners, general practitioners). However, they only provided sensitivity and (scarce) specificity data on nine studies on ACL testing and four on meniscal tests. Unfortunately, the studies did not describe how the tests were performed. The tests were conducted on patients known to have the injury, hence specificities could not be derived. Tests of heterogeneity were not performed. However, they explain that they used ROCs rather than weighted sensitivity and specificity information to overcome varying test cutoffs used in the studies. Indeed, ROCs are useful at converting dichotomous data into continuous data by allowing a comparison of diagnostic tests at different thresholds of test positivity [13]. LRs were reported only for the composite ACL and PCL examinations (Table 32.1) and not for the individual tests. The LRs reported for the meniscal tests show that while a positive McMurray test can rule in the meniscal injury, a negative test does not provide enough confidence to rule out the lesion. Joint line tenderness is not sufficiently useful to rule in or rule out a meniscal lesion.

Malanga et al., in their extensive review of the knee examination, attempted to standardize all the diagnostic tests as they were originally described [14]. Of the ligament tests, the Lachman and pivot shift were most accurate in identifying ACL tears. The accuracy of the posterior drawer test is also good and it can be augmented with the posterior sag sign. The quadriceps active test did not perform as well due to limited data. There is a lack of studies on collateral ligament testing, the accuracy of this test is unknown. Of the patellar tests, there are no studies to support the patellar grind test. In fact, the correlation between the test and pathological findings of chondromalacia patella are poor. The apprehension test to diagnose patellar dislocation, done at 30° of flexion, also performed poorly when done on patients in the operating room under anesthesia with a history of patellar dislocation. The sensitivity of this test was higher at 70–80° of knee flexion. For meniscal tears, as also shown in the above meta-analyses, the specificity of the McMurray test is good but it lacks sensitivity, whereas the reverse is true for joint line tenderness [8,10,11,14].

A study by Bansal et al. showed that in 50 acute knee-injured patients, the triad of effusion, locking and joint line tenderness was 100% sensitive at predicting a mechanical cause (meniscal lesion, loose body, cyclops cruciate tear). Further, they recommended immediate referral to an orthopedic clinic for arthroscopy [7].

As stated earlier, the majority of papers reporting on knee examinations have been performed by orthopedic surgeons. While ED data have validated the precision and reliability of some knee examination signs elicited by emergency physicians, similar research has not yet been done among orthopedic surgeons. For example, in the Ottawa Knee Rules work [15–17], some well-accepted maneuvers for knee examination were found to be unreliable (e.g., detection of effusion using the sweep test, kappa (κ) = 0.46), while others were highly reliable ($\kappa > 0.8$) and could be used (e.g. tenderness at head of fibula). Overall, the available literature is incompletely applicable to the emergency setting. Studies indicate that no physical examination maneuver is sufficiently accurate to reliably rule in or rule out ligamentous or meniscal knee injuries, and a low threshold for specialist referral is appropriate. The emergency physician must be adept at performing a standardized physical exam of the knee. In acute knee injuries, this becomes more difficult in the setting of an inflammatory effusion, pain and/or a mechanical block to range-of-motion assessment. The pre-test probability of an injury based on the mechanism of injury derived from the history should be emphasized even though there are no studies on the accuracy of the history in acute knee trauma.

In summary, the history and composite knee examination rather than any individual test should guide further imaging and/or management.

Question 2: In adults with acute knee injuries (population), are there valid and reliable clinical criteria (clinical prediction guides) that can direct radiography to rule out a fracture (outcome)?

Search strategy

- PubMed – search: knee injuries AND clinical prediction rules AND imaging

The literature on clinical prediction rules with respect to knee radiographs in the ED has been dominated by the Ottawa Knee Rule (OKR). This rule was derived, tested and validated using standard techniques for clinical decision rules [15–18]. This rule has been validated in many clinical settings and is thus considered the standard of care for decision making on when to order knee radiographs.

In their derivation study [17], Stiell et al. demonstrated that although 68% of patients presenting with acute knee injuries underwent radiography, only 6.6% of patients had a clinically important fracture identified. Derivation of this rule included 1054 non-pregnant adults presenting for the first time to EDs for a knee injury within the last 7 days. Patients were also excluded if they were paraplegic, had superficial skin injuries only, multiple trauma or an altered level of consciousness.

Multiple predictor variables for knee injury were studied, comprising patient characteristics, history and physical exam features. The reliability of each variable was assessed statistically using the proportion of potential agreement beyond chance (κ). Variables that had the highest agreement among physicians, and were strongly associated with fracture, were used to develop a decision rule with a sensitivity of 100% and the highest specificity possible. The higher the κ, the better the agreement between physicians for that physical or historical finding. Agreement for tenderness at the head of the fibula was highest at 0.92, and the lowest score included in the rules was 0.59 for both isolated tenderness of the patella and flexion of less than 90°. Inability to weight bear both immediately and in the department had an agreement score of 0.75. All of these factors were significantly correlated with fracture.

Using this methodology, the authors concluded that a knee radiograph was only required for patients with acute knee injury with one or more of the listed findings related to age, tenderness or function (Box 32.1). The decision rule had 100% sensitivity but a specificity of only 54% in the derivation sample. Emergency physicians were reassured that no clinically significant knee fractures would be missed using the rule; however, radiography of those patients meeting the criteria will still often be normal.

This rule has been validated in multiple settings, and the reliability of the physical exam findings have been reproduced in the validation study by Stiell et al. [17]. A recent systematic review [18,19] pooled data from six studies containing a total of 4249 patients who met the inclusion criteria. This review showed a pooled sensitivity of 98.5% (95% CI: 93% to 100%) and a pooled

Box 32.1 Ottawa knee radiograph decision rule: if any of these findings are present, a radiograph of the knee is recommended.

- Age 55 years or older
- Tenderness at head of fibula
- Isolated tenderness of patella*
- Inability to flex to 90°
- Inability to bear weight both immediately and in the emergency department (four steps)†

*No bone tenderness of knee other than patella.
†Unable to transfer weight twice onto each lower limb regardless of limping.

---

specificity of 48.6% (95% CI: 43% to 51%). The pooled negative LR was 0.05 (95% CI: 0.02 to 0.23). Assuming a fracture prevalence of 7%, the probability of a patient having a fracture when the knee rule is negative is approximately 0.37% (four in 1000).

An implementation trial ($N = 3907$) compared intervention sites to control sites and showed a 26% decrease in the use of radiography and a mean of 33 minutes less in the ED without compromising patient safety or satisfaction [15]. The OKR is easy to apply, and can accurately determine the need for radiography in patients presenting to the ED with blunt knee trauma.

In most cases, emergency physicians should use this rule to decide on radiography; however, as in any decision aid, the knee decision rule results should not supersede clinical judgment. Moreover, despite a negative OKR result or radiography, there is considerable work remaining to ensure patients recover from their injuries as quickly as possible.

Question 3: In adults with an acute knee injury (population), does MRI (intervention) identify injuries and predict the need for subsequent treatment/arthroscopy (outcome) better than history and directed physical examination (control)?

Search strategy

- MEDLINE, EMBASE, Cochrane Library and Sport Discus: (magnetic resonance imaging OR MRI) AND (knee injuries [MeSH] OR knee injuries [text]) AND arthroscopy [MeSH]

If the emergency physician rules out a knee fracture with the OKR, a significant soft tissue injury cannot be ruled out in the patient encountered at the beginning of this chapter. Most patients (93.5%) have soft tissue rather than bony injuries in the ED [17]. Your preliminary diagnosis of an ACL tear and a possible medial meniscal tear is based on the high prevalence of these injuries in skiers, the mechanism of injury and your clinical examination. Balancing the costs and safety of arthroscopy compared to MRI, you feel screening MRI is a cost-effective non-invasive method to distin-

guish patients who require follow-up with an orthopedic surgeon from those who do not. Your literature search, however, reveals only one study performed in an acute ED setting [20].

This randomized study compared history, clinical examination and plain radiography with the addition of low magnetic field MRI to this standard diagnostic work-up. The outcome variable was the difference in treatments received between the two groups at 6 months' follow-up. Surprisingly, the MRI result had no added predictive power compared to the standard diagnostic approach to knee trauma. In fact, as in the clinical examination, the accuracy of MRI in the diagnosis of internal knee pathology with an acute knee hemarthrosis is limited. MRI is also unreliable in patients who have had previous knee surgery [21,22] and in multiply injured knees. There is no role for MRI in the acutely injured knee.

Most of the literature on MRI in comparison to clinical diagnosis suffers from the same limitations as that for the clinical examination alone; over-inflation of the accuracy of the clinical examination due to non-acute presentations in patients referred to non-blinded specialists [21,23,24]. A blinded trial done in the UK [22] compared the diagnostic accuracy of chronic knee injuries in 144 patients referred from the ED among an orthopedic fellow, a consultant orthopedic surgeon and a musculoskeletal radiologist. All patients received a magnetic resonance image and were then managed as usual for 12 months. The orthopedists and the radiologist were blinded to the initial diagnosis and to each other's diagnoses. After 1 year, two of the study researchers (not involved with the initial examination) compared the hospital records or surgical notes to the original diagnoses made by the three clinicians. They found that the more junior orthopedist was less accurate (44% correct) than the radiologist (68%) and consultant orthopedist (72%) in their original diagnoses. Other trials have also demonstrated that the clinical examination is as good as the MRI in predicting the need for further treatment in experienced hands. Thus, the decision on whether to proceed with arthroscopy should be based on the history, physical exam and radiographs. MRI should be reserved for those cases where the clinical findings are equivocal or the initial treatment has failed. Remember, however, that these results cannot be generalized to emergency physicians whose accuracy in clinical examination of the knee has not been assessed.

A more recent meta-analysis performed for 29 trials on MRI focused on the diagnosis of meniscal, ACL or PCL tears, or a combination of these tears, in knee trauma compared to the gold standard of arthroscopy [25]. The results show that MRI is highly accurate for the diagnosis of these injuries (>90%). The pooled weighted sensitivities were similar for the cruciates and medial meniscus; however, diagnosis of the lateral meniscus was less sensitive but more specific. The role of arthroscopy as the reference standard for internal knee derangements has been criticized since it is operator dependent and misses lesions in the posterior meniscal horns and PCL. These lesions cannot be directly visualized but are diagnosed by probing. Thus, false-negative arthroscopy results could still result in positive magnetic resonance images. Overall, MRI is a suitable screening tool in reducing the need for diagnostic arthroscopy in cruciate and meniscal tears after the acute hemarthrosis has resolved in knee trauma; however, its role in the ED is limited. Since increasing age is significantly associated with an abnormal meniscal signal on MRI, this needs to be factored into the treatment plan.

An acute knee dislocation after a fall from a height, motor vehicle collision or contact sports may not be appreciated in the ED since most are spontaneously reduced and radiographs may be normal. However, these injuries represent true orthopedic emergencies due to nerve and arterial injury in which magnetic resonance angiography may aid diagnosis. Popliteal artery injury is common and as many as one-third may require below-knee amputation if not recognized acutely (<6 hours). MRI is also useful in assessing multiple ligament ruptures in these cases [26].

Magnetic resonance imaging does not perform as well as in cruciate and meniscal lesions, for collateral ligament tears and for patellar or articular cartilage defects. It has comparable accuracy to a triple phase bone scan in detecting occult bony trauma and for guiding healing of these lesions [26]. These lesions are usually treated non-operatively, but diagnosis is still important to guide non-operative management which will be discussed in the next section.

Question 4: In adults with acute knee injuries and negative radiographs (population), does ice (intervention) allow earlier return to work/play (outcome) compared to treatment without ice (control)?

Search strategy

- MEDLINE, EMBASE, Cochrane Library and Sport Discus: (cryotherapy [MeSH] OR ice [MeSH]) AND soft tissue injuries [MeSH]

Ice is often recommended immediately after musculoskeletal injury to produce vasoconstriction and reduce metabolic rate, thereby reducing further injury. Later in rehabilitation, ice is considered beneficial because it allows earlier range of motion and activity. This section investigates the benefits of such cryotherapy.

This search revealed one systematic review of RCTs comparing ice to no ice and concluded further studies are needed on the use of ice in the treatment of soft tissue injuries [27]. This review included 22 RCTs in the English language literature involving 1469 patients with a variety of non-fracture injuries. It included studies on cryotherapy with or without other treatments. Outcomes included at least one measure of function, pain, swelling or range of motion.

Overall, the methodological quality of the trials was not high. Many of the trials used adequate randomization methods; however, blinding was often not performed, and only one study used an intention-to-treat analysis. Wide variation in icing protocols

occurred among trials; methods varied from crushed ice to cold compressive devices, and the duration and frequency of therapy also varied. Such a wide spectrum of treatment methods makes assessment of efficacy difficult. No study included patients with muscle contusions or strains. It is important to recognize that several studies were performed on post-operative patients who may vary significantly from the ED population, making generalization to the emergency setting difficult.

A single study showed that ice combined with exercise therapy was more effective than heat after ankle injury [27]. Another study comparing patients post arthroscopic knee surgery showed a significant reduction in reported pain and less analgesic use with the application of ice before physiotherapy. In addition, ice in combination with compression showed benefit in decreasing pain more than ice alone or placebo. The authors of this review note that it may be difficult to randomize patients to no ice or compression only since these modalities have frequently already been applied by the patient prior to entry into the study.

Adverse effects from ice application only included one reported case of nerve palsy in this review. There were no reports of skin burns. At this time, there is some evidence to support the use of ice in acute soft tissue injuries, especially in combination with compression; however, the optimal duration, frequency and temperature of cooling have yet to be determined.

Question 5: In adults with acute knee injuries and negative radiographs (population), does treatment with non-steroidal anti-inflammatory drugs (NSAIDs) (intervention) reduce pain and swelling (outcome) faster and more completely compared to acetaminophen with or without a narcotic (control)?

Search strategy

- MEDLINE, EMBASE, Cochrane Library and Sport Discus: knee injuries/therapy AND drug therapy AND acetaminophen [MeSH] AND musculoskeletal diseases [MeSH] AND anti-inflammatory [MeSH]

Most of the literature on analgesics in musculoskeletal pain comes from the rheumatological literature in patients with osteoarthritis. Only a few RCTs have been performed on patients with acute soft tissue injury.

In the most recent RCT, Woo et al. enrolled 300 patients with either acute soft tissue injury or fractures of a limb [28,29]. The patients were randomized to one of four arms: acetaminophen (1 g), indomethacin (25 mg), diclofenac (25 mg), or diclofenac (25 mg) plus acetaminophen (1 g). It is important to recognize that these NSAID doses are lower than the recommended doses. The patients were given a placebo tablet in addition to the tablet in their designated group (except for the combined group to maintain blinding). Pain scores were recorded at 30, 60, 90 and

120 minutes after analgesia was given and three times daily for 3 days afterwards. Follow-up was obtained 5–8 days after study enrollment. Outcomes were measured on a validated visual analog scale (VAS) pain score. The results showed no improvement in pain until 90 minutes, when all groups had clinically significant reductions in VAS score; however, there were no statistically significant differences among the groups. There was never a statistically significant difference among groups either in the ED or on follow-up; however, there was a trend towards superiority in the combination therapy group. Conversely, this group also had the highest rate of minor side-effects. It is unclear why the investigators chose to include patients with fractures since this group would presumably require more analgesia. It is also uncertain whether there was an appropriate distribution of injury severity amongst the four groups. Future studies should address one injury category and account for injury severity [29].

Acetaminophen with oxycodone has been compared to valdecoxib in an RCT [30]. This double-blind study looked at a convenience sample of patients presenting to an ED with musculoskeletal pain including chronic and atraumatic cases. Fifty-one enrolled patients recorded their VAS score at 30 and 60 minutes after administration of a single dose of either valdecoxib or acetaminophen with oxycodone. All participants were then discharged home with two doses of 400 mg ibuprofen and no further doses of the study drugs. A follow-up phone call at 24 hours was made to determine if rescue analgesics were necessary or side-effects had occurred. There was no difference in pain between the groups at 30 or 60 minutes. At 24-hour follow-up, however, patients using valdecoxib were less likely to require rescue medication than the acetaminophen/oxycodone group. While the use of a convenience sample has the potential to introduce selection bias, the randomization process should ensure these results are valid. Of note, valdecoxib has since been removed from the market due to deleterious cardiovascular side-effects. Newer coxibs are currently being marketed with a better safety profile; moreover, established NSAIDs can be used as alternatives.

There is more evidence on the efficacy of topical than oral NSAIDs in acute musculoskeletal pain (less than 1 week). A recent meta-analysis from the UK included 36 RCTs with over 3000 patients comparing: (i) various topical NSAIDs to placebo (ii) topical NSAIDs to oral NSAIDs with or without placebo; or (iii) two different topical NSAIDs [31]. The authors performed a sensitivity analysis to account for this heterogeneity; however, the trials had large variations in treatment formulations, schedules and study sizes so this was still a problem. Overall, 3.8 people needed to be treated with a topical NSAID compared to placebo to show a 50% reduction in pain at 7 days. Oral and topical NSAIDs had equivalent efficacy but there was a trend toward less gastrointestinal side-effects with topical agents.

In summary, the use of anti-inflammatories for musculoskeletal pain is a common practice in many EDs. There is no convincing evidence showing the superiority of one anti-inflammatory over another or to acetaminophen. Further research is needed to determine the optimal analgesic for acute musculoskeletal injuries.

Question 6: In adults with acute knee injuries and negative radiographs (population), does physiotherapy (intervention) allow earlier return to work/play (outcome) compared to a period of immobilization or no treatment period (control)?

Search strategy

- MEDLINE, EMBASE, Cochrane Library and Sport Discus: immobilization AND knee injury/therapy AND prognosis [MeSH] AND physical therapy modalities [Majr]

No high-quality literature was found investigating the physiological role of immobilization for acute knee injuries without a fracture [32]. Given the proliferation of bracing companies in the last 20 years, some readers may be surprised by this result. Thus, the use of braces in acute knee injuries can only be recommended on an empirical basis.

A Cochrane review of the use of exercise in treating adults with isolated ACL injuries [33] includes both post-operative patients and those undergoing non-operative treatment. Of nine trials, only two included patients who were undergoing conservative treatment, resulting in small patient numbers. In addition, this review excluded trials that specifically considered bracing, cryotherapy, electrotherapy and continuous passive motion, which may be included in many physiotherapy treatments. This may make results difficult to generalize to emergency medicine patients who are sent for physiotherapy.

The two trials reporting conservative rehabilitation were considered separately. Eighty-two percent of the 76 participants in these studies were male. These studies examined additional proprioceptive training, otherwise known as perturbation training, in addition to a conventional physiotherapy program. There was no significant difference between treatment groups receiving this additional proprioceptive training; however, the total sample is small. Perturbation training showed an earlier return to sport at 6 months, but this trial included only 26 patients. Neither study included a control group.

At the present time there is little evidence to support any physiotherapy program over another in the treatment of ACL ruptures. There are no quality studies that investigate the role of physiotherapy compared to no physiotherapy.

Patients with patellofemoral pain due to subluxation or previous dislocation are usually treated non-surgically. In a Cochrane review of 12 trials addressing the role of exercise in the treatment of patellofemoral pain, heterogeneity precluded meaningful pooled data analysis [34]. One high-quality RCT showed that differences in pain reduction were not significant at 3 months between patients attending physiotherapy compared to those that were not; however, the number of patients satisfied with their results was significantly greater for the group that exercised. Another trial used a device designed to apply gradually increased resistance during activities of daily living. Patients treated with this device showed improved functional ability after 4 weeks. Another low-quality trial showed that both static and isokinetic exercise showed little improvement over the control group who were awaiting physiotherapy. This evidence suggests that exercise shows some benefit for patients suffering from patellofemoral pain, however more research is needed.

Overall, the current evidence suggests that physiotherapy and bracing may improve patient satisfaction; however, there is limited outcome evidence for using these modalities.

Question 7: In adults with knee injuries (population), does early referral to an orthopedic surgeon or musculoskeletal specialist (intervention) reduce morbidity and complications (outcomes) compared to usual care (control)?

Search strategy

- MEDLINE, EMBASE, Cochrane Library and Sport Discus: referral and consultation [MeSH] AND knee injuries [MeSH]

There was only one US study [35] identified that compared the diagnosis and management plan of patients with knee injuries referred by non-orthopedic practitioners to orthopedists. The non-orthopedic physicians consisted of pediatricians, family practitioners, general internists and physician assistants supervised by family practitioners. These physicians acted as "gatekeepers", meaning they were responsible for referring patients to orthopedists if deemed necessary. The purpose of a "gatekeeper" in primary care is to reduce the number of referrals to specialists in order to reduce health care costs in a managed care system. In many countries, patients are usually seen by their family physicians or an emergency physician, who then decides on appropriate orthopedic (or other musculoskeletal specialist) referral. Some patients self-refer to sports medicine physicians who have specialty training in musculoskeletal problems. The accuracy of sports medicine specialists compared to orthopedists has not been studied.

The findings of Rupp's 2-year chart review concluded that the generalists missed 50% of clinically important knee diagnoses that were found by the orthopedists, some of which were confirmed by MRI or arthroscopy. Overall, 85% and 50% of ACL and meniscal tears, respectively, were missed by the primary physicians. The morbidity and future prognosis of a persistent meniscal lesion cannot be quantified. However, missing the diagnosis of an unstable knee and allowing the patient to return to sports or occupational activities can lead to further injury and can delay recovery. Two quadriceps ruptures and one case of tibial osteomyelitis were also missed, which resulted in permanent disability. Not all missed injuries required orthopedic assessment, such as patellofemoral pain and tendinopathies. Primary care physicians should be comfortable in managing these disorders.

This study has several limitations. Orthopedists have the advantage of assessing patients after their acute hemarthrosis and painful guarding have resolved. Also, the retrospective design and reliance on medical charts may reflect poor documentation, not reality. Lastly, the author of this study is an orthopedic surgeon and thus bias cannot be ruled out. Nevertheless, this study highlights the importance of accurate and timely diagnosis of knee injuries by primary care physicians and acknowledges that there is room for improvement in medical education.

Conclusions

The patient above was placed in a straight leg splint and given crutches instructing her not to walk on the affected leg until seen by an orthopedic surgeon the following week. The reason for this was that acute injuries of the knee are better examined after a period of treatment with rest, ice, and anti-inflammatory agents. Moreover the effusion suggested she likely had an ACL tear and the locked knee suggested a meniscal tear, both of which warrant orthopedic consultation.

The following is a summary of evidence and recommendations for future research [36].

- *Good evidence* exists for the Lachman test for diagnosing subacute ACL tears when the pain and swelling have subsided. The OKR is 100% sensitive at ruling out acute knee fractures in the ED. It has been validated in several settings; however, it is a guideline and clinical judgment must prevail. Topical and oral NSAIDs are effective in acute knee injuries treated non-operatively; however, topical agents produce less frequent side-effects.

- *Expert opinion* suggests that history, mechanism of injury and the composite exam should assist clinicians in making a diagnosis of internal knee pathology. MRI is an appropriate screening test, especially for ACL and medial meniscal tears, and should be used when the clinical examination is equivocal. Referral to an orthopedic surgeon should be considered for the following internal knee lesions: ACL, PCL, menisci and posterolateral complex tears (or combination). Collateral ligament injuries do not require surgery unless there is a suspicion of a combined tear, and suspected knee dislocations should have pulse verification and timely referral.

- *Fair evidence* exists for the use of braces or physiotherapy (except for proprioceptive training) in conservative management. There is some evidence that icing in combination with compression decreases pain in acute knee injuries. There is no evidence that RICE (rest, ice, compression, elevation) is otherwise effective.

References

1 Centers for Disease Control and Prevention. *Preventing Injuries in Sports, Recreation, and Exercise.* Available at www.cdc.gov/ncipc/pub-res/research_agenda/05_sports.htm (accessed July 9, 2006).

2 Majewski M, Susanne H, Klaus S. Epidemiology of athletic knee injuries: a 10-year study. *Knee* 2006;**13**(3):184–8.

3 Burt CW, Overpeck MD. Emergency visits for sports-related injuries. *Ann Emerg Med* 2001;**37**(3):301–8.

4 Atkinson T, Atkinson P. Knee injuries in motor vehicle collisions: a study of the National Accident Sampling System database for the years 1979–1995. *Accid Anal Prev* 2000;**32**(6):779–86.

5 Yawn BP, Amadio P, Harmsen WS, Hill J, Ilstrup D, Gabriel S. Isolated acute knee injuries in the general population. *J Trauma* 2000;**48**(4):716–23.

6 Canadian Resident and Interns Matching Service (CaRMS). Family Medicine Program brochures. CaRMS, 2007.

7 Bansal P, Deehan DJ, Gregory RJ. Diagnosing the acutely locked knee. *Injury* 2002;**33**(6):495–8.

8 Scholten RJ, Opstelten W, van der Plas CG, Bijl D, Deville WL, Bouter LM. Accuracy of physical diagnostic tests for assessing ruptures of the anterior cruciate ligament: a meta-analysis. *J Fam Pract* 2003;**52**(9):689–94.

9 Scholten RJ, Opstelten W, van-der-Plas CG, Bijl D, Deville WL, Bouter LM. Accuracy of physical diagnostic tests for assessing ruptures of the anterior cruciate ligament: a meta-analysis (Structured abstract). *Cochrane Database Syst Rev* 2007;**1**:DARE20031991.

10 Scholten RJ, Deville WL, Opstelten W, Bijl D, van der Plas CG, Bouter LM. The accuracy of physical diagnostic tests for assessing meniscal lesions of the knee: a meta-analysis. *J Fam Pract* 2001;**50**(11):938–44.

11 Solomon DH, Simel DL, Bates DW, Katz JN, Schaffer JL. The rational clinical examination. Does this patient have a torn meniscus or ligament of the knee? Value of the physical examination. *JAMA* 2001;**286**(13):1610–20.

12 Jackson JL, O'Malley PG, Kroenke K. Evaluation of acute knee pain in primary care. *Ann Intern Med* 2003;**139**(7):575–88.

13 Thompson SG, Higgins JP. How should meta-regression analyses be undertaken and interpreted? *Stat Med* 2002;**21**(11):1559–73.

14 Malanga GA, Andrus S, Nadler SF, McLean J. Physical examination of the knee: a review of the original test description and scientific validity of common orthopedic tests. *Arch Phys Med Rehabil* 2003;**84**(4):592–603.

15 Stiell IG, Wells GA, Hoag RH, et al. Implementation of the Ottawa Knee Rule for the use of radiography in acute knee injuries. *JAMA* 1997;**278**(23):2075–9.

16 Stiell IG, Greenberg GH, Wells GA, et al. Prospective validation of a decision rule for the use of radiography in acute knee injuries. *JAMA* 1996;**275**(8):611–15.

17 Stiell IG, Greenberg GH, Wells GA, et al. Derivation of a decision rule for the use of radiography in acute knee injuries. *Ann Emerg Med* 1995;**26**(4):405–13.

18 Bachmann LM, Haberzeth S, Steurer J, ter Riet G. The accuracy of the Ottawa Knee Rule to rule out knee fractures (Structured abstract). *Cochrane Database Syst Rev* 2007;**1**:DARE 20048087.

19 Bachmann LM, Haberzeth S, Steurer J, ter R,G. The accuracy of the Ottawa Knee Rule to rule out knee fractures: a systematic review. *Ann Intern Med* 2004;**140**(2):121–4.

20 Oei EH, Nikken JJ, Ginai AZ, et al. Acute knee trauma: value of a short dedicated extremity MR imaging examination for prediction of subsequent treatment. *Radiology* 2005;**234**:125–33.

21 Miller GK. A prospective study comparing the accuracy of the clinical diagnosis of meniscus tear with magnetic resonance imaging and its effect on clinical outcome. *Arthroscopy* 1996;**12**(4):406–13.

22 Bryan S, Weatherburn G, Bungay H, et al. The cost-effectiveness of magnetic resonance imaging for investigation of the knee joint. *Health Technology Assessment* 2001; **5**(27).

23 Rose NE, Gold SM. A comparison of accuracy between clinical examination and magnetic resonance imaging in the diagnosis of meniscal and anterior cruciate ligament tears. *Arthroscopy* 1996;**12**(4):398–405.

24 Muellner T, Weinstabl R, Schabus R, Vecsei V, Kainberger F. The diagnosis of meniscal tears in athletes. A comparison of clinical and magnetic resonance imaging investigations. *Am J Sports Med* 1997;**25**(1):7–12.

25 Oei EH, Nikken JJ, Verstijnen AC, Ginai AZ, Myriam Hunink MG. MR imaging of the menisci and cruciate ligaments: a systematic review. *Radiology* 2003;**226**(3):837–48.

26 American College of Radiology (ACR). *Expert Appropriateness Criteria for Acute Trauma to the Knee.* American College of Radiology, Reston, VA, 2005.

27 Bleakley C, McDonough S, MacAuley D. The use of ice in the treatment of acute soft-tissue injury: a systematic review of randomized controlled trials. *Am J Sports Med* 2004;**32**(1):251–61.

28 Woo WW, Man SY, Lam PK, Rainer TH. Randomized double-blind trial comparing oral paracetamol and oral nonsteroidal antiinflammatory drugs for treating pain after musculoskeletal injury. *Ann Emerg Med* 2005;**46**(4):352–61.

29 Hart L. NSAID compared with paracetamol for pain after traumatic musculoskeletal injury (Editorial). *Clin J Sport Med* 2006;**16**(4):379–81.

30 Lovell SJ, Taira T, Rodriguez E, Wackett A, Gulla J, Singer AJ. Comparison of valdecoxib and an oxycodone-acetaminophen combination for acute musculoskeletal pain in the emergency department: a randomized controlled trial. *Acad Emerg Med* 2004;**11**(12):1278–82.

31 Mason L, Moore RA, Edwards JE, Derry S, McQuay HJ. Topical NSAIDs for acute pain: a meta-analysis. *BMC Fam Pract* 2004;**5**:10.

32 Cawley PW, France EP, Paulos LE. The current state of functional knee bracing research. A review of the literature. *Am J Sports Med* 1991;**19**(3):226–33.

33 Trees AH, Howe TE, Dixon J, White L. Exercise for treating isolated anterior cruciate ligament injuries in adults. *Cochrane Database Syst Rev* 2005;**4**:CD005316.

34 Heintjes E, Berger MY, Bierma-Zeinstra SM, Bernsen RM, Verhaar JA, Koes BW. Exercise therapy for patellofemoral pain syndrome. *Cochrane Database Syst Rev* 2003;**4**:CD003472.

35 Rupp RE. Evaluation of knee consultations to a referral-only orthopedic clinic in a managed care system. *Orthopedics* 2001;**24**(2):153–6.

36 Robb G. General practitioner diagnosis and management of acute knee injuries: summary of an evidence-based guideline. *NZ Med J* 2007;**120**(1249):1–13.

33 Wrist Injuries

Sandy L. Dong & Brian H. Rowe

Department of Emergency Medicine, University of Alberta, Edmonton, Canada

Clinical scenario

A 30-year-old healthy male presents to the emergency department (ED) after suffering from a fall onto an outstretched hand. He complains of pain and swelling in his right wrist. On examination, he has tenderness to the anatomic snuff box and axial loading of the thumb. There is minimal swelling and the hand is neurovascularly intact. Plain radiographs of the wrist with scaphoid views are unremarkable.

Due to the clinical suspicion of a scaphoid injury, the patient's wrist is immobilized with a cast that includes the thumb ("thumb spica"). He is instructed to follow up with his family physician in 10–14 days for reassessment and repeat radiographs. The patient wishes to know if the cast is necessary if the radiographs are normal.

Background

The wrist comprises the distal radioulnar joint, the radiocarpal joint and the midcarpal joints. It includes the distal radius, distal ulna, scaphoid, lunate, triquetrum, pisiform, trapezium, trapezoid, capitate and hamate. It is a complex joint capable of flexion, extension and medial and lateral deviation, and is involved in both pronation and supination. The complex articulations and strength of the joint are dependent on the integrity of the bones, ligaments and articulations.

Acute wrist injuries usually result from a fall onto an outstretched hand, with either hyperflexion or hyperextension of the wrist joint, and may be combined with supination or pronation. Although most wrist fractures are evident on either clinical or plain radiographic examination, some can provide a diagnostic challenge. According to one study from Northern Ireland, most wrist injuries occur in males, with two peaks – between 11 and 15

years and between 21 and 25 years of age [1]. There was an even distribution between right and left limb, although the dominant limb was more commonly injured.

An emergency physician, with orthopedic follow-up, can manage most closed wrist injuries; however, complex, penetrating and open fractures of the wrist should be managed aggressively by hand/orthopedic specialists. Displaced wrist fractures usually require some form of procedural sedation, manipulation in the ED and close follow-up, usually with orthopedic specialists.

This chapter focuses on several of the common wrist injuries seen in the ED.

Clinical questions

1 In patients with a painful traumatic wrist injury (population), what is the sensitivity and specificity (diagnostic test characteristics) of plain radiographs (test) to detect acute scaphoid fractures (outcome)?

2 In patients with a suspected scaphoid fracture (population), does the use of advanced imaging (intervention) reduce the need for casting and improve quality of life (outcomes) compared to conservative casting and 10–14-day follow-up (control)?

3 In patients with a painful traumatic wrist injury (population), is magnetic resonance imaging (intervention) as sensitive as a bone scan (control) for detecting acute scaphoid fractures?

4 In patients with a painful traumatic wrist injury (population), is there a valid clinical decision rule (test/rule) sufficiently sensitive and specific (diagnostic test characteristics) to guide clinicians in the evaluation of a possible scaphoid fracture (outcome)?

5 In patients with radiographically negative but clinically suspected scaphoid fractures (population), does thumb immobilization (intervention) reduce the pain and improve functional outcomes (outcomes) compared to conservative measures without immobilization (control)?

6 In patients with a displaced fracture of the distal radius (population), which method of analgesia (intervention/control) is most effective?

Evidence-based Emergency Medicine. Edited by Brian H. Rowe
© 2009 Blackwell Publishing, ISBN: 978-1-4051-6143-5.

7 In patients with a displaced fracture of the distal radius (population), are specific maneuvers (interventions) more successful at achieving adequate reduction (outcome) than others (control)?

8 In patients with a displaced fracture of the distal radius (population), does operative management (intervention) reduce pain and disability and improve time to normal activities (outcomes) compared to closed reduction and casting (control)?

9 In older patients (>59 years) with a displaced fracture of the distal radius (population), does facilitated management (intervention) improve osteoporosis-preventive practices and reduce future fractures (outcomes) compared to regular return to orthopedic or primary care clinics (control)?

General search strategy

The literature search will start with the common electronic medical databases such as MEDLINE and EMBASE. These databases will be searched to answer questions of therapy, diagnostic accuracy and for clinical decision rules. The Cochrane Library will also be searched for questions related to therapeutic alternatives.

Critical review of the literature

Question 1: In patients with a painful traumatic wrist injury (population), what is the sensitivity and specificity (diagnostic test characteristics) of plain radiographs (test) to detect acute scaphoid fractures (outcome)?

Search strategy

- MEDLINE and EMBASE: (scaphoid AND sensitivity and specificity) OR (scaphoid AND radiography)

Most emergency medicine texts report that plain radiographs can fail to detect scaphoid fractures and recommend immobilization for 10–14 days with a repeat examination at that time [2]. Lozano-Calderòn et al. compared plain scaphoid radiographs read by senior hand residents, hand fellows and attending surgeons to a combined gold standard of wrist arthroscopy, radiographs and computerized tomography (CT) read by a musculoskeletal radiologist and the treating surgeon. The sensitivity of the radiographs was only 75% (95% CI: 67% to 88%) and the specificity was only 64% (95% CI: 52% to 70%) [3]. These numbers equate to a positive likelihood ratio of 2.08 and a negative likelihood ratio of 0.39; neither of these values would be sufficient to rule in or rule out the diagnosis. It is unclear how an emergency physician would compare to trained hand surgeons when reading the plain radiographs; however, we would not expect emergency physicians to be markedly better than hand consultants.

Annamalai and Raby evaluated two indirect signs of scaphoid injury (scaphoid and pronator fat stripes) on scaphoid radiographs, read by a musculoskeletal radiologist. The gold standard in this study was magnetic resonance imaging (MRI). All radiographs were obtained from patients with clinically suspected scaphoid fractures but with normal radiographs as interpreted by the emergency physician and radiologist. The scaphoid fat stripe had a sensitivity and a specificity of 50%, leading to positive and negative likelihood ratios of 1.00. The pronator fat stripe had a sensitivity of 26% and a specificity of 70%. The positive likelihood ratio was 0.87 and the negative likelihood ratio was 1.06, suggesting that these two indirect radiographic signs should not be used to evaluate a possible occult scaphoid injury [4].

The evidence suggests that plain radiographs are inadequately sensitive to rule out a scaphoid fracture when clinical suspicion is present. The current practice of immobilization and follow-up re-evaluation should not be changed based on the current evidence.

Question 2: In patients with a suspected scaphoid fracture (population), does the use of advanced imaging (intervention) reduce the need for casting and improve quality of life (outcomes) compared to conservative casting and 10–14-day follow-up (control)?

Search strategy

- MEDLINE and EMBASE: (scaphoid bone OR carpal bones) AND (radionucleotide imaging OR magnetic resonance imaging)
- Cochrane Library: scaphoid fracture

One trial randomized 28 patients with clinical suspicion of scaphoid fracture but normal radiographs to either early (within 5 days) MRI or standard of care, which was immobilization and follow-up. The MRI group had a significant decrease in the number of days until a diagnosis of scaphoid fracture was made and a significant decrease in the number of unnecessary days in a cast. The MRI group demonstrated a non-significant increase in health care costs [5].

There were no studies evaluating outcomes with bone scans. Overall, more sophisticated tests for a scaphoid fracture do not exist. At the present time, there is insufficient evidence to suggest all patients with a suspected scaphoid fracture with a negative radiograph should be offered a special/confirmatory radiographic imaging modality.

Question 3: In patients with a painful traumatic wrist injury (population), is magnetic resonance imaging (intervention) as sensitive as a bone scan (control) for detecting acute scaphoid fractures?

Search strategy

- MEDLINE and EMBASE: (scaphoid OR carpal bones) AND (radionucleotide imaging OR magnetic resonance imaging)

A best evidence topic (BestBETs) report was identified [6]. It identified four studies comparing MRI to bone scanning in patients with suspicion of acute scaphoid fractures but normal radiographs. The authors conclude that MRI is slightly superior to bone scan, unless the patient is claustrophobic, in which case a bone scan would be preferred. No other studies were found that were not identified in the report.

Overall, MRI may be a more valid approach to confirming of the presence of a scaphoid fracture. At the present time, there is insufficient evidence to suggest all patients with a suspected scaphoid fracture with a negative radiograph should be offered a special/confirmatory radiographic imaging modality.

Question 4: In patients with a painful traumatic wrist injury (population), is there a valid clinical decision rule (test/rule) sufficiently sensitive and specific (diagnostic test characteristics) to guide clinicians in the evaluation of a possible scaphoid fracture (outcome)?

Search strategy

- MEDLINE and EMBASE: scaphoid AND sensitivity AND specificity

Two studies were identified, both describing the same clinical decision tool for suspected scaphoid fractures. The prospective derivation study evaluated 18 clinical tests for scaphoid fracture, with a subset of seven of these factors used in a combination clinical decision protocol [7]. The scaphoid decision protocol is outlined in Table 33.1. The protocol determines that initial scaphoid radiographs are necessary if the patient scores ≥ 5 points. Patients who qualified for radiographs but had no fracture identified were managed with a bandage and the same clinical protocol was repeated after 2 weeks with further advanced imaging if necessary. Unfortunately, one of the major weaknesses of the study was that patients with less than 5 points on the protocol were discharged and not followed up in the study.

Table 33.1 Scaphoid decision protocol [7]. A positive score is considered to be ≥ 5 points.

Clinical tests	Points
Less of the concavity of the anatomic snuff box	1
The "clamp" sign (the patient marks the most scaphoid area as the most painful spot with a pencil)	4
Palmar tenderness of the scaphoid	2
Tenderness on axial compression of the thumb along the longitudinal axis	2
Pain on resisted supination	3
Pain on ulnar deviation, from a position of full pronation	4
Snuffbox tenderness	1

In the second pilot study with 31 patients, the reported sensitivity of the clinical decision rule was 100% [8]; however, the specificity was only 12.5%. In this pilot validation study, two patients initially had less than 5 points on the protocol but had other fractures identified on plain radiographs. Sixteen of the remaining patients had evidence of scaphoid fractures on radiographs, and the remaining 13 patients were followed after 2–3 weeks. Six of these 13 patients no longer had clinical signs of scaphoid fractures and were discharged without further imaging. The remaining seven patients underwent the scaphoid decision protocol again. Five of these seven had less than 5 points, but two had other fractures that were missed on the initial films. The remaining two patients, with 5 or more points on the protocol, underwent bone scans.

The derivation of this clinical decision protocol differs from that of other clinical decision rules [9]. First, the samples were small. Second, the failure to apply a "gold standard" test to rule out scaphoid fractures in all patients needs to be addressed. We await the results of a larger validation study of this clinical decision rule, with complete follow-up of all patients enrolled, regardless of the number of points achieved on the protocol. Until then, this clinical decision rule cannot be recommended.

Question 5: In patients with radiographically negative but clinically suspected scaphoid fractures (population), does thumb immobilization (intervention) reduce the pain and improve functional outcomes (outcomes) compared to conservative measures without immobilization (control)?

Search strategy

- MEDLINE: scaphoid AND immobilization
- EMBASE: (scaphoid fracture OR scaphoid bone) AND (fracture immobilization OR immobilization)

Current emergency medicine texts advise the use of a thumb spica as the method of immobilization for suspected scaphoid fractures [2]. In a study conducted by Clay et al., 392 patients with acute scaphoid fractures were randomized to either a thumb spica or a forearm gauntlet (described as a Colles' cast) that did not immobilize the thumb. Of the 292 (74%) patients followed for 6 months, there was no difference in the rate of scaphoid non-union [10]. The major drawback to the study is the loss of 100 patients to follow-up. However, since the patients in this study all had known scaphoid fractures, this practice is likely safe in patients with suspected scaphoid fractures, who would have a much lower incidence of disease and, potentially, any fracture would be less severe, since these would be not seen on the initial scaphoid views. Furthermore, healthy volunteers given a thumb spica had diminished hand function based on a standard hand function test when compared to a Colles' cast [11]. In summary, the evidence for the use of a Colles' cast is promising, and further research is needed.

Until such time, patient and provider preference should dictate the approach.

Question 6: In patients with a displaced fracture of the distal radius (population), which method of analgesia (intervention/control) is most effective?

Search strategy

- MEDLINE and EMBASE: (radius fracture OR wrist injuries) AND (anesthetics OR anesthesia OR analgesia)
- Cochrane Library: radius fracture AND analgesia

A Cochrane review was identified that examined the evidence for the relative effectiveness of the main methods of anesthesia, associated physical techniques and medications used to manipulate distal radius fractures in adults [12]. The anesthetic interventions considered were hematoma block, intravenous regional anesthesia, regional nerve block, sedation and general anesthesia. The review found 18 studies, all with poor methodological quality, mainly due to lack of confirmed concealed allocation and deficiencies in outcome assessment. Five trials provided evidence to support intravenous regional block over hematoma block in terms of better analgesia during the procedure and easier fracture reduction. The hematoma blocks were found to be quicker, easier to perform and less resource intensive. There was inadequate evidence to support any of the other methods in terms of relative effectiveness. Studies evaluating different physical techniques (e.g., injection site for intravenous regional anesthesia, technique for brachial plexus block) did not demonstrate improved effectiveness or safety.

No pooling of data was possible due to the different comparisons made (e.g., intravenous regional anesthesia vs hematoma block and sedation vs hematoma block) and incompatible outcome measures. The authors concluded that there was some indication that intravenous regional anesthesia provided superior analgesia to hematoma block, and recommended further research on the topic. In many EDs, procedural sedation is becoming a more common approach to achieving anesthesia for painful procedures such as fracture reduction [13]. Further research should include these methods.

Question 7: In patients with a displaced fracture of the distal radius (population), are specific maneuvers (interventions) more successful at achieving adequate reduction (outcome) than others (control)?

Search strategy

- MEDLINE and EMBASE: (radius fracture OR wrist injuries) AND (clinical trials OR randomized controlled trials)
- Cochrane Library: radius fracture

In summary, the evidence from different non-operative interventions for closed distal radius fractures fails to identify a superior approach. Until further evidence is available, emergency physicans should continue to attempt closed reduction and casting for the majority of these patients. Two systematic reviews were identified on this topic, one involving closed reduction and the other involving conservative treatment of distal radius fractures. Both reviews found that distal radius fractures most commonly occurred in elderly women [14,15]. The first systematic review focused on closed reduction methods for distal radius fractures and found insufficient evidence from randomized controlled trials to establish the relative effectiveness of different techniques [15]. Overall, there were three trials involving 404 patients. The three trials compared different novel reduction methods with manual reduction. The heterogeneity of the studies prevented a combination of results.

The second review examined conservative (non-surgical) techniques for treating distal radius fractures, including no reduction, closed reduction and delayed reduction, and different immobilization techniques [14]. Overall, there were 37 trials involving 4215 patients. The authors found poor study quality, and heterogeneity in terms of patient characteristics, interventions compared and outcomes. There was insufficient evidence to recommend one conservative method over another.

It is clear from these systematic reviews that study quality is a problem, as is heterogeneity in terms of patient selection, intervention and outcomes reported. A uniform reporting method and agreed-upon outcome measures would be beneficial to advance this area of research.

Question 8: In patients with a displaced fracture of the distal radius (population), does operative management (intervention) reduce pain, reduce disability and improve time to normal activities (outcomes) compared to closed reduction and casting (control)?

Search strategy

- MEDLINE and EMBASE: (radius fracture OR wrist injuries) AND (clinical trials OR randomized controlled trials)
- Cochrane Library: radius fracture

One systematic review was identified on this topic [16]. This review of English language studies excluded pediatric and geriatric age groups, but did not limit itself to comparisons of closed reduction methods. Overall, there were 31 articles identified. Two were prospective, randomized, comparative trials and two were non-randomized comparative trials. The remaining 27 papers were case series. The review could not perform a meta-analysis on the included studies because of poor study quality and lack of a uniform outcome assessment. However, the authors concluded that the comparative studies found that external fixation was favored over closed reduction with casting in this population. Additionally, one of the case series suggested that external fixation was superior to internal fixation.

Question 9: In older patients (>59 years) with a displaced fracture of the distal radius (population), does facilitated management (intervention) improve osteoporosis-preventive practices and reduce future fractures (outcomes) compared to regular return to orthopedic or primary care clinics (control)?

Search strategy

- MEDLINE and EMBASE: (radius fractures OR wrist injuries) AND osteoporosis
- Cochrane Library: radius fractures

Many patients who suffer a distal wrist fracture have suffered a "fragility" fracture – that is, one which would not have occurred in the setting of younger age and stronger bones. These patients are at risk for osteoporosis and future fractures (e.g., of the hip, spine or wrist) [17]. Moreover, there are a number of safe and effective treatments that reduce the risk of recurrent fracture by 40–60%. Despite this, studies indicate that only up to a half of women and men who suffer distal radius fractures are counseled to reduce the risk of osteoporotic fractures [18–23].

One potentially useful strategy would be to identify injured patients with typical osteoporosis-related fractures in the ED and target them for interventions. Since several osteoporotic fractures require hospitalization (e.g., hip, spine), the preventive care becomes the responsibility of the consulting physician and the patient's primary care provider. In wrist fractures, however, the role of the emergency physician or ED may be more important, since this population is at the greatest risk of future fracture and perhaps derives the greatest benefit from preventive treatment.

In a controlled clinical trial in two Canadian EDs, 102 patients (age > 49 years) with fragility distal forearm fractures were enrolled and followed to determine if osteoporosis testing and treatment increased with an enhanced intervention [24]. The enhanced intervention consisted of mailed physician reminders (containing treatment guidelines endorsed by local opinion leaders) and osteoporosis patient education pamphlets in the ED delivered by orthopedic technicians. Control patients received usual care including specific recommendations about fall prevention. Overall, the intervention increased bone mineral density testing rates from 17% to 62% ($P < 0.001$) and osteoporosis treatment rates from 10% to 40% ($P = 0.001$) within 6 months of fracture. Overall, this study demonstrated that a simple, yet multifaceted, intervention directed at patients and primary care physicians can increase the proportion of patients receiving osteoporosis testing and treatment after a fragility fracture. The intervention did not change the fracture rate in these patients; however, this study was not designed to determine the effectiveness of osteoporosis management

(considered already proven) and was limited to a short-term follow-up period.

In another US randomized controlled trial, patient-specific post-fracture advice was provided to the primary care provider via an electronic medical record and resulted in 51.5% of patients receiving bone densitometry and osteoporosis medication, compared to 5.9% in the control group ($P < 0.001$) [25]. A third group of patients, who received a specific patient education letter on osteoporosis as well as the electronic medical record notification to their primary care provider, experienced a 43.1% rate of bone densitometry and osteoporosis therapy ($P = 0.88$, compared to the electronic medical record group).

The implications for EDs are that post-fracture programs of these types may improve the overall health of the community, and should be considered part of our link to chronic disease management.

Conclusions

The patient described in the scenario should either be immobilized with repeat assessment in 10–14 days, or receive an early (within 5 days) MRI to rule out a scaphoid fracture. If the former approach is chosen, the patient would benefit from having a simple Colles' cast over a thumb spica.

Wrist injuries are common presentations to the ED, and two of the most common problems are Colles fractures of the wrist and scaphoid injuries. In most injuries, decision rules are not sufficiently developed to be useful and plain radiography is indicated, including dedicated scaphoid views when indicated. Patients with displaced scaphoid fractures should be casted for 6 weeks and followed by specialists for non-union. Patients with "clinical" scaphoid fractures should be casted for 10–14 days and if suspicion of fracture remains after casting, more advanced testing should be considered. When identified, Colles fractures should be reduced using regional anaesthesia or PSA. External fixation should be reserved for poor reductions and intra-articular fractures in young patients. Further evaluation of this question in an active area of research.

Acknowledgments

The authors would like to acknowledge Dr. Helen H. G. Handoll for providing suggestions for the manuscript.

Conflicts of interest

None were declared by Dr. Dong. Dr. Rowe was a co-investigator on the Majumdar paper [24].

References

1 Hill C, Riaz M, Mozzam A, Brennen MD. A regional audit of hand and wrist injuries. A study of 4873 injuries. *J Hand Surg* (Br) 1998;**23**(2):196–200.

2 Woolfrey KGH, Eisenhauer MA. Wrist and forearm. In: Marx JA, Hockberger RS, Walls RM, eds. *Rosen's Emergency Medicine: Concepts and clinical practice*, 6th edn. Mosby, St. Louis, 2006.

3 Lozano-Calderòn S, Blazar P, Zurakowski D, Lee SG, Ring D. Diagnosis of scaphoid fracture displacement with radiography and computed tomography. *J Bone Joint Surg Am* 2006;**88**(12):2695–703.

4 Annamalai G, Raby N. Scaphoid and pronator fat stripes are unreliable soft tissue signs in the detection of radiographically occult fractures. *Clin Radiol* 2003;**58**(10):798–800.

5 Brooks S, Cicuttini FM, Lim S, Taylor D, Stuckey SL, Wluka AE. Cost effectiveness of adding magnetic resonance imaging to the usual management of suspected scaphoid fractures. *Br J Sports Med* 2005;**39**(2):75–9.

6 Foex B, Speake P, Body R. Best evidence topic report. Magnetic resonance imaging or bone scintigraphy in the diagnosis of plain x ray occult scaphoid fractures. *Emerg Med J* 2005;**22**(6):434–5.

7 Steenvoorde P, Jacobi C, van der Lecq A, van Doorn L, Kievit J, Oskam J. Development of a clinical decision tool for suspected scaphoid fractures. *Acta Orthop Belg* 2006;**72**(4):404–10.

8 Steenvoorde P, Jacobi C, van Doorn L, Oskam J. Pilot study evaluating a clinical decision tool on suspected scaphoid fractures. *Acta Orthop Belg* 2006;**72**(4):411–14.

9 Stiell IG, Wells GA. Methodologic standards for the development of clinical decision rules in emergency medicine. *Ann Emerg Med* 1999;**33**(4):437–47.

10 Clay NR, Dias JJ, Costigan PS, Gregg PJ, Barton NJ. Need the thumb be immobilised in scaphoid fractures? A randomised prospective trial. *J Bone Joint Surg Br* 1991;**73**(5):828–32.

11 Karantana A, Downs-Wheeler MJ, Webb K, Pearce CA, Johnson A, Bannister GC. The effects of scaphoid and Colles' casts on hand function. *J Hand Surg* (Br) 2006;**31**(4):436–8.

12 Handoll HH, Madhok R, Dodds C. Anaesthesia for treating distal radial fracture in adults. *Cochrane Database Syst Rev* 2002;**3**:CD003320.

13 Godwin SA, Caro DA, Wolf SJ, et al. Clinical policy: procedural sedation and analgesia in the emergency department. *Ann Emerg Med* 2005;**45**(2):177–96.

14 Handoll HH, Madhok R. Conservative interventions for treating distal radial fractures in adults. *Cochrane Database Syst Rev* 2003;**2**:CD000314.

15 Handoll HH, Madhok R. Closed reduction methods for treating distal radial fractures in adults. *Cochrane Database Syst Rev* 2003;**1**:CD003763.

16 Paksima N, Panchal A, Posner MA, Green SM, Mehiman CT, Hiebert R. A meta-analysis of the literature on distal radius fractures: review of 615 articles. *Bull Hosp Jt Dis* 2004;**62**(1–2):40–46.

17 Cuddihy MT, Gabriel SE, Crowson CS, O'Fallon WM, Melton LJ, III. Forearm fractures as predictors of subsequent osteoporotic fractures. *Osteoporos Int* 1999;**9**(6):469–75.

18 Feldstein A, Elmer PJ, Orwoll E, Herson M, Hillier T. Bone mineral density measurement and treatment for osteoporosis in older individuals with fractures: a gap in evidence-based practice guideline implementation. *Arch Intern Med* 2003;**163**(18):2165–72.

19 Castel H, Bonneh DY, Sherf M, Liel Y. Awareness of osteoporosis and compliance with management guidelines in patients with newly diagnosed low-impact fractures. *Osteoporos Int* 2001;**12**(7):559–64.

20 Cuddihy MT, Gabriel SE, Crowson CS, et al. Osteoporosis intervention following distal forearm fractures: a missed opportunity? *Arch Intern Med* 2002;**162**(4):421–6.

21 Khan SA, de Geus C, Holroyd B, Russell AS. Osteoporosis follow-up after wrist fractures following minor trauma. *Arch Intern Med* 2001;**161**(10):1309–12.

22 Freedman BA, Potter BK, Nesti LJ, Cho T, Kuklo TR. Missed opportunities in patients with osteoporosis and distal radius fractures. *Clin Orthop Relat Res* 2007;**454**:202–6.

23 Hooven F, Gehlbach SH, Pekow P, Bertone E, Benjamin E. Follow-up treatment for osteoporosis after fracture. *Osteoporos Int* 2005;**16**(3):296–301.

24 Majumdar SR, Rowe BH, Folk D, et al. A controlled trial to increase detection and treatment of osteoporosis in older patients with a wrist fracture. *Ann Intern Med* 2004;**141**(5):366–73.

25 Feldstein A, Elmer PJ, Smith DH, et al. Electronic medical record reminder improves osteoporosis management after a fracture: a randomized, controlled trial. *J Am Geriatr Soc* 2006;**54**(3):450–57.

34 Shoulder Injuries

Jenn Carpenter,[1] Marcel Emond[2] & Rob Brison[1]

[1] Departments of Emergency Medicine *and* Community Health and Epidemiology, Queen's University, Kingston, Canada
[2] Departments of Emergency Medicine and Family Medicine, Laval University, Quebec, Canada

Clinical scenarios

A 24-year-old hockey player arrived in the emergency department (ED) stating that he was checked into the boards. He was experiencing severe pain and very limited mobility in his right shoulder and said that his fingers had become "tingly". There was no obvious deformity of his shoulder, and distal strength and sensation testing were normal. The patient was tender both at the acromioclavicular (AC) and posterior shoulder and a full assessment was limited by pain. Radiographs of the shoulder and AC joints were normal. You suspected a rotator cuff tear and wondered about the best method to diagnose and manage such an injury.

A 50-year-old woman arrived in the ED complaining of left shoulder pain after a fall. On examination, her shoulder was swollen and diffusely tender. There appeared to be a "step" at her glenohumeral joint. The X-ray demonstrated an anterior glenohumeral joint dislocation. Your resident asked you whether the radiograph was required in the first place, what the best way to reduce the shoulder would be and what post-reduction management and follow-up he should suggest.

An 80-year-old woman arrived in the ED after a fall. She complained of left shoulder pain. On examination the shoulder was very swollen and diffusely tender and a radiograph demonstrated a proximal humeral fracture.

Background

Shoulder injuries are common presentations to the ED and often result in long-term disability. Injuries of the shoulder may involve damage to any of the structures in this very complex joint. The three most common injuries are a glenohumeral joint dislocation, acromioclavicular joint separation and a rotator cuff tear. This chapter will explore the diagnosis and management of two groups of shoulder injuries: fracture-dislocations and soft tissue injuries.

Anatomy overview

The shoulder is one of the most intricate joints in the body and is the most flexible. It owes its flexibility to the elaborate coordination of its bones, ligaments and muscles (Figs 34.1–34.3). Three bones compose the shoulder girdle: the scapula, the proximal humerus and the clavicle. Four articular surfaces are formed by these bones: the glenohumeral, acromioclavicular, scapulothoracic and sternoclavicular. The shallowness of the glenohumeral joint, which provides the joint's great flexibility, is stabilized by the cartilaginous labrum, the glenohumeral ligament and the rotator cuff. The rotator cuff, the dynamic portion of the stabilization, is comprised of four muscles (subscapularis, supraspinatus, infraspinatus, teres minor). These muscles also provide for the majority of the movement of the joint. Two other muscles of note are the biceps, whose long tendon runs in the groove between the greater and lesser tubercles of the humerus, and the deltoid, the most superficial muscle of the shoulder, which provides for the majority of the joint's abduction.

The diarthrodial AC joint only permits 5–8° of motion and is reinforced by both static and dynamic stabilizers [1]. The static ligaments that support the joint are: the AC ligaments (posterior, anterior, superior, inferior), the coracoclavicular (CC) ligaments (trapezoid and conoid) and the coracoacromial (CA) ligaments (Fig. 34.4). The muscles around the AC joint that permit stability and movement are the trapezius and the deltoid.

Shoulder dislocations

A shoulder dislocation is an important cause of shoulder injuries seen in EDs [2]. It is the most frequent dislocation reduced by emergency physicians [3] and most patients (70%) present with a first episode of anterior shoulder dislocation [4]. The reported prevalence in the general population is approximately 1.7% [5]. More than 95% of patients suffer an anterior shoulder dislocation; the posterior and erecta luxatio are seen rarely ($\leq 5\%$) and will not be dealt with in this chapter [6].

Evidence-based Emergency Medicine. Edited by Brian H. Rowe
© 2009 Blackwell Publishing, ISBN: 978-1-4051-6143-5.

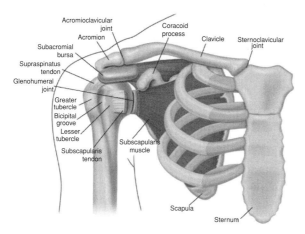

Figure 34.1 Anterior view of the shoulder. (Reproduced with permission from Anderson & Anderson [74], © 2007 UpToDate.)

Numerous investigators have described risk factors for shoulder dislocations among patients presenting in the ED. In particular, patient age seems to affect the incidence of shoulder dislocations [2,7,8]. A recent review series on shoulder dislocation dichotomized the management by using age 40 years or older as a meaningful cut-off based on associated injuries such as brachial plexus injury, rotator cuff tear or axillary artery injury [9,10]. Recently, age 40 and older has been also related to the presence of important fracture-dislocation [11].

Conservative ED and orthopedic management had advocated the use of pre- and post-reduction radiographs of the shoulder to

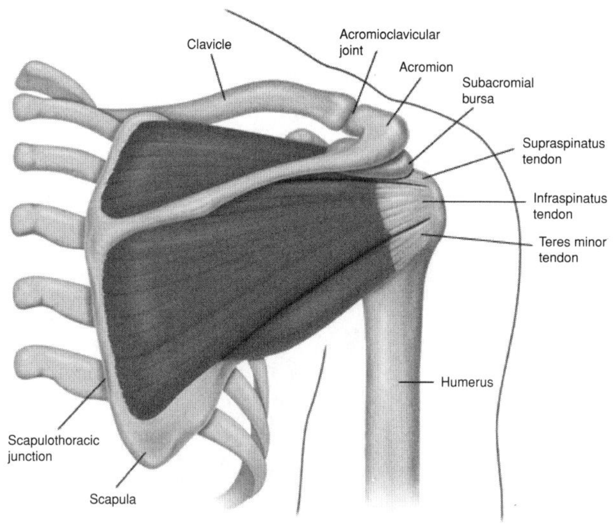

Figure 34.3 Posterior view of the shoulder. (Reproduced with permission from Anderson & Anderson [74], © 2007 UpToDate.)

confirm the diagnosis of shoulder dislocation and to identify any associated fractures [3,12–14]. In 2006, a survey of the management of first-time acute anterior shoulder dislocation confirmed use of this conservative approach [15], although this practice has been challenged recently [6,16,17].

Different techniques of reduction are available to emergency physicians confronted with an acute anterior shoulder dislocation [18]. Currently, the vast majority of patients have a closed

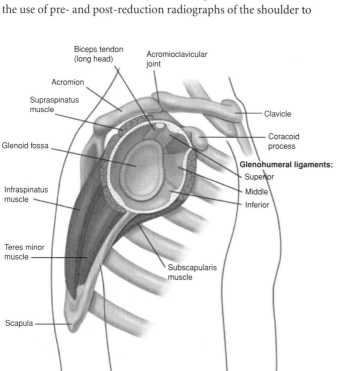

Figure 34.2 Lateral view of the shoulder. (Reproduced with permission from Anderson & Anderson [74], © 2007 UpToDate.)

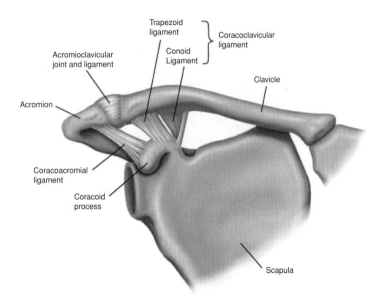

Figure 34.4 Normal shoulder ligaments. (Reproduced with permission from Koehler [75], © 2007 UpToDate.)

reduction under conscious sedation in the ED and then discharge with an appropriate follow-up plan [15]. Only patients with associated humeral neck fracture or irreducible dislocation will need open reduction by an orthopedic surgeon [19,20]. Associated fractures are diagnosed in about 6–25% of acute anterior shoulder dislocations [6,11,16,21,22].

Acromioclavicular joint separations

Injuries of the AC are now classified into six types. Types I, II and III were initially described by Tossy et al. and the classification system was finalized by Rockwood [23]. Type I is a minor injury in which the joint integrity is left intact. Type II injuries involve rupture of the AC ligaments, with maintenance of CC integrity. In type III injuries both the CC and the AC ligaments are torn, which allows complete dislocation of the joint. Type IV injuries have posterior dislocation of the clavicle with penetration of the trapezius fascia by the clavicle. Type V dislocations are superior but involve significant disruption of the deltotrapezial fascia. Finally, in type VI injuries, the clavicle dislocates inferiorly into the subacromial or subcoracoid positions.

Soft tissue injuries

Shoulder disorders are very common. Kuijpers et al. have quoted 1-year prevalence rates of anywhere between 5% and 47% in the general population [24]. The intricacy of the structures involved and the patient's intolerance to the physical exam due to acute pain often make specific diagnosis difficult in the ED. In the ED, identifying the specific soft tissue injury is often difficult, particularly for rotator cuff injuries. Patients are often in too much discomfort to fully partake in the physical examination required to determine the diagnosis, and conventional radiographs are often unhelpful. Many attempts have been made to find specific maneuvers that accurately differentiate which specific anatomic structures are

injured; however, to date, the literature has been conflicted as to the usefulness of such maneuvers.

When history and physical exam are inadequate to classify the injury, and when specific diagnosis of the injury is felt to be clinically important, radiological investigations can be employed. Since conventional radiographs are unhelpful in the diagnosis of soft tissue injuries, the most common modalities used in the diagnosis of soft tissue injuries of the shoulder are ultrasound and magnetic resonance imaging (MRI).

The correct management of suspected rotator cuff injuries has also long been elusive. As with undifferentiated soft tissue injuries of the shoulder, clinicians have long debated which management techniques would be most helpful, such as immobilization, physiotherapy and intra-articular or oral steroids. The management of AC joint injuries has also been the subject of much debate over the years. In addition to the management questions that characterize all soft tissue injuries of the shoulder – such as whether to mobilize or immobilize, the role of physiotherapy, and the role of steroids and non-steroidal agents – AC joint injuries raise the question of the appropriate indications for surgery.

Humeral fractures

Proximal humeral fractures account for 5% of all fractures and are about half as common as hip fractures. The incidence rapidly increases with age, and women are affected over twice as often as men [25]. Many patients who sustain a proximal humeral fracture are elderly. Recently published studies found that more than 80% of these fractures in adults resulted from falls from a standing height [26,27]. Bone quality also influences the appropriateness of any intervention and hence long-term clinical outcome. The majority of proximal humeral fractures are not displaced or only minimally displaced. For these fractures, conservative treatment is generally the preferred option. The arm is immobilized to maintain fracture stability. However, no specific period of time has been determined for these fractures. This is usually followed by physiotherapy and exercises aimed at restoring function and mobility. Hence, most patients are evaluated in the ED and discharged with an appropriate follow-up plan. Surgery is usually reserved for displaced and unstable fractures.

Clinical questions

In order to address the issues of most relevance to your patients above and to help in searching the literature for the evidence regarding these issues, you structure your clinical questions as recommended in Chapter 1.

1 In ED patients with shoulder injuries (population), are there any key features of the history or physical exam (tests) which are sensitive and specific enough (diagnostic test characteristics) to determine the presence of rotator cuff tears and labral tears (outcomes)?

2 In patients with suspected acute rotator cuff tears (population), what imaging modalities (tests) are the most sensitive and specific (diagnostic test characteristics) for confirming rotator cuff tears (outcome)?

3 In patients with confirmed acute rotator cuff tears (population), does any treatment (e.g., surgery or physiotherapy) (intervention) improve quality of life, reduce duration of pain and hasten return to activities (outcomes) compared to conservative management (control)?

4 In patients with confirmed AC joint separation (population), does early physiotherapy (intervention) improve quality of life, reduce intensity and duration of pain, and hasten return to activities (outcomes) compared to conservative management (control)?

5 In adults with a suspected acute anterior shoulder dislocation (population), which patients should have pre- and post-reduction radiographs in the ED (intervention) without missing any important fracture-dislocation (outcome)?

6 In patients with confirmed anterior shoulder dislocation (population), which method for reduction (intervention) is the most effective and has the lower rate of iatrogenic fracture (outcomes)?

7 In patients with a reduced, non-complicated shoulder dislocation (population), how long should the immobilization be for and which technique should be used (intervention) to prevent recurrence and provide recuperation of shoulder function (outcomes)?

8 In adults with a proximal undisplaced humeral fracture (population), does early mobilization (intervention) improve post-fracture shoulder function (outcome) compared to standard delayed mobilization (intervention)?

General search strategy

In order to address the specific questions on this topic, you search the Cochrane Library, MEDLINE and EMBASE database looking specifically for publications on shoulder injuries, including dislocation, AC joints, humeral factures and soft tissue injuries. Your interest was devoted to the diagnostic test characteristics of various imaging modalities for shoulder injuries or systematic reviews of those studies, as well as clinical prediction rules for patients with possible shoulder injuries. The Cochrane Library has only a few systematic reviews in those trauma topics. The Cochrane Library is useful for questions on therapy of some shoulder injuries; however, this area is not particularly well covered in the Library's databases. When a systematic review is identified, you also search for recent updates on the Cochrane Library and also search MEDLINE and EMBASE to identify randomized controlled trials (RCTs) that became available after the publication date of the systematic review.

Critical appraisal of the literature

Question 1: In ED patients with shoulder injuries (population), are there any key features of the history or physical exam (tests) which are sensitive and specific enough (diagnostic test characteristics) to determine the presence of rotator cuff tears (outcome)?

> **Search strategy**
>
> • Cochrane Library: (rotator cuff OR soft tissue shoulder) AND diagnosis
> • MEDLINE, EMBASE and EBM Reviews: (rotator cuff OR (soft tissue AND shoulder) OR shoulder injury OR shoulder joint OR shoulder pain) AND physical examination

Once fractures and glenohumeral dislocations have been ruled out in the patient presenting with acute shoulder injury, the clinician may find it difficult to differentiate what type of soft tissue injury has been sustained, often because the patient's acute pain limits the exam. If there were signs and symptoms that ruled in or out rotator cuff injury, it would make it worthwhile performing the full exam despite the discomfort that it would entail.

In his 2004 book, Luime presented a systematic review of studies describing historical features and/or clinical tests for the diagnosis of rotator cuff injuries [28]. His review was critically assessed in the Database of Abstracts of Review of Effects (DARE) [29]. There were 20 clinical tests reviewed in six studies. Though the evidence was limited, three tests may provide reasonable sensitivity and specificity. The Hornblower's test, which involves an inability to externally rotate the elevated arm, and the dropping sign, which is an inability to hold the affected arm in a position of 0° abduction and 45° external rotation with the elbow flexed at 90°, each have greater than 90% sensitivity and specificity for teres minor and infraspinatus tears. The internal rotation lag sign, which has the patient holding their arm behind the back with the palm facing outward without touching their back while the examiner supports only their elbow, had greater than 90% sensitivity and specificity for partial or full tears of the supraspinatus and/or infraspinatus.

A study by Litaker et al. [30] in which one orthopedic surgeon examined 448 patients prior to double-contrast arthroscopy, showed no correlation for individual tests. Using logistic regression, the authors determined that a combination of age over 65 years, night pain and weakness on external rotation was highly suggestive of rotator cuff injury, but this study was not conducted on patients in the acute phase of their injury and therefore is of little use to the emergency physician.

Murrell and Walton [31] published a two-part study in the *Lancet* in 2001 in which an orthopedic surgeon examined 400 patients with and without rotator cuff injuries and identified three clinical tests that were predictive of rotator cuff injury: supraspinatus weakness, weakness of external rotation, and impingement in internal and/or external rotation). They then validated their predictive rule and found that patients with all three positives, or two positives and age over 60 years, had a 98% chance of having a rotator cuff injury. The absence of these signs ruled out the diagnosis.

This information must also be considered with caution as many other studies [32,33] and reviews [34] have demonstrated very low accuracy of the physical exam to differentiate shoulder disorders, and only poor to moderate inter-observer agreement in the performance of the physical exam [35].

In summary, there is very little consistent evidence supporting the use of specific clinical tests in the diagnosis of rotator cuff injuries, especially in the acute phases of injury. Tests that have been found to have both excellent specificity and sensitivity are the Hornblower test, the dropping sign and the internal rotation lag test. Two studies performed by orthopedic surgeons [30,31] both identified advanced age and weakness on external rotation as important components of their clinical diagnosis. Although these findings are encouraging, their clinical significance is unclear. At present, because of conflicting evidence, and because most research in the area has been conducted once the acute phase of the injury has subsided, the authors cannot highly recommend the use of any specific physical tests for diagnosis or to rule out soft tissue injuries of the shoulder by the emergency physician.

Question 2: In patients with suspected acute rotator cuff tears (population), what imaging modalities (tests) are the most sensitive and specific (diagnostic test characteristics) for confirming rotator cuff tears (outcome)?

Search strategy

- Cochrane Library: (rotator cuff OR soft tissue shoulder) AND diagnosis
- MEDLINE, EMBASE and EBM Reviews: (rotator cuff OR (soft tissue AND shoulder) OR shoulder injury OR shoulder joint OR shoulder pain) AND (tests OR ultrasound OR magnetic resonance)

As described in the previous section, diagnosis of shoulder pain and disability after injury begins with a careful history and physical exam. This clinical evaluation, however, is limited in the ED due to lack of sensitivity and specificity of the various elements of the evaluation and because patients can rarely tolerate a detailed physical examination acutely after an injury. Because of these facts, radiological tests provide an attractive addition to the task of diagnosis.

Once bony injury has been eliminated with clinical evaluation and/or plain radiographs, the diagnosis of rotator cuff tear may become a concern. Ultrasonography, MRI and magnetic resonance arthrography (MRA) may all be potential secondary imaging modalities for ED consideration. A 2003 systematic review examined the evidence for various diagnostic tests in the setting of soft tissue shoulder pain (Table 34.1) [36]. Reviewing 38 cohort studies, they found that ultrasound had a sensitivity of 0.87 (95% CI: 0.84 to 0.89) and a specificity of 0.96 (95% CI: 0.94 to 0.97) for full thickness tears. For partial tears, the sensitivity was reduced to 0.67 (95% CI: 0.61 to 0.73); however, the specificity remained high at 0.94. In 29 cohort studies MRI was found to have a pooled sensitivity of 0.89 (95% CI: 0.86 to 0.92) and a specificity of 0.95 (95% CI: 0.91 to 0.95). Using six cohort studies, they found that MRA had a sensitivity of 0.95 (95% CI: 0.82 to 0.98) and specificity of 0.93 (95% CI: 0.84 to 0.97). Considering the invasiveness and difficulty obtaining MRA in most centers, the modest increases in sensitivity and specificity will be outweighed in most instances.

In summary, both MRI and ultrasound are reasonable choices when the emergency clinician is faced with a patient in whom they suspect rotator cuff injury. Availability and preference at each center will surely play a role in decision making. Given the lower cost and increased sensitivity in partial tears, ultrasound should be preferable when both ultrasound and MRI are equally accessible. Because of the invasiveness, MRA should most likely be reserved to the discretion of the treating orthopedic surgeon.

Question 3: In patients with confirmed acute rotator cuff tears, does any treatment (e.g., surgery or physiotherapy) (intervention) improve quality of life, reduce duration of pain and hasten return to activities (outcomes) compared to conservative management (control)?

Search strategy

- Cochrane Library: rotator cuff tears AND treatment
- MEDLINE, EMBASE and EBM Reviews: (rotator cuff OR (soft tissue AND shoulder) OR shoulder injury OR shoulder joint OR shoulder pain) AND (treatment OR surgery OR physiotherapy)

A recent Cochrane systematic review examined the evidence for the various methods of treating rotator cuff tears [37]. Eight studies fit their inclusion criteria and involved the following interventions: dexamethasone injections, physiotherapy, acupuncture,

	Full thickness rotator cuff tear		Partial thickness tear	
	Sensitivity (95% CI)	Specificity (95% CI)	Sensitivity (95% CI)	Specificity (95% CI)
Ultrasound	0.87 (0.84 to 0.89)	0.96 (0.94 to 0.97)	0.67 (0.61 to 0.73)	0.94 (0.92 to 0.96)
MRI	0.89 (0.86 to 0.92)	0.95 (0.91 to 0.95)	0.44 (0.36 to 0.51)	0.95 (0.87 to 0.92)
MRA	0.95 (0.82 to 0.98)	0.93 (0.84 to 0.97)	N/A	N/A

Table 34.1 Sensitivities and specificities of diagnostic modalities in full and partial thickness rotator cuff tears.

MRA, magnetic resonance arthrography; MRI, magnetic resonance imaging.

nerve blocks, arthroscopic subacromial decompression, open repair, splinting in abduction and passive range of motion (ROM) exercises. Unfortunately, there were no studies that compared surgical to non-surgical interventions. The outcomes examined were varied, but all eight studies included pain and ROM as outcome. The only evidence that showed any difference between interventions was found by pooling data looking at arthroscopic versus open repair of rotator cuff tears. Although the evidence was weak, it did suggest some benefit to open repair when compared to arthroscopic repair. No other type of intervention showed any benefit over others studied. The authors commented on "non controlled open studies" that suggest that conservative treatment is better than surgical, but highlight that there is still no sound evidence for this. Another systematic review, which included observational studies in addition to trials [38], found some very weak evidence supporting the use of exercise therapy in shoulder injuries. They also suggested possible support for acupuncture, electrotherapy and steroid injections; however, the patient populations included in these studies appear to be those with chronic pain rather than injuries.

In summary, there is insufficient evidence to support the use of any specific interventions in rotator cuff tears, except possibly exercise therapy. The emergency physician should institute interventions such as non-steroidal anti-inflammatory drugs (NSAIDs), ice and physiotherapy because they are less invasive and expensive. In cases of significant pain and/or disability, it is reasonable to order imaging and refer to an orthopedic consultant on an outpatient basis for consideration of surgical repair until the literature provides more definitive evidence to guide our management.

Question 4: In patients with confirmed AC joint separation, does surgical management (intervention) improve quality of life, reduce intensity and duration of pain, and hasten return to activities (outcomes) compared to conservative management (control)?

Search strategy

- Cochrane Library: rotator cuff tears AND treatment
- MEDLINE, EMBASE and EBM Reviews: (acromioclavicular joint OR (soft tissue AND shoulder) OR shoulder injury OR shoulder joint OR shoulder pain) AND (treatment OR surgery OR physiotherapy)

Despite some weak observational evidence that between 14% and 30% of patients with grade I and II AC separations continue to have pain or disability 1 year after injury [39,40], there has not been much controversy in the literature for the non-operative treatment of type I and II AC separations. This treatment usually involves a period of ice and short-term immobilization in a sling, followed by progressive ROM and strengthening exercises [1]. Types IV, V and VI injuries do not incite any controversy either. The literature has been clear that these injuries require prompt referral to orthopedic surgeons for operative repair (despite a paucity of true evidence).

The management of type III injuries, however, has remained controversial. A 1998, somewhat limited, review of the literature by Phillips et al. [41] reviewed 24 studies involving 1172 patients. Of these studies, only two were RCTs, three were non-randomized trials of conservative (C) versus surgical (S) management; 14 studies only included S management and five included only C management. The systematic review concluded that outcomes were deemed satisfactory in 88% of the S group and 87% of the C group. The C group had a lower occurrence of long-term pain (4% vs 7%) and better ROM at outcome (95% vs 86% were normal or near normal). Strength was also deemed to be better in the C group (92% vs 87% had normal or near normal power). They determined that the three most common complications were need for further surgery (59% S vs 6% C), infection (6% S vs 1% C) and deformity (3% S vs 37% C). The "meta-analysis" of four of the five trials directly comparing conservative to surgical management demonstrated a non-statistical trend towards better outcome with conservative management.

It is important to bear in mind that this systematic review contains limitations because of the lack of appropriate randomized trials and because no heterogeneity was assessed. Two comparison studies are noteworthy, both of which were included in the meta-analysis. The first, a prospective randomized trial performed by Larsen et al. [42], demonstrated that outcomes were similarly good in most subjects in both the conservative and surgical groups. The second, performed by Bannister et al. [43], demonstrated an earlier return to work with conservative management.

In summary, it appears that conservative management including such modalities as immobilization, physiotherapy, NSAIDs and strengthening exercises are warranted for the majority of grade I, II and III AC separations. Because the evidence is still controversial for grade III injuries, the authors suggest referring these patients for outpatient orthopedic consultation when they are athletes (especially throwing athletes), when the injury involves their dominant extremity, and when cosmesis is a substantial concern. Grades IV, V and VI should always be referred to orthopedics.

Question 5: In adults with a suspected acute anterior shoulder dislocation (population), which patients should have pre- and post-reduction radiographs in the ED (intervention) without missing any important fracture-dislocation (outcome)?

Search strategy

- Cochrane Library: shoulder dislocation AND humeral fracture
- MEDLINE: (shoulder dislocation AND radiography [MeSH]) OR (shoulder dislocation AND therapy [MeSH]). Limits: adults, English or French, clinical trial or practice guidelines or randomized control trial or review, and humans
- EMBASE: equivalent search terminology as for MEDLINE was used

The investigation of patients with acute anterior shoulder dislocations seems to vary in different countries [11,15,44]; however, the use of both pre- and post-reduction radiographs has been advocated on both legal and patient care grounds [9,10,12–14]. The largest clinician survey of first-time anterior shoulder dislocation management confirms such practice [15].

The pre-reduction films may not always be needed if the physician is able to perform an appropriate clinical diagnosis. When experienced physicians are certain of their clinical diagnosis, radiographic findings are concordant [45]. Prospective validation of the emergency physicians' ability to perform adequate clinical diagnosis has been examined [6] by dichotomizing in two subgroups: recurrent and first-time dislocations. Accuracy of confident assessments was 100% (95% CI: 92% to 100%) and 98% (95% CI: 94% to 100%, respectively. Furthermore, those publications reported similar findings for the appropriateness of reduction diagnosis. Even though the latest studies were limited by lack of standardization and inter-observer agreement, evidence suggests that both set of radiographs are not essential when physicians are certain of their clinical diagnosis. Avoiding unnecessary radiographs will avoid inappropriate radiation exposure and shorten ED visit times [46].

Moreover, retrospective chart reviews demonstrated that newly visualized fractures were identified on post-reduction radiographs in only 2.8–8% of cases [16,17] – mainly Hill-Sach's deformities, which did not change the ED treatment. Furthermore, 1.7% of new avulsion fractures were detected in one retrospective cohort ($n = 131$); however, review by a second-blinded radiologist noted those fractures on the pre-reduction films [17]. A post-reduction radiograph rarely revealed any clinically significant abnormality and treating physicians should question such practice. From the patient care perspective, the radiographs are used to: (i) confirm humeral head position; and (ii) identify associated fractures that may alter management in the ED.

To date, only one retrospective derivation study has identified a set of factors linked to clinically important fractures associated with dislocation (excluding the Hill-Sach's deformity). The following set of clinical factors was associated with fracture and mandate pre-reduction radiographs [11]: age >40 years (OR = 5.18; 95% CI: 2.74 to 9.78), first episode of dislocation (OR = 4.23; 95% CI: 1.82 to 9.87) and injury mechanism (fight or assault/fall greater than 2.4 m (8 feet)/motor vehicle crash, OR = 4.06; 95% CI: 1.95 to 8.48). A predictive model using any one of the three factors achieved a sensitivity of 97.7% (95% CI: 91.8% to 99.4%), a specificity of 22.9% (95% CI: 18.1% to 28.5%) and a negative predictive value of 96.6% (95% CI: 88.3% to 99.6%). Although this rule offers a safe reduction of pre-reduction radiographs by more than 20% while missing less than 5% of significant associated injury, it needs further prospective validation.

Two clinical algorithms have been suggested for investigation of acute shoulder dislocation (Figs 34.5, 34.6). While the Banff guideline (Fig. 34.5) lacks generalizability, it has been prospectively validated in a single rural community hospital with a convenience sample of young athletic patients by "experienced" physicians. Utilization of such an algorithm is not recommended until further prospective validation is completed [47,48].

The Hendey algorithm (Fig. 34.6) has been validated in a trauma center with a consecutive study population (mean age = 34 years), a 60% recurrent dislocation rate and few associated fracture-dislocations (7%). The algorithm was widely used by trainees and emergency physicians and reported an overall radiograph reduction of 46% without missing any significant injuries. It is the best evidence available for the investigation of patients sustaining acute shoulder dislocations. Without multi-center validation, however, this algorithm should be used with caution and only in settings with similar populations [47,48].

In summary, algorithms do exist for the approach to radiography for shoulder dislocations. However, until further validation research is complete, their employment should be used with caution and only in settings with similar populations.

Question 6: In patients with confirmed anterior shoulder dislocation (population), which method for reduction (intervention) is the most effective and has the lower rate of iatrogenic fracture (outcomes)?

Search strategy

- Cochrane Library: shoulder dislocation AND shoulder reduction
- MEDLINE (1966–2007): shoulder dislocation/therapy [MeSH]. Limits: adults, English or French, clinical trial or practice guidelines or randomized control trial or review, and humans
- EMBASE: shoulder dislocation AND (therapy OR reduction)

Over the years, many reduction techniques have been described for the treatment of shoulder dislocations – the Kocher, Milch,

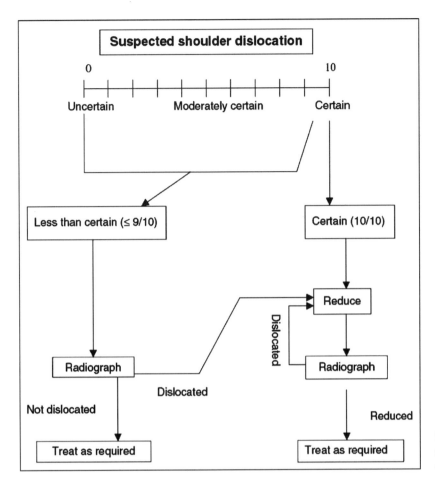

Figure 34.5 Banff shoulder dislocations guide. (Reproduced with permission from Shuster et al. [46], courtesy of the *Canadian Journal of Emergency Medicine*.)

Stimson, scapular manipulation, external rotation, Spaso and Zahiri methods have encompassed some of these procedures [49–60]. (Descriptions of these techniques are available in the previous references.) To date, no systematic review exists that assesses the success and iatrogenic fracture rates of all the available procedures.

Table 34.2 summarizes all the evidence on the most frequently used reduction methods in the recent literature: Kocher [61], Milch [62], scapular manipulation [60], external rotation [53] and traction–counter-traction. Only one study compared two reduction methods (Kocher vs Milch) [64] and it failed to identify a difference in success rates. Although this was an RCT with crossover design, it was methodologically flawed [68], did not complete the procedure using procedural sedation and analgesia as is the current norm [15], and for the most part did not reflect current practice of limited radiography and maneuvers.

In summary, there is no good evidence to support one maneuver over another in shoulder dislocation. Emergency physicians should become familiar with several approaches to shoulder reduction.

Question 7: In patients with a reduced, non-complicated shoulder dislocation (population), how long should immobilization be for and which techniques should be used (intervention) to prevent recurrence and provide recuperation of shoulder function (outcomes)?

Search strategy

- Cochrane Library: shoulder dislocation AND shoulder immobilization
- MEDLINE: shoulder dislocation/therapy [MeSH]. Limits: adults, English or French, clinical trial or practice guidelines or randomized control trial or review, and humans
- EMBASE: shoulder dislocation AND (therapy OR immobilization)

In 2004, a survey of European physicians revealed that most patients were immobilized in a internal rotation position for a mean duration of 4 weeks (range, 1 to 12 weeks) following shoulder dislocations [15]. Some evidence suggests that 1 week was

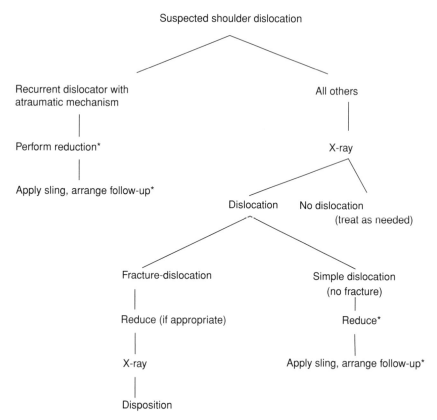

Suspected shoulder dislocation

Recurrent dislocator with atraumatic mechanism

All others

Perform reduction*

X-ray

Apply sling, arrange follow-up*

Dislocation

No dislocation (treat as needed)

Fracture-dislocation

Simple dislocation (no fracture)

Reduce (if appropriate)

Reduce*

X-ray

Apply sling, arrange follow-up*

Disposition

Figure 34.6 Suggested Hendey algorithm for the management of patients with suspected should dislocation. (Reproduced with permission from Hendey [6], courtesy of the *Annals of Emergency Medicine*.)

*If the physician is uncertain of dislocation or relocation, obtain radiographs

sufficient to prevent recurrence in patients older than 30 years, and 3 weeks in younger patients [69]. However, a 10-year observational report showed no effect of type or duration of immobilization [7]. A Cochrane Library search revealed one systematic review on the subject, published in 2006; the authors found no randomized or quasi-randomized studies on post-reduction duration of immobilization [70].

In 2007, an RCT of 198 patients experiencing an acute anterior shoulder were randomized to receive either internal or external rotation immobilization (Fig. 34.7) for 3 weeks [71]. The inclusion criteria were: (i) an initial anterior dislocation caused by a substantial traumatic event; (ii) presentation within 3 days after the dislocation; and (iii) no associated fractures of the shoulder detectable on routine radiographic examination. Compliance was 53% in the internal rotation group and 72% in the external rotation group ($P = 0.013$), and external rotation immobilization was preferred by patients. The external rotation group experienced significantly fewer recurrences than the internal rotation group (RR = 0.62; 95% CI: 0.40 to 0.96) – a relative risk reduction of 38% (number needed to treat (NNT) = 7; 95% CI: 4 to 62).

In summary, the external rotation immobilization method provides the best therapeutic evidence available; however, it should be investigated further before widespread use.

Question 8: In adults with a proximal undisplaced humeral fracture (population), does early mobilization (intervention) improve post-fracture shoulder function (outcome) compared to standard delayed mobilization (intervention)?

Search strategy

- Cochrane Library: humeral fracture AND immobilization
- MEDLINE (2003–2007): humeral fracture OR shoulder fracture [MeSH]. Limits: English or French, and clinical trial or randomized control trial
- EMBASE (2003–2007): (humeral fracture OR shoulder fracture) AND (therapy OR immobilization)

The care of proximal undisplaced fractures varies greatly among emergency and orthopedic physicians. A systematic review in the Cochrane Library reviewed the treatment of humeral fractures [72], and no other published article was identified since that review. Only one RCT, evaluating the length of immobilization [73], compared commencing physiotherapy within 1 week of fracture versus delayed physiotherapy after 3 weeks of immobilization in

Table 34.2 Summary of the techniques, evidence and success rates reported to reduce shoulder dislocations.

Methods	Success rate	Iatrogenic fracture rate	Type of evidence	Comments
Kocher	83%	Not reported	Small (n = 12) case series [63]	No sedation was administered; 50% had a recurrent dislocation
	80.9%	Not reported	Consecutive prospective case series [56]	
	77%	Not reported	RCT with crossover design [64]	Main outcome of study was the comparison of two different procedural sedation protocols
Milch and variants	94.5%	None	Case series [50]	No sedation was administered
	75%	Not reported	RCT with crossover design [64]	
Scapular manipulation and variants	79%	None	Prospective case series [52]	50% of patients had recurrent dislocation. No pre-medication in half of the patients
	92%	Not reported	Case series [60]	
	96%	None	Prospective consecutive case series [65]	58% had past episodes of dislocation
	90.5%	None	Prospective consecutive case series [66]	17.5% had recurrent dislocation and only 10% had procedural sedation
External rotation and variants	87.5%	None	Small (n = 18) prospective case series [58]	This variant involved vertical traction and external rotation
	90%	None	Prospective case series [49]	Unsuccessful in all cases of associated tuberosity fracture
Traction- or counter-traction variants	72%	None	Prospective case series [67]	No sedation. Analgesia with intramuscular NSAIDs

NSAIDs, non-steroidal anti-inflammatory drugs; RCT, randomized controlled trial.

a collar and cuff sling of 86 patients with undisplaced fractures. The study population included patients over 40 years old, with minimally displaced two-part fractures (Neer fractures), including isolated fractures of the greater tuberosity. The authors found that patients given early physiotherapy required fewer treatments

(mean difference = −5 sessions; 95% CI: −8.25 to −1.75) until independent shoulder function had been achieved (Fig. 34.8). At 16 weeks, patients in the early group had significantly better health-related quality-of-life scores in two sub-domains of a valid instrument. Shoulder function, relative to the unaffected shoulder, as

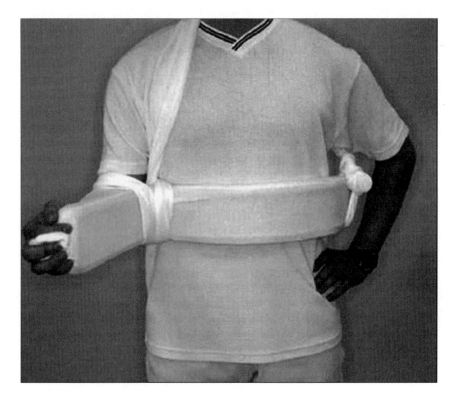

Figure 34.7 External rotation immobilization. (Reproduced with permission from Itoi et al. [71], courtesy of the *Journal of Bone and Joint Surgery, America*.)

Review: Interventions for treating proximal humeral fractures in adults

Comparison: 01 Early mobilization within I week vs immobilization for 3 weeks

Outcome: 01 Number of treatment sessions

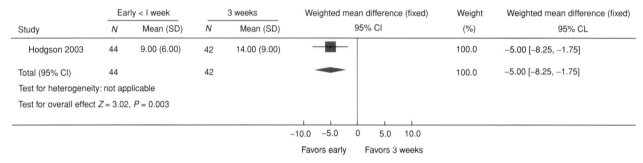

Figure 34.8 The effect of early mobilization on the number of physiotherapy sessions needed. (From Handoll et al. [72].)

measured with a pathology-specific score was statistically significantly better at 8 and 16 weeks.

In summary, early mobilization after 1 week benefits patients in the short term, but therapy results are similar after 1–2 years.

Conclusions

The 24-year-old hockey player had a rotator cuff tear diagnosed by ultrasound, and was referred to orthopedics for conservative management.

The 50-year-old woman had a left anterior shoulder joint dislocation demonstrated on radiography and the question was whether that radiograph could be deferred in favor of expedited management of the dislocation. For most shoulder injuries, it would be wise to confirm a dislocation prior to reduction efforts and identification of a concomitant fracture, which may alter management. However, many emergency physicians might elect to reduce the shoulder prior to radiography in well-documented recurrent dislocations. To date, an algorithm dictating the use of pre- and post-reduction radiographs lacks multi-center validation, but the application of Hendey's algorithm (see Fig. 34.6) would mandate such films. The patient's dislocation was reduced with procedural sedation (e.g., fentanyl and propofol) using the scapular rotation technique. As this was the patient's first episode, immobilization in external rotation was advocated for 3 weeks.

The 80-year-old woman with the humeral fracture was treated non-operatively, with immobilization, analgesics and early physiotherapy to avoid a frozen shoulder.

Overall, shoulder injuries are common presentations to the ED. Injuries can range from a contusion/soft tissue injury to rotator cuff strains; more severe injuries can include humeral fracture, AC joint separation or glenohumeral dislocation. This chapter reviewed the evidence-based diagnostic approach to these injuries and the unique features associated with treatment and follow-up.

Conflicts of interest

None were declared by Drs Carpenter and Brison; Dr. Emond has been involved in one of the studies cited in this chapter.

References

1 Bishop JY, Kaeding C. Treatment of the acute traumatic acromioclavicular separation. *Sports Med Arthroscopy Rev* 2006;**14**(4):237–45.

2 Kroner K, Lind T, Jensen J. The epidemiology of shoulder dislocations. *Arch Orthop Trauma Surg* 1989;**108**(5):288–90.

3 Mohamud D. Shoulder. In: Marx J, ed. *Rosens's Emergency Medicine: Concepts and clinical practice.* Mosby, St. Louis, 2002:576–606.

4 Hovelius L, Lind B, Thorling J. Primary dislocation of the shoulder. Factors affecting the two-year prognosis. *Clin Orthop* 1983;**176**: 181–5.

5 Hovelius L. Incidence of shoulder dislocation in Sweden. *Clin Orthop* 1982;**166**: 127–31.

6 Hendey GW. Necessity of radiographs in the emergency department management of shoulder dislocations. *Ann Emerg Med* 2000;**36**(2):108–13.

7 Hovelius L, Augustini BG, Fredin H, et al. Primary anterior dislocation of the shoulder in young patients. A ten-year prospective study. *J Bone Joint Surg Am* 1996;**78**(11):1677–84.

8 Simonet WT, Cofield RH. Prognosis in anterior shoulder dislocation. *Am J Sports Med* 1984;**12**(1):19–24.

9 Cleeman E, Flatow EL. Shoulder dislocations in the young patient. *Orthop Clin North Am* 2000;**31**(2):217–29.

10 Stayner LR, Cummings J, Andersen J, et al. Shoulder dislocations in patients older than 40 years of age. *Orthop Clin North Am* 2000;**31**(2):231–9.

11 Emond M, Le Sage N, Lavoie A, et al. Clinical factors predicting fractures associated with an anterior shoulder dislocation. *Acad Emerg Med* 2004;**11**(8):853–8.

12 Blake R, Hoffman J. Emergency department evaluation and treatment of the shoulder and humerus. *Emerg Med Clin North Am* 1999;**17**(4):859–76, vi.

13 Uehara D, Rudzinski J. Injuries to the shoulder complex and humerus. In: Tintinalli J, ed. *Emergency Medicine. A comprehensive study guide.* McGraw-Hill, New York, 1999:1783–91.

14 Wirth AM, Rockwood CA. Subluxations and dislocations about the glenohumeral joint. In: *Rockwood and Green's Fractures in Adults.* Lippincott-Raven, 2001:1100–140.

15 Chong M, Karataglis D, Learmonth D. Survey of the management of acute traumatic first-time anterior shoulder dislocation among trauma clinicians in the UK. *Ann R Coll Surg Engl* 2006;**88**(5):454–8.

16 Harvey RA, Trabulsy ME, Roe L. Are postreduction anteroposterior and scapular Y views useful in anterior shoulder dislocations? *Am J Emerg Med* 1992;**10**(2):149–51.

17 Hendey GW, Kinlaw K. Clinically significant abnormalities in postreduction radiographs after anterior shoulder dislocation. *Ann Emerg Med* 1996;**28**(4):399–402.

18 Zahiri CA, Zahiri H, Tehrany F. Anterior shoulder dislocation reduction technique – revisited. *Orthopedics* 1997;**20**(6):515–21.

19 Ferkel RD, Hedley AK, Eckardt JJ. Anterior fracture-dislocations of the shoulder: pitfalls in treatment. *J Trauma* 1984;**24**(4):363–7.

20 Hersche O, Gerber C. Iatrogenic displacement of fracture-dislocations of the shoulder. A report of seven cases. *J Bone Joint Surg Br* 1994;**76**(1):30–3.

21 Hovelius L, Eriksson K, Fredin H, et al. Recurrences after initial dislocation of the shoulder. Results of a prospective study of treatment. *J Bone Joint Surg Am* 1983;**65**(3):343–9.

22 Simonet WT, Melton LJ, III, Cofield RH, et al. Incidence of anterior shoulder dislocation in Olmsted County, Minnesota. *Clin Orthop* 1984;**186**:186–91.

23 Rockwood CA, Jr. Injuries to acromioclavicular joints. In: Rockwood CA, Jr., Green DP, eds. *Fractures in Adults*, Vol. 1, 2nd edn. JB Lippincott, Philadelphia, 1984:860–910, 974–82.

24 Kuijpers T, van der Windt DA, van der Heijden GJ, et al. Systematic review of prognostic cohort studies on shoulder disorders. *Pain* 2004;**109**(3):420–31.

25 Lind T, Kroner K, Jensen J. The epidemiology of fractures of the proximal humerus. *Arch Orthop Trauma Surg* 1989;**108**(5):285–7.

26 Lind T, Kroner K, Jensen J. The epidemiology of fractures of the proximal humerus. *Arch Orthop Trauma Surg* 1989;**108**(5):285–7.

27 Court-Brown CM, Garg A, McQueen MM. The epidemiology of proximal humeral fractures. *Acta Orthop Scand* 2001;**72**(4):365–71.

28 Luime J. *Shoulder Complaints: The occurrence, course and diagnosis.* Optima BV, Rotterdam, 2004:109–32.

29 Centre for Reviews and Diagnostic evaluation of shoulder pain: a systematic review on the accuracy of signs and symptoms related to rotator cuff disorders (Structured abstract). *Database Abstracts Rev Effects* 2007;**1**.

30 Litaker D, Pioro M, El Bilbeisi H, et al. Returning to the bedside: using the history and physical examination to identify rotator cuff tears. *J Am Geriatrics Soc* 2000;**48**(12):1633–7.

31 Murrell GA, Walton JR. Diagnosis of rotator cuff tears. *Lancet* 2001;**357**(9258):769–70 (erratum in *Lancet* 2001;**357**(9266):1452).

32 Naredo E, Aguado P, De Miguel E, et al. Painful shoulder: comparison of physical examination and ultrasonographic findings. *Ann Rheum Dis* 2002;**61**(2):132–6.

33 Riddle D. Individual tests from the history and physical examination are inaccurate in diagnosing rotator cuff tears. *Aust J Physiother* 2001;**47**(4):297–8.

34 Marx RG, Bombardier C, Wright JG. What do we know about the reliability and validity of physical examination tests used to examine the upper extremity? *J Hand Surg Am* 1999;**24**(1):185–93.

35 de Winter AF, Jans MP, Scholten RJ, et al. Diagnostic classification of shoulder disorders: interobserver agreement and determinants of disagreement. *Ann Rheum Dis* 1999;**58**(5):272–7.

36 Dinnes J, Loveman E, McIntyre L, et al. The effectiveness of diagnostic tests for the assessment of shoulder pain due to soft tissue disorders: A systematic review. *Health Technology Assessment* 2003;**7**(2).

37 Ejnisman B, Andreoli CV, Soares BGO, et al. Interventions for tears of the rotator cuff in adults. *Cochrane Database Syst Rev* 2007;**1**.

38 Grant HJ, Arthur A, Pichora DR. Evaluation of interventions for rotator cuff pathology: a systematic review. *J Hand Ther* 2004;**17**(2):274–99.

39 Mouhsine E, Garofalo R, Crevoisier X, et al. Grade I and II acromioclavicular dislocations: results of conservative treatment. *J Shoulder Elbow Surg* 2003;**12**(6):599–602.

40 Shaw MB, McInerney JJ, Dias JJ, et al. Acromioclavicular joint sprains: the post-injury recovery interval. *Injury* 2003;**34**(6):438–42.

41 Phillips AM, Smart C, Groom AF. Acromioclavicular dislocation. Conservative or surgical therapy. *Clin Orthop Relat Res* 1998;**353**:10–17.

42 Larsen E, Bjerg-Nielsen A, Christensen P. Conservative or surgical treatment of acromioclavicular dislocation. A prospective, controlled, randomized study. *J Bone Joint Surg Am* 1986;**68**(4):552–5.

43 Bannister GC, Wallace WA, Stableforth PG, et al. The management of acute acromioclavicular dislocation. A randomised prospective controlled trial. *J Bone Joint Surgery Br* 1989;**71**(5):848–50.

44 Hendey GW, Chally MK, Stewart VB. Selective radiography in 100 patients with suspected shoulder dislocation. *J Emerg Med* 2006;**31**(1):23–8.

45 Shuster M, Abu-Laban RB, Boyd J. Prereduction radiographs in clinically evident anterior shoulder dislocation. *Am J Emerg Med* 1999;**17**(7):653–8.

46 Shuster M, Abu-Laban R, Boyd J, et al. Prospective evaluation of a guideline for the selective elimination of pre-reduction radiographs in clinically obvious anterior shoulder dislocation. *Can J Emerg Med* 2002;**4**(4):257–62.

47 McGinn TG, Guyatt GH, Wyer PC, et al. Users' guides to the medical literature. XXII. how to use articles about clinical decision rules. Evidence-Based Medicine Working Group. *JAMA* 2000;**284**(1):79–84.

48 Stiell IG, Wells GA. Methodologic standards for the development of clinical decision rules in emergency medicine. *Ann Emerg Med* 1999;**33**(4):437–47.

49 Eachempati KK, Dua A, Malhotra R, et al. The external rotation method for reduction of acute anterior dislocations and fracture-dislocations of the shoulder. *J Bone Joint Surg Am* 2004;**86A**(11):2431–4.

50 Garnavos C. Technical note: modifications and improvements of the Milch technique for the reduction of anterior dislocation of the shoulder without premedication. *J Trauma* 1992;**32**(6):801–3.

51 Kothari RU, Dronen SC. The scapular manipulation technique for the reduction of acute anterior shoulder dislocations. *J Emerg Med* 1990;**8**(5):625–8.

52 McNamara RM. Reduction of anterior shoulder dislocations by scapular manipulation. *Ann Emerg Med* 1993;**22**(7):1140–44.

53 Mirick MJ, Clinton JE, Ruiz E. External rotation method of shoulder dislocation reduction. *Jacep* 1979;**8**(12):528–31.

54 O'Connor DR, Schwarze D, Fragomen AT, et al. Painless reduction of acute anterior shoulder dislocations without anesthesia. *Orthopedics* 2006;**29**(6):528–32.

55 Ufberg JW, Vilke GM, Chan TC, et al. Anterior shoulder dislocations: beyond traction-countertraction. *J Emerg Med* 2004;**27**(3):301–6.

56 Uglow MG. Kocher's painless reduction of anterior dislocation of the shoulder: a prospective randomised trial. *Injury* 1998;**29**(2):135–7.

57 Westin CD, Gill EA, Noyes ME, et al. Anterior shoulder dislocation. A simple and rapid method for reduction. *Am J Sports Med* 1995;**23**(3):369–71.

58 Yuen MC, Yap PG, Chan YT, et al. An easy method to reduce anterior shoulder dislocation: the Spaso technique. *Emerg Med J* 2001;**18**(5):370–72.

59 Zahiri CA, Zahiri H, Tehrany F. Anterior shoulder dislocation reduction technique – revisited. *Orthopedics* 1997;**20**(6):515–21.

60 Anderson D, Zvirbulis R, Ciullo J. Scapular manipulation for reduction of anterior shoulder dislocations. *Clin Orthop Relat Res* 1982(164): 181–3.

61 Kocher T. Eine neue reductions methode fur schulter verrenking. *Berlin Klin* 1870;**7**(101).

62 Milch H. Pulsion-traction in the reduction of dislocations or fracture dislocations of the humerus. *Bull Hosp Joint Dis* 1963;**24**:147–52.

63 Chitgopkar SD, Khan M. Painless reduction of anterior shoulder dislocation by Kocher's method. *Injury* 2005;**36**(10):1182–4.

64 Beattie TF, Steedman DJ, McGowan A, et al. A comparison of the Milch and Kocher techniques for acute anterior dislocation of the shoulder. *Injury* 1986;**17**(5):349–52.

65 Kothari RU, Dronen SC. Prospective evaluation of the scapular manipulation technique in reducing anterior shoulder dislocations. *Ann Emerg Med* 1992;**21**(11):1349–52.

66 Baykal B, Sener S, Turkan H. Scapular manipulation technique for reduction of traumatic anterior shoulder dislocations: experiences of an academic emergency department. *Emerg Med J* 2005;**22**(5):336–8.

67 Noordeen MH, Bacarese-Hamilton IH, Belham GJ, et al. Anterior dislocation of the shoulder: a simple method of reduction. *Injury* 1992;**23**(7):479–80.

68 Ashton HR, Hassan Z. Best evidence topic report. Kocher's or Milch's technique for reduction of anterior shoulder dislocations. *Emerg Med J* 2006;**23**(7):570–71.

69 Kiviluoto O, Pasila M, Jaroma H, et al. Immobilization after primary dislocation of the shoulder. *Acta Orthop Scand* 1980;**51**(6):915–19.

70 Handoll HH, Hanchard NC, Goodchild L, et al. Conservative management following closed reduction of traumatic anterior dislocation of the shoulder. *Cochrane Database Syst Rev* 2006;**1**:CD004962.

71 Itoi E, Hatakeyama Y, Sato T, et al. Immobilization in external rotation after shoulder dislocation reduces the risk of recurrence. A randomized controlled trial. *J Bone Joint Surg Am* 2007;**89**(10):2124–31.

72 Handoll HH, Gibson JN, Madhok R. Interventions for treating proximal humeral fractures in adults. *Cochrane Database Syst Rev* 2003;**4**:CD000434.

73 Hodgson SA, Mawson SJ, Stanley D. Rehabilitation after two-part fractures of the neck of the humerus. *J Bone Joint Surg Br* 2003;**85**(3):419–22.

74 Anderson BC, Anderson RJ. Evaluation of the patient with shoulder complaints. In: Rose BD, ed. *UpToDate*. UpToDate, Waltham, MA, 2007.

75 Koehler SM. Acromioclavicular injuries. In: Rose BD, ed. *UpToDate*. UpToDate, Waltham, MA, 2007.

35 Chest Trauma

Shahriar Zehtabchi & Richard Sinert

Department of Emergency Medicine, Downstate Medical Center, State University of New York, New York, USA

Case scenario

A 23-year-old man was brought to the emergency department (ED) after being involved in a high-speed motor vehicle crash. The patient was not wearing a seat belt. According to emergency medical services (EMS) staff, the patient had to be extricated from the car, the front windshield was shattered, and the steering wheel was damaged. The patient experienced loss of consciousness (LOC) for an estimated 3 minutes. On arrival to the ED, the patient was on a backboard with a cervical collar. He was alert and oriented. His airway was patent and he had normal breath sounds. Radial pulses were palpable but fast bilaterally. There was no midline neck tenderness. There was a bruise on the anterior chest wall right on the sternum, which was tender to palpation. The abdomen was soft and non-tender. There was no obvious deformity in the extremities. The neurological examination was normal, with a Glasgow Coma Score (GCS) of 15. The patient was hypotensive (blood pressure = 95/68 mmHg), tachycardic (heart rate = 120 beats/min), tachypnic (respiratory rate = 20 breaths/min) and afebrile. Oxygen saturation (SaO_2) on room air was 93%.

Treatment included two large-bore antecubital intravenous catheters and initiation of a normal saline infusion. The patient was placed on 100% oxygen via a face mask. A chest radiograph revealed a small patchy infiltrate in the right lower lung field and fractures of two anterior ribs (first and second ribs). No pneumo- or hemothorax were identified and the mediastinum was not wide. An electrocardiogram (ECG) demonstrated sinus tachycardia with no ST-T abnormalities. A FAST (focused assessment with sonography for trauma) ultrasound exam revealed no pericardial effusion. Bedside echocardiography was performed and failed to reveal wall motion abnormalities or pericardial effusion. Serum cardiac markers were normal.

The care of this patient was assumed by the trauma team and your shift ended. During the sign out, a medical student asked whether you were confident that you had ruled out cardiac contusion, aortic rupture and diaphragmatic injuries. Another medical student was interested to know if simple observation would have been adequate for management of pneumothorax in this patient instead of inserting a chest tube. The student also asked about the role of antibiotic prophylaxis after chest tube insertion to prevent any infection.

Background

Trauma is the leading cause of death among persons less than 35 years old and the fourth leading cause of death of all ages in the United States [1]. Almost 25% of these trauma-related deaths, approximately 16,000 deaths per year, are due to thoracic injuries [2]. The majority of thoracic injuries occur following blunt trauma from motor vehicle crashes.

Intrathoracic injuries following chest trauma may occur in the chest wall, lungs and pleura, great vessels, trachea, bronchus, heart, diaphragm and esophagus. The extent of these problems and the great possibility of associated injuries call attention to the importance of complete evaluation, timely diagnosis and proper management of such injuries in ED trauma patients. Interestingly, the majority of intrathoracic injuries that occur after chest trauma are treated non-operatively by the appropriate application of the essential principles of trauma management, which are generally started in the ED (e.g., airway management, tube thoracostomy). Timely evaluation of these patients and utilizing appropriate diagnostic tests will also identify patients with serious injuries requiring operative management.

Clinical questions

In order to address the issues of most relevance to your patient and to help in searching the literature for the evidence regarding these

Evidence-based Emergency Medicine. Edited by Brian H. Rowe
© 2009 Blackwell Publishing, ISBN: 978-1-4051-6143-5.

issues, you structure your clinical questions as recommended in Chapter 1.

1 In ED patients with blunt chest trauma (population), what are the sensitivities and specificities (diagnostic test characteristics) of electrocardiogram, cardiac biomarkers and echocardiography (tests) for identifying cardiac contusion (outcome).

2 In ED patients with blunt chest trauma (population), what is the sensitivity and specificity (diagnostic test characteristics) of plain chest radiography (test) in identifying traumatic aortic rupture (outcome)?

3 In ED patients with blunt chest trauma (population), what is the sensitivity and specificity (diagnostic test characteristics) of plain chest radiography (test) in identifying pulmonary contusion (outcome)?

4 In ED patients with small (occult) traumatic pneumothoraces (population), does treatment with observation alone (intervention) lead to less pain, improved quality of life or fewer complications (outcomes) compared to chest tube insertion (control)?

5 In ED patients with thoracic trauma requiring chest tube insertion for hemo- or pneumothorax (population), do prophylactic antibiotics (intervention) prevent infection (outcome) compared to standard care (control)?

6 In ED patients with blunt thoracic trauma (population), what is the sensitivity and specificity (diagnostic test characteristics) of a computerized tomography scan (test) in identifying diaphragmatic injuries (outcome) compared to chest radiography (control)?

7 In ED patients with blunt thoracic trauma (population), what is the sensitivity and specificity (diagnostic test characteristics) of ultrasound (test) in detecting pericardial effusions and tamponade (outcome)?

General search strategy

You begin to address these questions by searching for evidence in the common electronic databases such as the Cochrane Library, MEDLINE and EMBASE, looking specifically for systematic reviews. When a systematic review is identified, you also search MEDLINE and EMBASE to identify randomized controlled trials (RCTs) that became available after the publication date of the systematic review. In addition, consensus statements on chest trauma from trauma organizations were used when other evidence was unavailable.

Critical review of the literature

Your search strategy for the Cochrane Library and MEDLINE identified several pertinent and relevant articles to this series of questions.

Question 1: In ED patients with blunt chest trauma (population), what are the sensitivities and specificities (diagnostic test characteristics) of electrocardiogram, cardiac biomarkers and echocardiography (tests) for identifying cardiac contusion (outcome).

> **Search strategy**
>
> - MEDLINE and EMBASE: (electrocardiography OR creatine kinase OR troponin OR echocardiography) AND sensitivity and specificity AND (cardiac OR heart OR myocardial) AND (contusion OR trauma OR injury)

Cardiac contusion (also called blunt cardiac injury) has been reported in approximately 9–76% of patients sustaining blunt chest trauma [3]. This broad range originates from the wide variety of diagnostic criteria and definitions which are used for the diagnosis. Cardiac injuries may cause important complications such as arrhythmias, hypotension or anatomic defects such as valvular, septal or free wall rupture [4].

Cardiac contusion has been the topic of controversy in the trauma literature for many decades. Clinically, there are few reliable signs and symptoms that are specific for cardiac contusion [5]. Patients may have evidence of external chest trauma such as fractures or ecchymosis at the site of impact (by the steering wheel or other objects). At the same time, well-defined and uniformly accepted diagnostic criteria do not exist. The lack of a gold standard test does not allow the evaluation of sensitivity and specificity of different diagnostic tests proposed to detect cardiac injury. In the literature, the criteria for diagnosis vary from clinical suspicion to criteria based on ECG findings, serum cardiac biomarker (creatine phosphokinase-MB isoenzyme (CPK-MB) and troponin) determination, radionuclear imaging and echocardiography [6].

This search identified one meta-analysis [7] evaluating the utility of serum CPK-MB and troponin, abnormal ECGs, radionuclide scans and echocardiograms to identify patients at risk of developing cardiovascular complications following blunt cardiac trauma. This meta-analysis suffered from several limitations including lack of pre-set inclusion criteria for a reference standard or outcome measure, limited description of search strategy and data retrieval, and lack of adequate reporting of some of the key elements of a systematic review. Due to these serious flaws, the results of this meta-analysis do not provide clarity with respect to the question above.

Electrocardiography

Electrocardiogram changes have been widely used for predicting cardiac contusion in trauma patients. Unfortunately, ECG abnormalities observed in patients with cardiac contusion are non-sensitive and non-specific and could be a reflection of a wide variety of non-cardiac metabolic and organic abnormalities. Several animal studies [8,9] have demonstrated that cardiac contusion can result in non-specific ST-T abnormalities as well as a spectrum of conduction abnormalities. Building on these findings, Potkin et al. [10] studied the ECG abnormalities in 100 patients with severe blunt chest trauma and demonstrated that ECG changes were not predictive of cardiac complications or of myocardial contusion at necropsy in patients who died from these injuries. On the other hand, several studies have advocated the use of ECG for diagnosing or ruling out cardiac contusion. Christensen and Sutton [11] reviewed 18 studies involving more than 5000 patients from 1986 through 1992, noting that 80% of all arrhythmias requiring treatment were present on the initial ECG obtained in the ED. However, the rate of ECG abnormalities in general was difficult to analyze because there was no uniform definition for an "abnormal" ECG. Based on such studies, the practice management guidelines for trauma published by the Eastern Association for the Surgery of Trauma recommend that an ECG should be performed on all patients suspected of having cardiac contusion (level I recommendation) and if the admission ECG is abnormal the patient should be admitted for continuous monitoring (level II recommendation). These guidelines also suggest that if the admission ECG is normal, the risk of cardiac contusion is low and therefore such a diagnosis should not be pursued (level II recommendation).

Serum CPK-MB

The overwhelming majority of studies conclude that elevation of CPK-MB has very low sensitivity and specificity and is of limited value for diagnosing cardiac contusion. [12–14]. For example, one study, which enrolled 128 patients with cardiac contusion (defined as abnormal echocardiogram consistent with cardiac contusion, or arrhythmia/conduction abnormalities on ECG, or hemoperi-cardium), reported a sensitivity of 21% and specificity of 74% for the CPK-MB index (CPK-MB/CPK $\geq$5%) for diagnosing cardiac contusion.

Serum troponin

Cardiac troponins appear to be very specific but relatively non-sensitive tests in diagnosing cardiac injury. One study that used abnormal echocardiographic or ECG findings as a reference standard (Table 35.1), revealed a sensitivity of 31% and a specificity of 91% for troponin T in identifying cardiac injury. Another study [15] that prospectively reviewed 115 cases of clinically significant cardiac trauma (defined as cardiogenic shock, arrhythmias requiring treatment, or structural cardiac abnormalities directly related to the cardiac trauma) reported a sensitivity of 68%, specificity of 85%, negative predictive value of 93% and positive predictive values 48% for troponin I (at admission, at 4 hours and at 8 hours). Rajan et al. [16] also showed that elevated troponin I at admission or 6 hours after admission could predict arrhythmia and ventricular dysfunction in patients with blunt chest trauma. Other studies have confirmed these findings as well (Table 35.1) [17,18].

The ideal timing of blood sampling for troponin assays for diagnosing cardiac contusion has not been determined. Troponin can reach peak values earlier following cardiac trauma than after myocardial infarction. Despite this fact, it has been recommended that a second measurement should be taken after

Table 35.1 Summary of studies evaluating the operating characteristics of serum troponin (with or without ECG) in detecting cardiac contusion.

| Study | Population | Outcome | Test | Operating characteristics of the test | | | | | |
				Sensitivity	Specificity	PPV	NPV	+LR	−LR
Ferjani et al. [14]	128 patients with significant blunt chest trauma	Cardiac contusion: abnormal ECHO consistent with cardiac contusion or arrhythmias or conduction abnormalities or hemopericardium	Elevated Tn T	31%	91%	16%	82%	3.4	0.76
Bertinchant et al. [18]	94 patients with blunt chest trauma	Cardiac contusion based on ECHO and ECG criteria	Elevated Tn I Elevated Tn T	23% 12%	97% 100%	75% 100%	77% 75%	7.7 —	0.79 0.88
Edouard et al. [17]	724 trauma patients admitted to surgical ICU	Cardiac contusion based on ECG criteria	Elevated Tn I	63%	98%	40%	98%	31.5	0.37
Salim et al. [15]	115 patients with significant blunt chest trauma	Cardiac contusion: arrhythmias requiring treatment, pericardial effusion, unexplained hypotension, cardiogenic shock	Elevated Tn I Abnormal ECG Both	68% 84% 100%	85% 56% 88%	48% 28% 62%	93% 95% 100%	4.5 1.9 8.3	0.38 0.29 —
Velmahos et al. [24]	333 patients with significant chest trauma	Cardiac contusion: unexplained hypotension or arrhythmias requiring treatment or post-trauma anatomic abnormalities on ECHO or decreased cardiac index (< 2.5 L/min/m^2 body surface area)	Elevated Tn I Abnormal ECG Both	73% 89% 100%	60% 67% 71%	21% 29% 34%	94% 98% 100%	1.82 2.7 3.4	0.45 0.16 —

ECG, electrocardiography; ECHO, echocardiography; ICU, intensive care unit; +LR, likelihood ratio of a positive test; −LR, likelihood ratio of a negative test; NPV, negative predictive value; PPV, positive predictive value; Tn, troponin.

4–6 hours if troponin concentrations are within normal ranges on admission.

Echocardiography

Contused myocardial tissue not only resembles infarcted myocardial tissue histologically but also functionally [19]. Therefore, transthoracic echocardiography (TTE) can detect wall motion abnormalities that could be due to cardiac contusion. Transesophageal echocardiography (TEE) is more reliable in diagnosing cardiac contusion than TTE [20,21]. In a study of 117 patients highly suspicious of having cardiac contusion based on clinical criteria, investigators identified ventricular dysfunction in 42% of patients who underwent TTE [22]. In another study, 27% of patients who were diagnosed with cardiac contusion based on abnormal findings on TEE did not survive [23]. Despite these findings, it has been recommended that echocardiography (TTE or TEE) should be reserved as a complementary test in selected patients, rather than a primary screening tool.

Combination testing

Recent studies have proposed using a combination of ECG and serum troponin level for ruling out cardiac injury in hemodynamically stable patients (see Table 35.1), [24].

Summary

In summary, using a combination of ECG and serum troponin level appears to maximize the sensitivity and specificity of cardiac contusion diagnosis. Perhaps echocardiography is best reserved for confirmation of myocardial dyskinesia for prognostic purposes. In the setting of suspected cardiac contusion, a normal ECG and a normal serum troponin level would produce a post-test probability of <5%.

Question 2: In ED patients with blunt chest trauma (population), what is the sensitivity and specificity (diagnostic test characteristics) of plain chest radiography (test) in identifying traumatic aortic rupture (outcome)?

Search strategy

- MEDLINE and EMBASE: (radiography OR X-rays) AND chest AND aorta AND wounds and injuries AND sensitivity and specificity

Andreas Vesalius in 1557 first described traumatic thoracic aortic rupture (TAR) (as cited by Sailer [25]). Today TAR is most commonly associated with motor vehicle crashes, falls from height and crushing chest injuries. Approximately 80–85% of patients with aortic rupture will die at the scene [26]. A meta-analysis of 1742 patients with TAR who arrived alive at the hospital experienced a 32% mortality rate; with one-third dying before reaching the operating room [27].

Table 35.2 Chest radiographs: findings associated with traumatic aortic rupture.

Signs of mediastinal hemorrhage
Widened mediastinum (>8.0 cm)*
M : C ratio (>0.25)**
Left mediastinal width†
Mediastinal width ratio‡
Abnormal contour of aortic knob
Aortopulmonary window opacification
Displaced paraspinal line (right or left)
Widening paratracheal stripe
Depression of left main bronchus
Tracheal deviation
Nasogastric tube shift
Left apical cap
Left hemothorax

Signs associated with severe blunt chest trauma
Lung contusion
1st or 2nd rib fracture
Multiple rib fractures with or without flail chest
Fracture of sternum

*Defined by a greater than 8.0 cm width at the level of the aortic arch on an anteroposterior supine chest radiograph taken at a distance of 100 cm.
**A ratio greater than 0.25 of the mediastinal (M) width across the aortic knob divided by the transverse width of the chest (C) from the inner ribs at the level of the aortic arch.
†Measured from the midline of the trachea to the left border of the mediastinum at the level of the aortic arch (>6.0 cm).
‡A ratio greater than 0.60 of the left mediastinal width to mediastinal width measured at the level of the aortic arch.

Clearly the early identification of such a life-threatening injury as TAR requires a rapid and easily obtainable screening test with excellent operating characteristics. The initial anteroposterior (AP) chest radiograph (CXR) has been extensively studied as such a screening test for TAR. Our literature search failed to find any meta-analyses, systematic reviews or RCTs of CXR in diagnosing TAR. We reviewed observational cohort studies of blunt trauma patients with and without TAR who received aortography, the gold standard for TAR [28]. The signs associated with TAR can be divided into those suggestive of mediastinal hemorrhage or diagnostic of other thoracic injuries indicative of severe blunt chest trauma (Table 35.2).

We were unable to identify any sign with sufficiently robust operating characteristics to obviate the need to rule out TAR by further testing while significantly decreasing the number of computerized tomography (CT) scans, echocardiography or aortography. The most widely tested CXR signs of mediastinal hemorrhage were an absolute widening of the mediastinum (a width greater than 8.0 cm at the level of the aortic arch on an AP supine CXR taken at a distance of 100 cm) [29] or an increase in the ratio of the width of the mediastinum to the width of the chest wall (the ratio of mediastinal width across the aortic knob divided by the transverse width of the chest from the inner ribs at the level of the aortic arch) [30]. The operating characteristics of an absolute widening of the mediastinum in diagnosing TAR range from a positive likelihood ratio (+LR) of 2.66 (95% CI: 2.14 to 3.30) and a negative likelihood ratio (–LR) of 0.22 (95% CI: 0.07 to 0.66) [31] to a +LR of 1.45 (95% CI: 1.28 to 1.65) and a –LR of 0.08 (95% CI: 0.00 to 6.04) [32]. A ratio of > 0.25 provides a +LR of 1.29 (95% CI: 1.02 to 1.62) and a –LR of 0.33 (95% CI: 0.05 to 2.28) for diagnosing TAR [33].

Ungar et al. [31] attempted to develop a clinical decision rule to exclude thoracic aortic imaging in patients with blunt trauma after motor vehicle crashes. This group studied 1096 patients with blunt thoracic trauma resulting from a motor vehicle crash. All patients underwent contrast-enhanced CT scans of the chest and/or aortography to evaluate TAR. TAR was diagnosed in 22 (2.0%; 95% CI: 1.2% to 3.0%) of their patients. Of the patients with TAR, 5% had a normal CXR. Displacement of the left paraspinal line had the best operating characteristics of any individual CXR finding (+LR = 16, –LR = 0.38). This was followed by an abnormal aortic knob (+LR = 7, –LR = 0.22) and a widened mediastinum (+LR = 6.0, –LR = 0.22). Putting these three signs in a classification and regression tree (CART) analysis created a model with the best operating characteristics (+LR = 3.8, 95% CI: 1.1 to 12.9; –LR = 0.18, 95% CI: 0.05 to 0.61). This model was then validated internally with a cross-validation technique. To date there has been no external validation of this clinical decision rule.

In summary, in patients suspected of traumatic aortic rupture, any of the findings listed in Table 35.2 should prompt further investigation. More importantly, any patient with a high pre-test probability of TAR requires further investigation even in the absence of any of these findings. CXR is not a reliable modality to exclude the possibility of traumatic aortic rupture.

Question 3: In ED patients with blunt chest trauma (population), what is the sensitivity and specificity (diagnostic test characteristics) of plain chest radiography (test) in identifying pulmonary contusion (outcome)?

Search strategy

- MEDLINE and EMBASE: (X-rays OR radiography) AND computed tomography AND sensitivity and specificity AND (pulmonary OR lung) AND (contusion OR laceration)

Pulmonary contusion is the most common cause of lung opacification in blunt chest trauma, occurring in 30–75% of patients with a mortality rate ranging from 14% to 40% [34]. Radiographically, pulmonary contusion is visualized as a focal or multi-focal area of ground glass opacity, not limited by segmental boundaries [34,35]. Frequently, these finding are accompanied by evidence of associated injuries such as rib or spine fractures [34]. The increased lung density is due to alveolar and distal bronchial hemorrhage and edema [35]; however, radiographic signs of pulmonary contusion may not be apparent until a few hours after the injury [35].

Computerized tomography of the chest is generally considered the gold standard for detecting pulmonary contusion [35]; however, this issue has not been adequately studied. Similarly, the value of CXR in detecting such injuries is controversial. Human studies evaluating the role of CXR in identifying pulmonary contusion have generally used chest CT scan as the reference standard. According to the four studies identified in the search above, the sensitivity of CXR for detecting pulmonary contusion ranges from 22% to 60% [36–39]. Calculation of specificity values was not possible based on the data provided in these studies. Only one experimental study [40] used the presence of pulmonary contusion on pathological examination as the reference standard. In this study, chest CT detected pulmonary contusion in 100% of cases compared with 37.5% by CXR. When CXR was repeated after 30 minutes, the sensitivity improved from 37% to 70%. CT also provided a better estimation of the size and extent of injury [40].

Although routine chest CT has been recommended by some authors for diagnosing pulmonary contusion [38,40], others have argued that CT findings not apparent on plain chest radiographs may not have any clinical impact on the management of these patients and, therefore, may not be clinically important [37,41].

In summary, the sensitivity and specificity of CXR in identifying pulmonary contusion remains unknown. In the absence of a large randomized trial and current guidelines comparing CXR to CT for diagnosing pulmonary contusion, it is reasonable to conclude that CXR could be used as a screen, and that CT be reserved for confirmation of the degree of injury or in patients with unexplained hypoxia/dyspnea with a normal CXR.

Question 4: In ED patients with small (occult) traumatic pneumothoraces (population), does treatment with observation alone (intervention) lead to less pain, improved quality of life or less complications (outcomes) compared to chest tube insertion (control)?

Search strategy

- MEDLINE and EMBASE: occult pneumothorax AND (observation OR conservative OR expectant) AND (management OR treatment OR therapy)

Proper ED management of occult pneumothoraces is controversial. Occult pneumothorax is defined as a pneumothorax that is detected on CT scan (chest or abdomen) but not on CXR [42]. Up to 70% of small pneumothoraces may not be apparent on initial CXR [43]. Management of pneumothoraces secondary to blunt trauma has traditionally been tube thoracostomy [44], fearing the progression of pneumothorax and the occurrence of serious complications such as tension pneumothorax. This recommendation has been emphasized for patients undergoing mechanical ventilation [44]. Tube thoracostomy is not benign; it has been associated with complications in as many as 21% of cases (e.g., pain, vascular injury, improper positioning, longer hospital stay, infections, etc.)

Table 35.3 Summary of studies evaluating the role of observation compared to tube thoracostomy in the management of occult pneumothorax.

Study	Study characteristics	Population	Outcomes	OBS results
Collins et al. [46]	Retrospective review of blunt trauma patients	24 patients with OPTX (11 OBS and 13 TT)	TT requirement, complications	No complications or TT requirement in OBS patients
Wolfman et al. [47]	Retrospective review of blunt trauma patients	25 patients with OPTX (11 OBS and 14 TT)	Resolving PTX, TT requirement	No complications or TT requirement in OBS patients
Enderson et al. [42]	Prospective, randomized study of blunt trauma patients	40 patients with OPTX (21 OBS and 19 TT)	Complications, progression or PTX, empyema, pneumonia	No complications or TT requirement in OBS patients
Wolfman et al [48]	Prospective (non-randomized) study of blunt trauma patients	35 patients with OPTX (27 OBS and 8 TT)	TT requirement, complications	No complications or TT requirement in OBS patients
Brasel et al. [49]	Retrospective review of blunt trauma patients > 18 years old	39 patients with OPTX (21 OBS and 18 TT)	Respiratory distress, progression of PTX, pneumonia, TT requirement	No complications or TT requirement in 21 OBS patients (including 9 patients on PPV)
Holmes et al. [43]	Retrospective review of children (< 16 years old) with blunt trauma	11 OPTX (1 TT and 10 OBS)	TT requirement, complications	No complications or TT requirement in OBS patients (including 2 on PPV)
Ball et al. [50]	Retrospective review of blunt trauma patients	89 patients with OPTX (26 OBS)	TT requirement, complications	Two patients required TT; the remaining 24 patients (including 2 on PPV) had no complications and did not require TT
Summary	Seven studies: two controlled clinical trials and five retrospective cohorts	263 patients (127 OBS)	At least: TT requirement, complications	Two of 127 (1.6%) patients required TT; remainder had no complications (including at least 13 on PPV)

OBS, observation; OPTX, occult pneumothorax; PPV, positive pressure ventilation; PTX, pneumothorax; TT, tube thoracostomy.

[45]. These complications can be avoided with improved technique and vigilant monitoring [42].

Using the search above, seven studies [42,43,46–50] were identified (two controlled clinical trials and five retrospective cohorts) involving 163 patients who had received observation only (without thoracostomy) for their occult pneumothorax. These studies have demonstrated that an occult pneumothorax resulting from blunt trauma in a hemodynamically stable patient can be safely managed with simple observation (Table 35.3). This strategy has been associated with minimal complications (~1% thoracostomy placement), even in patients who require mechanical ventilation.

Some investigators have suggested that expectant management in patients with occult pneumothoraces should be based on criteria developed on the basis of size [51] or location [48] of the pneumothorax on CT scan. The long-term follow-up and recurrence rate of this therapeutic modality has not been reported. It must be noted that such management may not apply to patients with penetrating trauma since the reviewed studies only included blunt trauma cases.

In summary, the evidence suggests that in selected hemodynamically stable patients, occult pneumothoraces resulting from blunt trauma can be managed conservatively with simple observation, without thoracostomy.

Question 5: In ED patients with thoracic trauma requiring chest tube insertion for hemo- or pneumothorax (population), do prophylactic antibiotics (intervention) prevent infection (outcome) compared to standard care (control)?

Search strategy

- MEDLINE and EMBASE: (chest tube OR tube thoracostomy) AND (antibacterial agents OR antibiotics)

The insertion of a chest tube for a hemopneumothorax after chest trauma is often a life-saving procedure, but is often complicated by empyema formation and pneumonia. The incidence of empyema and pneumonia have been reported to be as high as 17.9% [52] and 35.1% [53], respectively. The question whether prophylactic antibiotics decrease the incidence of these complications has been the subject of many studies.

A systematic review by Sanabria et al. [54] in 2006 addressed the efficacy of prophylactic antibiotics for thoracic trauma patients after chest tube insertion. Five RCTs were included, involving a total of 614 patients, of whom 315 were given antibiotics with 263 placebo controls. The primary outcome tested was thoracic trauma patients who developed an empyema or pneumonia after chest tube insertion. The antibiotics that were tested consisted of first- and second-generation cephalosporins and clindamycin. Their review concluded that both empyema and pneumonia were less likely if the patients were given antibiotics at the time of chest tube insertion. An empyema occurred in 1.1% of the antibiotic group versus 7.6% of the placebo group, and pneumonia was noted in 6.6% of the antibiotic group versus 16% of the placebo group. The use of prophylactic antibiotics reduced the development of empyema (RR = 0.19; 95% CI: 0.07 to 0.5) and pneumonia (RR = 0.44; 95% CI: 0.27 to 0.73).

In summary, this systematic review supports the Eastern Association for the Surgery of Trauma (EAST) guideline advocating the use of prophylactic antibiotics after chest tube insertion [55].

Question 6: In ED patients with blunt thoracic trauma (population), what is the sensitivity and specificity (diagnostic test characteristics) of a computerized tomography scan (test) in identifying diaphragmatic injuries (outcome) compared to chest radiography (control)?

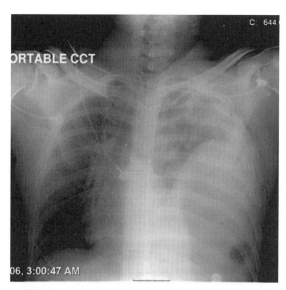

Figure 35.1 Herniation of stomach into the thoracic cavity following traumatic diaphragm rupture in a victim of a motor vehicle crash.

Search strategy

- MEDLINE and EMBASE: diaphragm AND (rupture OR laceration OR injury) AND (X-ray OR radiograph) AND (computed tomography OR CT) AND sensitivity and specificity

---

Traumatic diaphragm rupture (TDR) is detected in up to 6% of patients suffering from blunt thoracic or abdominal trauma undergoing laparoscopy or laparotomy [56]. TDR resulting from penetrating trauma is far more common (ratio of 2:1), and the majority of TDRs involve the left hemidiaphragm [56]. This predominance is attributed to the protective effect of the liver as well as under-diagnosis of right-sided TDRs [57]. The detection of TDR mandates operative repair of the injured diaphragm since undiagnosed herniation of abdominal contents into the thorax through the diaphragmatic defect is associated with high morbidity and mortality (Fig. 35.1) [56]. Therefore, using an appropriate and reliable imaging technique to identify TDR significantly impacts clinical management.

The supine CXR is commonly used as the screening tool in patients with thoraco-abdominal trauma. Radiographic findings associated with TDR include intrathoracic herniation of an abdominal organ and the presence of the nasogastric tube above the left hemidiaphragm [58]. Other radiographic findings that are suggestive of TDR include elevation of the hemidiaphragm, obliteration of the diaphragm outline and contralateral shift of the mediastinum [57]. Unfortunately, the initial CXR is normal or unclear in up to 50% of patients with TDR [56]. The diagnostic yield of chest radiographs is even less in patients with right-sided TDRs [56]. In general, CXR demonstrates a low sensitivity (46%

for left-sided TDR; 17% for right-sided TDR) for identifying TDR [57].

Older studies evaluating the diagnostic performance of CT scans (mostly single-detector or helical CT) in identifying TDR reported poor sensitivity (ranging from 54% to 73%) and reasonable specificity (ranging from 86% to 90%) [58–60]. Advances in CT technology, especially multi-detector CT (MDCT), have shown promising results in diagnosing TDR in small studies [56]. MDCT obtains thinner sections with greater speed, provides better quality axial images, and non-axial reformations, compared to the conventional or single-detector CT [56,58]. The sensitivity and specificity of MDCT in detecting TDR, however, has not been studied in any large trial.

Diagnostic signs of TDR by CT include visualization of the diaphragm tear, visualization of herniated abdominal contents above the diaphragm (collar sign), and direct contact between the herniated viscera and posterior chest wall (dependent viscera sign) [57,61]. The CT "collar sign" has been reported as 100% specific, but with a limited sensitivity of 60% for diagnosing TDR [59].

In summary, although MDCT has improved the accuracy of CT for identifying TDR, both CXR and CT are not sensitive enough to rule out TDR. In cases of a high index of suspicion (e.g., blunt abdominal trauma with presence of intra-abdominal organ injuries), magnetic resonance imaging (MRI) and or laparotomy should be considered.

Question 7: In ED patients with blunt thoracic trauma (population), what is the sensitivity and specificity (diagnostic test characteristics) of ultrasound (test) in detecting pericardial effusions and tamponade (outcome)?

Table 35.4 Echocardiography for diagnosing hemopericardium after penetrating chest trauma.

Study	Total penetrating chest trauma (n)	Incidence of hemopericardium (n; %)	Operating characteristics (95% CI)			
			Sensitivity	Specificity	+LR	−LR
Jimenez et al. [63]	74	10; 13.5%	90%	87%	29 (7.25 to 114)	0.10 (0.02 to 0.66)
Freshman et al. [64]	36	4; 11.1%	100%	100%	Infinite	0.00 (0.01 to 1.41)
Meyer et al. [65]	105	9; 8.6%	56%	93%	8.0 (1.63 to 39)	0.47 (0.13 to 1.67)
Rozycki et al. [66]	261	29; 11.1%	100%	96.9	33 (15 to 62)	0.00 (0.00 to 0.27)
Summary	N = 446	8.6% to 13.5%	56% to 100%	87% to 100%	> 8.0	< 0.47

Search strategy

- MEDLINE and EMBASE: (echocardiography OR ultrasound OR sonography) AND thoracic injuries AND sensitivity and specificity

Hemopericardium and tamponade are important concerns for emergency physicians dealing with penetrating chest trauma. In the past, emergency physicians relied on injury mechanism, clinical signs and symptoms to diagnose hemopericardium. For example, chest trauma associated with pulsus paradoxus > 10 mmHg, low voltage electrocardiography, jugular venous distension and hypotension would strongly suggest a diagnosis of pericardial tamponade [62]. In more subtle cases, however, advanced imaging to identify patients with these important findings was required which led to diagnostic delays and poor outcomes. The diagnosis of pericardial effusion and tamponade has more recently been aided by the use of portable ultrasound devices [62].

The above search identified no systematic reviews on the role of portable ultrasound in the diagnosis of pericardial effusion and tamponade. The evidence for this question was assembled from four studies of patients with penetrating chest trauma (Table 35.4) [63–66]. Three of the four studies show that ultrasound has excellent operating characteristics in identifying hemopericardium in patients with penetrating chest trauma. The one discordant study by Meyer et al. [65] found that the presence of a massive hemothorax significantly degraded ultrasound imagining of hemopericardium. In a subgroup analysis of those patients without a hemothorax, the authors demonstrated that ultrasound had a sensitivity and specificity consistent with the other three studies (100% and 94%, respectively) [65].

In summary, in the hands of minimally trained physicians, portable ultrasound devices are invaluable in assisting the clinician with a rapid diagnosis of pericardial effusion and tamponade. This is with the caveat that, in the setting of a hemothorax, ultrasound may be unreliable.

Conclusions

The patient identified above was seen urgently and received fluid resuscitation which improved the patient's vital signs to a blood pressure of 123/79 mmHg, respiratory rate of 20 breaths/min, pulse rate of 100 breaths/min and SaO_2 (on 100% oxygen) to 100%. The patient underwent CT scan imaging of the chest and abdomen. The CT confirmed the presence of pulmonary contusions and rib fractures and also identified a small left-sided pneumothorax. There were no other obvious injuries and a left-sided chest tube was inserted; the patient was admitted to the surgical intensive care unit.

Overall, chest trauma is a common ED presentation and significant injuries to the heart, lung and other intrathoracic organs may occur following such trauma. Many aspects of thoracic trauma have not been adequately studied. The evidence assembled in this chapter suggests that a combination of clinical judgment, high index of suspicion and the use of available tests should all be used in combination for rapid identification and treatment of significant chest injuries.

References

1 Web-based Injury Statistics Query and Reporting System (WISQARS). US Department of Health and Human Services, Center for Disease Control, National Centre for Injury Prevention and Control, Atlanta, 2002.

2 LoCicero J, III, Mattox KL. Epidemiology of chest trauma. *Surg Clin North Am* 1989;**69**:15-19.

3 Pretre R, Chilcott M. Blunt trauma to the heart and great vessels. *N Engl J Med* 1997;**336**:626–32.

4 Lindstaedt M, Germing A, Lawo T, et al. Acute and long-term clinical significance of myocardial contusion following blunt thoracic trauma: results of a prospective study. *J Trauma* 2002;**52**:479–85.

5 Bokhari F, Brakenridge S, Nagy K, et al. Prospective evaluation of the sensitivity of physical examination in chest trauma. *J Trauma* 2002;**53**:1135–8.

6 Pasquale M, Fabian TC. Practice management guidelines for trauma from the Eastern Association for the Surgery of Trauma. *J Trauma* 1998;**44**:941–56.

7 Maenza RL, Seaberg D, D'Amico F. A meta-analysis of blunt cardiac trauma: ending myocardial confusion. *Am J Emerg Med* 1996;**14**:237–41.

8 Schick TD, van der Zee H, Powers SR, Jr. Detection of cardiac disturbances following thoracic trauma with high-frequency analysis of the electrocardiogram. *J Trauma* 1977;**17**:419–24.

9 Viano DC, Artinian CG. Myocardial conducting system dysfunctions from thoracic impact. *J Trauma* 1978;**18**:452–9.

10 Potkin RT, Werner JA, Trobaugh GB, et al. Evaluation of noninvasive tests of cardiac damage in suspected cardiac contusion. *Circulation* 1982;**66**:627–31.

11 Christensen MA, Sutton KR. Myocardial contusion: new concepts in diagnosis and management. *Am J Crit Care* 1993;**2**:28–34.

12 Biffl WL, Moore FA, Moore EE, et al. Cardiac enzymes are irrelevant in the patient with suspected myocardial contusion. *Am J Surg* 1994;**168**: 523–7.

13 Swaanenburg JC, Klaase JM, DeJongste MJ, et al. Troponin I, troponin T, CKMB-activity and CKMB-mass as markers for the detection of myocardial contusion in patients who experienced blunt trauma. *Clin Chim Acta* 1998;**272**:171–81.

14 Ferjani M, Droc G, Dreux S, et al. Circulating cardiac troponin T in myocardial contusion. *Chest* 1997;**111**:427–33.

15 Salim A, Velmahos GC, Jindal A, et al. Clinically significant blunt cardiac trauma: role of serum troponin levels combined with electrocardiographic findings. *J Trauma* 2001;**50**:237–43.

16 Rajan GP, Zellweger R. Cardiac troponin I as a predictor of arrhythmia and ventricular dysfunction in trauma patients with myocardial contusion. *J Trauma* 2004;**57**:801–8.

17 Edouard AR, Felten ML, Hebert JL, et al. Incidence and significance of cardiac troponin I release in severe trauma patients. *Anesthesiology* 2004;**101**:1262–8.

18 Bertinchant JP, Polge A, Mohty D, et al. Evaluation of incidence, clinical significance, and prognostic value of circulating cardiac troponin I and T elevation in hemodynamically stable patients with suspected myocardial contusion after blunt chest trauma. *J Trauma* 2000;**48**:924–31.

19 Tenzer ML. The spectrum of myocardial contusion: a review. *J Trauma* 1985;**25**:620–27.

20 Chirillo F, Totis O, Cavarzerani A, et al. Usefulness of transthoracic and transoesophageal echocardiography in recognition and management of cardiovascular injuries after blunt chest trauma. *Heart* 1996;**75**: 301–6.

21 Karalis DG, Victor MF, Davis GA, et al. The role of echocardiography in blunt chest trauma: a transthoracic and transesophageal echocardiographic study. *J Trauma* 1994;**36**:53–8.

22 Garcia-Fernandez MA, Lopez-Perez JM, Perez-Castellano N, et al. Role of transesophageal echocardiography in the assessment of patients with blunt chest trauma: correlation of echocardiographic findings with the electrocardiogram and creatine kinase monoclonal antibody measurements. *Am Heart J* 1998;**135**:476–81.

23 Weiss RL, Brier JA, O'Connor W, et al. The usefulness of transesophageal echocardiography in diagnosing cardiac contusions. *Chest* 1996;**109**:73–7.

24 Velmahos GC, Karaiskakis M, Salim A, et al. Normal electrocardiography and serum troponin I levels preclude the presence of clinically significant blunt cardiac injury. *J Trauma* 2003;**54**:45–50.

25 Sailer S. Dissecting aneurysm of the aorta. *Arch Pathol* 1942;**23**:704.

26 Parmley LF, Mattingly TW, Manion WC, et al. Nonpenetrating traumatic injury of the aorta. *Circulation* 1953;**17**:1086–101.

27 von Oppell UO, Dunne TT, De Groot MK, et al. Traumatic aortic rupture: twenty-year metaanalysis of mortality and risk of paraplegia. *Ann Thorac Surg* 1994;**58**:585–93.

28 Sturm JT, Hankins DG, Young G. Thoracic aortography following blunt chest trauma. *Am J Emerg Med* 1990;**8**:92–6.

29 Marsh DG, Sturm JT. Traumatic aortic rupture: roentgenographic indications for angiography. *Ann Thorac Surg* 1976;**21**:337–40.

30 Seltzer SE, D'Orsi C, Kirshner R, et al. Traumatic aortic rupture: plain radiographic findings. *Am J Roentgenol* 1981;**137**:1011–14.

31 Ungar TC, Wolf SJ, Haukoos JS, et al. Derivation of a clinical decision rule to exclude thoracic aortic imaging in patients with blunt chest trauma after motor vehicle collisions. *J Trauma* 2006;**61**:1150–55.

32 Wong YC, Ng CJ, Wang LJ, et al. Left mediastinal width and mediastinal width ratio are better radiographic criteria than general mediastinal width for predicting blunt aortic injury. *J Trauma* 2004;**57**:88–94.

33 Cook AD, Klein JS, Rogers FB, et al. Chest radiographs of limited utility in the diagnosis of blunt traumatic aortic laceration. *J Trauma* 2001;**50**:843–7.

34 Costantino M, Gosselin MV, Primack SL. The ABCs of thoracic trauma imaging. *Semin Roentgenol* 2006;**41**:209–25.

35 Mirvis SE. Diagnostic imaging of acute thoracic injury. *Semin Ultrasound CT MR* 2004;**25**:156–79.

36 Traub M, Stevenson M, McEvoy S, et al. The use of chest computed tomography versus chest X-ray in patients with major blunt trauma. *Injury* 2007;**38**:43–7.

37 Smejkal R, O'Malley KF, David E, et al. Routine initial computed tomography of the chest in blunt torso trauma. *Chest* 1991;**100**:667–9.

38 Trupka A, Waydhas C, Hallfeldt KK, et al. Value of thoracic computed tomography in the first assessment of severely injured patients with blunt chest trauma: results of a prospective study. *J Trauma* 1997;**43**: 405–11.

39 Soldati G, Testa A, Silva FR, et al. Chest ultrasonography in lung contusion. *Chest* 2006;**130**:533–8.

40 Schild HH, Strunk H, Weber W, et al. Pulmonary contusion: CT vs plain radiograms. *J Comput Assist Tomogr* 1989;**13**:417–20.

41 Omert L, Yeaney WW, Protetch J. Efficacy of thoracic computerized tomography in blunt chest trauma. *Am Surg* 2001;**67**:660–64.

42 Enderson BL, Abdalla R, Frame SB, et al. Tube thoracostomy for occult pneumothorax: a prospective randomized study of its use. *J Trauma* 1993;**35**:726–9.

43 Holmes JF, Brant WE, Bogren HG, et al. Prevalence and importance of pneumothoraces visualized on abdominal computed tomographic scan in children with blunt trauma. *J Trauma* 2001;**50**:516–20.

44 American College of Surgeons, Committee on Trauma. *Advanced Trauma Life Support Course for Doctors: Instructors course manual.* American College of Surgeons, Chicago, 1997.

45 Etoch SW, Bar-Natan MF, Miller FB, et al. Tube thoracostomy. Factors related to complications. *Arch Surg* 1995;**130**:521–5.

46 Collins JC, Levine G, Waxman K. Occult traumatic pneumothorax: immediate tube thoracostomy versus expectant management. *Am Surg* 1992;**58**:743–746.

47 Wolfman NT, Gilpin JW, Bechtold RE, et al. Occult pneumothorax in patients with abdominal trauma: CT studies. *J Comput Assist Tomogr* 1993;**17**:56–59.

48 Wolfman NT, Myers WS, Glauser SJ, et al. Validity of CT classification on management of occult pneumothorax: a prospective study. *Am J Roentgenol* 1998;**171**:1317–20.

49 Brasel KJ, Stafford RE, Weigelt JA, et al. Treatment of occult pneumothoraces from blunt trauma. *J Trauma* 1999;**46**:987–90.

50 Ball CG, Kirkpatrick AW, Laupland KB, et al. Incidence, risk factors, and outcomes for occult pneumothoraces in victims of major trauma. *J Trauma* 2005;**59**:917–24.

51 Garramone RR, Jr., Jacobs LM, Sahdev P. An objective method to measure and manage occult pneumothorax. *Surg Gynecol Obstet* 1991;**173**:257–61.

52 LoCurto JJ, Jr., Tischler CD, Swan KG, et al. Tube thoracostomy and trauma – antibiotics or not? *J Trauma* 1986;**26**:1067–72.

53 Grover FL, Richardson JD, Fewel JG, et al. Prophylactic antibiotics in the treatment of penetrating chest wounds. A prospective double-blind study. *J Thorac Cardiovasc Surg* 1977;**74**:528–36.

54 Sanabria A, Valdivieso E, Gomez G, et al. Prophylactic antibiotics in chest trauma: a meta-analysis of high-quality studies. *World J Surg* 2006;**30**:1843–7.

55 Eastern Association for the Surgery of Trauma. Practice management guidelines for prophylactic antibiotic use in tube thoracostomy for traumatic hemopneumothorax: the EAST Practice Management Guidelines Work Group. *J Trauma* 2000;**48**(4):753–7.

56 Hanmuganathan K, Mirvis SE, Chiu WC, et al. Triple-contrast helical CT in penetrating torso trauma: a prospective study to determine peritoneal violation and the need for laparotomy. *Am J Roentgenol* 2001;**177**:1247–56.

57 Gelman R, Mirvis SE, Gens D. Diaphragmatic rupture due to blunt trauma: sensitivity of plain chest radiographs. *Am J Roentgenol* 1991;**156**:51–7.

58 Mirvis SE. Imaging of acute thoracic injury: the advent of MDCT screening. *Semin Ultrasound CT MR* 2005;**26**:305–31.

59 Murray JG, Caoili E, Gruden JF, et al. Acute rupture of the diaphragm due to blunt trauma: diagnostic sensitivity and specificity of CT. *Am J Roentgenol* 1996;**166**:1035–9.

60 Killeen KL, Mirvis SE, Shanmuganathan K. Helical CT of diaphragmatic rupture caused by blunt trauma. *Am J Roentgenol* 1999;**173**:1611–16.

61 Bergin D, Ennis R, Keogh C, et al. The "dependent viscera" sign in CT diagnosis of blunt traumatic diaphragmatic rupture. *Am J Roentgenol* 2001;**177**:1137–40.

62 Roy CL, Minor MA, Brookhart MA, et al. Does this patient with pericardial effusion have cardiac tamponade? *JAMA* 2007;**297**:1810–18.

63 Jimenez E, Martin M, Krukenkamp I, et al. Subxiphoid pericardiotomy versus echocardiography: a prospective evaluation of the diagnosis of occult penetrating cardiac injury. *Surgery* 1990;**108**:676–9.

64 Freshman SP, Wisner DH, Weber CJ. 2-D echocardiography: emergent use in the evaluation of penetrating precordial trauma. *J Trauma* 1991;**31**:902–5.

65 Meyer DM, Jessen ME, Grayburn PA. Use of echocardiography to detect occult cardiac injury after penetrating thoracic trauma: a prospective study. *J Trauma* 1995;**39**:902–7.

66 Rozycki GS, Feliciano DV, Ochsner MG, et al. The role of ultrasound in patients with possible penetrating cardiac wounds: a prospective multicenter study. *J Trauma* 1999;**46**:543–51

36 Hemorrhagic Shock

Dennis Djogovic,[1] Jonathan Davidow[1] & Peter Brindley[2]

[1]Department of Emergency Medicine, University of Alberta, Edmonton, *and* Division of Critical Care Medicine, University of Alberta Hospital, Edmonton, Canada
[2]Division of Critical Care Medicine, University of Alberta Hospital, Edmonton, Canada

Clinical scenario

A 74-year-old female was an unrestrained driver in a single vehicle rollover at highway speed. She was ejected 40 m from her car and found in a roadside ditch. Initial vital signs were: blood pressure 80/60 mmHg, heart rate 123 beats/min and respiratory rate 25 breaths/min. The patient was moaning and only moved limbs to deep pain stimulus.

Emergency medical services (EMS) secured two large-bore peripheral intravenous sites and instituted a crystalloid bolus (2 L). Oxygen by non-rebreather mask and cervical spine collar were applied and the patient was immobilized on a spinal board. The decision was made to "scoop and run" by ground ambulance to the nearest emergency department (ED) 25 minutes away. The ambient temperature of the ambulance was increased for transport.

EMS arrived with the patient to your tertiary center ED. Her blood pressure improved transiently to 105/62 mmHg after the intravenous crystalloid; however, on ED arrival her vitals were BP of 89/54 mmHg with a heart rate of 119 beats/min. There had been no improvement in her level of consciousness. As the primary physician responsible for her care, you feel that she is suffering from hemorrhagic shock as a result of blunt trauma. How will you treat her?

Background

Every year, thousands of people of all ages suffer injury due to both blunt and penetrating trauma. Many deaths occur in the prehospital setting when catastrophic injuries preclude survival. Within health care institutions, many of the patients that survive to ED arrival die from hemorrhagic shock. Management of traumatic hemorrhagic shock lies in rapid recognition, investigation

and management of injuries and their antecedent complications. Knowledge of available evidence can assist in treatment success.

The resuscitation of hemorrhagic shock is complicated by many variables, such as trauma type (blunt, penetrating), treatment setting (prehospital, ED, operating room, intensive care unit), resuscitation fluid type (crystalloids, colloids, blood products), resuscitation fluid amount (small volume, large volume) and resuscitation timing (early or delayed). Add to these factors the varied resuscitation targets (controlled hypotension, "normal range" vitals, supraphysiological vitals) and the landscape indeed becomes confusing and very heterogeneous. Debate exists between the systemic complications of unmitigated shock that can occur with hypotension (acidosis, end organ ischemia) versus the risk of inducing dilutional coagulopathy and even dislodging clot formation when resuscitating to normotension.

The varied presentation is no doubt in part why hemorrhagic shock is a killer, not only in trauma but in other conditions (massive gastrointestinal bleed, hemoptysis, etc.) too. The creation of the advance trauma life support (ATLS) [1] course by the American College of Surgeons was meant to educate large numbers of trauma care practitioners across North America in order to elevate the baseline of expected care in the trauma patient. The ATLS guidelines for resuscitation utilize a four-part classification of shock based on consensus agreement. Since its inception, it has become the prerequisite for almost all staff now working within the acute care setting caring for trauma.

Clinical questions

In order to address the issues of most relevance to your patient and to help in searching the literature for the evidence regarding hemorrhagic shock, you structure your clinical questions as recommended in Chapter 1.

1 In the hemorrhagic shock patient seen in the ED (population), does low volume/delayed resuscitation (intervention) improve mortality (outcome) compared to resuscitation to "normal" vital signs (control)?

Evidence-based Emergency Medicine. Edited by Brian H. Rowe
© 2009 Blackwell Publishing, ISBN: 978-1-4051-6143-5.

2 In the hemorrhagic shock patient seen in the ED (population), does the use of colloids (intervention) improve mortality (outcome) compared to using crystalloids (control)?

3 In the hemorrhagic shock patient seen in the ED (population), does the use of hypertonic saline (intervention) improve mortality (outcome) compared to using crystalloids (control)?

4 In the hemorrhagic shock patient seen in the ED (population), does the use of recombinant activated factor VIIa (intervention) improve mortality and reduce bleeding (outcomes) compared to using crystalloids (control)?

5 In the hemorrhagic shock patient seen in the ED (population), does the use of pharmacological hemostatic agents (intervention) decrease mortality (outcome) compared to using crystalloids (control)?

6 In multi-trauma patients (population), does the use of focused assessment with sonography for trauma (FAST) (intervention) reduce delays in treatment and improve outcomes compared to computerized tomography (control)?

7 In the hemorrhagic shock patient seen in the ED with pelvic trauma (population), does the use of external pelvic stabilization or internal blood vessel control (intervention) improve mortality (outcome) compared to using crystalloids (control)?

General search strategy

Trauma is a broad term which generally signifies major injury and high mortality, as compared to injury, which encompasses all events where some form of energy is transferred to the body, regardless of the severity. Searching for trauma can be difficult and a variety of medical subject headings (MeSH) may be required. The Cochrane Library, MEDLINE and EMBASE were searched for relevant systematic reviews and meta-analyses using the MeSH and text words "trauma". CENTRAL and MEDLINE (PubMed) were then searched for randomized clinical trials. Since evidence is occasionally sparse in this topic area, MEDLINE was also eventually used to identify consensus statements, clinical practice guidelines, or large cohort or retrospective studies that have infiltrated commonly accessed journals.

Critical review of the literature

Question 1: In the hemorrhagic shock patient seen in the ED (population), does low volume/delayed resuscitation (intervention) improve mortality (outcome) compared to resuscitation to "normal" vital signs (control)?

Search strategy

- MEDLINE and Cochrane Library: trauma [MeSH or text] AND (blunt OR penetrating) AND resuscitation AND (goal OR endpoint OR delayed)

The ATLS guidelines for resuscitation suggest that shock with ongoing tachycardia or hypotension should be treated with fluid (crystalloid or blood) replacement in a pre-operative setting. Although adopted almost universally, there are no randomized controlled trials (RCTs) upon which these resuscitation parameters were based, and they seem to be mainly consensus driven.

Randomized controlled trials have been performed that attempted to address the issue of endpoints and resuscitation strategies. The first trial that assessed early versus delayed prehospital fluid replacement suggested that resuscitation should be less aggressive, in fact, allowing for permissive hypotension in order to decrease time to definitive treatment in the operating room [2]. A relative risk of death of 1.26 and prolongation of prothrombin time (PT) and partial thromboplastin time (PTT) were found. However, this trial looked only at penetrating torso trauma, in a single tertiary care institution with short prehospital transport times, and suffered from bias potential due to poor randomization, protocol violations and lack of blinding. A larger and very high-quality study [3] assessing early or no/delayed fluid resuscitation in the prehospital setting showed no significant mortality difference (RR of death = 1.06) with adequate randomization, but assessed both blunt and penetrating trauma collectively. Other studies that assessed small- versus large-volume fluid resuscitation [4–6] failed to show significant mortality differences as well. These studies were complicated by small numbers (ranging from 24 to 110 patients) with varying mortality rates (25% vs 31%, 7.3% vs 7.3%, and 0% vs 0%, respectively). A Cochrane review assessing early versus delayed and small- versus large-volume resuscitation was not able to conduct a meta-analysis or study pooling due to the considerable clinical and statistical heterogeneity of available trials, and the lack of high-quality RCTs [7].

Until higher quality studies examining more homogeneous populations and resuscitation strategies are produced, a clear set of evidence-based physiological goals for traumatic shock resuscitation remains elusive. While it is clear that resuscitation to supraphysiological values is not necessary, resuscitation allowing permissive hypotension in penetrating trauma patients cannot be recommended with confidence.

Question 2: In the hemorrhagic shock patient seen in the ED (population), does the use of colloids (intervention) improve mortality (outcome) compared to using crystalloids (control)?

Search strategy

- MEDLINE: (fluid resuscitation OR hemorrhagic shock [MeSH or text]) AND (colloids OR crystalloids OR albumin OR saline). Limited to human and English language

A variety of types of fluids or combinations are available with which to treat shock patients (Table 36.1). Crystalloids such as normal saline (NS) and Ringer's lactate are inexpensive and readily

	Favorable	Unfavorable
Physiology:		
Colloids	Oncotic pressure $\geq$ 30 mOsm/L Increased vascular expansion Reduction of interstitial edema	?Coagulopathy with starches ?Reduced renal function with starches ?Fever and chills with albumin
Crystalloids	Extensive experience with normal saline Extensive experience with Ringer's lactate No clear side-effects, drug interactions	<40 cm^3 plasma expansion/500 cm^3 saline Interstitial expansion Non-anion gap acidosis with large volume
Delivery/cost:		
Colloids	Usually limited to 20 ml/g for starches	Up to 50 times cost of a similar volume of crystalloid
Crystalloids	No upper limit for volume; inexpensive	Interstitial edema
Clinical data:		
Colloids	SAFE trial [15]: 4% albumin and 0.9% saline equivalent	Cochrane Group [9]: Increased mortality with albumin
Crystalloids	SAFE trial [15]: Trend towards worse outcome in trauma	SAFE trial [15]: Trend towards worse outcome in sepsis

Table 36.1 Evidence supporting fluid resuscitation in hemorrhagic shock.

available; however, some argue that they fail to provide important intravascular expansion, and in large amounts may cause interstitial expansion that can worsen lung oxygenation, intracranial pressure and slow recovery. Colloids are more expensive, may have side-effects such as anaphylaxis or coagulation disturbance, and may contribute to renal insufficiency; however, they do provide greater volume expansion when compared to crystalloids.

A series of meta-analyses [8–11] looking at albumin efficacy and safety – most notably one from the Cochrane Group (of 30 RCTs and >1400 patients) [9] – have markedly altered practice. Higher mortality was identified with albumin when compared to crystalloids (particularly in trauma) and it was suggested that "administration of albumin be halted" [12]. Counter arguments included: the omission of relevant trials; heterogeneity of included trials; inadequate assessment of trial quality; inadequate knowledge of the microcirculation; and unclear etiology for harm. Subsequent meta-analyses found no difference in mortality with albumin [13,14].

The multi-center randomized SAFE trial compared 4% albumin with NS in almost 7000 intensive care unit patients and found no significant difference in 28-day mortality (RR = 0.99; 95% CI: 0.91 to 1.09) or morbidity (e.g., length of stay, need for mechanical ventilation, need for dialysis) [15]. Since 4% albumin is an atypical choice in North America, this study may not change opinions: albumin proponents argue it shows no harm; opponents argue no benefit, just extra cost; and others that it says little about starches.

While albumin may be safe in a heterogeneous population, experts argue it may not be safe for all patients. Notably, a SAFE subgroup analysis showed a trend towards higher mortality in almost 1200 trauma patients (RR = 1.36; 95% CI: 0.99 to 1.86). This effect disappears if trauma with brain injury is excluded; however,

the authors emphasized that the SAFE trial was not powered for secondary analyses.

In summary, the collective evidence suggests that fluid choice following hemorrhagic shock is still empirical rather than clearly evidence based. What is clear, however, is that fluid resuscitation following trauma should not delay medical and surgical hemostasis. In addition, it also represents only one component of a well-orchestrated resuscitation.

Question 3: In the hemorrhagic shock patient seen in the ED (population), does the use of hypertonic saline (intervention) improve mortality (outcome) compared to using crystalloids (control)?

Search strategy

- MEDLINE: hypertonic saline [MeSH or text] AND (hemorrhage OR hemorrhagic shock OR trauma). Limited to human and English language

Evidence questioning the safety of blood products has redoubled efforts to minimize transfusion. Hypertonic (7.5%) saline (HS) has been proposed where there are inadequate donors (developing world), poor refrigeration (disaster medicine), insufficient time for large volumes (prehospital) or difficulty carrying volume (military casualties) [16]. There are theoretical rationales for using HS; however, insufficient clinical evidence currently exists to support widespread use (Table 36.2). HS is most commonly used in traumatic brain injury, where small human trials have shown it to lower intracranial pressure [17]. Even in traumatic brain injury, however, an RCT ($n = 266$) failed to show improved survival [18].

Table 36.2 Theoretical benefits of hypertonic saline in hemorrhagic shock.

Hypertonic (7.5%) saline	
Theoretical benefits	Reduced need to carry large fluid volumes
	Reduced need for blood donors
	Reduced need for refrigeration
	Reduced time required to infuse volume [16]
Clinical data	Decreased interstitial edema and intracranial pressure [17,18]
	Increases plasma volume up to 10 times the equivalent volume of NS [19]
	Decreased blood transfusion [18,19]
	Improves cardiac output and hypotension for hours
	Trend towards improved survival in hemorrhagic shock [21]
	No clear harm; potential benefit; but more study required

Table 36.3 Summary of evidence supporting the role of factor VIIa in hemorrhagic shock.

Mechanism	Binds exposed tissue factor
	Facilitates a thrombin burst
	Decreases fibrinolysis
Clinical safety data	Safe (and beneficial) in >400,000 hemophilia patients
	1–2% thromboembolism rate in non-hemophilia patients [22,26]
	Trend towards increased myocardial infarction and cerebral infarction in a hemorrhagic stroke trial [23]
Clinical outcome data	No clear mortality benefit [22,24,26]
	Blunt trauma: significant reduction in PRBC transfusion and need for massive transfusion [24]
	Penetrating trauma: non-significant trend towards decreased PRBC transfusion and massive transfusion [24]
	Optimal dose unclear: range from 40 to 200 μg/kg

PRBC, packed red blood cell.

A multi-centre trauma trial suggested HS can increase plasma volume by more than 10 times that achieved using a similar volume of NS [19]. It may also decrease blood transfusion, decrease interstitial edema, and normalize base excess, lactate and pH [18,19]. Potential side-effects include hyperosmolarity, hypernatremia and central pontine myelinolysis. While prospective and blinded human clinical trials involving >1000 patients have shown HS to be relatively safe [17–21], these potential side-effects have hampered trial enrollment and hence more definitive conclusions. HS has, however, reached a low-level expert recommendation level [8,21].

A meta-analysis compared HS and NS in 230 patients with hemorrhagic shock following penetrating torso trauma [21]. They found a non-significant trend towards improved survival in HS patients (HS = 82.5% vs NS = 75.5%, $P = 0.19$) and improved survival for the 68% requiring surgery (84.5% vs 67.1%, $P = 0.01$).

Overall, while evidence suggests that HS is not harmful and may have application in a variety of clinical situations, until larger clinical studies show clear benefit its use should remain restricted.

Question 4: In the hemorrhagic shock patient seen in the ED (population), does the use of recombinant activated factor VIIa (intervention) improve mortality and reduce bleeding (outcomes) compared to using crystalloids (control)?

Search strategy

- MEDLINE: (factorVII OR factor VIIa OR NiaStase OR NovoSeven [MeSH or text]) AND (hemorrhagic shock OR trauma)

Recombinant factor VIIa (RFVIIa) was approved in 1999 for hemophilia treatment. In terms of its use following trauma, 2006 European recommendations summarized grade B evidence for its use as adjunct therapy in blunt hemorrhagic shock [22]. While several phase III trials are underway, their results are not expected to be available for years.

Recombinant factor VIIa binds to exposed tissue factor to create a "thrombin burst" and decrease fibrinolysis of immature clots (Table 36.3). A trend towards increased thromboembolic events, mainly myocardial or cerebral infarction, was reported in a placebo-controlled, randomized trial of RFVIIa for acute intracerebral hemorrhage (7% vs 2% at 90 days, $P = 0.12$) [23]. This is presumably from TF exposure at sites other than tissue injury (e.g., unstable coronary plaques). It also suggests risk increases with age and dose.

Guidelines emphasize that RFVIIa is not first-line therapy and that coagulation and surgical bleeding should be concomitantly optimized. They suggest a hematocrit of >24%, platelets >50,000 × 10^9/L and fibrinogen >0.5–1.0g/L should be targeted. Moreover, the "lethal triad" of hypothermia, acidosis and coagulopathy should be corrected such that pH is >7.20, temperature is >32°C and iCalcium level is >0.8 mmol/L [8,22].

In 2002, a multi-center, randomized, double-blinded, placebo-controlled study enrolled 301 blunt and penetrating trauma patients to either three doses of RFVIIa (200 μg/kg then 100 μg/kg at 1 hour and 100 μg/kg at 3 hours) or placebo in addition to standard treatment. [24]. Over the subsequent 48 hours, 143 blunt trauma patients had a significant reduction in packed red blood cells (PRBCs) (–2.6 units, $P = 0.02$). The need for massive transfusion (>20 units PRBCs) was also reduced (14% vs 33% of patients, $P = 0.03$). For penetrating trauma ($n = 134$), however, a non-significant trend towards decreased transfusion (–1.0 units, $P = 0.1$) and massive transfusion was reported (7% vs 19%, $P = 0.08$). This is presumably because RFVIIa cannot "plug large holes" [25]. Both groups showed only a trend towards reduced mortality. Adverse events were evenly distributed.

Recombinant factor VIIa's volume of distribution and clearance is variable in hemorrhagic shock. As such, optimal dosing is unclear. Retrospective review of 29 patients who received only

40 µg/kg (repeated once if needed), and matched to placebo by injury severity score, showed no mortality benefit but significantly less additional PRBCs (8.5 ± 9.6 vs 2.4 ± 6.2, $P = 0.001$), platelets ($P = 0.01$) and cryoprecipitate ($P = 0.006$) for the 72 hours following RFVIIa [25]. RFVIIa is not repeated unless bleeding is ongoing; however, that endpoint is clinically judged. For this reason most studies focus on the need for blood products, rather than time to bleeding cessation. Equally, RFVIIa is usually only released following hematology/hematopathology consultation.

In summary, RFVIIa can be considered for any salvageable patient with massive hemorrhage not resolved by medical, surgical and transfusion therapy. However, the optimal dose is unclear, with recommendations ranging from 40 µg/kg [25] to 200 µg/kg [22,26]. Furthermore, the use of RFVIIa is largely to save scarce blood products as no consistent mortality benefit has yet been shown.

Question 5: In the hemorrhagic shock patient seen in the ED (population), does the use of pharmacological hemostatic agents (intervention) decrease mortality (outcome) compared to using crystalloids (control)?

Search strategy

- MEDLINE and Cochrane Library: trauma AND (hemorrhage$ OR bleed OR blood transfusion) AND (aprotinin OR tranexamic acid OR aminocaproic OR desmopressin OR ddavp OR deamino-8-D-arginine vasopressin)

Antifibrinolytic drugs promote blood clotting by preventing fibrinolysis and have been extensively used in major surgery to minimize blood loss [26,27]. Examples of these agents include aprotinin, tranexamic acid (TXA) and ε-aminocaproic acid (EACA). Aprotinin is a serine protease inhibitor which forms irreversible inhibitory complexes with several serine proteases, particularly with plasmin. TXA (*trans*-4-aminomethylcyclohexane-1-carboxylic acid) is a synthetic lysine analog that is a competitive inhibitor of plasmin and plasminogen. EACA is also a synthetic lysine analog, but has one-tenth the potency of TXA.

Coats et al. performed a Cochrane systematic review of RCTs evaluating the use of antifibrinolytics in trauma [27]. Unfortunately, they found only two trials, which enrolled a total of 97 participants; the authors concluded that insufficient evidence exists to either support or refute a clinically important treatment effect. They called for further RCTs of antifibrinolytic agents in trauma patients. The efficacy of TXA in trauma will be evaluated by the Clinical Randomization of an Antifibrinolytic in Significant Hemorrhage (CRASH II) study currently in progress [28]. In this international study, 20,000 trauma patients are being randomized to 1 g TXA over 10 minutes followed by a 1 g infusion over 8 hours versus placebo. The primary outcomes are mortality, transfusion requirements and incidence of vascular events.

A recent systematic review [29] of RCTs of antifibrinolytics in elective surgical patients showed that antifibrinolytics reduced the rate of packed red blood cell transfusion by one-third, reduced the volume needed per transfusion by 1 unit, and cut the need for further surgery to control bleeding by 50%. The risk of precipitating thrombosis with the use of antifibrinolytic agents has been of concern; however, the Cochrane review of antifibrinolytics cites studies that included over 8000 patients and demonstrated no increased risk of either arterial or venous thrombotic events [30]. Since the coagulopathy that occurs after injury is similar to that seen after surgery, it is possible that antifibrinolytic agents might also reduce blood loss, the need for transfusion, and mortality following trauma. As such, the European guidelines for management of bleeding following major trauma suggest that antifibrinolytic agents be considered in the bleeding trauma patient, but therapy should be continued only until bleeding has been adequately controlled [26]. An ongoing study involving 25 Canadian centers comparing the three agents head-to-head on reducing the need for transfusion in cardiac surgery may shed light on which of them is superior [30].

Desmopressin or 1-deamino-8-D-arginine vasopressin (DDAVP) is an analog of arginine vasopressin that functions by releasing endothelial stores of von Willebrand's factor, increasing the activity of factor VIII and causing platelet adhesion and aggregation [31]. There is a paucity of evidence surrounding the use of DDAVP in trauma. However, a Cochrane review of the use of desmopressin in reducing peri-operative blood loss and the need for transfusion has been performed [32]. The review included 18 trials involving 1295 patients and concluded that there was no evidence that DDAVP reduced peri-operative blood transfusion. Hypotension can occur with intravenous infusion, and there were slight, non-significant increases in stroke, non-fatal myocardial infarction and intravascular thrombosis [31,32].

In summary, evidence for the use of fibrinolytics is mixed. To date the evidence is suggestive of a positive effect; however, pending trials will clarify this situation. Due to concerns with a risk of anaphylaxis, stroke and renal failure with aprotinin, TXA appears to be a safer choice currently [26]. Given the lack of evidence of efficacy and potential for harm, the use of DDAVP to decrease bleeding in trauma patients without congenital bleeding disorders cannot be supported.

Question 6: In multi-trauma patients (population), does the use of focused assessment with sonography for trauma (FAST) (intervention) reduce delays in treatment and improve outcomes compared to computerized tomography (control)?

Search strategy

- MEDLINE and Cochrane Library: trauma AND (investigation OR CT OR FAST OR radiology OR sonography OR ultrasound)

Trauma patients require a rapid and thorough clinical assessment to determine stability and injuries. The appropriate use of radiological investigations can aid with this assessment. Each has its own merits and drawbacks, and varying levels of accuracy. The most common investigations currently utilized for investigation of the hemorrhagic trauma patient are computerized tomography (CT) and focused assessment with sonography for trauma (FAST). The ideal test is rapid, repeatable, accurate and all-encompassing, easy to perform, cheap and poses no risk to the patient. Unfortunately, this ideal test does not yet exist. Debate continues as to which test or tests should be used, for which of blunt or penetrating, stable or unstable patients, in which order, and for what circumstances.

Computerized tomography can be relatively quick, can assess head, spine, chest and abdominal injuries, including the retroperitoneum, and can be repeated and evaluated by multiple physicians, yet requires movement of the patient to a poorly monitored area that is not conducive to ongoing resuscitation, requires contrast and radiation exposure, and is expensive. The FAST exam has been developed as a rapid and non-invasive bedside screening test for the detection of hemopericardium and hemoperitoneum. It consists of four sonographic views: pericardiac, perihepatic (Morison's pouch), perisplenic and pelvic (pouch of Douglas) [33]. FAST can detect free fluid within the abdomen and pericardium, is quickly completed, can be repeated, and does not require the patient to be moved from the ED, but it is dependent on the user's skills and cannot diagnose the type of injury or assess aortic root involvement.

Several prospective observational studies have assessed the sensitivity and specificity of ultrasound in detecting abdominal free fluid or organ damage after trauma. There is considerable heterogeneity in the techniques used, definitions of positive and negative studies, operator training and methodological quality. These studies have observed a high specificity (range 0.97–1.0) and a high accuracy (range 0.92–0.99), yet variable sensitivity (range 0.56–0.99) of initial FAST examination for the detection of intra-abdominal injury [34,35]. A retrospective study by Rozycki et al. of 1540 patients (1227 blunt and 313 penetrating trauma), showed that FAST examination performed by surgeons had a sensitivity and specificity close to 100% among patients who were hypotensive [36]. This finding has also been replicated in other similar studies [37,38]. Observational literature also suggests that emergency physicians and trauma surgeons can accurately detect hemoperitoneum [39,40], use focused sonography comparably with other specialties [39,41], and acquire the skills reasonably quickly [42,43].

A recent Cochrane systematic review [44] revealed only two RCTs and two quasi-RCTs of sufficient quality assessing outcomes of FAST scans in torso trauma. They were able to pool data from a total of 1037 patients for the primary endpoint of mortality. There was a non-significant trend towards increased mortality in the ultrasound group (RR = 1.40; 95% CI: 0.94 to 2.08). There was a non-significant trend towards reduction in ordering of CT scans. Their ultimate conclusion was that there is insufficient evidence from RCTs to justify promotion of ultrasound-based clinical pathways in diagnosing patients with suspected blunt abdominal trauma [44]. Unfortunately, the data were erroneously entered

in the review and when it is corrected, the FAST group shows a mortality reduction.

Since the publication of the Cochrane review, the Sonography Outcomes Assessment Program (SOAP) trial has been published ($n = 217$) [45]. To date, this is the only randomized trial to show improvement in clinically important outcomes. The primary outcome in this trial was time to transfer to operating room. They reported that trauma patients receiving a FAST scan during resuscitation were transferred to the operating room 64% sooner than the control group. In addition, all of the secondary outcome variables – CT use, length of stay, complications (including mortality as part of a composite) and hospital costs – had clinically significant odds ratios favoring the FAST group.

Studies of CT are notoriously difficult to compare for as time progresses technology improves, and, with it, accuracy and utility. In 1995, a prospective cohort study of 1600 trauma patients found that less than 30% of CT scans contributed to patient management and 6% of scans had false-positive findings [46]. By 2000, a large retrospective chart review of over 8000 patients showed that the new technology of helical CT was accurate for diagnosis of blunt bowel mesenteric injuries, previously deemed difficult to diagnose without laparotomy [47]. A prospective trial of 200 patients with penetrating injury, previously diagnosed by laparotomy or serial physical exams, found high accuracy with helical CT and triple contrast (intravenous, oral, rectal) administration [48]. The reliance on CT scan has extended to the investigation of stable trauma patients with suspicious mechanism of injury, where a prospective trial resulted in a change in treatment plan in 19% of the 592 patients [49]. Not one of these studies was a high-quality RCT, and yet most trauma practitioners have embraced CT technology as part of their overall trauma approach [49].

In summary, both FAST and CT are promising investigations of the hemorrhagic trauma patient. Clarification is needed regarding which investigation should be used and when. In the hemodynamically unstable patient, FAST may be ideal to allow screening for injuries and bleeding source, without exposing the patient to the risk of transport to the CT suite. In the stable patient, insufficient high-grade evidence exists to ascertain whether CT or FAST, or both, should be used in patient investigation.

Question 7: In the hemorrhagic shock patient seen in the ED with pelvic trauma (population), does the use of external pelvic stabilization or internal blood vessel control (intervention) improve mortality (outcome) compared to using crystalloids (control)?

Search strategy

- MEDLINE and Cochrane Library: trauma AND pelvic AND (treatment OR stabilization OR fixator OR angiography OR binding)

Major trauma may result in pelvic injuries that can be life- and limb-threatening. Proximity to intra-abdominal organs, lower extremities, pelvic organs and a rich neurovascular network within the pelvis all make for a complicated scenario. Trauma to the pelvis can result in significant bleeding due to the rich venous plexi within the pelvis, the ability for bidirectional blood flow due to a lack of vein valves, and the existence of retroperitoneal blood collection, which is difficult to access and diagnose via investigations such as ultrasound and deep peritoneal lavage. The unique pelvic bone anatomy is easily disrupted by trauma, and laceration and crush damage to blood vessels can result in significant mortality.

Treatment approaches to halt pelvic bleeding can be broadly categorized by external and internal techniques. External mechanical stabilization of pelvic anatomy can be achieved with towel tie and clamp and similar compressive devices, and orthopedically placed external fixator apparatus. Internal interventions include pelvic packing, ligation of internal iliac arteries and, most commonly, pelvic angiography and embolization of bleeding areas. While the topic of pelvic trauma and bleeding has been covered at length in surgical and trauma literature, no RCTs, systematic reviews or meta-analyses exist. Most studies consist of retrospective chart reviews of trauma databases, or expert and experience-derived consensus protocols.

Indications for angiography and embolization are frequently quoted as: (i) >4 units of PRBCs transfused in <24 hours; (ii) >6 units PRBCs transfused in <48 hours; (iii) large pelvic hematoma seen on CT scan; (iv) negative deep peritoneal lavage with undiagnosed etiology of hemodynamic instability; and (v) large expanding retroperitoneal hematoma evident on laparotomy [50]. These criteria were not derived with evidence-based methods; they represent local consensus at the institution that published the related article.

The determination of which treatment modality or therapeutic approach to use is unclear due to lack of strong evidence. A retrospective chart review spanning 7 years in a major tertiary care center suggests that non-responders to initial resuscitation have a higher incidence of arterial bleeding that requires early angiography, rather than being delayed for external fixation [51]. Institutional guidelines for pelvic bleeding treatment show promise [52] and the most ambitious multidisciplinary practice guideline to date reviewed over 88 articles spanning 1970 to 2002 [53]. Again, without proper studies it is impossible to recommend a unified approach to the treatment of hemorrhagic traumatic shock due to pelvic bleeding.

Conclusions

In our elderly blunt trauma patient, it is evident that she is suffering from hemorrhagic shock. Rapid resuscitation to normotension with crystalloids or colloids and emergent surgical consultation should be completed. If instability persists, FAST may be used as a screening tool for hemoperitoneum or hemopericardium. If significant pelvic disruption has occurred, internal or external control methods may be required. RFVIIa is a potential agent should hemorrhage continue after adequate resuscitation and coagulation, acidosis and hypothermia correction, and surgical intervention. In the future, if the promising trends continue in research into the use of hypertonic saline and hemostatic agents, these treatments may also make their way into the standard treatment armamentarium.

Overall, the treatment of hemorrhagic shock has advanced over the past two decades. Excellent evidence exists to not resuscitate to supraphysiological goals and that colloids and crystalloids are equally safe. Good evidence exists for permissive hypotension in penetrating trauma, and the use of hypertonic saline, RFVIIa, hemostatic agents, FAST, CT and internal and external pelvic bleeding control methods in hemorrhagic shock. These interventions, however, require higher level evidence or clearer recommendations for safe and effective use.

References

1 American College of Surgeons Committee on Trauma. *Advanced Trauma Life Support for Doctors Student Course Manual.* American College of Surgeons, Chicago, 1997.

2 Bickell WH, Wall MJ, Pepe PE, et al. Immediate versus delayed fluid resuscitation for hypotensive patients with penetrating torso injuries. *N Engl J Med* 1994;**331**(17):1105–9.

3 Turner J, Nicholl J, Webber L, et al. A randomised controlled trial of pre-hospital intravenous fluid replacement therapy in serious trauma. *Health Technology Assessment* 2000;**4**(31).

4 Dunham CM, Belzberg H, Lyles R, et al. The rapid infusion system: a superior method for the resuscitation of hypovolemic patients. *Resuscitation* 1991;**21**(2–3):207–27.

5 Dutton RP, MacKenzie CF, Scalea TM. Hypotensive resuscitation during active haemorrhage: impact on in-hospital mortality. *J Trauma* 2002;**52**:1141–6.

6 Fortune JB, Feustel PJ, Saifi J, Stratton HH, Newell JC, Shah DM. Influence of hematocrit on cardiopulmonary function after acute hemorrhage. *J Trauma* 1987;**27**(3):243–9.

7 Kwan I, Bunn F, Roberts I. Timing and volume of fluid administration for patients with bleeding. *Cochrane Database Syst Rev* 2003;**3**:CD002245.

8 Spahn DR, Cerny V, Coats T, et al. Management of bleeding following major trauma: a European Guideline. *Crit Care* 2007;**11**:R17.

9 Schierhout G, Roberts I. Fluid resuscitation with colloid or crystalloid solutions in critically ill patients: a systematic review of randomized trials. *BMJ* 1998;**316**:961–4.

10 Cochrane Injuries Group Albumin Reviewers. Human albumin administration in critically ill patients; systematic review of randomized controlled trials. *BMJ* 1998;**317**:235–40.

11 Choi PT, Yip G, Quinonez LG, Cook DJ. Crystalloids vs. colloids in fluid resuscitation: a systematic review. *Crit Care Med* 1999;**27**:200–210.

12 Offringa M. Excess mortality after human albumin administration in critically ill patients. Clinical and pathophysiological evidence suggests albumin is harmful. *BMJ* 1998; **317**: 223–4.

13 Wilkes MM, Navickis RJ. Patient survival after human albumin administration: a meta-analysis of randomized, controlled trials. *Ann Intern Med* 2001;**135**:149–64.

14 Roberts I, Alderson P, Bunn F, Chinnock P, Ker K, Schierhout G. Colloids versus crystalloids for fluid resuscitation in critically ill patients. *Cochrane Database Syst Rev* 2004;**4**:CD000567.

15 Finfer S, Bellomo R, Boyce N, French J, Myburgh J, Norton R. A comparison of albumin and saline for fluid resuscitation in the intensive care unit. *N Engl J Med* 2004;**350**:2247–56.

16 Brindley PG. Fluid resuscitation: theory and practice. In: Neilipovitz DT, ed. *Acute Resuscitation and Acute Crisis Management.* University of Ottawa Press, Ottawa, 2005:167–77.

17 Battision C, Andrew PJ, Graham C, Petty T. Randomized controlled trial on the effect of a 20% mannitol solution and a 7.5% saline/6% dextran solution on increased intracranial pressure after brain injury. *Crit Care Med* 2005,**33**:196–202 (discussion 257–8).

18 Cooper DJ, Myles PS, McDermott FT, et al. Prehospital hypertonic saline resuscitation of patients with hypotension and severe traumatic brain injury: a randomized controlled trial. *JAMA* 2004;**291**:1350–57.

19 Vassar MJ, Fischer RP, O'Brien PE, Bachulis BL, Chambers JA, Hoyt DB. A multicenter trial for resuscitation of injured patients with 7.5% sodium chloride. The effect of adding dextran 70. The Multicenter Group for the Study of Hypertonic Saline in Trauma Patients. *Arch Surg* 1993;**128**:1003–11 (discussion 1011–13).

20 Simma B, Burger R, Falk M, Sacher P, Fanconi S. A prospective randomized and controlled study of fluid management in children with severe head injury: lactated Ringer's solution versus hypertonic saline. *Crit Care Med* 1998;**26**:1265–70.

21 Wade CE, Grady JJ, Kramer GC. Efficacy of hypertonic saline dextran fluid resuscitation for patients with hypotension from penetrating trauma. *J Trauma* 2003;**54**:S144–8.

22 Vincent JL, Rossaint R, Riou B, Ozier Y, Zideman D, Spahn DR. Recommendations on the use of recombinant activated factor VII as an adjunctive treatment for massive bleeding – a European perspective. *Crit Care* 2006;**10**:R120.

23 Mayer SA, Brun NC, Begtrup K, et al. Recombinant activated factor VII for acute intra cerebral hemorrhage. *N Engl J Med* 2005;**352**: 777–85.

24 Boffard KD, Riou B, Warren B, et al. Recombinant factor VIIa as adjunctive therapy for bleeding control in severely injured trauma patients: two parallel randomized, placebo-controlled, double-blind clinical trials. *J Trauma* 2005;**59**:8–18.

25 Harrison TD, Laskosky J, Jazaeri O, Pasquale MD, Cipolle M. "Low-dose" recombinant activated factor VII results in less blood and blood product use in traumatic hemorrhage. *J Trauma* 2005;**59**:150–54.

26 Spahn DR, Cerny B, Coats TJ, et al. Management of bleeding following a major trauma: a European guideline. *Crit Care* 2007;**11**:R17 (doi:10.1186/cc5686).

27 Coats T, Roberts I, Shakur H. Antifibrinolytic drugs for acute traumatic injury. *Cochrane Database Syst Rev* 2004;**4**:CD004896 (doi: 10.1002/14651858.CD004896.pub2).

28 Clinical Randomization of an Antifibrinolytic in Significant Hemorrhage study. Available at www.CRASH2.LSHTM.ac.uk.

29 Henry DA, Moxey AJ, Carless PA, et al. Anti-fibrinolytic use for minimising perioperative allogeneic blood transfusion. *Cochrane Database Syst Rev* 1999;**4**:CD001886 (doi: 10.1002/14651858.CD001886).

30 BART study. Available at http://www.ohri.ca/programs/clinical_epidemiology/thrombosis_group/studies/bart.asp.

31 Mannucci PM. Drug therapy: hemostatic drugs (Review). *N Engl J Med* 1998;**339**(4):245–53.

32 Carless PA, Henry DA, Moxey AJ, et al. Desmopressin for minimising perioperative allogeneic blood transfusion. *Cochrane Database Syst Rev* 2004;**1**:CD001884 (doi: 10.1002/14651858.CD001884.pub2).

33 Scalea TM, Rodriguez A, Chiu WC, et al. Focused assessment with sonography for trauma (FAST): results from an international consensus conference. *J Trauma* 1999;**46**:466–72.

34 Spahn DR, Cerny B, Coats TJ, et al. Management of bleeding following a major trauma: a European guideline. *Crit Care* 2007;**11**:R17 (doi:10.1186/cc5686).

35 Stengel D, Bauwens K, Sehouli J, et al. Systematic review and meta-analysis of emergency ultrasonography for blunt abdominal trauma. *Br J Surg* 2001;**88**:901–12.

36 Rozycki GS, Ballard RB, Feliciano DV, Schmidt JA, Pennington SD. Surgeon-performed ultrasound for the assessment of truncal injuries. Lessons learned from 1,540 patients. *Ann Surg* 1998;**228**:557–67.

37 Farahmand N, Sirlin CB, Brown MA, et al. Hypotensive patients with blunt abdominal trauma: performance of screening US. *Radiology* 2005;**235**:436–43.

38 Wherrett LJ, Boulanger BR, McLellan BA, et al. Hypotension after blunt abdominal trauma: the role of emergent abdominal sonography in surgical triage. *J Trauma* 1996;**41**:815–20.

39 Branney SW, Wolfe RE, Moore EE, et al. Quantitative sensitivity of ultrasound in detecting free intraperitoneal fluid. *J Trauma* 1995;**39**:375–80.

40 Jehle D, Guarino J, Karamanoukian H. Emergency department ultrasound in the evaluation of blunt abdominal trauma. *Am J Emerg Med* 1993;**11**:342–6.

41 Ma OJ, Mateer JR, Ogata M, et al. Prospective analysis of a rapid trauma ultrasound examination performed by emergency physicians. *J Trauma* 1995;**38**:879–85.

42 Smith RS, Kern SJ, Fry WR, et al. Institutional learning curve of surgeon-performed trauma ultrasound. *Arch Surg* 1998;**133**:530–35.

43 Shackford SR, Rogers FB, Osler TM, et al. Focused abdominal sonogram for trauma: the learning curve of nonradiologist clinicians in detecting hemoperitoneum. *J Trauma* 1999;**46**:553–64.

44 Stengel D, Bauwens K, Sehouli J, et al. Emergency ultrasound-based algorithms for diagnosing blunt abdominal trauma. *Cochrane Database Syst Rev* 2005;**2**:CD004446 (doi: 10.1002/14651858.CD004446.pub2).

45 Melniker LA, Leibner E, McKenney LG, Lopez P, Briggs WM, Mancuso CA. Randomized controlled clinical trial of point-of-care, limited ultrasonography for trauma in the emergency department: the first Sonography Outcomes Assessment Program Trial. *Ann Emerg Med* 2006; **48**(3):227–35.

46 Rizzo A, Steinberg SM, Flint LM, et al. Prospective assessment of the value of computed tomography for trauma. *J Trauma Injury Infect Crit Care* 1995;**38**(3):338–43.

47 Malhotra A, Fabian TC, Katsi SB, et al. Blunt bowel and mesenteric injuries: the role of screening computed tomography. *J Trauma Injury Infect Crit Care* 2000;**48**(6):991–1000.

48 Shanmuganathan K, Mirvis SE, Chiu WC, et al. Penetrating torso trauma: triple-contrast helical CT in peritoneal violation and organ injury – a prospective study in 200 patients. *Radiology* 2004;**231**:775–84.

49 Salim A, Sangthong B, Martin M, et al. Whole body imaging in blunt multisystem trauma patients without obvious signs of injury. *Arch Surg* 2006;**141**:468–75.

50 Henry SM, Tornetta P, Scalea TM. Damage control for devastating pelvic and extremity injuries. *Surg Clin North Am* 1997;**77**:879.

51 Miller PR, Moore PS, Mansell E, et al. External fixation or arteriogram in bleeding pelvic fracture: initial therapy guided by markers of arterial hemorrhage. *J Trauma* 2003;**54**:437–43.

52 Balogh Z, Caldwell E, Heetveld M, et al. Institutional practice guidelines on management of pelvic fracture-related hemodynamic instability: do they make a difference? *J Trauma* 2005;**58**:778–82.

53 Heetveld MJ, Harris I, Schlaphoff G, et al. Guidelines for the management of haemodynamically unstable pelvic fracture patients. *Aust NZ J Surg* 2004;**74**:520–29.

6 Genitourinary and Abdominal

37 Acute Appendicitis

James A. Nelson & Stephen R. Hayden

Department of Emergency Medicine, University of California at San Diego, San Diego, USA

Case scenario

A 20-year-old man presented to the emergency department (ED) with 1 day of progressive abdominal pain that had migrated to the right lower quadrant, associated with nausea and vomiting. He appeared alert and attentive, with a rectal temperature of 37.7°C (99.8°F) and a heart rate of 84 beats/min. His physical examination was normal except for the abdominal examination, which showed tenderness to palpation of the right lower quadrant and a positive Rovsing's sign. There was localized peritoneal tenderness to percussion over this area, and guarding but no rigidity. The medical student placed acute appendicitis as the primary diagnostic possibility, and suggested a call to the general surgeon to assess for immediate operative intervention. The general surgeon was in the operating room at an outside hospital, and requested that laboratory and imaging studies be completed before she consulted.

Laboratory studies were pending, and radiology was called for an abdominal computerized tomography (CT) scan. The radiologist asked whether you wanted the scan to be performed with oral or intravenous contrast. You requested an unenhanced CT, but you wondered whether the addition of contrast might offer any additional benefit. You also wondered whether a delay in surgery would increase the patient's risks for morbidity.

Background

Abdominal pain is a common presentation to the ED. Although most cases ultimately prove to be benign, those with emergent medical conditions need to be identified. Acute appendicitis is a consideration in most differential diagnoses. It is the most common cause of the acute abdomen today, with a lifetime incidence of 7% [1]. It is thought to arise from luminal obstruction, which leads to venous engorgement, bacterial invasion, tissue ischemia and, eventually, necrosis and perforation. Unperforated appen-

dicitis carries a low mortality rate of 0.1%, but this increases to 4% with perforation. Short-term morbidity from appendicitis includes abdominal abscess, sepsis and surgical wound infection; long-term morbidity from appendicitis includes adhesions and bowel obstructions. It is generally understood that patients who present later in the course of their illness tend to fare worse. It is therefore important to ensure that our practice habits reflect rapid, efficient diagnosis as well as optimal therapy.

Clinical questions

In order to optimize your diagnostic strategy as well as management of the patient with suspected appendicitis, you structure your literature search strategy according to the principles described in Chapter 1.

1 In patients with confirmed appendicitis receiving antibiotics (population), does a delay in surgery (intervention) increase morbidity or mortality (outcomes) compared to patients who receive surgery promptly (control)?

2 In adult patients with suspected appendicitis (population), what is the sensitivity and specificity (diagnostic test performance) of physical examination findings (test) in detecting acute appendicitis (outcome)?

3 In undifferentiated ED patients with suspected appendicitis (population), what is the sensitivity and specificity (diagnostic test performance) of laboratory markers of inflammation (test) in detecting acute appendicitis (outcome)?

4 In adult patients with suspected acute appendicitis (population), what are the sensitivity and specificity (diagnostic test performance) of thin-section helical CT scanning without contrast (test) for appendicitis (outcome)?

5 In patients with suspected acute appendicitis (population), does enhanced CT scanning with oral, rectal or intravenous contrast (test) improve sensitivity and specificity (diagnostic test performance) for appendicitis (outcome) compared to non-contrast studies (control)?

6 In patients with suspected appendicitis (population), is ultrasound (diagnostic test) as sensitive and specific (diagnostic test performance)

Evidence-based Emergency Medicine. Edited by Brian H. Rowe as CT (diagnostic test control) in the diagnosis of appendicitis (outcome)?

7 In pregnant patients with suspected appendicitis (population), does CT (intervention) cause teratogenesis, carcinogenesis or mutagenesis (outcomes) compared to clinical diagnosis (control)?

8 In pregnant patients suspected of having acute appendicitis (population), are there safe and effective alternatives to CT (test) to confirm or exclude appendicitis (diagnostic test performance)?

General search strategy

You search for answers to these questions by searching MEDLINE clinical queries for appendicitis under the "diagnosis" protocol, as well as searching for systematic reviews and meta-analyses. When these are located, you also search for more recent prospective studies addressing the same topic. You search EMBASE for similar topics. You also check the National Guideline Clearinghouse (www.guideline.gov) for any clinical practice guidelines and the Cochrane Library for systematic reviews in the Cochrane Database of Systemic Reviews (CDSR) or the Database of Abstracts of Reviews of Effects (DARE).

Searching for evidence synthesis: primary search strategy
- Cochrane Library: appendicitis
- MEDLINE: appendicitis AND (systematic review OR meta-analysis OR meta-analysis) AND (topic)
- EMBASE: appendicitis AND (systematic review OR meta-analysis OR meta-analysis) AND (topic)
- Guideline.gov: appendicitis

Critical review of the literature

Your search strategy for the Cochrane Library and guideline.gov website did not reveal any articles relevant to your questions. Your search of MEDLINE and EMBASE, however, identified several pertinent and interesting articles.

Question 1: In patients with confirmed appendicitis receiving antibiotics (population), does a delay in surgery (intervention) increase morbidity or mortality (outcomes) compared to patients who receive surgery promptly (control)?

Search strategy

- MEDLINE and EMBASE: appendicitis AND antibiotics; appendectomy AND delay

The natural history and surgical treatment of acute appendicitis was described long before the advent of intravenous antibiotics, and this understanding forms the background of how we view appendicitis [2]. It has traditionally been considered a potentially lethal illness which, untreated, progresses inexorably to perforation and either abscess or peritonitis, depending on whether the infection is contained. Prompt appendectomy has been considered the most important intervention in acute appendicitis. Delays in surgical care often arouse concern among emergency physicians that the patient may suffer preventable harm. It is generally thought that patients who present later to the ED do in fact experience a greater degree of morbidity, as do patients in whom the diagnosis is delayed [3]. Due to logistical constraints, however, sometimes the surgeon is unable to perform appendectomy immediately and a delay results.

A number of retrospective reviews have determined that selected adults as well as children with delayed appendectomy have the same rate of complications as patients with prompt surgery [4–7]. One retrospective observational study concluded that only after a delay of 24 hours does the rate of complications increase [8]. Another reported that delays do in fact increase the rate of complications [9]. No prospective studies have addressed this question and such studies are unable to definitively answer the question of whether a delay increases morbidity. As noted earlier, however, complication rates do rise significantly following appendiceal perforation [1], an event generally felt to be preventable with timely surgical intervention. This suggests that delay beyond the point of perforation should be assiduously avoided. However, there is at present insufficient evidence to directly answer the question of whether a delay in surgical therapy increases the rate of complications.

Prospective studies have asked the question of whether surgery in the acute appendicitis patient offers any benefit over antibiotic therapy. These studies were motivated by prior reports of US Navy submariners treated solely with antibiotics, as well as a case series of 471 patients [10,11]. A randomized controlled trial of appendectomy versus antibiotic therapy for acute appendicitis was published in 1995 [12]. The same group subsequently published a much larger ($n = 252$) prospective, multi-center, randomized controlled trial of appendectomy versus antibiotic therapy for acute appendicitis, and they found no significant difference in the rate of complications [13]. However, the group treated with antibiotics did suffer a 14% rate of recurrence during the following year. Women and patients with suspected perforation were excluded from this study.

In summary, the paucity of evidence precludes at this time a definitive answer to the question of whether surgical delay results in important deleterious clinical effects. The decision to allow delayed surgery for appendicitis remains an individual one based on the many factors that arise in each case. One innovative prospective, randomized study suggests that in male patients with no evidence of perforation, surgery offers no immediate advantage over intravenous antibiotics. This suggests that in selected patients with no evidence of perforation, surgical delays are probably safe when these conditions are met and the patient is receiving intravenous antibiotics. However, this will need to be validated in a generalized population before changing the routine practice of performing appendectomy as promptly as possible. Local resources and surgeon preference will likely continue to direct the timing of surgical intervention. For the emergency physician, it is important to promptly consult an appropriate surgeon or immediately transfer a patient to a facility where surgical consultation is available.

Question 2: In adult patients with suspected appendicitis (population), what is the sensitivity and specificity (diagnostic test performance) of physical examination findings (diagnostic test) in detecting acute appendicitis (outcome)?

Search strategy

- MEDLINE (PubMed): appendicitis AND physical examination AND (sensitivity and specificity OR likelihood). Limited to systematic review

The diagnostic process for a patient with suspected appendicitis involves a series of decisions using imperfect laboratory and imaging tests to raise or lower one's pre-test probability of disease. The usefulness of these tests rests upon the accuracy of the clinician's pre-test probability. Therefore it is worth pursuing excellence in evaluating the historical and physical findings in the patient with suspected appendicitis. This clinical excellence is grounded in knowledge of which of the many features of physical diagnosis have high positive likelihood ratios (+LRs) or powerful negative likelihood ratios (−LRs).

A systematic review of the likelihood ratios of signs and symptoms in patients with suspected appendicitis was published as part of the Rational Clinical Examination Series in the *Journal of the American Medical Association* in 1996 [14]. Features of the history and physical examination from the 10 studies retrieved were assessed. Findings with significantly +LRs include right lower quadrant (RLQ) pain (+LR = 8.0; 95% CI: 7.3 to 8.5), rigidity (+LR = 4.0; 95% CI: 3.0 to 4.8) and migration of initial periumbilical pain to the RLQ (+LR = 3.1; 95% CI: 2.4 to 4.2). Findings with powerful −LRs include the absence of RLQ tenderness (−LR = 0.2; 95% CI: 0.0 to 0.3) and the previous presence of similar pain (−LR = 0.3; 95% CI: 0.25 to 0.42) (Table 37.1). This review is limited by the quality of the studies, most of which have important limitations, such as restricting their focus to patients who were admitted or had undergone surgery.

A more recent large prospective study suggests that individual aspects of the history and physical examination each have rela-

Table 37.1 Likelihood ratios of clinical signs in suspected appendicitis.

Sign	+LR	−LR
Right lower quadrant pain	8.0	0.2
Rigidity	+4.0	NA
Migration	+3.1	NA
Similar pain in the past	NA	0.3

Table 37.2 Likelihood ratios for rebound tenderness and guarding in suspected appendicitis.

	+LR when moderate	+LR when strong
Rebound tenderness	+2.8	+7.9
Guarding	+5.2	+7.5

tively small diagnostic utility, but that their combination is useful. Independent predictors of acute appendicitis included rebound tenderness (+LR = 2.8 when moderate; 95% CI: 2.1 to 3.8; +LR = 7.9 when strong; 95% CI: 3.6 to 17.1) and guarding (+LR = 5.2 when moderate; 95% CI: 3.3 to 8.1; +LR = 7.5 when strong; 95% CI: 2.7 to 20.7) (Table 37.2). Another meta-analysis supports these findings [15].

In summary, although eliciting and interpreting the history and physical examination remains an art, and an intuition about the patient based on the constellation of clinical findings remains fundamental to the practice of medicine, it behooves the clinician to know which findings carry the strongest weight. Current data suggest that RLQ pain or guarding, rigidity and peritoneal signs are associated with useful +LRs. The absence of RLQ tenderness and a history of similar pain in the past argue against appendicitis. These values, when employed with the Fagan nomogram, can be used to calculate the post-test probability of disease [16]. For example, in an ED population in which 5% of patients with abdominal pain have acute appendicitis (a prior probability of 5%), the finding of RLQ pain alone raises the posterior probability to 30%.

Question 3: In undifferentiated ED patients with suspected appendicitis (population), what is the sensitivity and specificity (diagnostic test performance) of laboratory markers of inflammation (test) in detecting acute appendicitis (outcome)?

Search strategy

- MEDLINE (PubMed): appendicitis AND (laboratory OR white blood cell) AND sensitivity and specificity

Appendicitis is an inflammatory condition, and laboratory markers of inflammation are part of the routine evaluation in patients with suspected appendicitis. Commonly used parameters include the white blood cell (WBC) count, the neutrophil percentage and the C-reactive protein (CRP). It is therefore worth evaluating the influence of each test on our estimate of the probability of the disease.

A number of studies have addressed this issue; however, few have addressed the population of most interest to emergency physicians in a prospective fashion, and those that have did not assess the neutrophil percentage or immature ("band") forms. One prospective observational study of 125 ED patients presenting with suspected appendicitis can be used to estimate likelihood ratios. For WBC

Table 37.3 Likelihood ratios for serum markers of inflammation in suspected appendicitis.

Laboratory test	+LR	−LR
WBC >10,000/mm³	2.1	0.37
CRP >10 mg/L	1.9	0.59
Both	2.9	NA
Neither	NA	0.23

CRP, C-reactive protein; WBC, white blood cell.

elevations >10,000/mm³, the +LR was 2.1 (95% CI: 1.5 to 2.9) and the −LR was 0.37 (95% CI: 0.2 to 0.6) [17]. For CRP (>10 mg/L), the +LR was 1.9 (95% CI: 1.3 to 2.8) and the −LR was 0.59 (95% CI: 0.4 to 0.8). The combination of both being elevated revealed a +LR of 2.9 (95% CI: 1.6 to 5.4). Using the elevation of either laboratory test, the −LR was 0.23 (95% CI: 0.1 to 0.5). This suggests that, when using specific cut-offs for elevation, laboratory studies are of only modest benefit in modulating one's pre-test probability of disease (Table 37.3); their ability to affect clinical decision making is probably limited. When both laboratory tests are elevated the probability of disease rises from a prior probability of 46% to a posterior probability of 71%, which is not sufficient to justify surgery without confirmatory testing. When neither are elevated, the probability of disease drops from 46% to 16%, which may not be considered sufficiently low for discharge without further testing.

A second prospective ED study using the same definition of "elevated" suggests less utility of the WBC count. Of 274 patients with suspected appendicitis, an elevated WBC count (>10,000 cells/mm³) was found to have a sensitivity of 76% and a specificity of 52%, corresponding to a +LR of 1.59 (95% CI: 1.31 to 1.93) and a −LR of 0.46 (95% CI: 0.31 to 0.67) [18].

In summary, these studies highlight that laboratory markers of inflammation are of limited value in the diagnostic testing for appendicitis. They should be cautiously used to raise or lower the clinician's pre-test probability of disease [15]. Although arguably not necessary, these markers of inflammation may sometimes serve as helpful adjuncts to diagnosis.

Question 4: In adult patients with suspected acute appendicitis (population), what are the sensitivity and specificity (diagnostic test performance) of thin-section helical CT scanning without contrast (test) for appendicitis (outcome)?

Search strategy

- MEDLINE (PubMed): unenhanced CT AND appendicitis AND specificity

Prior to the advent of CT, patients with acute appendicitis were evaluated clinically, and decisions to perform laparotomy were based on the history and physical and laboratory examinations. This traditionally yielded a negative laparotomy rate of approximately 20% [19]. The advent of CT appears to have improved diagnostic accuracy, but there is no consensus on the optimal scanning strategy. Unenhanced CT scanning is employed as a matter of routine at many centers, and it is worth reviewing its clinical utility.

Although many studies have been performed in the past 10 years using different protocols for CT scanning, few have prospectively evaluated the use of unenhanced CT scanning. Our search identified a small number of observational studies that have prospectively evaluated whether unenhanced CT scanning is sufficient to exclude appendicitis. One study of 103 adult patients showed that unenhanced CT compared to gold standard laparoscopy had a sensitivity of 95.4%, a specificity of 100%, with the +LR approaching infinity (95% CI: 2.0 to 472) and the −LR equal to 0.05 (95% CI: 0.02 to 0.14) [20]. Unfortunately, this study is limited by selection bias, in that only patients scheduled for surgery based on clinical examination were enrolled, and the prevalence of disease in this population was 85%, which is well above the rate reported for a general population presenting to the ED with undifferentiated abdominal pain. Another study of 130 ED patients identified a sensitivity of 94.7% and a specificity of 91.7% [21]. The calculated +LR is 11 (95% CI: 3.8 to 34) and the −LR is 0.06 (95% CI: 0.02 to 0.14). Another group studying thin-slice CT of the RLQ on 296 patients reported a sensitivity of 96% and specificity of 98% [22]. The calculated +LR was 60 (95% CI: 20 to 186) and the −LR was 0.04 (95% CI: 0.01 to 0.04). These last two studies were limited by incorporation bias, or a lack of blinding, such that surgeons incorporated the results of the diagnostic test in question to decide whether to employ the gold standard diagnostic confirmation – surgery (Table 37.4).

Some limitations should be borne in mind. First, the clinician must consider how the quality of his or her scanner and radiology department would compare to those at the research institutions in the above studies. Second, the studies described above are subject to publication bias. Other studies addressing different questions have reported lower sensitivity and specificity, as described below [23].

In summary, these studies have methodological limitations, but they support the assertion that CT scanning can significantly lower the posterior probability of disease in patients with low to moderate suspicion of disease. Assuming the reported −LR of 0.05 is

Table 37.4 Likelihood ratios for unenhanced abdominal CT in suspected appendicitis in different studies.

Study	+LR	−LR
in't Hof et al. [20]	Infinity	0.05
Cakirer et al. [21]	11	0.06
Ege et al. [22]	60	0.04

accurate, and accepting a missed appendicitis rate of 5%, a patient with a 50% prior probability of disease would have a posterior probability of 4%, which, under the appropriate clinical circumstances, can be sufficient to allow a patient to be discharged from the ED.

Question 5: In patients with suspected acute appendicitis (population), does enhanced CT scanning with oral, rectal or intravenous contrast (test) improve diagnostic accuracy (diagnostic test performance) for appendicitis (outcome) compared to non-contrast studies (control)?

Search strategy

- MEDLINE (PubMed) and EMBASE: appendicitis AND CT AND sensitivity and specificity

There is presently no consensus on the optimal imaging technique for patients with suspected appendicitis. Strategies to optimize CT scanning are diverse, and include the use of contrast to opacify the bowel – whether given orally or rectally – as well as the use of intravenous contrast. Disadvantages of rectal contrast include patient discomfort and logistical challenges to the radiology technicians. Disadvantages to oral contrast include time delay and discomfort associated with the prevalence of concomitant nausea in patients with suspected appendicitis. Disadvantages to intravenous contrast include the risk of nephrotoxicity and anaphylactoid reactions. Advantages might include the potential for improved diagnostic accuracy.

No prospective randomized controlled trials on adults were found that compared unenhanced CT to CT enhanced with either oral or intravenous contrast. One study of 288 patients comparing oral alone to oral and intravenous contrast found that the sensitivity of the former was 71–83%, whereas the latter was 92–98% [23], suggesting that intravenous contrast may have some added utility. Taking the reader with lowest sensitivity, the +LR for the unenhanced scan was 35 (95% CI: 14 to 88) and that for the enhanced scan was 29 (95% CI: 14 to 61). The −LR for the scan with oral contrast only was 0.30 (95% CI: 0.2 to 0.45) and that for oral and intravenous contrast was 0.12 (95% CI: 0.06 to 0.26). For the highest sensitivity reader, the +LR of the unenhanced scan was 12 (95% CI: 7.3 to 19) and for the enhanced study was 15 (95% CI: 9.3 to 26). The −LR for the unenhanced scan was 0.18 (95% CI: 0.10 to 0.34) and for the enhanced scan was 0.07 (95% CI: 0.03 to 0.20). The summary of these findings seems to indicate that the addition of intravenous contrast allowed the reader to exclude appendicitis with better discrimination (Table 37.5).

As for oral contrast, a systematic review using a pooled analysis found that use of oral contrast itself has negative utility, with the non-contrast CT yielding a +LR of 32 and a −LR of 0.05 and the use of oral contrast showing a +LR of 15 and a −LR of 0.09 [24]. However, confidence intervals were not able to be calculated.

Table 37.5 The degree of improved accuracy with intravenous contrast.

	−LR of oral contrast only	−LR of oral and IV contrast
Lowest sensitivity reader	0.30	0.12
Highest sensitivity reader	0.18	0.07

This study has many confounding variables, including the heterogeneous use of intravenous contrast among the included scans.

One study of 91 patients compared rectal contrast only to scans done with rectal, oral and intravenous (triple) contrast, and showed no statistically significant benefit from the addition of IV contrast [25]. A second study detailed an imaging protocol whereby unenhanced CT was the study of choice, and in cases of diagnostic uncertainty intravenous and sometimes oral or rectal contrast were employed. It found that the addition of contrast improved sensitivity for appendicitis, but because there was no control, it is not known whether the added benefit accrued simply from repeating the scan after a delay, regardless of the addition of contrast [26]. Additionally, lack of standardization of the use of contrast limits our ability to assess the study protocol.

In summary, studies of the added benefit of enhanced CT scanning are limited by the large variation in type of enhancement employed and demonstrate varying results. Any combination of oral, IV or rectal contrast may be employed and have all been studied. Because of the heterogeneity of methodology, and variability in results, few conclusions can be drawn at this time. Given the necessity of accurate diagnosis, it is reasonable for clinicians to employ unenhanced CT scanning as a matter of routine, with repeat scanning with intravenous and possibly rectal or oral contrast for cases in which there is diagnostic uncertainty and where the clinical suspicion remains significant. No definite recommendations can be made, however, until enhanced and unenhanced CT scanning are compared to each other in a randomized prospective trial.

Question 6: In patients with suspected appendicitis (population), is ultrasound (diagnostic test) as sensitive and specific (diagnostic test performance) as CT (diagnostic test control) in the diagnosis of appendicitis (outcome)?

Search strategy

- MEDLINE (PubMed) and EMBASE: appendicitis AND ultrasound AND computed tomography. Limited to systematic review

Ultrasonography for the diagnosis of acute appendicitis has appeal because of its safety profile and speed of acquisition. A search for systematic reviews yields two recent articles addressing this issue. A meta-analysis of 57 studies separately analyzed the 31 that were restricted to adults, and the pooled sensitivity and specificity for adult ultrasound was 83% and 93%, respectively. The

Table 37.6 Likelihood ratios of computerized tomography (CT) and ultrasound for suspected appendicitis in two studies.

Study	+LR	−LR
Doria et al. [27]		
Ultrasound	12	0.18
CT	16	0.06
Terasawa et al. [28]		
Ultrasound	3.4	0.26
CT	15	0.09

corresponding +LR and −LR for ultrasound are 12 (95% CI: 8.7 to 16) and 0.18 (95% CI: 0.15 to 0.22), respectively. For CT scanning, the sensitivity and specificity were both 94% [27]. The corresponding +LR and −LR are 16 (95% CI: 11 to 22) and 0.06 (95% CI: 0.04 to 0.09), respectively. No attempt was made to use a consistent method of CT scanning, whether with delivery of contrast, thickness of slices or number of detectors.

Another review reported that the sensitivity and specificity of ultrasound for diagnosing appendicitis in adults were 81% and 80%, respectively. This corresponds to a +LR of 3.4 (95% CI: 2.2 to 5.1) and a −LR of 0.26 (95% CI: 0.12 to 0.58) [28]. For CT scanning, reported in the same review, the sensitivity and specificity was 94% and 95%, respectively. This corresponds to a +LR of 15 (95% CI: 9.4 to 22) and a −LR of 0.09 (95% CI: 0.09 to 0.14) (Table 37.6).

Both articles were limited by the studies they assessed, many of which suffered from methodological weaknesses, including incomplete blinding. By necessity, only positive results were assessed by the gold standard – removal and examination of the appendix (negative results were assessed by clinical follow-up). None the less, the diagnostic superiority of CT scanning over ultrasound has been consistently supported. Use of ultrasound scanning for suspected appendicitis is reasonable as long as the clinician is aware of its limitations. It is probably more useful as a potentially time- and radiation-sparing measure for confirming the diagnosis in patients with a high probability of disease, or for excluding it in those with a low probability of disease. Those with a moderate to high suspicion of disease and a negative or equivocal result will need further testing or observation.

Question 7: In pregnant patients with suspected appendicitis (population), does CT (intervention) cause teratogenesis, carcinogenesis or mutagenesis (outcomes) compared to clinical diagnosis (control)?

Search strategy

- MEDLINE (PubMed): appendicitis AND pregnan* AND (filter) radiation

No outcomes-based studies were identified that could confirm or refute the hypothesis that fetal exposure to CT causes malforma-

tion, teratogenesis, malignancy or intellectual impairment. Some evidence-based reviews were identified that also describe being unable to find relevant studies addressing this question [29].

Our current understanding of the teratogenic risk of ionizing radiation to the fetus is extrapolated from population studies of pregnant women exposed to nuclear radiation during the atomic bombing of Hiroshima and Nagasaki in 1945. Offspring were found to have microcephaly and mental retardation, although most of these were believed to have had 10–100 rad (100–1000 mGy) of fetal exposure. For a relative perspective, the fetal dose of a chest radiograph is 0.00007 rad, that of an acute abdominal series is 0.245 rad, that of a chest CT is estimated at less than 0.10 rad, and that of an abdominal CT is 2.60 rad [30]. Additionally, most of these untoward events were related to exposure during organogenesis, that stage of fetal development between 8 and 15 weeks of gestation.

Our understanding of the carcinogenic risk of ionizing radiation to the fetus comes from retrospective reviews [31]. The risk of leukemia after CT scanning of the fetus has been estimated as similar to the risk of exposure to CT during childhood, a relative risk of approximately 1.4 [32].

The International Commission on Radiologic Protection concludes, "Prenatal doses from most properly done diagnostic procedures present no measurably increased risk of prenatal death, malformation, or impairment of mental development" [33]. The American College of Obstetricians and Gynecologists has stated that exposure of up to 5 rad (50 mGy) is not believed to cause fetal anomalies [33].

In the absence of good prospective data, it is possible that clinicians and patients may continue to be wary of the use of CT [34]. This has the unfortunate potential to lead to morbidity due to delays in diagnosis and should be approached cautiously with the best available evidence. If a clinician chooses to recommend CT, discussion should probably take place with the mother in which the benefits, risks and alternatives are discussed (including other imaging modalities). If the decision is made to proceed with CT scanning, this can be done knowing that our best assessments of risk suggest that abdominal CT in the pregnant patient is a very low-risk procedure, and that many national and international organizations have spoken in support of the practice when medically indicated.

Question 8: In pregnant patients suspected of having acute appendicitis (population), are there safe and effective alternatives to CT (test) to confirm or exclude appendicitis (diagnostic test performance)?

Search strategy

- MEDLINE and EMBASE: pregnant appendicitis AND sensitivity and specificity

A search strategy was employed evaluating the specificity of diagnostic tests for appendicitis in the pregnant patient. In a retrospective observation of 45 pregnant patients with suspected appendicitis, ultrasound was shown to have a sensitivity and specificity of 100% and 96%, respectively, corresponding to a +LR of 25 (95% CI: 4 to 78) and a −LR of 0.0 (95% CI: 0.0 to 0.45) [35]. However, in addition to the problematic issues attendant with retrospective design, this study was flawed in that it excluded analysis of subjects in whom the operator had difficulty performing the examination due to the third-trimester gravid uterus. Furthermore, because only 16 patients had acute appendicitis, the power of this study is limited.

Largely based on theoretical understandings, magnetic resonance imaging (MRI) has been reported as safe in pregnancy, although it has not been prospectively studied [36]. A retrospective review of 51 subjects (though only four with appendicitis) reports MRI as being 100% sensitive and 94% specific, corresponding to a +LR of 17 (95% CI: 4 to 38) and a −LR of 0.0 (96% CI: 0.01 to 1.47). Further search for related articles reveals similar design and sample size limitations, but points out the advantage of MRI in diagnosing other pathology, including ovarian torsion, uterine pathology and other inflammatory conditions [37].

Technetium-99 tagged WBC scanning was retrospectively reviewed in 13 pregnant patients with suspected acute appendicitis, and was found to have poor sensitivity (50%) as well as specificity (73%) [38]. This limited study found no relationship between the tagged WBC scan and the presence of acute appendicitis.

In summary, the pregnant patient with lower abdominal pain will continue to offer a diagnostic challenge. The literature at this time is limited, and merely offers suggested courses of action. Ultrasonography may be useful in competent and experienced hands; however, this remains unproven, and while human fetal radiation risks have been quantified to some degree, little is known about the fetal impact of magnetic resonance exposure. CT, however, has demonstrated high sensitivity and specificity for the detection of appendicitis and appears to be safe based on all available data. Regardless of modality, prudent consideration of laparoscopy, extended observation or close follow-up should be given to pregnant patients with suspected appendicitis in whom the diagnostic process of choice does not yield a definitive answer.

Conclusions

The patient mentioned above was found to have a WBC count of 11,000/mm^3. Computerized tomography performed without contrast revealed a 1 cm appendix with periappendiceal inflammation. Antibiotics were started and the surgeon removed the appendix 6 hours later. Pathology confirmed the diagnosis of unruptured appendicitis. The patient recovered well and was discharged home the following day without complications.

Appendicitis continues to offer diagnostic challenges for emergency physicians. Knowledge of diagnostic options and their likelihood ratios allows the clinician to intelligently weigh the benefits and drawbacks of various approaches. These options rest on our ability to formulate an accurate pre-test probability based on the history and physical examination. At this time the findings of RLQ pain, rigidity and peritoneal signs have most consistently been demonstrated to support appendicitis. Laboratory adjuncts such as the WBC count and C-reactive protein have limited value; however, they might prove useful in helping to confirm appendicitis in the patient with a high prior probability of disease, or in helping to exclude it in the patient with a low prior probability of disease.

Computerized tomography has been consistently shown to be the most accurate imaging study for appendicitis, and unenhanced CT scanning has been shown to have powerful positive and negative likelihood ratios. If the patient's diagnosis remains uncertain after unenhanced scanning, the use of intravenous contrast enhancement is supported by the literature to improve the negative likelihood ratio. There is currently no clear evidence on when to use oral and rectal contrast. Ultrasound is inferior to CT, but may be sufficient to confirm or exclude the diagnosis in patients with respectively high or low prior probability of disease.

Flexibility in approaching each patient with suspected appendicitis is wise. Depending on the particular patient's history and findings, different approaches are reasonable as long as they are based on an impression of prior probability of disease and knowledge of the power of each test to modulate this and produce a posterior probability. The traditional negative laparotomy rate of 20% is probably much lower at this time, due to the many excellent diagnostic options available to the clinician.

References

1 Wolfe JM, Henneman PL. Acute appendicitis: In: Marx JA, Hockberger RS, Walls RM, eds. *Rosen's Emergency Medicine: Concepts and clinical practice.* Mosby, Philadelphia, 2006:1451–1460.

2 Fitz RH. Perforating inflammation of the vermiform appendix. *Am J Med Sci* 1886; **92**:321–46.

3 Paulson EK, Kalady MF, Pappas TN. Clinical practice: suspected appendicitis. *N Engl J Med* 2003;**348**:236–42.

4 Eldar S, Nash E, Sabo E, et al. Delay of surgery in acute appendicitis. *Am J Surg* 1997;**173**:194–8.

5 Yardeni D, Hirschl RB, Drongowski RA, et al. Delayed versus immediate surgery in acute appendicitis: do we need to operate during the night? *J Pediatr Surg* 2004;**39**:464–9.

6 Taylor M, Emil S, Nguyen N, et al. Emergent vs urgent appendectomy in children: a study of outcomes. *J Pediatr Surg* 2005;**40**:1912–15.

7 Abou-Nukta F, Bakhos C, Arroyo K, et al. Effects of delaying appendectomy for acute appendicitis for 12 to 24 hours. *Arch Surg* 2006;**141**:504–7.

8 Omundsen M, Dennett E. Delay to appendicectomy and associated morbidity: a retrospective review. *Aust NZ J Surg* 2006;**76**:153–5.

9 Ditillo MF, Dziura JD, Rabinovici R. Is it safe to delay appendectomy in adults with acute appendicitis? *Ann Surg* 2006;**244**:656–60.

10 Coldrey E. Five years of conservative treatment of acute appendicitis. *J Int Coll Surg* 1959;**32**:255–61.

11 Adams ML. The medical management of acute appendicitis in a nonsurgical environment: a retrospective case review. *Milit Med* 1990;**155**:345–7.

12 Eriksson S, Granstrom L. Randomized controlled trial of appendicectomy versus antibiotic therapy for acute appendicitis. *Br J Surg* 1995;**82**:166–9.

13 Styrud J, Erikkson S, Nilsson I, et al. Appendectomy versus antibiotic treatment in acute appendicitis: a prospective multicenter randomized controlled trial. *World J Surg* 2006;**30**:1033–7.

14 Wagner JM, McKinney WP, Carpenter JL. Does this patient have appendicitis? *JAMA* 1996;**276**:1589–94.

15 Andersson REB. Meta-analysis of the clinical and laboratory diagnosis of appendicitis. *Br J Surg* 2004;**91**:28–37.

16 Fagan TJ. Nomogram for Bayes theorem (Letter). *N Engl J Med* 1975;**293**:257.

17 Kessler N, Cyteval C, Gallix B, et al. Appendicitis: evaluation of sensitivity, specificity, and predictive values of US, Doppler US, and laboratory findings. *Radiology* 2004;**230**:472–8 (Epub December 19, 2003).

18 Cardall T, Glasser J, Guss DA. Clinical value of the total white blood cell count and temperature in the evaluation of patients with suspected appendicitis. *Acad Emerg Med* 2004;**11**:1021–7.

19 Andersson RE, Hugander AP, Ghazi SH, et al. Why does the clinical diagnosis fail in suspected appendicitis? *Eur J Surg* 2000;**166**:796–802.

20 in't Hof KH, van Lankeren W, Krestin GP, et al. Surgical validation of unenhanced helical computed tomography in acute appendicitis. *Br J Surg* 2004;**91**:1641–5.

21 Cakirer S, Basak M, Colakoglu B, et al. Diagnosis of acute appendicitis with unenhanced helical CT: a study of 130 patients. *Emerg Radiol* 2002;**9**:155–61 (Epub May 4, 2002).

22 Ege G, Akman H, Sahin A, et al. Diagnostic value of unenhanced helical CT in adult patients with suspected acute appendicitis. *Br J Radiol* 2002;**75**: 721–5.

23 Jacobs JE, Birnbaum BA, Macari M, et al. Acute appendicitis: comparison of helical CT diagnosis focused technique with oral contrast material versus nonfocused technique with oral and intravenous contrast material. *Radiology* 2001;**220**:683–90.

24 Anderson BA, Salem L, Flum DR. A systematic review of whether oral contrast is necessary for the computed tomography diagnosis of appendicitis in adults. *Am J Surg* 2005;**190**:474–8.

25 Mittal VK, Goliath J, Sabir M, et al. Advantages of focused helical computed tomographic scanning with rectal contrast only vs triple contrast in the diagnosis of clinically uncertain acute appendicitis: a prospective randomized study. *Arch Surg* 2004;**139**:495–500.

26 Tamburrini S, Brunetti A, Brown M, et al. Acute appendicitis: diagnostic value of nonenhanced CT with selective use of contrast in routine clinical settings. *Eur Radiol* 2007;**17**:2055–61 (Epub Dec 16, 2006).

27 Doria AS, Moineddin R, Kellenberger CJ, et al. US or CT for diagnosis of appendicitis in children and adults? A meta-analysis. *Radiology* 2006;**241**:83–94.

28 Terasawa T, Blackmore CC, Bent S, et al. Systematic review: computed tomography and ultrasonography to detect acute appendicitis in adults and adolescents. *Ann Intern Med* 2004;**141**:537–46

29 Smits AK, Paladine HL, Judkins DZ, et al. Clinical inquiries. What are the risks to the fetus associated with diagnostic radiation exposure during pregnancy? *J Fam Pract* 2006;**55**:441–4.

30 Toppenberg KS, Hill DA, Miller DP. Safety of radiographic imaging during pregnancy. *Am Fam Physician* 1999;**59**:1813–20.

31 Doll R, Wakeford R. Risk of childhood cancer from fetal irradiation. *Br J Radiol* 1997;**70**:130–39.

32 Valentin J, ed. *Pregnancy and Medical Radiation, International Commission on Radiological Protection*, Vol. 30, No. 1. Annals of the ICRP, Publication No. 84. Pergamon, Elsevier Science, Tarrytown, NY, 2000.

33 American College of Obstetricians and Gynecologists, Committee on Obstetric Practice. Guidelines for Diagnostic Imaging during Pregnancy. ACOG Committee Opinion No. 158. American College of Obstetricians and Gynecologists, Washington, 1995.

34 Ratnapalan S, Bona N, Chandra K, Koren G. Physicians' perceptions of teratogenic risk associated with radiography and CT during early pregnancy. *Am J Roentgenol* 2004;**182**:1107–9.

35 Lim HK, Bae SH, Seo GS. Diagnosis of acute appendicitis in pregnant women: value of sonography. *Am J Roentgenol* 1992;**159**:539–42.

36 Birchard KR, Brown MA, Hyslop WB, et al. MRI of acute abdominal and pelvic pain in pregnant patients. *Am J Roentgenol* 2005;**184**: 452–8.

37 Oto A, Ernst RD, Shah R, et al. Right-lower-quadrant pain and suspected appendicitis in pregnant women: evaluation with MR imaging – initial experience. *Radiology* 2005;**234**:445–51.

38 Stewart D, Grewal N, Choi R, et al. The use of tagged white blood cell scans to diagnose appendicitis in pregnant patients. *Am Surg* 2006;**72**: 894–6.

38 Ectopic Pregnancy

Heather Murray & Elisha David Targonsky

Departments of Emergency Medicine *and* Community Health and Epidemiology, Queen's University, Kingston, Canada

Clinical scenario

A 32-year-old female presented to the emergency department (ED) triage desk with a history of vaginal bleeding. She was approximately 7 weeks' pregnant and this was her first pregnancy, diagnosed after a positive home pregnancy test 1 week previously. She complained of vaginal spotting for 2 days and some diffuse abdominal cramping starting 2 hours prior to arrival. She was an otherwise healthy woman with no previous medical problems, denied any medication use and was a non-smoking, local teacher.

On examination, she appeared in no distress and her vital signs were a pulse of 90 beats/min and blood pressure of 110/70 mmHg (left = right arm) with no postural changes noted. Her abdomen was soft and non-tender and her pelvic examination revealed a closed cervix with some blood at the cervical os. There were no adnexal masses detected and mild cervical motion tenderness was identified.

It is examination time for her grade 12 class, and she wishes to go back to classes as soon as possible.

Background

Women with first trimester bleeding or pain presenting to the ED are common, and all should be assessed for the possibility of an ectopic pregnancy. An ectopic pregnancy is any gestation that occurs outside the uterine cavity, and it is both a life- and fertility-threatening condition. The incidence in the United States is on the rise, with approximately 2% of pregnancies falling into this category [1,2]. Outcomes from ectopic pregnancy are variable and dependent on the stage at diagnosis. Recent advances in the diagnostic approach to symptomatic first trimester pregnancies have led to earlier detection and an overall reduction in the

mortality and morbidity associated with ectopic pregnancy; the incidence of death has declined from 35.5 per 10,000 in 1970 to 3.8 per 10,000 in 1989 [2]. Among pregnant ED patients with first trimester vaginal bleeding and/or abdominal pain, the diagnosis of ectopic pregnancy should be strongly considered, as the prevalence among this population ranges from 6% to 16% [3].

Clinical questions

In order to address the issues of most relevance to your patient and to help in searching the literature for the evidence regarding these issues, you structure your clinical questions as recommended in Chapter 1.

1 In pregnant patients with first trimester abdominal pain and/or vaginal bleeding (population), what are the sensitivity and specificity (diagnostic test characteristics) of various historical risk factors and physical examination findings (tests) in the diagnosis of ectopic pregnancy (outcome)?

2 In pregnant patients with first trimester symptoms (population), what is the diagnostic value (diagnostic test characteristic) of single and serial measurements of serum β-human chorionic gonadotrophin (test) in identifying an ectopic pregnancy (outcome)?

3 In pregnant patients with first trimester symptoms (population), what are the sensitivity and specificity (diagnostic test characteristics) of formal ultrasound (test) for the diagnosis of ectopic pregnancy (outcome)?

4 In pregnant patients with first trimester symptoms (population), what are the sensitivity and specificity (diagnostic test characteristics) of ED targeted ultrasound (EDTU) (test) for the diagnosis of intrauterine pregnancy (outcome)?

5 In patients with possible ectopic pregnancy (population), does EDTU (test) influence clinical outcomes such as time to diagnosis, tubal rupture, costs and length of stay in the ED (outcomes) compared to use of standard ultrasound (comparison)?

6 In patients with documented non-ruptured ectopic pregnancy (population), what is the effectiveness of methotrexate

Evidence-based Emergency Medicine. Edited by Brian H. Rowe
© 2009 Blackwell Publishing, ISBN: 978-1-4051-6143-5.

(intervention) in preventing rupture, reducing hospitalization and improving patient well-being (outcomes) compared to surgical treatment (control)?

General search strategy

You begin to address the topic of ectopic pregnancy by searching for evidence in the common electronic databases such as MEDLINE and EMBASE, looking specifically for prospective studies of diagnostic test strategies and systematic reviews and randomized controlled trials in therapy. In addition, you search the Cochrane Library looking specifically for systematic reviews of treatment strategies in ectopic pregnancy. When a systematic review is identified, you also search for recent updates on the Cochrane Library and also search MEDLINE and EMBASE to identify randomized controlled trials that became available after the publication date of the systematic review.

Critical appraisal of the literature

Question 1: In patients with first trimester abdominal pain and/or vaginal bleeding (population) what are the sensitivity and specificity (diagnostic test characteristics) of various historical risk factors and physical examination findings (tests) in the diagnosis of ectopic pregnancy (outcome)?

Search strategy

- MEDLINE and EMBASE (risk factors): *explode* ectopic pregnancy AND (risk factors OR risk factors.mp) AND clinical trial AND case–control studies AND cohort studies AND meta-analysis
- Hand-searching (risk factors): references listed in the articles obtained

The clinical picture of patients with ectopic pregnancy depends to some extent on whether or not there is tubal rupture. Unruptured ectopic pregnancy has been characterized to have a "classic triad" of amenorrhea, abdominal pain and vaginal bleeding [4]. A ruptured ectopic pregnancy may be more obvious to the clinician, presenting with signs of hemodynamic compromise such as orthostasis, hypotension or shock. Two prospective studies have specifically examined the predictive ability of the elements in the "classic triad". A large study by Stovall et al. [4] found that while common in ruptured ectopic pregnancies, symptoms of abdominal pain, vaginal bleeding and amenorrhea were present in only 30%, 39% and 51% of the 100 unruptured ectopic pregnancies, respectively. According to a study by Buckley et al. [5], the presence of abdominal pain is 97.4% sensitive and vaginal bleeding 69.2% sensitive for ectopic pregnancy. These symptoms are not specific (15.3% and 26.2%, respectively) and are often found in

the presence of other gynecological and surgical conditions. Kaplan et al. [6] found that the overall physical exam had a sensitivity of only 36%. The sensitivity of the combined history and physical exam was even lower (18.5%) in a study by Barnhart et al. [7]. Reliance on the presence of the signs and symptoms in the classic triad will clearly result in missed cases of ectopic pregnancy.

A large number of epidemiological studies have investigated possible causative factors in the development of ectopic pregnancy. Several meta-analyses and case–control studies have addressed a wide range of possible risk factors thought to be responsible for the development of ectopic pregnancy (Table 38.1). The most important risk factors indicate the presence of altered Fallopian tube anatomy or physiology. A history of prior ectopic pregnancy [8–11,13], tubal surgery [8–10,12–14], documented tubal pathology [8], previous pelvic inflammatory disease (PID) [8–11,15] and infertility [8,9,12,13,15] are associated with greatest risk. A history of sexually transmitted infections, in particular by *Chlamydia trachomatis*, appears to be of significance, although to a lesser extent when it has not progressed to PID [8,11,16]. One historical factor traditionally considered a risk factor is the presence of an intrauterine device at the time of conception. Although this device reduces the overall risk of pregnancy, patients who become pregnant with a device in place are at greater risk of ectopic pregnancy [9,11,12,14,17,18]. Interestingly, smoking also appears to be a risk factor [8–10,15,67], perhaps due to a direct alteration of normal tubal physiology [19,20]. Identification of patient risk factors may aid in enhancing the clinician's suspicion. For the emergency physician, however, the identification of risk factors is only useful if their presence (or absence) changes the likelihood of ectopic pregnancy. A 1994 study of ED patients with positive urine pregnancy tests demonstrated that traditional risk factors were absent in 46% of unruptured ectopic pregnancies [4]. Absence of risk factors does not appear to translate into absence of risk.

Several studies have investigated the utility of the physical examination in identifying patients at increased risk for ectopic pregnancy (Table 38.2). Although the presence of hemodynamic instability in the setting of early pregnancy represents an ectopic pregnancy until proven otherwise, the performance of other physical findings in identifying patients with non-ruptured ectopic pregnancy has been disappointing. The presence of cervical motion tenderness has been shown in several studies [5,6,12,21,22] to be strongly associated with ectopic pregnancy; however, the likelihood ratios are still lower than required to satisfactorily rule in or rule out ectopic pregnancy. It must be noted that the presence or absence of a mass on digital pelvic examination does not appear in the list of useful or potentially relevant physical findings shown in Table 38.2.

In summary, a large body of evidence suggests that the history and physical examination are of limited predictive value for identifying ectopic pregnancy. The presence of risk factors may heighten the clinical suspicion of an ED physician, but risk factors are often absent in patients harboring ectopic pregnancies. The clinical examination has not been shown to be helpful in the detection of unruptured ectopic pregnancy and no combination of risk factors

Table 38.1 Summary of studies examining risk factors associated with ectopic pregnancy.

Risk factor	OR (95% CI) in different studies					
	Ankum et al. [8]*	Ankum et al. [8]†	Mol et al. [14]	Xiong et al. [17]	Dart et al. [12]	Case-controls with OR range [studies]
Prior EP	8.3 (6.0 to 11.5)					2.98 to 13.3 [9–11,13]
Past smoker	2.5 (1.8 to 3.4)					0.7 to 1.5 [9,15]
Current smoker	2.3 (2.0 to 2.8)					1.0 to 3.9 [9,10,15,67]
≥2 prior spontaneous abortions		.				1.5 to 3.0 [9,13,15]
Prior pelvic or abdominal surgery	0.93 to 3.8‡	1.5 (1.1 to 2.6)			2.0 (1.0 to 4.3)	0.95 to 3.0 [11, 13]
Prior tubal surgery**	21 (9.3 to 47)		9.3 (4.9 to 18)		18 (3.0 to 139)	4.0 to 5.1 [9,10,13]
Prior STI	2.8 to 3.7					0.97 to 1.4 [11,16]
Prior PID	2.5 (2.1 to 3.0)	5.7 (2.5 to 13)				1.5 to 4.7 [9–11,15]
Documented tubal pathology	3.5 to 25					
History of infertility	2.5 to 21	2.0 (1.2 to 3.4)			5.0 (1.1 to 28)	1.3 to 4.7 [9,13,15]
Current or past IUD use			4.2 to 45^B	6.37 (4.09 to 9.92)^A	5.0 (1.1 to 2.8)^B	1.06 to 3.5^A [9,11,18]
In utero DES exposure		5.6 (2.4 to 13)				

*Meta-analysis of case–control studies.
† Meta-analysis of prospective studies.
‡ Where 95% CI is omitted, the OR is presented as a range from multiple studies due to study heterogeneity.
**Includes tubal ligation.
A, past IUD use; B, current IUD use.
CI, confidence interval; DES, diethylstilbestrol; EP, ectopic pregnancy; IUD, intrauterine device; OR, odds ratio; PID, pelvic inflammatory disease; STI, sexually transmitted infection.

and physical findings has been shown to accurately and consistently rule out or confirm ectopic pregnancy in ED patients. Given the high prevalence of ectopic pregnancy in ED patients, further investigation to confirm pregnancy location is warranted in all ED patients with first trimester bleeding or pain.

Question 2: In pregnant patients with first trimester symptoms (population), what is the diagnostic value (diagnostic test characteristic) of single and serial measurements of serum β-human chorionic gonadotrophin (test) in identifying an ectopic pregnancy (outcome)?

Search strategy

- MEDLINE and EMBASE: *explode* ectopic pregnancy AND (chorionic gonadotropin.mp OR chorionic gonadotropin OR beta hCG) AND (sensitivity and specificity OR diagnostic accuracy.mp OR diagnostic accuracy)

- Hand-searching: reference lists were used to identify additional articles of interest

- Inclusion: articles were required to provide adequate descriptions of the parameters explored (e.g., discriminatory zones or 48-hour rise of <66%)

Assays for serum β-human chorionic gonadotrophin (β-hCG) have evolved and are now sensitive enough to detect levels as low as 5 IU/L [23]. Urine assays are less sensitive than serum tests; however they can still detect levels of 20–50 IU/L, depending on the concentration of the urine specimen [23]. For the most part, screening for pregnancy using a urine test will be adequate to confirm or refute pregnancy. Serum testing will be definitive if pregnancy is strongly suspected in the setting of a negative urine

Table 38.2 Predictive value of various physical findings in diagnosing ectopic pregnancy.

Study	Physical finding	Predictive value (95% CI)		LR (+) (95% CI)
		Sensitivity	Specificity	
Dart et al. [12]	Moderate to severe pain intensity	57.9 (45 to 69.8)	63.5 (58.6 to 68.2)	1.6 (1.2 to 2.0)
	CMT	31.6 (21 to 44.5)	86.6 (82.8 to 89.7)	2.4 (1.5 to 3.7)
	Positive peritoneal signs	12.3 (6.1 to 23.3)	96.6 (94.3 to 98)	3.6 (1.5 to 8.6)
	Lateral or bilateral abdominal tenderness	47.4 (35.0 to 60.1)	66.9 (62.0 to 71.5)	1.4 (1.1 to 2.0)
	Lateral or bilateral pelvic tenderness	50.9 (38.3 to 63.4)	68.2 (63.4 to 72.7)	1.6 (1.2 to 2.2)
Mol et al. [21]	Rebound tenderness	20.7 (14.3 to 28.9)	94.4 (90.9 to 96.6)	3.7 (2.0 to 6.7)
	Muscular rigidity on abdominal examination	6.0 (3.0 to 11.9)	99.3 (97.3 to 99.8)	8.0 (1.7 to 38)
	Digital vaginal exam inconclusive due to pain	25.0 (18.0 to 33.6)	96.6 (93.7 to 98.2)	7.4 (3.6 to 15.1)
Buckley et al. [22]	Peritoneal irritation on abdominal examination or definite CMT	32 (17 to 49)	95 (92 to 97)	6.1*
Buckley et al. [5]	Abdominal peritoneal signs	23.1 (12.7 to 38.3)	94.9 (92.4 to 96.6)	4.5 (2.2 to 9.0)
	Definite CMT	23.1 (12.7 to 38.3)	97.3 (95.4 to 98.5)	8.6 (3.9 to 19.1)
Kaplan et al. [6]	Adnexal tenderness	64.3 (51.2 to 75.5)	50.7 (45.7 to 55.6)	1.3 (1.0 to 1.6)
	CMT	54.5 (40.1 to 68.3)	80.7 (76.4 to 84.3)	2.8 (2.0 to 4.0)

*95% CI not provided.
CI, confidence interval; CMT, cervical motion tenderness; LR, likelihood ratio.

test and while this is reported in the literature it is relatively and reassuringly uncommon.

Single serum levels of β-hCG cannot confirm pregnancy location. Although patients with ectopic pregnancy tend to have lower β-hCG levels than those with intrauterine pregnancies, there is considerable overlap (Table 38.3). A low β-hCG level (usually less than 1000–1500 IU/L, although various thresholds have been tested) increases the relative risk of both ectopic pregnancy and abnormal intrauterine pregnancy, but cannot reliably distinguish between them [6]. Very few ectopic pregnancies exceed the threshold of >40,000 IU/L, and two retrospective studies have suggested that a single high level could be used to rule out ectopic pregnancy [24,25]. Importantly, very low-level serum β-hCG values have not been able to predict a benign clinical course, as ruptured ectopic pregnancies have been reported with serum levels below 100 IU/L

and even as low as 10 IU/L [7,26]. Single β-hCG measurements in the absence of diagnostic imaging are not helpful in clinical decision making.

Repeated or serial β-hCG measurements offer valuable information about fetal viability, but are not useful in determining the location of the gestation in the absence of diagnostic imaging. During the first trimester, β-hCG values approximately double every 2 days in women with healthy intrauterine pregnancies [27]. Pregnant patients whose β-hCG levels do not follow this trend may be presumed to have abnormal gestations [27], but the precise threshold for "abnormal doubling" is a matter of some debate. Failure of β-hCG levels to increase at least by 50–66% in 48 hours has been used as a diagnostic test for ectopic pregnancy in several studies [28–30]. Most (but not all) ectopic pregnancies in these studies had plateaued or subnormal doubling times and this failure to

Table 38.3 Sensitivity and specificity of serum β-human chorionic gonadotrophin (β-hCG) values in detecting ectopic pregnancy.

Study	N	Type of study	β-hCG threshold or range	Predictive value (95% CI)		+LR
				Sensitivity	Specificity	
Kohn et al. [24]	730	Retrospective	≤1500 IU/L	41.7 (32.3 to 51.7)	81.4 (78.2 to 84.2)	2.24
			>1500 to <40000 IU/L	57.3 (47.3 to 66.7)	54.6 (50.7 to 58.4)	1.26
Kaplan et al. [6]	439	Prospective	≤1000 IU/L	37.5 (26.0 to 50.6)	90.3 (87.0 to 92.9)	3.86
Cacciatore et al. [33]	200	Prospective	<1000 IU/L	33.8 (23.7 to 45.7)	82.6 (75.2 to 88.1)	1.94

CI, confidence interval; +LR, positive likelihood ratio.

Table 38.4 Sensitivity and specificity of serum β-human chorionic gonadotrophin (β-hCG) values used in combination with an ultrasound that is either negative for IUP or indeterminate for EP/IUP.

Study	N	Type of study	β-hCG threshold or range	Predictive value (95% CI)		+LR
				Sensitivity	Specificity	
Condous et al. [67]	527	Prospective	>1000 IU/L, indeterminate TVUS	21.7 (12.3 to 35.6)	87.3 (84.1 to 90)	1.71
			>1500 IU/L, indeterminate TVUS	15.2 (7.6 to 28.2)	93.4 (90.8 to 95.3)	2.30
			>2000 IU/L, indeterminate TVUS	10.9 (4.73 to 23.0)	95.2 (92.9 to 96.8)	2.27
Dart et al. [29]	307	Retrospective	48 hour rise of <66%, empty uterus on TVUS	39.4 (24.7 to 56.3)	97.4 (94.8 to 98.8)	15.4
Mol et al. [30]	354	Prospective	>2000 IU/L, no IUP on TVUS	38.1 (27.1 to 50.4)	98.5 (95.7 to 99.5)	25.4
			>2000 IU/L, no IUP + ectopic mass or fluid in pouch of Douglas on TVUS	54.6 (42.6 to 66.0)	96.2 (81.1 to 99.3)	14.37
			48 hour rise <50%, no IUP on TVUS	39.5 (25.6 to 55.3)	87.9 (81.9 to 92.1)	3.26
Barnhart et al. [7]	?†	Prospective	≥1500 IU/L, no IUP on TVUS	81.6*	100*	∞
Ankum et al. [32]	208	Prospective	>1500 IU/L (initial value), no IUP on TVUS *Or* >1000 IU/L (after 4 days), no IUP on TVUS	96.6 (90.6 to 98.9)	95.0 (89.4 to 97.7)	19.32
Cacciatore et al. [33]	200	Prospective	>1000 IU/L, no IUP on TVUS	66.2 (54.3 to 76.3)	100 (93.6 to 100)	∞
Aleem et al. [28]	58	Prospective	48 hour rise of <66%, TAUS scan indeterminate	85.0 (64.0 to 94.8)	71.1 (55.2 to 83.0)	2.94

*Confidence intervals not provided for this study.
CI, confidence interval; EP, ectopic pregnancy; IUP, intrauterine pregnancy; +LR, positive likelihood ratio; TAUS, transabdominal ultrasonography; TVUS, transvaginal ultrasonography.
†Unnumbered subset of larger study population.

increase had a high association with ectopic pregnancy. Non-viable intrauterine pregnancies exhibit the same β-hCG pattern, however, and are biochemically indistinguishable from ectopic pregnancies although the treatment requirements are clearly very different. Thus important therapeutic decisions cannot be made on the basis of subnormal doubling alone. Using even a conservative threshold of a 66% increase over 48 hours may occasionally result in the inadvertent termination of a normal pregnancy if clinicians proceed with dilation and curettage, or methotrexate administration. One study identified several patients with serum levels that increased by less than 66% (53% in one case) who went on to have healthy intrauterine pregnancies [31]. In summary, a patient exhibiting normal doubling of serum β-hCG levels over 48 hours has a viable fetus in an unknown location (intrauterine or ectopic). Patients with serum levels that fail to reach 50% over 48 hours are at high risk of ectopic pregnancy but may also have a non-viable intrauterine pregnancy. Falling levels are indicative of non-viable pregnancy, but do not rule out ectopic pregnancy.

Serum β-hCG levels are most helpful when used in combination with ultrasonography. The usefulness of the discriminatory threshold (the serum β-hCG level at which a normally developing intrauterine gestational sac can be visualized on ultrasound imaging) in clinical decision making has improved in concert with advances in ultrasound technology. The discriminatory threshold has dropped from 6500 IU/L using a transabdominal ultrasound (TAUS) approach to between 1000 and 2000 IU/L with transvaginal imaging. This threshold may change somewhat from institution to institution as it is somewhat user and machine dependent; more experienced sonographers using better quality machines will have lower discriminatory thresholds. Several studies have explored the predictive value of different β-hCG thresholds when no intrauterine pregnancy can be detected on ultrasound (Table 38.4).

In summary, serial β-hCG levels rising above 1500 IU/L in the absence of sonographic signs of early pregnancy can be considered presumptive evidence of an ectopic pregnancy, with exceedingly high likelihood ratios in several studies [7,30,32,33].

Question 3: In pregnant patients with first trimester symptoms (population), what are the sensitivity and specificity (diagnostic test characteristics) of formal ultrasound (test) for the diagnosis of ectopic pregnancy (outcome)?

Search strategy

- MEDLINE and EMBASE: *explode* ectopic pregnancy AND ultrasonography AND ultrasonography.mp AND ultrasound.mp AND transvaginal.mp AND endovaginal.mp AND (sensitivity and specificity OR diagnostic accuracy.mp)
- Hand-searching: reference lists from articles were used to identify additional articles

Improvements in ultrasonographic technology have revolutionized the diagnosis of ectopic pregnancy. Studies assessing the utility of ultrasound have explored a variety of aspects, ranging from the sensitivity and specificity of detecting an intrauterine pregnancy at different β-hCG thresholds to the predictive value of different sonographic findings suggestive of ectopic pregnancy. With the advent of transvaginal ultrasonography (TVUS), visualization of intrauterine or ectopic pregnancies can occur as early as 5 weeks gestational age [28,34]; 1–2 weeks earlier than with a transabdominal approach. The identification of an intrauterine pregnancy with TVUS (gestational sac with yolk sac ± cardiac activity) virtually rules out an ectopic pregnancy, as heterotopic pregnancies (simultaneous intrauterine and ectopic pregnancies) are extremely rare in patients not undergoing fertility treatments [35,36].

A number of specific criteria have been suggested for making a sonographic diagnosis of ectopic pregnancy (Table 38.5). A 1994 meta-analysis of 10 studies [34] assessed the sensitivity and specificity of four TVUS findings: (i) adnexal embryo with heart beat; (ii) adnexal mass containing yolk sac or embryo; (iii) adnexal mass with central anechoic area and hyperechoic ring or containing yolk sac or embryo; and (iv) any adnexal mass other than a simple cyst or intraovarian lesion (in the absence of intrauterine pregnancy). Criteria (iv), the least stringent, had the highest sensitivity (84.4%), with a specificity of 98.9%. The remaining three criteria had specificities of 99.5–100%, but sensitivities of only 20.1–64.6%. The authors conclude that the detection of any non-cystic or non-intraovarian adnexal mass in the absence of intrauterine pregnancy should be taken as strong evidence for ectopic pregnancy [34]. The presence of free pelvic fluid in the cul de sac (pouch of Douglas), especially in conjunction with other findings such as adnexal masses or no visible intrauterine pregnancy, is highly associated with ectopic pregnancy [6,32,37–40]. Although operator dependent, the majority of studies have reported the specificity of TVUS to be at least 95% [6,7,28,32,33,38,39,41]. Figures 38.1–38.3 demonstrate TVUS images of an empty uterus with intrauterine fluid and a non-specific echogenic focus (a pseudogestational sac), an early intrauterine pregnancy and an ectopic pregnancy, respectively.

In summary, ultrasound has proved an excellent tool for the assessment of women in early stages of pregnancy. The presence of an intrauterine pregnancy is reassuring that an ectopic pregnancy is unlikely. The absence of an intrauterine pregnancy should be taken as strong evidence for an ectopic pregnancy, and other ultrasound findings (e.g., adnexal mass, free pelvic fluid in the cul de sac, and so forth) have been identified that will assist in making the diagnosis. The importance of near 100% specificity cannot be stressed enough, as it is essential to avoid potential surgical or medical intervention (and thus termination) of a possibly viable, early, normal intrauterine pregnancy.

Question 4: In patients suspected of having ectopic pregnancy (population), what are the sensitivity and specificity (diagnostic test characteristics) of ED targeted ultrasound (test) for the diagnosis of intrauterine pregnancy (outcome)?

Search strategy

- MEDLINE and EMBASE: *explode* ectopic pregnancy AND pregnancy trimester, first AND (ultrasonography OR ultrasound.mp) AND (emergency service, hospital OR emergency medicine OR emergency physician.mp)
- Hand-searching: reference lists from identified articles were used to identify additional articles
- Inclusion: articles containing data addressing diagnostic value (sensitivity and specificity) of ED targeted ultrasound in identifying intrauterine pregnancy to rule out ectopic pregnancy or its value in outcomes such as time to diagnosis, risk of rupture, costs and length of stay in the ED

Emergency department targeted ultrasound (EDTU), performed by an emergency physician at the patient's bedside in the ED, has dramatically decreased the time to diagnosis for medical emergencies such as thoracic/abdominal trauma, cardiac arrest, pericardial effusions and abdominal aortic aneurysms [42–44]. EDTU differs from "formal ultrasound" (performed by radiologists or radiology technologists and interpreted by radiologists) in its limited and goal-directed approach. In the setting of symptomatic first trimester pregnancy, this approach involves answering two "yes/no" questions: (i) is there an intrauterine pregnancy; and (ii) is there free pelvic fluid [3]? Answering these questions allows the emergency physician to either quickly identify patients at increased risk of ectopic pregnancy, or to obtain valuable information on the viability of a visualized intrauterine pregnancy.

To date, six studies, using either one or both of TAUS and TVUS, have explored the use of EDTU in identifying intrauterine pregnancies in this patient population (Table 38.6). The sensitivity of EDTU in detecting any intrauterine pregnancy (including both viable and non-viable) ranged from 54% to 99%, with five of the six studies reporting a sensitivity of 82% or greater, and four of the six reporting a sensitivity exceeding 92% [45–50]. The specificity of EDTU for intrauterine pregnancies was greater than 92% in five of these studies, and greater than 98% in four. Two studies showed that emergency physicians could also detect adnexal signs consistent with ectopic pregnancy (outside the traditional "targeted question" role of EDTU) with reasonable accuracy [47,50]. The transvaginal approach was superior to the transabdominal approach in all studies.

In summary, EDTU has proved an excellent bedside tool for the assessment of women in early stages of pregnancy. These findings demonstrate that emergency physicians can use transabdominal or transvaginal EDTU to identify the presence or absence of intrauterine pregnancy accurately following a brief training program. As

Table 38.5 Predictive value of formal ultrasound in the diagnosis of ectopic pregnancy.

Study	n	Study details	Specific criteria	Predictive value (95% CI)		
				Sensitivity	Specificity	LR (+)
Barnhart et al. [41]	333	Retrospectively assessed accuracy of formal TVUS when β-hCG values were above and below 1500 IU/L	IUP >1500 IU/L	98.4 (95 to 99)	90.1 (81 to 96)	9.9
			IUP <1500 IU/L	33.3 (10 to 65)	98.1 (90 to 100)	17.5
			EP >1500 IU/L	80 (52 to 96)	98.1 (90 to 100)	42.1
			EP <1500 IU/L	25 (5 to 57)	96.2 (87 to 99)	6.6
Shalev et al. [68]	840	Prospectively assessed accuracy of formal TVUS in diagnosis of EP. Criteria for EP: no IUP and one of: β-hCG >1500 IU/L, >1000 ml fluid, fetal cardiac activity		87.1 (83.4 to 90.1)	94.2 (91.7 to 96.0)	15.0
Dart et al. [37]	111	Retrospectively assessed accuracy of formal TAUS and/or TVUS. Criteria for EP: any of: EUGS ± yolk sac or fetal pole, complex mass discrete from ovary, and large amount of fluid in the cul de sac		39.1%	—	—
Kaplan et al. [6]	439	Prospectively assessed formal TAUS or TVUS. Criteria for EP: adnexal sac-like ring with fetal pole or fetal heart beat; findings highly suggestive of EP: adnexal sac-like ring, complex or cystic mass ± cul de sac fluid; also evaluated value of indeterminate ultrasound when β-hCG ≤1000 IU/L	Ultrasound at initial visit	68.8 (54.7 to 80.1)	98.3 (90.9 to 99.7)	40.5
			Indeterminate ultrasound with β-hCG ≤1000 IU/L	66.7 (41.7 to 84.8)	73.7 (61.0 to 83.4)	2.5
Sadek & Schiotz [38]	525	Prospectively assessed TVUS by gynecology. Criteria for EP: assessed utility of "free pelvic fluid" and "tubal mass" when no IUP present	Free fluid	96.2 (87.3 to 99.0)	99.4 (98.2 to 99.8)	160.3
			Tubal mass	81.1 (68.6 to 89.4)	99.6 (98.5 to 99.9)	202.8
			Free fluid or mass	100 (93.2 to 100)	99.2 (97.8 to 99.7)	125.0
Barnhart et al. [7]	?*	Prospective assessment accuracy of formal TVUS. Criteria for EP: no IUP present or β-hCG of >1500 IU/L		81.6	100	∞
Braffman et al. [69]	1427	Prospective assessment of formal TAUS and TVUS. Criteria for EP: "definite EP" (detection of EUGS) also assessed utility of "indeterminate scan" and "complex adnexal mass" in indeterminate scans	Definite + indeterminate scans	99.0 (94.7 to 99.8)	84.3 (82.2 to 86.2)	6.3
			Complex adnexal mass	46.2 (35.0 to 58.2)	92.2 (87.6 to 95.1)	5.9
Ankum et al. [32]	208	Prospective assessment of TVUS by gynecology. Criteria for EP: no IUP when initial β-hCG >1500 IU/L or >1000 IU/L after 4 days		96.6 (90.6 to 98.9)	95.0 (89.4 to 97.7)	19.3
Ankum et al. [70]	208	Prospective assessment of TVUS by gynecology. Criteria for EP: absence of IUP; also assessed utility of adnexal findings (EUGS, ectopic mass with free fluid) when IUP absent	No IUP	98.9 (93.9 to 99.8)	41.2 (32.7 to 50.2)	1.7
			Adnexal findings	55.7 (45.3 to 65.6)	98.6 (92.3 to 99.8)	39.8
Cacciatore et al. [33]	200	Prospective assessment of TVUS. Criteria for EP: assessed utility of adnexal mass or GS-like ring ± fetal pole, or no IUP when β-hCG >1000 IU/L plus adnexal mass	Adnexal mass	92.7 (83.9 to 96.8)	99.2 (95.8 to 99.9)	115.9
			No IUP, mass + β-hCG >1000 IU/L	97.1 (89.9 to 99.2)	99.2 (95.8 to 99.9)	121.4
Aleem et al. [28]	58	Prospective assessment TAUS or TVUS by radiology or gynecology. Criteria for EP: assessed utility of complex adnexal mass		55.2 (42.5 to 67.3)	96.6 (88.3 to 99.1)	16.2
Timor-Tritsch et al. [39]	132	Prospective assessment of TVUS after indeterminate TAUS. Criteria for EP: no IUP plus (i) GS and/or yolk sac or ectopic fetal and (ii) complex free fluid ± thickened tube	TVUS only	100 (92.9 to 100)	97.8 (88.7 to 99.6)	45.5
			TAUS + TVUS	100 (93.0 to 100)	98.8 (93.3 to 99.8)	83.3
Dashefsky et al. [40]	53	Retrospective and prospective assessment of formal TAUS and TVUS. Criteria for EP: ectopic cardiac activity. Secondary criteria: absence of IUP with adnexal non-cystic mass or free adnexal fluid	No IUP	100	74	3.8
			No IUP + mass	67	94	11.2
			No IUP + fluid	83	91	9.2

β-hCG, β-human chorionic gonadotrophin; CI, confidence interval; EP, ectopic pregnancy; EUGS, extrauterine gestational sac; GS, gestational sac; IUP, intrauterine pregnancy; +LR, positive likelihood ratio; TAUS, transabdominal ultrasonography; TVUS, transvaginal ultrasonography.
* Un-numbered subset of larger population study.

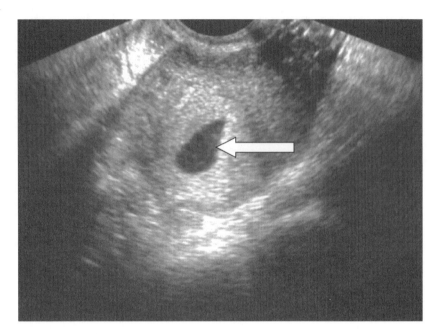

Figure 38.1 Transvaginal ultrasound with arrow showing intrauterine fluid collection without yolk sac or fetal pole (pseudosac).

the familiarity and experience with EDTU grows, the diagnostic accuracy of EDTU will likely improve.

Question 5: In patients with possible ectopic pregnancy (population), does EDTU (test) influence clinical outcomes such as time to diagnosis, risk of rupture, costs and length of stay in the ED (outcomes) compared to use of standard ultrasound (comparison)?

Search strategy

- MEDLINE and EMBASE: *explode* ectopic pregnancy AND pregnancy trimester, first AND (ultrasonography OR ultrasound.mp) AND (emergency service, hospital OR emergency medicine OR emergency physician.mp)
- Hand-searching: reference lists from identified articles were used to identify additional articles
- Inclusion: articles containing data addressing diagnostic value (sensitivity and specificity) of ED targeted ultrasound in identifying intrauterine pregnancy to rule out ectopic pregnancy or its value in outcomes such as time to diagnosis, risk of rupture, costs and length of stay in the ED

The introduction of EDTU has also had a significant impact on other important patient outcomes such as time to diagnosis, length of stay (LOS) in the ED and the risk of ectopic pregnancy rupture. When EDTU is available in the ED, the detection of an intrauterine pregnancy frequently allows the emergency physician to rapidly arrange patient disposition and follow-up without the need for further consultation or imaging. Two prospective studies have investigated the impact of EDTU on LOS. Shih [48] demonstrated that patients who underwent EDTU had an average LOS of 60

minutes, compared to 180 minutes for patients without EDTU. This difference was most significant in the group of patients with viable intrauterine pregnancies. A prospective randomized study by Pierce et al. [51] showed that time to disposition was 3.3 hours for EDTU patients whereas those not receiving EDTU stayed for 5.4 hours, with a higher rate of obstetrics consultation in the latter group. EDTU showed 100% accuracy in those patients where follow-up was obtained. In a retrospective study by Blaivas et al. [52], LOS was 59 minutes less (21%) when a live intrauterine pregnancy was confirmed by EDTU. Jang and Aubin [53] showed that resident-performed EDTU reduced the average LOS of symptomatic first trimester pregnancies by 149 minutes ($P < 0.05$) compared to patients needing consultation with obstetrics. There was no significant difference in the subgroup of patients diagnosed with ectopic pregnancy; however, all patients receiving only EDTU had diagnosis confirmed at follow-up, and no ectopic pregnancies were missed. An earlier study demonstrated a 70 minute (30%) shorter stay when patients with ectopic pregnancy underwent transvaginal EDTU compared to TVUS by obstetrics/gynecology [54]. No ectopic pregnancies were missed in this study.

Another improved outcome associated with EDTU is the reduction in time to treatment. Rodgerson et al. [55] assessed the utility of EDTU in expediting treatment for patients with ruptured ectopic pregnancies, specifically focusing on scans of the right upper quadrant for fluid in Morison's pouch. The authors found that EDTU reduced both time to diagnosis and time to treatment by 149 minutes and 211 minutes, respectively. A separate study looked at the time from the ED to the operating room in patients requiring surgery for ectopic pregnancy [56]. Patients scanned by emergency physicians had a mean time of 4 hours and 35 minutes, compared to 6 hours and 58 minutes for those scanned by radiology. Incidence of blood in the abdomen

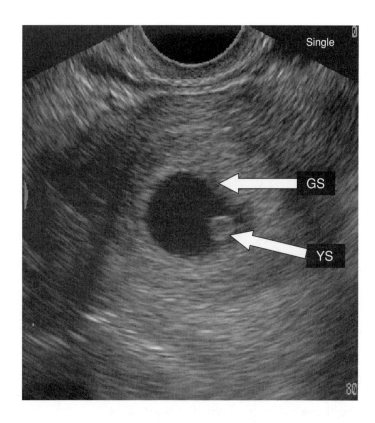

Figure 38.2 Transvaginal ultrasound showing early intrauterine gestational sac (GS) with yolk sac (YS).

and length of hospital stay, however, did not differ between the groups.

Two studies have reported the benefit of EDTU in reducing treatment costs. One prospective randomized study [51] found that bill charges in patients receiving EDTU averaged US$535.30, compared to $926.47 for patients randomized to the non-EDTU arm. This difference, however, was not statistically significant ($P = 0.18$). Another study [46] found that for each ectopic pregnancy diagnosed, emergency physician ultrasonography saved an average of 15.9 scans by medical imaging and 9.7 call-ins for ultrasound technicians. The authors determined that the estimated cost savings per ectopic pregnancy diagnosed ranged from $229 to $1244. However, the authors of this study stress the importance of radiology consultation for all EDTU scans that are indeterminate or fail to show an intrauterine pregnancy.

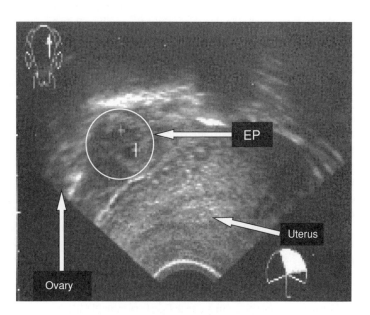

Figure 38.3 Transvaginal ultrasound showing an empty uterus and complex adnexal mass (ectopic pregnancy, EP) separate from the ovary.

Table 38.6 Sensitivity and specificity of emergency department targeted ultrasound in detecting intrauterine pregnancy.

Study	n	Study details	Predictive value (95% CI)		
			Sensitivity	Specificity	LR (+)
Todd et al. [45]	215	Prospective study using TAUS	54.2 (46.0 to 62.1)	98.5 (92.0 to 99.7)	36.2
Durston et al. [46]	921	Retrospective study using TAUS and TVUS	98.4 (96.9 to 99.2)	100 (98.3 to 100)	∞
Durham et al. [47]	125	Prospective study using TAUS and TVUS	99.0 (94.5 to 99.8)	88.9 (71.9 to 96.2)	8.9
Shih [48]	74	Prospective study using TAUS and TVUS	94 (82 to 98)	100 (83 to 100)	∞
Mateer et al. [49]	300	Prospective study using TVUS	92.9 (88.8 to 95.7)	98.8 (93.7 to 99.8)	79.9
Wong et al. [50]	143	Prospective study using TAUS	82 (76 to 88)	92 (88 to 96)	6.7

CI, confidence interval; ED, emergency department; TAUS, transabdominal ultrasonography; TVUS, transvaginal ultrasonography.

In summary, EDTU reduces LOS, leads to earlier treatment and reduces costs when compared to standard care with traditional ultrasound.

Question 6: In patients with documented non-ruptured ectopic pregnancy (population), what is the effectiveness of methotrexate (intervention) in preventing rupture, reducing hospitalization and improving patient well-being (outcomes) compared to surgical treatment (control)?

Search strategy

- Cochrane: ectopic pregnancy

The evolution of surgical techniques has allowed the minimally invasive laparoscopic technique to supplant the traditional open salpingectomy approach in the surgical therapy of ectopic pregnancy. Salpingosomy, which attempts to preserve tubal patency and future fertility, has evolved into the surgical management of choice for unruptured ectopic pregnancy, although there is the potential for retention of trophoblastic tissue and recurrence of clinical symptoms [57]. Methotrexate is a folic acid antagonist, and inhibits DNA synthesis in rapidly dividing cells. Methotrexate has been used to treat unruptured ectopic pregnancies for more than two decades, via local injection during laparoscopic surgery, locally via ultrasound guidance or systemically in the form of one or more intramuscular injections. There have been several direct comparisons of the effectiveness of systemic methotrexate when compared to standard surgical intervention.

Four studies examined different outcomes when comparing a fixed multiple-dose regimen of methotrexate (1 mg/kg IM on days 0, 2, 4 and 6, alternating with oral folinic acid 0.1 g/kg on days 1, 3, 5 and 7) [58–61]. Patients were eligible for the trials regardless of the size of the ectopic pregnancy and the level of serum β-hCG. No

significant differences between surgical and medical therapy were observed in the rate of treatment success, subsequent tubal patency and long-term fertility outcomes. The multiple-dose methotrexate regimen, however, caused significantly more toxicity, with 61% of patients reporting side-effects (vs 12% in the surgical group) and a significant decrease in many of the indices for health-related quality of life.

This observed toxicity in the multiple fixed-dose regimen has led to investigation of reduced doses of methotrexate. Five studies have examined methotrexate administered in a variable-dose intramuscular regimen (single dose of 50 mg/m^2 intramuscularly or 1 mg/kg body weight without folinic acid) compared to laparoscopic salpingostomy [62–66]. This regimen is often referred to as "variable dose" rather than "single dose" since a repeat dose is administered if the serum β-hCG levels fail to decline appropriately within 4–7 days ("acceptable decline" is generally felt to be at least 15% from baseline; some centers have a more stringent criterion of 25%) [3,57]. Additional doses may be given weekly for inappropriate decline.

A single dose of 50 mg/m^2 was shown to be significantly less successful than laparoscopic salpingostomy in the elimination of non-ruptured tubal ectopic pregnancy (OR = 0.38; 95% CI: 0.20 to 0.71) [57]. Treatment success rises with additional administration of methotrexate (variable-dose protocol) in response to inadequately declining serum levels, and the outcomes using this regimen are no different from those observed with laparoscopic salpingostomy (OR = 1.1; 95% CI: 0.52 to 2.3) [57]. There was substantial clinical and statistical heterogeneity within the four studies pooled, particularly with respect to study eligibility. Different thresholds of serum β-hCG were used (<5000 IU/L [65], <10,000 IU/L [66]) and the size of tubal ectopic pregnancy varied (<3.5 cm [63,65], <4 cm [66]). Three of the studies required that the ectopic pregnancy did not have visible cardiac activity [63,65,66]. The variable-dose methotrexate regimen showed very few toxic side-effects, and women who received methotrexate in this regimen reported better physical functioning compared with laparoscopic salpingostomy [57]. No differences were observed in future fertility and tubal patency rates in follow-up.

In summary, the administration of methotrexate in a fixed-dose or variable-dose schedule to women with unruptured tubal ectopic pregnancy appears to have equivalent outcomes to laparoscopic salpingostomy, with the variable-dose regimen demonstrating better tolerance and fewer side-effects. Careful observation of serum β-hCG levels is mandatory, however, as many patients will require additional doses of methotrexate. Patients continue to be at risk for complications after methotrexate administration, including tubal rupture, and it is important for emergency physicians to be vigilant in their assessment of these patients.

Conclusions

You decide to use the ED ultrasound probe to evaluate the status of your patient's pregnancy. Using the transvaginal probe, you see some intrauterine fluid, but are not confident of a gestational sac, and there is clearly no fetal pole. You deem her ultrasound indeterminate for an intrauterine pregnancy, and order a serum β-hCG level, which returns at 3500 IU/L. You are concerned about the possibility of ectopic pregnancy and arrange a formal ultrasound, which indeed shows no intrauterine pregnancy and a complex adnexal mass separate from the ovary. You diagnose her with a probable tubal ectopic pregnancy and refer her to the gynecologist on call for further assessment and consideration of treatment. In consultation with a gynecological consultant, she undergoes treatment with methotrexate, and her serum β-hCG levels rise slightly over the first 7 days of treatment, so she receives a second dose at day 7. She recovers completely without further intervention.

Ectopic pregnancy is a common and serious problem frequently encountered by emergency physicians. Many patients present without either risk factors or suspicious physical examination findings, thus ultrasound imaging of all patients with symptomatic early pregnancy is prudent. Serum β-hCG levels in combination with ultrasound imaging (both EDTU and formal ultrasound) are most useful in determining pregnancy location, particularly if patient stability allows repeated or serial measurements. EDTU is becoming an essential part of the emergency physicians' skill set, and has been shown to be accurate and to reduce time to disposition, time to treatment and costs for women with threatened abortion and ectopic pregnancies. Treatment with methotrexate has allowed non-invasive management of unruptured ectopic pregnancies, with equivalent outcomes to laparoscopic salpingostomy when serum β-hCG levels are conscientiously followed and repeated injections are given as needed for suboptimal decline.

Acknowledgement

The authors would like to acknowledge the invaluable assistance of Dr Andrew McRae with questions 4 and 5 of this chapter.

References

1 Centers for Disease Control and Prevention. Ectopic pregnancy – United States, 1990–1992. *MMWR* 1995;**44**(3):46–8.

2 Goldner TE, Lawson HW, Xia Z, Atrash HK. Surveillance for ectopic pregnancy – United States, 1970–1989. *MMWR CDC Surveill Summ* 1993;**42**(6):73–85.

3 Murray H, Baakdah H, Bardell T, Tulandi T. Diagnosis and treatment of ectopic pregnancy. *Can Med Assoc J* 2005;**173**(8):905–12.

4 Stovall TG, Kellerman AL, Ling FW, Buster JE. Emergency department diagnosis of ectopic pregnancy. *Ann Emerg Med* 1990;**19**(10):1098–103.

5 Buckley RG, King KJ, Disney JD, Ambroz PK, Gorman JD, Klausen JH. Derivation of a clinical prediction model for the emergency department diagnosis of ectopic pregnancy. *Acad Emerg Med* 1998;**5**(10):951–60.

6 Kaplan BC, Dart RG, Moskos M, et al. Ectopic pregnancy: prospective study with improved diagnostic accuracy. *Ann Emerg Med* 1996;**28**(1):10–17.

7 Barnhart K, Mennuti MT, Benjamin I, Jacobson S, Goodman D, Coutifaris C. Prompt diagnosis of ectopic pregnancy in an emergency department setting. *Obstet Gynecol* 1994;**84**(6):1010–15.

8 Ankum WM, Mol BW, van der Veen F, Bossuyt PM. Risk factors for ectopic pregnancy: a meta-analysis. *Fertil Steril* 1996;**65**(6):1093–9.

9 Bouyer J, Coste J, Shojaei T, et al. Risk factors for ectopic pregnancy: a comprehensive analysis based on a large case–control, population-based study in France. *Am J Epidemiol* 2003;**157**(3):185–94.

10 Coste J, Job-Spira N, Fernandez H, Papiernik E, Spira A. Risk factors for ectopic pregnancy: a case–control study in France, with special focus on infectious factors. *Am J Epidemiol* 1991;**133**(9):839–49.

11 Barnhart KT, Sammel MD, Gracia CR, Chittams J, Hummel AC, Shaunik A. Risk factors for ectopic pregnancy in women with symptomatic first-trimester pregnancies. *Fertil Steril* 2006;**86**(1):36–43.

12 Dart RG, Kaplan B, Varaklis K. Predictive value of history and physical examination in patients with suspected ectopic pregnancy. *Ann Emerg Med* 1999;**33**(3):283–90.

13 Michalas S, Minaretzis D, Tsionou C, Maos G, Kioses E, Aravantinos D. Pelvic surgery, reproductive factors and risk of ectopic pregnancy: a case controlled study. *Int J Gynaecol Obstet* 1992;**38**(2):101–5.

14 Mol BW, Ankum WM, Bossuyt PM, van der Veen F. Contraception and the risk of ectopic pregnancy: a meta-analysis. *Contraception* 1995;**52**(6):337–41.

15 Parazzini F, Tozzi L, Ferraroni M, Bocciolone L, La Vecchia C, Fedele L. Risk factors for ectopic pregnancy: an Italian case–control study. *Obstet Gynecol* 1992;**80**(5):821–6.

16 Bakken IJ, Skjeldestad FE, Nordbo SA. *Chlamydia trachomatis* infections increase the risk for ectopic pregnancy: a population-based, nested case–control study. *Sex Transm Dis* 2007;**34**(3):166–9.

17 Xiong X, Buekens P, Wollast E. IUD use and the risk of ectopic pregnancy: a meta-analysis of case–control studies. *Contraception* 1995;**52**(1):23–34.

18 Parazzini F, Ferraroni M, Tozzi L, Benzi G, Rossi G, La Vecchia C. Past contraceptive method use and risk of ectopic pregnancy. *Contraception* 1995;**52**(2):93–8.

19 Stergachis A, Scholes D, Daling JR, Weiss NS, Chu J. Maternal cigarette smoking and the risk of tubal pregnancy. *Am J Epidemiol* 1991;**133**(4):332–7.

20 Saraiya M, Berg CJ, Kendrick JS, Strauss LT, Atrash HK, Ahn YW. Cigarette smoking as a risk factor for ectopic pregnancy. *Am J Obstet Gynecol* 1998;**178**(3):493–8.

21 Mol BW, Hajenius PJ, Engelsbel S, et al. Should patients who are suspected of having an ectopic pregnancy undergo physical examination? *Fertil Steril* 1999;**71**(1):155–7.

22 Buckley RG, King KJ, Disney JD, Gorman JD, Klausen JH. History and physical examination to estimate the risk of ectopic pregnancy: validation of a clinical prediction model. *Ann Emerg Med* 1999;**34**(5):589–94.

23 Brennan DF. Ectopic pregnancy – Part I: Clinical and laboratory diagnosis. *Acad Emerg Med* 1995;**2**(12):1081–9.

24 Kohn MA, Kerr K, Malkevich D, O'Neil N, Kerr MJ, Kaplan BC. Beta-human chorionic gonadotropin levels and the likelihood of ectopic pregnancy in emergency department patients with abdominal pain or vaginal bleeding. *Acad Emerg Med* 2003;**10**(2):119–26.

25 Marill KA, Ingmire TE, Nelson BK. Utility of a single beta HCG measurement to evaluate for absence of ectopic pregnancy. *J Emerg Med* 1999;**17**(3):419–26.

26 Saxon D, Falcone T, Mascha EJ, Marino T, Yao M, Tulandi T. A study of ruptured tubal ectopic pregnancy. *Obstet Gynecol* 1997;**90**(1):46–9.

27 Kadar N, Caldwell BV, Romero R. A method of screening for ectopic pregnancy and its indications. *Obstet Gynecol* 1981;**58**(2):162–6.

28 Aleem FA, DeFazio M, Gintautas J. Endovaginal sonography for the early diagnosis of intrauterine and ectopic pregnancies. *Hum Reprod* 1990;**5**(6):755–8.

29 Dart RG, Mitterando J, Dart LM. Rate of change of serial beta-human chorionic gonadotropin values as a predictor of ectopic pregnancy in patients with indeterminate transvaginal ultrasound findings. *Ann Emerg Med* 1999;**34**(6):703–10.

30 Mol BW, Hajenius PJ, Engelsbel S, et al. Serum human chorionic gonadotropin measurement in the diagnosis of ectopic pregnancy when transvaginal sonography is inconclusive. *Fertil Steril* 1998;**70**(5):972–81.

31 Barnhart KT, Sammel MD, Rinaudo PF, Zhou L, Hummel AC, Guo W. Symptomatic patients with an early viable intrauterine pregnancy: HCG curves redefined. *Obstet Gynecol* 2004;**104**(1):50–55.

32 Ankum WM, van der Veen F, Hamerlynck JV, Lammes FB. Laparoscopy: a dispensable tool in the diagnosis of ectopic pregnancy? *Hum Reprod* 1993;**8**(8):1301–6.

33 Cacciatore B, Stenman UH, Ylostalo P. Diagnosis of ectopic pregnancy by vaginal ultrasonography in combination with a discriminatory serum hCG level of 1000 IU/l (IRP). *Br J Obstet Gynaecol* 1990;**97**(10):904–8.

34 Brown DL, Doubilet PM. Transvaginal sonography for diagnosing ectopic pregnancy: positivity criteria and performance characteristics. *J Ultrasound Med* 1994;**13**(4):259–66.

35 Reece EA, Petrie RH, Sirmans MF, Finster M, Todd WD. Combined intrauterine and extrauterine gestations: a review. *Am J Obstet Gynecol* 1983;**146**(3):323–30.

36 Albayram F, Hamper UM. First-trimester obstetric emergencies: spectrum of sonographic findings. *J Clin Ultrasound* 2002;**30**(3):161–77.

37 Dart RG, Kaplan B, Cox C. Transvaginal ultrasound in patients with low beta-human chorionic gonadotropin values: how often is the study diagnostic? *Ann Emerg Med* 1997;**30**(2):135–40.

38 Sadek AL, Schiotz HA. Transvaginal sonography in the management of ectopic pregnancy. *Acta Obstet Gynecol Scand* 1995;**74**(4):293–6.

39 Timor-Tritsch IE, Yeh MN, Peisner DB, Lesser KB, Slavik TA. The use of transvaginal ultrasonography in the diagnosis of ectopic pregnancy. *Am J Obstet Gynecol* 1989;**161**(1):157–61.

40 Dashefsky SM, Lyons EA, Levi CS, Lindsay DJ. Suspected ectopic pregnancy: endovaginal and transvesical US. *Radiology* 1988;**169**(1):181–4.

41 Barnhart KT, Simhan H, Kamelle SA. Diagnostic accuracy of ultrasound above and below the beta-hCG discriminatory zone. *Obstet Gynecol* 1999;**94**(4):583–7.

42 Rose JS. Ultrasound in abdominal trauma. *Emerg Med Clin North Am* 2004;**22**(3):581–99, vii.

43 Tayal VS, Kline JA. Emergency echocardiography to detect pericardial effusion in patients in PEA and near-PEA states. *Resuscitation* 2003;**59**(3):315–18.

44 Tayal VS, Graf CD, Gibbs MA. Prospective study of accuracy and outcome of emergency ultrasound for abdominal aortic aneurysm over two years. *Acad Emerg Med* 2003;**10**(8):867–71.

45 Todd WM, Moore CL, O'Brien E. Risk stratification of suspected ectopic pregnancy by transabdominal emergency physician-performed ultrasonography. *Ann Emerg Med* 2004;**44**(4):S82–3.

46 Durston WE, Carl ML, Guerra W, Eaton A, Ackerson LM. Ultrasound availability in the evaluation of ectopic pregnancy in the ED: comparison of quality and cost-effectiveness with different approaches. *Am J Emerg Med* 2000;**18**(4):408–17.

47 Durham B, Lane B, Burbridge L, Balasubramaniam S. Pelvic ultrasound performed by emergency physicians for the detection of ectopic pregnancy in complicated first-trimester pregnancies. *Ann Emerg Med* 1997;**29**(3):338–47.

48 Shih CH. Effect of emergency physician-performed pelvic sonography on length of stay in the emergency department. *Ann Emerg Med* 1997;**29**(3):348–51.

49 Mateer JR, Valley VT, Aiman EJ, Phelan MB, Thoma ME, Kefer MP. Outcome analysis of a protocol including bedside endovaginal sonography in patients at risk for ectopic pregnancy. *Ann Emerg Med* 1996;**27**(3):283–9.

50 Wong TW, Lau CC, Yeung A, Lo L, Tai CM. Efficacy of transabdominal ultrasound examination in the diagnosis of early pregnancy complications in an emergency department. *J Accid Emerg Med* 1998;**15**(3):155–8.

51 Pierce DL, Friedman KD, Killan A, Stahmer SA. Emergency department ultrasonography (EUS) in symptomatic first-trimester pregnancy. *Acad Emerg Med* 2001;**8**:546.

52 Blaivas M, Sierzenski P, Plecque D, Lambert M. Do emergency physicians save time when locating a live intrauterine pregnancy with bedside ultrasonography? *Acad Emerg Med* 2000;**7**(9):988–93.

53 Jang TB, Aubin CD. Resident ultrasonography in symptomatic first-trimester pregnancy and department length of stay. *Ann Emerg Med* 2003;**42**(4):S89–90.

54 Burgher SW, Tandy TK, Dawdy MR. Transvaginal ultrasonography by emergency physicians decreases patient time in the emergency department. *Acad Emerg Med* 1998;**5**(8):802–7.

55 Rodgerson JD, Heegaard WG, Plummer D, Hicks J, Clinton J, Sterner S. Emergency department right upper quadrant ultrasound is associated with a reduced time to diagnosis and treatment of ruptured ectopic pregnancies. *Acad Emerg Med* 2001;**8**(4):331–6.

56 Blaivas M, Bell G. Benefit from emergency physician identified ectopic pregnancy using bedside ultrasound. *Acad Emerg Med* 2000;**7**:500.

57 Hajenius PJ, Mol F, Mol BW, Bossuyt PM, Ankum WM, van der Veen F. Interventions for tubal ectopic pregnancy. *Cochrane Database Syst Rev* 2007;**1**:CD000324.

58 Hajenius PJ, Engelsbel S, Mol BW, et al. Randomised trial of systemic methotrexate versus laparoscopic salpingostomy in tubal pregnancy. *Lancet* 1997;**350**(9080):774–9.

59 Nieuwkerk PT, Hajenius PJ, Ankum WM, van der Veen F, Wijker W, Bossuyt PM. Systemic methotrexate therapy versus laparoscopic salpingostomy in patients with tubal pregnancy. Part I. Impact on patients' health-related quality of life. *Fertil Steril* 1998;**70**(3):511–17.

60 Mol BW, Hajenius PJ, Engelsbel S, et al. Treatment of tubal pregnancy in the Netherlands: an economic comparison of systemic methotrexate

administration and laparoscopic salpingostomy. *Am J Obstet Gynecol* 1999;**181**(4):945–51.

61 Dias PG, Hajenius PJ, Mol BW, et al. Fertility outcome after systemic methotrexate and laparoscopic salpingostomy for tubal pregnancy. *Lancet* 1999;**353**(9154):724–5.

62 Fernandez H, Yves Vincent SC, Pauthier S, Audibert F, Frydman R. Randomized trial of conservative laparoscopic treatment and methotrexate administration in ectopic pregnancy and subsequent fertility. *Hum Reprod* 1998;**13**(11):3239–43.

63 Saraj AJ, Wilcox JG, Najmabadi S, Stein SM, Johnson MB, Paulson RJ. Resolution of hormonal markers of ectopic gestation: a randomized trial comparing single-dose intramuscular methotrexate with salpingostomy. *Obstet Gynecol* 1998;**92**(6):989–94.

64 Sowter MC, Farquhar CM, Gudex G. An economic evaluation of single dose systemic methotrexate and laparoscopic surgery for the treatment of unruptured ectopic pregnancy. *Br J Obstet Gynaecol* 2001;**108**(2):204–12.

65 Sowter MC, Farquhar CM, Petrie KJ, Gudex G. A randomised trial comparing single dose systemic methotrexate and laparoscopic surgery

for the treatment of unruptured tubal pregnancy. *Br J Obstet Gynaecol* 2001;**108**(2):192–203.

66 El-Sherbiny MT, El-Gharieb IH, Mera IM. Methotrexate versus laparoscopic surgery for the management of unruptured tubal pregnancy. *Middle East Fertil Soc J* 2003;**8**(3):256–62.

67 Condous G, Kirk E, Lu C, et al. Diagnostic accuracy of varying discriminatory zones for the prediction of ectopic pregnancy in women with a pregnancy of unknown location. *Ultrasound Obstet Gynecol* 2005;**26**(7):770–5.

68 Shalev E, Yarom I, Bustan M, Weiner E, Ben Shlomo I. Transvaginal sonography as the ultimate diagnostic tool for the management of ectopic pregnancy: experience with 840 cases. *Fertil Steril* 1998;**69**(1):62–75.

69 Braffman BH, Coleman BG, Ramchandani P, et al. Emergency department screening for ectopic pregnancy: a prospective US study. *Radiology* 1994;**190**(3):797–802.

70 Ankum WM, van der Veen F, Hamerlynck JV, Lammes FB. Transvaginal sonography and human chorionic gonadotrophin measurements in suspected ectopic pregnancy: a detailed analysis of a diagnostic approach. *Hum Reprod* 1993;**8**(8):1307–11.

Acute Ureteric Colic

Andrew Worster

Emergency Medicine, Clinical Epidemiology & Biostatistics, McMaster University, Hamilton, Canada

Clinical scenario

A 52-year-old man walked into the emergency department (ED) complaining of left flank pain radiating to the ipsilateral groin. The pain developed suddenly while the patient was sitting at his computer 4 hours ago. It has been continuous, without any relieving or aggravating factors, and reached maximum intensity one hour previously. The patient complained of nausea but no vomiting or diarrhea. He denied any fever, chills or urinary symptoms but admitted to having darker than normal urine for the last 12 hours. He denied never experiencing anything similar previously or any medical problems, medications or allergies to medications.

Examination revealed a white male who appeared his stated age but was slightly pale and in obvious discomfort. He was alert and oriented with the following vital signs: temperature $37.1°C$ (oral); pulse 88 beats/min, respiration 20 breaths/min and blood pressure 166/96 mmHg (right arm). Chest examination was unremarkable. The patient's abdomen was moderately obese but otherwise normal in appearance; on palpation, it was soft and non-tender without any palpable masses. He had normal bowel sounds and percussion of the left costovertebral angle caused moderate discomfort. The genitourinary exam was normal; specifically, his testicles were non-tender and in normal position.

The patient appeared to be suffering from a first episode of acute ureteric caculus. His pain decreased following analgesics and antiemetics intravenously; he was comfortable and waiting patiently while you and the radiologist decided which method of diagnostic imaging to perform. The nurse requested an order for intravenous fluid and ongoing analgesia. The patient asked what medication the nurse gave him for the pain and what he could do to prevent it from recurring.

Evidence-based Emergency Medicine. Edited by Brian H. Rowe
© 2009 Blackwell Publishing, ISBN: 978-1-4051-6143-5.

Background

Acute ureteric colic is the pain resulting from the presence of a stone in the urinary tract, often resulting in partial or complete ureteral obstruction. This disease has many names including urolithiasis, ureteric calculi, kidney stones and renal colic. The term "colic" describes the unrelenting, crampy, waxing and waning characteristic of the pain caused by a stone once it enters the ureter. Most, but not all, episodes are painful, thereby forcing patients to seek medical care. Because patients can remain asymptomatic during an episode, the true incidence of this condition is not known; however, in the industrialized world the prevalence ranges from 1% to 10% [1]. This is a disease primarily striking young, healthy adults; the incidence peaks in males at age 30 and in females at age 35 and 55 years. Incidentally, 1–2% of the affected Western population is children [1,2]. Finally, emergency physicians are often challenged to ensure patients presenting with symptoms of renal colic are not suffering from other, potentially more serious conditions, including ruptured aortic aneurysm, appendicitis and pyelonephritis. In women, ovarian pathology (e.g., cyst, torsion, rupture) and ectopic pregnancy must be ruled out; similarly in men, testicular torsion, prostatitis and epididymitis must be ruled out. This being said, renal colic is a common diagnosis in the ED and emergency physicians must become familiar with its diagnosis and treatment.

Due to the nature of the presentation (e.g., nausea, vomiting, diaphoresis, severe abdominal pain), management is often urgent and aggressive. The primary management approach is to relieve the pain and nausea; the secondary issues are investigation of the patient, and then finally the elimination of the ureteric foreign body. The American Urologic Association recommends conservative management for small (≤ 5 mm) calculi in the distal ureter as 98% of these will pass spontaneously [3]. This describes the findings in the majority of patients seen in the ED with ureteric colic. Invasive definitive therapy is indicated for patients with urinary tract infection, renal function impairment and prolonged duration of symptoms [3].

To date, ED management has been limited to confirmatory diagnosis and symptomatic treatment ending with discharge and appropriate follow-up. In many hospitals, newer imaging modalities are replacing intravenous urography (IVU) or pyelography (IVP) as the gold or reference standard of diagnostic imaging, Treatment now includes initiation of stone expulsion therapy. In this chapter, the evidence for ED management of suspected acute ureteric colic will be reviewed.

Clinical questions

1 In patients with suspected ureteric calculi (population), what is the likelihood ratio (diagnostic test characteristic) of computerized tomography (test) in diagnosing acute ureteric colic (outcome) compared to IVU/IVP (reference standard)?

2 In patients with suspected ureteric calculi (population), does computerized tomography (intervention) provide any benefit (outcome) in the diagnostic imaging of ED patients compared to IVU/IVP testing (comparison)?

3 In patients with ureteric calculi (population), do non-steroidal anti-inflammatory drugs (intervention) relieve pain more effectively (outcome) compared to routine care with narcotic analgesics (control)?

4 In patients with ureteric calculi (population), do antimuscarinic agents (interventions) effectively relieve pain (outcome) compared to routine care with narcotic analgesics (control)?

5 In patients with ureteric calculi (population), do diuretics and/or intravenous fluids (intervention) facilitate the passage of acute ureteric calculi (outcome) compared to routine care with analgesics (control)?

6 In patients with ureteric calculi (population), do calcium channel and/or α-adrenergic antagonists (interventions) safely facilitate the passage of ureteric calculi (outcome) compared to routine care with analgesics (control)?

7 In patients with ureteric calculi (population), does drinking large volumes of water (intervention) reduce recurrent ureteric calculi (outcome) compared to no change in water intake (control)?

General search strategy

PubMed is a free, web-based (http://www.ncbi.nlm.nih.gov/entrez/query.fcgi?DB=pubmed) search engine providing access by the National Library of Medicine to MEDLINE and the most recent completed reviews in the Cochrane Database of Systematic Reviews (CDSR). This is a powerful tool, albeit with some database limitations, that can identify the most recent and highest level of published evidence on any medical subject from any internet-connected computer. As with any tool, the amount of time spent using it for a particular task is inversely proportional to the amount of time spent learning how to use it. For example, the fastest and most effective search strategy to find systematic reviews or ran-

domized controlled trials (RCTs) is to go to the left-hand tool bar, and under "PubMed services" click on the "clinical queries" tab and follow the simple directions. As with any literature search, multiple synonymous terms may have to be employed to find all of the relevant articles.

Critical review of the literature

Question 1: In patients with suspected ureteric calculi (population), what is the likelihood ratio (diagnostic test characteristic) of computerized tomography (test) in diagnosing acute ureteric colic (outcome) compared to IVU/IVP (reference standard)?

> **Search strategy**
>
> • PubMed – clinical queries in systematic review: intravenous urography

Intravenous urography, also known as intravenous pyelography or excretory urography, has been the gold standard of diagnostic imaging for the investigation of patients with suspected acute ureteric colic since the middle of the last century [4]. The advent of spiral or helical computerized tomography (CT), a modification of standard CT in that it performs continuous data acquisition, has increased the resolution of CT to include the detection of miniscule (1 mm) objects such as ureteral calculi. This has led to the introduction of non-contrast or unenhanced helical CT in 1994 as a possible replacement for IVU in the investigation of patients with suspected acute urolithiasis [5]. There are multiple advantages of CT imaging over standard IVU, of which the most appealing is the elimination of patient exposure to intravenous contrast material. Other advantages include visualization of radiolucent calculi, detection of ureteric inflammation during and immediately after stone passage, more widespread availability, detection of pathology outside of the urinary tract, less pain and shorter examination times [5–10]. CT also has its limits such as: distorted images in the presence of metallic prostheses (e.g., Harrington rods, surgical clips) and concerns that the radiation exposure may actually be higher than for IVU.

The apparent advantages of CT outweigh the disadvantages as long as the diagnostic performance is as good as IVU. This was addressed by multiple, small, observational studies of varying quality that all reported CT to be more accurate than IVU; however, the small sample sizes and correspondingly large confidence intervals around the summary measures precluded any single study from providing unequivocal evidence favoring CT. This led to a meta-analysis of studies identified through standard systematic review methods from computerized searches of MEDLINE and EMBASE, combined with hand reviews of major journals and of articles from reference lists [11]. Two reviewers independently assessed study eligibility using a priori inclusion criteria. The results of the four selected studies, involving a total of 296 patients, were combined in a meta-analysis. The pooled positive likelihood ratios (+LRs) for CT and IVU were 23.15 (95% CI: 11.53 to 47.23) and 9.32 (95% CI: 5.23 to 16.61), respectively. The pooled negative likelihood ratios (−LRs) for CT and IVU were 0.05 (95% CI: 0.02 to 0.15) and 0.33 (95% CI: 0.23 to 0.48), respectively, with no statistically significant differences among trials. The results can be interpreted as CT being statistically significantly superior to IVU in accurately diagnosing acute urolithiasis. Moreover, the LRs of CT are both in the clinically significant range (i.e., +LR =>10 and −LR = <0.1), making this an important diagnostic tool for emergency physicians.

In summary, if a clinician suspects a diagnosis of ureteric stone, following a thorough history and physical exam, and confirmation of blood in the urine, the preferred approach for confirming the location and size of the ureteric stone is a non-enhanced abdominal CT scan.

Question 2: In patients with suspected ureteric calculi (population), does computerized tomography (intervention) provide any benefit (outcome) in the diagnostic imaging of ED patients compared to IVU/IVP testing (comparison)?

Search strategy

- PubMed – clinical queries in clinical study type: intravenous urography AND diagnosis AND narrow, specific search

While diagnostic accuracy is an important measure of a test's performance, it is not the only criterion upon which the choice of diagnostic test is made. Associated with each test are direct and indirect costs, risks such as exposure to radiation or complications if the procedure is invasive, and impact on patient management. Although a systematic review has demonstrated CT to be superior to IVU in accurately diagnosing acute ureteric colic, the comparative risks and benefits should also be considered [11].

At the time of writing, there were no published systematic reviews comparing the risks and benefits of CT and IVU. However, the three published RCTs agree that the two forms of diagnostic imaging for suspected acute ureteric colic have similar costs, although CT was faster and had a higher associated radiation dose exposure [12–14]. These studies also report, as previously mentioned, the higher risk of complication associated with the contrast used in IVU and the increased detection of non-urological causes of symptoms with CT. These are clearly patient-important outcomes. One single-center medical record review specifically examined patient outcomes and reported that replacing IVU with CT scanning for the investigation of suspected acute ureteric colic did not result in significantly shorter stays, reduced hospital admissions or fewer interventions for patients [15]. Clearly, these findings need to be confirmed in prospective studies at other centers.

In summary, the current evidence suggests that replacing IVU with CT scanning for the investigation of suspected acute ureteric colic confers, at the least, some important patient-specific outcomes, including lower risk of complication and increased detection of non-urological causes of symptoms.

Question 3: In patients with ureteric calculi (population), do non-steroidal anti-inflammatory drugs (intervention) relieve pain more effectively (outcome) compared to routine care with narcotic analgesics (control)?

Search strategy

- PubMed – clinical queries in systematic review: renal colic

Symptomatic, acute ureteric colic typically presents as unilateral flank pain often radiating to the ipsilateral groin. As the calculus descends the ureter, the patient develops symptoms of cystitis. Nulliparous patients complain that the pain of ureteric colic is second to none and their primary objective for an ED visit is pain relief. Opioids have long served as the analgesic of choice by these patients and their attending emergency physicians. Opioids act on the central nervous system to reduce the perception of pain. Impressive doses are often required to reach the desired effect and are associated with vomiting and decreased level of consciousness. While often effective, opioids do not address the etiological mechanisms of the pain associated with renal colic.

We now know that the pain of acute ureteric colic is prostaglandin-mediated: local prostaglandin synthesis and release occur as a result of the irritation and increased tension to the ureteral wall and renal pelvis [16,17]. The effects of the prostaglandins are ureteral smooth muscle spasm and vasodilation. The latter in turn causes diuresis, which again increases the tension to the ureteral wall and renal pelvis. Non-steroidal anti-inflamatory drugs (NSAIDs) and cyclooxygenase-2 (COX-2) inhibitors interfere with prostaglandin synthesis and release and, therefore, should effectively reduce the associated pain of acute ureteric colic by blocking the mechanism of action [16,17]. A Cochrane systematic review of RCTs compared any opioid with any NSAID for acute ureteric colic without restriction on doses and routes of administration [17]. The authors identified 20 trials involving a total of 1613 participants; however, they were unable to pool the results of all 20 trials because of heterogeneity. Despite this concern, they reported some clinically important findings: both NSAIDs and opioids reduced patient-reported pain scale scores, although patients receiving NSAIDs reported lower pain scores, (Fig. 39.1; analysis 01.02 [17]), were significantly less likely to require rescue medication (Fig. 39.2; analysis 01.06 [17]) and were less likely to vomit than those receiving opioids.

The opiate studies most commonly used meperidine (pethidine, demerol) and so the effects attributed to opiates might in

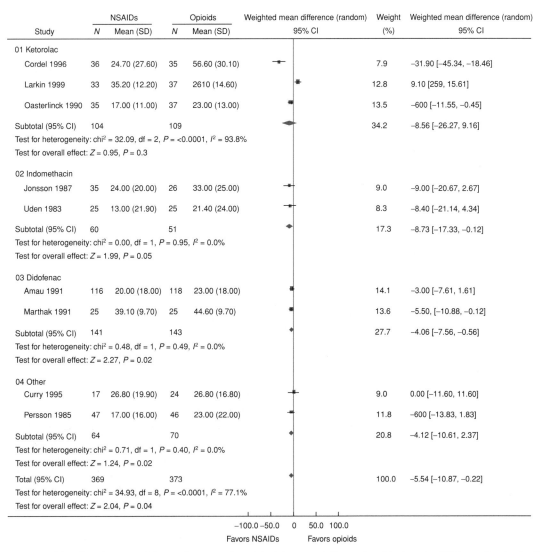

	NSAIDs		Opioids		Weighted mean difference (random)	Weight	Weighted mean difference (random)
Study	N	Mean (SD)	N	Mean (SD)	95% CI	(%)	95% CI
01 Ketorolac							
Cordel 1996	36	24.70 (27.60)	35	56.60 (30.10)		7.9	−31.90 [−45.34, −18.46]
Larkin 1999	33	35.20 (12.20)	37	2610 (14.60)		12.8	9.10 [259, 15.61]
Oasterlinck 1990	35	17.00 (11.00)	37	23.00 (13.00)		13.5	−600 [−11.55, −0.45]
Subtotal (95% CI)	104		109			34.2	−8.56 [−26.27, 9.16]
Test for heterogeneity: chi² = 32.09, df = 2, P = <0.0001, I² = 93.8%							
Test for overall effect: Z = 0.95, P = 0.3							
02 Indomethacin							
Jonsson 1987	35	24.00 (20.00)	26	33.00 (25.00)		9.0	−9.00 [−20.67, 2.67]
Uden 1983	25	13.00 (21.90)	25	21.40 (24.00)		8.3	−8.40 [−21.14, 4.34]
Subtotal (95% CI)	60		51			17.3	−8.73 [−17.33, −0.12]
Test for heterogeneity: chi² = 0.00, df = 1, P = 0.95, I² = 0.0%							
Test for overall effect: Z = 1.99, P = 0.05							
03 Didofenac							
Amau 1991	116	20.00 (18.00)	118	23.00 (18.00)		14.1	−3.00 [−7.61, 1.61]
Marthak 1991	25	39.10 (9.70)	25	44.60 (9.70)		13.6	−5.50 [−10.88, −0.12]
Subtotal (95% CI)	141		143			27.7	−4.06 [−7.56, −0.56]
Test for heterogeneity: chi² = 0.48, df = 1, P = 0.49, I² = 0.0%							
Test for overall effect: Z = 2.27, P = 0.02							
04 Other							
Curry 1995	17	26.80 (19.90)	24	26.80 (16.80)		9.0	0.00 [−11.60, 11.60]
Persson 1985	47	17.00 (16.00)	46	23.00 (22.00)		11.8	−600 [−13.83, 1.83]
Subtotal (95% CI)	64		70			20.8	−4.12 [−10.61, 2.37]
Test for heterogeneity: chi² = 0.71, df = 1, P = 0.40, I² = 0.0%							
Test for overall effect: Z = 1.24, P = 0.02							
Total (95% CI)	369		373			100.0	−5.54 [−10.87, −0.22]
Test for heterogeneity: chi² = 34.93, df = 8, P = <0.0001, I² = 77.1%							
Test for overall effect: Z = 2.04, P = 0.04							

−100.0 −50.0   0   50.0 100.0
Favors NSAIDs   Favors opioids

Figure 39.1 Comparison of the effect of non-steriodal anti-inflammatory drugs (NSAIDs) versus opioids on pain at 30 minutes by NSAID type. (Reprinted with permission from Holdgate & Pollock [17], © Wiley, Cochrane Library.)

fact be meperidine-specific. It should also be noted that the two most common and serious adverse events attributed to NSAIDs, gastrointestinal bleeding and renal impairment, were not reported. An RCT published after the systematic review compared morphine with the NSAID, ketorolac, versus both for the treatment of ureteric colic pain [18]. The combination of an opioid and NSAID was found to have an additive analgesic effect that was greater than either medication alone.

Since many patients with renal colic have associated nausea and vomiting and cannot tolerate oral medications, ketorolac is often the NSAID that many North American emergency physicians prescribe in the ED because it can be delivered parenterally. Rectal indomethacin is a less expensive option to intravenous ketorolac and, although the efficacy of the two has never been directly compared, it has been reported to be as effective as intravenous indomethacin for ureteric colic. Moreover, there is no obvious

difference in efficacy seen from the systematic review comparing NSAIDs to opioids (Fig. 39.1) [19].

Parenthetically, the most effective pain-relieving medications for acute ureteric colic might prove to be neither NSAIDs nor opiates but rather medications that induce rapid stone passage thereby eliminating the cause of the pain altogether. See the answer to Question 6 below for further details.

In summary, the combination therapy of NSAIDs with opiates provides more effective analgesia than either medication alone and is an appropriate management approach to employ in the acute setting.

Question 4: In patients with ureteric calculi (population), do antimuscarinic agents (intervention) effectively relieve pain (outcome) compared to routine care with narcotic analgesics (control)?

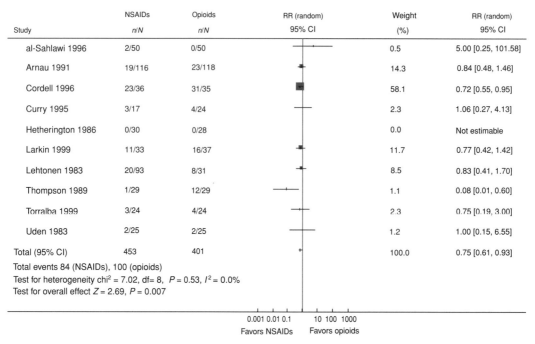

Study	NSAIDs n/N	Opioids n/N	RR (random) 95% CI	Weight (%)	RR (random) 95% CI
al-Sahlawi 1996	2/50	0/50		0.5	5.00 [0.25, 101.58]
Arnau 1991	19/116	23/118		14.3	0.84 [0.48, 1.46]
Cordell 1996	23/36	31/35		58.1	0.72 [0.55, 0.95]
Curry 1995	3/17	4/24		2.3	1.06 [0.27, 4.13]
Hetherington 1986	0/30	0/28		0.0	Not estimable
Larkin 1999	11/33	16/37		11.7	0.77 [0.42, 1.42]
Lehtonen 1983	20/93	8/31		8.5	0.83 [0.41, 1.70]
Thompson 1989	1/29	12/29		1.1	0.08 [0.01, 0.60]
Torralba 1999	3/24	4/24		2.3	0.75 [0.19, 3.00]
Uden 1983	2/25	2/25		1.2	1.00 [0.15, 6.55]
Total (95% CI)	453	401		100.0	0.75 [0.61, 0.93]

Total events 84 (NSAIDs), 100 (opioids)
Test for heterogeneity chi^2 = 7.02, df= 8, P = 0.53, I^2 = 0.0%
Test for overall effect Z = 2.69, P = 0.007

0.001 0.01 0.1   10 100 1000
Favors NSAIDs   Favors opioids

Figure 39.2 Comparison of the effect of non-steriodal anti-inflammatory drugs (NSAIDs) versus opioids on the need for rescue analgesia. (Reprinted with permission from Holdgate & Pollock [17], © Wiley, Cochrane Library.)

Search strategy

- PubMed – clinical queries in "clinical study category": renal colic AND therapy AND narrow, specific search

Ureteral smooth muscle spasm is believed to be a primary cause of the pain from acute ureteric colic and this is the basis for antispasmodic treatment in the form of antimuscarinics. There are currently no published systematic reviews evaluating the analgesic effectiveness of antimuscarinics in this condition; however, there are two RCTs. The first RCT evaluated the efficacy of a single sublingual dose of 0.125 mg of hyoscyamine sulfate compared to placebo [20]. All patients in both arms received intravenous ketorolac. In the 43 patients analyzed, there was no clinically important difference in change of pain scores at 30 minutes. A subsequent trial sought to determine whether the addition of hyoscine butylbromide (Buscopan) reduced the amount of opioid needed to achieve pain relief and subsequent need for rescue opioid analgesia [21]. ED patients with acute ureteric colic were randomized to receive Buscopan or placebo in addition to IV fluids and morphine, administered in 2.5 mg increments until pain relief was achieved. Indomethacin was given to those with no contraindications to NSAIDs and so the groups were stratified based on whether or not they received NSAIDs in addition to the antispasmodic. Recordings of hourly pain scores were ceased at 4 hours or upon ED discharge. The data were analyzed on an intention-to-treat basis. Of the 192 patients randomized, data were available for 85 of the patients who received Buscopan and 93 of those who received placebo. The me-

dian amount of morphine required was 0.12 mg/kg by patients who received Buscopan and 0.11 mg/kg for those who did not (P = 0.4). These two trials used different medications by different routes, on geographically different ED populations, and both studies reported no detectable improvement in pain relief when antimuscarinics are administered in addition to standard therapy to ED patients suffering from suspected acute ureteric colic.

In summary, the use of antimuscarinics for the treatment of pain from acute ureteric colic secondary to ureteral smooth muscle spasm might be theoretically sound but has no basis in clinical evidence. Their use in this setting should be discouraged.

Question 5: In patient with ureteric calculi (population), do diuretics and/or intravenous fluids (intervention) facilitate the passage of acute ureteric calculi (outcome) compared to routine care with analgesics (control)?

Search strategy

- PubMed – clinical queries in systematic review: renal colic AND fluids

The ED treatment of acute ureteric colic is primarily focused on pain control and secondarily on replacement of fluid loss from vomiting and/or reduced oral intake. The latter is typically achieved with IV fluid at maintenance volumes. Given that most ureteral stones are small enough to pass spontaneously, it is postulated that high-volume fluid therapy and/or diuretics in the acute setting might theoretically facilitate stone migration because of the associated increased hydrostatic pressure within the ureter forcing the stone into the bladder. More rapid stone elimination would not only reduce the duration of symptoms and associated adverse effects, it would cure the patient of an acute episode. However, the risk of high-volume fluid in the ureter and associated rapid increase in pressure could cause irreversible renal impairment and/or ureteric rupture. A Cochrane systematic review was conducted to examine the benefits and harms of high volume (above maintenance) and/or diuretics in acute ureteric colic to determine the effectiveness in facilitating stone passage with minimal risk of renal impairment [22]. The search identified only one study [23]. In this single-center RCT, 60 patients were randomized to receive 3 L of IV fluids or no fluids over a 6-hour period. The outcomes were difference in pain at 6 hours (RR = 1.06; 95% CI: 0.71 to 1.57), the proportion who underwent stone extraction (RR = 1.20; 95% CI: 0.41 to 3.51) and the proportion who underwent manipulation by cystoscopy (RR = 0.67; 95% CI: 0.21 to 2.13). Given that the confidence intervals around the summary measures all include a value of 1.0, there is no statistically significant difference between the hydrated and non-hydrated groups with respect to any of the outcomes. The authors of the Cochrane review concluded that there was no evidence supporting either diuretics or high-volume fluid therapy to facilitate stone passage in acute ureteric colic.

A subsequent RCT in which 43 patients received 2 L of normal saline intravenously over 2 hours or 20 ml/h of IV normal saline for 4 hours following IV analgesia, revealed no difference in baseline characteristics, no difference in narcotic requirement, no difference in hourly visual analog pain scale score, and no difference in stone passage rates between the two groups ($P > 0.05$) [24]. The findings of this trial independently confirm that of the systematic review to the extent that there is no evidence supporting high-volume fluid therapy to facilitate stone passage in acute ureteric colic. Furthermore, it appears that aggressive hydration does not contribute to pain relief. Since neither of the cited studies reported adverse events associated with diuretics or high-volume fluid therapy, we cannot know how frequently these occur.

In summary, the potential harm caused by adverse events and the lack of evidence supporting high-volume fluid therapy, indicate that this is not a suitable treatment for patients with acute ureteric colic.

Question 6: In patients with ureteric calculi (population), do calcium channel and/or α-adrenergic antagonists (interventions) safely facilitate the passage of ureteric calculi (outcome) compared to routine care with analgesics (control)?

Search strategy

- PubMed – clinical queries in systematic review: stone passage AND medical therapy

As stated previously, medical therapies that reduce the time to calculus elimination and, therefore, have the potential to reduce the duration of the symptoms and associated hardships, reduce repeated physician visits and hospital admissions, and preclude invasive rescue procedures, would provide considerable advantages for patients with renal calculi. Until recently, there were no ED medical treatments that could provide this degree of benefit.

A systematic review of RCTs evaluating calcium channel blockers or α-blockers for the treatment of ureteral stones reported pooled data from nine trials involving 693 patients [25]. The authors used a comprehensive search of electronic databases to avoid publication and selection biases and their main outcome was the proportion of patients who passed stones. The interventions were α-blockers with and without corticosteroids, α-blockers with and without diazepam, and calcium channel blockers with and without corticosteroids. They found that patients given α-blockers or calcium channel blockers had a 65% (absolute risk reduction (ARR) = 0.31; 95% CI: 0.25 to 0.38) greater likelihood of stone passage than those who were not (RR = 1.65; 95% CI: 1.45 to 1.88). Side-effects were insignificant as only four (0.6%) of all 693 patients discontinued the treatment before the end of their respective study. The authors concluded that "medical therapy is an option for facilitation of urinary-stone passage for patients amenable to conservative management, potentially obviating the need for surgery". While this conclusion may eventually be proved accurate, it is also worth noting that none of the trials in the review utilized blinding methods, therefore all subjects and treating physicians were aware of therapy and group assignments. This serves to explain why the validated Jadad scoring system indicated only moderate quality of the included studies. Nonetheless, expulsive therapy did appear to confer a consistent benefit in these non-blinded study settings. The authors also demonstrated the costs compared to other therapies. Their institutional cost of 6 weeks of treatment of tamulosin hydrochloride (Flomax, Flomaxtra, Urimax) was US$104.41. Using their calculated number needed to treat (NNT) of 4, the expulsion of one stone by medical therapy would cost approximately $417.64 compared to >$2000 for ureteroscopy and >$4000 for shockwave lithotripsy, assuming that each has an NNT of 1 and no associated complications.

In summary, although the effectiveness of these therapies needs to be confirmed through RCTs in multiple centers, the results are very promising for ED patients suffering acute ureteric colic and provides emergency physicians with an opportunity to extend their evidence-based care for this population.

Question 7: In patients with ureteric calculi (population), does drinking large volumes of water (intervention) reduce recurrent ureteric calculi (outcome) compared to no change in water intake (control)?

Search strategy

- PubMed – clinical queries in systematic review: calculi AND water

Increased water intake has long been prescribed as a preventive measure for ureteric colic based on the belief that calculi will not form in patients who are well hydrated [26]. A Cochrane review was undertaken to access the effectiveness of this practice of increased water intake for the prevention of urinary calculi [27]. Once again, the authors used a comprehensive search of electronic databases without any language restriction to avoid publication and selection biases for relevant RCTs and quasi-RCTs of increased water intake for the prevention and/or recurrence of urinary calculi and found only one RCT that fulfilled the inclusion criteria [25]. This trial randomized 220 patients to either a high water intake, which would give a urine volume equal to or greater than 2 L/day (intervention), or "usual" water intake (control). After a follow-up of 5 years, data were available for 99 patients in the intervention group and 100 in control group. There was no information about the method of randomization, the allocation concealment or blinding, and no intention-to-treat analysis was performed. The recurrence rate of ureteric colic was lower in the intervention group than the control group (RR = 0.45; 95% CI: 0.24 to 0.84) with an average interval for recurrences of 3.23 ± 1.1 years and 2.09 ± 1.37 years (weighted mean difference (WMD) = 1.14; 95% CI: 0.33 to 1.95) in the intervention and control groups, respectively, and there were no reported complications in either group. The NNT was 6.7 (95% CI: 4.1 to 25.7). The review authors concluded that "there is suggestive, but inconclusive evidence of the benefit of increasing water intake for the secondary prevention of urinary calculi".

In summary, based on this information, it is reasonable to suggest that patients increase their non-alcoholic fluid intake in order to avoid future episodes of ureretic calculi as this is unlikely to be harmful and is possibly beneficial.

Conclusions

The patient described above received an IV infusion of normal saline at maintenance rate and IV morphine and ketorolac (he refused the indomethacin suppository) for his pain. He underwent a non-contrast helical CT of his abdomen that demonstrated a 3 mm calculus in the distal ureter without evidence of hydronephrosis. His treatment consisted of pain relief, and 3 days following discharge he passed the stone. He now drinks water regularly in the hope of never having to suffer a similar event.

In conclusion, patients with ureteric colic are frequently seen in the ED. Most patients will have small stones <5 mm that will pass spontaneously and, therefore, require only analgesia. For those with larger stones or evidence of complete obstruction, a urological consult is required. Treatment consists of narcotic analgesics, NSAIDs and perhaps agents to increase the passage of stones following ED discharge, such as calcium channel blockers or α-blockers. Urinary tract infection in the presence of ureteric calculi is a true urological emergency.

Acknowledgments

Dr. Worster's research is supported in part by the Hamilton Health Sciences Corporation. Thanks to Brian Rowe for giving me the opportunity to contribute to the dissemination of evidence-based emergency medicine.

Conflicts of interest

Dr. Worster has never received funding or gifts from any of the manufacturers of the therapeutic agents listed in this article.

References

1 Ramello A, Vitale C, Marangella M. Epidemiology of nephrolithiasis. *J Nephrol* 2000;**13**(Suppl 3):40–50.

2 Asplin JR, Favus MJ, Coe FL. Nephrolithiasis. In: Brenner BM, ed. *Brenner and Rector's: The Kidney*, 5th edn. WB Saunders, Philadelphia, 1996:1893–935.

3 Segura JW, Preminger GW, Assimos DG, et al. Ureteral Stones Clinical Guidelines Panel summary report on the management of ureteral calculi. The American Urological Association. *J Urol* 1997;**158**(5):1915–21.

4 Osborne ED, Sutherland CG, Scholl AJ, et al. Landmark article February 10, 1923: Roentgenography of urinary tract during excretion of sodium iodide. *JAMA* 1983;**250**:2848–53.

5 Smith RC, Rosenfield AT, Choe KA, et al. Acute flank pain: comparison of non-contrast-enhanced CT and intravenous urography. *Radiology* 1995;**194**:789–94.

6 Levine JA, Neitlich J, Verga M, et al. Ureteral calculi in patients with flank pain: correlation of plain radiography with unenhanced helical CT. *Radiology* 1997;**204**:27–31.

7 Vieweg J, The C, Freed K, et al. Unenhanced helical computerized tomography for the evaluation of patients with acute flank pain. *J Urol* 1998;**160**:679–84.

8 Smith RC, Verga M, McCarthy S, et al. Diagnosis of acute flank pain: value on unenhanced helical CT. *Am J Roentgenol* 1996;**166**:97–101.

9 Katz DS, Lane MJ, Sommer FG. Unenhanced helical CT of ureteral stones: incidence of associated urinary tract findings. *Am J Roentgenol* 1996;**166**:1319–22.

10 Dalrymple NC, Verga M, Anderson KR, et al. The value of unenhanced helical computerized tomography in the management of acute flank pain. *J Urol* 1998;**159**:735–40.

11 Worster A, Preyra I, Weaver B, Haines T. The accuracy of noncontrast helical computed tomography versus intravenous pyelography in the diagnosis of suspected acute urolithiasis: a meta-analysis. *Ann Emerg Med* 2002;**40**(3):280–86.

12 Pfister SA, Deckart A, Laschke S, et al. Unenhanced helical computed tomography vs intravenous urography in patients with acute flank pain: accuracy and economic impact in a randomized prospective trial. *Eur Radiol* 2003;**13**(11):2513–20.

13 Thomson JM, Glocer J, Abbott C, Maling TM, Mark S. Computed tomography versus intravenous urography in diagnosis of acute flank pain from urolithiasis: a randomized study comparing imaging costs and radiation dose. *Australas Radiol* 2001;**45**(3):291–7.

14 Homer JA, Davies-Payne DL, Peddinti BS. Randomized prospective comparison of non-contrast enhanced helical computed tomography and intravenous urography in the diagnosis of acute ureteric colic. *Australas Radiol* 2001;**45**(3):285–90.

15 Worster A, Haines T. Does replacing intravenous pyelography with non-contrast helical computed tomography benefit patients with suspected acute urolithiasis? *Can Assoc Radiol J* 2002;**53**(3):144–8.

16 Teichman JM. Clinical practice. Acute renal colic from ureteral calculus. *N Engl J Med* 2004;**350**(7):684–93.

17 Holdgate A, Pollock T. Nonsteroidal anti-inflammatory drugs (NSAIDs) versus opioids for acute renal colic. *Cochrane Database Syst Rev* 2005;**2**:CD004137.

18 Safdar B, Degutis LC, Landry K, Vedere SR, Moscovitz HC, D'Onofrio G. Intravenous morphine plus ketorolac is superior to either drug alone for treatment of acute renal colic. *Ann Emerg Med* 2006;**48**(2):173–81.

19 Lee C, Gnanasegaram D, Maloba M. Best evidence topic report. Rectal or intravenous non-steroidal anti-inflammatory drugs in acute renal colic. *Emerg Med J* 2005;**22**(9):653–4.

20 Jones JB, Giles BK, Brizendine EJ, Cordell WH. Sublingual hyoscyamine sulfate in combination with ketorolac tromethamine for ureteral colic: a randomized, double-blind, controlled trial. *Ann Emerg Med* 2001;**37**(2):141–6.

21 Holdgate A, Oh CM. Is there a role for antimuscarinics in renal colic? A randomized controlled trial. *J Urol* 2005;**174**(2):572–5; discussion: 575.

22 Worster A, Richards C. Fluids and diuretics for acute ureteric colic. *Cochrane Database Syst Rev* 2005;**3**:CD004926.

23 Edna TH, Hesselberg F. Acute ureteral colic and fluid intake. *Scand J Urol Nephrol* 1983;**17**(2):175–8.

24 Springhart WP, Marguet CG, Sur RL, et al. Forced versus minimal intravenous hydration in the management of acute renal colic: a randomized trial. *J Endourol* 2006;**20**(10):713–16.

25 Hollingsworth JM, Rogers MA, Kaufman SR, et al. Medical therapy to facilitate urinary stone passage: a meta-analysis. *Lancet* 2006;**368**(9542):1171–9.

26 Borghi L, Meschi T, Amato F, Briganti A, Novarini A, Giannini A. Urinary volume, water and recurrences in idiopathic calcium nephrolithiasis: a 5-year randomized prospective study. *J Urol* 1996;**155**(3):839–43.

27 Qiang W, Ke Z. Water for preventing urinary calculi. *Cochrane Database Syst Rev* 2004;**3**:CD004292.

40 Urinary Tract Infection

Rawle A. Seupaul, Chris McDowell & Robert Bassett

Department of Emergency Medicine, Indiana University School of Medicine, Indianapolis, USA

Clinical scenario

During a busy shift in an urban emergency department (ED), a 22-year-old woman presented with a complaint of "pain with urination." She reported 3 days of dysuria and urinary frequency despite drinking cranberry juice. She denied fevers, nausea, vomiting or vaginal symptoms. Her past medical, surgical, family and social histories were unremarkable. Further questioning revealed that she had no primary care doctor and attends the ED whenever she has a health concern. Her vital signs were all within normal limits. Her physical exam was notable only for mild suprapubic tenderness.

Background

In the United States, acute urinary tract infections (UTIs) account for nearly 6 million physician visits per year. Over 1 million of these are seen in EDs [1]. It is estimated that 20% of women between the ages of 20 and 65 years experience a UTI every year. Moreover, approximately 50% of women will experience a UTI in their lifetime [2]. Therefore, the emergency physician must be comfortable with the diagnosis and management of these infections. In this chapter the authors address several pertinent questions regarding the management and treatment of acute uncomplicated UTIs.

Clinical questions

In order to optimize your diagnostic strategy as well as management of the patient with suspected urinary tract infection, you structure your literature search strategy according to the principles described in Chapter 1.

Evidence-based Emergency Medicine. Edited by Brian H. Rowe
© 2009 Blackwell Publishing, ISBN: 978-1-4051-6143-5.

1 In patients with symptoms suggestive of a UTI (population), what is the sensitivity and specificity (diagnostic test performance) of the urine dipstick test (diagnostic test) to determine the presence of UTI (outcome)?

2 In adult females with symptoms suggestive of a UTI (population), what is the sensitivity and specificity (diagnostic test performance) of clinical criteria (diagnostic test) for determining the presence of bacterial infection (outcome)?

3 In adult females with UTIs (population), are short-course (3 days) antimicrobial regimens (intervention) associated with similar bacteriological or clinical cure rates and less adverse events (outcomes) than long-course (5 days or more) antimicrobial regimens (comparison)?

4 In adult females with UTIs (population), are single-dose antimicrobial regimens (intervention) associated with improved bacteriological or clinical cure rates (outcomes) compared to multi-dose antimicrobial regimens (comparison)?

5 In adult females with UTIs (population), does the use of fluoroquinolones (intervention) confer a therapeutic or financial advantage (outcomes) compared to trimethoprim/sulfamethoxazole (control)?

6 In adults at risk for a UTI (population), does ingestion of cranberry juice (intervention) prevent UTIs compared to placebo or water (control)?

7 In adults with a documented acute UTI (population), does the addition of pyridium (intervention) safely reduce symptoms (outcome) compared to standard treatment with antibiotics alone (control)?

General search strategy

You search for answers to these questions by searching MEDLINE clinical queries for urinary tract infection or UTI under the "diagnosis" protocol, as well as searching for systematic reviews and meta-analyses. When these are located, you also search for more recent prospective studies addressing the same topic. You search EMBASE for similar topics. You also check the National Guideline Clearinghouse (http://www.guideline.gov) for any clinical practice guidelines on urinary tract infections and the Cochrane Library for systematic reviews (in the Cochrane Database of

Table 40.1 Likelihood ratios and diagnostic odds ratios for testing positive for nitrites on a urine dipstick. (Adapted from Deville et al. [3].)

	+LR (95% CI)	−LR (95% CI)	Diagnostic odds ratio (95% CI)
Population			
All patients	2.78 (1.52 to 11.6)	0.61 (0.44 to 0.79)	11 (6 to 21)
Children	6.25 (3.23 to 30)	0.54 (0.41 to 0.67)	34 (12 to 97)
Pregnant women	23 (1.81 to 56)	0.55 (0.44 to 0.78)	165 (73 to 372)
Elderly	17.75 (5.56 to α)	0.3 (0 to 0.55)	108 (10 to 1165)
Urology	19.67 (8.83 to α)	0.42 (0.34 to 0.5)	64 (19 to 216)
Surgery	13.5 (5.57 to 74)	0.48 (0.26 to 0.66)	34 (25 to 47)
Setting			
Family physician	4.42 (2.32 to 16.25)	0.53 (0.36 to 0.69)	12 (7 to 21)
Outpatient	11.25 (4.63 to 56)	0.57 (0.44 to 0.68)	87 (38 to 198)
Emergency	9.33 (4 to 40.5)	0.47 (0.19 to 0.67)	34 (10 to 112)
Inpatient	3.87 (1.96 to 33.5)	0.49 (0.34 to 0.66)	23 (10 to 54)

Systematic Review (CDSR) or Database of Reviews of Effectiveness (DARE)).

Searching for evidence synthesis: primary search strategy

- Cochrane Library: urinary tract infection OR UTI
- MEDLINE: (urinary tract infection OR UTI) AND (systematic review OR meta-analysis OR meta-analysis) AND (topic)
- EMBASE: (urinary tract infection OR UTI) AND (systematic review OR meta-analysis OR meta-analysis) AND (topic)
- Guideline.gov: urinary tract infection OR UTI

Critical review of the literature

Your search strategy for the Cochrane Library and guideline.gov website did not reveal any articles relevant to your questions. Your search of MEDLINE and EMBASE, however, identified several pertinent and interesting articles.

Question 1: In patients with symptoms suggestive of a UTI (population), what is the sensitivity and specificity (diagnostic test performance) of the urine dipstick test (diagnostic test) to determine the presence of UTI (outcome)?

Search strategy

- MEDLINE, Cochrane database and Cochrane DARE: urine dipstick AND accuracy

Given the large number of patients that present to the ED with urinary symptoms, rapid identification of infection or a high likelihood of infection is necessary. This is usually accomplished with a thorough history and diagnostic testing. The most commonly used diagnostic test is the urine dipstick. While the dipstick contains multiple components, two are relevant for the diagnosis of acute infection: nitrites and leukocyte-esterase. Thus, specimens can be reported in three categories: negative for both nitrites and leukocyte-esterase, positive for either, or positive for both. Clinicians use these results to diagnose acute infection, consider further testing and guide their management plans.

The utility of urine dipstick testing has been the subject of considerable debate in the ED and infectious disease literature. A number of trials have been conducted over the past 15 years attempting to clarify the diagnostic utility of this test. In 2004, a meta-analysis by Deville et al. addressed this question directly, identifying 72 studies for inclusion [3]. The studies included patients from a variety of clinical practice settings: family physician outpatients, inpatients and EDs; as well as various demographic groups: children, pregnant females, the elderly, and surgical and urology patients. The authors analyzed the diagnostic value of nitrites alone and combined with leukocyte-esterase (Tables 40.1, 40.2).

The authors note that there was variance in the diagnostic odds ratio dependent on both patient population and the clinical setting. They found that negative test results for leukocyte-esterase and nitrites sufficiently excluded infection in all populations studied, while the presence of nitrites had a sufficiently high predictive value only in pregnant women and the elderly. The predictive value of positive leukocyte-esterase alone was low across all patient subgroups [3].

The authors concluded that in all patients, the absence of leukocyte-esterase and nitrites was sufficient to exclude the presence of a UTI and to examine alternative diagnoses for the symptoms. The presence of positive nitrites alone suggested infection and was sufficiently predictive to diagnose infection in elderly patients. Overall the presence of leukocyte-esterase in combination with nitrites predicted infection but not strongly enough to preclude confirmatory tests [4].

When analyzing this data using likelihood ratios (Tables 40.1, 40.2), similar conclusions can be drawn. In general, the pre-test probability in the ED can be described as low (<25%), moderate (25–70%) or high (>70%). The presence of nitrates alone has a moderate to significant increase in the likelihood that the patient

	+LR (95% CI)	−LR (95% CI)	Diagnostic odds ratio (95% CI)
Population			
General	2.5 (1.65 to 4.23)	0.36 (0.09 to 0.62)	12 (6 to 22)
Children	5.53 (3.71 to 9.89)	0.2 (0.12 to 0.28)	46 (23 to 95)
Pregnant women	5.23 (3.05 to 9.75)	0.37 (0.24 to 0.52)	17 (10 to 30)
Elderly	2.83 (1.64 to 3.17)	0.25 (0.11 to 0.47)	16 (8 to 34)
Surgery	6.14 (5.25 to 6.77)	0.16 (0.14 to 0.19)	43 (22 to 85)
Urology	6.77 (4.47 to 11.11)	0.14 (0 to 0.29)	52 (48 to 56)
Setting			
Family physician	2.57 (2.28 to 2.97)	0.15 (0.12 to 0.18)	18 (13 to 25)
Outpatient	4.17 (3 to 6.31)	0.3 (0.21 to 0.4)	18 (12 to 27)
Emergency department	5.41 (4.53 to 6.53)	0.1 (0.02 to 0.17)	54 (25 to 117)
Hospital inpatient	3.43 (2.3 to 5.69)	0.27 (0.11 to 0.44)	25 (14 to 46)

Table 40.2 Likelihood ratios and diagnostic odds ratios for combined nitrites and leukocyte-esterase results (one or both positive). (Adapted from Deville et al. [3].)

has a UTI (positive likelihood ratio, +LR = 9.33; 95% CI: 4 to 40.5) and would result in a post-test likelihood in these three groups of 75.7%, 90.3% and 95.6%, respectively. The absence of both nitrates and leukocyte-esterase is sufficient to exclude the diagnosis (negative likelihood ratio, −LR = 0.1; 95% CI: 0.02 to 0.4) and would result in a post-test likelihood in these three groups of 3.2%, 9.1% and 18.9%, respectively.

In summary, emergency physicians assessing patients for suspected uncomplicated UTIs should attempt to place patients into general pre-test probabilities (e.g., low, moderate, high) based on their clinical experience and the patient's symptoms. Once this has been completed, the use of the urine dipstick results, especially nitrates and leukocyte-esterase, can guide decision making. For example, urine negative for both tests effectively rules out a UTI, and mandates a search for an alternative diagnosis. Furthermore, urine positive for both tests, or urine nitrates alone, effectively rules in a UTI, and suggests treatment can be initiated without further testing.

Question 2: In adult females with symptoms suggestive of a UTI (population), what is the sensitivity and specificity (diagnostic test performance) of clinical criteria (diagnostic test) for determining the presence of bacterial infection (outcome)?

Search strategy

- MEDLINE, Cochrane database and Cochrane DARE: urine dipstick AND accuracy

Distinguishing a simple UTI from other disorders such as a sexually transmitted disease (STD) by presenting symptoms can be difficult. It has been well documented that there is considerable overlap in symptoms between these two disease entities [5]. In a recent and substantial literature review of female patients presenting with symptoms suggestive of UTI, Bent et al. found that 50%

Table 40.3 Summary likelihood ratios for each sign and symptom. (Reproduced with permission from Aubin [1].)

Signs and symptoms	+LR (95% CI)	−LR (95% CI)
Symptom		
Dysuria	1.5 (1.2 to 2.0)*	0.5 (0.3 to 0.7)*
Frequency	1.8 (1.1 to 3.0)*	0.6 (0.4 to 1.0)
Hematuria	2.0 (1.3 to 2.9)*	0.9 (0.9 to 1.0)
Back pain	1.6 (1.2 to 2.1)*	0.8 (0.7 to 0.9)*
Vaginal discharge (absence)	3.1 (1.0 to 9.3)	0.3 (0.1 to 0.9)*
Vaginal irritation (absence)	2.7 (0.9 to 8.5)	0.2 (0.1 to 0.9)*
Low abdominal pain	1.1 (0.9 to 1.4)	0.9 (0.8 to 1.1)
Flank pain	1.1 (0.9 to 1.4)	0.9 (0.8 to 1.1)
Self-diagnosis	4.0 (2.9 to 5.5)*	0.1 (0.0 to 0.1)*
Sign		
CVA tenderness	1.7 (1.1 to 2.5)*	0.9 (0.8 to 1.0)
Vaginal discharge (absence)	1.1 (1.0 to 1.2)	0.7 (0.5 to 0.9)*
Fever	1.6 (1.0 to 2.6)	0.9 (0.9 to 1.0)
Urine dipstick†	4.2 (n/a)	0.3 (n/a)
Symptom combinations		
+Dysuria, +frequency, −Discharge, −irritation	24.6 (n/a)	−
−Dysuria, +discharge or irritation	0.3 (n/a)	−
+Dysuria or frequency, + +Discharge or irritation	0.7 (n/a)	−

*95% CI not crossing 1.0.
†Positive was considered leukocyte-esterase *or* nitrite positive and negative was considered both leukocyte-esterase *and* nitrite negative.
CI, confidence interval; n/a, not available due to lack of raw data.

of patients actually had a UTI. In the subset of patients without vaginal irritation or discharge, the prevalence of UTI increased to 90% [2]. Based on his findings, Bent suggests that women with vaginal symptoms should be evaluated for gonorrhea, *Chlamydia* or other vaginal infections, although the absence of vaginal symptoms does not rule out sexually transmitted or vaginal infections (Table 40.3).

In a retrospective chart review of an urban teaching hospital population, Berg et al. reported that more than half of the women discharged with the diagnosis of UTI alone were found to have an occult STD [6]. A prospective cohort study published in 2005 found that 17.3% of patients with symptoms of a simple UTI *also* had an STD. Secondly, 13.9% of patients who presented with simple UTI symptoms but were culture-negative for bacterial cystitis had a laboratory-proven STD infection [7].

These findings suggest that a significant number of cases of concomitant infections are mislabeled as simple cystitis while others with an isolated STD are misdiagnosed as having a UTI. After retrospective analysis, the only variables reported to be significant in predicting patients with an STD were "the number of sexual partners over the last year" and "a new sex partner within the last 90 days" [7,8]. Although a large well-designed study is needed to fully identify the prevalence of these misdiagnosis phenomena, additional screening in this patient population should be considered. With the advent of urine DNA ligase testing for both *Neisseria gonorrhea* and *Chlamydia trachomatis*, screening for these common STD pathogens may become easier and more practical [9].

In summary, ED physicians should be aware of the coincidence of STDs in patients presenting with urinary tract symptoms. More specifically, if a patient presents with vaginal itching, vaginal discharge or the absence of dysuria *and* urinary frequency (having only one of this pair is not sufficient), STD testing should be strongly considered.

Question 3: In adult females with UTIs (population), are short-course (3 days) antimicrobial regimens (intervention) associated with similar bacteriological or clinical cure rates and less adverse events (outcomes) than long-course (5 days or more) antimicrobial regimens (comparison)?

Search strategy

- MEDLINE and Cochrane database: urinary tract infections AND treatment duration

Various treatment courses have been suggested for uncomplicated UTIs, ranging from a single dose to 14 days of antibiotic therapy. Addressing the question of treatment duration requires a specifically defined treatment goal: symptomatic relief, culture-based eradication of the organism, or both. Multiple studies have attempted to answer these questions by comparing the same antibiotics, different doses of the same antibiotic, and different antibiotics on the basis of treatment duration.

Traditionally, physicians treated patients who presented with a UTI with at least a week of antibiotic therapy; however, shorter courses have been proposed as a method to reduce side-effects such as yeast vaginitis. A meta-analysis of 32 clinical trials comparing the efficacy and safety of 3-day versus longer course therapy (>5 days) was performed by Milo et al. in 2005 [10]. Comparisons

between 3-day and longer treatment courses were made on the basis of both symptomatic and bacteriological failure. The relative risk for short-term symptomatic failure was 1.16 (95% CI: 0.96 to 1.41), while for long-term symptomatic failure the relative risk was 1.17 (95% CI: 0.99 to 1.38) [11], indicating no clinically significant difference between the treatment courses. The authors also assessed treatment course efficacy compared to longer durations of therapy, demonstrating superiority of longer therapy for bacterial eradication. This difference persisted in follow-up as far out as 10 weeks, with a relative risk of 1.27 (95% CI: 1.09 to 1.47) favoring prolonged treatment courses [11].

In summary, 3-day treatment regimens provide efficacious and symptomatic relief for most patients. In addition, these regimens are less likely to result in significant adverse reactions. Although short-course antibiotic therapy provides significant symptomatic relief that is comparable to longer regimens, this regimen is not as efficacious at preventing asymptomatic bacteriuria. Therefore, in patient populations where bacterial eradication is important (e.g., patients who are immunocompromised, planning pregnancy or who suffer from recurrent infections) a longer antibiotic course may be more appropriate.

Question 4: In adult females with UTIs (population), are single-dose antimicrobial regimens (intervention) associated with improved bacteriological or clinical cure rates (outcomes) compared to multi-dose antimicrobial regimens (comparison)?

Search strategy

- MEDLINE and Cochrane database: urinary tract infections AND treatment duration

Since short-course antibiotics have been shown to maintain excellent cure rates and reduce side-effects, interest in single-dose therapy has been high. A Cochrane meta-analysis investigated the efficacy of single-dose regimens compared to multi-day regimens (3–14 days) in elderly women [12]. Although the methodological quality of the included studies was determined to be poor, the results suggest that while single-dose therapy seemed to demonstrate a slight (and statistically non-significant) decrease in effectiveness, increased compliance was noted in this group.

Single-dose therapy for UTIs has also been investigated, particularly for those patients in whom compliance is considered potentially problematic. It has been suggested that patient compliance is inversely proportional to length of treatment [13]. In its most recent clinical practice guideline for the treatment of urinary tract infections, the Infectious Disease Society of America (IDSA) addressed single-dose therapy, asserting that no trial or meta-analysis of sufficient power had demonstrated equivalence between single and multi-day regimens [14]. Two meta-analyses, one published in 1991 and the other in 2007, appear to support the IDSA's guideline [12,15]. However, two large (*n* = > 1000), randomized, multi-center trials published after the IDSA's guideline reported similar efficacy between single-dose gatifloxacin and 3-day ciprofloxacin therapy, suggesting that in selected population- single dose therapy may be safe and effective [16,17].

In summary, single-dose treatment for UTIs may be a viable option for select patient populations (e.g., those with a history of poor medication compliance, the indigent, or patients with ineffective/no primary care follow-up). This method of therapy can be especially relevant for ED populations. It should be noted, however, that the bulk of evidence suggests that longer courses of treatment (at least 3 days) have proven therapeutic benefit.

Question 5: In adult females with UTIs (population), does the use of fluoroquinolones (intervention) confer a therapeutic or financial advantage (outcomes) compared to trimethoprim/sulfamethoxazole (control)?

Search strategy

- Cochrane Library and MEDLINE: cystitis AND trimethoprim/sulfamethoxazole AND fluoroquinolones

Fluoroquinolones and trimethoprim/sulfamethoxazole (TMP/SMX) are commonly accepted 3-day regimens for the treatment of uncomplicated UTIs in adult women. Few guidelines formally prioritize either treatment option with respect to efficacy, cost or patient compliance. Four randomized controlled trials have addressed the question of short-course TMP/SMX versus short-course quinolone therapy [18–21]. In terms of antimicrobial efficacy, the fluoroquinolones studied were as efficacious as co-trimoxazole in all four trials. In the best powered study, McCarty et al. examined three treatment regimens in 687 patients. The authors found that 3-day treatment regimens with either TMP/SMX (160 mg/800 mg), ciprofloxacin (100 mg) or ofloxacin (200 mg) had similar efficacies for the treatment of acute, uncomplicated, symptomatic cystitis in women (Table 40.4) [21].

Patient compliance with treatment can be improved by choosing agents that are inexpensive, safe and easy to administer. Since both TMP/SMX and fluoroquinolones are dosed similarly, variables of interest include cost and side-effect profile. McCarty et al. reported that overall adverse events were greater in the TMP/SX group ($P < 0.05$) and in the ofloxacin group ($P = 0.05$) when compared to those treated with ciprofloxacin [21]. Also, adverse events were responsible for premature discontinuation of therapy more often in TMP/SX-treated patients ($n = 9$) than patients given ciprofloxacin ($n = 2$) or ofloxacin ($n = 1$; $P = 0.02$) [21]. In terms of cost, it was noted that the higher wholesale acquisition cost per unit dose for ciprofloxacin (US$2.40) as compared to TMP/SX ($0.34) may be mitigated by decreased morbidity, treatment failures and adverse events [21]. The meta-analysis used in the IDSA guidelines also found a significant reduction in adverse

events with shorter courses of therapy (11% vs 28%, $P < 0.001$) [13].

In summary, when deciding between these two agents, emergency medicine physicians will need to consider the needs of their individual patient. If cost is not a significant factor in treatment compliance, a fluoroquinolone may be appropriate. In situations where the use of fluoroquinolones is prohibitive, TMP/SX should be prescribed.

Question 6: In adults at risk for a UTI (population), does ingestion of cranberry juice (intervention) prevent UTIs compared to placebo or water (control)?

Search strategy

- MEDLINE, Cochrane database and Cochrane DARE: cranberry juice AND urinary tract infection

Patients with UTIs may ask about the role of cranberry juice as a method of prevention or cure. Despite the interest of the lay public, high-quality literature regarding cranberries' role in prevention or treatment is sparse [22,23].

The understanding of the mechanism behind cranberries and UTI has changed over the years and is currently focused on two mechanisms. Cranberries acidify the urine via the excreted metabolite hippuric acid. Hippuric acid has inherent bacteriostatic activity against *Escherichia coli*. However, in vivo studies found large doses of cranberry juice ($\sim$4 L) did not result in enough hippuric acid secretion to reach bacteriostatic levels [24].

Other investigators demonstrated that cranberry ingestion diminished *E. coli* adherence to the uroepithelium. Raz et al. identified two substances in cranberries, fructose and proacthocyanidin, that inhibit *E. coli* adhesions [24]. These molecules work at the level of the fimbria to inhibit bacterial adherence. Therefore, cranberries may directly prevent adherence and indirectly select for less adherent strains of *E. coli* [24].

Although the mechanisms by which cranberries work may have been elucidated, there is a dearth of evidence to support any clinical correlation in the setting of acute infection or prophylactic use. A Cochrane review failed to identify any randomized controlled trials of UTI treatment that met their inclusion criteria [23]. On the subject of UTI prophylaxis in high-risk individuals, however, the Cochrane review suggested that there may be some benefit in preventing recurrence (Fig. 40.1) [22].

In summary, these findings suggest that counseling patients at high risk for UTI (e.g., those with indwelling urinary catheters or recurrent UTI) to increase or initiate cranberry juice intake is appropriate, particularly given the lack of evidence to suggest harm or significant risk associated with this strategy.

Table 40.4 Summary of evidence table for trials comparing fluoroquinolones and co-trimoxazole in the treatment of adult females with an uncomplicated urinary tract infection [18–21].

Study	Design	Trial features	Results			Conclusions
Grubbs et al. [19]	Single-center RCT	Drug	Ciprofloxacin	TMP/SMZ		Ciprofloxacin and TMP/SMX are equally effective. Ciprofloxacin was associated with fewer adverse reactions
		Dose	250 mg bid	160 mg/800 mg bid		
		Rx duration	10 days	10 days		
		Study size	$n = 76$	$n = 68$		
		Microbiology				
		E. coli	$n = 61, 80\%$	$n = 64, 95\%$		
		Other Gram-negatives	$n = 10, 13\%$	$n = 2, 3\%$		
		S. saprophyticus	$n = 5, 7\%$	$n = 2, 3\%$		
		Rx success	$n = 69, 91\%$	$n = 62, 91\%$		
		Adverse drug reaction	17%	32%		
		Drug discontinued	1.9%	6%		
Cox et al. [18]	Multi-center RCT	Drug	Ofloxacin	TMP/SMZ		A 3-day course of ofloxacin is as effective as TMP/SMX. Ofloxacin is better tolerated than TMP/SMX
		Dose	200 mg QD	160 mg/800 mg bid		
		Rx duration	3 days	7 days		
		Study size	$n = 75$	$n = 66$		
		Microbiology				
		E. coli	$n = 56, 75\%$	$n = 52, 79\%$		
		K. pneumoniae	$n = 6, 8\%$	$n = 4, 6\%$		
		S. saprophyticus	$n = 2, 3\%$	$n = 0, 0\%$		
		Other	$n = 11, 15\%$	$n = 12, 19\%$		
		Rx success	$n = 73, 97.\%$	$n = 66^*, 97\%$		
		Adverse drug reaction	5%	15%		
		Drug discontinued	0%	5%		
McCarty et al. [20]	Multi-center RCT	Drug	Ofloxacin	TMP/SMZ	Ciprofloxacin	3-day courses of ciprofloxacin, ofloxacin and TMP/SMX had similar efficacies
		Dose	200 mg QD	160 mg/800 mg bid	100 mg bid	
		Rx duration	3 days	3 days	3 days	
		Study size	$n = 230$	$n = 229$	$n = 228$	
		Microbiology				
		E. coli	$n = 183, 79\%$	$n = 184, 80\%$	$n = 188, 83\%$	
		K. pneumoniae	$n = 11, 5\%$	$n = 9, 4\%$	$n = 10, 4\%$	
		S. saprophyticus	$n = 16, 7\%$	$n = 13, 6\%$	$n = 16, 7\%$	
		Other	$n = 20, 9\%$	$n = 23, 10\%$	$n = 14, 6\%$	
		Rx success	96%	95%	93%	
		Adverse drug reaction	39%	41%	31%	
		Drug discontinued	0.4%	4%	1%	
Henry et al. 1986	Single-center RCT	Drug	Ciprofloxacin	TMP/SMZ		Ciprofloxacin is as effective and less toxic than co-trimoxazole
		Dose	250 mg bid	160 mg/800 mg bid		
		Rx duration	10 days	10 days		
		Study size	$n = 31$	$n = 34$		
		Microbiology				
		E. coli	$n = 28, 90\%$			
		Coag. neg. Staph.	$n = 1, 3\%$	$n = 31, 90\%$		
		S. saprophyticus	$n = 1, 3\%$	$n = 1, 3\%$		
		Proteus	$n = 1, 3\%$			
		K. pneumoniae	$n = 0, 0\%$			
		Rx success[†]	$n = 29, 93\%$	$n = 1, 3\%$		
		Adverse drug reaction	$n = 3, 10\%$	$n = 28, 82\%$		
		Drug discontinued	$n = 0, 0\%$	$n = 10, 29\%$		

[*] Although there were 66 in this cohort, the cure rate was not 100% because one subject was infected with multiple pathogens making the number of patients 66, but the number of pathogens 68.

[†] Treatment success did not demonstrate a statistically significant difference.

bid, twice daily; Coag. neg. Staph., coagulase-negative Staphylococci; E. coli, Escherichia coli; K. pneumoniae, Klebsiella pneumoniae; Rx, treatment; Staphylococcus saprophyticus, TMP/SMZ, trimethoprim/sulfamethoxazole.

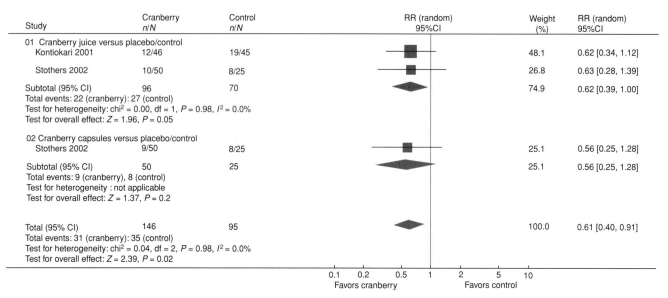

Figure 40.1 Summary data for the benefit of cranberry products in preventing urinary tract infection (UTI) recurrence. (Reprinted with permission from Jepson et al. [22], © Cochrane database, Wiley.)

Question 7: In adults with a documented acute UTI (population), does the addition of pyridium (intervention) safely reduce symptoms (outcome) compared to standard treatment with antibiotics alone (control)?

Search strategy

• MEDLINE and EMBASE: pyridium (phenazopyridine) AND urinary tract infection

Phenazopyridine (pyridium) is a treatment option used in the management of some urinary tract infections. As a urinary analgesic, this agent may be used as an adjunct with appropriate antibiotics for the early management of UTIs associated with dysuria. Although phenazopyridine use is reported, the extent of its use in the ED is unknown.

Extensive searching for evidence on the use of phenazopyridine revealed one review, which summarized the evidence for the use of this agent in patients with UTIs [25]. The authors conducted an English-language search of MEDLINE seeking evidence for the safety and efficacy of phenazopyridine in the treatment of UTIs. The review concluded that the few studies that reported the use of phenazopyridine examined variable populations, used weak designs, infrequently involved comparisons relevant to current UTI treatment, reported various outcomes, and provided conflicting results. Overall, the review concluded that evidence for the beneficial role of phenazopyridine was lacking. More importantly, the review identified impressive side-effects including gastrointestinal symptoms in over 10% of patients prescribed this agent. While rare, phenazopyridine can also cause some serious adverse effects such

as hemolytic anemia, renal failure and met-hemoglobinemia. The authors suggested that a definitive trial was required to determine the safety and efficacy of antibiotics compared to a combination of antibiotics and phenazopyridine in UTIs; however, the search described above failed to identify the existence of such a trial since the publication of this review in 1996.

In summary, these findings suggest that treating patients who have a UTI with phenazopyridine is not based on evidence. Given the lack of evidence to suggest benefit, and the potential for harm, physicians should abandon the use of phenazopyridine in the ED treatment of UTIs.

Conclusions

A urine dipstick and pregnancy test was performed on the patient described above. She was not pregnant and her dipstick was positive for both leukocyte-esterase and nitrites. Given the potential for poor medication compliance and the lack of a primary care physician, she received a single dose of ciprofloxacin (500 mg) before being discharged home with a prescription to complete a 3-day course. She returned for an unrelated reason 2 weeks later and reported that her UTI symptoms resolved within 2 days after her initial visit despite the fact that she did not fill her antibiotics prescription.

In conclusion, patients with suspected UTIs are frequently seen in the ED. The diagnosis is suggested by symptoms and can be quickly and effectively confirmed with the urine dipstick test. In patients whose urine dipstick test is negative, alternative diagnoses and investigations should be considered. Patients with an uncomplicated UTI can be effectively treated with a short course (3 days) of either TMP/SMX or a fluoroquinolone. Given the diversity of patients encountered in the ED, creativity with dosing regimens is encouraged. As exemplified in the patient scenario above, a combination of therapies may prove the best option.

Conflicts of interest

None were reported.

References

1 Aubin C. Does this woman have an acute uncomplicated urinary tract infection? *Ann Emerg Med* 2007;**49**(1):106–8.

2 Bent S, Nallamothu BK, Simel DL, Fihn SD, Saint S. Does this woman have an acute uncomplicated urinary tract infection? *JAMA* 2002;**287**(20):2701–10.

3 Deville WLJM, Yzermans JC, van Duijn NP, Bezemer PD, van der Windt DAWM, Bouter LM. The urine dipstick test useful to rule out infections. A meta-analysis of the accuracy. *BMC Urol* 2004;**4**:4.

4 Centre for Reviews and Dissemination. The urine dipstick test useful to rule out infections: a meta-analysis of the accuracy (Structured abstract). *Database Abstr Rev Effects* 2007;**1**.

5 Komaroff AL. Acute dysuria in women. *N Engl J Med* 1984;**310**(6):368–75.

6 Berg E, Benson DM, Haraszkiewicz P, Grieb J, McDonald J. High prevalence of sexually transmitted diseases in women with urinary infections. *Acad Emerg Med* 1996;**3**(11):1030–34.

7 Shapiro T, Dalton M, Hammock J, Lavery R, Matjucha J, Salo DF. The prevalence of urinary tract infections and sexually transmitted disease in women with symptoms of a simple urinary tract infection stratified by low colony count criteria. *Acad Emerg Med* 2005;**12**(1):38–44.

8 Mehta SD, Rothman RE, Kelen GD, Quinn TC, Zenilman JM. Unsuspected gonorrhea and chlamydia in patients of an urban adult emergency department: a critical population for STD control intervention. *Sex Transm Dis* 2001;**28**(1):33–9.

9 Shafer MA, Pantell RH, Schachter J. Is the routine pelvic examination needed with the advent of urine-based screening for sexually transmitted diseases? *Arch Pediatr Adolesc Med* 1999;**153**(2):119–25.

10 Milo G, Katchman EA, Paul M, Christiaens T, Baerheim A, Leibovici L. Duration of antibacterial treatment for uncomplicated urinary tract infection in women. *Cochrane Database Syst Rev* 2005;**2**:CD004682.

11 Katchman EA, Milo G, Paul M, Christiaens T, Baerheim A, Leibovici L. Three-day vs longer duration of antibiotic treatment for cystitis in women: systematic review and meta-analysis. *Am J Med* 2005;**118**(11):1196–207.

12 Lutters M, Vogt-Ferrier NB. Antibiotic duration for treating uncomplicated, symptomatic lower urinary tract infections in elderly women (Systematic review) *Cochrane Database Syst Rev* 2007;**1**:CD001535.

13 Kruse W, Eggert-Kruse W, Rampmaier J, Runnebaum B, Weber E. Dosage frequency and drug-compliance behaviour – a comparative study on compliance with a medication to be taken twice or four times daily. *Eur J Clin Pharmacol* 1991;**41**(6):589–92.

14 Warren JW, Abrutyn E, Hebel JR, Johnson JR, Schaeffer AJ, Stamm WE. Guidelines for antimicrobial treatment of uncomplicated acute bacterial cystitis and acute pyelonephritis in women. Infectious Diseases Society of America (IDSA). *Clin Infect Dis* 1999;**29**(4):745–58.

15 Leibovici L, Wysenbeek AJ. Single-dose antibiotic treatment for symptomatic urinary tract infections in women: a meta-analysis of randomized trials. *Q J Med* 1991;**78**(285):43–57.

16 Naber KG, Allin DM, Clarysse L, et al. Gatifloxacin 400 mg as a single shot or 200 mg once daily for 3 days is as effective as ciprofloxacin 250 mg twice daily for the treatment of patients with uncomplicated urinary tract infections. *Int J Antimicrob Agents* 2004;**23**(6):596–605.

17 Richard GA, Mathew CP, Kirstein JM, Orchard D, Yang JY. Single-dose fluoroquinolone therapy of acute uncomplicated urinary tract infection in women: results from a randomized, double-blind, multicenter trial comparing single-dose to 3-day fluoroquinolone regimens. *Urology* 2002;**59**(3):334–9.

18 Cox CE, Serfer HS, Mena HR, et al. Ofloxacin versus trimethoprim/sulfamethoxazole in the treatment of uncomplicated urinary tract infection. *Clin Therapeut* 1992;**14**(3):446–57.

19 Grubbs NC, Schultz HJ, Henry NK, Ilstrup DM, Muller SM, Wilson WR. Ciprofloxacin versus trimethoprim-sulfamethoxazole: treatment of community-acquired urinary tract infections in a prospective, controlled, double-blind comparison. *Mayo Clin Proc* 1992;**67**(12):1163–8.

20 Henry NK, Schultz HJ, Grubbs NC, Muller SM, Ilstrup DM, Wilson WR. Comparison of ciprofloxacin and co-trimoxazole in the treatment of uncomplicated urinary tract infection in women. *J Antimicrob Chemother* 1986;**18**(Suppl D):103–6.

21 McCarty JM, Richard G, Huck W, et al. A randomized trial of short-course ciprofloxacin, ofloxacin, or trimethoprim/sulfamethoxazole for the treatment of acute urinary tract infection in women. Ciprofloxacin Urinary Tract Infection Group. *Am J Med* 1999;**106**(3):292–9.

22 Jepson RG, Mihaljevic L, Craig J. Cranberries for preventing urinary tract infections. Update of Cochrane Database Syst Rev 2004;1:CD001321; PMID: 14973968. *Cochrane Database Syst Rev* 2004;**2**:CD001321.

23 Jepson RG, Mihaljevic L, Craig J. Cranberries for treating urinary tract infections. *Cochrane Database Syst Rev* 2000;**2**:CD001322.

24 Raz R, Chazan B, Dan M. Cranberry juice and urinary tract infection. *Clin Infect Dis* 2004;**38**:1413–19.

25 Zelenitsky SA, Zhanel GG. Phenazopyridine in urinary tract infections. *Ann Pharmacother* 1996;**30**:866–8.

41 Pelvic Inflammatory Disease

Linda Papa[1] & Kurt Weber[2]

[1]Department of Emergency Medicine, Orlando Regional Medical Center, Orlando *and* Department of Emergency Medicine, College of Medicine, University of Florida, Gainesville *and* Florida State University College of Medicine, Tallahassee, USA
[2]Department of Emergency Medicine, Orlando Regional Medical Center, Orlando *and* Florida State University College of Medicine, Tallahassee, USA

Clinical scenario

A 27-year-old female presents to the emergency department (ED) with a complaint of non-radiating right lower quadrant abdominal pain that has been worsening over 2 days. On exam the patient was alert and oriented but appears to be very uncomfortable from pain and is vomiting. You administer some intravenous analgesics and anti-emetics and proceed with the history. Upon review of systems the patient reports no previous surgeries or hospitalizations. She denies fever, chills, urinary symptoms and diarrhea; she has minimal vaginal discharge and has vomited twice in 24 hours. She had a normal menstrual period 1 week previously and is monogamous with her current partner of 6 months. Examination reveals vital signs of: pulse 105 beats/min, respiratory rate 16 breaths/min, blood pressure 110/65 mmHg, temperature 37.6°C (oral) and oxygen saturation 99%. Her abdominal exam reveals the presence of bowel sounds with moderate right lower quadrant pain together with guarding and rebound. The pelvic exam revealed normal external genitalia, a small amount of whitish cervical discharge on speculum exam, and right adnexal tenderness on bimanual palpation. The rest of the physical examination is unremarkable for any other abnormalities. Her microscopic urinalysis and urine pregnancy test are negative. Your differential diagnosis includs pelvic inflammatory disease (PID) and appendicitis.

A computerized tomography (CT) scan of the abdomen and pelvis is performed and identifies no abnormalities (including a normal appendix) except for a small amount of free fluid in the cul de sac. Your presumptive diagnosis following these tests is PID. The intern asks if further testing is warranted and about the certainty of this diagnosis. Upon discussing the diagnosis with the patient, she asks if her current partner needs to be treated and if this could affect her ability to have children. Soon after, the nurse approaches and asks if you are planning to discharge the patient.

Background

Pelvic inflammatory disease is a term that encompasses a range of pelvic infections of the upper genital tract. This includes any combination of endometritis, salpingitis or pyosalpinx, which in severe cases can be complicated by tubo-ovarian abscess and pelvic peritonitis [1,2]. The annual incidence of PID in women of reproductive age is 8%, affecting approximately 1 million American women each year [1]. The average per person lifetime cost of PID ranges between US$1060 and $3180 [3] and it generates direct and indirect annual health care costs of about $4.2 billion in the USA alone [4,5].

Accurate diagnosis of PID can be difficult, many episodes of PID may be sub-clinical and many may go unrecognized [6–8]. Often, women with PID have subtle or mild symptoms. Although some cases are asymptomatic, others are undiagnosed because the patient or the health care provider fails to recognize the implications of mild or non-specific symptoms or signs (e.g., abnormal bleeding, dyspareunia, vaginal discharge) [6,8]. The clinical presentation of PID can mimic acute appendicitis and abdominal ectopic pregnancy, as well as pain from liver, gallbladder or renal etiologies [2,9,10]. Furthermore, secondary PID may also arise following a puerperal infection, abortion, appendicitis or diverticulitis [11].

A large prospective cohort study has established risk factors for PID, such as prior sexually transmitted disease (STD) infection and smoking; however, these are non-specific and generally lack predictive power [1,12]. While PID is commonly thought of as an STD, it is now recognized as having poly-microbial etiology. Gonorrhea and *Chlamydia* have a higher prevalence in patients with common STD risk factors, such as no barrier protection, multiple sex partners, and so forth. However, in

Evidence-based Emergency Medicine. Edited by Brian H. Rowe
© 2009 Blackwell Publishing, ISBN: 978-1-4051-6143-5.

clinical trials the incidences of these bacteria vary, while other pathogens, including Gram-negative pathogens and anaerobes, become more common [13,14]. Despite the fact that ascending infections of *Chlamydia trachomatis* or *Neisseria gonorrhea* are commonly found in the pelvic area of women experiencing PID, the presence of either bacterium is not required for the development and manifestation of PID to occur. Microorganisms that comprise the vaginal flora (e.g., anaerobes, *Gardnerella vaginalis*, *Haemophilus influenzae*, enteric Gram-negative rods and *Streptococcus agalactiae*) have also been associated with PID. In addition, cytomegalovirus (CMV), *Mycoplasma hominis* and *Ureaplasma urealyticum* may be the etiologic agents in some cases of PID [6].

The diagnosis of PID is often challenging. Laparoscopy has been used as a diagnostic aid and as a reference standard for acute PID since 1960 [15]; however, laparoscopy is expensive, invasive, and impractical in the outpatient setting [16]. Laparoscopic examination may not detect endometritis or subtle inflammation of the Fallopian tubes [17] and is subject to intra-observer and inter-observer variability [18].

Timely diagnosis of PID is critical to improving and preserving the overall health of the patient. Delay in diagnosis and effective treatment probably contributes to inflammatory sequelae in the upper reproductive tract and can result in complications such as tubal scarring and infertility, chronic pelvic pain and/or ectopic pregnancy [19,20]. Although early diagnosis and treatment are known to effectively reduce the incidence of complications associated with known PID [19], the optimal treatment regimen and long-term outcome of early treatment of women with asymptomatic or atypical PID are widely debated. While the majority of patients with PID are treated as outpatients, some experts advocate inpatient parenteral therapy in cases where future fertility is of particular risk, for instance nulligravid teenagers [21].

What is also not clear is the best route of administering treatment as no efficacy data have compared parenteral with oral regimens [6]. The efficacy of both parenteral and oral regimens has been shown in many randomized trials [22]. While most trials have used parenteral treatment for at least 48 hours after clinical improvement, this time designation is arbitrary [6].

The focus of this chapter will be the presentation and discussion of evidence-based information to arm the physician with the tools and knowledge to best diagnose and treat PID in a timely manner within the ED setting.

Clinical questions

In order to address the issues of most relevance to your patient and to help in searching the literature for the evidence regarding these issues, you structure your clinical questions as recommended in Chapter 1.

1 What is the reference standard for diagnosing pelvic inflammatory disease? What is the sensitivity and specificity of this technique?

2 In female patients with pelvic complaints (population), what are the sensitivity, specificity and likelihood ratios (diagnostic test characteristics) of the history, physical examination and laboratory elements (diagnostic tests) in determining the likelihood of acute pelvic inflammatory disease compared to laparoscopy (reference standard)?

3 In female patients with pelvic complaints (population), what are the sensitivity, specificity and likelihood ratios (diagnostic test characteristics) of radiological tests (diagnostic tests) in determining the likelihood of pelvic inflammatory disease compared to laparoscopy (reference standard)?

4 In female patients with lower abdominal pain (population), what clinical and laboratory factors (diagnostic tests) have diagnostic or discriminatory utility (diagnostic test characteristics) in distinguishing between appendicitis and pelvic inflammatory disease compared to laparoscopy (reference standard)?

5 In women diagnosed with acute pelvic inflammatory disease (patients), which antibiotics (intervention, comparison) result in the highest clinical and microbiological cure rate (outcome)?

6 In women diagnosed with acute pelvic inflammatory disease (patients), does hospitalization (intervention) reduce long-term sequelae (e.g., infertility, chronic pelvic pain) (outcome) compared to outpatient management (comparison)?

General search strategy

You begin to address the topic of PID by searching for evidence in the common electronic databases such as MEDLINE looking specifically for systematic reviews and randomized controlled trials. This topic is covered by a large body of evidence from disparate sources; consequently, few meta-analyses have been published, and no Cochrane reviews were identified for the questions above. Finally, access to relevant, updated, evidence-based clinical practice guidelines (CPGs) on PID are accessed to determine the consensus rating of areas lacking evidence.

Specific search strategy

- Cochrane Library: (pelvic inflammatory disease OR PID OR salpingitis) AND (topic)
- MEDLINE: (systematic review OR meta-analysis OR metaanalysis) AND (pelvic inflammatory disease OR PID OR salpingitis) AND (topic)
- MEDLINE: (pelvic inflammatory disease OR PID OR salpingitis) AND diagnosis AND (sensitivity and specificity [MeSH] OR likelihood ratio [MeSH])
- MEDLINE: (pelvic inflammatory disease OR PID OR salpingitis) AND therapy

Critical review of the literature

Question 1: What is the reference standard for diagnosing pelvic inflammatory disease? What is the sensitivity and specificity of this technique?

Search strategy

- MEDLINE: (pelvic inflammatory disease OR PID OR salpingitis) AND (diagnosis OR (sensitivity and specificity [MeSH])

Laparoscopic diagnosis of acute salpingitis is recognized as a reference standard for PID as the procedure allows direct visualization of the ovaries, uterus, Fallopian tubes and other abdominal structures. The sensitivity and specificity, however, have yet to be established, partly due to lack of an alternate, highly accurate, diagnostic technique [23]. Inflammatory responses in biopsies and cytology smears from women with clinical PID but negative laparoscopy have been examined; however, standards defining the histopathological diagnosis have not been established either [17,23].

The first large published series using laparoscopy in women with lower abdominal pain, in 1969 [15], studied 814 women over 8 years with clinical suspicion of PID. Patients were included if they had lower abdominal pain and at least two of: (i) abnormal vaginal discharge; (ii) fever; (iii) vomiting; (iv) menstrual irregularities; (v) urinary symptoms; (vi) proctitis symptoms; (vii) marker tenderness of pelvic organs on bimanual exam; (viii) palpable adnexal mass or swelling; and (ix) an erythrocyte sedimentation rate of ≥ 15 mm/h. Of these, only 523 (65%) were examined laparoscopically. No pathological changes were found in 23% of those undergoing laparoscopy, while 12% demonstrated other pathological changes including acute appendicitis, ectopic pregnancy, endometriosis and other non-specific pelvic disorders.

Sellors et al. [24] performed laparoscopy on women with acute pelvic pain in whom PID was suspected. The diagnosis of PID was based on combined laparoscopic and histopathological findings. In this study, laparoscopy missed 50% of those with histopathological confirmation of salpingitis. Of those thought to have salpingitis by laparoscopy, the diagnosis was histopathologically confirmed in only 65%. Similarly, Bevan et al. evaluated women with acute abdominal pain and clinical signs of acute salpingitis microbiologically and laparoscopically and found that only 70% had acute salpingitis diagnosed at laparoscopy [25]. In summary, these and other studies have demonstrated the complexity of defining both an appropriate reference standard, and the disease itself. Emergency physicians should be aware that laparoscopy will likely not detect subtle disease and is usually reserved for difficult diagnostic cases or cases that require intra-operative management.

Question 2: In female patients with pelvic complaints (population), what are the sensitivity, specificity and likelihood ratios (diagnostic test characteristics) of the history, physical examination and laboratory elements (diagnostic tests) in determining the likelihood of acute pelvic inflammatory disease compared to laparoscopy (reference standard)?

Search strategy

- MEDLINE: (pelvic inflammatory disease OR salpingitis) AND diagnosis AND (sensitivity and specificity [MeSH] or likelihood ratio [MeSH])

In 1991, Kahn et al. [26] conducted a systematic review of the English-language literature for the period 1969 through 1990 to examine the accuracy of existing diagnostic indicators for PID. Diagnostic findings were divided into four categories: historical (symptoms), clinical examination (signs), laboratory, and combinations of the first three (Table 41.1). No single or combination diagnostic indicator was found to reliably predict PID [26].

Since this systematic review we identified six additional studies that evaluated the accuracy of the clinical diagnosis of acute PID; the evidence is summarized in Table 41.2 [14,24,27–30]. There are a number of methodological limitations to these studies, including the variability of the inclusion criteria, sampling bias and the definition of the outcome measure used to confirm the presence of PID.

In summary, the frequency of clinical and laboratory manifestations of PID varies widely. The only physical finding that appears consistently across studies is abdominal tenderness and/or adnexal tenderness. Laboratory tests can be helpful but are often non-specific. Emergency physicians should ensure that they maintain a high clinical suspicion for milder and more atypical presentations of the disease.

Question 3: In female patients with pelvic complaints (population), what are the sensitivity, specificity and likelihood ratios (diagnostic test characteristics) of radiological tests (diagnostic tests) in determining the likelihood of pelvic inflammatory disease compared to laparoscopy (reference standard)?

Search strategy

- MEDLINE and Cochrane: (PID OR pelvic inflammatory disease) AND (ultrasound OR sonography) OR (CT OR computerized tomography) OR (MRI OR magnetic resonance imaging) OR leukocyte scintigraphy

A variety of radiographic approaches can be employed when investigating women with abdominal and/or pelvic pain, including

Table 41.1 Sensitivity and specificity of PID diagnostic indicators. (Reprinted with permission from Kahn [26].)

Criterion	Study	Sensitivity (%)	Specificity (%)
History			
Duration of lower abdominal pain >4 days	Wolner-Hanssen et al. [55]	76	54
		80	54
7–14 days	Wolner-Hanssen et al. [55]	33	89
	Wasserheit et al. [56]	§	§
Irregular menses		50	82
		47	82
	Jacobson and Westrom [15]	36	57
	Hadgu et al. [57]	40	60
Fever/chills	Jacobson and Westrom [15]	41	80
	Hadgu et al. [57]	34	75
Sexual contact with a known gonorrhea carrier	Tavelli and Judson [58]	40	82
History of use of an intrauterine device	Wolner-Hanssen et al. [55]	34	67
	Tavelli and Judson [58]	13	88
	Wolner-Hanssen et al. [55]	36	86
Urinary symptoms	Tavelli and Judson [58]	32	83
	Jacobson and Westrom [15]	19	80
	Hadgu et al. [57]	20	78
	Wolner-Hanssen et al. [55]	21	64
≥4 symptoms	Jacobson and Westrom [15]	20	89
Proctitis symptoms	Jacobson and Westrom [15]	7	97
	Hadgu et al. [57]	7	97
Age	Hadgu et al. [57]	§	§
	Tavelli and Judson [58]	§	§
Marital status	Hadgu et al. [57]	§	§
Clinical Examination			
Abnormal vaginal discharge	Jacobson and Westrom [15]	63	75
Purulent vaginal discharge	Hadgu et al. [57]	81	42
	Tavelli and Judson [58]	26	83
	Wolner-Hanssen et al. [55]	68	43
Palpable mass	Jacobson and Westrom [15]	49	76
	Hadgu et al. [57]	48	74
	Wolner-Hanssen et al. [55]	24	79
	Westrom [60]	§	§
≥4 signs	Jacobson and Westrom [15]	39	91
Temperature >38°C	Jacobson and Westrom [15]	33	86
	Hadgu et al. [57]	35	85
	Westrom [60]	40	80
	Wolner-Hanssen et al. [55]	24	79
	Wasserheit et al. [56]	§	§
Laboratory finding			
C-reactive protein	Jacobson et al. [15]	92	50
	Lehtinen et al. [61]	74	67
	Wasserheit et al. [56]	85	90
	Hemila et al. [62]	93	83
Antichymotrypsin	Jacobson et al. [15]	92	56
Orosomucoid	Jacobson et al. [15]	88	77
Endometrial biopsy	Paavonen et al. [64]	69	67
	Wasserheit et al. [56]	70	89

(Continued)

Table 41.1 (*Continued*)

Criterion	Study	Sensitivity (%)	Specificity (%)
Erythrocyte sedimentation rate	Jacobson and Westrom [15]	76	47
>15 mm/h	Westrom [60]	75	25
	Lehtinen et al. [61]	81	57
>20 mm/h	Wolner-Hanssen et al. [55]	76	69
		64	69
	Hadgu et al. [57]	81	43
>25 mm/h	Wasserheit et al. [56]	55	84
Positive gonococcal *Chlamydia* test any site	Wasserheit et al. [56]	77	77
Fallopian tubes and endometrium	Wasserheit et al. [56]	55	100
Positive gonoccocal culture	Hadgu et al. [57]	§	§

ultrasound, computerized tomography (CT), magnetic resonance imaging (MRI) and leukocyte scintigraphy. The respective approaches will be evaluated in detail below.

Ultrasound

The MEDLINE search uncovered six articles relating the diagnostic test characteristics of pelvic ultrasound relative to laparoscopy. Kupesic and colleagues in 1995 compared transvaginal color and pulsed Doppler (TVCD), laparoscopic and clinical findings in 102 women with proven PID [31]. Seventy-two of them had acute symptoms, 11 presented with chronic pelvic pain and 19 patients were infertility cases suspected of tubal etiology. Color flow was obtained in all six patients presenting with ovarian enlargement, in 12 (54.5%) of those presenting with tubular adnexal structure, and in 56 (75.7%) of those with complex adnexal mass. Ovarian morphology was clearly delineated from adnexal mass in 59 patients (55.9%). The ipsilateral ovarian flow was altered in 50 of them (84.7%). The mean resistance index (RI) in patients with acute symptoms was 0.53 ± 0.09 (RI $\pm$ SD). It significantly differed from those obtained in patients with chronic pelvic pain (RI $= 0.71 \pm 0.07$) and infertility cases (RI $= 0.73 \pm 0.09$). The authors concluded that TVCD was a useful additional tool in the diagnosis and treatment monitoring in patients with PID [31].

In 1995 Taipale et al. used transvaginal sonography (TVS) in the evaluation of clinically suspected PID. The diagnosis of PID was confirmed in 37% of patients by laparoscopy, laparotomy or positive cervical culture of *Chlamydia trachomatis* or *Neisseria gonorrhea*. In the remainder, the diagnosis was based on tenderness of the uterus, fever and lower abdominal pain that responded rapidly to antibiotics. C-reactive protein concentrations and sedimentation rate values correlated positively with the ultrasonically determined volumes of pyosalpinx/pyoovaries, cul de sac fluid and ovaries [32].

In 1990, results of pre-operative pelvic examination and ultrasound examination were correlated with laparoscopic findings in 133 women with acute pelvic pain. If ultrasound findings were abnormal the results at laparoscopy were also abnormal in 90% of cases. However, a normal ultrasound examination did not exclude abnormal laparoscopic findings and the predictive value of a normal ultrasound was 50% [33].

During that same period Patten correlated endovaginal ultrasound (EVUS) results with laparoscopic findings in 16 patients with operatively confirmed acute PID to evaluate the sensitivity and accuracy of EVUS for the identification of uterine and adnexal pathology. Laparoscopy confirmed prospective sonographic abnormalities in 25 of 27 inflamed Fallopian tubes (sensitivity 93%) and in 19 of 21 ovaries with periovarian inflammation (sensitivity 90%). Overall accuracy for EVUS prediction of periovarian or tubal disease was 91% and 93%, respectively. However, EVUS was less sensitive to uterine abnormalities and detected inflammatory changes in only three of 12 confirmed cases (25%). EVUS also failed to demonstrate small quantities of purulent fluid (less than 20 cm^3) in the pelvic cul de sac in six of nine cases [34].

Papadimitriou evaluated the efficacy of power Doppler sonography in depicting soft tissue hyperemia in pelvic inflammatory conditions in 31 patients [35]. All the women underwent laparoscopy after 10 days. Soft tissue hyperemia was seen on power Doppler sonograms in 22 of the symptomatic patients. Specificity was 52.4%, sensitivity 47.1% and the positive predictive value was 53.2%. Power Doppler sonography showed hyperperfusion in many cases associated with pelvic inflammatory pathology and may be a useful adjunct to standard color Doppler imaging in the depiction of vascular flow [35].

In 2001, Molander et al. evaluated the usefulness of power Doppler TVS in the diagnosis of PID and assessed the diagnostic reliability of specific sonographic findings [36]. Thirty women admitted for suspected acute PID were compared to 20 controls with known hydrosalpinx. Conventional TVS and power Doppler TVS (to assess vascularity) were performed on all patients, and those patients with suspected acute PID underwent diagnostic laparoscopy. Laparoscopy confirmed the diagnosis of PID in 20 (67%) of the 30 women with clinically suspected acute PID. Specific TVS findings,

Table 41.2 Summary of evidence table of studies examining the sensitivity, specificity and likelihood ratios/relative risk of the history, physical examination and laboratory elements.

Study	Sample size	Setting	Design	Outcome measure	Effect measure	Comments
Kahn et al. [26]	12 studies	MEDLINE search English-language literature	Systematic review from 1969 to 1990	PID confirmed by strict clinical criteria or laparoscopy	See sensitivity and specificity in Table 41.1 Sensitivity and specificity were extracted using raw data. Results were grouped by a quality rating based on subject selection, definition of PID, data analysis and other measures	Historical findings were usually not significant predictors. Clinical findings were somewhat more sensitive and just as specific Several lab tests had reasonably high sensitivity and specificity
Sellors et al. [24]	95 subjects	Sample of pre-menopausal women referred from family physician offices and ED for laparoscopy	Prospective cohort of referrals to three gynecologists	PID confirmed by laparoscopy and histopathology	Divorced: RR = 2.3 (95% CI: 1.82 to 2.92) Days of pain: 14.8 (+PID) vs 26.5 (−PID) (P = 0.007) Gravida >3 births: RR = 2.06 (95% CI: 1.44 to 2.94) History of abortion: RR = 1.66 (95% CI: 1.1 to 2.49) Current IUD use: RR = 2.06 (95% CI: 1.44 to 2.94) Lower abdominal guarding: RR = 1.79 (95% CI: 1.12 to 2.84) ESR (mm/h): 21.2 (+PID) vs 12.8 (−PID) (P = 0.006) CRP (mg/L): 59.4 (+PID) vs 20.1 (−PID) (P < 0.001)	In the study no cut-offs were used to assess days of pain, ESR or CRP
Morcos et al. [27]	176 subjects	Women included if admitted for diagnostic laparoscopy Single hospital Tested 21 clinical indicators using logistic regression	Retrospective chart review from 1983 to 1990	PID confirmed by laparoscopy	Logistic model I: (i) Adnexal tenderness (ii) Lower abdominal pain of < 1 week's duration (iii) Elevated serum WBC counts If all present: Sensitivity = 87% Specificity = 46% PPV = 84% NPV = 52% Logistic model II: (i) Cervical motion tenderness (ii) Adnexal tenderness (iii) Lower abdominal tenderness If all present: Sensitivity = 82% Specificity = 29% PPV = 78% NPV = 33%	
Miettinen et al. [28]	72 subjects	ESR and CRP were measured at admission	Prospective cohort at a single university center	PID confirmed by laparoscopy and endometrial histopathology	ESR ≥ 40 mm/h: OR = 17.1 (95% CI: 4.35 to 67.6) CRP ≥ 60 mg/L: OR = 6.66 (95% CI: 1.72 to 25.7) ESR ≥ 40 mm/h *and* CRP ≥ 60 mg/L: Sensitivity = 97% Specificity = 61% NPV = 96% PPV = 70%	

(Continued)

Table 41.2 (*Continued*)

Study	Sample size	Setting	Design	Outcome measure	Effect measure	Comments
Bevan et al. [25]	147 studies	Consecutive women with clinical signs of acute salpingitis in an inner city teaching hospital	Prospective longitudinal cohort	PID confirmed by laparoscopy	Never pregnant: RR = 0.78 (95% CI: 0.63 to 0.97) Urinary symptoms: RR = 1.36 (95% CI: 1.11 to 1.66) Mucopurulent vaginal discharge: RR = 2.2 (95% CI: 1.5 to 3.2) ESR >15 mm/h: RR = 1.38 (95% CI: 1.14 to 1.66) ESR elevated: RR = 2.98 (95% CI: 1.3 to 6.96)	Women with moderate or severe disease were more likely to have an ESR > 15 mm/h than women with mild disease RR = 2.49 (95% CI: 1.4 to 4.4)
Peipert et al. [29]	120 studies	Women aged 18–45 with either CDC PID criteria or other signs of upper genital tract infection such as atypical pelvic pain or cervicitis	Prospective cohort from 1993 to 1995	PID confirmed by positive histology or positive cultures from either endometrial biopsy and/or laparoscopy	Serum WBC counts >10,000/mm³: Sensitivity = 57% Specificity = 88% OR = 9.97 (95% CI: 3.72 to 29.03) Vaginal WBC counts >3 WBCs/hpf: Sensitivity = 78% Specificity = 39% OR 2.23 (95%CI 0.83-0.654) ESR > 15 mm/h: Sensitivity = 70% Specificity = 52% OR = 2.51 (95% CI: 1.05 to 6.28) CRP >5 mg/dl: Sensitivity = 71% Specificity = 66% OR = 4.56 (95% CI: 1.87 to 11.72)	If any one criterion present: Sensitivity = 100% Specificity = 18% If all present: Sensitivity = 29% Specificity = 95% Vaginal WBC count most sensitive and serum WBC count most specific. Not one test was pathognomonic
Cibula et al. [30]	141 studies	Consecutively hospitalized patients with at least one prior episode of PID	Prospective cohort from 1995 to 1999	PID confirmed by laparoscopy	Temperature ≥ 37.2°C: PPV = 86% NPV = 19% Serum WBC counts > 10,000/μl: PPV = 95% NPV = 15% ESR > 15 mm/h: PPV = 63% NPV = 59% CRP > 5 mg/dl: PPV = 92% NPV = 29%	Assessed clinical accuracy in recurrent PID If any one of the following is present: (i) Temperature ≥ 37.2°C (ii) Serum WBC counts > 10,000/μl (iii) ESR > 15 mm/h (iv) CRP > 5 mg/dl then: PPV = 54% NPV = 78%

including wall thickness >5 mm, the cog-wheel sign, incomplete septa and the presence of cul de sac fluid, discriminated women with acute PID from the control women with hydrosalpinx. Power Doppler TVS revealed hyperemia in all women with acute PID, but in only two women with hydrosalpinx ($P = 0.01$). Power Doppler TVS was 100% sensitive and 80% specific in the diagnosis of PID (overall accuracy 93%) [36].

Computerized tomography

Although ultrasound is the primary imaging modality of choice in the radiological evaluation of the female patient with acute

pelvic pain, the role of CT in the evaluation of abdominal and pelvic pain continues to expand as many other diseases that cause acute pelvic pain (e.g., uterine disorders, ovarian disorders, endometriosis, appendicitis, post-operative or post-partum complications) often demonstrate characteristic CT findings [37].

Remarkably, although the ultrasound findings in PID are well documented, there have been relatively few studies regarding the CT appearance of this prevalent disease [38]. A MEDLINE search retrieved no studies that compared CT features of PID to laparosopy. In non-complicated acute salpingitis, CT findings are

Table 41.2 (*Continued*)

Study	Sample size	Setting	Design	Outcome measure	Effect measure	Comments
Simms et al. [14]	623 studies	Women with lower abdominal pain with suspected first episode of PID based on clinical criteria	Retrospective database analysis at Lund University from 1960 to 1969	PID confirmed by laparoscopy	Vaginal discharge: Sensitivity = 74% Specificity = 24% LR 0.98 Fever: Sensitivity = 47% Specificity = 64% LR = 1.30 Vomiting: Sensitivity = 14% Specificity = 88% LR = 1.11 Menstrual irregularity: Sensitivity = 45% Specificity = 57% LR = 1.04 Ongoing bleeding: Sensitivity = 25% Specificity = 77% LR = 1.12 Urinary symptoms: Sensitivity = 35% Specificity = 64% LR = 0.98 Proctitis symptoms: Sensitivity = 10% Specificity = 92% LR = 1.31 Pelvic organ tenderness on bimanual exam: Sensitivity = 99% Specificity = 0.01% LR = 1.00 Adnexal swelling/mass: Sensitivity = 52% Specificity = 70% LR = 1.73 ESR $\geq$ 15 mm/h: Sensitivity = 81% Specificity = 33% LR = 1.2	Forward stepwise discriminant analysis yielded three predictors. If all three of the following are present: (i) ESR (ii) Fever (iii) Adnexal tenderness then: Sensitivity = 65% Specificity = 66% PPV = 87% NPV = 33% LR = 1.3(95% CI: 1.19 to 1.44) Tenderness of pelvic organs on bimanual palpation and ESR very sensitive but non-specific. Proctitis symptoms and vomiting were specific but not sensitive

CDC, Centers for Disease Control and Prevention; CI, confidence interval; CRP, C-reactive protein; ESR, erythrocyte sedimentation rate; hpf, high powered field; IUD, intrauterine device; LR, likelihood ratio; NPV, negative predictive value; OR, odds ratio; PID, pelvic inflammatory disease; PPV, positive predictive value; RR, relative risk; WBC, white blood cell.

most often normal or demonstrate a small amount of fluid in the cul de sac. With progression to tubo-ovarian abscess, CT findings include bilateral, thick-walled, low-attenuation adnexal masses with thick septations and often with an associated serpiginous structure corresponding to a dilated, pus-filled Fallopian tube [37].

Magnetic resonance imaging

In 1999 Tukeva et al. assessed the value of MRI in the diagnosis of pelvic PID and compared MRI with TVS and laparoscopy [39]. Thirty consecutive patients hospitalized due to clinical suspicion of PID underwent TVS in the ED, done by the gynecologist, and MRI followed by laparoscopy. PID was laparoscopically proven in

21 (70%) patients. The MRI diagnosis agreed with laparoscopy in 20 (95%) of the 21 patients with PID, whereas findings at TVS agreed with those at laparoscopy in 17 (81%) of the 21 patients with PID. The sensitivity of MRI in the diagnosis of PID was 95%, the specificity was 89%, and the overall accuracy was 93%. For TVS, the corresponding values were 81%, 78% and 80%, respectively [39]. It appears that MRI demonstrated a higher sensitivity and specificity than TVS and may be an important diagnostic tool if validated in future prospective studies.

Leukocyte scintigraphy

Leukocyte scintigraphy is a non-invasive, safe and physiological procedure for the diagnosis of PID. The MEDLINE search found two studies that used radionuclide scintigraphy preceded by the injection of 99m-technetium hexamethylpropylenamine oxime-labeled autologous leukocytes to detect PID and tubo-ovarian abscess (TOA). The sample sizes were small and the patients selected had very severe disease. The results were promising; however, the results likely suffer from selection bias and need to be confirmed in larger samples.

In a prospective study, Mozas and colleagues assessed the performance of pelvic leukocyte scintigraphy for the diagnosis of PID [40]. The results of radionuclide scintigraphy in 20 women with PID confirmed laparoscopically were compared with the findings in 20 others hospitalized for suspected PID but with PID ruled out later by laparoscopy. The proportion of radionuclide scintigraphic findings demonstrating increased uptake in the genital region, compatible with an inflammatory process, was significantly larger ($P < 0.001$) in patients with PID (95%) than in those without PID (15%). The sensitivity of the technique was 95% and specificity was 85%; in all, 90% of the patients were correctly classified [40].

Similarly, Rachinsky et al. assessed 20 women undergoing confirmatory laparoscopy with suspected TOA using leukocyte scintigraphy [41]. The sensitivity of leukocyte scintigraphy in detecting TOA was 100%, specificity was 91.6%, the positive predictive value was 89% and the overall accuracy was 95%. Leukocyte scintigraphy is a non-invasive, safe, physiological and accurate procedure for the diagnosis of TOA. The 24-hour scan is crucial, since in some cases the abscess was not clearly visualized on the early scan. Leukocyte scintigraphy may reduce the need for CT, diagnostic laparoscopy and unnecessary invasive surgical procedures [41].

Moreover, Uslu et al. evaluated leukocyte scintigraphy in the early diagnosis of women with PID of child-bearing age [42]. Fifteen women with suspicion of pyogenic PID based on gynecological examinations, clinical findings and blood tests were included in this study. Ten of the patients were then evaluated by abdominal or transvaginal ultrasound, four by CT, and two by both ultrasound and CT. The final diagnosis was made by surgical intervention. Scintigraphy had a sensitivity of 100%, specificity of 90%, overall accuracy of 93%, positive predictive value of 83% and negative predictive value of 100% [42].

Summary

In summary, ultrasound remains the mainstay of the diagnosis and evaluation of PID. Ultrasound offers ready availability, low cost and lack of ionizing radiation but it requires technical expertise to reach its full diagnostic potential. MRI has the potential to demonstrate inflammatory changes in the pelvis (perhaps more than ultrasound) and does not emit ionizing radiation; however, it is still an expensive and a not always available diagnostic tool with some contraindications for use. While CT and leukocyte scintigraphy show promise as diagnostic alternatives, they result in greater radiation exposure, provide minimally higher sensitivities and are more costly.

Question 4: In female patients with lower abdominal pain (population), what clinical and laboratory factors (diagnostic tests) have diagnostic or discriminatory utility (diagnostic test characteristics) in distinguishing between appendicitis and pelvic inflammatory disease compared to laparoscopy (reference standard)?

Search strategy

- MEDLINE: (PID OR pelvic inflammatory disease) AND appendicitis AND (sensitivity and specificity [MeSH] OR likelihood ratio [MeSH])

The MEDLINE search retrieved three studies that compared diagnostic factors that have discriminatory utility in distinguishing PID from appendicitis. In 1985 Bongard et al. prospectively assessed 118 women of childbearing age who were admitted with a diagnosis of appendicitis versus PID over a 1 year period [43]. Appendicitis was determined by histopathology of the removed appendix in 36 (30.5%) and PID was diagnosed either via laparoscopy or by clinical improvement after antibiotics in 45 (38.1%), and other diagnoses were given in 37 (31.7%) patients. The criteria found to favor PID over appendicitis included: (i) longer duration of symptoms for PID (32 vs 65 hours); (ii) less nausea and/or vomiting for PID compared to appendicitis; (iii) previous history of STD; (iv) cervical motion tenderness; (v) adnexal tenderness; and (vi) diffuse lower abdominal tenderness rather than isolated peritoneal signs in the right lower quadrant (which occurred more frequently in appendicitis) [43]. The study is limited by its sampling bias, as it only included patients who were admitted, by the fact that PID was determined by laparoscopy and clinical grounds, and by the lack of multivariate data analyses.

In 1993 Webster et al. retrospectively evaluated the usefulness of various historical, clinical and laboratory findings in differentiating acute appendicitis from PID in women of childbearing age over a 2-year period [44]. The records were reviewed of all female patients presenting to the ED with abdominal pain who were found to have histologically proven appendicitis ($n = 80$) or PID confirmed by Centers for Disease Control and Prevention Criteria (clinical

Table 41.3 Summary of evidence table of predictors of pelvic inflammatory disease versus appendicitis in women of childbearing years.

Study	Statistical analysis	N	P vs R	Predictors	Outcome
Morishita et al. [10]	Multivariate	181	R	• No migration of pain • Bilateral abdominal tenderness • Absence of nausea and vomiting	Clinical diagnosis or imaging or laparoscopy
Webster et al. [44]	Univariate	151	R	• History of vaginal discharge • Urinary symptoms • Prior PID • Tenderness outside the right lower quadrant • Cervical motion tenderness • Vaginal discharge on pelvic examination • Positive urinalysis	Endocervical culture or imaging or clinical diagnosis or laparoscopy
Bongard et al. [43]	Univariate	118	P	• Longer duration of symptoms • Lack of nausea and/or vomiting • History of STD • Cervical motion tenderness • Adnexal tenderness • Diffuse lower abdominal tenderness instead of isolated right lower quadrant	Clinical diagnosis or laparoscopy

P, prospective; PID, pelvic inflammatory disease; R, retrospective; STD, sexually transmitted disease.

criteria with endocervical culture and/or laparoscopy ($n = 71$). Clinically useful indicators favoring appendicitis included the presence of anorexia and the onset of pain later than day 14 of the menstrual cycle. Indicators favoring PID included: (i) a history of vaginal discharge; (ii) urinary symptoms; (iii) prior PID; (iv) tenderness outside the right lower quadrant; (v) cervical motion tenderness; (vi) vaginal discharge on pelvic examination; and (vii) positive urinalysis [44]. This study is limited by its retrospective nature, lack of validation and lack of gold standard for determining PID.

In 2007, Morishita's study derived (but did not validate) a clinical decision rule for predicting PID by reviewing the medical records of female patients of childbearing age presenting with abdominal pain at an ED over 4 years who had a final diagnosis of either appendicitis ($n = 109$) or PID ($n = 72$) [10]. The diagnosis of appendicitis was based on histopathology and the diagnosis of PID was based on a clinical diagnosis or imaging or laparoscopy. Predictors of PID were derived using recursive partitioning and included: no migration of pain (OR = 4.2; 95% CI: 1.5 to 11.5), bilateral abdominal tenderness (OR = 16.7; 95% CI: 5.3 to 50.0) and absence of nausea and vomiting (OR = 8.4; 95% CI: 2.8 to 24.8). These factors were able to distinguish appendicitis from PID with a sensitivity of 99% (95% CI: 94% to 100%). The study is limited by its retrospective nature, lack of validation and lack of gold standard for determining PID.

Table 41.3 summarizes the variables from each study that were found to distinguish PID from appendicitis. These criteria are limited by the study designs and lack of gold standard for determining PID.

Question 5: In women diagnosed with acute pelvic inflammatory disease (patients), which antibiotics (intervention, comparison) result in the highest clinical and microbiological cure rate (outcome)?

Search strategy

• MEDLINE and Cochrane: (PID OR pelvic inflammatory disease) AND antibiotics

Antibiotics remain the mainstay of initial treatment in patients diagnosed with PID. The antibiotic choice has been repeatedly debated as the microbiology of PID has been clarified. Although *Neisseria gonorrhea* and *Chlamydia trachomatis* remain prevalent, clinical trials have demonstrated Gram-negative and anaerobic etiologies in as many as 40% of cases [45]. Other pathogenic bacteria implicated include *Mycoplasma*, streptococci species and coagulase-negative staphylococci [46]. Therefore, PID may best be thought of as a poly-microbial infection, suggesting the need for broad-spectrum antibiotics.

A Cochrane database search failed to reveal a systematic review of therapy for PID. A number of controlled trials of antibiotics were found in the Cochrane Central Register of Controlled Trials (CENTRAL). A meta-analysis published in 1993 critically appraised 21 treatment studies representing a variety of antimicrobial regimens [22]. Quantitative analyses of short-term outcomes, resolution of symptoms (clinical) and eradication of bacteria (microbiological) were performed (Figs 41.1, 41.2). Overall,

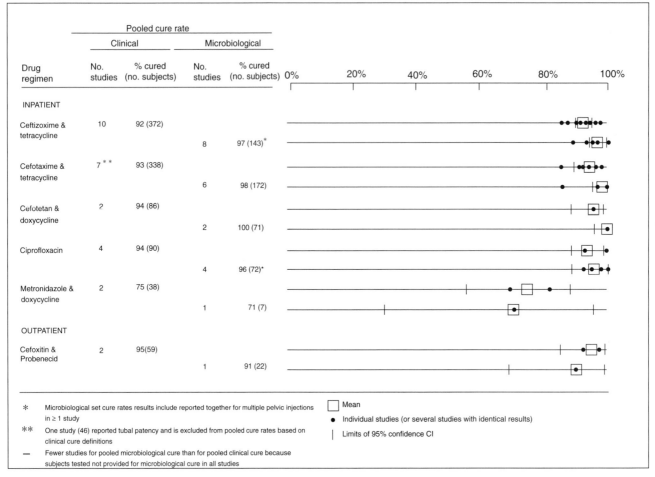

Figure 41.1 Pooled cure rates for antibiotics with more than one study included in the meta-analysis. (Reprinted with permission from Walker et al. [22].)

clinical cure ranged from 75% (metronidazole + doxycycline) to 95% (cefoxitin + probenocid + doxycycline); microbiological cure ranged from 71% (metronidazole + doxycycline) to 100% (multiple regimens).

Subsequent to this meta-analysis, there have been five published randomized controlled trials evaluating different antibiotics in acute PID. All studies were prospective, randomized, comparator trials; four involved outpatients and one was restricted to inpatients [13,47–50]. These trials reported excellent clinical efficacy with cure rates between 72% and 100%. Moreover, the antibiotic regimens, where reported, proved to be microbiologically efficacious (Table 41.4).

The best available clinical evidence does not appear to support the current CDC recommendations for providing anaerobic coverage, as high clinical cure rates have been demonstrated with regimens lacking intrinsic anaerobic activity [13,48]. No trials have demonstrated the superiority of courses of therapy that have anaerobic coverage. Expert consensus remains, however, in support of broad-spectrum coverage, including anaerobes – which are believed to potentially cause sub-clinical salpingitis, which may result in continual damage with long-term sequelae [13,22,46].

The CDC no longer recommends fluoroquinolones for the treatment of gonococcal infections in any group of patients, strengthening previous guidance against use in high-risk groups [51]. A parenteral, third-generation cephalosporin is now considered the treatment of choice. This guideline change is based on surveillance data from 2005 and 2006 showing an increase in fluoroquinolone-resistant *Neisseria gonorrhea* (QRNG) to 7% in heterosexual populations and 38% in groups of men who have sex with men [51]. Importantly, the published clinical trials do not comment on the number of QRNG isolates. Most of these trials were completed before the emergence of QRNG and it is possible subsequent studies will see an increasing prevalence.

In summary, emergency physicians have many antibiotic choices for treatment of patients with acute PID and must keep in mind the diverse etiology. A third-generation cephalosporin should always be used for treatment of *Neisseria gonorrhea*. *Chlamydia trachomatis* must always be treated with azithromycin, doxycycline or quinolones. These antibiotics have the added benefit of covering the other aerobic bacteria implicated in PID pathogenesis. Anaerobic flora may play some part in PID, yet studies do not show a clear benefit to their treatment, thus the decision to provide coverage is left at the discretion of the treating physician. When desired,

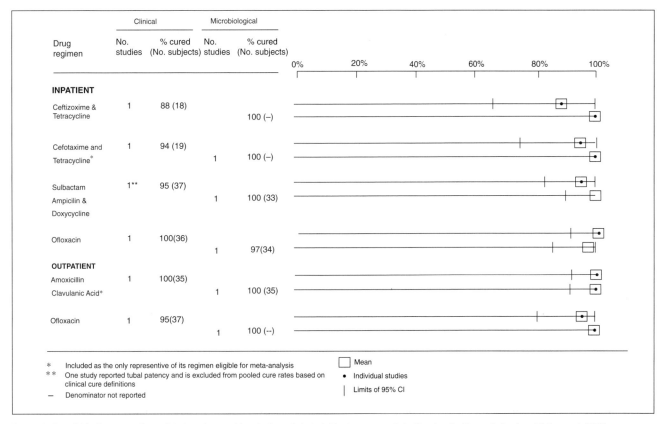

Drug regimen	Clinical		Microbiological		
	No. studies	% cured (No. subjects)	No. studies	% cured (No. subjects)	
INPATIENT					
Ceftizoxime & Tetracycline	1	88 (18)		100 (−)	
Cefotaxime and Tetracycline*	1	94 (19)	1	100 (−)	
Sulbactam Ampicilin & Doxycycline	1**	95 (37)	1	100 (33)	
Ofloxacin	1	100(36)	1	97(34)	
OUTPATIENT					
Amoxicillin Clavulanic Acid*	1	100(35)	1	100 (35)	
Ofloxacin	1	95(37)	1	100 (--)	

* Included as the only representive of its regimen eligible for meta-analysis
** One study reported tubal patency and is excluded from pooled cure rates based on clinical cure definitions
— Denominator not reported

☐ Mean
● Individual studies
| Limits of 95% CI

Figure 41.2 Individual cure rates for antibiotic regimens with a single study included in the meta-analysis. (Reprinted with permission from Walker et al. [22].)

flagyl and moxifloxacin have demonstrated efficacy in anaerobic infections.

Question 6: In women diagnosed with acute pelvic inflammatory disease (patients), does hospitalization (intervention) reduce long-term sequelae (e.g., infertility, chronic pelvic pain) (outcome) compared to outpatient management (comparison)?

Search strategy

- MEDLINE and Cochrane: (PID OR pelvic inflammatory disease) AND prognosis [MeSH]

In the ED, treatment of acute PID consists of antibiotics and analgesia to provide immediate symptomatic relief and a short-term clinical cure. However, there are long-term consequences from acute pelvic infections that should be considered with all patients. Cohort studies provide evidence of the sequelae of PID. A 24-year prospective cohort study from Sweden [52] showed that severity and recurrence of PID were associated with lower birth rates. Patients with severe, recurrent PID were eight times as likely to fail to achieve a live birth compared to single episodes of mild disease (RR = 8.1; 95% CI: 3.0 to 22.2). Another retrospective cohort study of 1355 women with acute PID showed an increase in chronic abdominal pain (RR = 4.75; 95% CI: 3.22 to 7.02) and ectopic pregnancy (RR = 11.88; 95% CI: 5.97 to 23.64) compared to the control population [53].

Although antibiotics are the mainstay of therapy in acute PID, there is controversy over the best route of administration. The efficacy of both parenteral and oral regimens have been examined in many randomized trials [22]. Although most trials have used parenteral treatment for at least 48 hours after the patient demonstrates substantial clinical improvement, this time designation is arbitrary [6].

The MEDLINE search above failed to reveal any prospectively studied clinical decision rules addressing route of antibiotic administration. A search of CENTRAL under the heading pelvic inflammatory disease identified 23 articles, only one of which studied long-term outcomes. In a randomized trial of 831 women diagnosed with PID, an initial 3-day hospitalization with parental antibiotics (cefoxitin + doxycycline) followed by outpatient therapy (doxycycline for 14 days in total) was compared to outpatient antibiotic therapy alone (cefoxitin IM for 1 day, then doxycycline for 14 days) [54]. Subjects were followed for a mean of 84 months and no differences were identified in the rates of pregnancy, live births and chronic pelvic pain. Ectopic pregnancies were observed more often in the outpatient group (five vs one); however, the overall incidence was low and this difference was not statistically significant.

Table 41.4 Summary of evidence table of antibiotic regimens and clinical and microbiological efficacy.

Study	Sample size	Design	Antibiotic (sample size per group)	Cure rate	
				Clinical	Microbiological
Outpatient					
Ross et al. [47]	564	RCT	Moxifloxacin ($n = 275$)	90%	88%
			vs		
			Ofloxacin + flagyl ($n = 289$)	90%	82%
Savaris et al. [48]	133	RCT	Ceftriaxone + azithromycin ($n = 62$)	90%	NR
			vs		
			Ceftriaxone + doxycycline ($n = 58$)	72%	NR
Martens et al. [13]	295	RCT	Ofloxacin ($n = 128$)	95%	NR
			vs		
			Cefoxitin + doxycycline ($n = 121$)	93%	NR
Arredondo et al. [49]	138	RCT	Clindamycin + ciprofloxacin ($n = 67$)	97%	NR
			vs		
			Ceftriaxone + doxycycline ($n = 64$)	95%	NR
Inpatient					
Hemsell et al. [50]	84	RCT	Meropenem ($n = 44$)	93%	96%
			vs		
			Clindamycin + gentamycin ($n = 40$)	100%	100%

NR, not reported; RCT, randomized controlled trial.

In summary, the evidence to answer this question is not robust. The single, relatively large randomized trial identified was well designed and enrolled the most common type of PID patient encountered by emergency physicians. The result suggests that hospitalization offers little or no benefit over outpatient antibiotic therapy with respect to long-term outcomes, although conclusions about ectopic pregnancy rates suffer from the study's lack of power to detect an important difference in this outcome. Unless patients with PID are toxic or unable to tolerate oral agents, they may be treated as outpatients.

Conclusions

Returning to the patient above, CT was an important test in order to rule out appendicitis, because of the location of the pain and tenderness. An ultrasound was ordered in this patient and demonstrated fluid in the cul de sac and endometritis. Due to the nature of the pain, the patient was administered ceftriaxone, azithromycin and metronidazole. She made an uneventful recovery, her partner was also treated, and she went on to have a live birth 1 year later.

Women with abdominal pain commonly present to the ED and the differential diagnosis is extensive. Emergency physicians need to obtain a thorough history searching for clues of PID, including: previous PID/STD, sexual contacts, duration of lower abdominal pain, irregular menses, urinary and proctitis symptoms, dyspareunia and fever. In addition, physicians need to conduct a thorough physical search for PID including abdominal and/or adnexal tenderness. Serum white blood cells, erythrocyte sedimentation rate and C-reactive protein may be used as diagnostic adjuncts in difficult cases. Radiological investigations should start with pelvic ultrasound, and treatment should follow accepted guidelines to cover the usual microbiological culprits. Most patients do not need to be hospitalized for treatment unless they appear toxic, have severe pain requiring intravenous analgesics or are vomiting; outcomes seem to be reasonable if the disease is diagnosed early.

References

1 Gray-Swain MR, Peipert JF. Pelvic inflammatory disease in adolescents. *Curr Opin Obstet Gynecol* 2006;**18**(5):503–10.

2 Hagen-Ansert SL. *Textbook of Diagnostic Ultrasonography*, 6th edn. Mosby Elsevier, St. Louis, 2006.

3 Yeh JM, Hook EW, III, Goldie SJ. A refined estimate of the average lifetime cost of pelvic inflammatory disease. *Sex Transm Dis* 2003;**30**(5):369–78.

4 Washington AE, Katz P. Cost of and payment source for pelvic inflammatory disease. Trends and projections, 1983 through 2000. *JAMA* 1991;**266**(18):2565–9.

5 Rein DB, Kassler WJ, Irwin KL, Rabiee L. Direct medical cost of pelvic inflammatory disease and its sequelae: decreasing, but still substantial. *Obstet Gynecol* 2000;**95**(3):397–402.

6 Centers for Disease Control and Prevention. Sexually transmitted diseases treatment guidelines 2002. *MMWR Recomm Rep* 2002;**51**(RR6):1–78.

7 Paavonen J. Immunopathogenesis of pelvic inflammatory disease and infertility – what do we know and what shall we do? *J Br Fertil Soc* 1996;**1**(1):42–5.

8 Wiesenfeld HC, Sweet RL, Ness RB, Krohn MA, Amortegui AJ, Hillier SL. Comparison of acute and subclinical pelvic inflammatory disease. *Sex Transm Dis* 2005;**32**(7):400–405.

9 Brandt AL, Tolson D. Missed abdominal ectopic pregnancy. *J Emerg Med* 2006;**30**(2):171–4.

10 Morishita K, Gushimiyagi M, Hashiguchi M, Stein GH, Tokuda Y. Clinical prediction rule to distinguish pelvic inflammatory disease from acute appendicitis in women of childbearing age. *Am J Emerg Med* 2007;**25**(2):152–7.

11 Ignacio EA, Hill MC. Ultrasound of the acute female pelvis. *Ultrasound Q* 2003;**19**(2):86–98; quiz: 108–110.

12 Ness RB, Smith KJ, Chang CC, Schisterman EF, Bass DC. Prediction of pelvic inflammatory disease among young, single, sexually active women. *Sex Transm Dis* 2006;**33**(3):137–42.

13 Martens MG, Gordon S, Yarborough DR, Faro S, Binder D, Berkeley A. Multicenter randomized trial of ofloxacin versus cefoxitin and doxycycline in outpatient treatment of pelvic inflammatory disease. Ambulatory PID Research Group. *South Med J* 1993;**86**(6):604–10.

14 Simms I, Warburton F, Westrom L. Diagnosis of pelvic inflammatory disease: time for a rethink. *Sex Transm Infect* 2003;**79**(6):491–4.

15 Jacobson L, Westrom L. Objectivized diagnosis of acute pelvic inflammatory disease. Diagnostic and prognostic value of routine laparoscopy. *Am J Obstet Gynecol* 1969;**105**(7):1088–98.

16 Ross J. Pelvic inflammatory disease. *Clin Evid* 2002;**8**:1649–54.

17 Paavonen J, Aine R, Teisala K, Heinonen PK, Punnonen R. Comparison of endometrial biopsy and peritoneal fluid cytologic testing with laparoscopy in the diagnosis of acute pelvic inflammatory disease. *Am J Obstet Gynecol* 1985;**151**(5):645–50.

18 Molander P, Finne P, Sjoberg J, Sellors J, Paavonen J. Observer agreement with laparoscopic diagnosis of pelvic inflammatory disease using photographs. *Obstet Gynecol* 2003;**101**(5 Part 1):875–80.

19 Patel DR. Management of pelvic inflammatory disease in adolescents. *Indian J Pediatr* 2004;**71**(9):845–7.

20 Henry-Suchet J, Catalan F, Loffredo V, et al. Microbiology of specimens obtained by laparoscopy from controls and from patients with pelvic inflammatory disease or infertility with tubal obstruction: *Chlamydia trachomatis* and *Ureaplasma urealyticum*. *Am J Obstet Gynecol* 1980;**138**(7 Part 2):1022–5.

21 Ness RB, Soper DE, Peipert J, et al. Design of the PID Evaluation and Clinical Health (PEACH) study. *Control Clin Trials* 1998;**19**(5):499–514.

22 Walker CK, Kahn JG, Washington AE, Peterson HB, Sweet RL. Pelvic inflammatory disease: metaanalysis of antimicrobial regimen efficacy. *J Infect Dis* 1993;**168**(4):969–78.

23 Wolner-Hanssen P. Pelvic inflammatory disease. *Curr Opin Obstet Gynecol* 1991;**3**(5):687–91.

24 Sellors J, Mahony J, Goldsmith C, et al. The accuracy of clinical findings and laparoscopy in pelvic inflammatory disease. *Am J Obstet Gynecol* 1991;**164**(1 Part 1):113–20.

25 Bevan CD, Johal BJ, Mumtaz G, Ridgway GL, Siddle NC. Clinical, laparoscopic and microbiological findings in acute salpingitis: report on a United Kingdom cohort. *Br J Obstet Gynaecol* 1995;**102**(5):407–14.

26 Kahn JG, Walker CK, Washington AE, Landers DV, Sweet RL. Diagnosing pelvic inflammatory disease. A comprehensive analysis and considerations for developing a new model. *JAMA* 1991;**266**(18):2594–604.

27 Morcos R, Frost N, Hnat M, Petrunak A, Caldito G. Laparoscopic versus clinical diagnosis of acute pelvic inflammatory disease. *J Reprod Med* 1993;**38**(1):53–6.

28 Miettinen AK, Heinonen PK, Laippala P, Paavonen J. Test performance of erythrocyte sedimentation rate and C-reactive protein in assessing the severity of acute pelvic inflammatory disease. *Am J Obstet Gynecol* 1993;**169**(5):1143–9.

29 Peipert JF, Boardman L, Hogan JW, Sung J, Mayer KH. Laboratory evaluation of acute upper genital tract infection. *Obstet Gynecol* 1996;**87**(5 Part 1):730–36.

30 Cibula D, Kuzel D, Fucikova Z, Svabik K, Zivny J. Acute exacerbation of recurrent pelvic inflammatory disease. Laparoscopic findings in 141 women with a clinical diagnosis. *J Reprod Med* 2001;**46**(1):49–53.

31 Kupesic S, Kurjak A, Pasalic L, Benic S, Ilijas M. The value of transvaginal color Doppler in the assessment of pelvic inflammatory disease. *Ultrasound Med Biol* 1995;**21**(6):733–8.

32 Taipale P, Tarjanne H, Ylostalo P. Transvaginal sonography in suspected pelvic inflammatory disease. *Ultrasound Obstet Gynecol* 1995;**6**(6):430–34.

33 Mikkelsen AL, Felding C. Laparoscopy and ultrasound examination in women with acute pelvic pain. *Gynecol Obstet Invest* 1990;**30**(3):162–4.

34 Patten RM, Vincent LM, Wolner-Hanssen P, Thorpe E, Jr. Pelvic inflammatory disease. Endovaginal sonography with laparoscopic correlation. *J Ultrasound Med* 1990;**9**(12):681–9.

35 Papadimitriou A, Kalogirou D, Antoniou G, Petridis N, Kalogirou O, Kalovidouris A. Power Doppler ultrasound: a potentially useful alternative in diagnosing pelvic pathologic conditions. *Clin Exp Obstet Gynecol* 1996;**23**(4):229–32.

36 Molander P, Sjoberg J, Paavonen J, Cacciatore B. Transvaginal power Doppler findings in laparoscopically proven acute pelvic inflammatory disease. *Ultrasound Obstet Gynecol* 2001;**17**(3):233–8.

37 Bennett GL, Slywotzky CM, Giovanniello G. Gynecologic causes of acute pelvic pain: spectrum of CT findings. *Radiographics* 2002;**22**(4):785–801.

38 Sam JW, Jacobs JE, Birnbaum BA. Spectrum of CT findings in acute pyogenic pelvic inflammatory disease. *Radiographics* 2002;**22**(6):1327–34.

39 Tukeva TA, Aronen HJ, Karjalainen PT, Molander P, Paavonen T, Paavonen J. MR imaging in pelvic inflammatory disease: comparison with laparoscopy and US. *Radiology* 1999;**210**(1):209–16.

40 Mozas J, Castilla JA, Alarcon JL, Ruiz J, Jimena P, Herruzo AJ. Diagnosis of pelvic inflammatory disease with 99mtechnetium-hexamethylpropylenamine-oxime-labeled autologous leukocytes and pelvic radionuclide scintigraphy. *Obstet Gynecol* 1993;**81**(5 Part 1):797–9.

41 Rachinsky I, Boguslavsky L, Goldstein D, et al. Diagnosis of pyogenic pelvic inflammatory diseases by 99mTc-HMPAO leucocyte scintigraphy. *Eur J Nucl Med* 2000;**27**(12):1774–7.

42 Uslu H, Varoglu E, Kadanali S, Yildirim M, Bayrakdar R, Kadanali A. 99mTc-HMPAO labelled leucocyte scintigraphy in the diagnosis of pelvic inflammatory disease. *Nucl Med Commun* 2006;**27**(2):179–83.

43 Bongard F, Landers DV, Lewis F. Differential diagnosis of appendicitis and pelvic inflammatory disease. A prospective analysis. *Am J Surg* 1985;**150**(1):90–96.

44 Webster DP, Schneider CN, Cheche S, Daar AA, Miller G. Differentiating acute appendicitis from pelvic inflammatory disease in women of childbearing age. *Am J Emerg Med* 1993;**11**(6):569–72.

45 Peipert JF, Sweet RL, Walker CK, Kahn J, Rielly-Gauvin K. Evaluation of ofloxacin in the treatment of laparoscopically documented acute pelvic inflammatory disease (salpingitis). *Infect Dis Obstet Gynecol* 1999;**7**(3):138–44.

46 Walker CK, Workowski KA, Washington AE, Soper D, Sweet RL. Anaerobes in pelvic inflammatory disease: implications for the Centers for

Disease Control and Prevention's guidelines for treatment of sexually transmitted diseases. *Clin Infect Dis* 1999;**28**(Suppl 1):S29–36.

47 Ross JD, Cronje HS, Paszkowski T, et al. Moxifloxacin versus ofloxacin plus metronidazole in uncomplicated pelvic inflammatory disease: results of a multicentre, double blind, randomised trial. *Sex Transm Infect* 2006;**82**(6):446–51.

48 Savaris RF, Teixeira LM, Torres TG, Edelweiss MI, Moncada J, Schachter J. Comparing ceftriaxone plus azithromycin or doxycycline for pelvic inflammatory disease: a randomized controlled trial. *Obstet Gynecol* 2007;**110**(1):53–60.

49 Arredondo JL, Diaz V, Gaitan H, et al. Oral clindamycin and ciprofloxacin versus intramuscular ceftriaxone and oral doxycycline in the treatment of mild-to-moderate pelvic inflammatory disease in outpatients. *Clin Infect Dis* 1997;**24**(2):170–78.

50 Hemsell DL, Martens MG, Faro S, Gall S, McGregor JA. A multicenter study comparing intravenous meropenem with clindamycin plus gentamicin for the treatment of acute gynecologic and obstetric pelvic infections in hospitalized women. *Clin Infect Dis* 1997;**24**(Suppl 2):S222–30.

51 Anon. Update to CDC's sexually transmitted diseases treatment guidelines, 2006. Fluoroquinolones no longer recommended for treatment of gonococcal infections. *MMWR* 2007;**56**(14):332–6.

52 Lepine LA, Hillis SD, Marchbanks PA, Joesoef MR, Peterson HB, Westrom L. Severity of pelvic inflammatory disease as a predictor of the probability of live birth. *Am J Obstet Gynecol* 1998;**178**(5):977–81.

53 Buchan H, Vessey M, Goldacre M, Fairweather J. Morbidity following pelvic inflammatory disease. *Br J Obstet Gynaecol* 1993;**100**(6):558–62.

54 Ness RB, Trautmann G, Richter HE, et al. Effectiveness of treatment strategies of some women with pelvic inflammatory disease: a randomized trial. *Obstet Gynecol* 2005;**106**(3):573–80.

55 Wolner-Hanssen P, Mardh PA, Svensson L, Westrom L. Laparoscopy in women with chlamydial infection and pelvic pain: a comparison of patients with and without salpingitis. *Obstet Gynecol* 1983;**61**(3):299–303.

56 Wasserheit JN, Bell TA, Kiviat NB, Wolner-Hanssen P, Zabriskie V, Kirby BD, Prince EC, Holmes KK, Stamm WE, Eschenbach DA. Microbial causes of proven pelvic inflammatory disease and efficacy of clindamycin and tobramycin. *Ann Intern Med* 1986;**104**(2):187–193.

57 Hadgu A, Westrom L, Brooks CA, Reynolds GH, Thompson SE. Predicting acute pelvic inflammatory disease. a multivariate analysis. *Am J Obstet Gynecol* 1986;**155**(5):954–960.

58 Tavelli BG, Judson FN. Comparison of the clinical and epidemiologic characteristics of gonococcal and nongonococcal pelvic inflammatory disease seen in a clinic for sexually transmitted diseases, 1978–1979. *Sex Transm Dis* 1986;**13**(3):119–122.

59 Wolner-Hanssen P, Svensson L, Mardh PA, Westrom L. Laparoscopic findings and contraceptive use in women with signs and symptoms suggestive of acute salpingitis. *Obstet Gynecol* 1985;**66**(2):233–238.

60 Westrom L. Clinical manifestations and diagnosis of pelvic inflammatory disease. *J Reprod Med* 1983;**28**(10 Suppl):703–708.

61 Lehtinen M, Laine S, Heinonen PK, Teisala K, Miettinen A, Aine R, Punnonen R, Gronroos P, Paavonen J. Serum C-reactive protein determination in acute pelvic inflammatory disease. *Am J Obstet Gynecol* 1986;**154**(1):158–159.

62 Hemila M, Henriksson L, Ylikorkala O. Serum CRP in the diagnosis and treatment of pelvic inflammatory disease. *Arch Gynecol Obstet* 1987;**241**(3):177–182.

63 Jacobson L, Laurell CB, Marholev K. Plasma protein changes induced by acute inflammation of the fallopian tubes. *Int J Gynaecol Obstet* 1975;**13**:249–252.

64 Paavonen J, Aine R, Teisala K, Heinonen PK, Punnonen R. Comparison of endometrial biopsy and peritoneal fluid cytologic testing with laparoscopy in the diagnosis of acute pelvic inflammatory disease. *Am J Obstet Gynecol* 1985;**151**(5):645–650.

42 Pregnancy

Ashley Shreves

Department of Emergency Medicine, St. Luke's–Roosevelt Hospital, New York, USA

Case scenario

A 25-year-old female presented to the emergency department (ED) complaining of a 1-day history of moderate vaginal bleeding. She thought her last menstrual period was 6 weeks ago and reported taking a home pregnancy test the day prior to ED presentation that was negative. On review of systems she reports nausea and vomiting daily for the past 2 weeks that has forced her to miss work and mild lower abdominal cramping for 3 days. She has no significant past medical or surgical history and takes no medications.

The patient's vital signs were normal: temperature 37°C (oral), heart rate 70 beats/min, respiratory rate 16 breaths/min and blood pressure 110/60 mmHg (left arm). Her abdomen was soft and nontender. On pelvic exam, blood clots were noted in the vaginal vault. The cervix was closed, and there were no adnexal tenderness or masses. The remainder of the physical exam was normal.

Point-of-care urine pregnancy testing performed in the ED revealed a positive result. The patient reported she had had several friends whose pregnancies have been missed by those over-the-counter tests. She asked if this bleeding is normal and what the chances are she is having a miscarriage. While in the room discussing these issues, she complained of nausea again and vomited. The nurse asked if you would like to administer anti-emetic medication, but on hearing this, the patient stated that she only wants something if it is absolutely safe for the baby.

Background

Pregnancy-related problems are common reasons for women to visit the ED. Accordingly, it is in the realm of the emergency medicine physician to both diagnose pregnancy and treat its inherent complications, ranging from simple nausea and vomiting to the seizing eclamptic patient. Complicating the issue, the overall prevalence of unrecognized pregnancy in the ED setting has been reported at 6%, so all women of childbearing age must be assumed by the emergency medicine physician to be pregnant and at risk for pregnancy-related complications until proven otherwise [1].

Clinical questions

In order to address the issues of most relevance to your patient and to help in searching the literature for the evidence regarding pregnancy issues, you structure your clinical questions as recommended in Chapter 1.

1 In pregnant patients with first trimester bleeding and a sonographic intrauterine pregnancy (population), what proportion of patients (prognosis) will progress to subsequent fetal loss (outcome)?

2 Following a first missed menstruation (population), what is the sensitivity and specificity (diagnostic test characteristics) of home urine pregnancy tests (tests) for detecting pregnancy (outcome)?

3 In pregnant patients with first trimester bleeding (population), what is the diagnostic accuracy (diagnostic test characteristics) of the history and physical examination for predicting pregnancy loss (outcome)?

4 In pregnant patients discharged from the ED with a diagnosis of a threatened abortion (population), does the use of maternal bed rest (intervention) compared to normal activity (control) decrease the rate of pregnancy loss (outcome) in this population?

5 For eclamptic pregnant patients in the ED setting (population), does intravenous magnesium sulfate reduce recurrent seizures or maternal mortality (outcome) compared to intravenous diazepam and/or phenytoin (control)?

6 For pregnant patients with nausea and vomiting (population), do anti-emetic treatments (intervention) provide safe and effective control of nausea and improve fetal outcomes (outcomes) compared to conservative treatment (control)?

7 In pregnant patients with severe or intractable hyperemesis gravidarum (population), do intravenous corticosteroids

Evidence-based Emergency Medicine. Edited by Brian H. Rowe
© 2009 Blackwell Publishing, ISBN: 978-1-4051-6143-5.

(intervention) improve oral intake and decrease readmission rates (outcomes) compared to anti-emetic administration alone (control)?

8 In pregnant patients with asymptomatic bacteriuria (population), does treatment with antibiotics (intervention) compared to no treatment or placebo (control) reduce the incidence of pyelonephritis, preterm and low birth weight delivery (outcomes)?

General search strategy

You begin to address these questions by searching for evidence in the common electronic databases such as the Cochrane Library and MEDLINE looking specifically for systematic reviews and meta-analyses. The Cochrane Library is particularly rich in high-quality systematic review evidence on numerous aspects of pregnancy and childbirth. In fact, this group's review productivity was the model for the development of the Cochrane Library. When a systematic review is identified, you also search for recent updates on the Cochrane Library and also search MEDLINE and EMBASE to identify randomized controlled trials that became available after the publication date of the systematic review. In addition, access to relevant, updated and evidence-based clinical practice guidelines (CPGs) on acute asthma are accessed to determine the consensus rating of areas lacking evidence.

Searching for evidence synthesis: primary search strategy

- Cochrane Library: pregnancy AND (topic)
- MEDLINE: pregnancy AND MEDLINE AND (systematic review OR meta-analysis OR metaanalysis) AND adult AND (topic)

Critical review of the literature

Question 1: In pregnant patients with first trimester bleeding and a sonographic intrauterine pregnancy (population), what proportion of patients (prognosis) will progress to subsequent fetal loss (outcome)?

Search strategy

- MEDLINE: (abortion, threatened OR abortion, incomplete OR abortion, spontaneous) AND uterine hemorrhage AND ultrasonography, prenatal

Up to 20% of pregnancies in the first trimester will be complicated by vaginal bleeding, and emergency practitioners should be prepared to offer cogent and accurate counsel on the risk of subsequent fetal loss for these commonly evaluated ED patients [2]. Evidence suggests that many women miscarry in the first trimester before a pregnancy is detected clinically, so truly estimating rates of first trimester fetal loss is challenging [3]. Patients with clinical

symptoms of a threatened abortion often suffer from considerable anxiety since the risk for subsequent miscarriage is high and parents are concerned about the effects of bleeding on a viable pregnancy. In 1997, Everett reported on a prospective cohort of first trimester patients with a diagnosis of threatened abortion and found a fetal loss rate of approximately 50% [2]. In this cohort, pregnancy was determined by a single positive pregnancy test result and no ultrasonographic information was utilized. Despite the questionable applicability of this figure to a general population and to current common practice, most texts and papers on the topic reference it.

Since the time of the study by Everett, ultrasound, where available, has become a routine diagnostic test used in the evaluation of pregnant first trimester patients with signs and symptoms of threatened abortion. This population usually has a transvaginal or transabdominal ultrasound evaluation at the time of their ED visit, and the status of their pregnancy is determined. In patients with a clinical diagnosis of threatened abortion but a confirmed live intrauterine pregnancy (IUP) by ultrasound, the risk for subsequent fetal loss has since been evaluated. Based on three recent, prospective studies, the fetal loss rates range from 0.5% to 14% [4–6]. While none of these studies was performed in an ED population, it seems reasonable to extrapolate these numbers as a conservative estimate for women presenting to the ED.

Most recently, first trimester patients with vaginal bleeding were assessed for both the amount of reported bleeding and their rates of subsequent fetal loss [4]. An overall miscarriage rate of 11.1% was reported, although "high risk" patients (age >35 years, history of more than two miscarriages) were excluded. Within this group, the variation in fetal loss ranged from 9% to 24%, based on the severity of the bleeding event. For example, women with light bleeding had a fetal loss rate of 9%, while those with moderate or heavy bleeding had a rate of 24%.

In a similar cohort of women with threatened miscarriage, an overall fetal loss rate of 14% was found [5]. In this population there was significant variation in rates of fetal demise based on gestational age at the time of presentation. For those with a clinical diagnosis of threatened miscarriage and an IUP at 5–6 weeks' gestational age (WGA), the subsequent rate of fetal loss was 29%, significantly higher than the 8% rate noted among those presenting between 7 and 12 WGA.

The largest single study to address the question of fetal loss after bleeding assessed over 16,000 patients with an IUP of between 10 and 14 WGA [6]. Subjects were enrolled prospectively and a self-reported history of vaginal bleeding in the previous 4 weeks was documented at that time. In those with self-reported heavy bleeding, the rate of loss was 1–2%, although no subgroup requiring ED evaluation for their bleeding episode was identified.

In summary, not all women who present to the ED with first trimester bleeding will suffer a spontaneous abortion; however, exact percentages have varied across studies. In addition, there are features that are more strongly associated with miscarriage at presentation, such as younger fetal gestational age and severity of blood loss.

Question 2: Following a first missed menstruation (population), what is the sensitivity and specificity (diagnostic test characteristics) of home urine pregnancy tests (tests) for detecting pregnancy (outcome)?

Search strategy

- MEDLINE: pregnancy test AND meta-analysis AND sensitivity and specificity

Many women present to the ED reporting a positive or negative pregnancy status based on the results of a home pregnancy test (HPT). Manufacturers of HPTs advertise that their tests are able to detect pregnancy at the first missed menstruation, with a sensitivity of 97–99% [7]. The validity of this claim becomes important for emergency physicians in judging when to trust patient-reported test results, determining if the test is worth repeating in the ED, and reconciling different results obtained in the ED versus the home setting. In evaluating manufacturers' claims of diagnostic test performance for HPTs, it is useful to first quantify the amount of human chorionic gonadotropin (hCG) in the urine of women at this early stage of pregnancy. Next, the detection limits of each test should be identified, and lastly, the accuracy of such tests in general usage by non-medical subjects should be assessed.

To address the first issue, a group of 25 women attending an infertility clinic who achieved clinical pregnancy were studied, 84% of whom proceeded to delivery [8]. Urine samples were analyzed for hCG concentrations at day 0, 1, 2 and 3 of missed menses. The median hCG at day 0 was 49 mIU/ml (95% CI: 12.4 to 241). They determined that to achieve 95% sensitivity at day 0, a HPT would need to reliably detect an hCG concentration of 12.4 mIU/ml, and by day 3 a level of 58 mIU/ml.

There have been three recent studies assessing diagnostic performances of over-the-counter HPTs in the period immediately following missed menstruation [8–10]. In the study noted above, 18 HPTs were evaluated, with an overall sensitivity of 0% (using a "clearly positive" test) for an hCG concentration of 12.5 mIU/ml [8]. At higher concentrations of 100 mIU/m, the overall sensitivity was 44%. In a follow-up study the next year, the in vitro sensitivity of seven HPTs was assessed. First Response was 95% sensitive at the low level of 6.3 mIU/ml, and Clearblue was 80% sensitive at 25 mIU/ml; however, the remaining five commercial tests only demonstrated 95% sensitivity when urine hCG concentrations were greater than 100 mIU/ml [9].

The above studies were performed in a laboratory setting; however, most significant for clinicians is the reliability of the test when performed by the general public. A meta-analysis addressed the diagnostic efficiency of HPT kits [11]. While this study does not seek to answer the specific question regarding the diagnostic accuracy at first missed menses, the results provide useful information about the test in the hands of non-health professionals. Included studies were conducted in both laboratory and home settings, using volunteers or patients, and comparing HPT results with a criterion standard (laboratory testing). While the authors found the overall sensitivity of HPTs was 91% (95% CI: 84% to 96%) in studies using volunteers, in studies of women who collected and tested their own samples the HPT performance dropped substantially, with an overall sensitivity of 75% (95% CI: 64% to 85%).

In conclusion, most over-the-counter HPT kits do not provide greater than 99% sensitivity in detecting pregnancy at the first missed menstruation. Further complicating the reliability of the test, HPTs do not seem to perform well in the hands of the average consumer. Self-reported test results by patients should be approached with caution. If there is a question of pregnancy, the test should be performed in the ED.

Question 3: In pregnant patients with first trimester bleeding (population), what is the diagnostic accuracy (diagnostic test characteristics) of the history and physical examination for predicting pregnancy loss (outcome)?

Search strategy

- MEDLINE: threatened abortion AND (physical exam OR signs OR symptoms)

As mentioned previously, many pregnant women present to the ED complaining of first trimester vaginal bleeding. In the absence of ultrasound, historical and diagnostic exam features are the only available diagnostic tools to assess the status of the patient's pregnancy. Today, physicians rely heavily on ultrasound for a definitive diagnosis in these patients; however, they are still performing a history and physical exam with uncertainty as to the prognostic significance of their findings.

There have been three recent studies that have investigated the diagnostic precision of signs and symptoms in this population. In a prospective cohort of 772 patients presenting to a clinic with symptoms of threatened abortion (<28 WGA), the ability of physicians to accurately diagnose a patient's pregnancy status was determined [12]. Physicians performed a structured history and physical exam and, after each step, recorded a presumed diagnosis (viable IUP, non-viable IUP, ectopic pregnancy, other gynecological condition, non-gynecological condition). The patient then underwent a transvaginal ultrasound exam, and the physician once again recorded a diagnosis, based on the ultrasonographic findings. Accuracy of the clinician's diagnosis at the different stages was expressed in kappa (κ) values. The physician's diagnosis after the history ($\kappa = 0.33$; 95% CI: 0.28 to 0.33) and physical exam ($\kappa = 0.57$; 95% CI: 0.52 to 0.62) proved unreliable, showing poor agreement with the final diagnosis.

In a similar study, general practitioners prospectively evaluated 204 first trimester patients with vaginal bleeding, performing a structured history and physical exam in addition to recording their estimate of probability of the pregnancy's viability, based on their findings [13]. All subjects were then referred to a hospital where a formal ultrasound was performed and a final, definitive diagnosis was made. Investigators found the physicians' initial diagnoses were inaccurate 58% of the time. Significant predictors of fetal loss included a history of increasing bleeding and visualized blood on speculum examination, though the actual likelihood ratios for each of these findings cannot be determined based on available study data.

In the largest prospective cohort, including 1000 patients, the relationship between signs and symptoms of first trimester patients being evaluated for threatened abortion and subsequent pregnancy loss was evaluated [14]. The design was similar to the above studies. The authors used logistic regression analysis to determine which features of the history and physical exam were independent predictors of pregnancy viability. A history of having passed clots (positive likelihood ratio, $+LR = 4.6$; 95% CI: 3.2 to 6.4) or fetal tissue vaginally ($+LR = 27.4$; 95% CI: 8.7 to 86.0) was significantly associated with a non-viable fetus. On exam, an open cervix was 100% specific (95% CI: 98.9% to 100%) while only 21.8% sensitive (95% CI: 18% to 26%) for fetal non-viability. The presence of blood in the vagina on exam had a likelihood ratio of 2.1 (95% CI: 1.8 to 2.5) in predicting fetal loss, while all 32 patients with both blood and products of conception on exam had a non-viable pregnancy (positive predictive value = 100%).

In summary, physician estimation of fetal loss was inaccurate; however, certain historical and physical findings were associated with outcome. While the above statistics can assist the practitioner in their discourse with patients, assessment of early pregnant patients with vaginal bleeding using historical and physical exam features only is unreliable. Ultrasonography information should be incorporated into the evaluation of these patients whenever available.

Question 4: In pregnant patients discharged from the ED with a diagnosis of a threatened abortion (population), does the use of maternal bed rest (intervention) compared to normal activity (control) decrease the rate of pregnancy loss (outcome) in this population?

Search strategy

- Cochrane: bed rest AND pregnancy

Miscarriage is defined as pregnancy loss before 23 WGA and occurs in up to 31% of pregnancies, 20% of which may be clinically unrecognized [3]. While maternal disease and placental dysfunction may contribute to the early loss of pregnancy, recent studies indicate two-thirds of spontaneous abortions are due to chromosomal abnormalities [15].

Bed rest has been suggested as an intervention to improve various reproductive outcomes, including reducing the risk of pregnancy loss in patients with threatened abortions. The reasoning behind such an intervention is that decreased physical activity might decrease the likelihood of pregnancy loss, though this logic

is called into question by the fact that most spontaneous abortions are secondary to genetic factors [16]. Complicating the issue, bed rest has been associated with adverse outcomes. Most dangerously, bed rest may increase the likelihood of thromboembolic disease [17]. There is also a significant financial burden to this intervention, with an estimated cost of US$1.03 billion in 1993 [18].

There are two relevant studies that compared clinical outcomes in pregnant women with a threatened abortion prescribed bed rest as compared to alternative care. Both studies included women with symptoms of a threatened abortion but live intrauterine pregnancies on ultrasound. A Cochrane review of these studies found that there was no significant difference in the risk of miscarriage in the comparison groups and that bed rest may actually increase the risk ($RR = 1.54$; 95% CI: 0.92 to 2.58) [16]. The total number of patients included in the review was very small, and the authors conclude that there is a lack of evidence regarding this clinical question. Neither study evaluated potential side-effects of bed rest.

In summary, there is no evidence to recommend the use of bed rest in women with threatened abortion to reduce the risk of subsequent fetal loss.

Question 5: For eclamptic pregnant patients in the ED setting (population), does intravenous magnesium sulfate reduce recurrent seizures or maternal mortality (outcome) compared to intravenous diazepam and/or phenytoin (control)?

Search strategy

- Cochrane and MEDLINE: eclampsia AND magnesium

Pre-eclampsia and eclampsia are referred to as the hypertensive disorders of pregnancy. In addition to elevations in blood pressure, pre-eclampsia is associated with proteinuria and often with pathological changes in the hepatic, renal, hematological and neurological systems. Eclampsia, the presence of seizures in conjunction with pre-eclampsia, is a relatively rare complication of pregnancy; however, it is associated with significant morbidity and mortality. Worldwide, eclampsia is responsible for about 50,000 deaths each year and 10% of maternal mortalities [19]. While the incidence of this disease is one in 100–1700 deliveries in low- and middle-income countries [20], eclampsia complicates fewer pregnancies in developed nations, with an incidence of one in 2000 deliveries and a reported mortality rate and major complication rate of 1.8% and 35%, respectively [21]. Maternal morbidity and mortality associated with eclampsia is directly caused by such problems as placental abruption, disseminated intravascular coagulation, acute renal failure, hepatocellular injury, liver rupture, blindness, cardiac arrest and, most commonly, cerebrovascular hemorrhage [22,23] Also of significance, perinatal mortality has been cited at 9–23% [21].

In evaluating any pregnant patient in their last trimester, it is important to obtain a blood pressure reading, since presentations

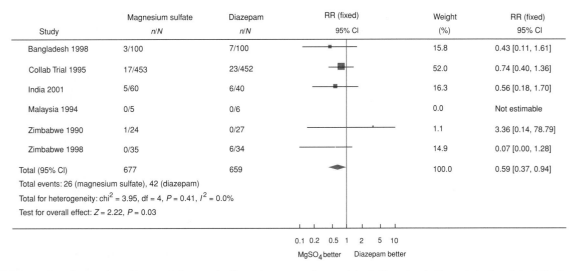

Figure 42.1 Comparison of magnesium sulfate versus diazepam, looking at the outcome of maternal death. (Reproduced with permission from Duley & Henderson-Smart [24], © Cochrane Collaboration.)

of pre-eclampsia can be non-specific (e.g., headache, abdominal pain, ankle swelling). The diagnosis of pre-eclampsia is usually made simply by blood pressure recording and urinalysis. However, it is important for emergency physicians to keep this diagnostic possibility in mind when evaluating pregnant patients, since its misdiagnosis can have serious consequences.

In evaluating an eclamptic patient in the ED, it is important to note the general management principles that should apply to this disease, including stabilization of maternal vital signs, control of maternal blood pressure, evaluation for prompt delivery and, relevant to this clinical question, control of seizure activity and prevention of recurrent seizures. The initial seizure of eclampsia is typically short lived, resolving without anticonvulsant intervention; however, 10–50% of eclamptic women will suffer from recurrent seizures, depending on which population and study is cited [21,23]. Accordingly, eclamptic women require anticonvulsant therapy as repeated seizure activity is associated with increased morbidity. Emergency physicians are accustomed to using benzodiazepines and phenytoin in epileptic and post-traumatic seizure management and so the substitution of magnesium sulfate ($MgSO_4$) for these more commonly used drugs may be met with hesitation.

The strongest evidence to support the usage of $MgSO_4$ over diazepam for eclamptic patients comes from a Cochrane systematic review that pooled the results of five high-quality randomized controlled trials. The review found significant decreases in the outcome of recurrent seizures (RR = 0.44; 95% CI: 0.34 to 0.57) and maternal death (RR = 0.59; 95% CI: 0.37 to 0.94) with use of $MgSO_4$ (Fig. 42.1) [24]. In comparing $MgSO_4$ to phenytoin, a second Cochrane systematic review, including five studies, found the use of $MgSO_4$ to be associated with a significant reduction in recurrent seizures (RR = 0.31; 95% CI: 0.2 to 0.47) and a non-significant reduction in maternal mortality (RR = 0.50; 95% CI: 0.24 to 1.05). The side-effect profiles of $MgSO_4$ include flushing,

some hypotension and loss of reflexes; however, side-effects are generally not severe and are self-limiting [25].

In summary, $MgSO_4$ is an inexpensive, safe, readily available and easy to use agent in the emergency setting. While its mechanism in the primary termination of seizures is not well defined, its overall benefit to eclamptic patients is supported by the evidence, making it the preferred first-line therapy over benzodiazepines and phenytoin in the treatment of eclampsia.

Question 6: For pregnant patients with nausea and vomiting (population), do anti-emetic treatments (intervention) provide safe and effective control of nausea and improve fetal outcomes (outcomes) compared to conservative treatment (control)?

Search strategy

- Cochrane and MEDLINE: nausea AND vomiting AND pregnancy AND therapy

Based on survey reports, nausea and vomiting in pregnancy (NVP) occur in up to 80% of all pregnancies, most often in the first trimester. These symptoms can be debilitating for women in early pregnancy, contributing to loss of employment time and leading to serious disruptions in everyday life [26]. At the same time, a large cohort study suggests that NVP does not increase the risk for adverse pregnancy outcomes, such as miscarriage, perinatal mortality and fetal anomalies [27]. When women visit the ED for NVP, initial goals include stabilization and resuscitation as necessary, confirmation of an IUP and the identification of hyperemesis gravidarum, typically defined by weight loss, ketonuria and varying degrees of electrolyte abnormalities. Once reassured that the patient's symptoms are not a sign of more severe pathology, the goals of treatment for NVP are ill defined. In the ED, there are numerous anti-emetics available for symptom control, but some question their safety and effectiveness in this population. Complicating the issue, there are no evidence-based or widely disseminated guidelines for the management of NVP [28].

The first question to address when prescribing any medication to pregnant women is whether the medicines are safe for the fetus. A qualitative and quantitative overview of observational controlled studies for anti-emetic drug safety in pregnancy was performed [29]. The authors referenced a meta-analysis of 24 controlled studies involving more than 200,000 first trimester exposures of antihistamines, with the summary odds ratio of major malformations associated with antihistamines taken during the first trimester of 0.76 (95% CI: 0.60 to 0.94) [30]. Of the dopamine antagonists (e.g., phenothiazines, droperidol and metoclopramide), the phenothiazines have been studied most extensively for evidence of teratogenicity. Prospective cohort, retrospective cohort, case–control and record linkage studies involving 2948 patients with exposures to phenothiazines have failed to show a risk for major malformation (RR = 1.03; 95% CI: 0.88 to 1.22) [29]. While metoclopramide, ondansetron and corticosteroids appear to be effective in managing NVP, there is a paucity of well-designed safety studies for these drugs [29].

A Cochrane review assessed the pooled effectiveness of all anti-emetic drugs (when compared to placebo) in reducing the incidence of nausea and vomiting in early pregnancy [31]. They found a beneficial reduction in these symptoms with the use of these drugs compared to placebo (OR = 0.16; 95% CI: 0.08 to 0.33), although there was considerable heterogeneity amongst the trials (Fig. 42.2). Primary outcomes were usually fairly subjective, related to a reduction in a nausea score. Of note, there were 12 included trials, and most assessed drugs less commonly used and prescribed as anti-emetics in the ED, such as dramamine, meclizine and hydroxizine. Only two trials assessed the use of phenothiazines in this population, and they found a non-significant benefit (OR = 0.09; 95% CI: 0.0 to 1.88). There is one randomized trial of intravenous ondansetron versus promethazine in subjects with hyperemesis gravidarum, the most severe form of NVP, but no significant difference between the treatment groups was identified (OR = 0.29; 95% CI: 0.03 to 3.12) [32].

Finally, a randomized trial assessing the effectiveness of three outpatient regimens in the management of NVP was performed [33]. First trimester patients with nausea and/or vomiting were randomized into three treatment groups: pyridoxine-metoclopramide, prochlorperazine or promethazine. All medications were administered orally, except for the pyridoxine, which was delivered as an intramuscular injection. For the primary outcome of decreased emesis at day 3, the group allocated to receive pyridoxine-metoclopramide had significantly fewer episodes than the other two groups, though the difference was small.

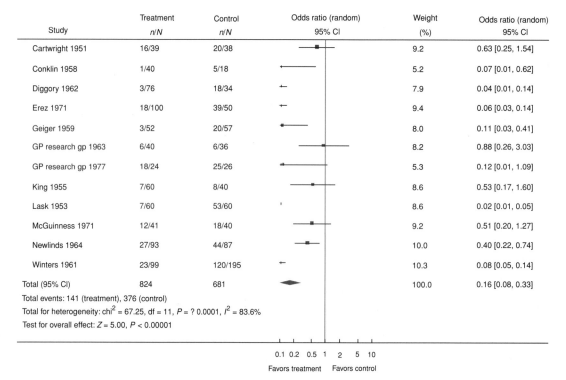

Figure 42.2 All anti-emetic medication compared with placebo for nausea and vomiting in early pregnancy, looking at the outcome of effect on nausea. (Reproduced with permission from Jewell & Young [31], © Cochrane Collaboration.)

In summary, NVP is a common presentation to the ED and management may include anti-emetic agents. As a group, the antihistamines and phenothiazines are best studied in terms of safety profiles in pregnancy, and drugs in these classes have proven benefit for NVP over placebo in a large meta-analysis. In general, emergency physicians should be cautious with medications in pregnant patients; however, in cases of NVP, they may be necessary.

Question 7: In pregnant patients with severe or intractable hyperemesis gravidarum (population), do intravenous corticosteroids (intervention) improve oral intake and decrease readmission rates (outcomes) compared to anti-emetic administration alone (control)?

Search strategy

- MEDLINE: hyperemesis gravidarum AND (steroids OR dexamethasone OR methlyprednisolone OR prednisone OR hydrocortisone)

While 50–90% of pregnancies are complicated by nausea and vomiting, the incidence of hyperemesis gravidarum is much lower, reported at one in 5000 deliveries [34]. There is no universally accepted definition for hyperemesis, but most studies evaluating the condition use persistent vomiting, a weight loss of more than 5% of pre-pregnancy weight, and large ketonuria to define the condition [35]. Maternal mortality is rare; however, morbidity can be significant, with complications ranging from electrolyte imbalances to Wernicke's encephalopathy and central pontine myelinolysis [36,37]. Standard resuscitation for such patients includes intravenous hydration and anti-emetic administration. For those pregnant patients with intractable symptoms, the role of corticosteroid therapy in reducing vomiting episodes and admission/readmission rates has been investigated.

There are two randomized, double-blinded studies comparing intravenous corticosteroids to standard anti-emetics (promethazine, metoclopramide) in an inpatient setting for patients with severe hyperemesis gravidarum. While often cited as showing a positive benefit to corticosteroid use in this setting, the first of these trials did not demonstrate improved efficacy of methylprednisolone over promethazine for the primary outcome of symptom improvement at day 2 [38]. For the secondary outcome of readmission rate, subjects sent home with oral steroids did better and had a 0% readmission rate, compared to 29% in the promethazine group ($P = 0.0001$). In the latter study, examining an intensive care unit population, in subjects randomized to intravenous hydrocortisone versus metoclopramide, vomiting episodes and readmission rates were both significantly reduced ($P < 0.0001$ for all comparisons) [39].

It has been proposed that corticosteroids could be given in addition to standard anti-emetic therapy. A randomized, placebo-controlled trial assessed the effectiveness of adjuvant intravenous methyl-prednisolone therapy versus placebo on readmission rates

[40]. There was no significant difference between groups (34 vs 35%, $P = 0.89$). In an outpatient setting, oral prednisone compared to promethazine was similarly ineffective [41].

In summary, while a single trial of intravenous corticosteroids suggests reductions in symptoms and need for readmission in an intensive care unit population of hyperemesis gravidarum patients, the remaining studies of outpatient and hospitalized subjects do not demonstrate a clear benefit. Routine use of this therapy can not be recommended based on available evidence.

Question 8: In pregnant patients with asymptomatic bacteriuria (population), does treatment with antibiotics (intervention) compared to no treatment or placebo (control) reduce the incidence of pyelonephritis, preterm and low birth weight delivery (outcomes)?

Search strategy

- Cochrane: asymptomatic bacteriuria AND pregnancy

Regardless of their chief complaint, many pregnant women presenting to the ED will have a urine dipstick test and/or official urinalysis performed. Interpreting the results of such tests in the context of a pregnant woman without complaints indicative of a urinary tract infection becomes problematic for the emergency medicine physician for several reasons that will be explored below.

The prevalence of asymptomatic bacteriuria in pregnancy is 2–10% [42], similar to the rates reported in non-pregnant women [43]. Bacteriuria is defined by the detection of more than 100,000 bacteria per milliliter in a single voided midstream urine, although the specificity of this test increases with two consecutive voided urine samples, which is recommended by the Infectious Diseases Society of America to make the diagnosis [43]. As in non-pregnant women, the most common uropathogen in this group is *Escherichia coli*.

It has been reported that up to 30% of pregnant women with asymptomatic bacteriuria will progress to pyelonephritis, as compared to 1.8% of non-bacteriuric pregnant patients [42]. The anatomic and physiological changes of pregnancy, such as smooth muscle relaxation and ureteral compression from an enlarging uterus, increase the likelihood that asymptomatic bacteriuria will progress to pyelonephritis. Pregnant women with pyelonephritis can have significant complications. A recent prospective study reported on a cohort of pregnant patients admitted with pyelonephritis and found the incidence of respiratory insufficiency, intensive care unit admission and septicemia in this group to be significant at 7%, 10% and 17%, respectively [44]. Accordingly, routine screening and treatment of asymptomatic bacteriuria has become standard in the obstetric community.

In addition to being associated with high rates of pyelonephritis, asymptomatic bacteriuria has been associated with low birth weight (LBW) and preterm delivery, although this link is somewhat controversial. A meta-analysis of cohort studies showed that

Table 42.1 Leukocyte-esterase and nitrite activity tests in identifying asymptomatic bacteriuria. (From Shelton et al. [47].)

	LE*	Nitrite†	LE or nitrite
Sensitivity (95% CI)	0.40% (0.19% to 0.64%)	0.15% (0.03% to 0.38%)	0.45% (0.23% to 0.68%)
Specificity (95% CI)	0.63% (0.56% to 0.70%)	0.99% (0.96% to 1.0%)	0.62% (0.55% to 0.69%)
PPV (95% CI)	0.11 (0.05 to 0.20)	0.60 (0.15 to 0.95)	0.12 (0.05 to 0.21)
NPV (95% CI)	0.90 (0.84 to 0.95)	0.91 (0.86 to 0.95)	0.91 (0.85 to 0.95)

*Positive LE = trace on urine dipstick analysis.
†Positive nitrite = positive value on dipstick analysis.
CI, confidence interval; LE, leukocyte-esterase; NPV, negative predictive value; PPV, positive predictive value.

untreated asymptomatic bacteriuria in pregnancy significantly increased rates of LBW and preterm delivery [45]. There is, however, evidence that asymptomatic bacteriuria is a surrogate marker for a truer predictor of LBW and preterm deliveries – lower socio-economic status. In a study comparing the incidence of asymptomatic bacteriuria and preterm delivery in three different socio-economic populations, lower socio-economic status rather than asymptomatic bacteriuria was associated with preterm delivery [46].

Taking all of these factors into consideration, the emergency medicine physician must, first, determine what defines asymptomatic bacteriuria in the ED setting, and, second, assess whether treating asymptomatic bacteria decreases the complications of pyelonephritis, LBW and preterm delivery. In regard to the first question, three recent studies evaluated the sensitivity and specificity of urine dipstick reagent strips and urinalysis in predicting asymptomatic bacteriuria in pregnant populations [47–49]. Overall, these tests perform poorly. In one study, the sensitivity and specificity of a positive leukocyte-esterase dipstick result was 40% (95% CI: 19% to 64%) and 63% (95% CI: 56% to 70%) (Table 42.1) [47]. For this reason, it is recommended that only urine culture tests be used for screening. Abnormal results on routine urinalysis and dipstick screening in asymptomatic pregnant patients are inadequately sensitive and specific to necessitate treatment and should be confirmed with culture testing.

If asymptomatic pregnant patients have urine culture tests sent from the ED that are confirmed positive as defined above, treatment with antibiotics is recommended based on a recent Cochrane review. Antibiotic therapy was effective in reducing the incidence of pyelonephritis in women with asymptomatic bacteriuria (RR = 0.23; 95% CI: 0.13 to 0.41) and LBW (RR = 0.66; CI: 0.49 to 0.89) [50]. However, there was no evidence of a reduction in preterm delivery. Of note, the authors conclude the overall quality of the included studies to be poor. In addition, there is no evidence to guide the appropriate antibiotic regimen for these patients, though the Infectious Diseases Society of America recommends 3–7 days of therapy [43].

In summary, pregnant women with asymptomatic bacteriuria should be treated with antibiotics as this seems to decrease the incidence of pyelonephritis and LBW infants in this population. In the ED, positive results on routine urinalysis and urine dipstick reagent strips should be confirmed with a positive urine culture (>100,000 bacteria/ml) before treatment is initiated.

Conclusions

The patient from this chapter was educated on the limitations of over-the-counter pregnancy tests in detecting early pregnancies. You explained that an ultrasound exam would be needed to determine the status of the pregnancy, and since a live intrauterine pregnancy was found on this exam, her risk of subsequent miscarriage would be low (approximately 10–15%). You advise the patient that while no study is perfect, the teratogenic potential of promethazine has never been shown in large evaluations of pregnant patients, and she chooses to receive the medication, which promptly gives her symptomatic relief.

In summary, pregnancy-related visits to the ED are common. Of those with threatened abortions, rates of subsequent fetal loss are likely lower than once estimated. Any first trimester patient with signs and symptoms of a threatened abortion should have a formal ultrasound evaluation as the history and physical exam is unreliable in differentiating between viable IUP, non-viable IUP and ectopic pregnancy. For those with a diagnosis of threatened abortion, bed rest is not recommended.

For the third trimester patient with eclampsia, magnesium sulfate is the drug of choice over diazepam and phenytoin. For those pregnant patients with nausea and vomiting, the antihistamines and phenothiazines are the best studied drugs in terms of safety profiles, so newer therapies such as metoclopramide and ondansetron should be used with caution. There may be some benefit to corticosteroids in those patients with hyperemesis gravidarum. Lastly, treatment of asymptomatic bacteriuria of pregnant women is recommended, but screening tests such as urinalysis and reagent strips are not reliable in detecting this condition and so culture testing is mandatory for the diagnosis.

Conflicts of interest

None were reported.

References

1 Stengel CL, Seaberg DC, MacLeod BA. Pregnancy in the emergency department: risk factors and prevalence among all women. *Ann Emerg Med* 1994;**24**:697–700.

2 Everett C. Incidence and outcome of bleeding before the 20th week of pregnancy: prospective study from general practice. *BMJ* 1997;**315**:32–4.

3 Wilcox, AJ, Weinberg CR, O'Connor JF, et al. Incidence of early loss of pregnancy. *N Engl J Med* 1989;**319**:189–94.

4 Poulouse T, Richardson R, Ewings P, Fox R. Probability of early pregnancy loss in women with vaginal bleeding and a singleton live fetus at ultrasound scan. *J Obstet Gynaecol* 2006;**26**:782–4.

5 Basama FMS, Crosfill F. The outcome of pregnancies in 182 women with threatened miscarriage. *Arch Gynecol Obstet* 2004;**270**:86–90.

6 Weiss JL, Fergal DM, Vidaver J, et al. Threatened abortion: a risk factor for poor pregnancy outcome, a population-based screening study. *Am J Obstet Gynecol* 2004;**190**:745–50.

7 Munroe WP. Home diagnostic kits. *Am Pharm* 1994;**NS34**:50–59.

8 Cole LA, Khanlian SA, Sutton JM, et al. Accuracy of home pregnancy tests at the time of missed menses. *Am J Obstet Gynecol* 2004;**190**:100–105.

9 Cole LA, Sutton-Riley JM, Khanlian SA, et al. Sensitivity of over-the-counter pregnancy tests: comparison of utility and marketing messages. *J Am Pharm* 2005;**45**:608–15.

10 Butler SA, Khanlian SA, Cole LA. Detection of early pregnancy forms of human chorionic gonadotropin by home pregnancy test devices. *Clin Chem* 2001;**47**:2131–6.

11 Bastian LA, Nanda K, Hasselblad V, Simel DL. Diagnostic efficiency of home pregnancy tests: a meta-analysis. *Arch Fam Med* 1998;**7**:465–9.

12 Yip SK, Sahota D, Cheung LP, et al. Accuracy of clinical diagnostic methods of threatened abortion. *Gynecol Obstet Invest* 2003;**56**:38–42.

13 Wieringa-de Waard M, Bonsel GJ, Ankum WM, et al. Threatened miscarriage in general practice: diagnostic value of history taking and physical examination. *Br J Gen Pract* 2002;**52**:825–9.

14 Chung TK, Sahota DS, Lau TK, et al. Threatened abortion: prediction of viability based on signs and symptoms. *Aust NZ J Obstet Gynaecol* 1999;**39**:443–7.

15 Menasha J, Levy B, Hirschhorn K, Kardon NB. Incidence and spectrum of chromosome abnormalities in spontaneous abortions: new insights from a 12-year study. *Genet Med* 2005;**7**:251–63.

16 Aleman A, Althabe F, Belizan J, Bergel E. Bed rest during pregnancy for preventing miscarriage (Cochrane review). *Cochrane Database Syst Rev* 2005;**2**:CD003576 (doi: 10.1002/14651858.CD003576.pub2).

17 Kovacevich GJ, Gaich SA, Lavin JP, et al. The prevalence of thromboembolic events among women with extended bed rest prescribed as part of the treatment for premature labor or preterm premature rupture of membranes. *Am J Obstet Gynecol* 2005;**182**:1089–92.

18 Goldenberg RL, Cliver SP, Bronstein J, et al. Bed rest in pregnancy. *Obstet Gynecol* 1994;**84**:131–6.

19 Duley L. Maternal mortality associated with hypertensive disorders of pregnancy in Africa, Asia, Latin America, and the Caribbean. *Br J Obstet Gynaecol* 1992;**99**:547–53.

20 Crowther C. Eclampsia at Harare Maternity Hospital. An epidemiological study. *South African Med J* 1985;**68**:927–9.

21 Douglas KA, Redman CWG. Eclampsia in the United Kingdom. *BMJ* 1994;**309**:1395–400.

22 Pritchard JA, Cunningham FG, Pritchard SA. The Parkland Memorial Hospital protocol for treatment of eclampsia: evaluation of 245 cases. *Am J Obstet Gynecol* 1984;**148**:951–60.

23 Mackay AP, Berg CJ, Atrash HK. Pregnancy-related mortality from preeclampsia and eclampsia. *Obstet Gynecol* 2001;**97**:533–8.

24 Duley L, Henderson-Smart D. Magnesium sulfate versus diazepam for eclampsia (Cochrane review). *Cochrane Database Syst Rev* 2003;**4**:CD000127 (doi: 10.1002/14651858.CD000127).

25 Duley L, Henderson-Smart D. Magnesium sulfate versus phenytoin for eclampsia (Cochrane review) *Cochrane Database Syst Rev* 2003;**4**:CD000128 (doi: 10.1002/14651858.CD000128).

26 Gadsby R, Barnie-Adshead AM, Jagger C. A prospective study of nausea and vomiting during pregnancy. *Br J Gen Pract* 1993;**43**:245–8.

27 Weigel MM, Weigel RM. Nausea and vomiting of early pregnancy outcome. An epidemiological study. *Br J Obstet Gynaecol* 1989;**96**:1304–11.

28 Mazzotta P, Magee L. A risk–benefit assessment of pharmacological and nonpharmacological treatments for nausea and vomiting in pregnancy. *Drugs* 2000;**59**:781–800.

29 Magee LA, Mazzotta P, Koren G. Evidence-based view of safety and effectiveness of pharmacologic therapy for nausea and vomiting of pregnancy (NVP). *Am J Obstet Gynecol* 2002;**186**:S256–61.

30 Seto A, Einarson T, Koren G. Pregnancy outcome following first trimester exposure to antihistamines: meta-analysis. *Am J Perinat* 1997;**14**:119–23.

31 Jewell D, Young G. Interventions for nausea and vomiting in early pregnancy (Cochrane review). *Cochrane Database Syst Rev* 2003;**4**:CD000145 (doi: 10.1002/14651858.CD000145).

32 Sullivan CA, Johnson CA, Roach H, et al. A pilot study of intravenous ondansetron for hyperemesis gravidarum. *Am J Obstet Gynecol* 1996;**174**:1565–8.

33 Bsat FA, Hoffman DE, Seubert DE. Comparison of three outpatient regimens in the management of nausea and vomiting in pregnancy. *J Perinat* 2003;**23**:531–5.

34 Bailit JL. Hyperemesis gravidarum: epidemiologic findings from a large cohort. *Am J Obstet Gynecol* 2005;**193**:811–14.

35 Goodwin TM. Hyperemesis gravidarum. *Clin Obstet Gynecol* 1998;**41**:597–605.

36 Wood P, Murray A, Sinha B, et al. Wernicke's encephalopathy induced by hyperemesis gravidarum: case reports. *Br J Obstet Gynaecol* 1983;**90**:583–6.

37 Peeters A, Van de Wyngaert F, Van Lierde M, et al. Wernicke's encephalopathy and central pontine myelinolysis induced by hyperemesis gravidarum. *Acta Neurol Belg* 1993;**93**:276–82.

38 Safari HR, Fassett MJ, Souter, IC, et al. The efficacy of methylprednisolone in the treatment of hyperemesis gravidarum: a randomized, double-blind, controlled study. *Am J Obstet Gynecol* 1998;**179**:921–4.

39 Bondok, RS, Sharnouby NME, Eid HE, Elmaksoud AMA. Pulsed steroid therapy is an effective treatment for intractable hyperemesis gravidarum. *Crit Care Med* 2006;**34**:2781–3.

40 Yost NP, McIntire DD, Wians FH, et al. A randomized, placebo-controlled trial of corticosteroids for hyperemesis due to pregnancy. *Obstet Gynecol* 2003;**102**:1250–54.

41 Ziaei S, Hosseiney FS, Faghihzadheh S. The efficacy of low dose prednisolone in the treatment of hyperemesis gravidarum. *Acta Obstet Gynecol Scand* 2004;**83**:272–5.

42 Whalley, P. Bacteriuria of pregnancy. *Am J Obstet Gynecol* 1967;**97**:723–38.

43 Nicolle LE, Bradley S, Colgan R, et al. Infectious Society of America guidelines for the diagnosis and treatment of asymptomatic bacteriuria in adults. *Clin Infect Dis* 2005;**40**:643–54.

44 Hill JB, Sheffield JS, McIntire DD, Wendel GD. Acute pyelonephritis in pregnancy. *Obstet Gynecol* 2005;**105**:18–23.

45 Romero R, Oyarzun E, Mazor M, et al. Meta-analysis of the relationship between asymptomatic bacteriuria and preterm delivery/low birth weight. *Obstet Gynecol* 1989;**73**:576–81.

46 Turck M, Goffe BS, Petersdorf RG. Bacteriuria in pregnancy: relation to socioeconomic factors. *N Engl J Med* 1962;**266**:857–60.

47 Shelton SD, Boggess KA, Kirvan K, et al. Urinary interleukin-8 with asymptomatic bacteriuria in pregnancy. *Obstet Gynecol* 2001;**97**:583–6.

48 Millar L, Debuque L, Leialoha C, et al. Rapid enzymatic urine screening test to detect bacteriuria in pregnancy. *Obstet Gynecol* 2000;**95**:601–4.

49 McNair RD, MacDonald SR, Dooley SL, Peterson L. Evaluation of the centrifuged and Gram-stained smear, urinalysis, and reagent strip testing to detect asymptomatic bacteriuria in obstetric patients. *Am J Obstet Gynecol* 2000;**182**:1076–9.

50 Smaill F, Vazquez JC. Antibiotics for asymptomatic bacteriuria in pregnancy (Cochrane review). *Cochrane Database Syst Rev* 2007;**2**:CD000490 (doi: 10.1002/14651858.CD000490.pub2).

43 Gastrointestinal Bleeding

Michael Bullard[1] & Justin Cheung[2]

[1]Department of Emergency Medicine, University of Alberta, Edmonton, Canada
[2]Division of Gastroenterology, Department of Medicine, University of Alberta, Edmonton, Canada

Clinical scenario

A 56-year-old male was brought to the emergency department (ED) complaining of passing very loose, dark red stools over the past 3 hours. He appeared pale, diaphoretic and was feeling faint at triage. He was moved onto an ED stretcher and continued with his history while the primary nurse obtained his vital signs and established a peripheral IV line. He was feeling well until today. He denied any abdominal pain. He was feeling nauseated but had not vomited. His past history revealed type 2 diabetes treated with metformin and he had suffered a myocardial infarct 1 year ago, following which he received a coronary stent. Since that time he had been on clopidogrel, metoprolol, lisinopril and lipitor. He stopped smoking a year ago and drinks socially, last at a party 2 nights prior to ED presentation.

His vital signs lying were: respiration 22 breaths/min, pulse 109 beats/min and blood pressure 114/76 mmHg (left arm). Upon sitting his pulse increased to 126 beats/min, his blood pressure fell to 92/60 mmHg and he felt faint.

Background

Gastrointestinal bleeding is a common ED presentation. The annual admission rate for upper gastrointestinal bleeding (UGIB) in the USA in the 1990s was 102 patients per 100,000, while in the UK during the same period the rate was reportedly 103 per 100,000 [1,2]. Almost 70% of admitted patients are over 70 years of age, with a 14% mortality rate – primarily among the elderly with associated co-morbidities [2]. The annual US incidence rate for non-variceal UGIB requiring hospitalization is reportedly between 30 and 100 per 100,000, with an estimated annual cost of greater than $2.5 billion [3,4]. A review of a Canadian national database found that the incidence of acute non-variceal UGIB between 1993 and 2003 decreased from 77.1 to 53.2 cases per 100,000 per year, while surgical interventions declined from 7.1% to 4.5% [5]. Therapeutic changes during that time period included: the introduction of proton pump inhibitors, antibiotic therapy for *Helicobacter pylori* infections in the early 1990s, improved access to endoscopic examinations in the ED, and additional interventions delivered endoscopically. The incidence of hospitalization for lower gastrointestinal bleeding (LGIB) is much lower at approximately 6–20 per 100,000 [6].

The main causes of UGIB admissions among UK EDs were reported as peptic ulceration (37%), erosive disease (11%), esophagitis (11%), Mallory–Weiss tear (6%), varices (4%), malignancy (4%) and none or "other" (29%) [2]. A recent US review article gave ranges for the most common causes of UGIB to be peptic ulcer (~50%), variceal bleeding (5–30%), Mallory–Weis tears (5–15%) and hemorrhagic and erosive gastropathy (gastritis) (up to 20%) [7]. The most common causes of LGIB are diverticulosis and angiodysplasia [6]. For the emergency physician, the primary goal after stabilization is to identify whether the bleeding source is upper or lower, as it not only influences therapy but also the diagnostic approach.

Clinical questions

1 In adults with acute gastrointestinal bleeding (population), what is the sensitivity/specificity (diagnostic test characteristics) of the clinical exam (test) for the determination of upper versus lower gastrointestinal bleeding (outcome)?

2 In adults with *Helicobacter*-positive peptic ulcers (population), does antibiotic therapy (intervention) compared to no antibiotic therapy (control) decrease gastrointestinal bleeding (outcome)?

Evidence-based Emergency Medicine. Edited by Brian H. Rowe
© 2009 Blackwell Publishing, ISBN: 978-1-4051-6143-5.

3 In adults with recent-onset anemia and normal-appearing stools (population), what is the sensitivity/specificity (diagnostic test characteristics) of stool occult blood testing (test) for detecting clinically important gastrointestinal bleeding (outcome)?

4 In adult patients with an acute upper gastrointestinal bleed (population), does immediate gastroscopy (intervention) compared to delayed gastroscopy (control) reduce inappropriate drug therapy and improve disposition-making (outcomes)?

5 In adult patients with clinical indications for Cox 1 non-steroidal anti-inflammatory drugs (NSAIDs) (population), do Cox 2 NSAIDs or the addition of acid suppression agents (interventions) compared to traditional NSAIDs alone (control) lead to fewer clinically important side-effects (outcomes)?

6 In adult patients with a suspected upper gastrointestinal bleed (population), what is the sensitivity/specificity (diagnostic test characteristics) of nasogastric tube insertion with gastric lavage (test) for detecting upper gastrointestinal bleeding (outcomes)?

7 In adults presenting with evidence of an acute upper gastrointestinal bleed (population), do parenteral proton pump inhibitors (intervention) compared to placebo (control) reduce further bleeding or need for transfusion or other morbidity (outcomes)?

8 In stabilized adult patients with a suspected lower gastrointestinal bleed (population), what initial diagnostic test (diagnostic test) provides the highest sensitivity and specificity (diagnostic test characteristics) to locate the source of bleeding (outcome)?

General search strategy

A large number of studies have been published in the area of UGIB and LGIB diagnosis and therapy. Consequently, a clinician looking for evidence-based resources must be organized and systematic or he/she could easily become overwhelmed with the search results. The first approach when examining a topic area with a large number of published papers is to search for a systematic review. Searching the Cochrane Library identified a number of relevant reviews for this chapter. Next, MEDLINE and EMBASE searches using terms for population (gastrointestinal bleeding) AND setting (terms for "emergency" or "acute") and exclusion of post-operative period identified the population. With each diagnosis question, diagnostic terms (e.g., UGIB OR LGIB) were matched to "sensitivity and specificity". With each question in treatment, terms for the treatment (e.g., proton pump inhibitors) restricted to "systematic reviews OR metaanalyses OR randomized controlled trials" (RCTs) was applied.

Clinical review of the literature

Question 1: In adults with acute gastrointestinal bleeding (population), what is the sensitivity/specificity (diagnostic test characteristics) of the clinical exam (test) for the determination of upper versus lower gastrointestinal bleeding (outcome)?

Search strategy

- MEDLINE, CENTRAL and EMBASE: (lower OR upper) AND gastrointestinal bleeds AND hemorrhage AND diagnosis AND (RCT OR sensitivity and specificity OR systematic review OR meta-analysis)

Emergency department patients with UGIB classically present with a history of bright red or coffee ground emesis associated with black or tarry stools [8]. Those with LGIB typically present with bright red rectal bleeding or hematochezia (bright red or maroon). In patients with very brisk UGIB the transit time is so short that melena does not have time to develop. From an investigative and therapeutic standpoint, pinpointing upper versus lower tract bleeding is important. Otherwise, the abdominal examination is generally benign and unhelpful.

Unfortunately, our search failed to identify any evidence-based medicine reviews on the diagnosis of UGIB; however, several diagnostic studies were identified and reviewed. One study enrolled 135 patients identified as having passed blood per rectum and undertook to evaluate the predictive validity of differences in stool color description by patients and physicians versus picking the best match from a five-color chart [9]. Color 1 and color 2 were both bright red shades, most consistent with blood, and color 4 was black, consistent with melena. Using the color chart physicians selecting color 2 (bright red) achieved a sensitivity of 0.33, a specificity of 0.98 and a positive likelihood ratio (+LR) of 16 (95% CI: 3.73 to 73) in predicting an LGIB site of bleeding. Selecting color 4 (melena) achieved a sensitivity of 0.49, a specificity of 0.98 and a +LR of 24 (95% CI: 3.48 to 172) in predicting a UGIB site. In two patients with massive gastrointestinal bleeding, both the patients and physicians pointed to the red color (1 or 2) on the chart. Numerous different terms were used by both parties to describe the stool color and in 22% of cases the color selected from the card did not appear to match the recorded description. The objective color chart was superior to written description for communicating information and predicting the bleeding site. Additional useful clinical information is the knowledge that melena on history or on rectal exam indicates blood that has spent at least 14 hours transiting the gastrointestinal tract [10]. A study of patients with acute gastrointestinal bleeding reported 31% presenting with orthostatic blood pressure changes or shock, much more commonly among UGIB patients ($P < 0.05$) [11].

In summary, clinical description of the color of the stool can assist the clinicians in understanding the location of the bleed. In addition, the presence of clinical signs of reduced blood volume may be helpful in indicating the degree and location of gastrointestinal bleeding.

Question 2: In adults with *Helicobacter*-positive peptic ulcers (population), does eradication therapy (intervention) compared to non-eradication therapy (control) decrease gastrointestinal bleeding (outcome)?

Search strategy

- MEDLINE, CENTRAL and EMBASE: (lower OR upper) AND gastrointestinal bleeds AND hemorrhage AND heliobacter pylori AND antibiotics AND (RCT OR systematic review OR meta-analysis)

A study looking at trends in the management and outcomes of acute non-variceal gastrointestinal bleeding in Canada from 1993 to 2003 noted a steady decline in both the incidence (from 52.4 to 34.3 cases per 100,000 per year) and requirements for surgical intervention (7.1% to 4.5%) [5]. The major therapeutic changes introduced during this period were an increased awareness and implementation of *Helicobacter pylori* antibiotic regimens and the introduction of more effective peptic acid suppression.

All RCTs comparing *H. pylori* eradication therapy plus ulcer healing drugs versus ulcer healing drugs alone have shown statistically significant benefit in favor of eradication. In this case, triple or dual therapy antibiotics for *H. pylori* infection are being evaluated. As an example, three RCTs that were identified reporting on peptic ulcer healing found eradication therapy led to a 13% reduction in unhealed ulcers (RR = 0.52; 95% CI: 0.31 to 0.85) with a number needed to treat (NNT) of 8 (95% CI: 4.5 to 50) [12]. Eradication therapy has also been shown to decrease ulcer rebleeding (Fig. 43.1): when compared to a non-eradication group without subsequent long-term antisecretory therapy the benefit was large (RR = 0.22; 95% CI: 0.12 to 0.40) with an NNT of 7 (95% CI: 5 to 11), and when compared to a non-eradication group with long-term maintenance antisecretory therapy the benefit was similarly effective (RR = 0.27; 95% CI: 0.09 to 0.77) with an NNT of 20 (95% CI: 12 to 100) [13]. In patients who require long-term nonsteroidal anti-inflammatory drug (NSAID) therapy after UGIB due to *H. pylori*-positive peptic ulcer disease, eradication therapy alone without long-term acid suppression is associated with a high recurrence of UGIB on NSAIDs [14]. Upon analysis, the majority of rebleeds were due to failure of eradication therapy or the use of NSAIDs. One study looked at the specific question "Does eradication therapy decrease gastrointestinal bleeding in patients with *H. pylori* infection and endoscopically proven duodenal ulcers?" The authors identified six upper gastrointestinal bleeds among the ranitidine group (257 patients), five among the omeprazole group (442 patients) and none among the clarithromycin and omeprazole group (441 patients) during the 1-year follow-up period [15].

In summary, clinicians should be familiar with a major contributor to UGIB (*H. pylori* microbial infection) and the need to treat this with antibiotics for best results. While antisecretory therapy does work, eradication therapy leads to a higher rate of ulcer healing and is more likely to limit recurrence.

Question 3: In adults with recent-onset anemia and normal-appearing stools (population), what is the sensitivity/specificity (diagnostic test characteristics) of stool occult blood testing (test) for detecting clinically important gastrointestinal bleeding (outcome)?

Search strategy

- MEDLINE, CENTRAL and EMBASE – search terms: (lower OR upper) AND gastrointestinal bleeds AND hemorrhage AND occult blood AND (RCT OR sensitivity and specificity OR systematic review OR meta-analysis)

The testing for fecal occult blood (FOB) is a common ED practice and requires an understanding of both the features of the test and the clinical situation to be able to interpret the results.

Hemoccult II is the most commonly used bedside test for FOB; however, in a study to detect FOB following the oral ingestion of 20 cm^3 of blood per day for three consecutive days it proved less sensitive (16%) when compared to Hemoccult II SENSA (64%) or HemoQuant (67%), with as little as 10–20 cm^3 detectable within the stool within 24 hours [16]. The sensitivities for the three tests were similar for ingestions of 60 cm^3 of blood. In a placebo-controlled study evaluating the risk of gastrointestinal bleeding during a 28-day course of ibuprofen (800 mg orally three times daily) using healthy volunteers, 21 of 31 subjects in the ibuprofen group had 2–7 episodes of microbleeding [17]. The volume of six of these microbleeds was greater than 15 cm^3 and would have been sufficient to produce a positive FOB test [17]. Confounders to test interpretation include the fact that gastric blood may take from 12 to 24 hours to reach the rectum, making early FOB testing likely to be negative. Moreover, the ingestion of red meat has been shown to lead to false-positive FOB tests for up to 3 days [18]. Two studies compared hemoccult-positive stools obtained by rectal examination to spontaneously passed stools and found no increase in false-positive results in detecting the presence of neoplastic lesions [18,19]. The sensitivity of a positive FOB test for the detection of cancer is reported to be around 50% but the specificity is only 10–15% [20].

In summary, in ED patients with acute-onset anemia from an acute bleed, the patient would be expected to show signs of hemodynamic compromise. If the history did not point to a specific cause and the rectal exam did not reveal melena, a negative FOB test would either indicate the blood had not yet transited the entire colon or the need to look for an alternate source of blood loss. A positive FOB test in the absence of melena would be noncontributory as it would not explain an acute hemoglobin drop.

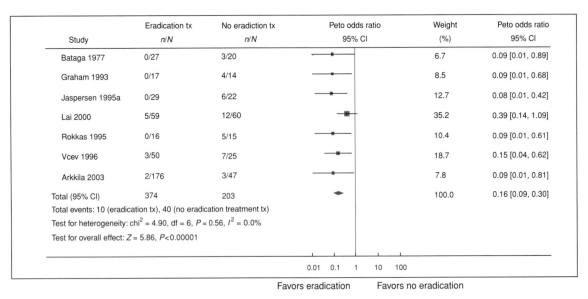

Study	Eradication tx n/N	No eradiction tx n/N	Peto odds ratio 95% CI	Weight (%)	Peto odds ratio 95% CI
Bataga 1977	0/27	3/20		6.7	0.09 [0.01, 0.89]
Graham 1993	0/17	4/14		8.5	0.09 [0.01, 0.68]
Jaspersen 1995a	0/29	6/22		12.7	0.08 [0.01, 0.42]
Lai 2000	5/59	12/60		35.2	0.39 [0.14, 1.09]
Rokkas 1995	0/16	5/15		10.4	0.09 [0.01, 0.61]
Vcev 1996	3/50	7/25		18.7	0.15 [0.04, 0.62]
Arkkila 2003	2/176	3/47		7.8	0.09 [0.01, 0.81]
Total (95% CI)	374	203		100.0	0.16 [0.09, 0.30]

Total events: 10 (eradication tx), 40 (no eradication treatment tx)
Test for heterogeneity: chi^2 = 4.90, df = 6, P = 0.56, I^2 = 0.0%
Test for overall effect: Z = 5.86, P<0.00001

0.01 0.1 1 10 100

Favors eradication   Favors no eradication

Figure 43.1 Comparison of eradication versus non-eradication therapy for recurrent bleeding, excluding non-steroidal anti-inflammatory drug users. (Reprinted with permission from Gisbert et al. [13], © Cochrane Library, Wiley.)

In a hemodynamically stable patient with age-indeterminate anemia and no clear history of gastrointestinal bleeding, a negative FOB test does not rule out gastrointestinal bleeds, since blood loss may be intermittent. Conversely, a positive test would not clearly support the need for endoscopic testing, recognizing some false-positive tests may be based on diet alone. In patients taking oral iron or bismuth presenting with black stools, a negative hemoccult test can provide reassurance that this is not melena [21].

Question 4: In adult patients with an acute upper gastrointestinal bleed (population), does immediate gastroscopy (intervention) compared to delayed gastroscopy (control) reduce inappropriate drug therapy and improve disposition-making (outcomes)?

Search strategy

- MEDLINE, CENTRAL and EMBASE – search terms: gastrointestinal hemorrhage AND upper gastrointestinal tract AND endoscopy AND (early OR delays OR timing)

While standards of practice vary among various jurisdictions, institutions and gastroenterology groups, and there are no RCTs to suggest that earlier endoscopy is associated with improved outcomes or cost-effectiveness, there appears to be broad consensus among gastrointestinal specialists that early endoscopy (within 24 hours) is beneficial [22–25]. No systematic review was identified for this topic; however, there were several RCTs. Da Silveira et al. noted some of the advantages of early endoscopy in non-variceal UGIB to include: rapid diagnosis, risk stratification, risk-based allocation of resources (e.g., early discharge for low-risk patients, lower level of care post treatment for intermediate risk, inten-

sive care unit admission for high-risk patients) and application of endoscopic hemostasis [26]. Patients found to have an ulcer with active bleeding or a non-bleeding visible vessel are considered high risk for rebleeding and should receive endoscopic therapy and an intravenous infusion of a proton pump inhibitor (PPI) for 72 hours post endoscopy. Patients with adherent clots should also receive IV infusion of a PPI, and many investigators suggest endoscopic therapy as well. Patients with flat pigmented spots and those with clean-based ulcers have minimal risk of rebleeding on oral PPI, and therefore do not require endoscopic therapy or IV PPIs; these patients can often be managed as an outpatient after endoscopic diagnosis [27,28].

In summary, despite the absence of RCTs to prove this, endoscopy is recommended as an appropriate diagnostic and potentially therapeutic intervention from an ED perspective. Endoscopy for UGIB should be viewed like any other diagnostic test: the sooner the better, to expedite disposition and provide optimal treatment based on a specific diagnosis.

Question 5: In adult patients with clinical indications for Cox 1 non-steroidal anti-inflammatory drugs (NSAIDs) (population), do Cox 2 NSAIDs or the addition of acid suppression agents (interventions) compared to traditional NSAIDs alone (control) lead to fewer clinically important side-effects (outcomes)?

Search strategy

- MEDLINE, CENTRAL and EMBASE: (lower OR upper) AND gastrointestinal bleeds AND hemorrhage AND NSAIDs AND Cox 2 inhibitors AND side effects AND (RCT OR systematic review OR meta-analysis)

Table 43.1 Cost-effectiveness analysis for preventing gastrointestinal events comparing Cox 1 non-steroidal anti-inflammatory drugs (NSAIDs) plus acid suppression options and Cox 2 NSAIDs. (From Brown et al. [30], © Queen's Printer and Controller of HMSO, 2006.)

Treatment arm vs NSAID	Cost per endoscopic ulcer avoided (£) (2.5th percentile, 97.5th percentile)	Cost per serious GI event averted (£) (2.5th percentile, 97.5th percentile)	Cost per LYG (£) (2.5th percentile, 97.5th percentile)
NSAID plus PPI	454 (251, 877)	5,744 (−99,537, 101,364)	3,204 (−55,521, 56,540)
NSAID plus H$_2$RA	−186 (−555, 804)	−4,477 (−9,718, 22,490)	−2,534 (−9,718, 22,490)
NSAID plus misoprostol	54 (−112, 238)	−2,550 (−21,103, 9,510)	−1,423 (−5,305, 11,771)
Cox 2 coxib inhibitor	301 (189, 418)	22,843 (10,742, 44,896)	12,742 (5,992, 25,093)
Cox 2 preferential inhibitor	263 (−570, 1280)	16,153 (−58,029, 104,973)	9,010 (−32,368, 58,553)

GI, gastrointestinal; H$_2$RA, H$_2$ receptor antagonist; LYG, life year gained; PPI, protein pump inhibitory. £ = UK pound sterling. Note 1 UK pound ~2.00 Canadian or US dollars (2008).

A 2002 Cochrane review of RCTs evaluating strategies to prevent NSAID-induced gastroduodenal ulcers, misoprostol, H$_2$ blockers and PPIs was analyzed. When taking NSAIDs, the addition of misoprostol significantly reduced gastric ulcer risk (RR = 0.26; 95% CI: 0.17 to 0.39) and duodenal ulcer risk (RR = 0.47; 95% CI: 0.33 to 0.69) when compared to placebo. While a dose of 800 μg/day provided the greatest benefit it also led to a greater incidence of diarrhea (RR = 3.25; 95% CI: 2.60 to 4.06) versus placebo (RR = 1.81; 95% CI: 1.52 to 2.16), leading to a greater drop-out rate. The NNT for misoprostol 800 μg/day to prevent one clinically important gastrointestinal event was 260; however, the NNT would be lower if applied to high-risk patients only. When taking NSAIDs, double-dose H$_2$ blockers significantly reduced both gastric (RR = 0.44; 95% CI: 0.26 to 0.74) and duodenal (RR = 0.26; 95% CI: 0.11 to 0.65) ulcers and abdominal pain (RR = 0.57; 95% CI: 0.33 to 0.98) compared to placebo with no increased adverse side-effects. PPIs significantly reduced gastric (RR = 0.40; 95% CI: 0.32 to 0.51) and duodenal (RR = 0.19; 95% CI: 0.09 to 0.37) ulcers while reducing symptoms of dyspepsia when compared to placebo. Factors putting patients at high risk for NSAID-related upper gastrointestinal toxicity include: age >65 years, previous peptic ulcer disease, co-morbid medical illness, and use of multiple NSAIDs or NSAIDs combined with corticosteroids [29].

A 2006 systematic review noted a decreased risk of developing a gastroduodenal ulcer by combining H$_2$ blockers with a Cox 1 NSAID (RR = 0.55; 95% CI: 0.44 to 0.70), with misoprostol (RR = 0.33; 95% CI: 0.27 to 0.41) or with a PPI (RR = 0.37; 95% CI: 0.30 to 0.46), and when using Cox 2 inhibitors versus Cox 1 NSAIDs (RR = 0.25; 95% CI: 0.21 to 0.30) [30]. In the same systematic review a comparison of Cox 2 to Cox 1 NSAIDs found a reduced risk of developing a serious gastrointestinal event (RR = 0.55; 95% CI: 0.38 to 0.80) and no increased risk for developing a serious cardiovascular or renal illness (RR = 1.19; 95% CI: 0.80 to 1.75). However, several RCTs have suggested that Cox 2 inhibitors may be associated with increased cardiovascular events [31–33]. Further studies specifically investigating the effects of Cox 2 inhibitors on cardiovascular events are underway. Based on economic modeling

some authors recommend against using NSAIDs alone [30]. The most cost-effective strategy to prevent one endoscopic ulcer is H$_2$ blockers + NSAIDs (<£750); NSAIDs + misoprostol would cost more (>£750) and have more drop-outs due to gastrointestinal side-effects and Cox 2s would cost >£3750 to prevent the same ulcer. Treatment with NSAIDs + PPI was never deemed the most cost-effective strategy (Table 43.1) [30].

In summary, some form of protection for patients at high risk for gastrointestinal bleeding seems reasonable. When receiving anti-inflammatory agents – given the similar effectiveness of comparisons between misoprostol, H$_2$ blockers, PPIs and Cox 2 inhibitors – cost and side-effect profile suggests the H$_2$ blockers warrant primary consideration.

Question 6: In adult patients with a suspected upper gastrointestinal bleed (population), what is the sensitivity/specificity (diagnostic test characteristics) of nasogastric tube insertion with gastric lavage (test) for detecting upper gastrointestinal bleeding (outcomes)?

Search strategy

- MEDLINE, CENTRAL and EMBASE – search terms: (lower OR upper) AND gastrointestinal bleeds AND hemorrhage AND nasogastric tube AND (RCT OR sensitivity and specificity OR systematic review OR meta-analysis)

A number of guidelines for the management of suspected gastrointestinal bleeding recommend nasogastric aspiration (NGA) as a diagnostic test to rule out an upper bowel source in patients with suspected LGIB and to confirm or prognosticate in patients with suspected UGIB [34–36]. This appears to have developed from a number of early studies indicating that few patients with NGA negative for blood had a UGIB source identified. In one study, however, 11% with UGIB severe enough to cause hematochezia had a negative nasogastric lavage [37]. An ED retrospective study of UGIB patients without hematemesis found a positive NGA had a sensitivity of 0.42 (95% CI: 0.32 to 0.51), a specificity of 0.91 (95% CI: 0.83 to 0.95), a +LR of 11 (95% CI: 4 to 30) and a negative likelihood ratio (−LR) of 0.6 (95% CI: 0.5 to 0.7) [38]. A large Canadian database review found that a bloody NGA achieved a sensitivity of 0.48 (95% CI: 0.40 to 0.57), a specificity of 0.76 (95% CI: 0.70 to 0.80) and a +LR of 2.0 (95% CI: 1.1 to 1.3); while combining bloody or coffee grounds and other (not clear or bile) NGAs achieved a sensitivity of 0.94 (95% CI: 0.88 to 0.97), a specificity of 0.16 (95% CI: 0.12 to 0.20), a +LR of 1.1 (95% CI: 1.0 to 1.2) and a −LR of 0.31 (95% CI: 0.17 to 0.57) for predicting a high-risk gastroduodenal lesion [39].

While the presence of blood in the NGA may help confirm a UGIB, it does not facilitate treatment nor adequately predict prognosis – gastroscopy is required for that. In addition, the fact that up to 16% of patients with clear or bile-tinged NGAs prove to have high-risk gastroduodenal lesions does not permit a negative test to direct ongoing management. Most importantly, patient discomfort (identified as the most painful commonly performed ED procedure) [40] and associated complications (e.g., epistaxis) represent an unacceptably high adverse events profile for a diagnostic test of low utility.

In summary, there is limited evidence for the role of NGA in the diagnosis of a gastrointestinal bleed. Until prospective trials are performed to determine the utility of NGA in the work-up of suspected UGIB patients, it should be abandoned [41].

Question 7: In adults presenting with evidence of an acute upper gastrointestinal bleed (population), do parenteral proton pump inhibitors (intervention) compared to placebo (control) reduce further bleeding or need for transfusion, or other morbidity (outcomes)?

Search strategy

- MEDLINE, CENTRAL and EMBASE – search terms: (lower OR upper) AND gastrointestinal bleeds AND hemorrhage AND proton pump inhibitors AND (RCT OR systematic review OR meta-analysis)

The rationale for trying to increase gastric pH is that gastric acid inhibits clot formation and promotes lysis and also promotes ongoing tissue damage [42]. In vitro studies demonstrate coagulation and platelet aggregation were reduced by 50% at a pH of 6.4, platelets increasingly disaggregate at a pH of 6.0, coagulation and platelet aggregation essentially stopped at a pH of 5.4, and fibrin clots dissolved at a pH of 4.0 [43]. In addition, increasing the pH above 4.0 virtually abolishes pepsin-induced clot lysis [44]. In vitro pepsins are able to break down the mucolytic barrier at pH < 5.0 [45] although in vivo studies are lacking.

Proton pump inhibitors only bind to actively secreting proton pumps [46]. The half-life of proton pumps in humans is 20–24 hours. As such, bolus therapy has proven ineffective in maintaining a gastric pH consistently above 4.0. To do so an initial bolus of 80 mg of omeprazole followed by 8 mg/h (HD-IV-PPI)

has proven effective in maintaining a pH above 6.0 [47,48]. Several RCTs of intravenous bolus followed by continuous infusion PPIs reported a decrease in the incidence of rebleeding plus decreased surgical interventions; however, no change in mortality was identified [49,50]. All three meta-analyses exploring the heterogeneous PPI studies concluded that overall these agents did decrease the incidence of rebleeding and need for surgical intervention [51–53]. The findings of these studies led to the recommendations from a consensus conference that PPI therapy may be effective and could be considered in the management of all patients with UGIB while awaiting endoscopy [54].

A closer look at the randomized clinical trial evidence only supports the efficacy of HD-IV-PPI if administered to patients with high-risk lesions, usually after successful endoscopic treatments. The concept that endoscopic therapy should be the mainstay of treatment with the decision whether or not to use PPI was emphasized in a 2003 study. The researchers noted that, in patients with a non-bleeding visible vessel or adherent clot lesions, the combination of endoscopic treatment (injection followed by thermal coagulation) followed by the administration of HD-IV-PPI was significantly superior to HD-IV-PPI alone in terms of rebleeding (0% and 9%, respectively, P = 0.01) but not mortality (2.6% and 5.1%, respectively, P > 0.20) [27]. There is no proven benefit of HD-IV-PPI in lesions at low risk for rebleed, information that can only be gleaned at endoscopy. In 2007, a placebo-controlled trial demonstrated that HD-IV-PPI infusion started prior to endoscopy in UGIB reduces the need for endoscopic therapy and the number of actively bleeding ulcers found at endoscopy [55]. More recent studies have examined the use of the oral rather than intravenous route to deliver these medications; however, further research is required to determine the role of this treatment.

In summary, based on current evidence, initiating HD-IV-PPI in patients who are unstable or suspected to be actively bleeding with a non-variceal UGIB is supported by the literature (Figs. 43.2, 43.3) [56]. For other patients the decision should be made at the time of endoscopy.

Question 8: In stabilized adult patients with a suspected lower gastrointestinal bleed (population), what initial diagnostic test (diagnostic test) provides the highest sensitivity and specificity (diagnostic test characteristics) to locate the source of bleeding (outcome)?

Search strategy

- MEDLINE, CENTRAL and EMBASE – search terms: (lower OR upper) AND gastrointestinal bleeds AND hemorrhage AND lower gastrointestinal tract AND (RCT OR sensitivity and specificity OR systematic review OR meta-analysis)

A systematic review of 13 studies using early colonoscopy as the diagnostic test of choice for LGIB found that a specific diagnosis was made 68% of the time (range 48% to 90%) with a 1.3%

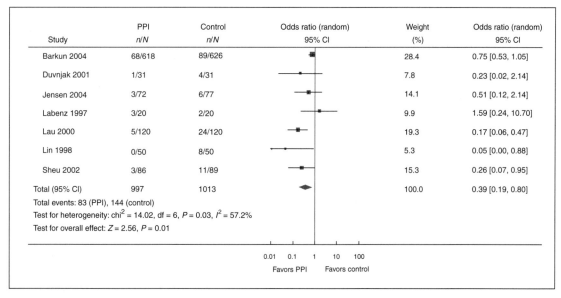

Figure 43.2 Comparison of rebleeding rates at 3 days for those patients receiving protein pump inhibitor (PPI) therapy versus placebo. (With permission from Leontiadis et al. [56], © Cochrane, Wiley.)

complication rate [57]. A review of four studies that evaluated colonoscopy as the initial investigation in LGIB evaluation found a diagnostic yield of 81% with a complication rate of 0.8% [58]. A review of 16 tagged erythrocyte studies (which may detect bleeds as small as 0.1–0.5 ml/min) on patients with clinical evidence of LGIB found a sensitivity of 0.78, a specificity of 0.73, a +LR of 2.89 (95% CI: 2.58 to 3.23) and a −LR of 0.30 (95% CI: 0.24 to 0.36) [57]. The major shortcoming of the tagged erythrocyte test was the

22% rate of inaccurate localization, making it unsafe to operate on the basis of this test alone. Angiography requires bleeding at a rate of 0.5–1.0 ml/min to allow detection of a lesion, and had a cumulative positive rate of 47% (range 27% to 77%) from 14 studies [57,58]. One study that compared both emergent endoscopy and angiography on the same 22 patients with severe hematochezia reported a diagnosis in 91% of endoscopies and only 14% of the angiograms [59].

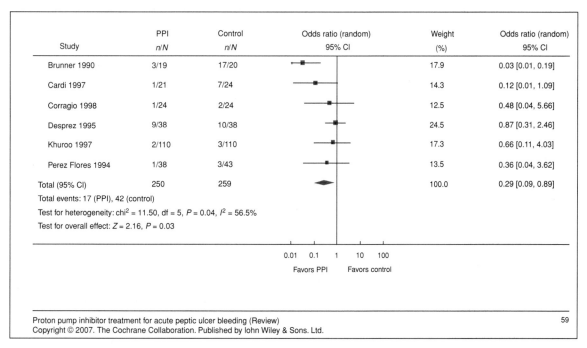

Figure 43.3 Comparison of the impact of protein pump inhibitor (PPI) therapy versus placebo on persistent peptic ulcer bleeding rates for patients still bleeding on arrival. (With permission from Leontiadis et al. [56], © Cochrane, Wiley.)

In an RCT comparing emergent colonoscopy to standard care for patients presenting with suspected LGIB, the mean time from presentation to procedure was 7.2 hours (4.2–7.6 hours) among those randomized to urgent colonoscopy, compared to 38.1 hours (27.2–74 hours) for those randomized to standard care. The likelihood of identifying a definite source of bleeding was greater in the urgent colonoscopy group (21 (42%) patients) than in the standard care group (11 (22%) patients); this represented a statistically significant increase in lesion identification (OR = 2.6; 95% CI: 1.1 to 6.2) [60].

In summary, like gastroscopy for UGIB, there appears to be a clear consensus that colonoscopy (following a colon prep) is the diagnostic test of choice for suspected LGIB. The one exception may be patients experiencing massive LGIB who are unable to safely undergo a timely colon prep for a colonoscopy; they may be best served by diagnostic angiography with embolization or immediate surgery [61].

Conclusions

The 56-year-old male described above who presented to the ED with a complaint of gastrointestinal bleeding has symptoms that suggest acute or chronic UGIB. Presenting at a convenient time, he underwent gastroscopy before leaving the ED. A duodenal ulcer with a visible vessel was identified and treated by epinephrine injection and thermal coagulation. He was admitted to hospital and treated with HD-IV-PPI. His *H. pylori* test was positive so he was started on eradication therapy and, after 48 hours with no evidence of rebleeding, was discharged on oral antibiotics and a PPI.

Gastrointestinal bleeding is a relatively common and important presentation in emergency medicine and determining the location of the bleed is an important step to managing these problems. Over the past decade, improvements in the diagnostic and treatment approach for gastrointestinal bleeding have been impressive. An organized approach using signs and symptoms, early endoscopy and a variety of treatments will lead clinicians to a more accurate and timely diagnosis of gastrointestinal bleeds.

Acknowledgments

The authors wish to thank Diane Milette for assistance with the manuscript preparations.

References

1 Longstreth GF. Epidemiology of hospitalizations for acute upper gastrointestinal hemorrhage: a population-based study. *Am J Gastroenterol* 1995;**90**:206–10.

2 Rockall TA, Logan RF, Devlin HB, Northfield TC. Incidence of and mortality from acute upper gastrointestinal haemorrhage in the United Kingdom. *BMJ* 1995;**311**:222–6.

3 Rollhauser C, Fleischer DE. Nonvariceal upper gastrointestinal bleeding: an update. *Endoscopy* 1997;**29**:91–105.

4 Wrenn KD, Thompson LB. Hemodynamically stable upper gastrointestinal bleeding. *Am J Emerg Med* 1991;**9**:309–12.

5 Targownik LE, Nabalamba A. Trends in the management and outcomes of acute nonvariceal upper gastrointestinal bleeding: 1993–2003. *Clin Gastro Hepatol* 2006;**4**:1459–66.

6 Longstreth GF. Epidemiology and outcome of patients hospitalized with acute lower gastrointestinal hemorrhage: a population-based study. *Am J Gastroenterol* 1997;**92**:419–24.

7 Laine L. Upper gastrointestinal bleeding. *Am Soc Gastro Endosc* 2007;**14**:1–4.

8 Witting MD, Magder L, Heins AE, Mattu A, Granja CA, Baumgarten M. ED predictors of upper gastrointestinal bleeding in patients without hematemesis. *Am J Emerg Med* 2006;**24**:280–85.

9 Zuckerman GR, Trellis DR, Sherman TM, Clouse RE. An objective measure of stool color for differentiating upper from lower gastrointestinal bleeding. *Dig Dis Sci* 1995;**40**:1614–21.

10 Hilsman JH. The color of blood-containing feces following the instillation of citrated blood at various levels of the small intestine. *Gastroenterology* 1950;**15**:131–4.

11 Peura DA, Lanza FL, Gostout CJ, Foutch PG. The American College of Gastroenterology Bleeding Registry: preliminary findings. *Am J Gastroenterol* 1997;**92**:924–8.

12 Ford AC, Delaney BC, Forman D, Moayyedi P. Eradication therapy for peptic ulcer disease in *Helicobacter pylori* positive patients. *Cochrane Database Syst Rev* 2006;**2**:CD003840 (doi:10.1002/14651858.CD003840.pub4).

13 Gisbert JP, Khorrami S, Carballo F, Calvert X, Gene E, Dominguez-Munoz JE. *H. pylori* eradication therapy vs. antisecretory non-eradication therapy (with or without longterm maintenance antisecretory therapy) for the prevention of recurrent bleeding from peptic ulcer (the Cochrane Collaboration). *Cochrane Database Syst Rev* 2004;**2**:CD004062 (doi: 10.1002/14651858.CD004062.pub2).

14 Lai KC, Lam SK, Chu KM, et al. Lansoprazole for the prevention of recurrences of ulcer complications from long-term low-dose aspirin use. *N Engl J Med* 2002;**346**:2033–8.

15 Sonnenberg A, Olson CA, Zhang J. The effect of antibiotic therapy on bleeding from duodenal ulcer. *Am J Gastroenterol* 1999;**94**:950–54.

16 Rockey DC, Auslander A, Greenberg PD. Detection of upper gastrointestinal blood with fecal occult blood tests. *Am J Gastroenterol* 1999;**94**:344–50.

17 Bowen B, Yuan Y, James C, Rashid F, Hunt RH. Time course and pattern of blood loss with ibuprofen treatment in healthy subjects. *Clin Gastro Hepatol* 2005;**3**:1075–82.

18 Feinberg EJ, Steinberg WM, Banks BL, Henry JP. How long to abstain from eating red meat before fecal occult blood tests. *Ann Intern Med* 1990;**113**:403–4.

19 Eisner MS, Lewis JH. Diagnostic yield of a positive fecal occult blood test found on digital rectal examination. *Arch Intern Med* 1991;**151**:2180–84.

20 Simon JB. Fecal occult blood testing: clinical value and limitations. *Gastroenterologist* 1998;**6**:66–78.

21 Coles EF, Starnes EC. Use of HemoQuant assays to assess the effect of oral iron preparations on stool hemoccult tests. *Am J Gastroenterol* 1991;**86**:1442–4.

22 Barkun A, Bardou M, Marshall JK. Consensus recommendations for managing patients with nonvariceal upper gastrointestinal bleeding. *Ann Intern Med* 2003;**139**:843–57.

23 Spiegel BM, Vakil NB, Ofman JJ. Endoscopy for acute nonvariceal upper gastrointestinal tract hemorrhage: is sooner better? A systematic review. *Arch Intern Med* 2001;**161**:1393–404.

24 Jiranek GC, Kozarek RA. A cost-effective approach to the patient with peptic ulcer bleeding. *Surg Clin North Am* 1996;**76**:83–103.

25 Cooper GS, Chak A, Connors AF, Harper DL, Rosenthal GE. The effectiveness of early endoscopy for upper gastrointestinal hemorrhage: a community-based analysis. *Med Care* 1998;**36**:462–74.

26 da Silveira EB, Lam E, Martel M, et al. The importance of process issues as predictors of time to endoscopy in patients with acute upper-GI bleeding using the RUGBE data. *Gastrointest Endosc* 2006;**64**:299–309.

27 Sung JJ, Chan FK, Lau JY, et al. The effect of endoscopic therapy in patients receiving omeprazole for bleeding ulcers with nonbleeding visible vessels or adherent clots: a randomized comparison. *Ann Intern Med* 2003;**139**:237–43.

28 Jensen DM, Kovacs TOG, Jutabha R, et al. Randomized controlled trial of medical therapy compared to endoscopic therapy for prevention of recurrent ulcer hemorrhage in patients with non-bleeding adherent clots. *Gastroenterology* 2002;**123**:407–13.

29 Rostom A, Dube C, Wells G, et al. Prevention of NSAID-induced gastroduodenal ulcers. Cochrane Database Syst Rev 2002;**4**:CD002296 (doi: 10.1002/14651858.CD002296).

30 Brown TJ, Hooper L, Elliott RA, Payne K, Webb R, Roberts C. A comparison of the cost-effectiveness of five strategies for the prevention of non-steroidal anti-inflammatory drug-induced gastrointestinal toxicity: a systematic review with economic modelling. *Health Technology Assessment* 2006;**10**(38).

31 Solomon SD, McMurray JJV, Pfeffer MA, et al. Cardiovascular risk associated with celecoxib in a clinical trial for colorectal adenoma prevention. *N Engl J Med* 2005;**352**:1071–80.

32 Bombardier C, Laine L, Reicin A, et al. Comparison of upper gastrointestinal toxicity of rofecoxib and naproxen in patients with rheumatoid arthritis. *N Engl J Med* 2000;**343**:1520–28.

33 Bresalier RS, Sandler RS, Quan H, et al. Cardiovascular events associated with rofecoxib in a colorectal adenoma chemoprevention trial. *N Engl J Med* 2005;**352**:1092–102.

34 Barkun A, Fallone CA, Chiba N, et al. A Canadian clinical practice algorithm for the management of patients with nonvariceal upper gastrointestinal bleeding. *Can J Gastroenterol* 2004;**18**(10):605–9.

35 Zuccaro GJ. Management of the adult patient with acute lower gastrointestinal bleeding. *Am J Gastroenterol* 1998;**93**:1202–8.

36 Al Qahtani AR, Satin R, Stern J, Gordon PH. Investigative modalities for massive lower gastrointestinal bleeding. *World J Surg* 2002;**26**:620–25.

37 Jensen DM, Machicado GA. Diagnosis and treatment of severe hematochezia. The role of urgent colonoscopy after purge. *Gastroenterology* 1988;**95**:1569–74.

38 Witting MD, Magder L, Heins AE, Mattu A, Granja CA, Baumgarten M. Usefulness and validity of diagnostic nasogastric aspiration in patients without hematemesis. *Ann Emerg Med* 2004;**43**:525–32.

39 Aljebreen AM, Fallone CA, Barkun AN. Nasogastric aspirate predicts high-risk endoscopic lesions in patients with acute upper gastrointestinal bleeding. *Gastrointest Endosc* 2004;**59**:172–8.

40 Singer AJ, Richman PB, Kowalska A, Thode HC. Comparison of patient and practitioner assessments of pain from commonly performed emergency department procedures. *Ann Emerg Med* 1999;**33**:652–8.

41 Leung FW. The venerable nasogastric tube (Editorial). *Gastrointest Endosc* 2004;**59**:255–60.

42 Kolkman JJ, Meuwissen SG. A review on treatment of bleeding peptic ulcer: a collaborative task of gastroenterologist and surgeon. *Scand J Gastroenterol* 1996;**218**:16–25.

43 Green FW, Kaplan MM, Curtis LE, et al. Effect of acid and pepsin on blood coagulation and platelet aggregation. *Gastroenterology* 1978;**74**:38–43.

44 Patchett SE, O'Donoghue DP. Pharmacological manipulation of gastric juice: thrombelastographic assessment and implications for treatment of gastrointestinal haemorrhage. *Gut* 1995;**36**:358–62.

45 Pearsson JP, Ward R, Allen A, Roberts NB, Taylor WH. Mucus degradation by pepsin: comparison of mucolytic activity of human pepsin 1 and pepsin 3: implications in peptic ulceration. *Gut* 1986;**27**:243–8.

46 Straathof JWA, Gielkens HAJ, Wurst W, et al. Pentagastrin enhances the effect of intravenous pantoprazole (Abstract). *Gastroenterology* 1997;**112**:A299.

47 Kiilerich S, Rannem T, Elsborg L. Effect of intravenous infusion of omeprazole and ranitidine or twenty-four-hour intragastric pH in patients with a history of duodenal ulcer. *Digestion* 1995;**56**:25–30.

48 Wilder-Smith CH, Bettschen H-U, Merki HS. Individual and group dose-responses to intravenous omeprazole in the first 24 h: pH-feedback-controlled and fixed-dose infusions. *Br J Clin Pharmacol* 1995;**39**:15–23.

49 Lau JYW, Sung JJY, Lee KKC, et al. Effect of intravenous omeprazole on recurrent bleeding after endoscopic treatment of bleeding peptic ulcers. *N Engl J Med* 2000;**343**:310–16.

50 Lin H-J, Lo W-C, Lee F-Y, Perng C-L, Tseng G-Y. A prospective randomized comparative trial showing that omeprazole prevents re-bleeding in patients with bleeding peptic ulcer after successful endoscopic therapy. *Arch Intern Med* 1998;**158**:54–8.

51 Selby NM, Kubba AK, Hawkby CJ. Acid suppression in peptic ulcer haemorrhage: a 'metaanalysis'. *Aliment Pharm Therap* 2000;**14**:1119–26.

52 Gisbert JP, Gonzalez L, Calvet X, et al. Proton pump inhibitors versus H2 antagonists: a meta-analysis of their efficacy in treating bleeding peptic ulcer. *Aliment Pharm Therap* 2001;**15**:917–26.

53 Zed PJ, Loewen PS, Slavik RS, et al. Meta-analysis of proton pump inhibitors in treatment of bleeding peptic ulcers. *Ann Pharmacother* 2001;**35**:1528–34.

54 Barkun A, Bardou M, Marshall JK. Consensus recommendations for managing patients with nonvariceal upper gastrointestinal bleeding. *Ann Intern Med* 2003;**139**:843–57.

55 Lau JY, Leung WK, Wu CJY, et al. Omeprazole before endoscopy in patients with gastrointestinal bleeding. *N Engl J Med* 2007;**356**:1631–40.

56 Leontiadis GI, Sharma VK, Howden CW. Proton pump inhibitor treatment for acute peptic ulcer bleeding. *Cochrane Database Syst Rev* 2006;**1**:CD002094 (doi: 10.1002/14651858.CD002094.pub3).

57 Zuckerman GR, Prakash C. Acute lower intestinal bleeding. Part I: Clinical presentation and diagnosis. *Gastrointest Endosc* 1998;**48**:606–17.

58 Bloomfeld RS, Rockey DC. Diagnosis and management of lower gastrointestinal bleeding. *Curr Opin Gastroenterol* 2000;**16**:89–97.

59 Jensen DM, Machicado GA. Colonoscopy for diagnosis and treatment of severe lower gastrointestinal bleeding: routine outcomes and cost analysis. *Gastrointest Endosc* 1997;**7**:477–98.

60 Green BT, Rockey DC, Portwood G, et al. Urgent colonoscopy for evaluation and management of acute lower gastrointestinal hemorrhage: a randomized controlled trial. *Am J Gastroenterol* 2005;**100**:2395–402.

61 Farrell JJ, Friedman LS. The management of lower gastrointestinal bleeding. *Aliment Pharm Therap* 2005;**21**:1281–98.

7 Neurosciences

44 Transient Ischemic Attack

Ted Glynn

Michigan State University, Emergency Medicine Residency, Lansing *and* Colleges of Human and Osteopathic Medicine, Michigan State University, East Lansing *and* Ingham Regional Medical Center, Lansing, USA

Case scenario

A 65-year-old diabetic male presents to the emergency department (ED) accompanied by his wife. The patient states that approximately 1 hour prior to arrival he experienced sudden right arm weakness and speech difficulty shortly after placing his entrée order at his favorite neighborhood restaurant. So as not to cause a scene, his wife sat next to him in the booth and immediately assessed his blood sugar via a glucometer with a result of 125 mg/dl (6.88 mmol/L). The patient and his wife stated that the symptoms appeared to have completely resolved after approximately 10–15 minutes, upon which they cancelled their order and proceeded to your ED for further evaluation.

Upon arrival in triage, the patient's vital signs were blood pressure 160/95 mmHg, pulse rate 65 beats/min, respiratory rate 16 breaths/min and temperature of 37.1°C (oral). The patient was well appearing, ambulatory and speaking clearly in full sentences. Upon entering the room, the patient stated that he felt "great" and was mistaken in rushing to the ED. He stated that he was embarrassed for taking up a bed and wasting your time; however, he was initially frightened by this spell, which he thought was a stroke. He convinced himself that it was just a matter of being "wiped out" following his golf outing this morning. You evaluate the patient and are concerned he may have experienced a transient ischemic attack (TIA). He appreciates your concern but would rather depart the chaotic ED environment and follow-up with his primary care doctor first thing next week.

Background

Transient ischemic attacks afflict an estimated 300,000 Americans every year [1,2]. Physicians practicing emergency medicine are faced with identifying and dispositioning patients presenting with

Evidence-based Emergency Medicine. Edited by Brian H. Rowe
© 2009 Blackwell Publishing, ISBN: 978-1-4051-6143-5.

symptoms suggestive of TIA on a daily basis. Traditionally, a focal neurological deficit lasting less than 24 hours defined a TIA. There has been a proposal to change the definition of a TIA to "a brief episode of neurological dysfunction caused by a focal disturbance of brain or retinal ischemia, with clinical symptoms typically lasting less than 1 hour, and without evidence of infarction" [3]. Thus a TIA should be considered akin to "unstable angina of the brain" and thus a near-term harbinger of subsequent stroke and its devastating consequences.

Approximately 700,000 people suffer a stroke each year in the USA, 23% of whom die within 1 year. Only 50–70% of stroke survivors regain functional independence, and 15–30% are permanently disabled. Institutional care is required by 20% of stroke survivors 3 months after onset. The cost of stroke in both human and economic terms is onerous and results in direct medical expenditures estimated to be around US$53 billion dollars a year [4]. Clearly, stroke is a disease where prevention is critically important. Therefore, TIAs should not be considered in isolation; instead TIAs should be viewed as part of an acute cerebrovascular ischemic continuum, which may ultimately result in a debilitating stroke. Thus it is paramount that the emergency medicine physician identifies such patients and facilitates timely diagnostic evaluation and preventive therapeutic interventions (both medical and surgical).

Despite the prevalence of cerebrovascular disease, as well as advances in imaging modalities of the brain, the clinical diagnosis of acute cerebrovascular ischemia (stroke and TIA) at times remains a challenge for physicians [5,6]. The use of computerized tomography (CT) of the brain in the acute setting has clear utility in excluding intracranial hemorrhage or mass lesions; however, CT does little to "rule in" or "rule out" a TIA. While perfusion and diffusion weighted magnetic resonance imaging (MRI) has provided further diagnostic capabilities in the setting of acute cerebrovascular ischemia, it still has limitations for use in the majority of EDs because of its lack of routine availability, examination time and patient cooperation.

The cumulative risk of stroke within the first 3 months after a TIA has been reported to be ~10% in selected populations [2,7–9]. More recently, several studies have revealed a significant risk of stroke within days of the sentinel TIA [10–13]. Therefore, properly identifying the patient with a TIA is essential and provides an opportunity to avert a completed stroke in a subset of patients at early risk of such an event. However, the exact nature, place and timing of interventions to reduce stroke risk in TIA patients have yet to be fully elucidated [1,14]. Patients with TIAs require prompt clinical evaluation to assess for potentially reversible underlying disease processes [15,16], which usually entails brain imaging (CT or MRI), electocardiogram (ECG), vascular imaging (i.e., carotid Doppler ultrasound, CT or magnetic resonance angiography) and possibly echocardiography [17]. Potential treatments include antiplatelet therapy, anticoagulation therapy and carotid endarterectomy or stent [15,16].

Ultimately, the emergency medicine physician must weigh competing factors when considering the degree and timing of further diagnostic evaluation despite the fact that in most cases the symptoms have completely resolved and the patient may appear remarkably well. The clinician must decide if this "spell" represented a TIA and, if so, attempt to quantify the patient's near-term risk of subsequent stroke. This prognostic information may guide the initial diagnostic work-up, therapy and appropriate disposition. This chapter examines the evidence for risk stratification of patients presenting with symptoms suggestive of TIA and the approach to the ED evaluation and management that may ultimately reduce the subsequent risk of completed stroke that this illness presages.

Clinical questions

1 In patients presenting to the ED with transient ischemic attack (population), what is the risk (prognosis) of subsequent cerebrovascular accident or stroke (outcomes) over the following 90 days (follow-up)?

2 In patients presenting to the ED with transient ischemic attack (population), are there valid and reliable clinical criteria (clinical prediction guides) that can accurately predict the risk of subsequent stroke (outcome)?

3 In patients diagnosed with transient ischemic attack (population), does aspirin combined with dipyridamole (treatment) result in lower morbidity and mortality (outcomes) than aspirin alone (control)?

4 In patients presenting to the ED with transient ischemic attack and evidence of carotid stenosis (population), does carotid endarterectomy (treatment) result in lower morbidity and mortality (outcomes) than medical therapy alone (control)?

5 In patients presenting to the ED with transient ischemic attack (population), does initiation of oral anticoagulation (treatment) result in lower morbidity and mortality (outcomes) than antiplatelet agents (control)?

6 In patients presenting to the ED with transient ischemic attack (population), does diffusion weighted MRI (intervention) identify patients at high risk for subsequent stroke over the following 90 days (outcome) more often than CT scan (control)?

7 In patients presenting to the ED with transient ischemic attack (population), does initiation of intravenous heparin or low molecular weight heparin (intervention) result in lower morbidity and mortality (outcomes) than standard care without anticoagulants (control)?

8 In patients presenting to the ED with transient ischemic attack (population), does urgent (within 48 hours) carotid imaging (intervention) identify patients at high risk for subsequent stroke over the following 90 days (outcome) more than delayed imaging (control)?

General search strategy

You begin to address these questions by searching for evidence in the common electronic databases such as the Cochrane Library, MEDLINE and EMBASE looking specifically for systematic reviews and meta-analyses. The Cochrane Database of Systematic Reviews (CDSR) includes high-quality systematic review evidence on therapy for TIAs. You also search the Cochrane Central Register of Controlled Trials (CENTRAL) and MEDLINE to identify randomized controlled trials (RCTs) that became available after the publication date of the systematic review or, if no systematic reviews were identified, to locate high-quality RCTs that directly address the clinical question. In addition, access to relevant, updated, evidence-based clinical practice guidelines (CPGs) on TIA are used to determine the consensus rating of areas lacking evidence.

Searching for evidence synthesis: primary search strategy
- Cochrane Library: transient ischemic attack OR TIA AND (topic)
- MEDLINE: transient ischemic attack OR TIA AND (systematic review OR meta-analysis OR metaanalysis) AND (topic)

Critical review of the literature

Your search strategy for the Cochrane Library and MEDLINE identified several pertinent and relevant articles to this series of questions.

Question 1: In patients presenting to the ED with transient ischemic attack (population), what is the risk of subsequent cerebrovascular accident or stroke over the following 90 days (outcome)?

Search strategy

- MEDLINE: risk of stroke after TIA OR risk of stroke after transient ischemic attack. Limited to English, published in the last 10 years, humans

Historically, patients presenting to the ED with symptoms suggestive of TIA have had varied work-ups and disposition. In the

1980s, the risk of subsequent stroke in the first year following a TIA was estimated to be between 6.6% for a hospital referred cohort [18] and 11.6% for a community-based cohort [19], and many practitioners deemed further evaluation via routine outpatient follow-up as adequate. Not until early in this decade did new data come to light that quantified the very early risk of stroke in patients following a sentinel TIA.

Several recent cohort studies [2,20–22] have confirmed that TIA patients have at least a 10% risk of stroke during the subsequent 90 days. A study by Johnston and colleagues [2] of 1707 TIA patients presenting to 16 EDs affiliated with a northern California health maintenance organization found the 90-day risk of stroke to be 10.5%, with half of the events occurring within the first 48 hours of ED presentation. Overall, one in four subjects had a major adverse event within 90 days. Three other population-based studies from Europe and the USA independently describe similar event rates (9.5–14.6%) [20–22].

This strikingly high risk of suffering a stroke (5%) within the first 48 hours following a TIA poses a dilemma for the emergency clinician. It is apparent that only the most robust and timely outpatient work-ups would capture those patients at very early, albeit high, risk of stroke. Despite the significant prognostic impact of TIAs, there is no definitive guidance concerning the early evaluation and disposition of patients presenting to the ED. The rationale for hospitalization of TIA cases is to expeditiously obtain diagnostic studies, evaluate risks, monitor for worsening symptoms, and to institute interventions including possible administration of thrombolytic therapy in instances of progression to stroke [14,23]. However, there are no prospective data supporting the inpatient evaluation of TIA patients, thus the major clinical guideline developed by the American Heart Association states that "the decision to hospitalize depends on the patient's individual circumstance" [1,15]. Recently, the National Stroke Association guidelines for the management of TIAs, published by an expert panel, state that "hospitalization should be considered for patients with their first transient ischemic attack within the past 24 to 48 hours to facilitate possible early deployment of lytic therapy and other medical management if symptoms recur and to expedite institution of definitive secondary prevention" [23]. However, this is a category 4 recommendation based on evidence drawn from descriptive case series and reports, ecological studies, cross-sectional studies, cohort studies using historical controls, expert medical opinion and general consensus [23].

In summary, considerable variation exists in terms of the decision for inpatient versus outpatient evaluation [24–26]. Even among hospitalized subjects there is considerable variability in the evaluations and treatments completed [26,27]. It is important to note that the approach of admitting all suspected TIA patients, as recommended by some authors [28,29], is not cost-effective [30]. Thus, in view of an absolute stroke risk of ~5% in the first 48 hours, the difficulty then arises in determining which TIA patients warrant expedited evaluation in the ED or inpatient admission.

Question 2: In patients presenting to the ED with transient ischemic attack (population), are there valid and reliable clinical criteria (clinical prediction guides) that can accurately predict the risk of subsequent stroke (outcome)?

Search strategy

- PubMed – clinical queries, search by clinical study category: risk of stroke after TIA. Category: prognosis; scope: narrow, specific search

Is there a decision tool based on historical and clinical findings that can reliably identify the 5–10% of patients who are at considerable short-term risk of stroke even before an expedited diagnostic evaluation can be accomplished? A clinical decision rule that allows emergency physicians to objectively quantify the risk for an individual patient might be useful when making the decision whether to admit or facilitate an outpatient evaluation. Not all clinical prediction rules are created equally and the clinician must consider the following when evaluating the potential impact of using prediction rules to make clinical decisions: reliability, validity, sensibility and impact potential [31].

Multiple investigators have previously used community-based studies to derive risk factors for subsequent stroke; however, they were unable to prospectively validate a clinical decision rule that accurately predicted the risk of subsequent stroke in patients with TIAs [32,33]. These early attempts failed to consistently identify the high-risk subgroup who might benefit from hospitalization for immediate work-up and monitoring. Further complicating the process is the fact that clinicians frequently struggle with uncertainty regarding the diagnosis of TIA. Despite the classic definition describing TIA as a sudden, focal neurological deficit lasting less than 24 hours, the duration of symptoms is typically <1 hour and thus patients are frequently asymptomatic upon ED evaluation [16,17,34]. TIA remains a clinical diagnosis [16,17] for the majority of ED physicians yet the inter-observer reliability concerning its diagnosis is often poor [35–38].

Two clinical prediction rules have been independently developed (Table 44.1). The California Rule [2] was derived by Johnston and colleagues as described above. In Europe, the ABCD Rule [39] was derived from a cohort with a first-ever probable or definite TIA who had been referred to a neurologist. Subsequent validation of the ABCD Rule involved two cohorts (clinic based and hospital referred). Investigators from both of these studies collaborated to derive a unified score optimized for prediction of 2-day stroke risk following presentation with a suspected TIA [40]. The ABCD^2 score (0–7 points) is calculated by evaluating five factors: **a**ge ($\geq$60 years, 1 point), **b**lood pressure at presentation ($\geq$140/90 mmHg, 1 point), **c**linical features (unilateral weakness, 2 points; speech disturbance without weakness, 1 point), **d**uration of symptoms ($\geq$60 minutes, 2 points; 10–59 minutes, 1 point) and **d**iabetes (1 point). Subsequent 2-day stroke risk based on the ABCD^2 score is 1% (0–3 points), 4% (4–5 points) or 8% (6–7 points). The ABCD^2

Table 44.1 California, ABCD and ABCD² scoring sytems, their components and stroke risks.

Scoring system	Derivation cohort (*N*)	Validation cohorts (*N*)	Outcome	Rule factors	Stroke risk (%) depending on risk score/points	
California	1707	None	90-day stroke risk	Age	Risk points[†]	%
				Diabetes	0	0
				Symptom duration	1	3
				Weakness	2	7
				Speech impaired	3	11
				(1 point/factor)	4	15
					5	34
ABCD	209	778	7-day stroke risk	Age	Risk score[‡]	%
				Blood pressure	(0–3)	0
				Clinical features	4	2
				Duration of	5	16
				symptoms	6	36
ABCD²	1916	2893	2-day stroke risk	Age	Risk score[*]	%
				Blood pressure	Low (0–3)	1
				Clinical features	Moderate (4–5)	4
				Duration of	High (6–7)	8
				symptoms		
				Diabetes		

[*]Ninety-day stroke risk.
[†]Seven-day stroke risk.
[‡]Two-day stroke risk.

score was retrospectively validated using the datasets from four previously conducted cohort studies [40].

In summary, there are no prospectively validated ED-based stratification tools to assist emergency clinicians to decide on the risk of immediate stroke following TIAs. The ABCD² score appears to be the best available tool in risk stratifying patients at short-term (2-day) risk of stroke after a suspected TIA. Patients identified as being high risk (score 6–7 points) by the ABCD² score are candidates for immediate evaluation to optimize stroke prevention and possibly therapeutic intervention should symptoms recur. Patients with a score <3 may be suitable for further outpatient evaluation following discharge on an antiplatelet agent, although this strategy has not been prospectively validated.

Question 3: In patients diagnosed with transient ischemic attack (population), does aspirin combined with dipyridamole (treatment) result in lower morbidity and mortality (outcomes) than aspirin alone (control)?

Search strategy

- PubMed – clinical queries, systematic reviews: (antiplatelet OR clopidogrel OR aspirin) AND (transient ischemic attack OR TIA)

Patients with TIA or non-disabling ischemic stroke have an annual risk of serious vascular events (death, stroke, myocardial infarction) of between 4% and 11% based on clinical trial cohorts and population-based studies [41,42]. A collaborative meta-analysis encompassing 287 randomized trials (both primary and secondary stroke prevention) and over 135,000 patients concluded that antiplatelet therapy provided absolute reductions in the risk of having a serious vascular event of 36 per 1000 treated for 2 years among those with previous stroke or TIA (number needed to treat (NNT) = 28) [43]. Twenty-one trials specifically evaluating any antiplatelet therapy versus control in high-risk patients with prior stroke or TIA revealed a 17% relative risk reduction (RRR) in subsequent serious vascular events (NNT = 28). The addition of dipyridamole to aspirin was associated with a nonsignificant 6% additional reduction in serious vascular events in comparison to aspirin alone [43]. The ESPS-2[a] randomized controlled trial enrolling patients with both stroke and TIA reported that combination treatment (aspirin + dipyridamole) resulted in an RRR of 22% (NNT = 35) for serious vascular events compared to aspirin alone [44]. However, it must be stressed that TIA-only patients accounted for only approximately 25% of the study subjects in this trial and results were not reported for this subgroup.

Another high-quality systematic review assessing the efficacy and safety of adding dipyridamole in the secondary prevention of stroke and other vascular events in patients with vascular disease included 27 trials and encompassed 20,242 patients [45]. There was no evidence of a mortality benefit, based on 11 trials, when evaluating combination therapy (dipyridamole + aspirin) versus aspirin alone. In the presence of aspirin, dipyridamole was associated with a significant reduction in vascular events (RR = 0.90;

95% CI: 0.82 to 0.97); this, however, became non-significant when the ESPS-2[a] trial data was excluded.

The ESPIRIT trial was an RCT evaluating aspirin plus dipyridamole versus aspirin alone and subsequent vascular events in patients who had suffered TIA or minor ischemic stroke in the preceding 6 months [46]. Overall, 2763 patients who had a minor ischemic stroke (66%), TIA (28%) or transient monocular blindness (5%) of presumed arterial origin in the preceding 6 months were randomized to either aspirin alone or aspirin once daily plus dipyridamole twice daily. Important exclusions in this study were patients with cardioembolic source and significant carotid disease. The main results at a mean follow-up of 3.5 years found a decrease in the risks for the composite endpoint (death from all vascular causes, stroke, myocardial infarction or major bleeding event) with an RRR of 19% (95% CI: 2% to 32%) and an NNT of 35 (95% CI: 20 to 347). ESPIRIT investigators updated a previously reported meta-analysis to include these data; based on six trials and over 7000 patients, the RR was 0.82 (95% CI: 0.74 to 0.91) for the composite outcome of vascular death, non-fatal stroke or non-fatal myocardial infarction [46].

In summary, when contraindications are absent, aspirin plus dipyridamole appears to be more effective than aspirin alone in preventing subsequent serious vascular events following TIA or minor ischemic stroke. Emergency physicians should consider this treatment if hemorrhagic stroke has been ruled out and patient bleeding risks have been assessed.

Question 4: In patients presenting to the ED with transient ischemic attack and evidence of carotid stenosis (population), does carotid endarterectomy (treatment) result in lower morbidity and mortality (outcomes) than medical therapy alone (control)?

Search strategy

- PubMed – clinical queries, systematic reviews: endarterectomy AND systematic AND (symptomatic OR TIA)

Carotid stenosis is an important cause of debilitating stroke. Patients who present with symptoms suggestive of cerebrovascular ischemia and found to have carotid stenosis have an annual stroke risk of approximately 6%. Even patients who are asymptomatic, yet harbor severe carotid stenosis, have an 11% risk of stroke over the subsequent 5 years.

Two large trials – NASCET (North American Symptomatic Carotid Endarterectomy Trial) and ECST (European Carotid Surgery Trial) – encompassing 5950 patients with symptomatic carotid stenosis who were randomized to best medical therapy with or without carotid endarterectomy, provide the bulk of the evidence supporting endarterectomy [47,48]. A systematic review [49] which included these two large trials revealed an RRR of 48% (95% CI: 27% to 73%) in the composite outcome of disabling stroke or death in patients with severe stenosis (ECST ≥80%

stenosis; NASCET ≥70%) undergoing carotid endarterectomy (NNT = 15). The degree of benefit is less for moderate stenosis (ECST = 70–79%; NASCET = 50–69%) (Fig. 44.1) and surgery was actually harmful in patients with lesser degrees of stenosis. Importantly, these outcomes were associated with patients who had reasonable pre-operative risk profiles and surgeons with complication rates of 6% or less.

In summary, patients presenting with symptomatic, moderate to severe carotid stenosis derive a significant reduction in disabling stroke or death by undergoing carotid endarterectomy in comparison to best medical therapy alone.

Question 5: In patients presenting to the ED with transient ischemic attack (population), does initiation of oral anticoagulation (treatment) result in lower morbidity and mortality (outcomes) than antiplatelet agents (control)?

Search strategy

- PubMed – clinical queries, systematic reviews: anticoagulants AND transient ischemic attack

There is an approximately 9% annual risk of serious adverse vascular events in patients who have suffered a TIA or minor stroke [42]. Aspirin plus dipyridamole provides a 19% RRR in untoward vascular events compared to aspirin alone [46]. The use of oral anticoagulants has been shown to provide significant clinical benefits following non-cerebrovascular events and thus may seem appealing in patients following TIA or minor stroke.

A systematic review [50], encompassing five trials and over 4000 patients, evaluated the use of oral anticoagulants versus antiplatelet therapy for secondary prevention of serious vascular events in patients following TIA or minor stroke. Medium- (international normalized ratio (INR) 2.1 to 3.6) to high-intensity (INR 3.0 to 4.5) anticoagulation did not offer any advantage over any antiplatelet therapy alone in important vascular endpoints or death (Fig. 44.2). High-intensity anticoagulation was associated with a significantly increased risk of major bleeding complications compared to any antiplatelet therapy (RR = 9.0; 95% CI: 3.9 to 21).

The WASID trial was a randomized, double-blind, multi-center trial evaluating medium-intensity anticoagulation (INR 2.0 to 3.0) versus aspirin in 569 patients following a TIA or stroke caused by an angiographically verified stenosis (>50%) of an intracranial artery [51]. Medium-intensity anticoagulation failed to reduce serious vascular events compared to aspirin and was associated with increased morbidity and all-cause mortality.

In summary, oral anticoagulation does not offer any advantage over aspirin alone and appears to be harmful with high-intensity anticoagulation (maintaining INR > 3.0). Emergency physicians should not consider routine anticoagulation of patients with stable TIAs.

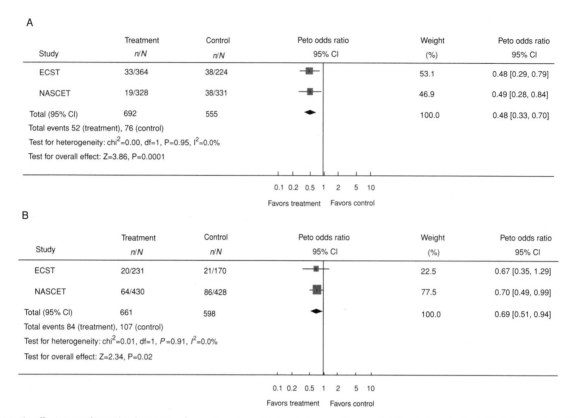

Figure 44.1 The effectiveness of carotid endarterectomy for symptomatic carotid stenosis for preventing any disabling stroke or death: A, 80–99% stenosis; B, 50–69% stenosis. INR, international normalized ratio. (Reproduced with permission from Cina et al. [49], © Wiley.)

Question 6: In patients presenting to the ED with transient ischemic attack (population), does initiation of intravenous heparin or low molecular weight heparin (intervention) result in lower morbidity and mortality (outcomes) than standard care without anticoagulants (control)?

Search strategy

- Cochrane Library (CDSR): anticoagulation AND (ischemic stroke OR transient ischemic attack)

The Cochrane reviews [52–55] identified 43 studies involving over 43,000 patients with ischemic stroke or TIA who received anticoagulation compared to placebo or antiplatelet therapy. Unfortunately, the reviews do not provide sufficient data on the outcomes for TIA patients specifically. While some of the trials included TIA patients, others did not, and outcomes are not provided for TIA subgroups. While direct evidence is not available for TIA, heparin does not provide an improvement in important outcomes in ischemic stroke and at the same time clearly increases morbidity due to an increase in bleeding complications.

In summary, emergency physicians should not consider routine anticoagulation with heparin or low molecular weight heparin in patients with TIA. Consensus recommendations suggest that patients with certain conditions may benefit from anticoagulation (e.g., cardioembolic TIAs); however, these decisions should be made following consultation with the appropriate neurosciences specialist(s).

Question 7: In patients presenting to the ED with transient ischemic attack (population), does diffusion weighted MRI (intervention) identify patients at high risk for subsequent stroke over the following 90 days (outcome) more often than CT scan (control)?

Search strategy

- PubMed – clinical queries, systematic reviews: MRI AND transient ischemic attack

Approximately 50% of TIA patients who undergo magnetic resonance diffusion weighted imaging (DWI) demonstrate a DWI abnormality [56]. The presence of multiple DWI lesions and lesions of varying ages have both been reported to portend a higher early risk of subsequent ischemic events [56]. The identification and quantification of DWI lesions may assist in the risk stratification of TIA patients.

In a prospective cohort of 83 ED patients with symptoms consistent with transient cerebral ischemia and a symptom duration

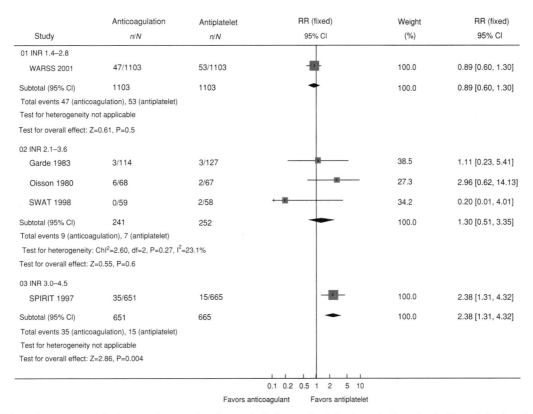

Study	Anticoagulation n/N	Antiplatelet n/N	RR (fixed) 95% CI	Weight (%)	RR (fixed) 95% CI
01 INR 1.4–2.8					
WARSS 2001	47/1103	53/1103		100.0	0.89 [0.60, 1.30]
Subtotal (95% CI)	1103	1103		100.0	0.89 [0.60, 1.30]
Total events 47 (anticoagulation), 53 (antiplatelet)					
Test for heterogeneity not applicable					
Test for overall effect: Z=0.61, P=0.5					
02 INR 2.1–3.6					
Garde 1983	3/114	3/127		38.5	1.11 [0.23, 5.41]
Oisson 1980	6/68	2/67		27.3	2.96 [0.62, 14.13]
SWAT 1998	0/59	2/58		34.2	0.20 [0.01, 4.01]
Subtotal (95% CI)	241	252		100.0	1.30 [0.51, 3.35]
Total events 9 (anticoagulation), 7 (antiplatelet)					
Test for heterogeneity: Chi²=2.60, df=2, P=0.27, I²=23.1%					
Test for overall effect: Z=0.55, P=0.6					
03 INR 3.0–4.5					
SPIRIT 1997	35/651	15/665		100.0	2.38 [1.31, 4.32]
Subtotal (95% CI)	651	665		100.0	2.38 [1.31, 4.32]
Total events 35 (anticoagulation), 15 (antiplatelet)					
Test for heterogeneity not applicable					
Test for overall effect: Z=2.86, P=0.004					

0.1 0.2 0.5 1 2 5 10

Favors anticoagulant   Favors antiplatelet

Figure 44.2 Anticoagulants versus antiplatelet agents for preventing all-cause death after transient ischemic attacks. (Reproduced with permission from Algra et al. [50], © Wiley.)

of >1 hour, the presence of a DWI abnormality was an independent predictor of a cerebrovascular ischemic event in the subsequent 90 days [57]. A systematic review involving 19 studies reported that the following clinical predictor variables were independently associated with DWI abnormality: symptom duration >60 minutes, dysphasia, dysarthria and motor weakness [58].

In summary, the presence of DWI abnormality in patients with symptoms of cerebrovascular ischemia may be useful in helping to predict subsequent stroke risk. Larger prospective studies will be required to validate whether the addition of MRI to detect DWI abnormalities will strengthen existing clinical prediction rules or alter clinical management in the ED setting.

Question 8: In patients presenting to the ED with transient ischemic attack (population), does urgent (within 48 hours) carotid imaging (intervention) identify patients at high risk for subsequent stroke over the following 90 days (outcome) more than delayed imaging (control)?

Search strategy

- PubMed and Cochrane Library – clinical queries: urgent carotid imaging

Despite extensive searching for research directly addressing this important clinical question, currently there is insufficient evidence to decide on the specific timing for carotid imaging after a TIA. Since carotid stenosis can be a cause of stroke, and some evidence suggests patients have a stroke soon after their TIA, it seems prudent to expedite carotid ultrasound or angiography for patients with TIA as soon as possible. This is especially so for those patients who are at the highest near-term risk of subsequent stroke as assessed by a clinical prediction rule such as the ABCD² score.

Conclusions

In the patient described above, there is a significant 8% risk of subsequent stroke (ABCD² score ≥ 6) in the next 48 hours. This patient would likely benefit from admission, allowing rapid evaluation to optimize stroke prevention and possible therapeutic intervention should stroke occur. If no contraindications are present, aspirin plus dipyridamole should be initiated. Diagnostic evaluation should include assessment for the presence of carotid stenosis and, if present, consultation for possible carotid endarterectomy. Warfarin or heparin anticoagulation would not appear to provide any benefit to our patient and would likely increase the risk of serious bleeding.

Overall, emergency physicians should consider TIAs to be a harbinger of near-term morbidity or mortality. Although most of these patients appear well and without symptoms at the time of ED evaluation, the emergency medicine physician must be diligent in guiding the initial diagnostic evaluation as well as ensuring an appropriate disposition. Utilizing evidence-based diagnostic and therapeutic regimens, the risk of subsequent serious vascular events may be significantly reduced in this high-risk group of patients.

References

1 Feinberg WM, Albers GW, Barnett HJ, et al. Guidelines for the management of transient ischemic attacks. From the Ad Hoc Committee on Guidelines for the Management of Transient Ischemic Attacks of the Stroke Council of the American Heart Association. *Circulation* 1994;**89**(6):2950–65.

2 Johnston SC, Gress DR, Browner WS, Sidney S. Short-term prognosis after emergency department diagnosis of TIA. *JAMA* 2000;**284**(22):2901–6.

3 Albers GW, Caplan LR, Easton JD, et al. for the TIA Working Group. Transient ischemic attack: proposal for a new definition. *N Engl J Med* 2002;**347**:1713–16.

4 American Heart Association. 2004 Heart and Stroke Statistical Update. American Heart Association, Dallas, TX, 2004.

5 Libman RB, et al. Conditions that mimic stroke in the emergency department. *Arch Neurol* 1995;**52**(11):1119.

6 Hand PJ, Kwan J, Lindley RI, Dennis MS, Wardlaw JM. Related articles. Links distinguishing between stroke and mimic at the bedside: the brain attack study. *Stroke* 2006;**37**(3):769–75 (Epub Feb 16, 2006).

7 Whisnant JP, Matsumot N, Elveback LR. Transient cerebral ischemic attacks in a community Rochester, Minnesota, 1955 through 1969. *Mayo Clinic Proc* 1973;**48**(3):194–8.

8 Dennis M, Bamford J, Sandercock P, Warlow C. Prognosis of transient ischemic attacks in the Oxfordshire Community Stroke Project. *Stroke* 1990;**21**(6):848–53.

9 Friedman GD, Wilson S, Mosier JM, Colandrea MA, Nichaman MA. Transient ischemic attacks in a community. *JAMA* 1969;**210**:1428–34.

10 Johnston SC, Gress DR, Browner WS, Sidney S. Short-term prognosis after emergency department diagnosis of TIA. *JAMA* 2000;**284**:2901–6.

11 Lovett J, Dennis M, Sandercock PAG, Bamford J, Warlow CP, Rothwell PM. The very early risk of stroke following a TIA. *Stroke* 2003;**34**:e138–e140.

12 Coull A, Lovett JK, Rothwell PM, on behalf of the Oxford Vascular Study. Early risk of stroke after a TIA or minor stroke in a population–based incidence study. *BMJ* 2004;**328**:326–8.

13 Hill MD, Yiannakoulias N, Jeerakathil T, Tu JV, Svenson LW, Schopflocher DP. The high risk of stroke immediately after transient ischemic attack. A population-based study. *Neurology* 2004;**62**:2015–20.

14 Ishimine P. Transient ischemic attack. In: Frank LR, Jobe KA, eds. *Admission and Discharge Decisions in Emergency Medicine*. Hanley and Belfus, Inc., Philadelphia, 2002.

15 Albers GW, Hart RG, Lutsep HL, Newell DW, Sacco RL. AHA Scientific Statement. Supplement to the guidelines for the management of transient ischemic attacks: a statement from the Ad Hoc Committee on Guidelines for the Management of Transient Ischemic Attacks, Stroke Council, American Heart Association. *Stroke* 1999;**30**(11):2502–11.

16 Johnston SC. Clinical practice. Transient ischemic attack. *N Engl J Med* 2002;**347**(21):1687–92.

17 Shah KH, Edlow JA. Transient ischemic attack: review for the emergency physician. *Ann Emerg Med* 2004;**43**(5):592–604.

18 Hankey GJ, Slattery JM, Warlow CP. The prognosis of hospital-referred transient ischaemic attacks. *J Neurol Neurosurg Psychiatry* 1991;**54**:793–802.

19 Dennis M, Bamford J, Sandercock P, Warlow C. Prognosis of transient ischemic attacks in the Oxfordshire Community Stroke Project. *Stroke* 1990;**21**:848–53.

20 Kleindorfer D, Panagos P, Pancioli A, et al. Incidence and shortterm prognosis of transient ischemic attack in a population–based study. *Stroke* 2005;**36**:720–23.

21 Lovett JK, Dennis MS, Sandercock PAG, Bamford J, Warlow CP, Rothwell PM. Very early risk of stroke after a first transient ischemic attack. *Stroke* 2003;**34**(8):e138–e140.

22 Hill MD, Yiannakoulias N, Jeerakathil T, Tu JV, Svenson LW, Schopflocher DP. The high risk of stroke immediately after transient ischemic attack – a population-based study. *Neurology* 2004;**62**(11):2015–20.

23 Johnston SC, Nguyen-Huynh MN, Schwarz ME, et al. National Stroke Association guidelines for the management of transient ischemic attacks. *Ann Neurol* 2006;**60**(3):301–13.

24 Naradzay JFX. Transient ischemic attack. *eMedicine* October 29, 2004.

25 Hassid E, *Clinical Pathway for the Evaluation and Management of Cerebral Ischemia.* BAMC Neurology Service, Fort Sam, TX, 1999.

26 Gladstone DJ, Kapral MK, Fang JM, Laupacis A, Tu JV. Management and outcomes of transient ischemic attacks in Ontario. *Can Med Assoc J* 2004;**170**(7):1099–104.

27 Chang E, Holroyd BR, Kochanski P, Kelly KD, Shuaib A, Rowe BH. Adherence to practice guidelines for transient ischemic attacks in an emergency department. *Can J Neurol Sci* 2002;**29**(4):358–63.

28 Henneman PL, Lewis RJ. Is admission medically justified for all patients with acute stroke or transient ischemic attack. *Ann Emerg Med* 1995;**25**(4):458–63.

29 Moss HE, Hill MD, Demchuk AM, et al. TIA reference unit: rapid investigation and management of TIA. *Stroke* 2003;**34**(1):310.

30 Gubitz G, Phillips S, Dwyer V. What is the cost of admitting patients with transient ischaemic attacks to hospital? *Cerebrovasc Dis* 1999;**9**(4):210–14.

31 Reilly BM, Evans AT. Translating clinical research into clinical practice: impact of using prediction rules to make decisions. *Ann Intern Med* 2006;**144**:201–9.

32 Ishimine P. Transient ischemic attack. In: Frank LR, Jobe KA, eds. *Admission and Discharge Decisions in Emergency Medicine*. Hanley and Belfus, Inc., Philadelphia, 2002.

33 Heyman A, Wilkinson WE, Hurwitz BJ, Haynes CS, Utley CM, Rosati RA, Burch JG, Gore TB, Risk of ischemic heart disease in patients with TIA. *Neurology* 1984;**34**:626–30.

34 Albers GW, Caplan LR, Easton JD, et al. Transient ischemic attack – proposal for a new definition. *N Engl J Med* 2002;**347**(21):1713–16.

35 Libman RB, Wirkowski E, Alvir J, Rao TH. Conditions that mimic stroke in the emergency department – implications for acute stroke trials. *Arch Neurol* 1995;**52**(11):1119–22.

36 Ferro JM, Falcao I, Rodrigues G, et al. Diagnosis of transient ischemic attack by the nonneurologist – a validation study. *Stroke* 1996;**27**(12):2225–9.

37 Calanchini PR, Swanson PD, Gotshall RA, et al. Cooperative study of hospital frequency and character of transient ischemic attacks. 4. Reliability of diagnosis. *JAMA* 1977;**238**(19):2029–33.

38 Dennis MS, Bamford JM, Sandercock PAG, Warlow CP. Incidence of transient ischemic attacks in Oxfordshire, England. *Stroke* 1989;**20**(3):333–9.

39 Rothwell PM, Giles MF, Flossmann E, et al. A simple score (ABCD) to identify individuals at high early risk of stroke after transient ischaemic attack. *Lancet* 2005;**366**:29–36.

40 Johnston SC, Rothwell PM, Nguyen-Huynh MN, et al. Validation and refinement of scores to predict very early stroke risk after transient ischaemic attack. *Lancet* 2007;**369**:283–92.

41 Antiplatelet Trialists' Collaboration. Collaborative overview of randomised trials of antiplatelet treatment. I. Prevention of death, myocardial infarction, and stroke by prolonged antiplatelet therapy in various categories of patients. *BMJ* 1994;**308**:81–106.

42 Warlow C. Secondary prevention of stroke. *Lancet* 1992;**339**:724–7.

43 Antithrombotic Trialists' Collaboration. Collaborative meta-analysis of randomized trials of antiplatelet therapy for prevention of death, myocardial infarction, and stroke in high risk patients. *BMJ* 2002;**324**:71–86.

44 Diener HC, Cunha L, Forbes C, Sivenius J, Smets P, Lowenthal A. European Stroke Prevention Study 2. Dipyridamole and acetylsalicylic acid in the secondary prevention of stroke. *J Neurol Sci* 1996;**143**:1–13.

45 De Schryver ELLM, Algra A, van Gijn J. Dipyridamole for preventing stroke and other vascular events in patients with vascular disease. *Cochrane Database Syst Rev* 2006;**2**:CD001820.

46 Halkes PH, van Gijn J, Kappelle LJ, Koudstaal PJ, Algra A. Aspirin plus dipyridamole versus aspirin alone after cerebral ischemia of arterial origin (ESPIRIT): randomized controlled trial. *Lancet* 2006;**367**:1665–73.

47 European Carotid Surgery Trialists' Collaborative Group (ECST). MRC European Carotid Surgery Trial: interim results for symptomatic patients with severe (70–99%) or with mild (0–29%) carotid stenosis. *Lancet* 1991;**337**:1235–43.

48 North American Symptomatic Carotid Endarterectomy Trial Collaborators (NASCET). Beneficial effect of carotid endarterectomy in symptomatic patients with high-grade carotid stenosis. *N Engl J Med* 1991;**325**:445–53.

49 Cina CS, Clase CM, Haynes RB. Carotid endarterectomy for symptomatic carotid stenosis. *Cochrane Database Syst Rev* 1999;**3**:CD001081 (doi: 10.1002/14651858.CD001081).

50 Algra A, De Schryver ELLM, van Gijn J, Kappelle LJ, Koudstaal PJ. Oral anticoagulants versus antiplatelet therapy for preventing further vascular events after transient ischaemic attack or minor stroke of presumed arterial origin. *Cochrane Database Syst Rev* 2006;**3**:CD001342.

51 Chimowitz MI, Lynn MJ, et al. Comparison of warfarin and aspirin for symptomatic intracranial arterial stenosis. *N Engl J Med* 2005;**352**(13):1305–16.

52 Sandercock P, Mielke O, Liu M, Counsell C. Anticoagulants for preventing recurrence following presumed non-cardioembolic ischaemic stroke or transient ischaemic attack. *Cochrane Database Syst Rev* 2003;**1**:CD000248 (doi: 10.1002/14651858.CD000248).

53 Gubitz G, Sandercock P, Counsell C. Anticoagulants for acute ischaemic stroke. *Cochrane Database Syst Rev* 2004;**3**:CD000024 (doi: 10.1002/14651858.CD000024.pub2).

54 Berge E, Sandercock P. Anticoagulants versus antiplatelet agents for acute ischaemic stroke. *Cochrane Database Syst Rev* 2002;**4**:CD003242 (doi: 10.1002/14651858.CD003242).

55 Sandercock P, Counsell C, Stobbs SL. Low-molecular-weight heparins or heparinoids versus standard unfractionated heparin for acute ischaemic stroke. *Cochrane Database Syst Rev* 2005;**2**:CD000119 (doi: 10.1002/14651858.CD000119.pub2).

56 Sylaja PN, Coutts SB, Subramaniam S, Hill MD, Eliasziw M, Demchuk AM; VISION Study Group. Acute ischemic lesions of varying ages predict risk of ischemic events in stroke/TIA patients. *Neurology* 2007;**68**(6):415–19.

57 Purroy F, Montaner J, Rovira A, Delgado P, Quintana M, Alvariz-Sabin J. Higher risk of further vascular events among transient ischemic attack patients with diffusion-weighted imaging acute ischemic lesions. *Stroke* 2004;**35**:2313–19.

58 Redgrave JN, Coutts SB, Schulz UG, Briley D, Rothwell PM. Systematic review of associations between the presence of acute ischemic lesions on diffusion-weighted imaging and clinical predictors of early stroke risk after transient ischemic attack. *Stroke* 2007;**385**:1482–8.

45 Stroke

William J. Meurer & Robert Silbergleit

Department of Emergency Medicine, University of Michigan, Ann Arbor, USA

Case scenario

A 75-year-old male arrived at the emergency department (ED) via ambulance. He reported a sudden onset of numbness and weakness of his left arm and leg 1 hour prior to arrival. This progressed over the next 30 minutes to total inability to move his left arm or leg. The patient had a history of hypertension and hyperlipidemia. His only medications were hydrochlorothiazide and niacin. He denied any recent surgery, trauma or gastrointestinal hemorrhage. His wife was present with him and confirmed the time of onset. Furthermore, she confirmed that at no point was there a loss of consciousness or seizure. The patient also denied any headache.

The stroke protocol was activated. His vital signs were blood pressure 176/100 mmHg (left arm), pulse 70 beats/min and respirations 16 breaths/min. He was alert and oriented. A subtle left facial droop was evident but his speech was normal. The left upper and lower extremities fell to the bed immediately when lifted and sensation was decreased on the left side of his body. He also demonstrated mild left-sided sensory neglect. The National Institute of Health Stroke Score (NIHSS) was 11. The patient was sent for an urgent non-contrast brain computerized tomography (CT) scan, which was interpreted promptly by a radiologist as being negative for any acute pathology. At this point in the scenario, the most likely diagnosis was acute ischemic stroke; based on the clinical presentation, subarachnoid hemorrhage was unlikely and there was no radiographic evidence of intracerebral hemorrhage.

Background

Stroke is the third leading cause of death [1] and the leading cause of disability in the United States; similar data exist for other developed countries [2]. The three major types of stroke are ischemic stroke, intracerebral hemorrhage and subarachnoid hemorrhage.

Evidence-based Emergency Medicine. Edited by Brian H. Rowe
© 2009 Blackwell Publishing, ISBN: 978-1-4051-6143-5.

The majority of patients who suffer a stroke will present to the ED; however, the amount of time from onset of symptoms to arrival is highly variable [3–5]. The initial recommended therapies for the three stroke subtypes are quite different [6–8] and the clinical history, exam and initial non-contrast brain CT provide the most important data in discriminating between them. Acute ischemic stroke (AIS) is the most common of these and is the focus of this chapter. Subarachnoid hemorrhage is covered in Chapter 46.

Clinical questions

1 In patients presenting to the ED with an acute neurological deficit (population), are there valid and reliable clinical criteria (clinical prediction guides) by which emergency physicians can accurately determine the pre-test probability of acute ischemic stroke (outcome)?

2 In patients with suspected acute ischemic stroke (population), what are the likelihood ratios (diagnostic test characteristics) of computerized tomography of the head performed within 3 or 6 hours of onset of symptoms (test) for the diagnosis of acute ischemic stroke (outcome)?

3 In patients with suspected acute ischemic stroke (population), what are the likelihood ratios (diagnostic test characteristics) of diffusion weighted magnetic resonance imaging of the head performed within 3 or 6 hours of onset of symptoms (test) for the diagnosis of acute ischemic stroke (outcome)?

4 In patients presenting to the ED with acute ischemic stroke (population), does initiation of aspirin or other antiplatelet agents in the ED (intervention) reduce morbidity and mortality (outcomes) compared to each other or to standard care without any antiplatelet agent (control)?

5 In patients presenting to the ED with acute ischemic stroke (population), does initiation of intravenous tissue plasminogen activator therapy at 0.9 mg/kg within 3 hours of the onset of symptoms (intervention) reduce morbidity and mortality (outcomes) compared to conservative care without thrombolysis (control)?

General search strategy

You have access to the Cochrane Database of Systematic Reviews (CDSR), the Cochrane Central Register of Controlled Trials (CENTRAL) and MEDLINE. You initially search the Cochrane database for meta-analyses and then systematic reviews. If a meta-analysis or systematic review is found, you then search for relevant controlled trials published after the most recent systematic review. In the absence of any systematic reviews or meta-analyses in the Cochrane Library, you then search MEDLINE with modifiers to first find meta-analyses, then systematic reviews, then published treatment trials or published diagnosis trials (depending on the clinical question) using the clinical queries feature of PubMed. If the "sensitive" search option yields an overwhelming number of hits, the search will be redone using the "specific" option. If a meta-analysis is found using MEDLINE, CENTRAL is searched for controlled trials published after the period covered in the meta-analysis. If no relevant trials or reviews are identified using any of the above methods, MEDLINE will be searched with the keywords listed and the results will be screened by title and then by abstract.

Primary search strategy

- Cochrane Database of Systematic Reviews – used title search: acute ischemic stroke AND (topic)
- MEDLINE – meta-analyses: acute ischemic stroke AND meta-analysis(SB) AND (topic)
- MEDLINE – systematic reviews: acute ischemic stroke AND systematic(SB) AND (topic)
- Cochrane Central Register of Controlled Trials: (randomized control trial.sd OR clinical control trial.sd) AND acute ischemic stroke AND (topic)
- MEDLINE – diagnosis: acute ischemic stroke AND specificity [title/abstract] AND (topic)
- MEDLINE – therapy: acute ischemic stroke AND (randomized controlled trial [publication type] OR randomized [title/abstract]) AND controlled [title/abstract] AND trial [title/abstract] AND (topic)
- MEDLINE: acute ischemic stroke AND (topic)

Critical review of the literature

Question 1: In patients presenting to the ED with an acute neurological deficit (population), are there valid and reliable clinical criteria (clinical prediction guides) by which emergency physicians can accurately determine the pre-test probability of acute ischemic stroke (outcome)?

Search strategy

- Cochrane and MEDLINE: systematic reviews AND clinical findings AND (stroke OR ischemic stroke OR CVA)

Despite advances in brain imaging, the ED determination of AIS remains a clinical diagnosis. The question implicit in every emergency physician's evaluation of a patient with acute focal neurological symptoms is straightforward: "Is this patient having a stroke?" Your search of the CDSR reveals no systematic reviews. When searching MEDLINE for systematic reviews you find 62 publications and scan the titles. No clinical prediction rules for stroke were identified but five potentially relevant reviews were found by scanning the titles [9–13]. Of these, the systematic review by Goldstein and Simel in 2005 as part of the Rational Clinical Examination Series in the *Journal of the American Medical Association* (*JAMA*) is most useful [12].

This article carefully reviews the use of screening tools designed for use by emergency medical personnel to identify patients at high risk of ischemic stroke, including the Cincinnati Prehospital Stroke Scale (CPSS) and the Los Angeles Prehospital Stroke Screen (LAPSS). Both scales were derived from recursive partitioning of extensive datasets to identify patient characteristics thought to be both high yield and reliable on repeated exams and between observers, and both have undergone subsequent validation. Not surprisingly, the CPSS and LAPSS are similar (Table 45.1). Both are three-item scales including facial paresis, arm drift and either abnormal speech (CPSS) or handgrip strength (LAPSS). The presence of any one of these findings as compared to none of these findings dramatically increases the probability of a subsequent final diagnosis of stroke with a positive likelihood ratio (+LR) of 5.2 (95% CI: 2.6 to 11). Having all three of these key clinical findings was uncommon but increased the +LR to 14 (95% CI: 1.6 to 121). If none of the three clinical findings are present, the +LR is 0.39 (95% CI: 0.25 to 0.61) when the CPSS is performed by physicians. Although some differences between paramedics and physicians have been demonstrated, both scales were generally reliable across providers [12].

Only two other articles identified by your search provide further information about the clinical diagnosis of stroke in the ED. In one study [14], all 446 patients evaluated in the ED of a university teaching hospital, and either admitted with a diagnosis of stroke, or subsequently discharged from the hospital with a diagnosis of stroke, over 14 months were studied. The final admitting diagnosis made by the emergency physician was compared with the final hospital discharge diagnosis, 95% of which were made by neurologists or neurosurgeons. Emergency physicians had a sensitivity of 98.6% and a positive predictive value of 94.8% for

Table 45.1 Prehospital stroke screening: Cincinnati Prehospital Stroke Scale (CPSS) and the Los Angeles Prehospital Stroke Screen (LAPSS).

CPSS	LAPSS
Unilateral facial paresis	Unilateral facial paresis
Unilateral arm weakness	Unilateral arm weakness
Abnormal speech	Abnormal grip strength

The presence of any one finding in either system is considered a positive screen.

diagnosing AIS. There were 19 patients with a variety of stroke mimics that included mostly "deficits of unclear etiology", seizure, neuropathy and complicated migraine [14]. Furthermore, the external validity of this study is unclear as it was conducted in an academic center with an ED dedicated to stroke research. This limitation is absent in the second study identified [15], which was performed as part of a population-based surveillance for acute stroke in an eastern Texas county without an academic medical center. Physicians staffing the ED had a sensitivity of 92% in identifying 1800 patients with acute stroke. Of the cases initially thought to be stroke, 11% were determined to have unspecified mimics, which were "mostly generalized neurologic and medical conditions" [15]. The study then went on to describe the diagnostic value of specific clinical criteria identified in the ED. False-positive ED diagnoses were significantly less likely in patients with motor symptoms (OR = 0.44; 95% CI: 0.32 to 0.62), as well as in those with sensory deficits (OR = 0.43; 95% CI: 0.28 to 0.66) and those with severe deficits (OR = 0.33; 95% CI: 0.14 to 0.78). Alternatively, a false-positive ED stroke diagnosis was more likely in patients with a prior history of stroke (OR = 1.72; 95% CI: 1.23 to 2.40) [15].

What is the diagnostic accuracy of emergency physicians in identifying stroke patients based on clinical criteria for an acute intervention, namely treatment with intravenous tissue-type plasminogen activator (t-PA)? Searching for "stroke" and "misdiagnosis" and "t-PA" you identify two articles including one relevant observational study of 151 consecutive stroke patients treated with t-PA by emergency physicians operating without an acute stroke team [16]. Based on discharge diagnosis, six patients (4%; 95% CI: 1% to 8%) had a stroke mimic, including four with conversion disorder, one with complex migraine and one with prolonged Todd's paralysis. There were no complications in this small number of mimics who received t-PA. Although limited, these data suggest that the diagnosis of stroke can be accurately made by emergency physicians using clinical criteria when it matters most.

In summary, no validated prediction rule exists for AIS. However, the CPSS or LAPSS are accurate and reliable screening tools that may be used in the prehospital or ED setting.

Question 2: In patients with suspected acute ischemic stroke (population), what are the likelihood ratios (diagnostic test characteristics) of computerized tomography of the head performed within 3 or 6 hours of onset of symptoms (test) for the diagnosis of acute ischemic stroke (outcome)?

Search strategy

- MEDLINE: meta-analyses AND acute ischemic stroke AND CT AND diagnosis
- CDSR: acute ischemic stroke AND CT AND diagnosis

Although the advent of CT in the 1970s revolutionized stroke diagnosis, non-contrast computerized tomography (NCCT) is still generally thought to be of limited utility in the ED management of the first few hours of AIS. There are initially no or few abnormalities on NCCT imaging immediately after the onset of stroke symptoms, but early infarct signs – relatively subtle findings – often develop within 3–6 hours. CT findings usually become quite apparent as the stroke progresses. Because early infarct signs are subtle, the evaluation of the utility of CT requires consideration of intra-observer reliability as well as the diagnostic test characteristics (likelihood ratios).

The searches above yielded 3 and 11 studies, respectively; however, none of these directly addressed the clinical question. When MEDLINE was searched for systematic reviews, 17 were identified on this subject. The abstracts were scanned for relevant studies and two were identified that addressed some portions of the question [17,18].

The most comprehensive of the two systematic reviews identified 15 studies, nine of which required that NCCT be performed within 6 hours of stroke onset, and six in which NCCT was obtained within 3 hours of onset [17]. This systematic review included 1300 NCCT scans from patients with AIS; however, the results are dominated by one study contributing 786 scans, with each of the others contributing 100 or fewer scans. The investigators found that the mean prevalence of early infarction signs was 57%. The focus of this review was on the reliability of readings of early infarct signs and the sensitivity and specificity against an expert or consensus review. The kappa (κ) statistics ranged from 0.20 to 0.62, and even for the most reliable early infarct sign, the hyper-attenuated artery sign, the κ value ranged from 0.36 to 1.00. The weighted mean sensitivity for early signs of infarction was 55% and the specificity was 80% (+LR = 2.8; negative likelihood ratio (−LR) = 0.56). This review suggests that the identification of early signs of infarction is not reliable, and the ability for early infarct signs to predict actual stroke is not supported by the existing data [17].

The other systematic review compared the test characteristics of NCCT and magnetic resonance imaging (MRI) used within the first 6 hours after stroke onset. Eight studies were identified including 909 subjects, almost all of whom had a final diagnosis of AIS [18]. Compared to final diagnosis, NCCT had a weighted mean sensitivity of 45.5% and specificity of 79.0% (+LR = 2.2; −LR = 0.69).

The MEDLINE search for primary studies yielded approximately 40 studies – most of which either failed to address the question or had been included in the above systematic reviews. Two studies published after the two systematic reviews provided additional insights. A systematic method for scoring early infarct signs on CT, called the Alberta Stroke Programme Early Computed Tomography Score (ASPECTS), was developed with the goal to improve both the inter-rater reliability and the accuracy of the modality. In 100 patients with stroke imaged within 6 hours of stroke onset by both NCCT and MRI, the NCCT using ASPECTS was 81% sensitive and 88% specific as compared to early MRI, and the inter-rater agreement was 80%. These results have not yet been externally validated in a patient population that includes both patients with and without stroke, and in a patient population consistently studied within 3 hours of symptom onset [19].

Surprisingly, the best data on this rather old question may be the most recent. A multi-center collaboration of stroke researchers reported on 356 patients with symptoms suspicious for AIS who underwent both NCCT and MRI, 217 of whom had a final diagnosis of stroke [20]. Of particular interest, a subgroup analysis of the 90 patients imaged within 3 hours of onset is reported. Median time of imaging for all patients was 6 hours from onset of symptoms. In this well-conducted study, the sensitivity of NCCT for a final diagnosis of AIS was 16%, with a specificity of 98%. Within 3 hours of stroke onset, the sensitivity dropped down to 12%, although specificity remained high (+LR = 5.9; −LR = 0.90) [20].

In summary, NCCT is clearly insensitive and unreliable in the diagnosis of AIS, especially within the first 3 hours of symptom onset. Use of a standardized scoring system appears to improve the reliability but not the sensitivity. Scanning articles to answer this question, however, demonstrates the increasing interest in using advanced contrast CT techniques such as CT cerebral angiography and perfusion CT to identify and stratify patients with acute stroke. At the present time, there is insufficient data available to evaluate these techniques.

Question 3: In patients with suspected acute ischemic stroke (population), what are the likelihood ratios (diagnostic test characteristics) of diffusion weighted magnetic resonance imaging of the head performed within 3 or 6 hours of onset of symptoms (test) for the diagnosis of acute ischemic stroke (outcome)?

Search strategy

- Cochrane: acute ischemic stroke AND MRI AND diffusion
- MEDLINE: meta-analyses AND acute ischemic stroke AND MRI AND diffusion

Unlike NCCT, MRI can identify physiological changes that usually occur rapidly after thrombotic or thromboembolic events in the cerebral vasculature and the development of brain ischemia. For example, decreased perfusion leads to differences in regional blood volume that can be detected by magnetic resonance techniques broadly designated as perfusion weighted. These techniques show relative differences in perfusion in one part of the brain as compared to another, but do not show absolute blood flow, or whether perfusion is adequate to prevent ischemia. When regions of the brain actually become ischemic, cells in those areas develop energy failure and begin to lose their ability to maintain ion gradients across their membranes, thus altering the diffusion of fluid into the cell. This change can be detected by MRI techniques broadly designated as diffusion weighted imaging (DWI). Images of acute stroke using DWI can be quite vivid, even on initial pre-

sentation; however, the issue for emergency physicians is whether this will impact the care provided in the ED setting. As discussed in the previous section, interpretation of cerebral imaging is partially subjective, and the reliability of the test between readers is an important consideration.

The search identified one systematic review which addressed the clinical question [21]. This review, performed in 2000, identified 47 studies reporting on 2436 patients. Unfortunately, the authors found that this body of literature, although tremendously enthusiastic, was so methodologically weak that it was not possible to determine any meaningful estimates of MRI performance. They concluded that false-negative and false-positive studies clearly occurred but with unknown frequency and they called for more research to address the question [21].

The MEDLINE search strategy produced 545 possible studies, so the search term "accuracy" was added. This yielded 21 studies for review, one of which appeared relevant to the search question. This was a study comparing three different DWI techniques, and determining their respective reliability [22]. The study included 75 patients imaged up to 24 hours from the onset of stroke symptoms, a quarter of whom were treated with thrombolysis, always prior to the MRI. Remarkably, as with the articles cited in the previous systematic review, the paper did not report how many of the patients ultimately had the final diagnosis of stroke by clinical criteria and follow-up imaging. Rather, the reference standard consisted of a panel of two expert neuroradiologists who determined whether or not the MRI showed findings consistent with stroke. This "reference standard" reading was compared to the readings of four other readers including two stroke clinicians and two different neuroradiologists. The expert panel determined that 67% of patients had lesions consistent with stroke on MRI; the diagnostic performance of the other readers ranged from a sensitivity of 82% to 84% and a specificity of 98% to 99%. Kappa statistics showed that both inter- and intra-rater reliability were 0.81 to 0.86, respectively, for the different techniques [22].

Having established that MRI-DWI has fair reliability, concern about its clinical utility remains, especially in the first few hours after stroke onset. In a German stroke center, 50 patients with a subsequent diagnosis of ischemic stroke and four with a final diagnosis of transient ischemic attack (TIA) who arrived within 6 hours of symptom onset had both CT and MRI-DWI performed within a 90-minute window [23]. Patients were randomized to the order of the two tests to eliminate potential bias related to changes in imaging over the 90-minute period. For MRI-DWI, the sensitivity compared to follow-up imaging and clinical course was 80% when all five expert readers read the test as positive, and was 91% on average for the five reviewers taken individually. The inter-rater reliability of expert readers was high ($\kappa = 0.84$); however, it varied with time from stroke onset. For patients imaged within 2 hours of stroke onset the κ statistic was only moderately good ($\kappa = 0.76$), but this increased with time from onset, and on those imaged at 6 hours there was perfect agreement ($\kappa = 1$) [23]. Because comparisons were made to repeat imaging and final diagnosis, and because four patients with TIA were also included, some inferences to the diagnostic performance of MRI-DWI can be made from this study. The sensitivity and specificity reported allows you to calculate a +LR of 18.2 and a −LR of 0.095. These estimates of test performance are likely inflated due to selection bias; the study population represented only those with severe disease since all patients without stroke or TIA (and many with TIA) were excluded.

Finally, you return to the Chalela article that was helpful in estimating CT performance [20]. As noted earlier, this study enrolled 356 consecutive patients presenting to the ED with symptoms concerning for stroke, of whom 217 had a final clinical diagnosis of AIS. Of particular interest is that the 90 patients evaluated within 3 hours of stroke onset are reported in a subgroup analysis. The advantage of this design over many of the others cited is that patients who were not ultimately found to have a stroke were included and it is more representative of the target population for which the test will be used in clinical practice. Overall, the investigators found that MRI-DWI had a sensitivity of 83% (95% CI: 77% to 88%) and a specificity of 96% (95% CI: 92% to 99%) compared to the discharge diagnosis. In the subgroup of patients with imaging performed within 3 hours of symptom onset, MRI-DWI sensitivity was only 73% (95% CI: 59% to 84%) and specificity was 92% (95% CI: 78% to 98%) [20]. Based on these data, when the MRI-DWI is performed within the first 3 hours of stroke symptoms, the +LR is 9.1 and the −LR is 0.3. Given a prevalence of stroke of 60% seen in this study, the post-test probability of stroke with a positive test is 93% and the post-test probability of stroke with a negative test is 31%. You conclude that MRI-DWI may be helpful in unusual cases when the clinical criteria for diagnosing stroke are unclear, but that diagnostic performance in acute stroke within 3 hours of stroke onset is no better, and likely worse, than diagnosis based on other clinical criteria. Overall, emergency physicians should not be demanding or required to obtain emergent MRI in patients suspected of acute ischemic stroke.

Question 4: In patients presenting to the ED with acute ischemic stroke (population), does initiation of aspirin or other antiplatelet agents in the ED (intervention) reduce morbidity and mortality (outcomes) compared to each other or to standard care without any antiplatelet agent (control)?

Search strategy

- Cochrane: anti-platelets AND acute ischemic stroke

Emergency physicians are well aware of the significant role of antiplatelet agents in the treatment of cardiovascular disease. In patients with acute myocardial infarction, provision of aspirin in the ED is often used as a critical marker of quality of care. It is therefore natural for us to wonder about the role of these agents in ED patients with cerebrovascular disease. Your search of the CDSR yielded four potentially relevant systematic reviews.

Sandercock et al. performed a systematic review in 2003 of trials that compared treatment with antiplatelet therapy (started within 2 weeks of the stroke) to controls in patients with ischemic stroke [24]. Nine trials involving 41,399 patients were included. Two trials that tested acetyl-salicylic acid (ASA) 160–300 mg once daily started within 48 hours of onset and contributed 98% of the data: the International Stroke Trial (IST) and the Chinese Acute Stroke Trial (CAST). One of these was a placebo-controlled trial, while the other was an open-label trial. With treatment, there was a small but statistically significant decrease in death or dependency at the end of follow-up (OR = 0.94; 95% CI: 0.91 to 0.98). ASA treatment also increased the odds of making a complete recovery from the stroke (OR = 1.06; 95% CI: 1.01 to 1.11). Overall, 100 stroke patients would need to be treated with ASA to produce one additional good outcome (NNT = 100). ASA also increased the rate of intracranial and other major hemorrhages, with a number needed to harm (NNH) of 166. Taken together, these outcomes suggest that ASA is modestly effective after ischemic stroke. Patients in these trials were generally enrolled and treated the day after their stroke; therefore, relevance to ED treatment is speculative. One other randomized controlled trial (RCT) designed to study efficacy (phase III) compared ASA to placebo with treatment initiated within 6 hours of treatment. In the 300 patients randomized in that trial (the Multicentre Acute Stroke Trial Italy, MAST-I), there were no statistically significant differences in any patient outcome. While this study was under-powered to demonstrate the small improvements seen in IST and CAST, the results demonstrate that ASA is not overwhelmingly more effective when given in the ED in the first 6 hours. Trials assessing other antiplatelet agents (ticlopidine, abciximab) given in the ED were mentioned in this review but provided no additional insight [24].

A subsequent systemic review from CDSR in 2006 specifically addressed the treatment of stroke patients with glycoprotein (GP) IIb-IIIa inhibitors within the first 6 hours after the onset of symptoms [25]. They identified two trials of abciximab versus placebo in 414 stroke patients and found non-significant improvements in outcome coupled with non-significant increases in bleeding. They noted that these phase II data had been considered encouraging and led to a larger phase III efficacy trial, which was terminated early because of an unacceptably high rate of intracranial hemorrhage in the treatment group. The review notes other ongoing trials of GP IIb-IIIa inhibitors for treatment of stroke patients in the ED including tirofiban and eptifibatide, so more information about emergently inhibiting platelet aggregation in stroke patients is likely to be forthcoming [25].

Three other systematic reviews were only tangentially relevant. One compared antiplatelet agents to anticoagulants, and concluded that anticoagulants offered no net advantages over antiplatelet agents in patients with AIS [26]. The other two reviewed the use of antiplatelet agents for secondary stroke prevention in patients with prior cardiac or cerebrovascular events, but the trials reviewed did not reflect acute ED care [27,28]. Time to recurrent stroke is better if antiplatelet therapy is initiated within 30 days of a stroke as compared to after 30 days; however, no effects of initiation relevant to emergency practice were considered. In particular, these reviews discuss the controversial trial results on combination antiplatelet therapy with clopidogrel and aspirin resulting from the CURE and CHARISMA trials. The authors concluded that despite some promising subgroup data, the potential benefits of combination therapy as compared to aspirin alone are not compelling for most patients with prior stroke [27,28]. Recent data from the MATCH trial similarly suggest that combination therapy is not better than clopidogrel alone [29].

Overall, existing acute stroke management guidelines support that antiplatelet agents should be administered within 48 hours of stroke onset, but should not be considered as an alternative to thrombolytic therapy [6,7]. This is important because guidelines for the use of thrombolytics in acute stroke, based upon the NINDS study protocol, all mandate that no antiplatelet agents be administered for 24 hours following the administration of the thrombolytic. There is no evidence suggesting that earlier administration of ASA, within 48 hours of stroke onset, is superior to initiation after hospital admission, but it is not unreasonable to initiate this in the ED in patients not receiving thrombolytics.

Question 5: In patients presenting to the ED with acute ischemic stroke (population), does initiation of intravenous tissue plasminogen activator therapy at 0.9 mg/kg within 3 hours of the onset of symptoms (intervention) reduce morbidity and mortality (outcomes) compared to conservative care without thrombolysis (control)?

Search strategy

- MEDLINE and Cochrane Library: (thrombolytics OR t-PA) AND acute ischemic stroke

The efficacy of thrombolysis in patients with AIS has, for a variety of reasons, become the most contentious issue in stroke care in the specialty of emergency medicine. How both advocates and critics reach differing conclusions using evidence-based approaches to the question illustrates a key concept in evidence-based medicine.

Your search of the Cochrane Library yielded two reviews [31,32] addressing the question. Wardlaw et al. performed an extensive review in 2003 that included studies of stroke patients receiving any thrombolytic agent, at any dose, and in any time window. The other was a systematic review of studies comparing different thrombolytic agents and different routes of administration.

Fortunately, the first review separately analyzed treatment with t-PA within 3 hours and reported on five blinded clinical trials with 930 subjects randomized to thrombolysis or placebo. When the results of the individual trials are considered separately, benefit from treatment was only statistically significant in the NINDS t-PA trial. However, as seen in Fig. 45.1, there is consistent improvement across the trials with minimal heterogeneity ($I^2 = 0\%$, $P = 0.77$) and the meta-analysis resulted in an odds ratio of 0.64 (95% CI: 0.50 to 0.83) for death or dependency at the end of follow-up. The composite OR was similar to the effect size seen in most of the individual trials, and is clinically and statistically significant. The rest of the systematic review shows that other agents given at

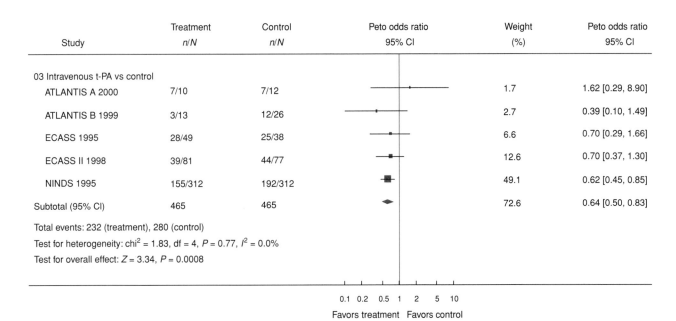

Study	Treatment n/N	Control n/N	Peto odds ratio 95% CI	Weight (%)	Peto odds ratio 95% CI
03 Intravenous t-PA vs control					
ATLANTIS A 2000	7/10	7/12		1.7	1.62 [0.29, 8.90]
ATLANTIS B 1999	3/13	12/26		2.7	0.39 [0.10, 1.49]
ECASS 1995	28/49	25/38		6.6	0.70 [0.29, 1.66]
ECASS II 1998	39/81	44/77		12.6	0.70 [0.37, 1.30]
NINDS 1995	155/312	192/312		49.1	0.62 [0.45, 0.85]
Subtotal (95% CI)	465	465		72.6	0.64 [0.50, 0.83]

Total events: 232 (treatment), 280 (control)
Test for heterogeneity: chi^2 = 1.83, df = 4, P = 0.77, I^2 = 0.0%
Test for overall effect: Z = 3.34, P = 0.0008

0.1 0.2 0.5 1 2 5 10
Favors treatment   Favors control

Note: CI = confidence interval; t-PA = tissue plasminogen activator.

Figure 45.1 Comparison of treatment with tissue plasminogen activator (t-PA) within 3 hours of stroke onset on death or dependency at the end of follow-up in randomized controlled trials [31].

later time points or by other routes are less consistently beneficial compared to placebo. Furthermore, the easily identified increased risks of treatment (symptomatic intracranial hemorrhage in particular) are consistent and not always offset by benefits. Direct comparisons of different doses and different routes of thrombolysis is the subject of the other Cochrane systematic review [32]. It does not provide any additional direct evidence of benefit beyond that provided by t-PA 0.9 mg/kg administered within the 3-hour window.

Your MEDLINE search for meta-analyses review yielded another two publications [33,34]. One focused on safety and included 2639 patients with stroke treated with t-PA from 15 prior post-marketing reports [35]. The meta-analysis demonstrated results consistent with, or better than, those seen in the NINDS t-PA study with favorable outcome in 37.1% (95% CI: 35.3% to 38.9%), symptomatic intracranial hemorrhage in 5.2% (95% CI: 4.3% to 6.0%) and death in 13.0% (95% CI: 11.7% to 14.3%). The second meta-analysis reported data from thrombolytic trials since 1992 as a cumulative time-series analysis, and concluded that the weight of accumulating evidence is failing to diminish uncertainty over time [33]. The authors of this meta-analysis concluded that further large-scale clinical trials of t-PA would be necessary to persuade clinicians to routinely use the therapy. Finally, another pooled analysis of the same t-PA trials was identified from the reference list in Wardlaw's Cochrane review [31]. This analysis extrapolated an efficacy–time curve in which efficacy is maintained within 3 hours, and then diminishes to zero in the following hours (Fig. 45.2) [34]. Although interesting, none of these add to the original RCT data presented in the CDSR.

How does one use evidence-based medicine to reconcile the apparent effectiveness of intravenous t-PA within 3 hours with inconsistent data regarding the efficacy of other thrombolytic strategies? In a landmark essay in *JAMA* in 1987, Browner and Newman argued that Bayesian processes, entirely analogous to those used by physicians to interpret diagnostic tests in clinical practice, are (and should be) used to interpret the results of clinical trials [36].

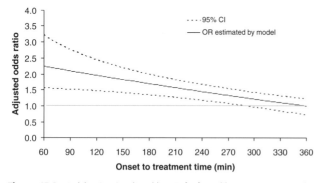

Figure 45.2 Model estimating the odds ratio for favorable outcome at 3 months, in tissue plasminogen activator-treated patients compared with control by onset to treatment time. Adjusted for age, baseline glucose concentration, baseline NIHSS measurement, baseline diastolic blood pressure, previous hypertension, and interaction between age and baseline NIHSS measurement. OR, odds ratio.

In their analogy, the significance of an RCT is analogous to the sensitivity of a diagnostic test, and the power of a trial is analogous to the specificity of a diagnostic test. The likelihood that a clinical trial's results are true is the same as the post-test probability of a disease given a positive diagnostic test result. This post-test (or post-trial) likelihood, in turn, depends on your assessment of the pre-test (or pre-trial) likelihood. A patient who tests positive for a common illness on a test that is 95% sensitive and 80% specific, probably has the illness. Similarly, a treatment that seemed likely to be effective and is tested and found effective in an RCT with significance of 95% and power of 80% probably is effective. Contrariwise, the positive diagnostic test and the positive clinical trial require confirmatory testing if the patient is at low risk for the illness, or the treatment studied in the RCT was without good supportive preliminary data.

This Bayesian process provides a way to explain differing expert interpretations of the clinical trial data on thrombolysis in patients with stroke. Many experts feel that the strong underlying physiological rationale of rapidly opening an acutely occluded artery, the weight of pre-clinical experimentation in the lab showing that efficacy is closely linked to early reperfusion, and the skillful execution of the NINDS trial in particular, combine to indicate a very high pre-test likelihood of t-PA being effective in patients with stroke provided they are treated within the narrow 3-hour window. Critics, on the other hand, feel that the larger number of negative or equivocal trials of thrombolysis with longer time windows and other agents, the methodological flaws in the positive trials like inadvertent imbalances of baseline severity, and the potentially high risk of being wrong given the clearly increased risk of hemorrhage, combine to indicate a much lower pre-test likelihood of t-PA being effective. The existing clinical trial data are supportive of treatment efficacy. Ultimately a judgment call is required to determine the need for a further confirmatory trial.

Conclusions

The patient described meets all three LAPSS criteria (+LR = 14) which significantly increases his probability of stroke. The patient also has both sensory and motor symptoms, so your clinical diagnosis of stroke is likely to be accurate. The NCCT, without evidence of hemorrhage or edema, further supports the diagnosis of acute ischemic stroke. You discuss the benefits and risk of thrombolysis with the patient and family and they quickly agree. The patient is treated 1 hour and 45 minutes after symptom onset and is admitted to the hospital's stroke unit. He does very well, and is discharged to home with minimal disability after staying in the hospital for 5 days. One year after you initially treated this patient you see him walking down the street with his wife.

Stroke is the third leading cause of death and the leading cause of disability in the United States. Currently available evidence confirms that the diagnosis of stroke can be accurately made on clinical criteria, especially in determining candidates for the use of intravenous thrombolytics. Early MRI is more accurate in stroke diagnosis than is early CT; however, both have limited reliability and the impact of these differences in diagnostic accuracy on ED care is uncertain. All patients with acute stroke benefit very modestly from antiplatelet agents such as aspirin (as long as they are not administered in the first 24 hours after thrombolysis) but these may be started at any time within 48 hours. Finally, clinical trial data demonstrate that intravenous t-PA given within 3 hours of symptom onset improves outcomes even after consideration of the associated risks of treatment. Alternate interpretations of the t-PA data are discussed.

Conflicts of interest

None were reported.

References

1 Miniño AM, Heron MP, Smith BL. Deaths: preliminary data for 2004. *Natl Vital Stat Rep* 2006;**54**(19):1–49.

2 Boerma T, Shibuya K, Pinchuk M, eds. *World Health Statistics*, 3rd edn. World Health Organization Press, Geneva, 2007.

3 Alberts MJ, Perry A, Dawson DV, Bertels C. Effects of public and professional education on reducing the delay in presentation and referral of stroke patients. *Stroke* 1992;**23**(3):352–6.

4 Engelstein E, Margulies J, Jeret JS. Lack of t-PA use for acute ischemic stroke in a community hospital: high incidence of exclusion criteria. *Am J Emerg Med* 2000;**18**(3):257–60.

5 Gebhardt JG, Norris TE. Acute stroke care at rural hospitals in Idaho: challenges in expediting stroke care. *J Rural Health* 2006;**22**(1):88–91.

6 Adams HP, Jr., Adams RJ, Brott T, et al. Guidelines for the early management of patients with ischemic stroke: a scientific statement from the Stroke Council of the American Stroke Association. *Stroke* 2003;**34**(4):1056–83.

7 Adams H, Adams R, Del Zoppo G, Goldstein LB. Guidelines for the early management of patients with ischemic stroke: 2005 guidelines update a scientific statement from the Stroke Council of the American Heart Association/American Stroke Association. *Stroke* 2005;**36**(4):916–23.

8 Broderick JP, Adams HP, Jr., Barsan W, et al. Guidelines for the management of spontaneous intracerebral hemorrhage: a statement for healthcare professionals from a special writing group of the Stroke Council, American Heart Association. *Stroke* 1999;**30**(4):905–15.

9 Wyer PC, Osborn HH. Recombinant tissue plasminogen activator: in my community hospital ED, will early administration of rt-PA to patients with the initial diagnosis of acute ischemic stroke reduce mortality and disability? *Ann Emerg Med* 1997;**30**(5):629–38.

10 Kwan J, Hand P, Sandercock P. Improving the efficiency of delivery of thrombolysis for acute stroke: a systematic review. *Q J Med* 2004;**97**(5):273–9.

11 Ferri M, De Luca A, Giorgi Rossi P, Lori G, Guasticchi G. Does a prehospital emergency pathway improve early diagnosis and referral in suspected stroke patients? Study protocol of a cluster randomised trial (ISRCTN41456865). *BMC Health Serv Res* 2005;**5**:66.

12 Goldstein LB, Simel DL. Is this patient having a stroke? *JAMA* 2005;**293**(19):2391–402.

13 Libman RB, Wirkowski E, Alvir J, Rao TH. Conditions that mimic stroke in the emergency department. Implications for acute stroke trials. *Arch Neurol* 1995;**52**(11):1119–22.

14 Kothari RU, Brott T, Broderick JP, Hamilton CA. Emergency physicians. Accuracy in the diagnosis of stroke. *Stroke* 1995;**26**(12):2238–41.

15 Morgenstern LB, Lisabeth LD, Mecozzi AC, et al. A population-based study of acute stroke and TIA diagnosis. *Neurology* 2004;**62**(6):895–900.

16 Scott PA, Silbergleit R. Misdiagnosis of stroke in tissue plasminogen activator-treated patients: characteristics and outcomes. *Ann Emerg Med* 2003;**42**(5):611–18.

17 Wardlaw JM, Mielke O. Early signs of brain infarction at CT: observer reliability and outcome after thrombolytic treatment (Systematic review). *Radiology* 2005;**235**(2):444–53.

18 Davis DP, Robertson T, Imbesi SG. Diffusion-weighted magnetic resonance imaging versus computed tomography in the diagnosis of acute ischemic stroke. *J Emerg Med* 2006;**31**(3):269–77.

19 Barber PA, Hill MD, Eliasziw M, et al. Imaging of the brain in acute ischaemic stroke: comparison of computed tomography and magnetic resonance diffusion-weighted imaging. *J Neurol Neurosurg Psychiatry* 2005;**76**(11):1528–33.

20 Chalela JA, Kidwell CS, Nentwich LM, et al. Magnetic resonance imaging and computed tomography in emergency assessment of patients with suspected acute stroke: a prospective comparison. *Lancet* 2007;**369**(9558):293–8.

21 Keir SL, Wardlaw JM. Systematic review of diffusion and perfusion imaging in acute ischemic stroke. *Stroke* 2000;**31**(11):2723–31.

22 Chen PE, Simon JE, Hill MD, et al. Acute ischemic stroke: accuracy of diffusion-weighted MR imaging – effects of b value and cerebrospinal fluid suppression. *Radiology* 2006;**238**(1):232–9.

23 Fiebach JB, Schellinger PD, Jansen O, et al. CT and diffusion-weighted MR imaging in randomized order: diffusion-weighted imaging results in higher accuracy and lower interrater variability in the diagnosis of hyperacute ischemic stroke. *Stroke* 2002;**33**(9):2206–10.

24 Sandercock P, Gubitz G, Foley P, Counsell C. Antiplatelet therapy for acute ischaemic stroke. *Cochrane Database Syst Rev* 2003;**2**:CD000029.

25 Ciccone A, Abraha I, Santilli I. Glycoprotein IIb-IIIa inhibitors for acute ischaemic stroke. *Cochrane Database Syst Rev* 2006;**4**:CD005208.

26 Berge E, Sandercock P. Anticoagulants versus antiplatelet agents for acute ischaemic stroke. *Cochrane Database Syst Rev* 2002;**4**:CD003242.

27 Hankey GJ, Sudlow CL, Dunbabin DW. Thienopyridine derivatives (ticlopidine, clopidogrel) versus aspirin for preventing stroke and other serious vascular events in high vascular risk patients. *Cochrane Database Syst Rev* 2000;**2**:CD001246.

28 Keller T, Squizzato A, Middeldorp S. Clopidogrel plus aspirin versus aspirin alone for preventing cardiovascular disease. *Cochrane Database Syst Rev* 2007;**3**:CD005158.

29 Hankey GJ, Eikelboom JW. Adding aspirin to clopidogrel after TIA and ischemic stroke: benefits do not match risks. *Neurology* 2005;**64**(7):1117–21.

30 Liu M, Wardlaw J. Thrombolysis (different doses, routes of administration and agents) for acute ischaemic stroke. *Cochrane Database Syst Rev* 2000;**2**:CD000514.

31 Wardlaw JM, Zoppo G, Yamaguchi T, Berge E. Thrombolysis for acute ischaemic stroke. *Cochrane Database Syst Rev* 2003;**3**:CD000213.

32 Mielke O, Wardlaw J, Liu M. Thrombolysis (different doses, routes of administration and agents) for acute ischaemic stroke. *Cochrane Database Syst Rev* 2004;**4**:CD000514.

33 Wardlaw JM, Sandercock PA, Berge E. Thrombolytic therapy with recombinant tissue plasminogen activator for acute ischemic stroke: where do

we go from here? A cumulative meta-analysis. *Stroke* 2003;**34**(6):1437–42.

34 Hacke W, Donnan G, Fieschi C, et al. Association of outcome with early stroke treatment: pooled analysis of ATLANTIS, ECASS, and NINDS rt-PA stroke trials. *Lancet* 2004;**363**(9411):768–74.

35 Graham GD. Tissue plasminogen activator for acute ishemic stroke in clinical practice: a meta-analysis of safety data. *Stroke* 2003;**34**:2847–50.

36 Browner WS, Newman TB. Are all significant P values created equal? The analogy between diagnostic tests and clinical research. *JAMA* 1987;**257**(18):2459–63.

46 Subarachnoid Hemorrhage

Jeffrey J. Perry

Department of Emergency Medicine, University of Ottawa, Ottawa, Canada

Clinical scenario

A 55-year-old woman was brought to the emergency department (ED) by ambulance. She was driving on the highway when she experienced a severe headache peaking within 5 minutes. She pulled over to the side of the road and called her friend, who told her to stay there and called an ambulance. On arrival at the ED she complained of nausea and had vomited several times en route to the hospital. She appeared to be in mild distress, noticeably photophobic; she denied any past medical problems, was not taking prescription medications and had no allergies.

Her vital signs were a pulse of 82 beats/min, respiration of 20 breaths/min, blood pressure of 170/90 mmHg (right arm) and a temperature of 37.5°C (oral). She was alert and oriented and her Glasgow Coma Score (GCS) was 15/15. She denied loss of consciousness, complained of pain involving her entire head, had no history of similar headaches, and no family history of cerebral aneurysms. Her examination was unremarkable with a normal neurological examination, no neck stiffness and normal cardiorespiratory examination.

Background

Headache is a common symptom, representing up to 4.5% of presenting complaints in the ED [1]. Although subarachnoid hemorrhage (SAH) is a relatively rare cause of headache, it is one of the most serious causes of headache. Hence emergency physicians go to great lengths to rule out this potentially catastrophic disease. SAH is generally classified as traumatic or non-traumatic. While traumatic SAH is more common, it typically is less serious and usually requires no surgical intervention. Non-traumatic SAH is most often caused by cerebral arterial aneurysms (80%) or arteri-

Evidence-based Emergency Medicine. Edited by Brian H. Rowe

ovenous malformations (10%). Non-traumatic SAH accounts for about 1% of all headaches seen in the ED [2–5].

Overall mortality of non-traumatic SAH is high, and of survivors, about one-third are left with neurological deficits [6]. Therefore, clinicians go to great lengths to exclude SAH including using computerized tomography (CT) scans and performing a lumbar puncture if the scan is negative [7]. Unfortunately, both of these tests have undesirable attributes. The use of CT exposes patients to radiation and increases health care costs. Lumbar puncture increases the time patients spend in the ED and causes pain and morbidity to patients, with many suffering post-lumbar puncture headaches [8]. Despite the low yield of testing, some patients with SAH are misdiagnosed on their first visit to a health care professional, which can lead to a poor outcome [9]. This may occur if they suffer a rebleed before they are seen and diagnosed by another health care provider. Hence, it is particularly important to diagnose patients who are alert, and neurologically intact, as these patients benefit most from prompt diagnosis and account for up to one-half of all SAH cases [10]. Such patients epitomize emergency medicine, as they can be difficult to diagnose and yet stand to lose the most by a missed diagnosis [11]. The crux to the problem for physicians is identifying which of these headache patients are at sufficient risk of SAH to warrant aggressive investigation and which are low enough risk that the costs and potential harms related to diagnostic testing make testing not worthwhile.

Clinical questions

1 In patients with an acute headache (population), are there reliable historical features (test) that are associated with subarachnoid hemorrhage (outcome)?

2 In patients with an acute headache (population), what are the likelihood ratios (diagnostic test characteristics) of physical exam findings (test) for the diagnosis of subarachnoid hemorrhage (outcome)?

3 In patients with acute headache (population), are there valid and reliable clinical criteria (clinical prediction guides) that can accurately

determine a patient's pre-test probability of subarachnoid hemorrhage (outcome)?

4 In patients with suspected subarachnoid hemorrhage (population), what are the likelihood ratios (diagnostic test characteristics) of brain computerized tomography for the diagnosis of subarachnoid hemorrhage (outcome)?

5 In patients with suspected subarachnoid hemorrhage (population), what are the likelihood ratios (diagnostic test characteristics) of cerebrospinal fluid analysis for the diagnosis of subarachnoid hemorrhage (outcome)?

6 Should spectrophotometry be used to identify xanthochromia in the cerebrospinal fluid?

7 In patients with confirmed subarachnoid hemorrhage (population), does lowering elevated blood pressure in the ED (treatment) result in lower mortality and morbidity (outcomes) compared to watchful waiting (control)?

8 In patients with confirmed subarachnoid hemorrhage (population), does the use of calcium channel blockers to prevent vasospasm (treatment) result in lower mortality and morbidity (outcomes) than placebo (control)?

9 In patients with confirmed subarachnoid hemorrhage (population), what is the risk (prognosis) of death or severe neurological deficit (outcomes) over the following year (follow-up)?

General search strategy

You begin to address these questions by searching for evidence in the common electronic databases such as the Cochrane Library and MEDLINE looking specifically for systematic reviews and meta-analyses. The Cochrane Library is particularly rich in high-quality systematic review evidence. When a systematic review is identified, you also search for recent updates on the Cochrane Library and also search MEDLINE to identify randomized controlled trials (RCTs) that became available after the publication date of the systematic review or for evidence where no previous systematic review is available. In addition, high-quality observational studies (i.e., prospective cohort studies) are accessed when no RCTs are available. Finally, in the absence of any evidence, summaries from clinical practice guidelines (CPGs) were sought.

Searching for evidence synthesis: primary search strategy
- Cochrane Library: subarachnoid hemorrhage AND (topic)
- MEDLINE: subarachnoid hemorrhage AND (systematic review OR meta-analysis) AND (topic)

Critical review of the literature

Question 1: In patients with an acute headache (population), are there reliable historical features (test) that are associated with subarachnoid hemorrhage (outcome)?

Search strategy

- Cochrane Library and MEDLINE: subarachnoid hemorrhage AND (risk factors OR clinical features)

Subarachnoid hemorrhage is a relatively rare cause of headache in ED patients, accounting for just 1% of all headaches. Despite being a rare cause of headache, it is arguably the most serious diagnosis to consider in patients with a complaint of headache. All patients with an altered mental status or a focal neurological deficit will be investigated for SAH. Therefore, it is only those patients presenting in an alert state without any neurological findings on physical examination with a severe headache who pose a diagnostic challenge. Given the limitations and side-effects of testing modalities, the first question to determine is which patients are at significant risk for SAH and warrant investigation. Much of this decision making is dependent on historical findings and eliciting risk factors.

A meta-analysis of risk factors associated with SAH included 14 longitudinal studies involving 892 patients and 23 case-controlled studies involving 3044 patients [12]. The review found that significant risk factors included: smoking (OR = 3.1; 95% CI: 2.7 to 3.5), hypertension (OR = 2.6; 95% CI: 2.0 to 3.1) and excessive alcohol intake (OR = 1.5; 95% CI: 1.3 to 1.8). These variables are prevalent among patients presenting to the ED and have not been assessed to determine how clinically useful they are for differentiating SAH from other headaches. Non-significant or equivocal findings included: race, oral contraceptives, hormone replacement therapy, diabetes or hypercholesterolemia.

A prospective study involving 1076 patients with SAH (mean age = 49 years) concluded that a provoking factor was present in 30% of cases, including intercourse in 5.5% of cases. Sixteen percent had a seizure, 31% were unconscious for greater than 1 hour and another 26% were unconscious for less than 1 hour [13]. Another prospective ED study enrolled 102 patients with a severe headache and found that seizure activity and temporary loss of consciousness were associated with SAH [14].

There are several studies that demonstrate an increased risk of SAH in patients whose first-degree relatives have had an SAH [4,15–22]. However, in a study that retrospectively identified patients who had suffered a fatal stroke, families were contacted to determine if they were able to identify correctly between an ischemic stroke, an intercerebral hemorrhage or an SAH. The families were not able to make this distinction; hence this may not be a reliable predictor [23].

Connective tissue disorders are also associated with an increased risk of SAH, including: Ehlers–Danlos syndrome type IV, autosomal dominant polycystic kidney disease, neurofibromatosis type I, α_1-antitrypsin deficiency and Marfan's syndrome [4]. People with these disorders, however, are very rare in the general population and these may not be useful for differentiating patients with SAH in the ED setting [24–29].

A prospective cohort study was conducted at three EDs in alert patients presenting with severe headache. This study enrolled 590 patients to identify high-risk historical features for SAH. Following multivariate logistic regression analysis, the following variables were significantly associated with SAH: age >50 years (OR = 7.8; 95% CI: 3.4 to 18.2), onset to peak headache in less than 10 minutes (OR = 1.4; 95% CI: 1.0 to 2.0), neck pain/stiffness (OR = 5.4; 95% CI: 2.1 to 13.5) and vomiting (OR = 2.7, 95% CI: 1.2 to 6.2). Of note, a headache described as the "worst headache of life" was not found to be significantly associated with SAH (adjusted OR = 1.9; 95% CI: 0.5 to 7.5) [30].

The inter-observer agreement of historical findings has only been reported in one abstract [31]. In this multi-center prospective cohort study, ED patients with a normal neurological exam and a complaint of a non-traumatic acute headache were enrolled. Two independent emergency physician assessments were completed prior to investigation. There were 204 assessments on 102 patients. There was substantial agreement (kappa (κ) > 0.6) for onset with headache awaking patient, transient loss of consciousness, sexual activity, vomiting, neck pain or stiffness, and onset with exertion. Factors that demonstrated insufficient agreement between reviewers (κ < 0.6) to be considered reliable predictors of SAH included isolated pain in occiput and worst headache of life.

In summary, SAH should be considered in patients with severe headache with a history of smoking, hypertension, heavy alcohol use, first-degree relative with SAH, connective tissue disorder, age over 50 years, provoking factor (e.g., physical exertion or sexual intercourse), loss of consciousness, neck pain or stiffness and/or vomiting.

Question 2: In patients with an acute headache (population), what are the likelihood ratios (diagnostic test characteristics) of physical exam findings (test) for the diagnosis of subarachnoid hemorrhage (outcome)?

Search strategy

- Cochrane Library and Medline: subarachnoid hemorrhage AND examination

No systematic reviews were identified for determining the accuracy of physical exam findings for SAH. Neck stiffness with flexion and extension has been frequently associated with the diagnosis of SAH and is cited in reviews of the topic [3,4,7]. Additional features associated with SAH include elevated systolic and diastolic blood pressure [3].

Kasner in 1997 and Garfinkle in 1992 discussed the ophthalmological findings in Terson's syndrome (intraocular hemorrhage in the unconscious patient with an anterior communicating artery aneurysmal hemorrhage). They describe subhyaloid hemorrhage as being a positive sign and intraocular blood being associated with greater mortality [32,33] These results, although interesting, do not occur in alert and conscious patients who are neurologi-

cally intact and are unlikely to prompt a treating physician to alter current management.

A prospective cohort study conducted at three university tertiary care EDs enrolled patients >15 years of age, with normal neurological examination, a GCS of 15 and a complaint of a non-traumatic acute headache over a 2-year period. Based on a study population of 589 patients, systolic blood pressure elevation demonstrated a weak association (OR = 1.02; 95% CI: 1.00 to 1.04) and neck stiffness a strong association (OR = 8.90; 95% CI: 3.9 to 20.2) with SAH.

In summary, any patients with global or focal neurological findings require investigations to identify SAH. In patients with a normal neurological exam, the presence of neck stiffness or increased blood pressure should increase your suspicion of SAH.

Question 3: In patients with acute headache (population), are there valid and reliable clinical criteria (clinical prediction guides) that can accurately determine a patient's pre-test probability of subarachnoid hemorrhage (outcome)?

Search strategy

- Cochrane Library and MEDLINE: subarachnoid hemorrhage AND (clinical decision rule OR prediction)

There are no validated clinical decision rules to safely rule out SAH. The only clinical rule developed to date categorizes neurologically intact, non-traumatic headache patients with headache peaking within 1 hour as either high or low risk [34]. While the rule shows promise, it must be validated prior to clinical use. This derivation study prospectively assessed 1993 ED headache patients including 128 (6.4%) SAH cases. The mean age was 43.4 years (standard deviation (SD) 17.1) with 60.5% of the patients being female. The median peak pain (0–10 scale) was 9 (inter-quartile range (IQR) = 8 to 10) and 78.5% reported the worst headache of their life. Of the 128 SAH cases, 80.3% underwent CT and 45.2% underwent lumbar puncture (LP). The proposed rule would stratify patients with any one of the following as high risk: arrived by ambulance, age ≥45 years, diastolic blood pressure ≥100 mmHg on arrival to ED or vomiting ≥1 time. In this derivation study, the rule was found to have a sensitivity of 100% (95% CI: 97% to 100%) and a specificity of 36% (95% CI: 34% to 39%) for SAH and would generate a 66% investigation rate [34].

Hence, while this proposed clinical decision rule should not be used to identify low-risk patients until prospectively validated, components of the rule could be used to identify high-risk patients. Patients with a severe headache, unlike previous headaches, peaking within 1 hour of onset with any of the high-risk features (i.e., arrived by ambulance, age ≥45 years, diastolic blood pressure ≥100 mmHg on arrival to ED, or vomiting) should have SAH considered in their differential diagnosis.

Question 4: In patients with suspected subarachnoid hemorrhage (population), what are the likelihood ratios (diagnostic test characteristics) of brain computerized tomography for the diagnosis of subarachnoid hemorrhage (outcome)?

Search strategy

- Cochrane Library and Medline: subarachnoid hemorrhage AND computed tomography

There was one systematic review identified which assessed the sensitivity of CT for SAH but was based on the results of only two studies [35]. One of the studies was retrospective ($N = 175$) [36] and the other was a prospective study of ED headache patients ($N = 51$) undergoing brain CT in less than 24 hours from headache onset with an SAH prevalence of 29% (15/51) [37]. The systematic review estimated that the sensitivity of brain CT for SAH was 93% (95% CI: 66% to 98%) [35].

The largest prospective cohort study identified in our search enrolled 1024 neurologically intact ED patients with rapidly peaking (<1 hour) headaches, including 83 (8.1%) patients with confirmed SAH [38]. In addition to the cases of SAH, there were 11 cases diagnosed with other serious illnesses with CT or LP: six with central nervous system neoplasm, four with other forms of cerebral hemorrhages and one with bacterial meningitis. The sensitivity of brain CT for SAH was 93% (95% CI: 85% to 97%), the specificity was 100% (95% CI: 99% to 100%) and the negative likelihood ratio was 0.072 (95% CI: 0.03 to 0.16); it was not possible to calculate the positive likelihood ratio due to zero false-positive scans in this study. The sensitivity for SAH in the a priori subgroup of patients with CT performed less than 6 hours from headache onset was 100% (95% CI: 94% to 100%) [38]. These data have only been published as an abstract and await full peer review publication.

An older prospective study, using second-generation CT technology, found overall sensitivity of brain CT for SAH to be 90.5% in less than 24 hours; however, when restricted to those with normal examinations, this sensitivity decreased to 80% [39].

Hence, it appears that the newer generation CT scanners have higher sensitivity and the sensitivity decreases as the time from headache onset increases. Although preliminary results indicate excellent sensitivity of brain CT scans performed within 6 hours of headache onset, the results are too imprecise to consider abandoning the current practice of performing routine LP for patients with negative brain CT scans.

Question 5: In patients with suspected subarachnoid hemorrhage (population), what are the likelihood ratios (diagnostic test characteristics) of cerebrospinal fluid analysis for the diagnosis of subarachnoid hemorrhage (outcome)?

Search strategy

- Cochrane Library and MEDLINE: subarachnoid hemorrhage AND (lumbar puncture OR cerebrospinal fluid)

Emergency medicine and neurosurgical dogma state that an LP is required for all patients with a negative CT scan to rule out SAH [40,41]. The rationale is that the sensitivity for SAH of CT is too low to be clinically acceptable (as discussed in Question 4). Despite the consensus, there is very little evidence to support this practice. Lumbar puncture is used to obtain cerebrospinal fluid. The fluid is examined for cell counts (number of red blood cells, white blood cells) and for the presence of xanthochromia (yellow pigment formed by the breakdown of red blood cells to oxyhemoglobin, bilirubin and methemoglobin within the cerebrospinal fluid).

The optimal test for the cerebrospinal fluid is uncertain; some have advocated testing the red blood cell count of the final tube of cerebrospinal fluid and others to check the supernatant for xanthochromia. An early retrospective study found that the red blood cell count was more sensitive than xanthochromia [42]. However, Vermeulen et al. refuted this by finding that xanthochromia by spectrophotometry was 100% sensitive in a retrospective study of 111 patients [43] and argued that the previous study had used visual inspection of the cerebrospinal fluid supernatant, which accounted for the lack of sensitivity of the xanthochromia test.

In a prospective cohort study of ED patients presenting with the worst headache of their lives (N = 107) 17% (18/107) were diagnosed with SAH [37]. Two patients were missed by brain CT but were diagnosed with SAH by having high red blood cells in the cerebrospinal fluid. There were many false-positive tests for xanthochromia using spectrophotometry [37]; however, neither of the two patients diagnosed with SAH solely by LP had an aneurysm identified despite repeated cerebral angiograms. Hence, it is unclear if these two cases represented false-positive tests or the so-called "angiogram-negative" SAH. Despite this uncertainty, the combined use of CT and LP (checking for both cell counts and xanthochromia) is thought to yield the highest sensitivity [7,44,45]. No studies determining the sensitivity of only using LP for diagnosis of SAH were found. However, there was one prospective study of 592 ED neurologically intact headache patients including 61 SAH cases which found that the strategy of performing a brain CT, and if normal, following it with an LP for visual xanthochromia or red blood cells, had a sensitivity of 100% (95% CI: 94% to 100%) and specificity of 67% (95% CI: 63% to 71%) for SAH, with a positive likelihood ratio (+LR) of 3.03 and a negative likelihood ratio (−LR) of <0.01 [46].

Cerebrospinal fluid has also been studied for D-dimers, bilirubin and ferritin. With the exception of an unblinded study with a small sample size, which claimed 100% sensitivity and specificity for SAH, the studies examining D-dimers did not add any information above that of the red blood cell count and the presence of xanthochromia [47]. This was also true of the studies testing for bilirubin and ferritin [48].

One novel study suggested that patients with a lone, acute, sudden headache and a normal examination should have an LP as the first investigation, and brain CT if this result was positive [49]. This study was based on a mathematical model and has not yet been prospectively validated. One potential criticism is whether or not it is safe to do an LP in the setting of SAH. The safety of performing an LP in patients with SAH was questioned in one study, which reported that seven out of 55 patients deteriorated after having an LP while being investigated for possible SAH [50]. These patients, however, all had focal deficits and/or neck stiffness. A subsequent observational study found that LP was safe; 91 patients without neurological deficits or neck stiffness underwent the procedure without adverse events [51]. Therefore, it is likely that this model is safe, albeit an incompletely proven approach. It does not, however, address the issue of which patients to test, the time delay with this test, or the morbidity involved with this procedure.

One problem with performing LP and examining the cerebrospinal fluid for blood is false-positive results. The main cause of false-positive red blood cells being present is a traumatic tap. This is a term that represents the presence of blood due to the spinal needle passing through a blood vessel prior to entering the subarachnoid space, causing the collection of blood (alone or mixed with cerebrospinal fluid) instead of cerebrospinal fluid only. Up to 25% of LPs result in a traumatic tap. Since this is fresh blood, it has been suggested that it should be negative for xanthochromia, which takes several hours to form. Many studies have tried to resolve this issue, however, none has been adequately proven to be accurate [52]. Hence, for cases with blood present in the cerebrospinal fluid without xanthochromia, the clinician must still use clinical judgment to determine if further investigation with angiography is justified based on their post-test probability of SAH.

In summary, until clarity emerges, the current standard of practice in modern EDs is to perform a brain CT scan followed by an LP to rule out SAH in patients with suspicious headaches.

Question 6: Should spectrophotometry be used to identify xanthochromia in the cerebrospinal fluid?

Search strategy

- Cochrane Library and MEDLINE: subarachnoid hemorrhage AND (spectrophotometry OR xanthochromia)

There are no systematic reviews assessing the accuracy of the presence of xanthochromia in cerebrospinal fluid in the diagnosis of SAH. Likewise, there are no randomized controlled studies in humans in which xanthochromia testing was compared to another standard approach to determine the impact of diagnostic testing on outcomes. Therefore, the only evidence available on this topic is based on several prospective cohort studies and in vitro laboratory studies.

Two laboratory studies where lysed red blood cells were artificially spiked into samples of cerebrospinal fluid have been conducted [53,54]. One of these studies concluded that visual detection of xanthochromia was only 27% sensitive and 98% specific for xanthochromia using spectrophotometry as the gold standard with the traditional definition of absorbance greater than 0.023 at 415 nm. This study demonstrated that oxyhemoglobin can be produced in vitro and that spectrophotometry is more sensitive to traces of pigment than the naked eye; their model is more relevant to red blood cells introduced into cerebrospinal fluid at the time of traumatic tap LP, and cannot estimate the diagnostic accuracy of spectrophotometry for SAH [53]. The second study added hemolysed blood and bilirubin to samples of cerebrospinal fluid [54]. The authors concluded that spectrophotometry is superior to visual inspection given that most cerebrospinal fluid samples are contaminated with oxyhemoglobin or only contain low levels of bilirubin. Neither study was conducted on cerebrospinal fluid samples of patients suspected of having SAH. Another laboratory study tested human cerebrospinal fluid samples that had bilirubin added to them to determine the sensitivity of physicians and medical students for visually detecting xanthochromia. They used spectrophotometry with an absorbance >0.05 at 450–460 nm as their gold standard. They found that visual detection of xanthochromia was very sensitive, with sensitivities of 100% for physicians ($N = 51$) and 99% for medical students ($N = 51$). They concluded that there was likely minimal benefit of spectrophotometry over visual inspection of cerebrospinal fluid for detecting xanthochromia [55].

A prospective Canadian study enrolled 220 acute headache patients with normal brain CT scans undergoing LP to rule out SAH. The cerebrospinal fluid was frozen and subsequently analyzed using spectrophotometry for four commonly accepted definitions of xanthochromia. The specificity of xanthochromia ranged from 97% (95% CI: 92% to 99%) for visual inspection down to 29% (95% CI: 23% to 35%) for two of the four spectrophotometric definitions tested. The introduction of spectrophotometry into routine practice would have resulted in 11–71% of all patients undergoing LP requiring cerebral angiography to rule out SAH. This study concluded that no proposed spectrophotometric definition was adequately specific for clinical practice. Because CT-negative patients undergoing LP have a low prevalence of SAH, utilizing spectrophotometry to identify xanthochromia would result in an unacceptably high rate of unnecessary cerebral angiography. Introducing spectrophotometry to "rule out" SAH can be expected to increase costs and potential harms associated with an invasive test such as cerebral angiography with little, if any, increase in diagnostic yield.

Furthermore, a retrospective case series of 189 patients with a normal brain CT scan who had cerebrospinal fluid analysis performed found that only one out of 60 positive cerebrospinal fluid results had an aneurysm [56]. Another retrospective case series was conducted involving 253 patients suspected of having an SAH with a normal brain CT scan [57]. Two of the included patients had an SAH (one aneurysm, one arteriovenous malformation) and the study determined that xanthochromia by spectrophotometry had a sensitivity of 100% and a specificity of 75%, which corresponded to a positive predictive value of just 3.3% in their patient population.

In summary, although spectrophotometry may be highly sensitive, it appears to lack adequate specificity to be clinically useful. The optimal analysis of cerebrospinal fluid appears to be assessing the cerebrospinal fluid for both visual xanthochromia or the presence of red blood cells.

Question 7: In patients with confirmed subarachnoid hemorrhage (population), does lowering elevated blood pressure in the ED (treatment) result in lower mortality and morbidity (outcomes) compared to watchful waiting (control)?

Search strategy

- Cochrane Library and MEDLINE: subarachnoid hemorrhage AND blood pressure control

Since many patients presenting to the ED with SAH have hypertension, uncertainty exists with respect to the role of hypertension in clinical outcome. A Cochrane systematic review published in 2001 examined interventions for deliberately altering blood pressure in acute stroke [58]. This review included four small studies of patients with ischemic and hemorrhagic stroke ($N = 153$) and reported 1-month mortality. None of the four studies individually had statistically significant improvement in outcome, nor did the combined outcome (OR = 1.10; 95% CI: 0.37 to 3.26).

In summary, in a patient diagnosed with SAH, there is no clear evidence to support acute blood pressure treatment in the ED. If

it is decided to treat an elevated blood pressure, this should be reserved for patients with severe hypertension [59].

Question 8: In patients with confirmed subarachnoid hemorrhage (population), does the use of calcium channel blockers to prevent vasospasm (treatment) result in lower mortality and morbidity (outcomes) than placebo (control)?

Search strategy

- Cochrane Library and MEDLINE: subarachnoid hemorrhage AND calcium antagonists

Cerebral vessel vasospasm is thought to contribute to the morbidity associated with SAH and efforts to reduce vasospasm have been the subject of considerable debate. Calcium antagonists may provide benefit to patients with an acute aneurysmal SAH by decreasing associated cerebral vessel vasospasm. A Cochrane systematic review found an overall benefit to the use of calcium channel antagonists [60]. There were 12 studies included in their analysis involving 2844 patients with aneurysmal SAH. These investigators found that the signs of secondary ischemia were less with calcium antagonists (RR = 0.67; 95% CI: 0.60 to 0.76) and the risk of infarction was lower (RR = 0.80; 95% CI: 0.71 to 0.89); however, there was no difference in mortality (RR = 0.90; 95% CI: 0.76 to 1.07). In the subgroup analysis including the five studies using nimodipine (either intravenous followed by oral, or oral only), there was a significant decrease in the risk of a poor outcome, defined as death, vegetative state or severe disability (RR = 0.73; 95% CI: 0.61 to 0.87) (Fig. 46.1).

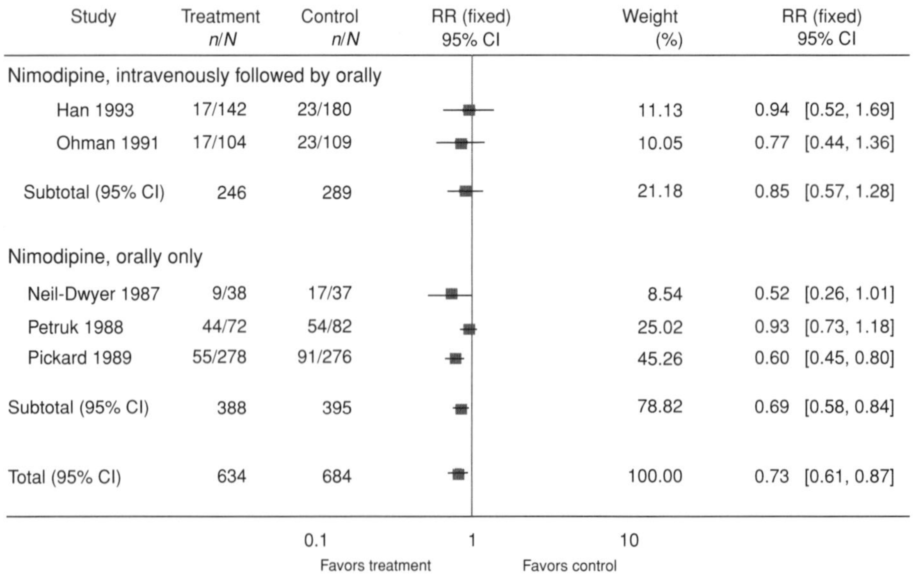

Study	Treatment n/N	Control n/N	RR (fixed) 95% CI	Weight (%)	RR (fixed) 95% CI
Nimodipine, intravenously followed by orally					
Han 1993	17/142	23/180		11.13	0.94 [0.52, 1.69]
Ohman 1991	17/104	23/109		10.05	0.77 [0.44, 1.36]
Subtotal (95% CI)	246	289		21.18	0.85 [0.57, 1.28]
Nimodipine, orally only					
Neil-Dwyer 1987	9/38	17/37		8.54	0.52 [0.26, 1.01]
Petruk 1988	44/72	54/82		25.02	0.93 [0.73, 1.18]
Pickard 1989	55/278	91/276		45.26	0.60 [0.45, 0.80]
Subtotal (95% CI)	388	395		78.82	0.69 [0.58, 0.84]
Total (95% CI)	634	684		100.00	0.73 [0.61, 0.87]

0.1   1   10
Favors treatment   Favors control

Figure 46.1 Poor outcome following the use of nimodipine between 3 and 6 months after subarachnoid hemorrhage [60].

Table 46.1 Classification, criteria, diagnosis and outcomes for patients with intracranial aneurysms according to surgical risk. (Adapted from Hunt & Hess [68], Chiang et al. [69] and Nina et al. [70].)

Category*	Criteria/diagnosis	Severe disability or mortality[†]	Treatment
Grade 1	Asymptomatic, or minimal headache and slight nuchal rigidity Both CT and LP usually required	Up to 16%	Expectant surgery
Grade 2	Moderate to severe headache, nuchal rigidity and no neurological deficit other than possible cranial nerve palsy Both CT and LP usually required	Up to 16%	Expectant surgery
Grade 3	Drowsiness, confusion or mild focal deficit CT usually positive	45–48%	Supportive care[‡]; surgery
Grade 4	Stupor, moderate to severe hemiparesis and possibly early decerebrate rigidity and vegetative disturbances CT always positive	79%	Supportive care; surgery
Grade 5	Deep coma, decerebrate rigidity and moribund appearance CT always positive	70–87%	Supportive care; coil embolization

*Serious systemic disease such as hypertension, diabetes, severe arteriosclersosis, chronic pulmonary disease and severe vasospasm, seen on angiography, result in placement of the patient in the next less favorable category.

[†]This assessment was based on the Hunt and Hess score on admission to hospital.

[‡]Supportive care = intracranial pressure monitor/ventricular drain, endotracheal intubation and blood pressure management as needed.

CT, computerized tomography of the head; LP, lumbar puncture.

Another meta-analysis included 10 studies using calcium channel blockers and three studies using magnesium infusions [61]. The authors concluded that only nimodipine has proven benefit to prevent vasospasm. Other calcium antagonists in this meta-analysis were nicardipine, an experimental drug labeled AT877, and magnesium; the benefit of any of these other agents was deemed to be inconclusive. A subsequent RCT that compared oral nimodipine to intravenous magnesium sulfate in 154 patients with SAH failed to identify a difference between the two treatment groups [62]. Another RCT comparing the combination of nimodipine and hypervolemic therapy to the same combination plus magnesium sulfate failed to identify a difference between treatments with respect to decreasing vasospasm frequency (RR = 1.21; 95% CI: 0.78 to 1.91) or survival (RR = 0.93; 95% CI: 0.76 to 1.14) [63]. A pilot study compared magnesium and nimodipine to nimodipine alone in 60 patients [64]. There was a trend towards a favorable outcome (defined by a Glasgow Outcome Scale score of 4 (moderate disability) or 5 (good recovery)) at 6 months in the magnesium group, which did not reach statistical significance (OR = 1.43; 95% CI: 0.68 to 3.06) [64].

The effectiveness of using calcium channel blockers for traumatic SAH is likely different than for SAH with non-traumatic etiology. A meta-analysis of 1074 traumatic SAH patients from five trials was completed in 2006 [65]. The risk of a poor outcome,

defined as death, vegetative state or severe disability, was similar with nimodipine compared to placebo (OR = 0.88; 95% CI: 0.51 to 1.54). When solely assessing survival, there was also no benefit to nimodipine (OR = 0.95; 95% CI: 0.71 to 1.26).

In summary, there is clear evidence to support the use of nimodipine in the setting of aneurysmal SAH although using nimodipine in traumatic SAH is not supported. Evidence is currently lacking for patients with non-traumatic SAH due to non-aneurysmal etiologies. Further study is required to determine if there is an advantage to using both nimodipine and magnesium.

Question 9: In patients with confirmed subarachnoid hemorrhage (population), what is the risk (prognosis) of death or severe neurological deficit (outcomes) over the following year (follow-up)?

Search strategy

- Cochrane Library and MEDLINE: subarachnoid hemorrhage AND prognosis

A meta-analysis of 21 population-based studies reported the range of case fatality rates to be between 32% and 67%, with the exception of one study with a fatality rate of 8% [6]. The outlier was an Italian study looking at all types of stroke and only included 12 cases of SAH, which is too small a sample size to draw any meaningful conclusions [66]. The meta-analysis found that the case fatality rate decreased by 0.5% per year from 1960 to 1992; however, this change was not statistically significant (95% CI: −0.1 to 1.2).

A second meta-analysis studied the proportion of patients with aneurysmal SAH who died prior to receiving medical attention. They included 18 studies between 1965 and 2001. The authors concluded that the overall risk of sudden death was 12.4% (95% CI: 11% to 14%) for anterior circulation aneurysmal SAH and 44.7% (95% CI: 7.4% to 86%) for posterior circulation aneurysms [67].

Based on a commonly used five-point clinical grading scale by Hunt and Hess, it has been estimated that survival to hospital discharge is 70% with grades 1–3 and less than 20% for grades 4 or 5 [68]. Subsequent studies have evaluated this scale on outcome with modern treatments (Table 46.1) [69,70]. Most overall prognosis studies report on death, but it is estimated that of survivors, approximately one-third require life-long assisted care [6].

In summary, the case fatality rate for SAH is high and efforts to detect and treat this disease are clearly warranted.

Conclusions

The 55-year-old patient with the rapidly peaking headache underwent an unenhanced brain CT scan which demonstrated diffuse SAH. She was referred to neurosurgery for consultation. Her cerebral angiogram demonstrated an 8 mm anterior communicating artery aneurysm. She was treated with nimodipine and went to the operating room to have the aneurysm clipped. She was subsequently discharged from the hospital with a good clinical outcome.

Subarachnoid hemorrhage is a devastating medical emergency with high morbidity and mortality. Patients with a more stable clinical condition (grades 1 and 2) have a much more favorable prognosis than those with more pronounced neurological deficits. Smoking, excessive alcohol intake, hypertension, family history and certain connective tissue disorders are risk factors for SAH. SAH should be considered in the differential diagnosis for patients presenting to the ED with severe headache and vomiting, elevated blood pressure, neck stiffness or if arriving by ambulance. The evaluation for possible SAH includes unenhanced brain CT and LP to analyze the cerebrospinal fluid for red blood cells and/or visual xanthochromia.

Acknowledgments

Dr. Perry's research is supported by the Ontario Ministry of Health and Long Term Care through a Career Scientist Award. The author wishes to thank Mrs. Irene Harris for her assistance with the completion of the manuscript.

Conflicts of interest

None were reported.

References

1 Ramirez-Lassepas M, Espinosa CE, Cicero JJ, Johnston KL, Cipolle RJ, Barber DL. Predictors of intracranial pathologic findings in patients who seek emergency care because of headache. *Arch Neurol* 1997;**54**: 1509.

2 Vermeulen M, van Gijn J. The diagnosis of subarachnoid haemorrhage. *J Neurol Neurosurg Psychiatry* 1990;**53**:365–72.

3 Edlow JA, Caplan LR. Avoiding pitfalls in the diagnosis of subarachnoid hemorrhage. *N Engl J Med* 2000;**342**:29–36.

4 Schievink WI. Intracranial aneurysms. *N Engl J Med* 1997;**336**:28–40.

5 Bonita R, Thomson S. Subarachnoid hemorrhage: epidemiology, diagnosis, management, and outcome. *Stroke* 1985;**16**:591–4.

6 Hop JW, Rinkel GJE, Algra A, van Gijn J. Case-fatality rates and functional outcome after subarachnoid hemorrhage – a systematic review. *Stroke* 1997;**28**:660–64.

7 Schull MJ. Headache and facial pain. In: Tintinalli JE, Kelen GD, Stapczynski JS, eds. *Emergency Medicine: A comprehensive study guide.* McGraw-Hill, New York, 2000:1427–8.

8 Perry JJ, Stiell IG, Wells GA, Spacek AM. Historical cohort study "use and yield of investigations for alert patients with possible subarachnoid hemorrhage". *Can J Emerg Med* 2002;**4**:333–7.

9 Vermeulen M, Schull M. Missed diagnosis of subarachnoid hemorrhage in the emergency department. *Stroke* 2007;**38**:1216–21.

10 Weir B. Headaches from aneurysms. *Cephalalgia* 1994;**14**:79–87.

11 Leicht MJ. Non-traumatic headache in the emergency department. *Ann Emerg Med* 1980;**9**:404–9.

12 Feigin VL, Rinkel GJE, Lawes CMM, et al. Risk factors for subarachnoid hemorrhage – an updated systematic review of epidemiological studies. *Stroke* 2005;**36**:2773–80.

13 Rosenorn J, Eskesen V, Schmidt K, et al. Clinical features and outcome in 1076 patients with ruptured intracranial saccular aneurysms: a prospective consecutive study. *Br J Neurosurgery* 1987;**1**:33–46.

14 Linn FHH, Rinkel GJE, Algra A, van Gijn J. Headache characteristics in subarachnoid haemorrhage and benign thunderclap headache. *J Neurol Neurosurg Psychiatry* 1998;**65**:791–3.

15 Leblanc R. Familial cerebral aneurysms. *Can J Neurol Sci* 1997;**24**:191–9.

16 Bromberg JEC, Rinkel GJE, Algra A, et al. Subarachnoid haemorrhage in first and second degree relatives of patients with subarachnoid haemorrhage. *BMJ* 1995;**311**:289.

17 Schievink WI, Schaid DJ, Michels VV, Piepgras DG. Familial aneurysmal subarachnoid hemorrhage: a community-based study. *J Neurosurg* 1995;**83**:426–9.

18 Schievink WI, Schaid DJ, Rogers HM, Piepgras DG, Michels VV. On the inheritance of intracranial aneurysms. *Stroke* 1994;**25**:2028–37.

19 Lozano AM, Leblanc R. Familial intracranial aneurysms. *J Neurosurg* 1987;**66**:522–8.

20 Norrgard O, Angquist K-A, Fodstad H, Forsell A, Lindberg M. Intracranial aneurysms and heredity. *Neurosurgery* 1987;**20**:236–9.

21 Ronkainen A, Hernesniemi J, Ryynanen M. Familial subarachnoid hemorrhage in East Finland, 1977–1990. *Neurosurgery* 1993;**33**:787–97.

22 Ronkainen A, Hernesniemi J, Tromp G. Special feature of familial intracranial aneurysms: report of 215 familial aneurysms. *Neurosurgery* 1995;**37**:43–7.

23 Bromberg JEC, Rinkel GJE, Algra A, Greebe P, Beldman T, van Gijn J. Validation of family history in subarachnoid hemorrhage. *Stroke* 1996;**27**:630–32.

24 Schievink WI, Prakash UBS, Piepgras DG, Mokri B. a1-antitrypsin deficiency in intracranial aneurysms and cervical artery dissection. *Lancet* 1994;**343**:452–3.

25 Schievink WI, Katzmann JA, Piepgras DG, Schaid DJ. Alpha-1-antitrypsin phenotypes among patients with intracranial aneurysms. *J Neurosurg* 1996;**84**:781–4.

26 Schievink WI, Michels VV, Piepgras DG. Neurovascular manifestations of heritable connective tissue disorders: a review. *Stroke* 1994;**25**:889–903.

27 Butler WE, Barker FG, Crowell RM. Patients with polycystic kidney disease would benefit from routine magnetic resonance angiographic screening for intracerebral aneurysms: a decision analysis. *Neurosurgery* 1996;**38**:506–16.

28 Chapman AB, Rubinstein D, Hughes R, et al. Intracranial aneurysms in autosomal dominant polycystic kidney disease. *N Engl J Med* 1992;**327**:916–20.

29 Wiebers DO, Torres VE. Screening for unruptured intracranial aneurysms in autosomal dominant polycystic kidney disease. *N Engl J Med* 1992;**327**:953–5.

30 Perry JJ, Stiell IG, Wells GA, et al. The value of history in the diagnosis of subarachnoid hemorrhage for emergency department patients with acute headache. *Acad Emerg Med* 2003;**10**:533.

31 Perry JJ, Stiell IG, Wells GA, et al. Interobserver agreement in the assessment of headache patients with possible subarachnoid hemorrhage. *Acad Emerg Med* 2006;**13**:S138.

32 Kasner SE, Liu GT, Galetta SL. Neuro-ophthalmologic aspects of aneurysms. *Neuroimag Clin North Am* 1997;**7**:679–92.

33 Garfinkle AM, Danys IR, Nicolle DA, Colohan RT, Brem S. Terson's syndrome: a reversible cause of blindness following subarachnoid hemorrhage. *J Neurosurg* 1992;**76**:766–71.

34 Perry JJ, Stiell IG, Wells GA, et al. A clinical decision rule to safely rule out subarachnoid hemorrhage in acute headache patients in the emergency department. *Acad Emerg Med* 2006;**13**:S9.

35 Edlow JA, Wyer PC. How good is a negative cranial computed tomographic scan result in excluding subarachnoid hemorrhage? *Ann Emerg Med* 2000;**36**:507–16.

36 van der Wee N, Rinkel GJE, Hasan D, van Gijn J. Detection of subarachnoid haemorrhage on early CT: is lumbar puncture still needed after a negative scan? *J Neurol Neurosurg Psychiatry* 1995;**58**:357–9.

37 Morgenstern LB, Luna-Gonzales H, Huber JC, Jr., et al. Worst headache and subarachnoid hemorrhage: prospective, modern computed tomography and spinal fluid analysis. *Ann Emerg Med* 1998;**32**:297–304.

38 Perry JJ, Stiell IG, Wells GA, et al. The sensitivity of computed tomography for subarachnoid hemorrhage for ED patients with headache. *Acad Emerg Med* 2004;**11**(5), 435.

39 Adams HP, Kassell NF, Torner JC, Sahs AL. CT and clinical correlations in recent aneurysmal subarachnoid hemorrhage: a preliminary report of the Cooperative Aneurysm Study. *Neurology* 1983;**33**:981–8.

40 Suarez JI, Tarr RW, Selman WR. Aneurysmal subarachnoid hemorrhage. *N Engl J Med* 2006;**354**:387–96.

41 Brisman JL, Song JK, Newell DW. Cerebral aneurysms. *N Engl J Med* 2006;**355**:928–39.

42 Macdonald A, Mendelow AD. Xanthochromia revisited: a re-evaluation of lumbar puncture and CT scanning in the diagnosis of subarachnoid haemorrhage. *J Neurol, Neurosurg Psychiatry* 1988;**51**:342–4.

43 Vermeulen M, Hasan D, Blijenberg BG, Hijdra A, van Gijn J. Xanthochromia after subarachnoid haemorrhage needs no revisitation. *J Neurol Neurosurg Psychiatry* 1989;**52**:826–8.

44 Tsementzis SA, Hitchcock ER, DeCothi A, Gill JS. Comparative studies of the diagnostic value of cerebrospinal fluid spectrophotometry and computed tomographic scanning in subarachnoid hemorrhage. *Neurosurgery* 1985;**17**:908–12.

45 Soderstrom CE. Diagnostic significance of CSF spectrophotometry and computer tomography in cerebrovascular disease. *Stroke* 1977;**8**:606–12.

46 Perry JJ, Spacek AM, Stiell IG, et al. Is a negative CT scan of the head and a negative lumbar puncture sufficient to rule out a subarachnoid hemorrhage? *Acad Emerg Med* 2005;**12**(5):53.

47 Lang DT, Berberian LB, Lee S, Ault M. Rapid differentiation of subarachnoid hemorrhage from traumatic lumbar puncture using the D-dimer assay. *Brief Sci Rep* 1990;**93**:403–5.

48 Page KB, Howell SJ, Smith CML, et al. Bilirubin, ferritin, D-dimers and erythrophages in the cerebrospinal fluid of patients with suspected subarachnoid haemorrhage but negative computed tomography scans. *J Clin Pathol* 1994;**47**:989.

49 Schull MJ. Lumbar puncture first: an alternative model for the investigation of lone acute sudden headache. *Acad Emerg Med* 1999;**6**:131–6.

50 Duffy GP. Lumbar puncture in spontaneous subarachnoid haemorrhage. *BMJ* 1982;**285**:1163–4.

51 Patel MK, Clarke MA. Lumbar puncture and subarachnoid hemorrhage. *Postgrad Med J* 1986;**62**:1021–4.

52 Buruma OJS, Janson HLF, Den Bergh FAJTM, Bots GT. Blood-stained cerebrospinal fluid: traumatic puncture or haemorrhage? *J Neurol Neurosurg Psychiatry* 1981;**44**:144–7.

53 Sidman R, Spitalnic S, Demelis M, Durfey N, Jay G. Xanthochromia? By what method? A comparison of visual and spectrophotometric xanthochromia. *Ann Emerg Med* 2005;**46**:51–5.

54 Petzold A, Keir G, Sharpe TL. Why human color vision cannot reliably detect cerebrospinal fluid xanthochromia. *Stroke* 2005;**36**:1295–7.

55 Linn FHH, Voorbij HAM, Rinkel GJE, Algra A, van Gijn J. Visual inspection versus spectrophotometry in detecting bilirubin in cerebrospinal fluid. *J Neurol Neurosurg Psychiatry* 2005;**76**:1452–4.

56 Foot C, Staib A. How valuable is a lumbar puncture in the management of patients with suspected subarachnoid haemorrhage? *Emerg Med* 2001;**13**:326–32.

57 Wood MJ, Dimeski G, Nowitzke AM. CSF spectrophotometry in the diagnosis and exclusion of spontaneous subarachnoid haemorrhage. *J Clin Neurosci* 2005;**123**:142–6.

58 Blood pressure in Acute Stroke Collaboration (BASC). Interventions for deliberately altering blood pressure in acute stroke (Review). *Cochrane Database Syst Rev* 2008;**2**:CD000039.

59 van Gijn J, Kerr R, Rinkel GJE. Subarachnoid haemorrhage. *Lancet* 2007;**369**:306–18.

60 Rinkel GJE, Feigin VL, Algra A, van den Bergh WM, Vermeulen M, van Gijn J. Calcium antagonists for aneurysmal subarachnoid haemorrhage (Review). *Cochrane Database Syst Rev* 2005;**1**:CD000277.

61 Weyer GW, Nolan CP, Macdonald RL. Evidence-based cerebral vasospasm management. *Neurosurg Focus* 2006;**21**:1–10.

62 Schmid-Elsaesser R, Kunz M, Zausinger S, Prueckner S, Briegel J, Steiger H-J. Intravenous magnesium versus nimodipine in the treatment of patients with aneurysmal subarachnoid hemorrhage: a randomized study. *Neurosurgery* 2006;**58**:1054–65.

63 Prevedello DM-S, Cordeiro JG, de Morais AL, Saucedo NS, Chen IB, Araujo JC. Magnesium sulfate: role as possible attenuating factor in vasospasm morbidity. *Surg Neurol* 2006;**65**:S1:14–S1:21.

64 Wong GKC, Chan MTV, Boet R, Poon WS, Gin T. Intravenous magnesium sulfate after aneurysmal subarachnoid hemorrhage: a prospective randomized pilot study. *J Neurosurg Anesthesiol* 2006;**18**:142–8.

65 Vergouwen MDI, Vermeulen M, Roos YBWEM. Effect of nimodipine on outcome in patients with traumatic subarachnoid haemorrhage: a systematic review. *Lancet Neurol* 2006;**5**:1029–32.

66 Lauria G, Gentile M, Fassetta G, et al. Incidence and prognosis of stroke in the Belluno Province, Italy. *Stroke* 1995;**26**:1787–93.

67 Huang J, Van Gelder JM. The probability of sudden death from rupture of intracranial aneurysms: a meta-analysis. *Neurosurgery* 2002;**51**:1101–7.

68 Hunt WE, Hess RM. Surgical risk as related to time of intervention in the repair of intracranial aneurysms. *J Neurosurg* 1968;**28**:14–20.

69 Chiang VLS, Claus EB, Awad IA. Toward more rational prediction of outcome in patients with high-grade subarachnoid hemorrhage. *Neurosurgery* 2000;**46**:28–36.

70 Nina P, Schisano G, Chiappetta F, et al. A study of blood coagulation and fibrinolytic system in spontaneous subarachnoid hemorrhage. Correlation with Hunt-Hess grade and outcome. *Surg Neurol* 2001;**55**:197–203.

47 Bacterial Meningitis

Cheryl K. Chang & Peter C. Wyer

Department of Medicine, Columbia University College of Physicians and Surgeons, New York, USA

Case scenario

A 19-year-old college freshman arrived in the emergency department (ED) accompanied by her roommate. She reported feeling poorly with subjective fevers and a headache with mild photophobia for 3 days. She complained of nausea and anorexia. She denied any past medical history, medication allergies or food allergies. Her past surgical history was significant for an appendectomy. Her medications included low-dose birth control pills.

Her friend brought her into the ED because she was concerned that the patient had not attended classes or eaten meals for the previous 4 days. She appeared diaphoretic and slightly unkempt, but answered all questions. Her vital signs were: pulse 102 beats/min, blood pressure 110/76 mmHg, respirations 14 breaths/min and temperature 39°C (oral). She was arousable, oriented and interacted appropriately. She was warm to the touch but did not have a skin rash; her abdominal and lung examinations were normal. Her heart exam was significant only for tachycardia. Head and neck examination identified slightly erythematous tonsils without exudates, shoddy anterior cervical lymph nodes, normal tympanic membranes and slight neck stiffness without true rigidity.

Your differential diagnosis included bacterial meningitis, and you were concerned about her drowsiness. After your team established intravenous access, drew blood and cultures, and monitored the patient, you prepared to perform a lumbar puncture (LP). The intern suggested initiation of empirical therapy with antibiotics and corticosteroids prior to the LP. Your resident recommended using a special type of spinal needle designed to decrease postpuncture headache.

Evidence-based Emergency Medicine. Edited by Brian H. Rowe
© 2009 Blackwell Publishing, ISBN: 978-1-4051-6143-5.

Background

Bacterial meningitis continues to affect children and adults in developed and developing nations alike. In developed countries, the incidence per year is estimated to be about 1–4 per 100,000 adults (prior to the meningococcal polysaccharide and conjugate vaccines, *Streptococcus pneumoniae* vaccine and *Haemophilus influenza* type b vaccine) and is many times higher in developing nations, such as in the African meningitis belt, an area of sub-Saharan Africa. About 80% of cases are caused by *S. pneumoniae* and *Neisseria meningitides* [1]. Because increasing vaccination rates in children has decreased the incidence of bacterial meningitis among children, there is a proportionally higher rate of infection in adults in developed countries. The case fatality rate for bacterial meningitis is 10–30% and long-term disability such as hearing loss occurs in up to 50% of patients [2].

As a high stakes disease, an accurate and rapid diagnosis of bacterial meningitis is crucial and treatment may be life saving. Diagnostic challenges include clinical selection, procedural technique and associated risks, and the interpretation of cerebral spinal fluid (CSF) results in patients who undergo LP. Therapeutic issues facing emergency practitioners pertain to choice of antibiotics and adjuvant therapy with corticosteroids in patients considered to be high risk.

In approaching an evidence-based review of our chosen questions, we have taken into account that much of the clinical research pertaining to bacterial meningitis has been done in preponderantly pediatric populations. Although the subject of our chapter is bacterial meningitis in adults, we have elected to consider studies done in pediatrics when no comparable studies in adults were available or when we considered the resulting evidence to be applicable to adult emergency care.

Clinical questions

In order to address the issues relevant to your patient and to help in searching the literature for the evidence regarding meningitis, the clinical questions are structured as recommended in Chapter 1.

1 In patients presenting to the ED with suspected bacterial meningitis (population), what are the likelihood ratios (diagnostic test characteristics) of biological markers on peripheral blood and CSF (tests) compared to CSF culture (criterion standard)?

2 In adults presenting to the ED with suspected bacterial meningitis (population), what are the sensitivity and specificity (diagnostic test characteristics) of clinical signs, patient symptoms or physical examination findings (tests) compared to CSF culture (criterion standard)?

3 In adults presenting to the ED with suspected bacterial meningitis (population), does early head computerized tomography (intervention) reduce the complications of lumbar puncture (outcome) compared to lumbar puncture without computerized tomography (comparison)?

4 In adults undergoing lumbar puncture (population), does the use of an "atraumatic" needle (intervention) compared to the use of a standard, cutting needle (comparison) decrease the incidence of post-lumbar puncture headache (outcome)?

5 In adult patients with bacterial meningitis (population), how do the third-generation cephalosporins (therapy) compare with the standard treatment of a penicillin with chloramphenicol (control) for reducing mortality and neurological sequelae (outcomes)?

6 In adult patients with bacterial meningitis (population), does fluid therapy (therapy) compared with fluid restriction (control) decrease mortality or neurological deficits (outcomes)?

7 In adult patients with bacterial meningitis (population), does adjuvant corticosteroid therapy plus appropriate antibiotics (therapy) compared to appropriate antibiotics alone (control) reduce mortality and neurological deficits (outcomes)?

General search strategy

Searching for systematic reviews, meta-analyses and randomized controlled trials, the initial search strategy for questions related to therapy and harm included the Cochrane Library, including the Cochrane Database of Systematic Reviews (CDSR) and the Cochrane Central Register of Controlled Trials (CENTRAL) and MEDLINE. For questions related to diagnosis, additional databases were searched including the Database of Abstracts of Reviews of Effects (DARE) within the Cochrane Library and bibliography reviews.

Critical appraisal of the literature

Question 1: In patients presenting to the ED with suspected bacterial meningitis (population), what are the likelihood ratios (diagnostic test characteristics) of biological markers on peripheral blood and CSF (tests) compared to CSF culture (criterion standard)?

Table 47.1 Predictors of bacterial etiology of meningitis in children with cerebrospinal fluid (CSF) pleocytosis. (Adapted from Nigrovic et al. [3].)

Criteria/factors
Bacterial organisms on CSF Gram stain
Absolute CSF neutrophil count > 1000 cells/μl
CSF protein > 80 mg/dl
Absolute peripheral blood neutrophil count > 10,000 cells/μl
Seizure before or at presentation

Search strategy

- OVID MEDLINE (1966–2007) and Cochrane: meningitis [MeSH] AND (specificity OR sensitivity [MeSH]) AND test* AND peripheral blood AND (cerebrospinal fluid OR CSF). Restricted to humans and English language

Lumbar puncture remains the diagnostic test of choice for ruling in or excluding bacterial meningitis. A MEDLINE search revealed an original validation study of a clinical decision rule for determining the risk of bacterial meningitis in pediatric patients [3] and one systematic review pertaining to the diagnosis of meningitis in adults [4]. Under the auspices of a pediatric emergency medicine research collaboration, Nigrovic et al. validated a previously derived clinical prediction rule for bacterial meningitis using a multi-center retrospective study of 3295 US children presenting to EDs and found to have CSF pleocytosis [3]. In this study, 3.7% (95% CI: 3.1% to 4.3%) of the children proved to have bacterial meningitis. Children who had none of the five predictors listed in Table 47.1 had a 0.12% (95% CI: 0.01% to 0.42%) risk of bacterial meningitis, yielding a likelihood ratio for a negative assessment of 0.03 (95% CI: 0.01 to 0.11).

The applicability of this prediction rule to adults is uncertain. Although Nigrovic et al. enrolled patients from 1 month to 19 years of age, the mean age was 4.6 years and most patients who ruled in for meningitis were less than a year old. On the other hand, the only cases of bacterial meningitis misclassified by the rule, both in the derivation and the validation studies, were among the very young (under 2 months old) [5]. Practitioners caring for adult patients may reasonably consider using the components of this rule in clinical decision making, but direct application of the rule itself cannot be recommended until studied in the adult population.

Straus et al. performed a systematic review of studies on techniques of LP and the interpretation of CSF results in relationship to bacterial meningitis in adults [4]. They examined published prediction models developed in adult populations and determined that no such model had been independently validated. They similarly found only poor-quality evidence regarding the performance of individual components of CSF analysis. In one retrospective study, CSF Gram stain was observed to have a positive likelihood ratio (+LR) of 737 and a negative likelihood ratio (−LR) of 0.14. However, the sensitivity of the Gram stain was reported to be substantially lower in two other studies that did not report full data. A CSF white blood cell (WBC) count of >500/μl or a CSF glucose to serum glucose ratio of <40% had substantial effects on increasing the likelihood of bacterial meningitis (+LR = 15 and 23, respectively), but only slightly decreased it (−LR = 0.30 and 0.50, respectively).

Other biological tests that have been used as markers for bacterial meningitis include CSF lactate [4], polymerase C reaction (PCR) [6] and serum procalcitonin [7]. The performance of these tests has not been as well studied as have the foregoing ones. Furthermore, although the PCR test is not affected by previous administration of antibiotics, in most hospital settings the turn around time is not rapid enough to be useful in emergency decision making.

In summary, valid criteria for interpreting CSF and other laboratory tests to distinguish between bacterial and viral meningitis have been reported in pediatric populations but not in adults with CSF pleocytosis. Studies of adults, however, indicate that CSF Gram stain, a glucose <40% of serum, and a CSF WBC count of >500/μl are relatively useful for this purpose.

Question 2: In adults presenting to the ED with suspected bacterial meningitis (population), what are the sensitivity and specificity (diagnostic test characteristics) of clinical signs, patient symptoms or physical examination findings (tests) compared to CSF culture (criterion standard)?

Search strategy

- OVID MEDLINE (1966–2007) and Cochrane: bacterial meningitis [MeSH] AND (cerebrospinal fluid OR CSF) AND (diagnosis OR physical examination). Restricted to humans and English language

A search of the literature revealed a systematic review published as part of the Rational Clinical Examination series in the *Journal of the American Medical Association* and a discussion [8,9] and two recent studies [10,11]. The authors selected studies that described the accuracy and precision of the clinical examination in the diagnosis of meningitis in adults, excluding studies involving immunocompromised patients, meningitis of a single specific microbial origin, tuberculous meningitis or metastatic meningitis. Ten studies enrolled 824 patients (ages 16 to 95 years). All but one were retrospective case series of confirmed meningitis based on chart review, and hence allowed the calculation of sensitivities of single or combined clinical criteria but not of specificities or likelihood ratios. This renders the evaluation of the utility of clinical findings incomplete. Meningitis was confirmed by LP or

autopsy and included both bacterial and viral acute infections of the meninges.

Elements of the clinical history, including headache, nausea and vomiting, and neck pain, have low sensitivity for the diagnosis of meningitis. The pooled sensitivity for headache was 50% (95% CI: 32% to 68%); however, for nausea and vomiting the pooled sensitivity was only 30% (95% CI: 22% to 38%). Although the absence of specificity data precludes a definitive conclusion, these results suggest that clinical history alone is not an adequate basis for excluding the diagnosis of bacterial meningitis.

Although none of the elements of the physical exam taken in isolation has sufficient sensitivity to rule out meningitis, based on the results of two studies the authors of the systematic review suggest that the absence of the clinical triad of fever, neck stiffness and altered mental status may allow the elimination of meningitis from the differential diagnosis (sensitivity, 99–100% for the presence of at least one of these findings). One small study ($n = 34$) suggests that the absence of jolt accentuation of headache in patients presenting with fever, headache and CSF pleocytosis was useful for eliminating the diagnosis of meningitis (sensitivity = 100%, specificity = 54%) [12]. This test required the patient to turn his or her head horizontally, back and forth, at a frequency of two to three rotations per second. Worsening of the existing headache was interpreted as a positive jolt accentuation test.

Fever alone, in the one prospective study, had a weak +LR (1.5) yet reasonably helpful −LR of 0.3 for the presence of either viral or bacterial meningitis [12]. The pooled sensitivity of 85% reported by the authors of the systematic review demonstrates why a relatively high sensitivity of a test does not guarantee clinical utility. A patient with a 50% likelihood of meningitis by other criteria would still have a 23% likelihood in the absence of fever. Neck stiffness had a pooled sensitivity of 70% (95% CI: 58% to 82%).

More recently, Dutch researchers conducted a retrospective study of 696 adults with community-acquired bacterial meningitis to determine clinical features and prognostic factors [10]. The classic triad of fever, stiff neck and altered mental status (14 points or fewer on the Glasgow Coma Scale) was found in only 44% of patients. However, at least one of the symptoms was present in 99% of patients, providing concordance with the results reported in the systematic review of Attia et al. [8,10].

The classic signs of Kernig and Brudzinski are unreliable in adults. In a study of adult patients suspected of having meningitis, only 5% of patients with and without meningitis demonstrated Kernig's or Brudzinski's signs [11].

In summary, history alone appears to be an inadequate basis for excluding bacterial meningitis. Absence of all of the components of the classic triad of fever, stiff neck and altered mental status is likely a sound basis for excluding the diagnosis of meningitis in immunocompetent adults. Existing clinical evidence does not provide strong guidance for patients with fever in the absence of the other two components of the triad.

Table 47.2 Summary of studies considering predictors of contraindications to lumbar puncture on routine computerized tomography (CT) imaging.

Study	Population	Candidate predictors	CT criteria	Operating characteristics of assessment				
				predictor	Sensitivity	Specificity	+LR	−LR
Gopal et al. [13]	113 adult patients presenting to the ED in a US teaching hospital with urgent need for LP, 37% to rule out meningitis	History/risk factors for HIV Other immune suppression Malignancy Head trauma within 72 hours History of CNS lesion Altered mental status Seizures within 72 hours Papilloedema Focal neurological findings Global clinical assessment	Midline shift Obliteration of cisterns Obliteration of fourth ventricle Any mass lesion	Papilloedema ≥ 1 abnormal historical or physical exam finding Global assessment	18% 100% 40%	87% 37% 96%	11 1.6 9	0.9 0 0.6
Hasbun et al. [14]	235 adults with suspected meningitis presenting to the ED in a US teaching hospital; 6% had bacterial meningitis	Wide range of historical, clinical and laboratory criteria. The NIH Stroke Scale was used to identify neurological deficits	Midline shift Obliteration of cisterns Focal abnormality without mass effect	Age > 60 years Immunocompromised state History of CNS disease Seizure <1 week Abnormal neurological finding	95%	52%	2.0	0.1

CNS, central nervous system; CT, computerized tomography; ED, emergency department; LP, lumbar puncture; +LR, positive likelihood ratio; −LR, negative likelihood ratio.

Question 3: In adults presenting to the ED with suspected bacterial meningitis (population) does early head computerized tomography (intervention) reduce the complications of lumbar puncture (outcome) compared to lumbar puncture without computerized tomography (comparison)?

Search strategy

- OVID MEDLINE (1966–2007) and Cochrane: bacterial meningitis [MeSH] AND (tomography OR CT) AND head AND (spinal OR lumbar OR LP) AND puncture. Restricted to humans and English language

Our search indirectly identified two prospective studies that addressed this question (Table 47.2) [13,14]. Of these, only Hasbun et al. confined their enrollment to patients with suspected meningitis [14]. The authors used logistic regression to identify a set of five characteristics (Table 47.2) that, if all were absent, lowered the likelihood of an abnormal head computerized tomography (CT) scan. Ninety-six of the 235 patients were negative with respect to all of these assessments, of whom three (negative predictive value = 3.1%; 95% CI: 0.7% to 8.9%) had an abnormal CT. Among the three patients, one had a focal abnormality, one had a non-focal abnormality and one had hydrocephalus with some mild mass effect. If CT positivity were restricted to mass effect, approximately

one in 100 patients would have been misclassified by applying the criteria. The derivation of Hasbrun's Clinical Prediction Rule requires prospective validation before widespread adoption into clinical practice [15].

Gopal et al. analyzed predictors of CT abnormality in an ED population of patients undergoing LP for any reason and also included the global clinical assessment (gestalt) of the examining physicians [13]. When an absolute contraindication to LP was used as the CT standard for positivity, global clinical judgment was 100% sensitive in identifying patients with such findings.

The prospective studies of Gopal and Hasbun supplant previous retrospective case series based on small numbers of patients of extreme severity who herniated around the time of lumbar puncture [16]. Although more compelling in their methodology, it is important to note that the more recent studies do not provide data regarding the actual risk of imminent herniation. Two patients in the study by Gopal et al. and none in that of Hasbun et al. were observed to have that outcome.

In summary, although brain herniation is a potentially devastating consequence of diagnostic LP, recent evidence supports the approach of performing LP without requiring an initial head CT in clinically stable immunocompetent patients with no history of central nervous system lesions or focal neurological deficit. The use of a prediction rule, however, should not override clinical judgment, particularly when independent validation studies have not been performed.

Question 4: In adults undergoing lumbar puncture (population), does the use of an "atraumatic" needle (intervention) compared to the use of a standard, cutting needle (comparison) decrease the incidence of post-lumbar puncture headache (outcome)?

Search strategy

- OVID MEDLINE (1966–2007) and Cochrane: (lumbar OR spinal [MeSH]) AND puncture AND needle*. Restricted to humans and English language

A search of the literature revealed one systematic review [4] and several randomized, controlled studies comparing standard LP needles versus "atraumatic" needles [17]. The etiology of post-LP headache has been attributed to CSF leakage. Many studies have compared the "atraumatic" needle, with or without an introducer, to the standard needle. The "atraumatic" needle has a pencil-point needle tip, with the eyelet lumen separated from the tip, and may require the use of a special introducer. The traditional Quincke needle has a beveled, sharp, needle tip.

Individual randomized trials have been done on non-emergent adult neurology patients comparing the incidence of post-LP headache when the atraumatic needle was used compared to the standard Quincke-type needle [17]. Strupp et al. found that the use of the atraumatic needle reduced the incidence of post-LP headache from 28/115 to 14/115 (RR = 0.50; 95% CI: 0.28 to 0.89); the number needed to treat in this study was eight. However, Straus et al. found significant heterogeneity among studies and reported a pooled absolute risk reduction of 12.3% (95% CI: −1.7% to 26%) which favors the atraumatic needle but is not definitive [4].

In summary, the atraumatic needle appears to decrease moderate to severe post-LP headache but the supporting evidence is variable in both quality and results. In addition, issues related to difficulty in use and failure rates are not adequately addressed, thus the generalizability and application to emergency care is questionable.

Question 5: In adult patients with bacterial meningitis (population), how do the third-generation cephalosporins (therapy) compare with the standard treatment of a penicillin with chloramphenicol (control) for reducing mortality and neurological sequelae (outcomes)?

Search strategy

- OVID MEDLINE (1966–2007) and Cochrane: bacterial meningitis [MeSH] AND (antibiotic* OR anti-bacterial agents). Restricted to humans and English language

The timing and selection of antibiotics for the treatment of meningitis are important considerations for emergency physicians. A Cochrane meta-analysis of 18 studies involving 993 patients compared the effectiveness of antibiotics to determine whether or not third-generation cephalosporins were safer and more effective than older, conventional antibiotics [2]. Half of the studies were from developed countries and the other half were from developing countries. Patient age ranged from 1 week to 59 years; four of the 18 studies included adults and only two studies were restricted to adults. The third-generation cephalosporins used in the studies included ceftriaxone, cefotaxime or ceftazidime. The comparison treatment regimens included various combinations of ampicillin, chloramphenicol, gentamicin and benzylpenicillin. Follow-up of the patients was as short as the length of the hospital stay in two studies, 1–2 weeks in four studies, more than 1 month in eight studies, and 3 months or more (12 months) in five studies. Mortality was more common in the developing countries.

Between the drug regimens, there was no difference in the risk of mortality, deafness or treatment failure [2]. Mortality in the third-generation cephalosporin group was 38 out of 503 patients compared with 38 out of 490 patients in the conventional antibiotic group (risk difference = −1%; 95% CI: −4% to 3%) (Fig. 47.1). Also, there was no significant difference in the risk of deafness between the two groups (risk difference = −4%; 95% CI: −9% to 1%). There was also no significant difference in the risk of treatment failure (risk difference = −2%; 95% CI: −5% to 2%). Diarrhea occurred more frequently in the cephalosporin group.

In summary, based on the best available systematic review evidence, there were no significant differences between third-generation cephalosporins and standard treatment with a penicillin and chloramphenicol in the risk of mortality, deafness or treatment failure. Appropriate choice of antibiotic may vary with geographical location and circumstances. Given the lack of definitive advantage between alternative regimens in major clinically important outcomes, less cost-intensive regimens may be appropriate in developing countries. Information on local antibiotic resistance should guide therapy whenever possible.

Question 6: In adult patients with bacterial meningitis (population), does fluid therapy (therapy) compared with fluid restriction (control) decrease mortality or neurological deficits (outcomes)?

Search strategy

- OVID MEDLINE (1966–2007) and Cochrane: bacterial meningitis [MeSH] AND (fluid therapy OR fluids). Restricted to humans and English language

A search of the literature revealed a systematic review related to our question [18]. Of the three trials included in the Cochrane review, all were performed in children. The review highlights a comparison of intravenous maintenance fluids versus fluid restriction in

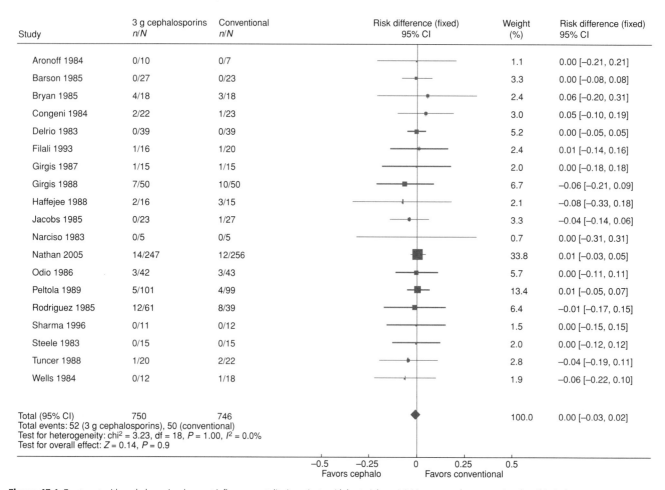

Study	3 g cephalosporins n/N	Conventional n/N	Risk difference (fixed) 95% CI	Weight (%)	Risk difference (fixed) 95% CI
Aronoff 1984	0/10	0/7		1.1	0.00 [−0.21, 0.21]
Barson 1985	0/27	0/23		3.3	0.00 [−0.08, 0.08]
Bryan 1985	4/18	3/18		2.4	0.06 [−0.20, 0.31]
Congeni 1984	2/22	1/23		3.0	0.05 [−0.10, 0.19]
Delrio 1983	0/39	0/39		5.2	0.00 [−0.05, 0.05]
Filali 1993	1/16	1/20		2.4	0.01 [−0.14, 0.16]
Girgis 1987	1/15	1/15		2.0	0.00 [−0.18, 0.18]
Girgis 1988	7/50	10/50		6.7	−0.06 [−0.21, 0.09]
Haffejee 1988	2/16	3/15		2.1	−0.08 [−0.33, 0.18]
Jacobs 1985	0/23	1/27		3.3	−0.04 [−0.14, 0.06]
Narciso 1983	0/5	0/5		0.7	0.00 [−0.31, 0.31]
Nathan 2005	14/247	12/256		33.8	0.01 [−0.03, 0.05]
Odio 1986	3/42	3/43		5.7	0.00 [−0.11, 0.11]
Peltola 1989	5/101	4/99		13.4	0.01 [−0.05, 0.07]
Rodriguez 1985	12/61	8/39		6.4	−0.01 [−0.17, 0.15]
Sharma 1996	0/11	0/12		1.5	0.00 [−0.15, 0.15]
Steele 1983	0/15	0/15		2.0	0.00 [−0.12, 0.12]
Tuncer 1988	1/20	2/22		2.8	−0.04 [−0.19, 0.11]
Wells 1984	0/12	1/18		1.9	−0.06 [−0.22, 0.10]
Total (95% CI)	**750**	**746**		**100.0**	**0.00 [−0.03, 0.02]**

Total events: 52 (3 g cephalosporins), 50 (conventional)
Test for heterogeneity: chi^2 = 3.23, df = 18, P = 1.00, I^2 = 0.0%
Test for overall effect: Z = 0.14, P = 0.9

−0.5 −0.25 0 0.25 0.5
Favors cephalo   Favors conventional

Figure 47.1 Treatment with cephalosporins does not influence mortality in patients with bacterial meninigitis compared to conventional antibiotic therapy.

bacterial meningitis in countries where mortality was high, and patients sought treatment late in the course of their disease. The largest study was performed in Papua New Guinea where one-quarter of the study population was malnourished and two-thirds of the patients had convulsions prior to presentation. The meta-analysis revealed no significant difference in mortality between the maintenance fluid and restricted fluid groups (RR = 0.82; 95% CI: 0.53 to 1.27), or in acute, severe or mild to moderate neurological sequelae (RR = 0.67; 95% CI: 0.41 to 1.08; and RR = 1.24; 95% CI: 0.58 to 2.68, respectively). However, further delineation of neu-rological sequelae demonstrated improved outcomes in patients receiving maintenance fluids with respect to spasticity (RR = 0.50; 95% CI: 0.27 to 0.93), seizure activity at 72 hours and at 14 days (RR = 0.59; 95% CI: 0.42 to 0.83; and RR = 0.19; 95% CI: 0.04 to 0.88, respectively) and long-term neurologic sequelae at 3 months (RR = 0.42; 95% CI: 0.20 to 0.89).

In summary, some evidence supports the use of intravenous maintenance fluids in preference to restricted fluid intake during the first 48 hours in patient populations with high mortality rates. Dehydration may be more of a factor in meningitis patients in developing countries where more aggressive fluid therapy may be more appropriate. The applicability of these findings to adults is uncertain.

Question 7: In adult patients with bacterial meningitis (population), does adjuvant corticosteroid therapy plus appropriate antibiotics (therapy) compared to appropriate antibiotics alone (control) reduce mortality and neurological deficits (outcomes)?

Search strategy

- OVID MEDLINE (1966–2007) and Cochrane: bacterial meningitis [MeSH] AND antibiotics [MeSH] AND corticosteroids [MeSH]. Restricted to humans and English language

Our search identified a Cochrane review that included published and unpublished randomized controlled trials on adjuvant use of corticosteroids in acute bacterial meningitis [19]. There was a

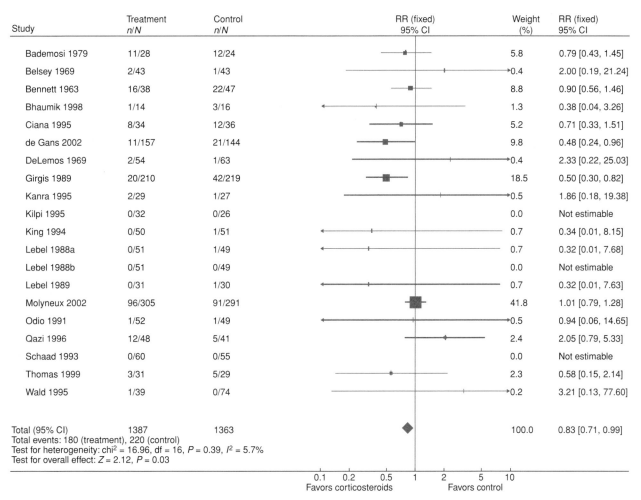

Study	Treatment n/N	Control n/N	RR (fixed) 95% CI	Weight (%)	RR (fixed) 95% CI
Bademosi 1979	11/28	12/24		5.8	0.79 [0.43, 1.45]
Belsey 1969	2/43	1/43		0.4	2.00 [0.19, 21.24]
Bennett 1963	16/38	22/47		8.8	0.90 [0.56, 1.46]
Bhaumik 1998	1/14	3/16		1.3	0.38 [0.04, 3.26]
Ciana 1995	8/34	12/36		5.2	0.71 [0.33, 1.51]
de Gans 2002	11/157	21/144		9.8	0.48 [0.24, 0.96]
DeLemos 1969	2/54	1/63		0.4	2.33 [0.22, 25.03]
Girgis 1989	20/210	42/219		18.5	0.50 [0.30, 0.82]
Kanra 1995	2/29	1/27		0.5	1.86 [0.18, 19.38]
Kilpi 1995	0/32	0/26		0.0	Not estimable
King 1994	0/50	1/51		0.7	0.34 [0.01, 8.15]
Lebel 1988a	0/51	1/49		0.7	0.32 [0.01, 7.68]
Lebel 1988b	0/51	0/49		0.0	Not estimable
Lebel 1989	0/31	1/30		0.7	0.32 [0.01, 7.63]
Molyneux 2002	96/305	91/291		41.8	1.01 [0.79, 1.28]
Odio 1991	1/52	1/49		0.5	0.94 [0.06, 14.65]
Qazi 1996	12/48	5/41		2.4	2.05 [0.79, 5.33]
Schaad 1993	0/60	0/55		0.0	Not estimable
Thomas 1999	3/31	5/29		2.3	0.58 [0.15, 2.14]
Wald 1995	1/39	0/74		0.2	3.21 [0.13, 77.60]
Total (95% CI)	**1387**	**1363**		**100.0**	**0.83 [0.71, 0.99]**

Total events: 180 (treatment), 220 (control)
Test for heterogeneity: chi^2 = 16.96, df = 16, P = 0.39, I^2 = 5.7%
Test for overall effect: Z = 2.12, P = 0.03

0.1 0.2 0.5 1 2 5 10
Favors corticosteroids   Favors control

Figure 47.2 Treatment with corticosteroids reduces mortality in patients with bacterial meninigitis compared to standard care.

significant decrease in mortality among those receiving corticosteroids (13.4%) versus the placebo group (16.1%) (RR = 0.83; 95% CI: 0.71 to 0.99) (Fig. 47.2). In adults, the use of corticosteroids was associated with reduced rates of severe hearing loss (RR = 0.65; 95% CI: 0.47 to 0.91) and reduced long-term neurological sequelae (RR = 0.67; 95% CI: 0.45 to 1.00). Adverse events were equal between the corticosteroid and the placebo groups. The risk of clinically evident gastrointestinal bleeding was not increased in patients treated with corticosteroids.

The corticosteroid dose most often used was a 4-day course of dexamethasone (about 10 mg in adults or 0.4–0.6 mg/kg/day) divided into four doses per day [19]. Subgroup analyses of the studies examining dexamethasone therapy initiated before or along with the first dose of antibiotics revealed no significant difference in administration timing. Based on the pooled analyses, the authors recommend initiation of dexamethasone (0.6 mg/kg/day) prior to the first dose of antibiotics in acute bacterial meningitis in adults and children in high-income countries. They also recommend that

if corticosteroids are initiated in a patient with suspected bacterial meningitis, the corticosteroids should be continued unless the diagnosis changes. No conclusions could be reached regarding the minimum length of corticosteroid therapy or the maximum length of time after initiation of antibiotic therapy for starting adjuvant corticosteroid therapy.

In summary, adults with acute bacterial meningitis benefit from adjuvant corticosteroid treatment with respect to mortality and neurological sequelae without an associated increase in adverse events.

Conclusions

The patient above was taken immediately to the CT scanner which failed to demonstrate a space-occupying lesion. Following her return to the ED, an LP was performed using an atraumatic needle without consequence. The CSF was cloudy, and the patient was empirically started on dexamethasone (10 mg IV) and ceftriaxone (1 g IV). The patient was admitted to the general internal medicine service; however, soon after admission she developed a petechial rash, hypotension and decreased level of consciousness. The patient was intubated and transferred to the intensive care unit.

Meningitis is a relatively uncommon, yet potentially fatal, ED diagnosis. The diagnosis cannot be determined by a single criterion; however, it should be suspected with a combination of classic clinical symptoms. CT scan should be reserved for those with neurological findings, and in their absence an LP should be performed urgently. Treatment with antibiotics and corticosteroids will reduce the risk of complications; however, fluid resuscitation is of limited value without a picture of sepsis.

References

1 Fitch MT, van de Beek D. Emergency diagnosis and treatment of adult meningitis. *Lancet Infect Dis* 2007;**7**(3):191–200.

2 Prasad K, Singhal T, Jain N, Gupta PK. Third generation cephalosporins versus conventional antibiotics for treating acute bacterial meningitis. *Cochrane Database Syst Rev.* 2004;**2**:CD001832.

3 Nigrovic LE, Kuppermann N, Macias CG, et al. Clinical prediction rule for identifying children with cerebrospinal fluid pleocytosis at very low risk of bacterial meningitis. *JAMA* 2007;**297**(1):52–60.

4 Straus SE, Thorpe KE, Holroyd-Leduc J. How do I perform a lumbar puncture and analyze the results to diagnose bacterial meningitis? *JAMA* 2006;**296**(16):2012–22.

5 Wyer PC. Bacterial meningitis score accurately predicts which children are at low risk. *J Pediatr* 2007;**151**(1):99–100.

6 Newcombe J, Cartwright K, Palmer WH, McFadden J. PCR of peripheral blood for diagnosis of meningococcal disease. *J Clin Microbiol* 1996;**34**(7):1637–40.

7 Dubos F, Moulin F, Gajdos V, et al. Serum procalcitonin and other biologic markers to distinguish between bacterial and aseptic meningitis. *J Pediatr* 2006;**149**(1):72–6.

8 Attia J, Hatala R, Cook DJ, Wong JG. The rational clinical examination. Does this adult patient have acute meningitis? *JAMA* 1999;**282**(2):175–81.

9 Newman DH. Clinical assessment of meningitis in adults. *Ann Emerg Med* 2004;**44**(1):71–3.

10 van de Beek D, de Gans J, Spanjaard L, Weisfelt M, Reitsma JB, Vermeulen M. Clinical features and prognostic factors in adults with bacterial meningitis. *N Engl J Med* 2004;**351**(18):1849–59.

11 Thomas KE, Hasbun R, Jekel J, Quagliarello VJ. The diagnostic accuracy of Kernig's sign, Brudzinski's sign, and nuchal rigidity in adults with suspected meningitis. *Clin Infect Dis* 2002;**35**(1):46–52.

12 Uchihara T, Tsukagoshi H. Jolt accentuation of headache: the most sensitive sign of CSF pleocytosis. *Headache.* 1991;**31**:167–171.

13 Gopal AK, Whitehouse JD, Simel DL, Corey GR. Cranial computed tomography before lumbar puncture: a prospective clinical evaluation. *Arch Intern Med* 1999;**159**(22):2681–5.

14 Hasbun R, Abrahams J, Jekel J, Quagliarello VJ. Computed tomography of the head before lumbar puncture in adults with suspected meningitis. *N Engl J Med* 2001;**345**(24):1727–33.

15 McGinn T, Guyatt GH, Wyer PC, et al. Users' Guides to the Medical Literature. XXIII. How to use articles about clinical prediction rules. *JAMA* 2000;**284**:79–84.

16 Durand ML, Calderwood SB, Weber DJ, et al. Acute bacterial meningitis in adults. A review of 493 episodes. *N Engl J Med* 1993;**328**(1):21–8.

17 Strupp M, Schueler O, Straube A, Von Stuckrad-Barre S, Brandt T. "Atraumatic" Sprotte needle reduces the incidence of post-lumbar puncture headaches. *Neurology* 2001;**57**(12):2310–12.

18 Oates-Whitehead RM, Maconochie I, Baumer H, Stewart ME. Fluid therapy for acute bacterial meningitis. *Cochrane Database Syst Rev.* 2005;**3**:CD004786.

19 van de Beek D, de Gans J, McIntyre P, Prasad K. Corticosteroids for acute bacterial meningitis. *Cochrane Database Syst Rev.* 2007;**1**:CD004405.

48 Migraine and Other Primary Headache Disorders

Benjamin W. Friedman

Department of Emergency Medicine, Albert Einstein College of Medicine, Montefiore Medical Center, New York, USA

Case scenario

A 25-year-old woman presents to the emergency department (ED) with a severe headache. She awoke 3 hours previously without pain; however, over the intervening time, the headache has gradually worsened. It is left-sided, frontal parietal, pounding, severe, "10 out of 10". She has been lying in bed all morning because moving around makes it worse. She reports no nausea or vomiting, and when asked if bright lights or loud noises bother her she replies, "Not really". Since age 15 she has experienced similar headaches about six times per year, typically waxing and waning over 48 hours, and often relieved with oral ibuprofen. Today she took 800 mg of ibuprofen without relief. A focused review of systems reveals no fever or chills, no neck pain or stiffness, no visual changes or disturbances, no sensory or motor abnormalities, and no ear, throat or tooth pain. She appears pale and uncomfortable; her vital signs and examination, including a focused neurological examination, are normal.

Review of her electronic medical record reveals three previous ED visits for severe headaches, which were successfully treated with intramuscular meperidine. She has never received a formal headache diagnosis, though her friend told her she had migraines. A computerized tomography (CT) scan of the head 4 years ago was normal. She says to you, "Please, give me anything, just get rid of this headache".

Background

Headaches are a common ED chief complaint, accounting for up to 5 million visits annually in the USA [1]. The majority of these headaches are acute exacerbations of chronic episodic primary headache disorders [2-4]. Episodic tension-type headache is ex- ceedingly common in the general population, though infrequently severe or functionally disabling [5], while migraine is less common, though still highly prevalent, and is the most common cause of an ED visit for headache [6]. Once malignant causes of headache have been excluded, especially subarachnoid hemorrhage, the goal of the emergency physician becomes the rapid alleviation of pain without causing unpleasant or debilitating side-effects.

No gold standard exists for the diagnosis of the primary headache disorders such as migraine, tension-type headache and cluster headache. Therefore, a manifestational definition of disease based on a constellation of symptoms has served as the de facto criterion standard; the International Headache Society (IHS) has refined and published The International Classification of Headache Disorders as a consensus guideline [7]. Using this guideline, specific primary headache disorders such as migraine with and without aura or tension-type headache may be diagnosed if secondary headache disorders have been excluded.

Many parenteral forms of general pain medications and headache-specific medications have demonstrated efficacy for acute primary headache disorders. Substantial variability in treatment exists among North American EDs [8]. National data show that emergency physicians commonly use two dozen different medications, or combinations of these medications, as treatment for headache [1]. As with other chronic, intermittent pain disorders, the ED attracts patients with frequent, severe exacerbations of their disease who prefer to dictate their own medical management. Guideline recommendations have been published that address the acute migraine attack in detail: the Canadian Association of Emergency Physicians published an ED-specific guideline statement [9] and the US Headache Consortium published a guideline for the treatment of acute migraine attacks [10]. Both these guidelines provide multiple options for treatment of the acute migraine attack, but there is uncertainty as to which medication should be first line.

The ideal headache medication would relieve pain quickly and completely and allow patients to promptly return to their work or usual daily activities. Side-effects of the treatment would be minimal, relapse would be prevented and a reasonable cost would

Evidence-based Emergency Medicine. Edited by Brian H. Rowe
© 2009 Blackwell Publishing, ISBN: 978-1-4051-6143-5.

make it accessible to all patients. Unfortunately, such a compound has been elusive for these patients and their physicians.

Clinical questions

1 In patients with an acute exacerbation of a primary headache disorder (population), what is the sensitivity and specificity (test characteristics) of clinical features test in predicting headache relief and future relapse (outcomes)?

2 In patients with an acute migraine (population), do parenteral opioid treatments (intervention) result in more effective pain relief or faster return to usual activities (outcomes) compared to placebo or other parenteral therapies (control)?

3 In patients with acute migraine (population), do parenteral sumatriptan treatments (intervention) result in more effective pain relief or return to usual activities (outcomes) compared to placebo or other parenteral therapies (control)?

4 In patients with an acute migraine (population), does use of injectable dihydroergotamine (intervention) lead to more effective pain relief or return to usual activities (outcomes) compared to placebo or other parenteral therapies (control)?

5 In patients with an acute migraine (population), does use of a parenteral anti-emetic (intervention) result in more effective pain relief or return to usual activities (outcomes) compared to placebo or other parenteral therapies (control)?

6 In patients with an acute migraine (population), does use of parenteral magnesium (intervention) lead to better pain relief or better return to usual activities (outcomes) than placebo or other parenteral therapies (control)?

7 In patients with an acute migraine (population), does use of parenteral ketorolac (intervention) lead to better pain relief or faster return to usual activities (outcomes) than placebo or other parenteral therapies (control)?

8 In headache patients who visit an ED more than two times per year (population), are there effective administrative or protocol-based management strategies (intervention) for decreasing ED visits, health care costs or patient suffering (outcomes)?

9 Do corticosteroids (intervention) decrease the frequency of post-discharge headache or functional impairment (outcomes) in patients with an acute migraine (population) when compared to placebo (control)?

General search strategy

You begin to address these questions by searching for evidence in the common electronic databases such as the Cochrane Library, MEDLINE and EMBASE looking specifically for systematic reviews and meta-analyses. The Cochrane Database of Systematic Reviews (CDSR) includes high-quality systematic review evidence on therapy for headache. You also search the Cochrane Central Register of Controlled Trials (CENTRAL), MEDLINE and

EMBASE to identify randomized controlled trials that became available after the publication date of the systematic review or, if no systematic reviews were identified, to locate high-quality randomized controlled trials that directly address the clinical question. In addition, access to relevant, updated, evidence-based clinical practice guidelines (CPGs) on headache are accessed to determine the consensus rating of areas lacking evidence.

Critical review of the literature

Question 1: In patients with an acute exacerbation of a primary headache disorder (population), what is the sensitivity and specificity (test characteristics) of clinical features test in predicting headache relief and future relapse (outcomes)?

Search terms

- MEDLINE: (migraine OR headache) AND (response to therapy OR outcome OR prognosis)

The traditional management of primary headache is based on the assumption that patients with migraine should be treated differently than patients with tension-type headache, who will be treated differently than patients with cluster headache. The detailed classification-based paradigm for treatment promulgated by the IHS's classification of headache disorders has allowed for the development of brief screening instruments, such as the Identification of Migraine screener [11], and high-yield questions that facilitate the diagnosis of migraine [12].

Does the IHS classification scheme help the ED clinician determine the optimal therapy for the individual patient? The classification scheme must create clinically relevant divisions, either with regard to outcome in the ED (prognosis and response to parenteral therapy) or with regard to longer term outcomes (medication needs after initial ED treatment). The classification should be reproducible among clinicians and comprehensive enough to be applicable to the majority of ED patients suspected of having a primary headache.

To date, there are insufficient data to address the clinical utility of the IHS classification scheme in the ED setting. There is evidence, however, to support the following:

1 There is overlap in response of both migraine and tension-type headache to parenteral anti-emetic medication [13–15]. Also, some patients with tension-type headache will respond to triptans [16,17].

2 Whether or not the diagnosis is migraine, many patients continue to suffer from their headache after discharge from the ED [18,19].

3 Once malignant secondary headaches have been excluded from the differential diagnosis, it can be difficult to assign a specific IHS diagnosis to every ED headache patient [3].

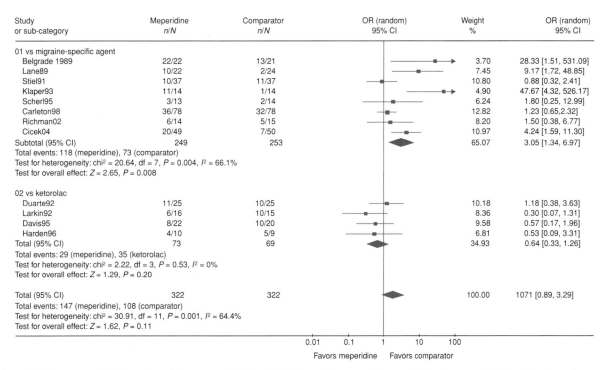

Study or sub-category	Meperidine n/N	Comparator n/N	OR (random) 95% CI	Weight %	OR (random) 95% CI
01 vs migraine-specific agent					
Belgrade 1989	22/22	13/21		3.70	28.33 [1.51, 531.09]
Lane89	10/22	2/24		7.45	9.17 [1.72, 48.85]
Stiel91	10/37	11/37		10.80	0.88 [0.32, 2.41]
Klaper93	11/14	1/14		4.90	47.67 [4.32, 526.17]
Scherl95	3/13	2/14		6.24	1.80 [0.25, 12.99]
Carleton98	36/78	32/78		12.82	1.23 [0.65, 2.32]
Richman02	6/14	5/15		8.20	1.50 [0.38, 6.77]
Cicek04	20/49	7/50		10.97	4.24 [1.59, 11.30]
Subtotal (95% CI)	249	253		65.07	3.05 [1.34, 6.97]
Total events: 118 (meperidine), 73 (comparator)					
Test for heterogeneity: chi² = 20.64, df = 7, P = 0.004, I² = 66.1%					
Test for overall effect: Z = 2.65, P = 0.008					
02 vs ketorolac					
Duarte92	11/25	10/25		10.18	1.18 [0.38, 3.63]
Larkin92	6/16	10/15		8.36	0.30 [0.07, 1.31]
Davis95	8/22	10/20		9.58	0.57 [0.17, 1.96]
Harden96	4/10	5/9		6.81	0.53 [0.09, 3.31]
Total (95% CI)	73	69		34.93	0.64 [0.33, 1.26]
Total events: 29 (meperidine), 35 (ketorolac)					
Test for heterogeneity: chi² = 2.22, df = 3, P = 0.53, I² = 0%					
Test for overall effect: Z = 1.29, P = 0.20					
Total (95% CI)	322	322		100.00	1071 [0.89, 3.29]
Total events: 147 (meperidine), 108 (comparator)					
Test for heterogeneity: chi² = 30.91, df = 11, P = 0.001, I² = 64.4%					
Test for overall effect: Z = 1.62, P = 0.11					

0.01   0.1   1   10   100

Favors meperidine   Favors comparator

Figure 48.1 Summary analysis: in patients with an acute migraine headache, is meperidine more likely to provide inadequate relief of headache than active comparators?

All of these issues have led some emergency medicine authors to suggest using the term "benign" headache, rather than attempting to differentiate among the various primary headache disorders in the acute care setting.

In summary, the criterion standard for the diagnosis of primary headache disorders is a consensus guideline, which divides primary headache disorders into subtypes such as migraine, tension-type headache and cluster headache. Its role in the ED has not been determined and the precise measurement of symptoms may not be clinically useful. Effective treatment can usually be delivered without assigning a specific primary headache disorder diagnosis, once life-threatening causes of headache are excluded from the differential diagnosis.

Question 2: In patients with acute migraine (population), do parenteral opioid treatments (intervention) result in more effective pain relief or faster return to usual activities (outcomes) compared to placebo or other parenteral therapies (control)?

Search terms

- MEDLINE: (migraine OR headache) AND (opioid OR narcotic OR meperidine OR morphine OR butorphanol OR hydromorphone)

Although guidelines recommend against their use, opioids are commonly used for the treatment of migraine and primary headaches in US and Canadian EDs [1,20]. The reason for the discrepancy between guidelines and practice is not clear; however, it is likely related to patient and practitioner preference and education. The relationship between opioids and "drug-seeking" behavior is often mentioned yet poorly quantified.

The search strategy listed above identified 85 studies. Of these, two systematic reviews and 12 randomized clinical trials were identified in which a parenteral opioid was compared to another agent or to placebo. From the 12 randomized trials, 14 different comparisons were identified between meperidine and placebo, meperidine and ketorolac, or meperidine and a parenteral migraine-specific agent such as a dopamine antagonist, dihydroergotamine (DHE), or a combination of these two [15,21–31]. Meperidine doses ranged from 50 mg to 1.5 mg/kg and were often co-administered with parenteral antihistamine. Obviously, a typical summary analysis is limited by this clinical heterogeneity among studies.

In general, meperidine did not outperform the migraine-specific analgesics in any of the eight comparisons. Among the individual studies, the effect estimates for inadequate relief with meperidine versus the active comparator ranged from showing no difference (OR = 0.88; 95% CI: 0.32 to 2.41) to demonstrating a strong trend towards inadequate relief (OR = 48; 95% CI: 4.3 to 526) (Fig. 48.1). Though limited by statistical heterogeneity among the trials, the best estimate of the number needed to harm (NNH) is 4 (95% CI: 2 to 16). When compared to parenteral ketorolac, a trend toward inadequate relief with ketorolac did not reach statistical significance (OR = 1.56; 95% CI: 0.79 to 3.03); inadequate relief occurred in 40% of meperidine patients and 51% of ketorolac patients (absolute risk reduction (ARR) = 11%; 95% CI: −4% to 28%). When compared to placebo, an analysis of 118 subjects with regard to inadequate relief failed to demonstrate the benefit of meperidine (OR = 1.72; 95% CI: 0.83 to 3.57). In this analysis, 41% of meperidine patients versus 54% of placebo patients suffered a poor pain outcome (ARR = 13%: 95% CI: −5% to 31%).

Return to normal functioning was assessed in two trials. In a trial of meperidine versus DHE ($n = 170$), 14% of the meperidine subjects returned to normal functioning by 1 hour versus 32% of the DHE group (ARR = 18%: 95% CI: 6% to 30%). In a small trial ($n = 31$), 25% of meperidine subjects reported complete absence of functional disability at 60 minutes versus none of the ketorolac patients. It is particularly noteworthy that the majority of patients in both of these trials did not return to normal functioning by 1 hour.

The US Headache Consortium guideline reports no statistical difference in relief of pain between parenteral meperidine and chlorpromazine or ketorolac or DHE [10]. Similarly, the Canadian Association of Emergency Physicians migraine guideline concludes that the results of controlled trials testing the therapeutic benefits of meperidine for acute migraines are mixed [9]. Importantly, a retrospective analysis of migraine headache treatment in a linked Canadian ED system reported significantly more relapses to the same ED with a headache within 7 days of the original visit ($P = 0.011$) for those treated with first-line narcotics (mainly meperidine) compared to non-narcotic therapies [20].

In summary, meperidine, as commonly administered, is less likely to provide adequate pain relief when compared to DHE, anti-emetics or a combination of these two classes of medication (NNH = 4). Meperidine does not provide substantially more headache relief than ketorolac or placebo, though the latter analysis is limited by fewer subjects. Limited evidence could be identified to support the notion that opioids, when used for treatment of episodic headache in the ED, cause ED recidivism or drug-seeking behavior. Therefore, opioids should not be withheld when needed in benign headache treatment, especially on the grounds of addiction. Because parenteral meperidine is less likely to result in adequate analgesia or rapid return to normal functioning, it should not be used routinely as first-line therapy. This evidence summary does not apply to intravenous morphine or hydromorphone, for which no randomized controlled trials could be found.

Question 3: In patients with acute migraine (population), do parenteral sumatriptan treatments (intervention) result in more effective pain relief or return to usual activities (outcomes) compared to placebo or other parenteral therapies (control)?

Search terms

- MEDLINE: (migraine OR headache) AND sumatriptan

Sumatriptan, the prototype of the serotonin 1B/1D agonist medications, has been available for almost 15 years and has had widespread success against migraine; however, the triptan class of medication is used infrequently in the ED setting [1]. Although multiple oral triptan options have been approved by the US Food and Drug Administration, subcutaneous sumatriptan remains the only injectable triptan available. We identified one meta-analysis in which subcutaneous sumatriptan is compared to placebo.

The meta-analysis from 2002 incorporated eight clinical trials involving 938 patients in which subcutaneous sumatriptan was compared to placebo [32]. Sumatriptan was almost 10 times as likely to relieve headache as placebo (OR = 9.74; 95% CI: 7.21 to 13.16) with an estimated number needed to treat (NNT) of 2. Sumatriptan was also shown to provide sustained pain-free response by attaining complete headache relief and maintaining it for 24 hours (OR = 4.46; 95% CI: 2.64 to 7.52). The US Headache Consortium guideline reports no added benefit of a second dose of subcutaneous sumatriptan [10]. In the only ED-based clinical trial of subcutaneous sumatriptan versus placebo identified, the median time to meaningful relief after subcutaneous sumatriptan was 34 minutes [33]; however, adverse effects were reported by 52% of the active arm versus 27% of the placebo group (NNH = 4; 95% CI: 2 to 11).

In summary, subcutaneous sumatriptan is an efficacious treatment of acute migraines, with an NNT of 2 relative to placebo for headache relief. In the patients in whom it is effective, it works quickly, allowing a rapid return to productivity and does not require the time and resources required for intravenous administration. Caution is warranted, since it is accompanied by adverse effects in 52% of patients, and it has a host of contraindications, many of which are difficult to assess completely in a patient suffering from acute pain. Sumatriptan is reasonable first-line therapy in patients who are known to tolerate it, but should be used cautiously in patients who are naïve to this medication.

Question 4: In patients with an acute migraine (population), does use of injectable dihydroergotamine (intervention) lead to more effective pain relief or return to usual activities (outcomes) compared to placebo or other parenteral therapies (control)?

Search terms

- MEDLINE: (migraine OR headache) AND dihydroergotamine

Dihydroergotamine was developed from ergotamine, an ancient migraine therapy, with the goal of increased tolerability. In current practice, it is often co-administered with an anti-emetic to ameliorate nausea. Multiple systematic reviews of DHE were identified. One that used a rigorous methodology of review and meta-analytical techniques is discussed here [34]. DHE was less effective than sumatriptan with regard to headache improvement (OR = 0.44; 95% CI: 0.25 to 0.77) and improvement in headache-related functional impairment (OR = 0.39; 95% CI: 0.22 to 0.69). Both medications were associated with an assortment of adverse events, including chest pain (more common with sumatriptan), nausea (more common with DHE), drowsiness, flushing, neck stiffness, vertigo, weakness and injection site reactions. When compared to chlorpromazine, DHE alone was more likely to result in use of rescue medication (OR = 3.80; 95% CI: 1.09 to 13.26) and less likely to result in complete resolution of migraine (OR = 0.60; 95% CI: 0.17 to 2.09).

In summary, dihydroergotamine is less efficacious than sumatriptan and probably less efficacious than chlorpromazine. Its use is often accompanied by unpleasant side-effects. Therefore, parenteral DHE should not be used routinely as a first-line therapy.

Question 5: In patients with an acute migraine headache (population), does use of a parenteral anti-emetic (intervention) result in more effective pain relief or return to usual activities (outcomes) compared to placebo or other parenteral therapies (control)?

Search terms

- MEDLINE: (migraine OR headache) AND (dopamine OR chlorpromazine OR prochlorperazine OR metoclopramide OR droperidol OR haloperidol OR trimethobenzamide OR methotrimeprazine)

Over the past 30 years, the anti-emetic dopamine antagonists have been used with increasing frequency as their efficacy against migraine has been realized. Although compelling mechanistic data are lacking, these agents probably antagonize dopamine receptors in pain-modulating regions of the brainstem. We identified one meta-analysis, multiple systematic reviews and 41 clinical trials in which a parenteral anti-emetic was compared to an active comparator or placebo. Metoclopramide was the subject of a Cochrane meta-analysis.

In the Cochrane meta-analysis, metoclopramide was more likely than placebo to lead to significant reductions in headache (OR = 2.84; 95% CI: 1.05 to 7.68; NNT = 4) [35]. Restlessness, drowsiness, dizziness and orthostatic hypotension were inconsistently reported as adverse effects. The effectiveness of metoclopramide compared to other anti-emetics is less clear, with some studies reporting benefit and others reporting comparability.

The US Headache Consortium identified 16 randomized trials comparing an anti-emetic to another agent and, based on a high-quality placebo-controlled trial, concluded that parenteral prochlorperazine may be the therapy of choice for migraine in the appropriate setting [10]. Granisetron and zatostetron did not demonstrate a statistically significant clinical benefit for headache relief. The Canadian Association of Emergency Physicians migraine guideline recommends chlorpromazine and methotrimeprazine as effective migraine abortive agents; however, the guideline cautioned against chlorpromazine due to hypotension, drowsiness and dysphoria [9].

We identified two randomized trials in which parenteral metoclopramide was compared to subcutaneous sumatriptan. In the first trial, patients received 10 mg of metoclopramide or 6 mg of subcutaneous sumatriptan [36]; the other trial used doses of up to 80 mg of metoclopramide, combined with diphenhydramine, versus the same dose of sumatriptan [37]. Sumatriptan was less likely to provide adequate headache relief (OR = 0.19; 0.06 to 0.65; NNH = 6). The most commonly encountered adverse effects, including weakness, dizziness and drowsiness, were evenly distributed between the two groups.

A recent study using droperidol 2.75 mg IM demonstrated benefit over placebo with respect to sustained pain-free response (NNT = 3) [38]. Malignant arrhythmias resulting from QT prolongation have been reported after this medication, so it has been suggested that patients administered droperidol should have an electrocardiogram and be monitored during therapy. Also, akathisia is reported in up to 31% of subjects who receive droperidol.

We identified six clinical trials in which an anti-emetic was compared to another anti-emetic. Patients receiving metoclopramide were less likely than those receiving prochlorperazine to achieve a favorable pain outcome (OR = 0.39; 95% CI: 0.20 to 0.76) and more likely to require rescue medication (OR = 2.74; 95% CI: 1.22 to 6.15) [39–41]. Patients receiving prochlorperazine were less likely than those receiving droperidol to achieve a favorable pain outcome (OR = 0.35; 95% CI: 0.20 to 0.63) though requirement of rescue medication was comparable (OR 1.28; 95% CI: 0.66 to 2.47) [42,43]. Chlorpromazine and metoclopramide had comparable efficacy outcomes and requirements of rescue medication [44].

In summary, although their mechanism of action is not yet understood, it appears that the anti-emetic dopamine antagonists are effective migraine therapy. Metoclopramide relieves migraine pain with an NNT of 4 versus placebo and an NNT of 6 versus sumatriptan. When choosing among the members of this class of medication, it is not yet clear which is the preferred therapy; however, droperidol relieves pain more frequently than prochlorperazine, which in turn appears to be more efficacious than metoclopramide; however, the side-effect profiles favor metoclopramide. The anti-emetic dopamine antagonist class of medication should be considered as first-line therapy for the ED-based treatment of migraine.

Question 6: In patients with an acute migraine (population), does use of parenteral magnesium (intervention) lead to better pain relief or better return to usual activities (outcomes) than placebo or other parenteral therapies (control)?

Search terms

• MEDLINE: (migraine OR headache) AND magnesium

Magnesium has been proposed as a treatment of migraine, though its mechanism of action is still theoretical. Magnesium is hypothesized to stabilize the hyperexcitable brain of a migraineur, possibly through modulation of NMDA (*N*-methyl-D-aspartic acid) receptors [45]. We identified four clinical trials, containing five comparisons, which fit our search strategy. Combining the results from two placebo-controlled trials, patients randomized to magnesium were less likely to require rescue medication (OR = 0.46; 95% CI: 0.26 to 0.83; NNT = 5), with a larger magnitude of effect in those patients with aura [45,46]. When compared to magnesium, prochlorperazine had greater efficacy with regard to headache relief (NNT = 3; 95% CI: 2 to 27), though metoclopramide and magnesium performed comparably with regard to need for rescue medication and change in pain intensity [46,47]. When used as part of a protocol-based treatment regimen containing 20 mg of metoclopramide administered every 15 minutes, adding magnesium to the regimen resulted in inferior pain relief (NNH = 4; 95% CI: 2 to 25) [48].

In summary, magnesium appears to be an effective treatment option for acute migraine; however, it should not be used as first-line therapy or in combination with metoclopramide.

Question 7: In patients with acute migraine (population), does use of parenteral ketorolac (intervention) lead to better pain relief or faster return to usual activities (outcomes) than placebo or other parenteral therapies (control)?

Search terms

• MEDLINE: (migraine OR headache) AND ketorolac

Over-the-counter and prescription non-steroidal anti-inflammatory drugs (NSAIDs) play a large role in the armamentarium against migraine. In the ED, parenteral ketorolac is widely used [1]. No systematic reviews were identified on this topic; however, seven randomized clinical trials in which parenteral ketorolac was compared to another active agent for the treatment of migraine in adults were identified [22,23,25,49–52]. Four of these trials compared ketorolac to meperidine and are discussed in the opioid section above. Ketorolac was compared to an anti-emetic in three small trials. Need for rescue medication occurred in more patients who received ketorolac than in an anti-emetic regimen (OR = 2.1; 95% CI: 0.8 to 5.5). In two of these studies, the anti-emetic regimen proved superior based on change in pain intensity scales and, in one trial, ketorolac performed comparably to the anti-emetic. Overall, the medications were well tolerated with few reports of adverse effects.

In summary, ketorolac is widely used for the treatment of migraine in the ED setting, although its precise role is not yet clear. In patients without contraindications to an NSAID, it can be considered as an alternative to parenteral opioids. It is likely to be less effective than the anti-emetic dopamine antagonists, and therefore should be used as an adjuvant or second-line migraine therapy.

Question 8: In headache patients who visit an ED more than two times per year (population), are there effective administrative or protocol-based management strategies (intervention) for decreasing ED visits, health care costs or patient suffering (outcomes)?

Search terms

• MEDLINE: emergency department AND (migraine OR headache) AND (frequent OR chronic OR drug seeking)

Although they represent fewer than 10% of all ED headache patients, frequent ED users account for 50% of all headache visits in some hospitals [53,54]. Why patients use the ED frequently is not well understood. It could represent "drug-seeking" behavior, although it more likely serves as a marker for poorly managed primary headache disorder. Headache patients who use the ED frequently tend to know their disease well and request specific medication, often opioids. Although randomized controlled trials testing the effectiveness of ED-based management strategies were not identified in our search, some have recommended a uniform departmental approach to the chronic pain patient that addresses not only the patient's pain, but also the social issues related to the repeat visits.

We identified three non-randomized clinical studies, all of which used a before–after design to demonstrate a decrease in the frequency of ED visits for chronic headache patients who participated in comprehensive headache management programs [55–57]. These programs offered headache education and interdisciplinary care. Although this type of study design based on historical controls is prone to confounding (lower level of evidence), these programs may decrease the burden of illness and health care costs in select patients with chronic headaches; further higher quality evidence is needed in this patient group.

In summary, we could not identify strong evidence to support ED-based strategies for dealing with frequent visitors. It is not clear if appropriate outpatient care or appropriate first-line therapy decreases ED recidivism.

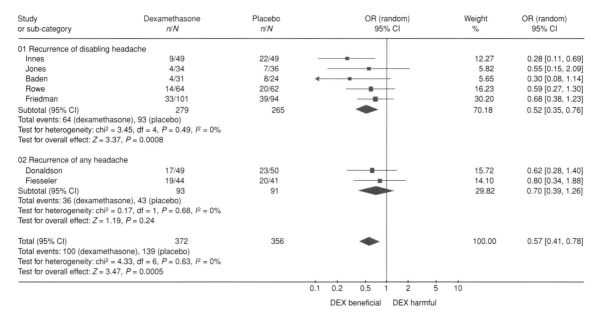

Study or sub-category	Dexamethasone n/N	Placebo n/N	OR (random) 95% CI	Weight %	OR (random) 95% CI
01 Recurrence of disabling headache					
Innes	9/49	22/49		12.27	0.28 [0.11, 0.69]
Jones	4/34	7/36		5.82	0.55 [0.15, 2.09]
Baden	4/31	8/24		5.65	0.30 [0.08, 1.14]
Rowe	14/64	20/62		16.23	0.59 [0.27, 1.30]
Friedman	33/101	39/94		30.20	0.68 [0.38, 1.23]
Subtotal (95% CI)	279	265		70.18	0.52 [0.35, 0.76]
Total events: 64 (dexamethasone), 93 (placebo)					
Test for heterogeneity: chi² = 3.45, df = 4, P = 0.49, I² = 0%					
Test for overall effect: Z = 3.37, P = 0.0008					
02 Recurrence of any headache					
Donaldson	17/49	23/50		15.72	0.62 [0.28, 1.40]
Fiesseler	19/44	20/41		14.10	0.80 [0.34, 1.88]
Subtotal (95% CI)	93	91		29.82	0.70 [0.39, 1.26]
Total events: 36 (dexamethasone), 43 (placebo)					
Test for heterogeneity: chi² = 0.17, df = 1, P = 0.68, I² = 0%					
Test for overall effect: Z = 1.19, P = 0.24					
Total (95% CI)	372	356		100.00	0.57 [0.41, 0.78]
Total events: 100 (dexamethasone), 139 (placebo)					
Test for heterogeneity: chi² = 4.33, df = 6, P = 0.63, I² = 0%					
Test for overall effect: Z = 3.47, P = 0.0005					

```
          0.1   0.2   0.5   1    2    5   10
             DEX beneficial    DEX harmful
```

Figure 48.2 Summary analysis: does dexamethasone (DEX) decrease the rate of poor pain and functional outcomes after initial treatment of an acute migraine headache in the ED setting when compared to placebo?

Question 9: Do corticosteroids (intervention) decrease the frequency of post-discharge headache or functional impairment (outcomes) in patients with an acute migraine (population) when compared to placebo (control)?

Search terms

- MEDLINE: (migraine OR headache) AND (corticosteroids OR dexamethasone)

Although often mentioned in guidelines and reviews, few published randomized clinical trials address the role of corticosteroids for acute migraine. Neurogenic inflammation is felt to be part of the pain-generating pathway in acute migraine. Theoretically, mitigating this inflammation could abort a migraine attack. We identified no systematic reviews and seven clinical trials in which dexamethasone was compared to placebo. In these seven trials, the dexamethasone dose ranged from 10 to 24 mg.

Five trials, involving 544 subjects provided data on the frequency of severe or disabling headache post-ED discharge [58–62]. Pooling the results of these trials, 23% of 279 patients had a severe or disabling post-ED discharge headache in the dexamethasone arm, versus 36% of 265 placebo subjects (OR = 0.52; 95% CI: 0.35 to 0.76; NNT = 7). The other two trials assessed any recurrent headache post-ED discharge and also found a trend toward benefit (Fig. 48.2). Few side-effects were reported in these trials.

In summary, it is likely that dexamethasone reduces severe headaches in patients with acute migraine following discharge; however, the optimal dose of this medication is not clear. Moreover, given the frequency of migraine presentation, care should be taken in administering repeated doses of systemic corticosteroids. Further research is needed to determine which subgroup of migraine sufferers is most likely to benefit from dexamethasone.

Conclusions

Acute migraine treatment described here is listed in a summary of effects table (Table 48.1). First-line parenteral treatment for acute migraine in the ED setting involves one of the dopamine antagonist anti-emetics. When choosing among the anti-emetics, droperidol and prochlorperazine are more effective than metoclopramide and chlorpromazine. Sumatriptan is an effective therapy, and might have a role in selected ED patients. Ketorolac is effective; however, it should only be used as a second-line therapy. Similarly, meperidine is less efficacious than other antimigraine agents and should not be used as first-line therapy. Though more effective than placebo, magnesium is less efficacious than other antimigraine agents and probably should not be combined with metoclopramide. Dexamethasone appears to modestly decrease the frequency of severe or disabling headache after ED discharge.

The young woman described in the case presentation probably has a migraine, but she does not meet IHS criteria for this disease. First-line treatment options are prochlorperazine IV, or droperidol

Table 48.1 Summary of evidence tables for acute migraine headache pharmacological treatments.*

Treatment	Control	Quality	Headache outcomes	Trials/ patients	Effect measure: OR (95% CI)	Heterogeneity	Summary (NNT)
Anti-emetics							
Droperidol	Placebo	High	Sustained pain free	1 RCT / 122 pts	4.94 (2.12 to11.47)	NA	Effective Rx NNT = 3
Droperidol	Prochlorperazine	High	Headache relief Need rescue medication	2 RCTs / 263 pts	2.86 (1.59 to 5.00) 0.78 (0.40 to 1.52)	$I^2 = 42.8\%$ $I^2 = 0\%$	Results mixed, droperidol better at relief of pain with NNT = 5
Metoclopramide	Placebo	High	Headache relief	3 RCTs / 185 pts	2.84 (1.05 to 7.68)	$I^2 = 59.3\%$	Effective Rx NNT = 4
Metoclopramide	Prochlorperazine	High	Headache relief Need rescue medication	3 RCTs / 178 pts	0.39 (0.20 to 0.76) 2.74 (1.22 to 6.15)	$I^2 = 0\%$ $I^2 = 0\%$	Prochlorperazine more effective with NNT = 5 for headache relief
Prochlorperazine	Placebo	High	Headache relief	3 RCTs / 185 pts	7.43 (3.72 to 14.80)	$I^2 = 0\%$	Effective Rx NNT = 2
Corticosteroids (dexamethasone)	Placebo + standard care	High	Disabling or recurrent post-discharge HA	7 RCTs / 728 pts	0.57 (0.41 to 0.78)	$I^2 = 0\%$	Effective Rx NNT = 8
DHE	Sumatriptan	Low	Headache relief	2 RCTs / 247 pts	0.44 (0.25 to 0.77)	Not reported	Sumatriptan more effective
Ketorolac	Anti-emetics	Mixed	Need rescue medication	3 RCTs / 112 pts	2.07 (0.78 to 5.51)	$I^2 = 59.7\%$	Inconclusive
Magnesium	Placebo	High	Need rescue medication	2 RCTs / 196 pts	0.46 (0.26 to 0.83)	$I^2 = 0\%$	Effective Rx NNT = 5
Meperidine	Placebo	High	Inadequate relief	2 RCTs / 118 pts	0.58 (0.28 to 1.20)	$I^2 = 0\%$	Inconclusive
Meperidine	Antimigraine agents (DHE, anti-emetics or both)	Mixed	Inadequate relief	8 RCTs / 502 pts	3.05 (1.34 to 6.97)	$I^2 = 66.1\%$	Meperidine less effective than antimigraine agents with NNH = 4 for inadequate relief
Meperidine	Ketorolac	High	Inadequate relief	4 RCTs / 142 pts	0.64 (0.33 to 1.26)	$I^2 = 64.4\%$	Inconclusive
Sumatriptan	Placebo	High	Headache relief Sustained pain free	8 RCTs / 938 pts 2 RCTs / 304 pts	9.74 (7.21 to 13.16) 4.46 (2.64 to 7.52)	Not reported	Effective Rx NNT = 2
Sumatriptan	Metoclopramide	Mixed	Headache relief	2 RCTs / 118 pts	0.19 (0.06 to 0.65)	$I^2 = 10.2\%$	Sumatriptan less effective NNT = 6

*Note that other considerations may outweigh the trial evidence in some situations (for example, the patient who does not want to experience akathisia may wish to avoid anti-emetics such as metoclopramide).

CI, confidence interval; DHE, dihydroergotamine; NNH, number needed to harm; NNT, number needed to treat; OR, odds ratio; pts, patients; RCT, randomized controlled trial; Rx, treatment.

IM or IV if the patient is not at risk of arrhythmia. Intravenous dexamethasone could be considered prior to discharge if this patient described frequent episodes of headache recurrence with her previous migraines.

References

1 Vinson DR. Treatment patterns of isolated benign headache in US emergency departments. *Ann Emerg Med* 2002;**39**(3):215–22.

2 Bigal M, Bordini CA, Speciali JG. Headache in an emergency room in Brazil. *Sao Paulo Med J* 2000;**118**(3):58–62.

3 Friedman BW, Hochberg ML, Esses D, et al. Applying the international classification of headache disorders to the emergency department: an assessment of reproducibility and the frequency with which a unique diagnosis can be assigned to every acute headache presentation. *Ann Emerg Med* 2007;**49**(4):409–19.

4 Luda E, Comitangelo R, Sicuro L. The symptom of headache in emergency departments. The experience of a neurology emergency department. *Ital J Neurol Sci* 1995;**16**(5):295–301.

5 Schwartz BS, Stewart WF, Simon D, Lipton RB. Epidemiology of tension-type headache. *JAMA* 1998; **279**(5):381–3.

6 Lipton RB, Diamond S, Reed M, Diamond ML, Stewart WF. Migraine diagnosis and treatment: results from the American Migraine Study II. *Headache* 2001;**41**(7):638–45.

7 International Headache Society. The International Classification of Headache Disorders, 2nd edn. *Cephalalgia* 2004;**24**(Suppl 1):1–151.

8 Vinson DR, Hurtado TR, Vandenberg JT, Banwart L. Variations among emergency departments in the treatment of benign headache. *Ann Emerg Med* 2003;**41**(1):90–97.

9 Ducharme J. Canadian Association of Emergency Physicians guidelines for the acute management of migraine headache. *J Emerg Med* 1999;**17**(1):137–44.

10 Matchar DB, Young WB, Rosenberg JA, et al. Evidence-based guidelines for migraine headache in the primary care setting: pharmological management of acute attacks. In: American Academy of Neurology Practice Guideline. Available at www.aan.com/professionals/practice/pdfs/gl0087.pdf (accessed July 28, 2004).

11 Lipton RB, Dodick D, Sadovsky R, et al. A self-administered screener for migraine in primary care: the ID Migraine(TM) validation study. *Neurology* 2003;**61**(3):375–82.

12 Detsky ME, McDonald DR, Baerlocher MO, Tomlinson GA, McCrory DC, Booth CM. Does this patient with headache have a migraine or need neuroimaging? *JAMA* 2006;**296**(10):1274–83.

13 Bigal ME, Bordini CA, Speciali JG. Intravenous chlorpromazine in the acute treatment of episodic tension-type headache: a randomized, placebo controlled, double-blind study. *Arq Neuropsiquiatr* 2002;**60**(3-A):537–41.

14 Bigal ME, Bordini CA, Speciali JG. Intravenous chlorpromazine in the emergency department treatment of migraines: a randomized controlled trial. *J Emerg Med* 2002;**23**(2):141–8.

15 Cicek M, Karcioglu O, Parlak I, et al. Prospective, randomised, double blind, controlled comparison of metoclopramide and pethidine in the emergency treatment of acute primary vascular and tension type headache episodes. *Emerg Med J* 2004;**21**(3):323–6.

16 Lipton RB, Stewart WF, Cady R, et al. 2000 Wolfe Award. Sumatriptan for the range of headaches in migraine sufferers: results of the Spectrum Study. *Headache* 2000;**40**(10):783–91.

17 Miner JR, Smith SW, Moore J, Biros M. Sumatriptan for the treatment of undifferentiated primary headaches in the ED. *Am J Emerg Med* 2007;**25**(1):60–64.

18 Ducharme J, Beveridge RC, Lee JS, Beaulieu S. Emergency management of migraine: is the headache really over? *Acad Emerg Med* 1998;**5**(9):899–905.

19 Friedman BW, Hochberg ML, Esses D, et al. Applying the International Classification of Headache Disorders to the emergency department: an assessment of reproducibility and the frequency with which a unique diagnosis can be assigned to every acute headache presentation. *Ann Emerg Med* 2007;**49**(4):409–19.

20 Colman I, Rothney A, Wright SC, Zilkalns B, Rowe BH. Use of narcotic analgesics in the emergency department treatment of migraine headache. *Neurology* 2004;**62**(10):1695–700.

21 Carleton SC, Shesser RF, Pietrzak MP, et al. Double-blind, multicenter trial to compare the efficacy of intramuscular dihydroergotamine plus hydroxyzine versus intramuscular meperidine plus hydroxyzine for the emergency department treatment of acute migraine headache. *Ann Emerg Med* 1998;**32**(2):129–38.

22 Davis CP, Torre PR, Williams C, et al. Ketorolac versus meperidine-plus-promethazine treatment of migraine headache: evaluations by patients. *Am J Emerg Med* 1995;**13**(2):146–50.

23 Duarte C, Dunaway F, Turner L, Aldag J, Frederick R. Ketorolac versus meperidine and hydroxyzine in the treatment of acute migraine headache: a randomized, prospective, double-blind trial. *Ann Emerg Med* 1992;**21**(9):1116–21.

24 Klapper JA, Stanton J. Current emergency treatment of severe migraine headaches. *Headache* 1993;**33**(10):560–62.

25 Larkin GL, Prescott JE. A randomized, double-blind, comparative study of the efficacy of ketorolac tromethamine versus meperidine in the treatment of severe migraine. *Ann Emerg Med* 1992;**21**(8):919–24.

26 Belgrade MJ, Ling LJ, Schleevogt MB, Ettinger MG, Ruiz E. Comparison of single-dose meperidine, butorphanol, and dihydroergotamine in the treatment of vascular headache. *Neurology* 1989;**39**(4):590–92.

27 Lane PL, McLellan BA, Baggoley CJ. Comparative efficacy of chlorpromazine and meperidine with dimenhydrate in migraine headache. *Ann Emerg Med* 1989;**18**(4):360–65.

28 Richman PB, Allegra J, Eskin B, Doran J, Reischel U, Kaiafas C, Nashed AH. A randomized clinical trial to assess the efficacy of intramuscular droperidol for the treatment of acute migraine headache. *Am J Emerg Med* 2002;**20**(1):39–42.

29 Scherl ER, Wilson JF. Comparison of dihydroergotamine with metoclopramide versus meperidine with promethazine in the treatment of acute migraine. *Headache* 1995;**35**(5):256–9.

30 Stiell IG, Dufour DG, Moher D, Yen M, Beilby WJ, Smith NA. Methotrimeprazine versus meperidine and dimenhydrate in the treatment of severe migraine: a randomized, controlled trial. *Ann Emerg Med* 1991;**20**(11):1201–5.

31 Tek D, Mellon M. The effectiveness of nalbuphine and hydroxyzine for the emergency treatment of severe headache. *Ann Emerg Med* 1987;**16**(3):308–13.

32 Oldman AD, Smith LA, McQuay HJ, Moore RA. Pharmacological treatments for acute migraine: quantitative systematic review. *Pain* 2002;**97**(3):247–57.

33 Akpunonu BE, Mutgi AB, Federman DJ, et al. Subcutaneous sumatriptan for treatment of acute migraine in patients admitted to the emergency department: a multicenter study. *Ann Emerg Med* 1995;**25**(4):464–9.

34 Colman I, Brown MD, Innes GD, Grafstein E, Roberts TE, Rowe BH. Parenteral dihydroergotamine for acute migraine headache: a systematic review of the literature. *Ann Emerg Med* 2005;**45**(4):393–401.

35 Colman I, Brown MD, Innes GD, Grafstein E, Roberts TE, Rowe BH. Parenteral metoclopramide for acute migraine: meta-analysis of randomised controlled trials. *BMJ* 2004;**329**(7479):1369–73.

36 Esteban-Morales A, Chavez PT, Martinez CGR, Zuniga AS. Respuesta clinica de metoclopramida en comparacion con sumatriptan en el tratamiento de ataques agudos de migrana. *Revista de la Sanidad Militar Mexico* 1999;**53**(1):36–40.

37 Friedman BW, Corbo J, Lipton RB, et al. A trial of metoclopramide vs sumatriptan for the emergency department treatment of migraines. *Neurology* 2005;**64**(3):463–8.

38 Silberstein SD, Young WB, Mendizabal JE, Rothrock JF, Alam AS. Acute migraine treatment with droperidol: a randomized, double-blind, placebo-controlled trial. *Neurology* 2003;**60**(2):315–21.

39 Coppola M, Yealy DM, Leibold RA. Randomized, placebo-controlled evaluation of prochlorperazine versus metoclopramide for emergency department treatment of migraine headache. *Ann Emerg Med* 1995;**26**(5):541–6.

40 Jones J, Pack S, Chun E. Intramuscular prochlorperazine versus metoclopramide as single-agent therapy for the treatment of acute migraine headache. *Am J Emerg Med* 1996;**14**(3):262–4.

41 Friedman BW, Esses D, Solorzano C, et al. A randomized controlled trial of prochlorperazine versus metoclopramide for treatment of acute migraine. *Ann Emerg Med* 2007 (Nov 12, Epub ahead of print).

42 Miner JR, Fish SJ, Smith SW, Biros MH. Droperidol vs. prochlorperazine for benign headaches in the emergency department. *Acad Emerg Med* 2001;**8**(9):873–9.

43 Weaver CS, Jones JB, Chisholm CD, et al. Droperidol vs prochlorperazine for the treatment of acute headache. *J Emerg Med* 2004;**26**(2):145–50.

44 Cameron JD, Lane PL, Speechley M. Intravenous chlorpromazine vs intravenous metoclopramide in acute migraine headache. *Acad Emerg Med* 1995;**2**(7):597–602.

45 Bigal ME, Bordini CA, Tepper SJ, Speciali JG. Intravenous magnesium sulphate in the acute treatment of migraine without aura and migraine with aura. A randomized, double-blind, placebo-controlled study. *Cephalalgia* 2002;**22**(5):345–53.

46 Cete Y, Dora B, Ertan C, Ozdemir C, Oktay C. A randomized prospective placebo-controlled study of intravenous magnesium sulphate vs. metoclopramide in the management of acute migraine attacks in the emergency department. *Cephalalgia* 2005;**25**(3):199–204.

47 Ginder S, Oatman B, Pollack M. A prospective study of i.v. magnesium and i.v. prochlorperazine in the treatment of headaches. *J Emerg Med* 2000;**18**(3):311–15.

48 Corbo J, Esses D, Bijur PE, Iannaccone R, Gallagher EJ. Randomized clinical trial of intravenous magnesium sulfate as an adjunctive medication for emergency department treatment of migraine headache. *Ann Emerg Med* 2001;**38**(6):621–7.

49 Harden RN, Gracely RH, Carter T, Warner G. The placebo effect in acute headache management: ketorolac, meperidine, and saline in the emergency department. *Headache* 1996;**36**(6):352–6.

50 Klapper JA, Stanton JS. Ketorolac versus DHE and metoclopramide in the treatment of migraine headaches. *Headache* 1991;**31**(8):523–4.

51 Seim MB, March JA, Dunn KA. Intravenous ketorolac vs intravenous prochlorperazine for the treatment of migraine headaches. *Acad Emerg Med* 1998;**5**(6):573–6.

52 Shrestha M, Singh R, Moreden J, Hayes JE. Ketorolac vs chlorpromazine in the treatment of acute migraine without aura. A prospective, randomized, double-blind trial. *Arch Intern Med* 1996;**156**(15):1725–8.

53 Chan BT, Ovens HJ. Chronic migraineurs: an important subgroup of patients who visit emergency departments frequently. *Ann Emerg Med* 2004;**43**(2):238–42.

54 Maizels M. Health resource utilization of the emergency department headache "repeater". *Headache* 2002;**42**(8):747–53.

55 Blumenfeld A, Tischio M. Center of excellence for headache care: group model at Kaiser Permanente. *Headache* 2003;**43**(5):431–40.

56 Harpole LH, Samsa GP, Jurgelski AE, Shipley JL, Bernstein A, Matchar DB. Headache management program improves outcome for chronic headache. *Headache* 2003;**43**(7):715–24.

57 Maizels M, Saenz V, Wirjo J. Impact of a group-based model of disease management for headache. *Headache* 2003;**43**(6):621–7.

58 Baden EY, Hunter CJ. Intravenous dexamethasone to prevent the recurrence of benign headache after discharge from the emergency department: a randomized, double-blind, placebo-controlled clinical trial. *Can J Emerg Med* 2006;**8**(6):393–400.

59 Innes G, Macphail I, Dillon E. Dexamethasone prevents relapse after emergency department treatment of acute migraine: a randomized clinical trial. *Can J Emerg Med* 1999;**1**(1):26–33.

60 Rowe BH, Colman I, Edmonds ML, Blitz S, Walker A, Wiens S. Randomized controlled trial of intravenous dexamethasone to prevent relapse in acute migraine headache. *Headache* 2008;**48**(3):333–40.

61 Friedman BW, Greenwald P, Bania TC, et al. Randomized trial of IV dexamethasone for acute migraine in the emergency department. *Neurology* 2007;**69**(22):2038–44.

62 Jones JS, Brown MD, Bermingham M, et al. Efficacy of parenteral dexamethasone to prevent relapse after emergency department treatment of acute migraine (Abstract). *Acad Emerg Med* 2003;**10**(5):542.

49 Seizures

Elizabeth B. Jones

Department of Emergency Medicine, University of Texas Health Science Center, Houston, USA

Clinical scenario

A 26-year-old man is brought to the emergency department (ED) by ambulance. His friend called the ambulance when the patient fell to the ground and experienced generalized tonic-clonic movements in all extremities. Emergency medical services (EMS) personnel were unable to arouse the patient. According to the patient's friend, the patient has no past medical history and is on no medications. The EMS staff placed him on oxygen and heart monitors and started an intravenous line. Rapid glucose measurement was 70 mg/dl (3.9 mmol/L). Two doses of 5.0 mg of diazepam did not terminate the seizure activity.

When the ambulance arrived at the ED, the triage nurse reported that the patient was unconscious and actively seizing. He had an abrasion on his right forehead. His vital signs were a pulse of 108 beats/min, blood pressure of 160/94 mmHg and oxygen saturation (SaO_2) of 95% on 100% O_2 by non-rebreather face mask; respiration was too difficult to count.

Background

A seizure is an acute change in behavior resulting from brain dysfunction. Seizures may be divided into epileptic seizures and non-epileptic seizures. Non-epileptic seizures may be physiological or psychogenic. Any condition that causes brain hypoperfusion or hypoxia may cause non-epileptic seizures. Other causes of non-epileptic seizures are hypoglycemia, hyponatremia, hypocalcemia, uremia, porphyria, hyperthyroidism, medications, stimulant drugs and drug overdose. Psychogenic non-epileptic seizures are commonly called pseudo-seizures. These seizures are associated with major emotional or psychological distress and may be difficult to distinguish clinically from other forms of seizures.

Evidence-based Emergency Medicine. Edited by Brian H. Rowe
© 2009 Blackwell Publishing, ISBN: 978-1-4051-6143-5.

Epileptic seizures are caused by abnormalities within the brain. These may be genetically determined or acquired brain abnormalities. Any structural change to the brain may cause epileptic seizures. Examples include stroke, intracranial hemorrhage, traumatic brain injury and brain infection such as meningitis, encephalitis or cystocercosis. Epilepsy is a condition of recurrent epileptic seizures.

The behavior seen during seizures is used to classify seizures as simple or complex, partial or generalized. In a simple seizure consciousness is maintained; in a complex seizure consciousness is impaired. Partial seizures originate in only part of the cortex, while generalized seizures start in almost all areas of the cortex. Physiological non-epileptic seizures are usually not associated with an aura and are usually generalized or complex partial seizures.

Generalized seizures are the most dramatic seizures and are the seizures most often treated acutely in the ED. Generalized seizures may be tonic, clonic, myoclonic or atonic. The generalized seizure may be preceded by an aura and begins with a sudden loss of consciousness. The skeletal muscles become tonic. The patient may appear cyanotic and pulse oximetry performed during this phase will demonstrate hypoxia. After approximately 1 minute, the muscles will jerk for 1–2 minutes. This jerking may be limited to jerking of the extraocular muscles resulting in twitching eye movements. After another few minutes, the jerking will abruptly cease and the post-ictal phase will begin. The post-ictal patient will initially be minimally responsive and display deep, snoring respirations. The patient's mouth may be full of secretions, which may be bloody due to tongue-biting during the seizure. Blood drawn during or immediately after the seizure may demonstrate a low bicarbonate level, due to lactic acidosis, that will typically resolve over the next minutes to hours. The post-ictal state may last from minutes to hours, but should be characterized by a progressive improvement in the level of consciousness. In some cases, patients present with stroke-like symptoms (e.g., hemiparesis), which may last from minutes to days (also called Todd's paralysis). Finally, patients with seizures can suffer a wide variety of injuries including lacerations, abrasions, fractures and head injuries from their falls and joint dislocations from the force of their convulsions.

Box 49.1 Drugs of use in epilepsy.

	Route	Adult dose
Diazepam	IV	5–10 mg
	PR (gel)	30 mg
Lorazepam	IV	0.05–0.1 mg/kg
Midazolam	IV	1–5 mg
	IM	0.07–0.08 mg/kg
Phenytoin	IV	10–15 mg/kg
	PO	300 mg every 2h × 2 doses
Fosphenytoin	IM, IV	10–15 pheny equivalent/kg
Phenobarbital	IV	20 mg/kg, up to 30 mg/kg total
Pentobarbital	IV	10–15 mg/kg over 1 hour, then 0.5–1 mg/kg/h
Propofol	IV	1–2 mg/kg, then 2–10 mg/kg/h
Valproic acid	IV	30 mg/kg

IM, intramuscular; IV, intravenous; PO, by mouth; PR, per rectum.

Status epilepticus is classically defined as convulsions lasting longer than 20–30 minutes or seizures that recur without full return of consciousness between seizures [1]. The 20–30-minute duration is based on estimates of the time likely to cause neurological damage [2]. Studies cited in the Cochrane review of anticonvulsant therapy for status epilepticus define status epilepticus as continuous or recurrent seizures lasting from 5 to 20 minutes, or as seizures unresponsive to benzodiazepines and phenytoin [3]. In the ED, it is often difficult to know the exact time of seizure onset and, consequently, the "working" ED definition of status epilepticus is often seizures that do not respond to initial therapy or recur frequently.

Epidemiology

There are approximately 2.5 million people with epilepsy in the USA and 150,000 patients are diagnosed with a seizure each year [4,5]. In the USA from 1988 to 1992, 466,000 patients were hospitalized for seizures [6]. Seizure-related complaints accounted for 1.2% of ED visits in one study of 12 EDs [7]. Population studies of the incidence of status epilepticus report an incidence of between 6.2 and 61 per 100,000 [8–13]. A recent retrospective study from California reported a case fatality rate of 10.7% among patients admitted for status epilepticus. Increasing age was found to be a significant predictor of mortality [8]. There are a variety of drugs used in ED treatment of epilepsy (Box 49.1). This chapter will examine the evidence-based medicine approach to seizures in the ED.

Clinical questions

1 In patients with a first seizure (population), what is the sensitivity and specificity (diagnostic test characteristics) of glucose and electrolyte assessment (tests) in the initial assessment of etiology (outcome)?

2 In patients with a first seizure (population), what is the sensitivity and specificity (diagnostic test characteristics) of neuroimaging (test) identifying a clinically significant lesion (outcome)?

3 In patients who are actively seizing in the ED (population), do systemic benzodiazepines (intervention) effectively terminate seizure activity (outcome) compared to placebo?

4 In patients who are actively seizing in the ED (population), do other anticonvulsant drugs (intervention) effectively terminate seizures (outcome) compared to additional therapy with benzodiazepines?

5 In patients needing non-emergent loading of phenytoin (population), which loading technique (intervention) delivers the shortest time to safe ED discharge with the fewest adverse effects and the lowest cost (outcomes)?

6 Following an uncomplicated first seizure (population), is discharge from the ED (intervention) safe and efficient (outcomes) compared to admission to the hospital (control)?

7 In the patient presenting to the ED with a possible seizure (population), what is the sensitivity and specificity (diagnostic test characteristic) of a prolactin level (test) used to differentiate seizure from syncope or pseudo-seizure (outcome)?

General search strategy

The Cochrane Library including the Cochrane Database of Systematic Reviews and the Database of Abstracts of Reviews of Effects (DARE) were searched for "seizure" and "status epilepticus". The same terms were used to search MEDLINE using the PubMed clinical queries search filters for randomized controlled trials and systematic reviews. In the event that evidence from clinical trials and systematic reviews was lacking, the results from a limited number of observational studies were reviewed. Articles were selected for full review and potential inclusion if the title and abstract appeared to address the clinical question. The bibliography of each included article was also reviewed for potential articles. Finally relevant, updated, evidence-based clinical practice guidelines (CPGs) on seizures were reviewed to determine the consensus rating of areas lacking evidence.

Question 1: In patients with a first seizure (population), what is the sensitivity and specificity (diagnostic test characteristics) of glucose and electrolyte assessment (tests) in the initial assessment of etiology (outcome)?

Search strategy

- MEDLINE: blood chemical analysis AND (epilepsy OR seizures)

As with all ED patients, laboratory evaluation should be guided by careful history and physical examination [14]. A comprehensive ED evaluation is indicated for all ED seizure patients with neurological abnormalities or persistent altered mental status. The more common diagnostic dilemma involves the work-up of a patient who has a normal history and physical examination following a seizure.

Four prospective studies have investigated the incidence of serum chemistry abnormalities following non-febrile seizures. Eisner et al. reported chemistry data from 163 patients with focal or generalized motor seizures including 30 children and 24 first-time seizures [15]. Many abnormalities were found; sodium bicarbonate was abnormal in 27%, potassium in 7%, glucose in 6%, sodium in 6%, chloride in 6%, calcium in 2% and blood urea nitrogen (BUN) in 2%. However, the only clinically significant abnormalities were two cases of hypoglycemia and one case of hyperglycemia. In a similar study, Turnbull et al. found eight cases of hyperglycemia, one case of hypomagnesemia and two cases of hypocalcemia among 147 adults and 16 children with seizure [16]. In 98 adults with a first seizure, Sempere et al. identified two patients with hyperglycemia and one with hyponatremia [17]. Retrospective studies support the low incidence of significant serum chemistry abnormalities in patient with seizures. Six retrospective studies document serum chemistries in 1001 patients over the age of 12 years experiencing first-time seizures [18–23]. Forty-seven of these patients (4.7%) had serum chemistry values identified by the authors as either causative or clinically significant.

The clinical practice guidelines that are available all stress the low yield of serum chemistry testing. The American College of Emergency Physicians (ACEP) clinical policy on adult seizures recommends only serum glucose and sodium testing for patients with a new-onset seizure and no co-morbidities who have returned to baseline mental status [14]. The practice parameter on first non-febrile seizures published by the American Academy of Neurology recommends that laboratory tests be ordered based on individual history and physical examination [24].

It is clear that the incidence of abnormal chemistries following seizure is low. As glucose is the most common significant abnormality, it is reasonable to consider a bedside glucose in all patients. It is also apparent that, in rare circumstances, routine chemistry tests do provide important information that is not clinically suspected. Because of the very low incidence of clinically significant laboratory abnormalities in the observational studies identified in our search, a high-risk subgroup of patients most likely to benefit from chemistry measurement has not been defined. However, blood testing poses little risk and is not expensive, so may be considered for patients thought to be at risk of laboratory abnormalities based on medication or medical history. Patients with recurrent seizures may benefit even less.

Question 2: In patients with a first seizure (population), what is the sensitivity and specificity (diagnostic test characteristics) of neuroimaging (test) identifying a clinically significant lesion (outcome)?

Search strategy

• MEDLINE: seizure AND (brain CT OR brain MRI)

Most patients require neuroimaging following a first-time non-physiological seizure [14]. While many EDs have access to computerized tomography (CT), the preferred technique for investigating seizures is magnetic resonance imaging (MRI). Brain MRI provides better images for identification of lesions such as tumors and vascular malformations. Two studies comparing MRI to CT in patients with first-time seizures found that MRI detected brain lesions 16% [17] and 22% [25] more often than did CT; however, none of the additional lesions changed management.

The goal in the ED, however, is to exclude all lesions that must be treated emergently. Head CT is more available in the ED setting and is able to identify lesions needing emergent treatment such as hemorrhage, swelling or mass effect. The ACEP clinical policy on seizures recommends emergent head CT following a first seizure in patients with new focal deficits, persistent altered mental status, fever, recent trauma, persistent headache, a history of cancer, a history of anticoagulation or suspicion of AIDS [14]. These indications for emergent head CT are not controversial. The more difficult question to answer is whether or not first-time seizure patients who have returned to baseline and have no other indication for emergent head CT require neuroimaging in the ED.

Table 49.1 presents data from class I and II studies of adults presenting to the ED with a first seizure without clear physiological cause such as hypoglycemia or anoxia. In the listed studies, 10–53% of patients had abnormal imaging studies, with 8–41% of patients having significant abnormalities. Thus, emergent neuroimaging is fairly productive in adults. The ACEP clinical policy recommends ED neuroimaging following a first-time seizure in adult patients who have returned to baseline [14]. This neuroimaging may be deferred when reliable follow-up is available.

In summary, MRI is the most sensitive test for the identification of brain abnormalities following seizure. If MRI is readily available in the ED, it may be preferable to CT; however, head CT will accurately identify lesions requiring emergent treatment following a first seizure [29]. All patients with persistent altered mental status, new focal neurological examination, persistent headache, focal seizure, bleeding diathesis, a history of cancer, anticoagulation, trauma or immunocompromise and fever (except children with simple febrile seizures) should have emergent neuroimaging following seizures. Adults with a first seizure who return to baseline quickly and have a normal history and physical exam may have neuroimaging deferred when follow-up is easily arranged.

Question 3: In patients who are actively seizing in the ED (population), do systemic benzodiazepines (intervention) effectively terminate seizure activity (outcome) compared to placebo?

Search strategy

• Cochrane Library and MEDLINE: seizures AND status epilepticus AND treatment

Table 49.1 Neuroimaging studies with first seizures in the ED.

Study	Class	Method	Number imaged	Number abnormal (%)	95% CI	Number of significant abnormalities (%)	95% CI	Number not suspected	95% CI
Schoenenberger & Heim [26]	I	CT	119	40 (34%)	30 to39	20 (17%)	12 to 29		
Sempere et al. [17]	I	CT/MRI	99	33 (33%)	28 to 38				
Gordon et al. [27]	I	CT	48	5 (10%)	6 to 16	4 (8%)	4 to 12	4 (8%)	4 to 12
Russo & Goldstein [28]	I	CT	62	29 (47%)	41 to 53	7 (11%)	2 to 15	0	0 to 3
Pesola & Westfal [23]	II	CT	121	31 (26%)	20 to 30				
Henneman et al. [21]	II	CT	325	169 (52%)	50 to 54	134 (41%)	39 to 43	28 (8.6%)	7.1 to 10.1
Tardy et al. [22]	II	CT	247	130 (53%)	50 to 56	38 (15%)	13 to 17		
Total			1021	437 (44%)	42 to 46	203/801 (25%)	22 to 27	32/435 (7%)	0 to 2

CT, computerized tomography; MRI, magnetic resonance imaging.

Many seizures terminate spontaneously. For example, in a prehospital study of status epilepticus, of 1623 "seizure" calls, in 1066 cases the seizure either stopped within 5 minutes spontaneously or was not witnessed by paramedics [30]. Seizures that continue require emergent intervention as status epilepticus may cause death or permanent neurological sequelae [2]. Despite the danger and relative frequency of status epilepticus, there are few treatment trials and no consensus as to the best treatment regimen [2,14,31].

A Cochrane review of anticonvulsant therapy for status epilepticus included 11 studies involving 2017 subjects [3]. To be included, participants were required to have premonitory or early-stage status epilepticus or established status epilepticus. The premonitory stage was defined as seizures that are becoming more frequent or severe, the early stage is the first 30 minutes of seizure activity, while established status epilepticus was defined as a seizure or a series of seizures without full recovery lasting more than 30 minutes [32]. The therapeutic interventions compared were diazepam (intravenous, rectal), lorazepam, midazolam (intravenous, intramuscular, rectal), clonazepam, paraldehyde (intramuscular, rectal), phenytoin, fosphenytoin, pentobarbitone, etomidate, propofol,

lignocaine, thiopentone and isoflurane. Outcomes used in the different studies were death, development or continuation of established status epilepticus, need for ventilatory support, incomplete return to baseline and long-term disabling sequelae.

Significant clinical and statistical heterogeneity was identified among the studies included in the systematic review; studies used different inclusion criteria, different interventions and different outcomes. Despite the difficulties comparing this heterogeneous group of studies, the authors of the Cochrane review were able to demonstrate that both lorazepam and diazepam were better than placebo for termination of seizure activity and lowering the risk of ventilatory support or further treatment. Lorazepam will terminate status epilepticus in 60–90% of patients [30,33–37] and is better than diazepam and phenytoin for the cessation of seizures (RR = 0.64; 95% CI: 0.45 to 0.90) (Fig. 49.1).

Lorazepam doses used in included studies were 2 mg for adults and 0.05–0.1 mg/kg for children. Diazepam gel 30 mg intrarectal stopped premonitory status epilepticus better than did 20 mg with no increase in side-effects. Definitive conclusions were not possible with other comparisons.

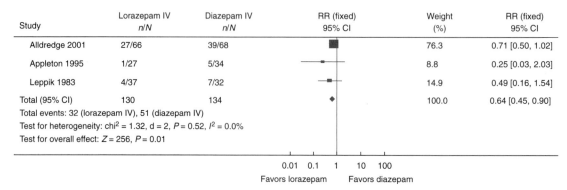

Figure 49.1 Comparison of IV lorazepam versus IV diazepam in acessing seizures. (Reproduced with permission from Prasad et al. [3]; data from Alldredge et al. [30], Appleton et al. [34] and Leppik et al. [35].)

In summary, first-line therapy with benzodiazepines is appropriate for patients in status epilepticus or with active seizures. The best evidence supports the use of lorazepam as the first therapy for premonitory, early-stage or established status epilepticus. When lorazepam is not available, intravenous diazepam should be used. When rectal diazepam is used in adults, 30 mg is the most effective dose.

Question 4: In patients who are actively seizing in the ED (population), do other anticonvulsant drugs (intervention) effectively terminate seizures (outcome) compared to additional therapy with benzodiazepines?

Search strategy

- Cochrane Library and MEDLINE: seizures AND status epilepticus AND treatment

No prospective, randomized controlled trial has compared treatments for seizures refractory to initial benzodiazepine treatment. While most published treatment guidelines recommend intravenous phenytoin as second-line treatment [1,38–40], very little data exist to support this recommendation. In one large randomized study comparing phenytoin, lorazepam and phenobarbital for first-line treatment of status epilepticus, phenytoin was the least effective treatment (terminating seizures in 43.6% of cases) [37]. In a retrospective case series of patients with status epilepticus refractory to benzodiazepine therapy, 54% of patients responded to second-line therapy, which was phenytoin in 84% of cases [40]. In a recent randomized, unblinded study of status epilepticus patients, 68 patients were randomized to receive either intravenous phenytoin or intravenous sodium valproate. Patients who continued to seize were given the other drug as second-line therapy. Phenytoin was effective as first-line therapy in 42% of patients and in 25% as second-line treatment (after sodium valproate) [41]. Intravenous sodium valproate was effective in 66% of patients when given initially and in 79% when given after phenytoin. In summary, although intravenous phenytoin is commonly used as the second agent in patients with refractory status epilepticus and will terminate seizures in 25–50% of patients, it may not be the most effective agent.

Status epilepticus will persist even after treatment with benzodiazepine and antiepileptic drug therapy in 9–31% of patients [36,40]. A systematic review assessing the effectiveness of therapy for refractory status epilepticus included 28 trials involving only 193 patients treated with midazolam, propofol or pentobarbital [42]. Pentobarbital appeared to be the most effective treatment; however, the clinical heterogeneity among studies and imprecision of point estimates make any conclusions difficult.

Given the paucity of data from clinical trials assessing the effectiveness of treatment of refractory status epilepticus, observations based on descriptive case series may provide the clinician with some insight. Both thiopental and pentobarbital appear to be effective. These agents almost always cause hypotension, but this is typically responsive to fluid or vasopressors [42,43]. Propofol terminates status epilepticus very quickly when it is administered in doses from 1 to 3 mg/kg followed by a maintenance infusion at 1–15 mg/kg/h [44,45]. In one small study of 16 patients with status epilepticus refractory to benzodiazepines, phenytoin and/or phenobarbitol, the mean time to seizure control was 2.6 ($\pm$0.75) minutes with propofol compared to 123 ($\pm$33) minutes with high-dose barbiturates [45]. Because propofol works more quickly than the barbiturates, it is reasonable to administer a trial of propofol in patients with refractory seizures. Pentobarbital or thiopental may be used if propofol is ineffective; however, these drugs are associated with prolonged recovery times [42,43]. Intravenous sodium valproate may be effective for refractory status epilepticus with reported termination rates of 63–86% [41,46,47].

In summary, for status epilepticus unresponsive to benzodiazepines, there are many treatment options, but none has been demonstrated to be superior. Concensus guidelines have recommended phenytoin as the preferred second-line treatment due to its familiarity and lack of respiratory depression. In patients whose seizures persist after adequate doses of benzodiazepine and phenytoin, anesthetic agents such as propofol or barbiturates should be considered.

Question 5: In patients needing non-emergent loading of phenytoin (population), which loading technique (intervention) delivers the shortest time to safe ED discharge with the fewest adverse effects and the lowest cost (outcomes)?

Search strategy

- Cochrane Library and MEDLINE: (phenytoin AND seizures) OR (fosphenytoin AND seizures)

While it is clear that phenytoin should be given intravenously in emergent situations, there is no standard loading method for the stable patient with a non-therapeutic phenytoin level. Only one randomized open-label trial has compared phenytoin-loading methods [48]. Overall, 45 patients were randomized to receive 20 mg/kg of oral phenytoin, 18 mg/kg of IV phenytoin at 50 mg/min or 18 mg/kg of IV fosphenytoin at 150 mg/min. Safe discharge from the ED was defined as a phenytoin level of >10 mg/L and the absence of any side-effects that would preclude discharge. Times to safe ED discharge were 1.7 $\pm$ 0.8 hours for IV phenytoin, 1.3 $\pm$ 1.0 hours for IV fosphenytoin and 6.4 $\pm$ 2.2 hours for oral phenytoin. The longer time to therapeutic concentration with oral loading is supported by many studies [49–54].

Adverse effects in the above trial were significantly lower in the oral loading group and were similar in both intravenous groups. The results are summarized in Table 49.2.

Of the four other trials that compared IV phenytoin to IV fosphenytoin, three found significantly fewer adverse events in the

Table 49.2 Adverse events with loading with IV phenytoin (IVP), IV fosphenytoin (IVF) and oral phenytoin (PO). (With permission from Swardon et al. [48].)

	IVP	IVF	PO	*P*-value
Number of patients	14	15	16	
Neurological*	14	11	15	n.s.
Nausea, vomiting	0	4	2	0.1
Hypotension	2	1	–	0.29
Tachycardia	0	1	–	0.36
Phlebitis	11	3	–	<0.001
Pruritus	0	12	–	<0.001

*Ataxia, disorientation, dizziness, headache and nystagmus.

fosphenytoin group [55–57], while the largest study found no significant difference in adverse event rates [58]. These differences may be due to different methods used for measurement of and reporting of side-effects. In all studies the incidence of phlebitis was higher with phenytoin and the incidence of pruritis was higher with fosphenytoin.

Cost-effectiveness studies comparing IV phenytoin and IV fosphenytoin have been mixed with two favoring fosphenytoin over phenytoin [59,60] and one with the opposite findings [61]. These differences are due to assumptions regarding the rates of adverse effects and costs. A cost-effectiveness analysis of the data from the open-label trial discussed in detail above found that oral phenytoin was the most cost-effective approach [60]. However, when the cost of increased time to ED discharge was considered, IV phenytoin cost only US$3.90 per hour of ED time saved over oral phenytoin, while IV fosphenytoin cost $387.27 per hour of ED time saved over IV phenytoin.

Oral phenytoin loading is safer and significantly less expensive than intravenous loading, but the time until therapeutic levels are achieved is substantially longer, which is important in the setting of ED overcrowding. Intravenous fosphenytoin is more expensive than IV phenytoin and no studies have definitively demonstrated that fosphenytoin is safer than phenytoin.

In summary, when rapid loading is needed in the patient with precarious IV access, intramuscular fosphenytoin may be considered; when time is not crucial, some patients may qualify for oral phenytoin loading.

Question 6: Following an uncomplicated first seizure (population), is discharge from the ED (intervention) safe and efficient (outcomes) compared to admission to the hospital (control)?

Search strategy

- Cochrane Library and MEDLINE: seizure(s) AND (hospital admission OR admission)

Seizure patients with signs of central nervous system infection, abnormal neurological exam, altered mental status or significant metabolic abnormalities require hospital admission [14]. The more difficult question is which patients with a first-time seizure who have returned to baseline can be safely discharged from the ED. Our search did not identify any clinical trials or prospective observational studies that specifically addressed disposition following a first-time seizure in the ED. We did identify two retrospective studies that assessed the risk of seizure recurrence in the first 24 hours following an uncomplicated first-time seizure in a patient population admitted to the hospital [21,62].

In the single adult study identified, recurrence rate was 19%; the highest recurrence rates were in patients with alcohol-related events and in those with focal lesions on head CT scan [21]. Similarly, the other applicable study, which included both adults and children, found a 19.8% recurrence rate [62]. Unfortunately, selection bias limits the applicability of these results to the ED population.

The ACEP seizure clinical policy recommends (level C) that patients with normal neurological examination may be discharged from the ED with outpatient follow-up [14]. Given the limited evidence available, it is reasonable to consider admission for the vulnerable patient population without access to physician follow-up and in those with higher than normal risk of recurrence from alcohol-related seizures or with focal findings on head CT scan. Given the recurrence risk may be as high as one in four, seizure precautions and observation by a reliable person are prudent for all discharged patients.

Question 7: In the patient presenting to the ED with a possible seizure (population), what is the sensitivity and specificity (diagnostic test characteristics) of a prolactin level (test) used to differentiate seizure from syncope or pseudo-seizure (outcome)?

Search strategy

- Cochrane Library and MEDLINE: prolactin AND (seizure OR status epilepticus OR epilepsy OR syncope OR pseudoseizure)

In the ED setting, seizures may be difficult to differentiate from pseudo-seizures or syncope. Pseudo-seizures are frequently repetitive and some patients may have both epileptic seizures and pseudo-seizures. The ED physician may suspect pseudo-seizure, but often cannot absolutely establish the diagnosis. Similarly, the history may suggest seizure versus syncope, but not definitively. It would be useful to have a test that could differentiate between these entities.

In 1978, Trimble demonstrated that prolactin was increased following a generalized tonic-clonic seizure, but not following psychogenic non-epileptic seizures [63]. Prolactin is released by the pituitary under stimulus from the hypothalamus and has since been investigated as a biomarker for epileptic seizures. It has been difficult to define an abnormal result given the circadian fluctuations in prolactin, differences in baseline levels among males and females, and higher baseline levels in people with epilepsy. Therefore, most studies define an elevated prolactin as two times the baseline for that individual. In the ED, one approach is to measure the baseline prolactin 6 hours after the event. In 2005, the American Academy of Neurology published a systematic review of the evidence supporting the use of prolactin in diagnosing epileptic seizures [64]. The pooled results of one class I and nine class II studies concluded that an elevated prolactin measured 10–20 minutes after an event probably indicates epileptic seizure, but a normal prolactin cannot rule out an epileptic event. The pooled specificity for generalized tonic-clinic seizure was 95.9% (95% CI: 91.4% to100%), while the pooled sensitivity was only 60% (95% CI: 48.9% to 71.1%).

Two small studies investigated whether prolactin increased following syncope [65,66]. In the 11 of 21 subjects who experienced syncope following 60° head-up tilt-table testing, prolactin was elevated, when measured 10 minutes after the event, in 82% [66]. Subjects who did not faint showed no significant changes in prolactin levels (0/10). Though these studies are small and were not ED-based, prolactin may be elevated following syncope and so cannot be used to differentiate between seizure and syncope.

When the ED physician cannot differentiate seizure from pseudo-seizure, a prolactin drawn 10–20 minutes after the event compared to a baseline level 6 hours later may help an admitting physician establish the correct diagnosis. Based on the evidence available, an elevated prolactin level (positive likelihood ratio = 12) significantly increases the probability that the patient had a seizure. If the pre-test probability for pseudo-seizure is very high (i.e., pre-test probability for true seizure is 10%) and there is no significant elevation in the prolactin level from baseline (negative likelihood ratio = 0.4), the post-test probability of the event representing a true seizure may be low enough (4%) to assume a pseudo-seizure.

Conclusions

Seizures are a common ED presentation associated with significant morbidity and mortality. A thorough history and physical examination should guide the laboratory and radiological evaluation of patients presenting with seizure. The evidence supports initial treatment with benzodiazepines such as lorazepam and loading with phenytoin intravenously to prevent further seizures if the patient has chronic epilepsy or status epilepticus. Disposition decisions should be based on the neurological examination of the patient and on the presence of other complicating conditions.

The patient in the clinical scenario was still seizing on arrival in the ED. He was placed on cardiac monitors and pulse oximetry. Intravenous lorazepam 4 mg was administered; however, the seizures continued. Phenytoin loading was initiated and a rapid sequence intubation was performed to protect his airway using lidocaine, etomidate and succinylcholine. Motor seizures ceased following administration of succinylcholine and did not recur. Head CT and serum electrolytes were normal. The patient's friend arrived at the ED and reported that the patient had been using cocaine prior to seizure onset. The patient was admitted to the intensive care unit and recovered uneventfully.

Conflicts of interest

Dr. Jones, research is supported by the NIH through the SPOTRIAS and NETT grant.

References

1 Lowenstein DH, Alldredge BK. Status epilepticus. *N Eng J Med* 1998;**338**:970–76.

2 Anon. Treatment of convulsive status epilepticus: recommendations of the Epilepsy Foundation of America's Working Group on Status Epilepticus. *JAMA* 1993;**270**:854–85.

3 Prasad K, Al-Roomi K, Krishnan PR, Sequeira R. Anticonvulsant therapy for status epilepticus. *Cochrane Database Syst Rev* 2005;**4**:CD003723 (doi: 10.1002/14651858.CD003723.pub2).

4 Hauser WA, Kurland LT. The epidemiology of epilepsy in Rochester, Minnesota, 1935 through 1967. *Epilepsia* 1975;**16**:1–66.

5 Begley CE, Annegers JF, Lairson DR, et al. Cost of epilepsy in the United States: a model based on incidence and prognosis. *Epilepsia* 2000;**41**:342–51.

6 Centers for Disease Control and Prevention. Hospitalization for epilepsy – United States, 1988–1992. *MMWR* 1995;**44**:818–21.

7 Huff JS, Morris DL, Kothari RU, Gibbs MA. Emergency department management of patients with seizures: a multicenter study. *Ann Emerg Med* 2001;**8**(6):622–8.

8 Wu YW, Shek DW, Garcia PA, et al. Incidence and mortality of generalized convulsive status epilepticus in California. *Neurology* 2001;**58**(7):1070–76.

9 DeLorenz RJ, Hauser WA, Towne AR, et al. A prospective, population-based study of status epilepticus in Richmond, Virginia. *Neurology* 1996;**46**:1029–1035.

10 Hesdorffer DC, Logroscino G, Cascino G, et al. Incidence of status epilepticus in Rochester, Minnesota, 1965–1984. *Neurology* 1996;**46**:1029–35.

11 Logroscino G, Hesdorffer DC, Cascino G, et al. Time trends in incidence, mortality, and case-fatality after first episode of status epilepticus. *Epilepsia* 2001;**42**:1031–5.

12 Knake S, Rosenow F, Vescovi M, et al. Incidence of status epilepticus in adults in Germany: a prospective, population-based study. *Epilepsia* 2001;**42**:714–18.

13 Coeytaux A, Jallon P, Galobardes B, Morabia A. Incidence of status epilepticus in French-speaking Switzerland (EPISTAR). *Neurology* 2000;**55**:693–7.

14 ACEP Clinical Policies Committee, Clinical Policies Subcommittee on Seizures. Clinical policy: critical issues in the evaluation and management of adult patients presenting to the emergency department with seizures. *Ann Emerg Med* 2004;**43**:605–25.

15 Eisner RF, Turnbull TL, Howes DS, Gold IW. Efficacy of a "standard" seizure work-up in the emergency department. *Ann Emerg Med* 1986;**15**:33–9.

16 Turnbull TL, Vandenhoek T, Howes DS, et al. Utility of laboratory studies in the ED patient with a new onset seizure. *Ann Emerg Med* 1990;**19**:373–7.

17 Sempere AP, Villaverde FJ, Martinez-Menendez B, et al. First seizure in adults: a prospective study from the emergency department. *Acta Neurol Scand* 1992;**86**:134–8.

18 Rosenthal RH, Helm ML, Waeckerle JF. First time major motor seizures in an emergency department. *Ann Emerg Med* 1980;**9**:242–5.

19 Powers RD. Serum chemistry abnormalities in adult patients with seizures. *Ann Emerg Med* 1985;**14**:416–20.

20 McKee PJ, Wilson EA, Dawson JA, et al. Managing seizures in the casualty department. *BMJ* 1990;**300**:978–9.

21 Henneman PL, DeRoos F, Lewis RJ. Determining the need for admission in patients with new onset seizures. *Ann Emerg Med* 1994;**24**:1108–14.

22 Tardy B, LaFond P, Convers P, et al. Adult first generalized seizure: etiology, biological tests, EEG, CT scan in an ED. *Am J Emerg Med* 1995;**13**:1–5.

23 Pesola GR, Westfal RE. New-onset generalized seizures in patients with AIDS presenting to an emergency department. *Acad Emerg Med* 1998;**5**:905–11.

24 Hirtz D, Ashwal S, Berg D, et al. Practice parameter: Evaluating a first nonfebrile seizure in children: Report of the Quality Standards Committee of the American Academy of Neurology, the Child Neurology Society, and the American Epilepsy Society. *Neurology* 2000;**55**:616–23.

25 Berg AT, Testa FM, Levy SR, Shinnar S. Neuroimaging in children with newly diagnosed epilepsy: a community-based study. *Pediatrics* 2000;**106**:527–32.

26 Schoenenberger RA, Heim SM. Indication for computed tomography of the brain in patients with first uncomplicated generalized seizure. *BMJ* 1994;**309**:986–9.

27 Gordon WH, Jabbari B, Dotty JR, Gunderson CH. Computed tomography and the first seizure of adults (Abstract). *Ann Neurol* 1985;**18**:153.

28 Russo LS, Goldstein KH. The diagnostic assessment of single seizures: is cranial computed tomography necessary? *Arch Neurol* 1983;**40**:744–6.

29 Dunn MJ, Breen DP, Davenport RJ, Gray AJ. Early management of adults with an uncomplicated first generalized seizure. *Emerg Med J* 2005;**22**:237–42.

30 Alldredge BK, Gelb AM, Isaacs SM, et al. A comparison of lorazepam, diazepam and placebo for the treatment of out-of-hospital status epilepticus. *N Eng J Med* 2001;**345**:631–7.

31 Working Group. Treatment of convulsive status epilepticus. Recommendations of the Epilepsy Foundation of America's Working Group on status epilepticus. *JAMA* 1993;**270**:854–9.

32 Shovron S. Tonic-clonic status epilepticus. *J Neurol Neurosurg Psychiatry* 1993;**56**:125–34.

33 Lowenstein DH, Alldredge BK, Gelb AM, et al. Results of a controlled trial of benzodiazepines for the treatment of status epilepticus in the prehospital setting. *Epilepsia* 1999;**40**:290–309.

34 Appleton R, Sweeney A, Choonara I, et al. Lorazepam verses diazepam in the acute treatment of epileptic seizures and status epilepticus. *Dev Med Child Neurol* 1995;**37**:682–8.

35 Leppik IE, Derivan AT, Homan RW, et al. Double-blind study of lorazepam and diazepam in status epilepticus. *JAMA* 1983;**249**:1452–4.

36 Shaner DM, McCurdy SA, Herring MO, Gabor AJ. Treatment of status, a prospective comparison of diazepam and phenytoin versus phenobarbitol and optional phenytoin. *Neurology* 1998;**38**:202–7.

37 Treiman DM, Meyers PD, Walton NY, et al. A comparison of four treatments for generalized convulsive status epilepticus. Veterans Affairs Status Epilepticus Cooperative Study Group. *N Engl J Med* 1998;**339**:779–84.

38 Status Epilepticus Working Party. The treatment of convulsive status epilepticus in children. *Arch Dis Child* 2000;**83**:415–19.

39 Walker M. Status epilepticus: an evidence based guide. *BMJ* 2005;**331**:673–7.

40 Mayer SA, Claassen J, Lokin J, et al. Refractory status epilepticus. Frequency, risk factors, and impact on outcome. *Arch Neurol* 2002;**59**:205–10.

41 Misra UK, Kalita J, Patel R. Sodium valproate vs phenytoin in status epilepticus: a pilot study. *Neurology* 2006;**67**:340–42.

42 Claassen J, Hirsch LJ, Emerson RG, Mayer SA. Treatment of refractory status epilepticus with pentobarbital, propofol, or midazolam: a systematic review. *Epilepsia* 2002;**43**:146–53.

43 Parviainen I, Uusaro A, Kälviäinen R, et al. High-dose thiopental in the treatment of refractory status epilepticus in the intensive care unit. *Neurology* 2002;**59**:1249–51.

44 Stecker MM, Kramer TH, Raps EC, et al. Treatment of refractory status epilepticus with propofol: clinical and pharmacokinetic findings. *Epilepsia* 1998;**39**:18–26.

45 Prasad A, Worrall BB, Bertram EH, Bleck TP. Propofol and midazolam in the treatment of refractory status epilepticus. *Epilepsia* 2001;**42**:380–86.

46 Limdi NA, Shimpi EF, Gomez CR, Burneo JG. Efficacy of rapid IV administration of valproic acid for status epilepticus. *Neurology* 2005;**64**:353–5.

47 Peters CN, Pohlmann-Eden B. Intravenous valproate as an innovative therapy in seizure emergency situations including status epilepticus – experience in 102 adult patients. *Seizure* 2005;**14**:164–9.

48 Swadron SP, Rudis MI, Azimian K, et al. A comparison of phenytoin-loading techniques in the emergency department. *Acad Emerg Med* 2004;**11**:244–52.

49 Wilder BJ, Serrano EE, Ramsay RE. Plasma diphenylhydantoin levels after loading and maintenance doses. *Clin Pharmacol Ther* 1973;**14**:797–801.

50 Lund L, Alvan G, Berlin A, Alexanderson B. Pharmacokinetics of single and multiple doses of phenytoin in man. *Eur J Clin Pharmacol* 1974;**7**:81–6.

51 Record KE, Rapp RP, Young AB, Kostenbauder HB. Oral phenytoin loading in adults: rapid achievement of therapeutic levels. *Ann Neurol* 1979;**5**:268–70.

52 Osborn HH, Zisfein J, Sparano R. Single-dose oral phenytoin loading. *Ann Emerg Med* 1987;**16**:407–12.

53 Van Der Meyden CH, Kruger AJ, Muller FO, et al. Acute oral loading of carbamazepine-CR and phenytoin in a double-blind randomized study of patients at risk of seizures. *Epilepsia* 1994;**35**:189–94.

54 Ratanakorn D, Kaojarern S, Phuapradit P, Mokkhavesa C. Single oral loading dose of phenytoin: a pharmacokinetics study. *J Neurol Sci* 1997;**147**:89–92.

55 Jamerson BD, Dukes GE, Brouwer KL, et al. Venous irritation related to intravenous administration of phenytoin versus fosphenytoin. *Pharmacotherapy* 1994;**14**:47–52.

56 Ramsay RE, DeToledo J. Intravenous administration of fosphenytoin: options for the management of seizures. *Neurology* 1996;**46**(Suppl 1):17S–19S.

57 Boucher BA, Feler CA, Dean JC, et al. The safety, tolerability and pharmacokinetics of fosphenytoin after intramuscular and intravenous administration in neurosurgery patients. *Pharmacotherapy* 1996;**16**:638–45.

58 Coplin WM, Rhoney DH, Debuck JA, et al. Randomized evaluation of adverse events and length-of-stay with routine emergency department use of phenytoin or fosphenytoin. *Neurol Res* 1996;**24**:842–8.

59 Touchette DR, Rhoney DH. Cost-minimization analysis of pheny-toin and fosphenytoin in the emergency department. *Pharmacotherapy* 2000;**20**:908–16.

60 Rudis MI, Touchette DR, Swadron SP, et al. Cost-effectiveness of oral phenytoin, intravenous phenytoin, and intravenous fosphenytoin in the emergency department. *Neurology* 2004;**43**:387–97.

61 Marchetti A, Magar R, Fischer J, et al. A pharmacoeconomic evaluation of intravenous fosphenytoin (Cerebyx®) versus phenytoin (Dilantin®) in hospital emergency departments. *Clin Ther* 1996;**18**:953–66.

62 Krumholz A, Grufferman S, Orr ST, Stern BJ. Seizures and seizure care in the emergency department. *Epilepsia* 1989;**30**:175–81.

63 Trimble MR. Serum prolactin in epilepsy and hysteria. *BMJ* 1978;**2**: 1682.

64 Chen DK, So YT, Fisher RS. Use of serum prolactin in diagnosing epileptic seizures. Report of the Therapeutic and Technology Assessment Subcommittee of the American Academy of Neurology. *Neurology* 2005;**65**:668–75.

65 Oribe E, Amini R, Nissenbaum E, Boal B. Serum prolactin concentrations are elevated after syncope. *Neurology* 1996;**47**:60–62.

66 Theodorakis GN, Markianos M, Miller M, et al. Hormonal responses during tilt-table test in neurally mediated syncope. *Am J Cardiol* 1997;**79**:1692–5.

50 The Agitated Patient

Michael S. Radeos[1] & Edwin D. Boudreaux[2]

[1]Department of Emergency Medicine, New York Hospital Queens, Flushing, USA
[2]Department of Emergency Medicine, Cooper University Hospital, Camden, USA

Case scenario

A 27-year-old male presented to the emergency department (ED) via ambulance from home where he was found by his girlfriend. He had been drinking earlier that evening; however, he was acting uncharacteristically angrily and threatening violence. The girlfriend immediately called emergency medical services (EMS). On arrival, they found the patient in a rage and they called local police for back-up. The police arrived and hog-tied (hands and feet tied together) the patient so that he could be transported to the hospital involuntarily. The girlfriend denied any ingestion of pills or other attempts at self-harm, nor was there a history of previous suicide attempts. The patient was previously healthy, had no known allergies and was not taking any prescribed medications. Apparently he had been depressed for the past year following the death of his mother from breast cancer and had been prescribed paroxetine. His girlfriend was not aware of the patient taking any illicit drugs and he only occasionally consumed alcohol. He had an uncle who committed suicide, but there were no other major medical problems in the family.

On arrival to the ED, he smelled slightly of alcohol, was screaming and swearing at the staff and refused to answer any questions or allow any vital signs to be recorded until he was untied. He was clearly straining at the ties that bound his hands and feet. The police asked if they could take their handcuffs and leave now that they had delivered the patient to the hospital.

Your first year resident was visibly frightened by this threatening patient and asked whether it was safe to approach him. He wanted to know if the patient could be left to "cool off" before a history and physical was performed. When you suggested that the patient may benefit from medication to reduce his agitation, the resident asked you whether this might be dangerous since the patient had been drinking. At the time, you elected to administer a combination of intramuscular lorazepam and haloperidol, place the patient in four-point leather restraints and order a cardiac monitor with pulse oximetry.

Background

The management of a violent or severely agitated patient (VSAP) who presents to the ED is fraught with difficult decisions. Fortunately, these cases are not common, and most patients can be persuaded to cooperate. The mere physical restraint of such patients has been associated with sudden death [1–5] as well as potential injury to the health care worker or law enforcement personnel [6–8]. Often, VSAPs are unwilling to cooperate with providing a history of present illness or permitting nursing and physician physical examination. When these patients present, the emergency physician must rapidly gain control of the situation to protect the patient as well as the staff.

Consensus guidelines have been promulgated by the American College of Emergency Physicians (ACEP) [9] as well as the American Association of Emergency Psychiatry (AAEP) [8,10]. The AAEP guidelines were developed using a consensus format, and involved 52 participants. Fifty of 52 (96%) selected experts responded to the survey on behavioral emergencies and their aggregate opinions were reflected in these guidelines. The written survey included 808 decision points and was scored using a modified RAND Corporation nine-point scale for rating appropriateness of medical decision making. These guidelines focus on care once the psychiatrist has assumed responsibility for the patient. Conversely, the ACEP guidelines were developed using a textual format, and involved seven participants – experts in emergency and/or psychiatric emergency care. They address four "critical" questions relating to general management of the psychiatric patient in the ED. One of these questions deals with pharmacological treatment of the agitated patient (chemical restraint). The other three questions related only to cooperative alert patients (what tests were appropriate to determine medical stability, and whether a urine drug screen or alcohol level were needed in the ED evaluation).

Physical and/or chemical restraints are a major issue for health care, and the use of restraints is a leading indicator for hospital accrediting bodies (e.g., the Joint Commission in the USA). Zun reviewed the experience of physical and chemical restraint at an inner-city teaching hospital for 1 year and found relatively few minor complications to this practice, none of them serious [11].

Once physical or chemical control has been employed, the primary issue of importance is the underlying diagnosis. For example, patients with mental health problems such as psychotic depression, psychosis and schizophrenia may make up many of the cases. Emergency physicians must also remember medical conditions such as severe hepatic failure, diabetic hypoglycemia, alcohol withdrawal, that may present with transient mental status changes that resolve with treatment of the medical disorder. Finally, abuse of drugs and alcohol may also result in agitated behavior that resolves once the agents have been metabolized.

Clinical questions

In order to address the issues of most relevance to your patient and to help in searching the literature for the evidence regarding these issues, you should structure your clinical questions as recommended in Chapter 1.

1 Among patients presenting to the ED with acute agitation (population), is physical restraint (intervention) safe and effective (outcomes) for restraining patients compared to isolation and medical management (comparison)?

2 Among patients presenting to the ED with acute agitation (population), what is the sensitivity and specificity (diagnostic test characteristics) of clinical criteria (tests) to diagnose depression in the ED (outcome)?

3 Among patients presenting to the ED with acute agitation (population), what are the likelihood ratios (diagnostic test characteristics) of clinical prediction guides (tests) to diagnose suicidal risk (outcome)?

4 Among patients presenting to the ED with acute agitation (population), does chemical restraint with phenothiazines (intervention) reduce risks and time to stabilization compared to benzodiazepines (comparison)?

5 Among patients presenting to the ED with acute agitation (population), does chemical restraint with newer agents (intervention) reduce risks and time to stabilization (outcomes) compared to benzodiazepines/phenothiazines (comparison)?

6 Among patients presenting to the ED with acute agitation (population), does psychiatric assessment (intervention) reduce recidivism and mortality (outcomes) compared to medical clearance alone?

7 Among patients presenting to the ED with acute agitation (population), is short-term hospitalization (intervention) effective and efficient (outcome) as a disposition strategy for determining suicide risk and/or major depression compared to outpatient assessment following medical clearance (comparison)?

8 Among adult patients presenting to the ED (population), can screening (intervention) identify depression and reduce recidivism/mortality (outcomes) compared to case finding alone (control)?

General search strategy

You begin to address these questions by searching for evidence in the common electronic databases, such as the Cochrane Library, MEDLINE and EMBASE, looking specifically for systematic reviews and meta-analyses. The Cochrane Library contains a number of high-quality systematic review with evidence on numerous aspects of psychiatric disease. When a systematic review is identified, you also search for recent updates on the Cochrane Library and search MEDLINE and EMBASE to identify randomized controlled trials (RCTs) that became available after the publication date of the systematic review. In addition, access to relevant, updated, and evidence-based clinical practice guidelines (CPGs) on acute agitation are accessed to determine the consensus rating of areas lacking evidence.

Searching for evidence synthesis: primary search strategy
- Cochrane Library: (agitation OR psychosis) AND (topic)
- MEDLINE: (agitation OR psychosis) AND MEDLINE AND (systematic review OR meta-analysis OR metaanalysis) AND adult AND (topic)
- EMBASE: (agitation OR psychosis) AND MEDLINE AND (systematic review OR meta-analysis OR metaanalysis) AND adult AND (topic)

Critical review of the literature

Question 1: Among patients presenting to the ED with acute agitation (population), is physical restraint (intervention) safe and effective (outcomes) for restraining patients compared to isolation and medical management (comparison)?

Search strategy

- MEDLINE (PubMed, 1950–2007): (agitat* OR psychosis) AND restrain* AND (isolation OR observation) (where * denotes the truncated wildcard)

The above search yielded 43 results, one of which related to the clinical question [12]. Damsa and colleagues performed an observational study of agitated patients in their psychiatric ED and found that involuntary parenteral injections were reduced by 27% – compared with historical controls – simply by using an agitation assessment tool (the positive and negative syndrome scale). Some centers use the positive and negative syndrome scale to measure symptom reduction in schizophrenia as well as to study psychosis in general. However, this study was not primarily designed to evaluate chemical restraint versus observation, and no outcomes in addition to providing chemical restraint were reported.

Searching the term "chemical restraint" and limiting the search to clinical trials, meta-analyses, practice guideline or randomized controlled trials, yielded 15 results, none of which were retrieved with the preceding search. Four were clinical trials and two were practice guidelines, one for children and adolescents [13] and one for adults [10]. Nobay and colleagues performed an RCT on VS-APs [14]. The investigators administered either midazolam (5 mg), lorazepam (2 mg) or haloperidol (5 mg) all by the intramuscular route, to a convenience sample of VSAPs who had been physically restrained but exhibited continued agitation. Midazolam resulted in a statistically shorter time to sedation (18.3 ± 14 minutes) compared with either haloperidol (28.3 ± 25 minutes) or lorazepam (32.2 ± 20 minutes). Adding the term "physical restraint" to this search yielded one systematic review related to physical restraint or seclusion. Sailas and Fenton performed a systematic review on a population of patients with serious mental illness, examining the published and unpublished literature for RCTs involving seclusion or restraint in patients with serious mental illness. The authors found no RCTs that "evaluated the value of seclusion or restraint in those with serious mental illness" [15].

In summary, although physical restraint of agitated patients may be required in order to control behavior, the efficacy and safety of such a strategy is unknown at this time. The ACEP guidelines did not address the issue of physical restraint in their recent clinical policy [9]. The AAEP guideline recommends physical restraint as a last resort when initial interventions (verbal intervention, voluntary medication, show of force, emergency medication, and offers of food, beverage or other assistance) fail [10].

Question 2: Among patients presenting to the ED with acute agitation (population), what is the sensitivity and specificity (diagnostic test characteristics) of clinical criteria (tests) to diagnose depression in the ED (outcome)?

Search strategy

- Cochrane Library, EMBASE (1980–2007) and MEDLINE (PubMed, 1950–2007): depression [MeSH] AND sensitivity and specificity [MeSH]

Certain behavioral and historical factors are associated with depression, although depression is common in all ages and both sexes. Patients become depressed for known and unknown reasons. For example, depression is seen during times of stress (e.g., marital break-up, job loss, war, illness), and may run in families. In addition, drugs and alcohol usually exacerbate depression and can make people appear more depressed than they normally are.

A variety of historical factors can point a physician towards the diagnosis of depression such as depressed mood and anhedonia.

A variety of decision aides and tools have been proposed for assessing patients in the ED with depression. The search above found 131 articles, two of which addressed the clinical question but did not provide estimates for sensitivity or specificity.

Kumar and colleagues [16] found that, after adjusting for age and sex, factors independently associated with depression were: less than high school education (OR = 2.37; 95% CI: 1.40 to 4.01), current smoking (OR = 2.36; 95% CI: 1.41 to 3.95), anxiety (OR = 9.26; 95% CI: 5.79 to 14.8), chronic fatigue (OR = 3.50; 95% CI: 1.91 to 6.40) and back problems (OR = 1.64; 95% CI: 1.02 to 2.62). Boudreaux and colleagues [17] found that, controlling for age and sex, variables independently associated with depression were: past psychiatric condition (OR = 6.8; 95% CI: 3.1 to 15.0), past substance abuse (OR = 3.9; 95% CI: 1.1 to 13.5) and past suicide attempt (OR = 3.2; 95% CI: 1.0 to 9.7).

In summary, despite the frequent presentation of patients with mental health issues to EDs across the world, clinical decision guides to identify depression in this setting have been derived but not validated. Studies do suggest that depression is likely to be associated with chronic medical, social and psychiatric factors.

Question 3: Among patients presenting to the ED with acute agitation (population), what are the likelihood ratios (diagnostic test characteristics) of clinical prediction guides (tests) to diagnose suicidal risk (outcome)?

Search strategy

- Cochrane Library, EMBASE (1980–2007) and MEDLINE (PubMed, 1950–2007): suicid* [MeSH] AND sensitivity and specificity [MeSH] AND (acute OR emerg*)

Certain risk factors are associated with suicide. For example, severe depression is closely associated with suicidal attempts. Suicidal attempts and success are also seen during times of loss (of job, self-worth, financial security, family, friends and partners). In addition, men tend to attempt suicide using more violent means and are more often successful. Finally, drugs and alcohol usually exacerbate depression and can make people attempt suicide who would not normally do so. A variety of mnemonics have been proposed for assessing patients in the ED with suicidal ideation. Mnemonics such as MASSALAD (which stands for: **m**ental status, **a**ffect, **s**ex, **s**upports, **a**ge, **a**ttempt, **l**osses, **a**lcohol and **d**rugs) and SADPERSONS (which stands for: **s**ex (male), **a**ge (very young or very old), **d**epression, **p**revious attempt, **e**thanol abuse, **r**ational thinking loss (psychosis), **s**ocial supports lacking, **o**rganized plan, **n**o spouse, **s**ickness (chronic illness)) have been used to weigh the risks of suicide in patients with mental health issues. The goal of

Table 50.1 Components of the Manchester Self Harm Rule. (Adapted from Copper et al. [18].

- History of self-harm?
- Previous psychiatric treatment?
- Current psychiatric treatment?
- Benzodiazepines taken as overdose?

Answering "yes" to any of these questions places patient at moderate/high risk for subsequent self-harm or suicide.

such tools is to remind physicians to examine a variety of different areas of the patient's life to determine decision making.

The search above identified 33 articles, of which one article addressed non-geriatric patients presenting to the ED. Cooper and colleagues studied 9068 patients who presented with self-harm to five EDs in England [18]. Using subjects from three of the five EDs, they derived a clinical prediction rule for repeat self-harm or completed suicide using recursive partitioning. The rule was then validated using subjects from the remaining two EDs. The resulting Manchester Self Harm Rule uses the following four factors: any history of self-harm, previous psychiatric treatment, benzodiazepine use in the index attempt, and any current psychiatric treatment. The presence of any of these four factors places the patient in the high-risk group (Table 50.1) [19]. This rule had a 94% sensitivity (95% CI: 92.1% to 95.0%) for identifying patients who attempted or completed suicide in the ensuing 6 months (Table 50.2). The positive likelihood ratio (+LR) for the rule was only 1.3 in both the derivation and validation sets [20]. However, the negative likelihood ratio (−LR) for the validation set was 0.12, a clinically useful −LR.

In summary, despite the frequent use of mnemonics to assess suicidal risk in the ED by clinicians, no guides have been externally validated. The Manchester Self Harm Rule has the potential to be a useful adjunct in the ED; however, it requires prospective validation, especially in non-UK centers.

Question 4: Among patients presenting to the ED with acute agitation (population), does chemical restraint with phenothiazines (intervention) reduce risks and time to stabilization compared to benzodiazepines (comparison)?

Table 50.2 Diagnostic accuracy of the Manchester Self Harm Rule in Predicting self-harm or suicide within 6 months in patients presenting to the emergency department with self-harm. (Adapted from Wills & Franklin [20].)

Dataset	Sensitivity (95% CI)	Specificity (CI)	+LR	−LR
Derivation	94% (92 to 95)	25% (24 to 27)	1.3	0.25
Validation	97% (95 to 98)	26% (24 to 29)	1.3	0.12

CI, confidence interval; +LR, likelihood ratio for a positive result; −LR likelihood ratio for a negative result.

Search strategy

- Cochrane Library, EMBASE (1980–2007) and MEDLINE (PubMed, 1950–2007): (phenothiazine* OR antipsychotic*) AND (agitation OR psychosis) AND (acute OR emerg*). Limited to clinical trials, meta-analysis, practice guidelines and randomized controlled trials

The search above yielded 261 articles. There were two systematic reviews related to this question. There were also 10 clinical trials and one clinical policy from the ACEP identified from this search. Gillies and colleagues reviewed the question of whether there was a difference between benzodiazepines alone or in combination with antipsychotic drugs in acute psychosis [21]. Based on two trials involving 216 patients with agitation, they found no statistically significant difference in the combination treatment versus benzodiazepines alone in achieving sedation (Fig. 50.1). This result produced wide confidence intervals to benefit (or harm) from either approach cannot be ruled out.

Carpenter et al. performed a systematic review on a population of patients with acute psychosis and found no advantage in using a newer antipsychotic (e.g., clotiapine) compared with "standard" antipsychotics (e.g., chlorpromazine, perphenazine, trifluoperazine) [22]. The review included three RCTs involving 83 patients and there was no difference between the two forms of therapy with respect to the primary outcome of "important global improvement" (RR = 0.82; 95% CI: 0.22 to 3.05; $I^2 = 58\%$) (Fig. 50.2). These results should be interpreted with caution since there was statistically significant heterogeneity demonstrated and the sample size upon which this analysis is based is small.

Binder et al. surveyed medical directors at 20 US psychiatric EDs on their choice of chemical restraint for patients who were agitated or were deemed to be at immediate risk for becoming combative [23]. The most commonly used chemical restraint was haloperidol plus lorazepam. Most respondents indicated that this combination was used intramuscularly and that the examination was conducted only when the patient had calmed down enough to make the exam feasible.

Droperidol has an advantage over haloperidol in quicker onset of action following intramuscular injection (10 minutes vs 30–60 minutes) [24]. However, the offset is also quicker (at 1 hour, the effect of haloperidol was still rising when the offset of droperidol was beginning) and may potentially jeopardize health care personnel as the effects of the chemical restraint wear off too soon. Furthermore, droperidol has been given a black box warning by the US Food and Drug Administration (FDA) in 2001 based upon reports of deaths associated with QT prolongation and torsades de pointes in patients treated with doses of droperidol above, within and even below the approved range. The controversy regarding the safety of droperidol continues, and physicians should be aware of this medico-legal issue.

In summary, chemical restraint with a phenothiazine agent is relatively safe, effective and rapid acting. There is no evidence to

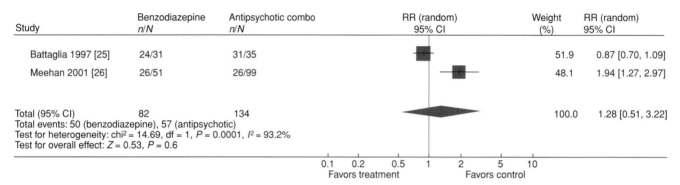

Figure 50.1 Medium-term need for additional medications (sedation failure) in acute psychosis when benzodiazepines alone are compared to combinations of benzodiazepines with antipsychotics. (Adapted with permission from Gillies et al. [21], © Cochrane Library.)

suggest one agent is better than another in this setting or that the newer antipsychotics are better than standard agents. Consequently, emergency physicians may use either a typical or atypical antipsychotic or a benzopdiazepine or a combination of both.

Question 5: Among patients presenting to the ED with acute agitation (population), does chemical restraint with newer agents (intervention) reduce risks and time to stabilization (outcomes) compared to benzodiazepines/phenothiazines (comparison)?

Search strategy

- Cochrane Library, EMBASE (1980–2007) and MEDLINE (PubMed, 1950–2007): (phenothiazine* OR antipsychotic*) AND (agitation OR psychosis) AND (acute OR emerg*). Limited to clinical trials, meta-analysis, practice guidelines and randomized controlled trials

Traditional treatment for agitated patients included benzodiazepines and/or the phenothiazine antipsychotic agents. More recently, newer agents (e.g., clotiapine, aripiprazole, clozapine, olanzipine, risperidone, ziprasidone) have been introduced into the pharmaceutical armamentarium. The advantage of the newer agents is more rapid onset of action and less frequent side-effects.

Using the search strategy above, several pieces of evidence emerged. In the systematic review by Carpenter et al. mentioned earlier [22], the authors identified only one trial involving 49 patients where newer agents were compared to standard antipsychotic agents. There was no difference in the hospital discharge rate in subjects treated with clotiapine compared with chlorpromazine (RR = 1.04; 95% CI: 0.96 to 2.12). Similarly among subjects with aggressive/violent outbursts, clotiapine, when compared with lorazepam (for people already treated with haloperidol), did not significantly improve mental state (weighted mean difference = −3.36; 95% CI: −8.09 to 1.37).

In summary, there is no evidence to suggest one agent is better than another in this setting or that the newer antipsychotics are better than standard agents. Consequently, emergency physicians may use either the typical or atypical antipsychotics with which they feel comfortable, pending future research in this area.

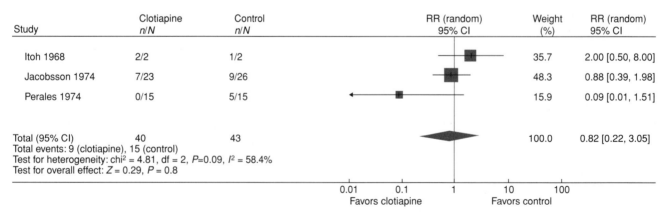

Figure 50.2 General clinical improvement is similar in patients with acute psychosis when clotiapine alone is compared to standard antipsychotic medications. (Adapted with permission from Carpenter et al. [22], © Cochrane Library.)

Question 6: Among patients presenting to the ED with acute agitation (population), does psychiatric assessment (intervention) reduce recidivism and mortality (outcomes) compared to medical clearance alone?

Search strategy

- Cochrane Library, EMBASE (1980–2007) and MEDLINE (PubMed, 1950–2007): psychiatr* AND medical clearance

This search yielded 14 articles, none of which were systematic reviews or clinical trials. One narrative review [27] dealt mainly with the medical assessment of the psychiatric patient, and provided only the following advice concerning psychiatric evaluation of such patients:

Indications for a psychiatric consultation include uncertainty about a patient's safety, diagnosis, or disposition, and assistance in determining inpatient versus outpatient management. If both the emergency medicine physician and the psychiatric consultant agree that the patient is not a threat to himself or herself or others, then outpatient treatment may be appropriate, providing close follow-up care is arranged. Even if the mental health consultant performs the psychosocial evaluation, the emergency physician shares responsibility for the safety of the patient. To arrange patient disposition most appropriately, the emergency physician must be aware of the available options for psychiatric treatment in his or her community and the laws governing voluntary psychiatric admission versus involuntary commitment in that state [27].

In summary, given the paucity of research evidence to guide clinical decision-making, it seems prudent to evaluate the need for formal psychiatric referral on a case-by-case basis.

Question 7: Among patients presenting to the ED with acute agitation (population), is short-term hospitalization (intervention) effective and efficient (outcome) as a disposition strategy for determining suicide risk and/or major depression compared to outpatient assessment following medical clearance (comparison)?

Search strategy

- Cochrane Library, EMBASE (1980–2007) and MEDLINE (PubMed, 1950–2007): behavioral disciplines and activities [MeSH] AND mortality [MeSH] AND (acute OR admit* OR admis*)

Disposition of VSAPs is often problematic, and physicians worry that, untreated, the patient will return with a similar ED

presentation or, worse, harm themselves or others. Given the discussion above suggesting that psychiatric assessment of patients with acute violent behavior is not always required, formal hospitalization of these patients would likely be rare. Certainly, the majority of hospitals in the 21st century are not equipped to admit all patients with transient violent, agitated or aggressive behavior. Moreover, since many of these patients behaving aggressively, violently or in an agitated state have formal chronic mental health issues restricted to drug and alcohol abuse, they would not benefit from hospitalization.

The search above identified 112 citations, of which two were highly relevant [28,29]. While neither article definitively answers the question, both are prospective cohort studies that followed patients who attempted suicide. Both authors suggest that psychiatric assessment may be beneficial in these patients.

In summary, while the evidence is rather weak, it seems impractical for patients with violent or severely agitated behavior to be admitted to hospital. Assuming most patients improve following observation and detoxification, then referral and hospitalization would be of limited value. If the violent behavior represents a less transient condition (e.g., psychotic depression, schizophrenia, and/or intoxication in the face of depression), then formal admission to a mental health program may be warranted in selected cases.

Question 8: Among adult patients presenting to the ED (population), can screening (intervention) identify depression and reduce recidivism/mortality (outcomes) compared to case finding alone (control)?

Search strategy

- Cochrane Library and MEDLINE (PubMed, 1950–2007): depression AND screening AND (emergency OR recidivism)

No studies were identified that directly compared differences in recidivism/mortality using depression screening versus case finding alone. There were several studies, however, examining prevalence rates of depressed mood in ED samples using standardized depression screening measures [16,17,30–35], and one study examining naturalistic observations of depression case finding during routine ED clinical encounters [34]. Another study examined predictors of ED recidivism in a sample of 1029 adult health maintenance organization (HMO) members visiting the ED for a psychiatric condition [35].

The available evidence suggests that depressed mood is highly prevalent in ED patients, ranging from 26% [31] to 34% [32]. In contrast, Rhodes et al. [34] studied audio-recorded ED visits for 871 females and found that only 70 (8%) contained any assessment of depression by ED clinical staff. This indirect comparison suggests that routine clinical case finding alone may miss the majority of patients with significant depression.

Kolbasovsky and Futterman [35] found that Medicaid insurance coverage and a history of inpatient admission for depression or substance abuse were significant predictors of ED recidivism in the 6 months after an index psychiatric ED visit. Assessing for a history of hospitalization for depression among patients presenting for psychiatric issues may help to identify those at higher risk for recidivism.

It is important to note that no published studies have validated a depression screening against a gold standard (i.e., structured clinical interview for the DSM-IV) in an ED sample. The screeners used in the existing literature are validated in general community samples, and other clinical samples, but not the ED. It is possible that screening instruments yield unacceptably high false-positive rates in ED patients.

In summary, there is not enough evidence to conclude that standardized screening for depression can reduce recidivism or mortality compared to case finding alone. Indirect evidence does suggest that case finding alone misses a large proportion of patients who endorse depressive symptoms, and that psychiatric patients with a history of inpatient hospitalization for depression are highly likely to make another emergency visit within 6 months after discharge.

Conclusions

After several hours, the patient described in the clinical scenario above awakened and wanted to go home. The laboratory tests demonstrated a slight elevated alcohol level (22 mmol/L), negative toxicology screen for acetaminophen and acetyl-salicylic acid (ASA), no anion or unaccounted osmol gap, and a normal electrocardiogram. Vital signs 6 hours later were pulse 80 beats/min, temperature 36.7°C (oral), respirations, 20 breaths/min, blood pressure 135/95 mmHg and SaO_2 98% on room air. The resident was eager to discharge his last patient of the night; however, you request a psychiatric consultation before releasing the patient. The psychiatrist diagnosed the patient with major depressive disorder and noted that he was suicidal. The psychiatrist admitted the suddenly tearful patient to the psychiatric ward.

Acute agitation is a relatively common presenting problem in most EDs. The differential diagnosis is wide and varied; however, most presentations are a result of drug/alcohol abuse or underlying psychiatric disorders such as schizophrenia or depression. Emergency physicians need to be vigilant in identifying the underlying disorders that may cause this problem, at the same time protecting the patient and staff from harm. A number of chemical and physical restraint options exist and physicians may choose to quickly calm the patient with midazolam (with or without haloperidol) or one of the newer antipsychotic medications. Subsequently, a low threshold for seeking psychiatric consultation may be useful in identifying potential depression or suicidal ideation in the patient. A psychiatric assessment may be beneficial in a subgroup of these patients by decreasing future complications; however, only a minority of these patients will require hospitalization.

Conflicts of interest

Dr. Radeos has received financial support for participation in consulting and medical research. These groups include Merck and Novartis. Dr. Radeos does not own stocks or other ownership interest in any of these companies.

References

1 Stratton SJ, Rogers C, Green K. Sudden death in individuals in hobble restraints during paramedic transport. *Ann Emerg Med* 1995;**25**:710–12.

2 Stratton SJ, Rogers C, Brickett K, Gruzinski G. Factors associated with sudden death of individuals requiring restraint for excited delirium. *Am J Emerg Med* 2001;**19**:187–91.

3 Chan TC, Vilke GM, Neuman T. Reexamination of custody restraint position and positional asphyxia. *Am J Forensic Med Pathol* 1998;**19**:201–5.

4 Pollanen MS, Chiasson DA, Cairns JT, Young JG. Unexpected deaths related to restraint for excited delirium: a retrospective study of deaths in police custody and in the community. *Can Med Am J* 1998;**158**:1603–7.

5 Hick JL, Smith SW, Lynch MT. Metabolic acidosis in restraint-associated cardiac arrest: a case series. *Acad Emerg Med* 1999;**6**:239–43.

6 Fernandes CM, Bouthillette F, Raboud JM, et al. Violence in the emergency department: a survey of health care workers. *Can Med Am J* 1999;**161**:1245–8.

7 Mechem CC, Dickinson ET, Shofer FS, Jaslow D. Injuries from assaults on paramedics and firefighters in an urban emergency medical services system. *Prehosp Emerg Care* 2002;**6**:396–401.

8 Cheney PR, Gossett L, Fullerton-Gleason L, Weiss SJ, Ernst AA, Sklar D. Relationship of restraint use, patient injury, and assaults on EMS personnel. *Prehosp Emerg Care* 2006;**10**:207–12.

9 Lukens TW, Wolf SJ, Edlow JA, et al. Clinical policy: critical issues in the diagnosis and management of the adult psychiatric patient in the emergency department. *Ann Emerg Med* 2006;**47**:79–99.

10 Allen MH, Currier GW, Hughes DH, Reyes-Harde M, Docherty JP, Expert Consensus Panel for Behavioral Emergencies. The Expert Consensus Guideline Series. Treatment of behavioral emergencies. *Postgrad Med* 2001;Special No:1–88.

11 Zun LS. A prospective study of the complication rate of use of patient restraint in the emergency department. *J Emerg Med* 2003;**24**:119–24.

12 Damsa C, Ikelheimer D, Adam E, et al. Heisenberg in the ER: observation appears to reduce involuntary intramuscular injections in a psychiatric emergency service. *Gen Hosp Psychiatry* 2006;**28**(5):431–3.

13 Masters KJ, Bellonci C, Bernet W, et al. Practice parameter for the prevention and management of aggressive behavior in child and adolescent psychiatric institutions, with special reference to seclusion and restraint. *J Am Acad Child Adolesc Psychiatry* 2002;**41**(Suppl 2):4S–25S.

14 Nobay F, Simon BC, Levitt MA, Dresden GM. A prospective, double-blind, randomized trial of midazolam versus haloperidol versus lorazepam in the chemical restraint of violent and severely agitated patients. *Acad Emerg Med* 2004;**11**:744–9.

15 Sailas E, Fenton M. Seclusion and restraint for people with serious mental illnesses. *Cochrane Database Syst Rev* 2008;**2**:CD00163.

16 Kumar A, Clark S, Boudreaux ED, Camargo CA. A multicenter study of depression among emergency department patients. *Acad Emerg Med* 2004;**11**:1284–9.

17 Boudreaux ED, Cagande C, Kilgallon H, Kumar A, Camargo CA. A prospective study of depression among adult patients presenting to the emergency department. *Prim Care Compan J Clin Psychiatry* 2006;**8**:66–70.

18 Cooper J, Kapur N, Dunning J, Guthrie E, Appleby L, Mackway-Jones K. A clinical tool for assessing risk after self-harm. *Ann Emerg Med* 2006;**48**:459–66.

19 Cooper J, Kapur N, Mackway-Jones K. A comparison between clinicians' assessment and the Manchester Self-Harm Rule: a cohort study. *Emerg Med J* 2007;**24**:720–1.

20 Wills CE, Franklin M. The Manchester Self Harm Rule had good sensitivity but poor specificity for predicting repeat self harm or suicide. *Evid Based Nurs* 2007;**10**:61.

21 Gillies D, Beck A, McCloud A, Rathbone J, Gillies D. Benzodiazepines alone or in combination with antipsychotic drugs for acute psychosis. *Cochrane Database Syst Rev* 2005;**4**:CD003079.

22 Carpenter S, Berk M, Rathbone J. Clotiapine for acute psychotic illness. *Cochrane Database Syst Rev* 2004;**4**:CD002304.

23 Binder RL, McNiel DE. Emergency psychiatry: contemporary practices in managing acutely violent patients in 20 psychiatric emergency rooms. *Psychiatr Serv* 1999;**50**(12):1553–4.

24 Thomas H, Schwartz E, Petrilli R. Droperidol versus haloperidol for chemical restraint of agitated and combative patients. *Ann Emerg Med* 1992;**21**:407–13.

25 Battaglia J, Moss S, Rush J, Kang J, Mendoza R, Leedom L, Dubin W, McGlynn C, Goodman L. Haloperidol, lorazepam, or both for psychotic agitation? A multicenter, prospective, double-blind, emergency department study. Am J Emerg Med. 1997 Jul; **15**(4):335–40. PMID: 9217519 [PubMed - indexed or MEDLINE].

26 Meehan K, Zhang F, David S, Tohen M, Janicak P, Small J, Koch M, Rizk R, Walker D, Tran P, Breier A. A double-blind, randomized comparison of the efficacy and safety of intramuscular injections of olanzapine, lorazepam, or placebo in treating acutely agitated patients diagnosed with bipolar mania. J Clin Psychopharmacol. 2001 Aug;**21**(4): 389–97. PMID: 11476123 [PubMed - indexed for MEDLINE].

27 Williams ER, Shepherd SM. Medical clearance of psychiatric patients. *Emerg Med Clin North Am* 2000;**18**:185–98.

28 Reith DM, Whyte I, Carter G, McPherson M, Carter N. Risk factors for suicide and other deaths following hospital treated self-poisoning in Australia. *Aust NZ J Psychiatry* 2004;**38**:520–5.

29 Suokas J, Suominen K, Isometsa E, Ostamo A, Lonnqvist J. Long-term risk factors for suicide mortality after attempted suicide – findings of a 14-year follow-up study. *Acta Psychiatr Scand* 2001;**104**:117–21.

30 Meldon SW, Emerman CL, Schubert DSP, Moffa DA, Etheart RG. Depression in geriatric ED patients: prevalence and recognition. *Ann Emerg Med* 1997;**30**:141–5.

31 Raccio-Robak N, McErlean MA, Fabacher DA, Milano PM, Verdile VP. Socioeconomic and health status differences between depressed and non-depressed ED elders. *Am J Emerg Med* 2002;**20**:71–3.

32 Rhodes KV, Lauderdale DS, Stocking CB, Howes DS, Roizen MF, Levinson W. Better health care while you wait: a controlled trial of a computer-based intervention for screening and health promotion in the emergency department. *Ann Emerg Med* 2001;**37**:284–91.

33 Schriger DL, Gibbons PS, Langone CA, Lee S, Altshuler LL. Enabling the diagnosis of occult psychiatric illness in the emergency department: a randomized, controlled trial of the computerized, self-administered PRIME-MD diagnostic system. *Ann Emerg Med* 2001;**37**:132–40.

34 Rhodes KV, Kushner HM, Bisgaier J, Prenoveau E. Characterizing emergency department discussions about depression. *Acad Emerg Med* 2007;**14**:908–11.

35 Kolbasovsky A, Futterman R. Predicting psychiatric emergency room recidivism. *Managed Care Interface* 2007;**20**(4):33–8.

8 ENT

51 Sore Throat

Benson Yeh[1] & Barnet Eskin[2]

[1]Department of Emergency Medicine, Brooklyn Hospital Center, New York, USA
[2]Department of Emergency Medicine, Morristown Memorial Hospital, Morristown, USA

Case scenario

A 23-year-old woman presented to the emergency department (ED) with a 4-day complaint of sore throat. She stated that she was having pain while swallowing; however, she was able to take both liquid and solids. The sore throat had worsened over the previous 24 hours and she stated that she would not be able to see her doctor for the next 2 weeks because his office was closed. She also complained of fever with swollen glands, and stated that her voice sounded slightly different than usual. She had no other complaints. She denied further having any past medical or surgical history. She was a 1 pack per day smoker and a recreational user of alcohol. On review of systems, she denied cough, difficulty breathing, rhinorrhea, headache, weight loss, anorexia, chest pain, abdominal pain or joint pains.

She was a well-nourished female in no acute distress and speaking full sentences. Vital signs were blood pressure 108/68 mmHg (right arm), pulse 98 beats/min, respiratory rate 16 breaths/min, temperature 38.1°C (oral) and pulse oximetry 99% on room air. She was able to swallow her own secretions. Her throat examination revealed injection of the left posterior pharynx with scant pus on the tonsils. The uvula was questionably deviated slightly to the right; however, no malodor was detected on her breath. Dentition was normal. She had both left submandibular and anterior neck shotty lymph nodes, which were tender and enlarged, but not fluctuant. The remainder of her examination, including cardiac, skin, joints and extremity examinations, was normal.

Background

Sore throat or pharyngitis accounts for 1–2% of all visits to EDs in North America [1]. While viruses represent the most common infectious etiology, 15% of cases in adults and 30% in children

are caused by group A β-hemolytic *Streptococcus* (GABHS) [2]. When faced with the acute sore throat, the emergency physician frequently faces both diagnostic and treatment dilemmas. Physicians wonder if patients have viral or bacterial infections, whether treatment with antibiotics for a potential streptococcal pharyngitis is appropriate, whether oral antibiotics will suffice or intravenous antibiotics are needed, and whether patients are harboring a peritonsillar abscess (PTA). These concerns result in various diagnostic and clinical challenges, the least of which is that the medical literature regarding these two diseases answer some questions well, others poorly and yet others not at all. While a separate entity, PTA is an uncommon complication of pharyngitis often assessed in the ED.

While GABHS is not the only causative bacteria for pharyngitis, it is the implicated etiology for the development of rheumatic fever, which occurs 10–21 days after virulent GABHS infection and can affect large joints, heart valves, the brain, skin and/or subcutaneous tissues [3]. Although it is the most important cause of acquired heart disease in children and young adults worldwide, it is very uncommon in developed countries. Treatment of GABHS pharyngitis with penicillin reduces the incidence of rheumatic fever about four-fold [4]. Other bacteria, such as group C, G and F streptococci, *Arcanbacterium haemolyticus*, *Mycoplasma pneumoniae*, *Chlamydia pneumoniae*, *Neisseria gonorrhea*, and *Corynebacterium diphtheriae*, are also known to cause pharyngitis, although at a much lower frequency. These other bacteria, however, are not associated with the development of rheumatic fever. Additionally, the vast majority of patients with pharyngitis have a self-limited disease that rarely produces significant sequelae [5]. Another potentially serious complication of GABHS-induced pharyngitis and tonsillitis is the development of acute glomerulonephritis, although treatment of pharyngitis with antibiotics does not prevent this complication [4]. Furthermore, pharyngitis may progress to the development of a PTA as well as other worrisome conditions such as septic shock, airway obstruction, deep neck space infections, sinusitis, mastoiditis, pneumonia, hemorrhagic tonsillitis and other vascular complications such as Lemierre's disease (jugular venous thrombophlebitis, which may lead to metastatic abscesses) [2].

Evidence-based Emergency Medicine. Edited by Brian H. Rowe
© 2009 Blackwell Publishing, ISBN: 978-1-4051-6143-5.

In the USA, children usually experience over five upper respiratory infections each year. On average, children have a streptococcal infection once every 4 years; adults have them once every 8 years [2]. PTA is much less common, with an incidence of approximately 30 per 100,000 people per year. The age group most commonly affected is from 15 to 35 years. The infecting organisms in PTA are usually Gram-positive aerobes and anaerobes with GABHS as the most common species. This chapter explores the diagnosis and treatment of sore throat in the ED setting.

Clinical questions

In order to address the issues of most relevance to your patient with sore throat and to help in searching the literature for the evidence regarding these, you should structure your questions as recommended in Chapter 1.

1 In patients with suspected streptococcal pharyngitis (population), what are the likelihood ratios (diagnostic test characteristics) of elements of the history and physical exam either in isolation or developed as clinical prediction rules (tests) in diagnosing streptococcal pharyngitis (outcome)?

2 In patients with suspected streptococcal pharyngitis (population), can rapid strep tests (intervention) reliably diagnose streptococcal pharyngitis and improve outcomes (outcomes) compared to a criterion standard (control)?

3 In patients with streptococcal pharyngitis (population), does giving antibiotics and other standard treatments (interventions) reduce morbidity and/or mortality (outcomes) compared to standard treatment alone (control)?

4 In patients with suspected streptococcal pharyngitis (population), does any specific analgesic (intervention) result in improved pain relief and/or more rapid resumption of activities of daily living without increased side-effects (outcomes) compared to another medication or placebo?

5 In patients with suspected peritonsillar abscess (population), what are the likelihood ratios (diagnostic test characteristics) of elements of the history and physical exam either in isolation or developed as clinical prediction rules (tests) in diagnosing peritonsillar abscess (outcome)?

6 In patients with suspected peritonsillar abscess (population), what are the likelihood ratios (diagnostic test characteristics) of computerized tomography scan, ultrasound, X-rays and aspiration (tests) in the correct diagnosis of peritonsillar abscess (outcome)?

7 For patients with suspected peritonsillar abscess (population), does needle aspiration (intervention) result in reduced rates of recurrence and increased overall resolution of the symptoms (outcomes) compared to formal incision and drainage (control)?

General search strategy

You begin to address these questions by searching for evidence in the common electronic databases such as the Cochrane Library and MEDLINE looking specifically for systematic reviews and meta-

---

Box 51.1 Databases in order of searching.

- Cochrane Database of Systemic Reviews (CDSR), Cochrane Database of Abstracts of Reviews of Effects (DARE) and Cochrane Central Register of Controlled Trials (CENTRAL) for treatment of pharyngitis and peritonsillar abscess
- PubMed's clinical queries of systematic reviews for the diagnosis of pharyngitis
- PubMed's clinical queries of diagnosis and therapy filters for pharyngitis
- PubMed's clinical queries of systematic reviews for the diagnosis of peritonsillar abscess
- PubMed's clinical queries of diagnosis and therapy filters for peritonsillar abscess
- PubMed's clinical queries of clinical prediction guides for pharyngitis (specific search)
- PubMed's clinical queries of clinical prediction guides for peritonsillar abscess (specific search)
- National Guideline Clearinghouse (www.guideline.gov)
MeSH terminology searches
- Pharyngitis
- Peritonsillar abscess
- Antibiotics

---

analyses. All MEDLINE searches were performed after 1950. The search terms were specific for and listed with each question. We also searched the Clinical Prediction Guides in the clinical queries section of MEDLINE using the terms, "pharyngitis" or "peritonsillar abscess" with the specific search scope (Box 51.1). For practical reasons, we did not search the old MEDLINE database. Finally, relevant, updated and evidence-based clinical practice guidelines (CPGs) on various terms for streptococcal pharyngitis and PTA were accessed to determine the consensus rating of areas lacking evidence. For example, we searched the Agency for Healthcare Research and Quality (AHRQ) website (National Guideline Clearinghouse, www.guideline.gov) for these guidelines.

Critical review of the literature

Question 1: In patients with suspected streptococcal pharyngitis (population), what are the likelihood ratios (diagnostic test characteristics) of elements of the history and physical exam either in isolation or developed as clinical prediction rules (tests) in diagnosing streptococcal pharyngitis (outcome)?

Search strategy

- MEDLINE: pharyngitis [MeSH] AND clinical prediction rule
- National Guideline Clearinghouse: pharyngitis

Table 51.1 The Centor score for determining the presence of streptococcal pharyngitis.

Number of variables	% patients with streptococcal infection (±SD)	Likelihood ratio	Post-test probability of GABHS infection assuming prevalence of 15% (%)
0	2.5 ± 3	0.13	2
1	6.5 ± 3	0.34	6
2	15 ± 5	0.80	12
3	32 ± 7	2.1	27
4	56 ± 10	5.8	51

GABHS, group A β-hemolytic *Streptococcus*; SD, standard deviation.

Table 51.3 The simplified Walsh rule for determining the presence of streptococcal pharyngitis.

Points	% patients with streptococcal infection (95% CI)	Likelihood ratio	Post-test probability of GABHS infection assuming prevalence of 15% (%)
−1	5 (0 to 12)	0.16	3
0	16 (7 to 30)	0.62	10
1	44 (28 to 62)	2.6	31
2	57 (29 to 82)	4.4	44
3	83 (36 to 100)	16	74

CI, confidence interval; GABHS, group A β-hemolytic *Streptococcus*.

The 2000 *Journal of the American Medical Association*'s Rational Clinical Examination Series, "Does this patient have strep throat?" reveals that no single element of history or physical examination can reliably rule in or out the diagnosis of streptococcal pharyngitis [6]. Despite these findings, the use of history and physical examination is helpful when combined in a variety of clinical prediction rules (CPRs). For example the Centor score [7] was judged to be simple to use and have discriminating ability for group A streptococcal pharyngitis compared with throat culture and is a level 2 CPR [8,9] (i.e., validated in one large prospective study including a broad spectrum of patients and clinicians, or in several smaller settings that differ from one another [10]).

The Centor score uses four variables (tonsillar exudates, swollen tender anterior cervical nodes, lack of a cough, and history of fever) (Table 51.1). To calculate the Centor score, one simply adds the number of variables present. The relationship between the number of variables and the probability of GABHS infection (using the criterion standard of a positive culture) is given in Table 51.1.

A modified Centor score has been developed and is also a level 2 CPR [11,12] (Table 51.2). In the modified Centor score all factors (e.g., history of fever or measured temperature >38°C, absence of cough, tender anterior cervical adenopathy, tonsilar swelling or exudates, and age less than 15 years) contribute a +1 to the score, except one (age at least 45 years), which results in a subtracted point.

Fischer Walker et al. [8] compared the two Centor scores in a validation study of children in Cairo, analyzing the results as

Table 51.2 Modified Centor score for determining the presence of streptococcal pharyngitis.

Points	% patients with streptococcal infection (±SD)	Likelihood ratio	Post-test probability of GABHS infection assuming prevalence of 15% (%)
−1 or 0	1 ± 0.8	0.05	1
1	10 ± 3	0.52	8
2	17 ± 4	0.95	14
3	35 ± 5	2.5	31
4 or 5	51 ± 6	4.9	46

GABHS, group A β-hemolytic *Streptococcus*; SD, standard deviation.

dichotomous data. Using the data from the original studies, positive and negative likelihood ratios (+LR and −LR) results were on average approximately 35% higher and 42% lower, respectively, for the Centor compared with the modified Centor scores. For the Cairo data, however, the differences were smaller (17% higher and 13% lower, respectively). For this calculation, the Centor score data for scoring points = 1 were excluded: the low specificity of 4% made the +LR very high and this result therefore appears to be an outlier. The clinical significance of these differences, however, is unclear. This is highlighted by examining Tables 51.1 and 51.2, where the post-test probabilities using the two scoring systems are clinically indistinguishable. Indeed, for either method, obtaining the lowest score makes streptococcal pharyngitis very unlikely, probably eliminating the need for further testing or treatment. It is, however, discouraging to find that several attempts to demonstrate an impact of the modified Centor score on clinician behavior yielded negative results [13]. Without a demonstrable impact on physician behavior, no CPR can effectively rule in or rule out disease in a wide spectrum of patients. Finally, other CPRs such as those of the World Health Organization, Breese, Wald, Steinhoff and Abu Reeseh do not appear to be applicable across a broad range of populations [8].

An additional CPR has been derived and validated (Table 51.3) [14]. In what is known as the simplified Walsh Rule, all factors (e.g., temperature >38.3°C, exposure to known strep pharyngitis contact, enlarged or tender nodes, pharyngeal or tonsillar exudates) contribute a +1 to the score, except one (recent cough), which results in a subtracted point. (An easy-to-use tool based on this rule can be found on the web at the following url: http://www.mssm.edu/medicine/general-medicine/ebm/CPR/strep_cpr.html, last accessed June 10, 2007). Recommendations for management are: for a score of −1, do nothing; for scores of 0 or 1, do a rapid strep test and treat if positive; for scores of 2 or 3, give empirical antibiotic therapy.

The acute pharyngitis guideline published by the American College of Physicians provides no explicit levels of evidence for their recommendations; however, they suggest that high-risk patients (3 or 4 positive Centor criteria findings) should be empirically treated with antibiotics [15]. The 2002 practice guideline of the Infectious Diseases Society of America states that, "the clinical diagnosis of group A beta-hemolytic streptococcal pharyngitis cannot be made with certainty even by the most experienced physicians, and bacteriologic confirmation is required" [16]. This recommendation is described as being derived from more than one well-designed non-randomized clinical trials or cohort or case-controlled types. However, others have commented that the value of bacteriological confirmation is limited by both false-positive as well as false-negative results [15], so this recommendation can be considered controversial (see below). Nevertheless, for the purposes of conducting studies that examine diagnostic testing strategies, a criterion standard is needed. Only two are available, namely culture and antistreptolysin O antibody titers. Although the latter may be preferred in theory, it is not without practical and other drawbacks and the former has a significant advantage of convenience of use.

In summary, there are a variety of clinical scoring systems available, and all provide modest to good positive and negative likelihood ratios for the diagnosis of streptococcal pharyngitis, and are thus useful guides to management. Some recommendations suggest that the diagnosis of streptococcal pharyngitis should be made by lab testing, not clinically [17,18]. These guidelines do confirm that the absence of these clinical factors (low scores) are useful to identify patients with exceedingly low risk of streptococcal infection who do not require further testing [19,20].

Question 2: In patients with suspected streptococcal pharyngitis (population), can rapid strep tests (intervention) reliably diagnose streptococcal pharyngitis and improve outcomes (outcomes) compared to a criterion standard (control)?

Search strategy

- MEDLINE: antigens, bacterial [MeSH] AND (immunologic tests [MeSH] OR enzyme-linked immunosorbent assay [MeSH]) AND sensitivity and specificity [MeSH] AND (streptococcus [MeSH] OR streptococcal infections [MeSH] OR streptococcus pyogenes [MeSH]) AND (pharyngitis [MeSH] OR tonsillitis [MeSH])
- National Guideline Clearinghouse: pharyngitis

As an adjunct to the aforementioned clinical scores, rapid streptococcal tests have been proposed. Most rapid strep tests currently in use are optical immunoassay tests although other technologies such as latex agglutination methods have been used in the past. Briefly, a throat swab sample is placed on a silicon wafer with an optical thin film to which an antibody to group A carbohydrate antigen is bound. The sample diffuses over the film and the antigen attaches to the antibody. A second reagent reacts with the antibody–antigen complex, which increases the thickness of the film, altering the reflected light path, which is visually observed as a color change [21].

No relevant meta-analysis was identified; however, seven relevant guidelines from the National Guideline Clearinghouse site and 10 relevant clinical trials were found that relate to rapid strep

tests. The guidelines [16–20,22,23] all recommend the performance of a rapid bedside test. They also state that the rapid test does not have sufficient sensitivity to be used alone and that cultures are the most sensitive test for GABHS. Further, they recognize that technique may limit the accuracy of results and suggest the test should be performed by touching both tonsillar pillars and the posterior pharynx with the swab, which may not be possible in all patients. The overall level of evidence for rapid bedside testing and culture for streptococcal pharyngitis is defined as either based on non-randomized trials with concurrent/historical controls, case–control studies, studies that determine the performance characteristics of a diagnostic test, or population-based descriptive studies.

Several guidelines suggest different age-specific testing algorithms. Children and adolescents with a negative rapid strep test require confirmation by culture since a significant proportion of negative rapid strep tests (7–27%) actually yield a positive culture [24–27]. This is not required in adults (and perhaps adolescents 16 years or older [19,20]) because of their lower incidence of streptococcal pharyngitis (5–10% vs 15–30% in pediatric patients) and very low risk for rheumatic fever [16]. Most guidelines state that their recommendations do not apply to children under 3 years old since they rarely contract streptococcal pharyngitis, although one guideline recommends that for these patients a rapid strep test should be done, but without culture confirmation if the rapid test is negative [18].

Since there is no clearly defined consensus on this topic, the various likelihood ratios for the rapid bedside tests extracted from the 10 relevant trials [28–37] are presented in Table 51.4.

In summary, there are a variety of rapid tests kits available to aid in the diagnosis of GABHS pharyngitis. Emergency physicians should be cautious and use these tests in conjunction with clinical symptoms and signs to increase their diagnostic accuracy. For example, a negative test in the setting of a low probability Centor score (score of <3: 2–12% probability) would likely exclude the diagnosis (post-test probability (PTP) <1%). A positive test in the setting of a moderate probability Centor score (score of 3: 27% probability) would change the PTP, yet insufficiently to confirm the diagnosis (LR = ~15; PTP = 85%). Alternatively, a positive test in the setting of a high probability Centor score (score of 4: 51% probability) would rule in the diagnosis (PTP = 97%).

Question 3: In patients with streptococcal pharyngitis (population), does giving antibiotics and other standard treatments (interventions) reduce morbidity and/or mortality (outcomes) compared to standard treatment alone (control)?

Search strategy

- MEDLINE: pharyngitis [MeSH]. Limited to practice guidelines or meta-analysis
- National Guideline Clearinghouse: pharyngitis

Table 51.4 Summary of evidence for the role of rapid strep tests for the diagnosis of GABHS pharyngitis.*

Study	Test	Study design	Number of patients	Sensitivity	Specificity	+LR	−LR
Araújo Filho et al. [28]	Strep A optical immunoassay system MAX	Consecutive patients vs culture	81	94	69	3.0	0.089
Nerbrand et al. [29]	One-step immunoassay kit (QuickVue In-Line® Strep A test)	Immunoassay vs culture	536	74	87	5.6	0.30
Roe et al. [30]	Strep A optical immunoassay system MAX	Pediatric ED children. Immunoassay vs culture	437	83	89	7.5	0.19
Anderson et al. [31]	Antigen immunoassay (Clearview)	Pediatric patients vs culture	353	67	95	13	0.35
Supon et al. [32]	Strep A optical immunoassay system MAX	Immunoassay vs culture	413	89	93	13	0.12
Schmuziger et al. [33]	Strep A optical immunoassay system MAX	Immunoassay vs culture	65	78	95	16	0.23
Gieseker et al. [34]	OSOM Ultra Strep A Test (rapid antigen test)	Two immunoassays vs culture	887	91	95	18	0.091
Heiter et al. [35]	Strep A optical immunoassay system MAX	Immunoassay vs culture	801	92	95	18	0.09
Roe et al. [30]	TestPack Plus Strep A (Abbott) immunoassay	Pediatric ED children. Immunoassay vs culture	459	82	96	20	0.19
Nerbrand et al. [29]	TestPack Plus Strep A (Abbott) immunoassay	Immunoassay vs culture	615	83	96	21	0.18
Gieseker et al. [34]	OSOM Ultra Strep A Test (rapid antigen test)	Pediatric patients. One immunoassay vs culture	887	88	96	23	0.12
Kuhn et al. [36]	Strep A optical immunoassay system MAX	Immunoassay vs culture	363	90	97	26	0.11
Chapin et al. [37]	Group A Streptococcus antigen testing (Thermobiostar)	Consecutive pediatric patients. Immunoassay vs 48-hour culture	520	86	97	30	0.14
Chapin et al. [37]	Direct probe test (Gen-Probe)	Consecutive pediatric patients. Immunoassay vs 48-hour culture	520	95	100	8	0.052
Schmuziger et al. [33.	Strep A Plus immunoassay	Immunoassay vs culture	65	78	100	8	0.22

*Tests arranged in ascending order of positive likelihood ratio.
GABHS, group A β-hemolytic Streptococcus; +LR, positive likelihood ratio; −LR, negative likelihood ratio.

The search described above yielded seven guidelines, one Cochrane systematic review and two Cochrane protocols. While antibiotics have been demonstrated to hasten the resolution of pain and fever in patients with streptococcal pharyngitis, one of the most feared sequelae of streptococcal pharyngitis is the development of rheumatic fever. In a Cochrane meta-analysis on antibiotics for sore throat, however, only studies done before 1975 demonstrated a benefit to antibiotic therapy in preventing rheumatic fever. Those conducted after 1975 showed no benefit since none of the patients in either the treatment or control arms developed rheumatic fever [4]. From these findings, there are three notes of caution that need to be considered. First, the 95% confidence interval around the 0% probability of developing rheumatic fever in the studies conducted after 1975 in patients not treated with antibiotics was actually 0.0–0.3%, so the risk might actually be as high as 0.3% or even greater. Second, sporadic outbreaks of rheumatic fever have been documented in various regions [38–40] so the clinician should maintain contact with local health officials regarding this possibility. Finally, clinical diagnosis of rheumatic fever may detect only 10% of those with echocardiographic evidence of the disease [41], so studies such as those included in the Cochrane review may have underestimated the number of patients that actually developed the sequelae of rheumatic fever as identified by echocardiography.

In cases where streptoccocal pharyngitis is diagnosed, there are multiple guidelines that support the use of penicillin as the first-line therapy, with erythromycin [15–17,42], clindamycin [22] or azithromycin [20] as an alternative in allergic patients. A number of these guidelines recommend a cephalosporin in penicillin-allergic patients, but this may not be acceptable to some clinicians. There are Cochrane protocols that hope to define the appropriate antibiotic use in streptococcal pharyngitis [43] and the appropriate selection and duration of treatment for streptococcal pharyngitis [44]; however, they have yet to be completed.

In summary, antibiotics should be used judiciously for sore throat, perhaps guided by clinical scores and local reports of rheumatic fever outbreaks.

Question 4: In patients with suspected streptococcal pharyngitis (population), does any specific analgesic (intervention) result in improved pain relief and/or more rapid resumption of activities of daily living without increased side-effects (outcomes) compared to another medication or placebo?

Search strategy

- MEDLINE: pharyngitis AND (pain [MeSH] OR pain measurement [MeSH]). Limited to randomized controlled trials
- MEDLINE: pharyngitis AND (prednisone OR prednisolone OR methylprednisolone OR dexamethasone OR betamethasone)
- National Guideline Clearinghouse: pharyngitis

While four guidelines recommend symptomatic treatment with tylenol, ibuprofen, naproxen, warm saline or ice water gargles, throat lozenges, lidocaine spray or gargle and/or popsicles, none of them detail the results of any studies that show the efficacy of these treatments [17,18,22,23].

Fifteen studies, which were blinded, randomized trials comparing non-steroidal anti-inflammatory drugs (NSAIDs), systemic corticosteroids, topical lozenges or herbal remedies with placebo, were identified and all showed superiority of treatment over placebo.

One additional study in Russian on NSAIDs compared flurbiprofen with acetaminophen [45]. According to the English language abstract, both medications had similar analgesic effects, although the flurbiprofen's onset of action was faster than that of acetaminophen (5–15 minutes vs 30–45 minutes, respectively). A second study comparing two doses of celecoxib (200 mg once or twice daily) with diclofenac (75 mg twice daily) found no difference in relief of throat pain or change in the patient's global assessment of disease activity [46]. The adverse side-effects (body as a whole, central and peripheral nervous system, gastrointestinal system and resistance mechanism) were more common in the diclofenac arm than in the combined celecoxib arms, with a number needed to harm for diclofenac compared to celecoxib of 11 (95% CI: 6 to 61).

Thus, a direct comparison between therapies is limited to only two studies.

A MEDLINE search combining the terms, "gargle" or "mouthwash" with "pharyngitis" yielded only two randomized controlled trials, both involving benzydamine hydrochloride (BH) gargle solution in patients with presumed viral pharyngitis. BH, which is a locally acting NSAID with local anesthetic and analgesic properties, relieves pain better than placebo (number needed to treat = 2; 95% CI: 1 to 4) [47]. It is somewhat inferior, however, to ketoprofen lysine mouthwash in terms of duration of symptom relief as well as the time course of pain intensity over several days [48].

Nine trials examined the use of corticosteroids to treat pharyngitis. No meta-analysis of these trials was identified. One trial was limited to patients with mononucleosis. For the other eight trials, antibiotics were given either to all patients or those for whom rapid and/or culture strep testing was positive. No trial reported significant side-effects of giving steroids; however, follow-up times, which varied from trial to trial, were between 1 and 7 days. One trial did not have a placebo arm since it examined the route of administration and found no difference between injected dexamethasone and oral prednisone for symptom relief [49]. One trial in adults did not report the time to relief of symptoms, but demonstrated a lower pain score for the prednisone compared to placebo arm at 12 and 24 hours, with no difference at 48 and 72 hours [50]. As for the remaining studies [51–56], the results are shown in Table 51.5.

Overall, the results provide compelling data on the role of corticosteroids in sore throat. Administering systemic corticosteroids reduced the average length of time to onset of relief of pain by an average of 6 ± 2 hours in the GABHS patients and 4 ± 8 hours in the GABHS-negative patients – overall by 5 ± 5 hours, a very modest effect. Such a small treatment effect may be of questionable value in this patient group, and systemic corticosteroids should be reserved for selected populations (e.g., severe pain, large tonsils, and so forth).

Question 5: In patients with suspected peritonsillar abscess (population), what are the likelihood ratios (diagnostic test characteristics) of elements of the history and physical exam either in isolation or developed as clinical prediction rules (tests) in diagnosing peritonsillar abscess (outcome)?

Search strategy

- MEDLINE: peritonsillar abscess [MeSH] AND (medical history taking [MeSH] OR physical examination [MeSH])
- National Guideline Clearinghouse: peritonsillar abscess

Using these search strategies, no studies of history taking or physical examination for the diagnosis of PTAs were identified, nor were any CPRs found. Three guidelines mention PTA as a complication

Table 51.5 Summary of evidence for the role of corticosteroids for treatment of GABHS pharyngitis.

| | | | Time to onset of pain relief (hours) | | | |
| | | | GABHS positive | | GABHS negative | |
Study	Group	Steroid	Steroid	Placebo	Steroid	Placebo
Niland et al. [51]	Children	Oral dexamethasone	24	48		
Olympia et al. [52]	Children	Oral dexamethasone	10	15	9	24
Bulloch et al. [53]	Children	Oral dexamethasone	6	12	13*	9*
Wei et al. [54]	Adults	IM or oral dexamethasone	7†	15†	8	10
Marvez-Valls et al. [55]	Adults	IM betamethasone	5	9	8	12
O'Brien et al. [56]	Adults	IM dexamethasone	6‡	12‡		

*Comparing steroid and placebo results, $P > 0.05$.
†"GABHS positive" included other pathogens (*Staphylococcus aureus, Haemophilus influenzae* and *H. parainfluenzae*) along with GABHS.
‡No GABHS testing was done.
GABHS, group A β-hemolytic *Streptococcus*; IM, intramuscular.

of pharyngitis. Symptoms suggesting the diagnosis include stridor, respiratory distress, air hunger, drooling, inability to swallow liquids, trismus, toxic appearance and severity of symptoms judged worrisome at triage [17,22,23].

Dunne et al. reported a prospective and retrospective observational study that examined the sensitivity of history and physical exam as compared with bilateral tonsillectomy for the diagnosis of PTA. A total of 142 patients were enrolled, of whom 89% had PTA confirmed at surgery. No specific clinical parameters for the history and physical exam were reported in the study [57]. Additionally, there are no studies that comment on the value of the presence or absence of pharyngeal bulging, trismus, tonsillar asymmetry or uvular deviation for distinguishing between PTA and peritonsillar cellulitis. Although both involve infections of the peritonsillar space, the difference between them is that a collection of pus is found in the former (usually by needle aspiration, ultrasound or computerized tomography (CT), see below), whereas no pus is found in the latter. Obviously, patients with an abscess may require aspiration or incision and drainage, whereas those with cellulitis do not.

Several articles from the ENT literature refer to needle aspiration as a means of diagnosing the disorder, but only one study found in our diagnostic testing question below (Question 6) reported the sensitivity and specificity of an otorhinolaryngologist's clinical diagnosis versus diagnostic testing [58]. Unfortunately, it suffers from small sample size ($N = 14$), and does not report the individual historical and physical findings of the patients. In addition, one patient had a pharyngeal abscess, but for our purposes here this will be considered as a positive finding since the important patient-related outcome was the need for surgery. Taking this into account and using the final diagnosis as the criterion standard, the pre-testing clinical diagnosis had a sensitivity, specificity, +LR and −LR of 0.80, 0.50, 1.6 and 0.40, respectively.

In summary, there is a dearth of evidence about which elements of the history and physical exam are useful for making the diagnosis

of PTA. No CPRs exist and emergency physicians must continue to rely on their expertise and experience.

Question 6: In patients with suspected peritonsillar abscess (population), what are the likelihood ratios (diagnostic test characteristics) of computerized tomography scan, ultrasound, X-rays and aspiration (tests) in the correct diagnosis of peritonsillar abscess (outcome)?

Search strategy

- National Guideline Clearinghouse: peritonsillar abscess
- MEDLINE: peritonsillar abscess (MeSH) AND ultrasound (MeSH) OR computerized tomography (MeSH)

The description of the procedure for using ultrasound for suspected PTA was derived as a synthesis of the procedures described in the references in Table 51.6 [58–61]. For the procedure, sit the patient up, visualize the oropharynx with the help of a tongue blade, then place a 5 or 10 MHz intracavatary or oral probe thinly coated with sterile gel and covered with a rubber sheath against the tonsil. Patients usually tolerate the procedure well without pre-treatment with topical anesthetic spray, but trismus and/or pain may limit the ability to do the procedure. Alternatively, transcutaneous ultrasound with a 5–7.5 MHz linear transducer close to the angle of the mandible with the patient supine and the head turned laterally away from the probe can be used [58–61].

A summary of the studies is shown in Table 51.6. In one study, a patient with a retropharyngeal abscess was considered as having the disease, since a surgical intervention was required. Additionally, a small number of patients (four in one study, one in another) could not have intra-oral ultrasound performed because of trismus.

In summary, both intra-oral and transcutaneous ultrasound as well as CT scanning had moderately good positive and negative

Study	Study type	Study size	Sensitivity (%)	Specificity (%)	+LR	−LR
Araújo Filho et al. [59]	Intra-oral US vs 3-needle aspiration (control)	35	95	79	4.4	0.061
Araújo Filho et al. [59]	Transcutaneous US vs 3-needle aspiration (control)	39	80	93	11	0.22
Scott et al. [58]	Intra-oral US vs final diagnosis	14	80	100	8	0.20
Scott et al. [58]	CT scan vs final diagnosis	14	90	75	3.6	0.13
Strong et al. [60]	Intra-oral US vs final diagnosis	16	89	83	5.3	0.13
Miziara et al. [61]	Intra-oral and transcutaneous US vs needle aspiration (control)	21	92	62	2.5	0.12

Table 51.6 Summary of evidence for the role of diagnostic testing for peritonsillar abscess.

CT, computerized tomography; +LR, positive likelihood ratio; −LR, negative likelihood ratio; US, ultrasound.

likelihood ratios, and so may assist in helping decide about further treatment of the patient with suspected PTA.

Question 7: For patients with suspected peritonsillar abscess (population), does needle aspiration (intervention) result in reduced rates of recurrence and increased overall resolution of the symptoms (outcomes) compared to formal incision and drainage (control)?

Search strategy

- National Guideline Clearinghouse: peritonsillar abscess
- MEDLINE including peritonsillar abscess [MeSH] AND incision and drainage OR needle aspiration

Both needle aspiration and incision and drainage are effective methods for treating PTA. We identified one systematic review on the treatment of PTA [62]. In an earlier article, Herzon [63] reported an unstructured narrative review that provides some information about the success rates of needle aspiration, summarized as follows: in nine international studies (USA, Israel, Finland and South Africa) published between 1961 and 1994, the needle aspiration was successful in 464 of 496 patients (94% success rate; Table 51.7). There was, however, considerable heterogeneity of the success rates among individual studies.

The systematic review by Johnson et al. [62] sought the answers to three clinical questions in patients with PTA: (i) do systemic corticosteroids plus standard care compared to standard care alone result in less morbidity and/or mortality; (ii) does needle aspiration compared to incision and drainage and/or immediate or delayed tonsillectomy result in better resolution of symptoms; and (iii) what are the recurrence rates over time? The search for articles was reproducible and detailed. Since the search was limited to English

language articles and the search terms did not include all possible descriptors of PTA, there is a strong suspicion of publication bias. For the question about recurrence rates, there were no randomized controlled trials comparing therapeutic strategies; all studies were retrospective, and most were case series. This review does not report any measures of the reproducibility of assessments of the studies. There is a registered protocol in the Cochrane Library [64]; however, there is no completed Cochrane review.

No studies were found addressing the question of whether corticosteroids are beneficial for PTA. In terms of resolution of symptoms, the only outcome reported was return to eating a regular diet. No statistically significant difference in this outcome was found between needle aspiration and incision and drainage; rates for initial successful abscess drainage were between 87% and 100% for both techniques in all studies (mean value for the studies: for needle aspiration, 92 ± 4%; for incision and drainage, 94 ± 5%). The

Table 51.7 Recurrent PTAs and failure rates.*

Study	Years	Place†	Patients	Recurrence	Failure rate
Herzon [63] Subtotal: 9 studies*	1972–1988	USA	684	69	10%
Johnson et al. [62] 19 studies	1970–1994	USA, Denmark, England, Finland, Israel	2083	272	13%

*Defined as recurrent abscess 2–3 months after first drainage with a minimum of 1-year follow-up.
†Data for the USA were homogeneous; outside the USA, the data were heterogeneous.

authors point out that the power of the studies to detect a difference in efficacy between the two techniques is low because of the small total number of patients studied, so that the results reported here would be unlikely to show a difference even if one existed. Although a summary recurrence rate for all the studies combined was not explicitly reported in the paper, the rates of recurrence of PTA were between 0% and 22% (mean value for the studies: 10 ± 8%). No specific complications of either procedure were reported. The most dreaded complication, injury to the carotid artery, has not been reported in recent literature [65].

In summary, the best initial approach to patients with a PTA appears to be needle aspiration since it is theoretically less invasive than incision and drainage. In terms of overall benefit, recurrences do not occur frequently and there is little or no evidence to distinguish between the two procedures in terms of outcome.

Conclusions

Following the initial assessment, you suspect a streptococcal pharyngitis with early PTA. The patient is reluctant to undergo a needle aspiration, and you elect to start intravenous antibiotics (penicillin G) through your outpatient antibiotic program. At that time, you suggest follow-up after 24 hours. At reassessment, the patient is no better, has mild trismus and is unable to swallow any fluid. On examination, features of a PTA are now more prominent. Needle aspiration following 4% xylocaine gargle and light 2% xylocaine spray to the affected area produced 4 cm^3 of yellow pustular fluid, which was sent off for culture. The patient was treated with IV antibiotics for 48 hours, and then changed to oral agents due to rapid improvement.

Sore throat is a common ED presentation, which infrequently requires hospitalization. The patient presented served to elucidate several potential problems related to the treatment of patients presenting with sore throat. There appears to be a great deal of variability in the ED approach to these patients. A variety of contributory factors have been identified, including a lack of consensus regarding diagnosis and management, gaps in knowledge among physicians and patients, and limitations in research.

Therapeutic strategies for the management of sore throat have been suggested largely on the basis of "clinical experience". Recommended treatment for GABHS pharyngitis consists of antibiotics [4,15–20,22,23]. Recommended treatment for a single occurrence of PTA consists of needle aspiration, incision and drainage, or for quinsy (i.e., PTA) tonsillectomy [62,63]. Tonsillectomy is considered curative and eliminates any chance of recurrence (10–15% chance); however, for the most part, it should be reserved for recurrent and severe cases [62,63].

Acknowledgments

We wish to thank our editors, Eddy Lang and Brian Rowe, for help editing this work.

Conflicts of interest

Drs Yeh and Eskin declare no conflicts of interest in the preparation of this chapter.

References

1 Schappert SM. *Ambulatory Care Visits to Physician's Offices, Hospital Outpatient Departments, and Emergency Departments: United States, 1996.* National Center for Health Statistics, Hyattsville, 1998.

2 Kazzi AA, Willis J. eMedicine: Emergency Medicine, Pharyngitis. Available at Emedicine.com (accessed March 11, 2007).

3 Manyemba J, Mayosi BM. Penicillin for secondary prevention of rheumatic fever. *Cochrane Database Syst Rev* 2002;**3**:CD002227 (doi: 10.1002/14651858.CD002227).

4 Del Mar CB, Glasziou PP, Spinks AB. Antibiotics for sore throat (Review). *Cochrane Database Syst Rev* 2006;**4**:CD000023 (doi: 10.1002/14651858.CD000023).

5 Cooper RJ, Hoffman JR, Bartlett JG, et al. Principles of appropriate antibiotic use for acute pharyngitis in adults: background. *Ann Emerg Med* 2001;**37**:711–19.

6 Ebell MH, Smith MA, Barry HC, Ives K, Carey M. The rational clinical examination: does this patient have strep throat? *JAMA* 2000;**13**:2912–18.

7 Centor RM, Witherspoon JM, Dalton HP, Brody CE, Link K. The diagnosis of strep throat in adults in the emergency room. *Med Decision Making* 1981;**1**:239–45

8 Fischer Walker CL, Rimoin AW, Hamza HS, Steinhoff MC. Comparison of clinical prediction rules for management of pharyngitis in settings with limited resources. *J Pediatr* 2006;**149**:64–71.

9 McIsaac WJ, Goel V, Slaughter PM, et al. Reconsidering sore throats. Part 2. Alternative approach and practical office tool. *Can Fam Physician* 1997;**43**:495–500.

10 Guyatt G, Drummon R, eds. *Users' Guide to the Medical Literature. A manual for evidence-based clinical practice.* AMA Press, Chicago, 2002.

11 McIsaac WJ, White D, Tannenbaum D, Low DE. A clinical score to reduce unnecessary antibiotic use in patients with sore throat. *Can Med Assoc J* 1998;**158**:75–83.

12 McIsaac WJ, Kellner JD, Aufricht P, Vanjaka A, Low DE. Empirical validation of guidelines for the management of pharyngitis in children and adults. *JAMA* 2004;**291**:1587–95.

13 McIsaac WJ, Goel V, To T, Low DE. The validity of a sore throat score in family practice. *Can Med Assoc J* 2000;**163**:811–15.

14 McGinn TG, Deluca J, Ahlawat SK, Mobo BH, Wisnivesky JP. Validation and modification of streptococcal pharyngitis clinical prediction rules. *Mayo Clin Proc* 2003;**78**:289–93.

15 Snow V, Mottur-Pilson C, Cooper RJ, Hoffman JR. Principles of appropriate antibiotic use for acute pharyngitis in adults. *Ann Intern Med* 2001;**134**:506–8.

16 Bisno AL, Gerber MA, Gwaltney JM, Kaplan EL, Schwartz RH. Practice guidelines for the diagnosis and management of group A streptococcal pharyngitis. *Clin Infect Dis* 2002;**35**:113–25.

17 Institute for Clinical Systems Improvement. *Acute Pharyngitis.* Institute for Clinical Systems Improvement, Bloomington, MN, 2005. Available at www.guideline.gov.

18 Finnish Medical Society Duodecim. *Tonsillitis and Pharyngitis in Children.* Wiley Interscience, Helsinki, 2005. Available at www.guideline.gov.

19 Michigan Quality Improvement Consortium. *Acute Pharyngitis in Children*. Michigan Quality Improvement Consortium, Southfield, MI, 2007. Available at www.guideline.gov.

20 University of Michigan Health System. *Pharyngitis*. University of Michigan Health System, Ann Arbor, 2000. Available at www.guideline.gov.

21 Harbeck RJ, Teague J, Crossen GR, Maul DM, Childers PL. Novel, rapid optical immunoassay technique for detection of group A streptococci from pharyngeal specimens: comparison with standard culture methods. *J Clin Microbiol* 1993;**31**:839–44.

22 Institute for Clinical Systems Improvement. *Diagnosis and Treatment of Respiratory Illness in Children and Adults*. Institute for Clinical Systems Improvement, Bloominton MN, 2007. Available at www.guideline.gov.

23 Finnish Medical Society Duodecim. Sore throat and tonsillitis. In: *EBM Guidelines. Evidence-based medicine*. Wiley Interscience, Helsinki, 2005. Available at www.guideline.gov.

24 Mirza A, Wludyka P, Chiu T, Rathore M. Throat culture is necessary after negative rapid antigen detection tests. *Clin Pediatr* 2007;**46**:241–6.

25 Armengol CE, Schlager TA, Hendley JO. Sensitivity of a rapid antigen detection test for group A streptococci in a private pediatric office setting: answering the Red Book's request for validation. *Pediatrics* 2004;**113**:924–6.

26 Anhalt JP, Heiter BJ, Numovitz DW, Bourbeau PP. Comparison of three methods for detection of group A streptococci in throat swabs. *J Clin Microbiol* 1992;**30**:2135–8.

27 Roosevelt GL, Kukarni MS, Shulman ST. Critical evaluation of a CLIA-waived streptococcal antigen detection test in the emergency department. *Ann Emerg Med* 2001;**37**:377–81.

28 Araújo Filho BC, Imamura R, Sennes LU, Sakae FA. Role of rapid antigen detection test for the diagnosis of group A beta-hemolytic streptococcus in patients with pharyngotonsillitis. *Rev Bras Otorrinolaringol* (English ed.) 2005;**71**:168–71.

29 Nerbrand C, Jasir A, Schalen C. Are current rapid detection tests for group A streptococci sensitive enough? Evaluation of 2 commercial kits. *Scand J Infect Dis* 2002;**34**:797–9.

30 Roe M, Kishiyama C, Davidson K, Schaefer L, Todd J. Comparison of BioStar Strep A OIA optical immune assay, Abbott TestPack Plus Strep A, and culture with selective media for diagnosis of group A streptococcal pharyngitis. *J Clin Microbiol* 1995;**33**:1551–3.

31 Andersen JB, Dahm TL, Nielsen CT, Frimodt-Moller N. Diagnosis of streptococcal tonsillitis in the pediatric department with the help of antigen detection test. *Ugeskr Laeger* 2003;**26**:2291–5.

32 Supon PA, Tunnell S, Greene M, Ostroff RM. Rapid detection of group A streptococcal antigen with a new optical immunoassay. *Pediatr Infect Dis J* 1998;**17**:349–51.

33 Schmuziger N, Schneider S, Frei R. Reliability and general practice value of 2 rapid *Streptococcus* A tests. *HNO* 2003;**51**:806–12.

34 Gieseker KE, Roe MH, MacKenzie T, Todd JK. Evaluating the American Academy of Pediatrics diagnostic standard for *Streptococcus pyogenes* pharyngitis: backup culture versus repeat rapid antigen testing. *Pediatrics* 2003;**111**(6 Pt 1):666–70.

35 Heiter BJ, Bourbeau PP. Comparison of two rapid streptococcal antigen detection assays with culture for diagnosis of streptococcal pharyngitis. *J Clin Microbiol* 1995;**33**:1408–10.

36 Kuhn S, Davies HD, Katzko G, Jadavji T, Church DL. Evaluation of the Strep A OIA assay versus culture methods: ability to detect different quantities of group A *Streptococcus*. *Diagn Microbiol Infect Dis* 1999;**34**:275–80.

37 Chapin KC, Blake P, Wilson CD. Performance characteristics and utilization of rapid antigen test, DNA probe, and culture for detection of group A streptococci in an acute care clinic. *J Clin Microbiol* 2002;**40**:4207–10.

38 Veasy LG, Wiedmeier SE, Orsmond GS, et al. Resurgence of acute rheumatic fever in the intermountain area of the United States. *N Engl J Med* 1987;**316**:421–7.

39 Barry DM, Eastcott RC, Reid PJ, Guillard BN, Martin DR. Rheumatic fever outbreak in a school associated with M type 5 streptococci. *NZ Med J* 1983;**96**:14–15.

40 Wong D, Bortolussi R, Lang B. An outbreak of acute rheumatic fever in Nova Scotia. *Can Commun Dis Rep* 1998;**24**:45–7.

41 Marijon E, Ou P, Celermajer DS, et al. Prevalence of rheumatic heart disease detected by echocardiographic screening. *N Engl J Med* 2007;**357**:470–76.

42 Singapore Ministry of Health. *Use of Antibiotics in Paediatric Care*. Singapore Ministry of Health, Singapore, 2002. Available at www.guideline.gov.

43 Van Driel ML, Habraken H, De Meyere M. Different antibiotic treatments for group A streptococcal pharyngitis. *Cochrane Database Syst Rev* 2003;**3**:CD004406 (doi: 10.1002/14651858.CD004406).

44 Altamimi SA, Milner RA, Pusic MV, Alothman MA. Short versus standard duration antibiotic therapy for acute streptococcal pharyngitis in children. *Cochrane Database Syst Rev* 2004;**3**:CD004872 (doi: 10.1002/14651858.CD004872).

45 Sedinkin AA, Balandin AV, Dimova AD. Results of an open prospective controlled randomized comparative trial of flurbiprofen and paracetamol efficacy and tolerance in patients with throat pain. *Ter Arkh* 2005;**77**:74–6.

46 Weckx LLM, Ruiz JE, Duperly J, et al. Efficacy of celecoxib in treating symptoms of viral pharyngitis: a double-blind, randomized study of celecoxib versus diclofenac. *J Int Med Res* 2002;**30**:185–94.

47 Whiteside MW. A controlled study of benzydamine oral rinse ("Difflam") in general practice. *Curr Med Res Opin* 1982;**8**:188–90.

48 Passali D, Volonte M, Passali GC, Damiani V, Bellussi L, MISTRAL Italian Study Group. Efficacy and safety of ketoprofen lysine salt mouthwash versus benzydamine hydrochloride mouthwash in acute pharyngeal inflammation: a randomized, single-blind study. *Clin Ther* 2001;**23**:1508–18.

49 Marvez-Valls EG, Stuckey A, Ernst AA. A randomized clinical trial of oral versus intramuscular delivery of steroids in acute exudative pharyngitis. *Acad Emerg Med* 2002;**9**:9–14.

50 Kiderman A, Yaphe J, Bregman J, Zemel T, Furst AL. Adjuvant prednisone therapy in pharyngitis: a randomised controlled trial from general practice. *Br J Gen Pract* 2005;**55**:218–21.

51 Niland ML, Bonsu BK, Nuss KE, Goodman DG. A pilot study of 1 versus 3 days of dexamethasone as add-on therapy in children with streptococcal pharyngitis. *Pediatr Infect Dis J* 2006;**25**:477–81.

52 Olympia RP, Khine H, Avner JR. Effectiveness of oral dexamethasone in the treatment of moderate to severe pharyngitis in children. *Arch Pediatr Adolesc Med* 2005;**159**:278–82.

53 Bulloch B, Kabani A, Tenenbein M. Oral dexamethasone for the treatment of pain in children with acute pharyngitis: a randomized, double-blind, placebo-controlled trial. *Ann Emerg Med* 2003;**41**:601–8.

54 Wei JL, Kasperbauer JL, Weaver AL, Boggust AJ. Efficacy of single-dose dexamethasone as adjuvant therapy for acute pharyngitis. *Laryngoscope* 2002;**112**:87–93.

55 Marvez-Valls EG, Ernst AA, Gray J, Johnson WD. The role of betamethasone in the treatment of acute exudative pharyngitis. *Acad Emerg Med* 1998;**5**:567–72.

56 O'Brien JF, Meade JL, Falk JL. Dexamethasone as adjuvant therapy for severe acute pharyngitis. *Ann Emerg Med* 1993;**22**:212–15.

57 Dunne AA, Granger O, Folz BJ, Sesterhenn A, Werner JA. Peritonsillar abscess – critical analysis of abscess tonsillectomy. *Clin Otolaryngol Allied Sci* 2003;**28**:420–24.

58 Scott PM, Loftus WK, Kew J, Ahuja A, Yue V, van Hasselt CA. Diagnosis of peritonsillar infections: a prospective study of ultrasound, computerized tomography and clinical diagnosis. *J Laryngol Otol* 1999;**113**:229–32.

59 Araújo Filho BC, Sakae FA, Sennes LU, Imamura R, de Menezes MR. Intraoral and transcutaneous cervical ultrasound in the differential diagnosis of peritonsillar cellulitis and abscesses. *Rev Bras Otorrinolaringol* (English ed.) 2006;**72**:377–81.

60 Strong EB, Woodward PJ, Johnson LP. Intraoral ultrasound evaluation of peritonsillar abscess. *Laryngoscope* 1995;**105**(8 Pt 1):779–82.

61 Miziara ID, Koishi HU, Zonato AI, Valentini M, Jr., Miniti A, de Menezes MR. The use of ultrasound evaluation in the diagnosis of peritonsillar abscess. *Rev Laryngol Otol Rhinol (Bord)* 2001;**122**:201–3.

62 Johnson RF, Stewart MG, Wright CC. An evidence-based review of the treatment of peritonsillar abscess. *Otolaryngol Head Neck Surg* 2003;**128**:332–43.

63 Herzon FS. Peritonsillar abscess: incidence, current management practices, and a proposal for treatment guidelines. *Laryngoscope* 1995;**105**(8 Pt 3, Suppl 74):1–17.

64 Keir J, Almeyda R, Bowyer DJ, Wilbourn MS, Burton MJ. Alternative strategies for drainage of peritonsillar abscess. *Cochrane Database Syst Rev* 2006;**4**:CD00628 (doi: 10.1002/14651858.CD006287).

65 Riviello RJ. Otolaryngologic procedures. In: Roberts JR, Hedges JR, eds. *Clinical Procedures in Emergency Medicine.* Saunders, Philadelphia, 2004:1280–316.

52 Rhinosinusitis

Errol Stern

Department of Family Medicine, McGill University, Montreal *and* Emergency Medicine, SMBD Jewish General Hospital, Montreal, Canada

Clinical scenario

A 48-year-old female presented to the emergency department (ED) with unilateral maxillary pain associated with purulent rhinorrhea and a low-grade fever of 37.9°C (oral). She was diagnosed with a previous episode of sinusitis last year. The patient reported that she had a viral illness 10 days ago. On physical exam, the patient was noted to have bilateral maxillary tenderness.

You suggested sinus radiographs, but the patient preferred not to have them and just wanted a prescription for antibiotics. The patient showed you an empty bottle of a levofloxacin prescribed last year for 7 days, which she stated worked quite well and would like a refill of the same antibiotic.

Background

Sinusitis refers to inflammation of the mucosa of the paranasal sinuses (maxillary, ethmoid, frontal, sphenoid). Since sinusitis is usually accompanied by inflammation of the nasal mucosa, the term rhinosinusitis is preferable. Rhinosinusitis is classified as acute (<4 weeks), sub-acute (4–12 weeks) and chronic (>12 weeks) [1]. Rhinosinusitis is the fifth most common diagnosis for which antibiotics are prescribed, with approximately $2 billion spent on prescription and non-prescription medication annually in the USA alone [2,3].

Acute rhinosinusitis is caused by allergens, environmental irritants, and viral and bacterial infections. Symptoms secondary to allergens and irritants are frequently self-diagnosed with recurrent presentations; exposure is often associated with itching and sneezing. Approximately 90% of patients with colds may have viral sinusitis and do not require antibiotic therapy [4]. Only 0.2–2% of adults with viral upper respiratory tract infections become infected with bacterial pathogens [5].

Evidence-based Emergency Medicine. Edited by Brian H. Rowe
© 2009 Blackwell Publishing, ISBN: 978-1-4051-6143-5.

The gold standard for the diagnosis of bacterial rhinosinusitis is aspiration of purulent secretions from a sinus cavity; however, it is seldom performed and is indicated only in complicated cases. *Streptococcus pneumonia* and *Haemophilus influenza* are common isolates from infected maxillary sinuses [6]. *Moraxella catarrhalis* is present in about 2–10% of aspirates in adults, and in 21–28% of aspirates in children [7]. *Streptococcus pyogenes* and anaerobic bacteria account for less than 8% of cases. Physicians often diagnose acute bacterial rhinosinusitis if the patient's symptoms last more than 7–10 days [8]. However, the signs and symptoms of acute bacterial rhinosinusitis and prolonged viral upper respiratory infection (URI) are similar, making it difficult to differentiate between them.

This chapter will review a series of questions pertaining to the diagnosis and treatment of acute rhinosinusitis.

Clinical questions

1 In patients with suspected rhinosinusitis (population), what is the sensitivity/specificity (diagnostic test accuracy) of the clinical exam (test) in establishing a diagnosis of acute bacterial rhinosinusitis (outcome)?

2 In patients with suspected rhinosinusitis (population), what is the sensitivity/specificity (diagnostic test accuracy) of sinus radiographs, sinus ultrasonography and computerized tomography scans (diagnostic tests) in establishing the diagnosis of acute bacterial rhinosinusitis (outcome)?

3 In patients with rhinosinusitis (population), do first-line (amoxicillin and folate inhibitors, e.g., trimethoprim/sulfimethoxazole) oral antibiotics (intervention) improve clinical cure (i.e., resolution of symptoms) and reduce complications (outcomes) compared to placebo or conservative management (control)?

4 In patients with rhinosinusitis (population), do newer broader spectrum antibiotics (intervention) improve clinical cure (i.e., resolution of symptoms) and reduce complications (outcomes) compared to first-line antibiotics (control)?

5 In patients with rhinosinusitis where antibiotics are indicated (population), do shorter duration antibiotic therapies (intervention) improve clinical cure (i.e., resolution of symptoms) and reduce complications (outcomes) compared to longer regimens (control)?

6 In patients with rhinosinusitis (population), do nasally inhaled corticosteroids (intervention) improve clinical cure (i.e., resolution of symptoms) and reduce complications (outcomes) compared to standard care (control)?

7 In patients with rhinosinusitis (population), do topical nasal decongestants (intervention) improve clinical cure (i.e., resolution of symptoms) and reduce complications (outcomes) compared to placebo (control)?

General search strategy

To address these questions, you specifically search for systematic reviews in electronic databases such as Cochrane Library, MEDLINE and the Rational Clinical Examination Series in the *Journal of the American Medical Association* (*JAMA*). You also search MEDLINE and EMBASE to find randomized controlled trials that have been published. In addition, sinusitis and/or rhinosinusitis consensus statements from infectious diseases and emergency medicine organizations should be considered.

Critical review of the literature

Question 1: In patients with suspected rhinosinusitis (population), what is the sensitivity/specificity (diagnostic test accuracy) of the clinical exam (test) in establishing a diagnosis of acute bacterial rhinosinusitis (outcome)?

Search strategy

- PubMed: sinusitis/diagnosis [Majr] AND physical examination [MeSH]
- *JAMA* Rational Clinical Examination Series: sinusitis/diagnosis

The search above revealed two recent review articles [9,10], both with excellent bibliographies. Relevant articles were further explored from these sources. A search of the Rational Clinical Examination Series revealed an article by Williams and Simel [11]. Berg and Carenfelt [12] examined 155 patients admitted to an ED with symptoms in the paranasal region. Patients were included if their symptoms were of <3 months' duration (longer than our current definition of acute rhinosinusitis), regardless of the intensity of their symptoms, and even if previously treated with antibiotic

therapy. This study compared 11 clinical findings by otolaryngologists with sinus X-rays and maxillary sinus aspiration. The study documented the clinician's empirical impression, as well as a risk score derived from four findings: purulent rhinorrhea with unilateral predominance, bilateral purulent rhinorrhea, the presence of pus in the nasal cavity, and local pain with unilateral predominance. Maxillary toothache was not studied. The overall empirical evaluation compared to sinus aspiration had a positive likelihood ratio (+LR) of 2.5 (95% CI: 1.8 to 3.5) and negative likelihood ratio (−LR) of 0.3 (95% CI: 0.2 to 0.5). With respect to the risk scores, if there were three or four findings, the +LR increased to 7.0 (95% CI: 3.9 to 12.8); for two findings the +LR was 1.3 (95% CI: 0.6 to 2.9), for one finding the +LR was 0.1 (95% CI: 0.03 to 0.4), and with none the +LR was 0.03 (95% CI: 0.01 to 0.2).

Lindbaek et al. [13] compared different symptoms and signs, as well as the erythrocyte sedimentation rate (ESR) and C-reactive protein (CRP) against the computerized tomography (CT) scan as the reference standard. Only fluid level or total opacification were used as hallmarks to confirm the diagnosis of sinusitis; however, CT findings with mucosal thickening of 5 mm or more in any sinus were recorded. A total of 201 primary care patients in Norway were evaluated in this standardized fashion. A total of 127 (63%) patients had a fluid level or total opacification in one or more sinuses. "Double sickening" (+LR = 2.1), purulent rhinorrhea (+LR = 1.5), purulent secretions in a cavum nasi (+LR = 5.5) and ESR >10 (+LR = 1.7) had the highest likelihood ratios and were independently associated with acute sinusitis. Patients with five or more sinus regions affected were more likely to have elevated ESR than patients with fewer sinus regions affected. On multivariate analysis, pain at bending, preceding common cold, age, gender, unilateral or bilateral maxillary pain, pain related to the teeth, nasal obstruction, nasal voice, hyposmia, unilateral frontal pain, swollen nasal mucosa, and CRP >10 were not found to be independently associated with acute sinusitis.

Williams et al. [14] studied 247 consecutive male patients seen in general medicine clinics who were symptomatic for less than 3 months, with rhinorrhea, facial pain or self-suspected sinusitis. This was a prospective comparison of clinical findings with radiographs. Patients were examined by the principal investigators, general internist or resident, or physician assistant blinded to the radiographic results. All examiners recorded 16 historical items, five physical examination findings, and the clinical impression of sinusitis (high, intermediate or low probability). The criteria standard was four-view sinus radiographs interpreted by a radiologist blinded to the clinical findings. Only 38% of patients had radiographically confirmed sinusitis. Five independent predictors of sinusitis were noted: maxillary toothache, transillumination, poor response to nasal decongestants or antihistamines, colored nasal discharge reported by the patient, or mucopurulence seen during examination (Table 52.1). The overall clinical impression was more accurate than any single findings: high probability, +LR = 4.7 (95% CI: 2.8 to 7.8), intermediate probability, +LR = 1.4

Table 52.1 Independent predictors of acute sinusitis. (Adapted with permission from Williams & Simel [11], Williams et al. [14] and Low et al. [15].)

Symptom or sign	Likelihood ratio (95% CI)	
	Positive	Negative
Maxillary toothache	2.5 (1.2 to 5.0)	0.9 (0.8 to 1.0)
Purulent secretion	2.1 (1.5 to 3.0)	0.7 (0.5 to 0.8)
Poor response to decongestants	2.1 (1.4 to 3.1)	0.7 (0.6 to 0.9)
Abnormal transillumination	1.6 (1.3 to 2.0)	0.5 (0.4 to 0.7)
History of colored nasal discharge	1.5 (1.2 to 1.9)	0.5 (0.4 to 0.8)

(95% CI: 0.9 to 1.9) and low probability, +LR = 0.4 (95% CI: 0.3 to 0.6).

Low et al. [15], in the Canadian guidelines for the diagnosis and treatment of acute rhinosinusitis, suggest William's criteria [11,14] are the best clinical predictors of acute sinusitis (Table 52.1). The authors rate this recommendation as level I evidence, using the Infectious Diseases Society of America–US Public Health Service Grading System for clinical guidelines [16]. In patients with four or more signs and symptoms, the likelihood of acute sinusitis is very high (Table 52.2), such that confirmation with X-ray is not necessary (high-level evidence). When fewer than two signs or symptoms are present, the likelihood of acute sinusitis is low enough that radiographs are also not required (low-level evidence). However, when the diagnosis is unclear (i.e., two or three of the above signs and symptoms), sinus radiography may be helpful (low-level evidence).

The Centers for Disease Control and Prevention (CDC) guideline [5,17] supports that the clinical diagnosis of acute bacterial rhinosinusitis should be reserved for patients with symptoms lasting 7 days or more, who have purulent nasal secretions and maxillary pain or tenderness in the face or teeth, especially when unilateral. Patients with symptoms lasting less than 7 days are unlikely to have bacterial infection, though rarely some patients may present with dramatic symptoms of unilateral maxillary pain, swelling and fever.

Table 52.2 Likelihood of acute sinusitis as determined by number of signs and symptoms present. (Adapted with permission from Williams & Simel [11], Williams et al. [14] and Low et al. [15].)

Number of signs and symptoms	Number of patients		Likelihood ratio
	With sinusitis	Without sinusitis	
4	16	4	6.4
3	29	18	2.6
2	27	39	1.1
1	14	48	0.5
0	2	32	0.1

Question 2: In patients with suspected rhinosinusitis (population), what is the sensitivity/specificity (diagnostic test accuracy) of sinus radiographs, sinus ultrasonography and computerized tomography scans (diagnostic tests) in establishing the diagnosis of acute bacterial rhinosinusitis (outcome)?

Search strategy

- PubMed: sinusitis/diagnosis [MeSH]. Limited to meta-analysis and human studies

Two systematic reviews on the diagnostic tests for acute sinusitis were identified [18,19]. Varonen et al. [18] searched MEDLINE, Medic, (Finnish medical database) as well as four important relevant journals. The target population studied had acute maxillary sinusitis (symptoms less than 3 months) in primary care settings Two authors independently rated the methodological quality of the studies with disagreements resolved by consensus. Although the authors illustrated the methodological characteristics of all included studies, they did include studies in which the test and reference standard were not measured independently and studies where even if the test was measured investigators were not blinded to the clinical information. With sinus punctures as a reference standard, they compared radiography with puncture [20–25], ultrasound compared to puncture [21–25], and as well as clinical examination compared to puncture [12,26]. Sinus radiographs were considered positive with air fluid levels, complete opacification or mucosal thickening of >6 mm. Ultrasound findings were considered positive if there was black wall echo greater than 3.5 cm from the initial echo. The authors analyzed the studies by weighted means of sensitivity, specificity and likelihood ratios. Furthermore, they used a Q* point [27], the point where the summary receiver operator characteristics (SROC) curve shoulders up to the desirable "northwest corner", and where the sensitivity and specificity are equal. They concluded that radiography was the most accurate diagnostic test for acute maxillary sinusitis (weighted mean +LR = 3.4, −LR = 0.03). The sensitivity was lower in the two primary care studies [23,25] than in the hospital-based studies, possibly a reflection of spectrum bias. Though significant heterogeneity was identified with ultrasonography, the overall results were not much weaker than radiography (weighted mean +LR = 2.8, −LR = 0.3). Finally, the clinical exam compared to puncture had a weighted mean +LR or 3.3 and −LR of 0.4; however, only two studies were included.

Under direction from the Agency for Healthcare Research and Quality (AHRQ), Engels et al. [19] conducted a meta-analysis of the diagnostic tests for acute sinusitis. They identified 4070 articles with a MEDLINE search, but included only studies that allowed estimation of sensitivity and specificity for at least one test in comparison to another. For each combination, they derived an SROC curve. They noted the criteria for positive test results and whether each diagnostic test was evaluated in a blinded manner. Unfortunately, some studies do not adequately describe the study populations, test methods or the criteria for a positive test, and some did not blind investigators to the results of the test when performing or interpreting another. Thirteen studies were included; five provide comparisons of more than two tests. The meta-analysis was conducted in five distinct groups: ultrasonography compared with puncture [21,22,24,25,28], ultrasonography compared with radiography [26,29,30], radiography compared with puncture [20–22,24,25,28], clinical examination with puncture [12] and clinical exam with radiography [14,31,32].

Five studies compared sinus ultrasonography with puncture/aspiration. Upon analyzing the sensitivity and specificity, points were poorly described on the SROC curve, implying variability in test performance. Performance was best in a study by Revonta [21] and poorest in the study by Laine et al. [25] in which untrained primary care physicians performed and interpreted the ultrasounds. The variability may arise from differences in medical personnel, ultrasonography techniques or patient populations. None the less, it seems that ultrasound is not reliable to diagnose sinusitis.

Six studies compared sinus radiograph with sinus punctures. The authors performed random effects estimates for summary measures of sensitivity and specificity. Using positive radiograph definitions as "fluid or opacity", sensitivity was 0.73 (95% CI: 0.60 to 0.83) and specificity was 0.80 (95% CI: 0.71 to 0.87); with +LR = 3.7 and −LR = 0.3. With positive radiographs defined as "sinus opacity" only, specificity increased only slightly to 0.85 (95% CI: 0.76 to 0.91), but sensitivity decreased dramatically to 0.41 (95% CI: 0.33 to 0.49); with +LR = 2.7 and −LR = 0.7. With the definition of positive radiograph "sinus fluid or opacity or mucous membrane thickening", the estimates for sensitivity increased to 0.90 (95% CI: 0.68 to 0.97) but specificity decreased to 0.61 (95% CI: 0.20 to 0.91); note the wide confidence intervals for the specificity for this last criterion, and thus the corresponding likelihood ratios of +LR = 2.3 and −LR = 0.2 are imprecise. The area under the weighted SROC curve for radiography compared to puncture is 0.83. In comparison the area under the SROC curve is 0.74 for the studies comparing clinical exam to radiography. Therefore, the authors state that it may be reasonable to defer radiographs if the clinical evaluation suggests sinusitis is unlikely. The clinical examination and risk scores offer a moderate ability to identify patients with positive radiographs, and could be used to determine which patients would benefit most from radiographs.

The authors concluded that additional work was needed to define and characterize the performance of diagnostic tests for acute rhinosinusitis. They also added that CT scans may identify abnormalities missed by conventional radiographs, but lack specificity since approximately 87% of patients with common colds have abnormalities of at least one maxillary sinus [4]. None the less, CT scans have the advantage of providing better views of the sphenoid and frontal sinuses. It is noteworthy that CT scans have never been compared against sinus aspiration.

In summary, there is little evidence to support the use of CT scans for routine diagnosis of sinusitis. The Canadian guideline suggests that CT scans are not cost-effective and should not be used routinely to diagnose acute sinusit (level II evidence) [15]. Noteworthy, the Canadian guideline (15) suggests that CT scans are not cost-effective and should not be used routinely to diagnose acute sinusitis (level II evidence, using the infectious Diseases Society of America-US Public Health Service Grading System for clinical guidelines [16]).

Question 3: In patients with rhinosinusitis (population), do first-line (amoxicillin and folate inhibitors, e.g., trimethoprim/sulfimethoxazole) oral antibiotics (intervention) improve clinical cure (i.e., resolution of symptoms) and reduce complications (outcomes) compared to placebo or conservative management (control)?

Search strategy

• Cochrane Database of Systematic Reviews: sinusitis

Williams et al. [33] published a Cochrane systematic review whose objective was to determine the effectiveness of antibiotics for acute sinusitis, and which antibiotic class is superior, if any. In this question, we will address the issue of antibiotic effectiveness, and in Question 4 we will address the issue of antibiotic classes.

The authors identified relevant studies from searches of MEDLINE and EMBASE, searched bibliographies of included studies, and contacted pharmaceutical companies. Primary outcomes were "clinical cure" and "clinical cure or improvement". Three studies [28,34,35] compared antibiotics to placebo, though Axelsson et al. [35] had no placebo, but compared antibiotics to topical decongestant. Using a modified intention to treat analysis, penicillin cured 35.4% of participants versus 19.2% of controls, had a relative risk of 1.72 (95% CI: 1.00 to 2.96) and a number needed to treat (NNT) of 7. For "cured or improved", 77.2% of penicillin-treated participants and 61.5% of control participants responded (RR = 1.24; 95% CI: 1.00 to 1.53; NNT = 7). Treatment with amoxicillin did not significantly improve cure rates (RR = 2.06; 95% CI: 0.65 to 6.53) or clinical cure or improvement rates (RR = 1.26; 95% CI: 0.91 to 7.94). This statistically insignificant result may be the result of the small sample (note the wide 95% confidence intervals); in addition, significant heterogeneity was identified. This heterogeneity may be due to the differences of diagnostic confirmation, CT scan [34] versus plain X-ray [28]. Patients with CT scan confirmation of sinusitis, with the more stringent diagnostic criteria of total opacification or air fluid levels, are probably more likely to have bacterial sinusitis compared to patients with plain X-ray demonstrating only mucosal thickening. This may explain the greater efficiency of amoxicillin in the CT scan study.

Similarly, if the diagnosis of sinusitis is based on clinical criteria rather than radiographic confirmation, the prevalence of bacterial sinusitis may be even lower, the treatment effect diluted, and the NNT greater than 7 [36]. Perhaps this phenomenon was responsible for the results of Merenstein et al. [37]. In this randomized

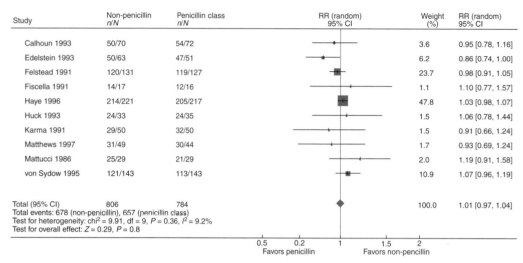

Study	Non-penicillin n/N	Penicillin class n/N	RR (random) 95% CI	Weight (%)	RR (random) 95% CI
Calhoun 1993	50/70	54/72		3.6	0.95 [0.78, 1.16]
Edelstein 1993	50/63	47/51		6.2	0.86 [0.74, 1.00]
Felstead 1991	120/131	119/127		23.7	0.98 [0.91, 1.05]
Fiscella 1991	14/17	12/16		1.1	1.10 [0.77, 1.57]
Haye 1996	214/221	205/217		47.8	1.03 [0.98, 1.07]
Huck 1993	24/33	24/35		1.5	1.06 [0.78, 1.44]
Karma 1991	29/50	32/50		1.5	0.91 [0.66, 1.24]
Matthews 1997	31/49	30/44		1.7	0.93 [0.69, 1.24]
Mattucci 1986	25/29	21/29		2.0	1.19 [0.91, 1.58]
von Sydow 1995	121/143	113/143		10.9	1.07 [0.96, 1.19]
Total (95% CI)	806	784		100.0	1.01 [0.97, 1.04]

Total events: 678 (non-penicillin), 657 (penicillin class)
Test for heterogeneity: chi^2 = 9.91, df = 9, P = 0.36, I^2 = 9.2%
Test for overall effect: Z = 0.29, P = 0.8

0.5 0.2 1 1.5 2
Favors penicillin   Favors non-penicillin

Figure 52.1 Clinical cure or improvement in sinusitis following treatment with penicillin compared to newer non-penicillin classes of antibiotics. (Reprinted with permission from Williams et al. [33], © Cochrane Library.)

controlled trial, 135 adults with clinical signs of bacterial sinusitis were treated with a 7–10-day course of amoxicillin or placebo. The study was performed in a sub-specialty population, and patients were required to have only one of four clinical features (purulent nasal discharge predominantly on one side, local facial pain predominately on one side, purulent bilateral nasal discharge, or pus in the nasal cavity). There was no statistical difference between groups for overall rate of improvement by 2 weeks; however, whether all the patients truly had sinusitis is an important consideration.

In summary, the evidence from the Cochrane review suggests a moderate benefit for patients with antibiotics for maxillary sinusitis confirmed radiographically. Given the small numbers of participants in the trials, a single, large, well-designed study could change the conclusion. Since most clinicians diagnose acute sinusitis clinically, the benefit may be even further diluted. It should be noted that these studies do not include isolated frontal, sphenoid or ethmoid sinusitis, and the results should not be generalized to patients with isolated, non-maxillary sinusitis.

Question 4: In patients with rhinosinusitis (population), do newer broader spectrum antibiotics (intervention) improve clinical cure (i.e., resolution of symptoms) and reduce complications (outcomes) compared to first-line antibiotics (control)?

Search strategy

- Cochrane Library: sinusitis
- *BMJ* Clinical Evidence (www.clinicalevidence.com): sinusitis
- National Guideline Clearinghouse (www.guideline.gov): sinusitis

Meta-analyses published to date have concluded that the newer broad-spectrum antibiotics are no more effective than amoxi-

cillin or folate inhibitors such as trimethoprim/sulfamethoxazole [2,33,38–40]. The Cochrane review of antibiotics for acute maxillary sinusitis [33] reported that there was no significant difference in cured/improved rate between newer non-penicillin antibiotics versus penicillins (RR = 1.01; 95% CI: 0.97 to 1.04) (Fig. 52.1) and newer non-penicillin antibiotics versus amoxicillin/clavulanate (RR = 0.98; 95% CI: 0.95 to 1.01). Drop-outs caused by adverse effects were significantly higher with amoxicillin/clavulanate than with cephalosporins. Relapse rates within 1 month were 5%, and did not differ significantly between antibiotic classes.

The AHRQ guideline assessed the evidence on the diagnosis and treatment of acute bacterial rhinosinusitis in 1999 [2,41]. *ACP Journal Club* [42] reviewed this publication, presenting the summary data of the 14 trials comparing amoxicillin to other antibiotics, and the nine trials comparing folate inhibitors to others. The weighted clinical failure rate of amoxicillin versus other antibiotics was not different (9% vs 11%); comparing folate inhibitors to other antibiotics also failed to identify a difference (13% vs 11%). Thus, they demonstrated no significant difference between the older and newer broad-spectrum antibiotics.

An update of the AHRQ publication in 2005 reviewed many more trials comparing different antibiotics published since the original publication [38,43]. The MEDLINE search identified a total of 39 studies that studied antibiotic comparisons in treating acute bacterial rhinosinusitis enrolling 15,739 subjects from 1997 to 2004. From the comparisons involving amoxicillin/clavulanate, it appears that this antibiotic is the preferred agent. It is more effective than the cephalosporin class of antibiotics in the treatment of sinusitis, reducing clinical failure rate by approximately 40% within 10–25 days of treatment initiation (RR = 1.41; 95% CI: 1.08 to 1.82). However, in absolute terms, for every 100 patients treated with a cephalosporin, only about 3.5% (95% CI: 0.9% to 6.0%) more clinical failures would occur than in patients treated with amoxicillin/clavulanate. The superiority in clinical efficacy of amoxicillin/clavulanate over cephalosporins disappears when patients are examined for recurrence 24–45 days after treatment initiation (RR = 1.10; 95% CI: 0.83 to 1.45). There was no consistent trend observed when comparing amoxicillin/clavulanate, cephalosporins or quinolones to the group encompassing macrolides, azalides and ketolides.

In summary, current evidence does not justify the use of newer antibiotics for treating uncomplicated, community-acquired, acute bacterial sinusitis. Serious complications of rhinosinusitis, such as meningitis, brain abscess and periorbital cellulites, are rare, and none were reported in the clinical trials examined. In all classes of antibiotics, gastrointestinal disturbances were most common, followed by headaches, skin rashes and vaginitis.

The recommendations are congruent with the recommendations of the Canadian Sinusitis Symposium [15]. This guideline concluded that amoxicillin therapy should be the first-line treatment for a duration of 10 days (level I evidence: Infectious Diseases Society of America–US Public Health Service Grading System for clinical guidelines [16]). Those not responding to first-line therapy should be treated with a second-line antimicrobial agent (i.e., any agent approved for treatment of acute bacterial sinusitis other than amoxicillin and folate inhibitors). Patients with recurrent episodes of acute sinusitis, who have been assessed and found not to have anatomic anomalies, may also benefit from second-line therapy.

A position paper endorsed by the CDC, the American Academy of Family Physicians, the American College of Physicians–American Society of Internal Medicine, and Infectious Diseases Society of America was published in 2001 [5,17]. For initial treatment amoxicillin is recommended, though the prescribing physician should consider factors that predispose patients to antibiotic-resistant bacteria, such as contact with children in day care centers or recent antibiotic use. It recommends symptomatic treatment and reassurance as the preferred initial management strategy for patients with mild symptoms of acute bacterial rhinosinusitis. Antibiotic therapy should be reserved for patients with specific findings of persistent purulent nasal discharge and facial pain or tenderness who are not improving after 7 days. Though the guidelines do not define severity, those with "severe" rhinosinusitis symptoms, regardless of duration, should be treated with antibiotics.

Question 5: In patients with rhinosinusitis where antibiotics are indicated (population), do shorter duration antibiotic therapies (intervention) improve clinical cure (i.e., resolution of symptoms) and reduce complications (outcomes) compared to longer regimens (control)?

Search strategy

- Cochrane Library: sinusitis
- *BMJ* Clinical Evidence (www.clinicalevidence.com): sinusitis
- National Guideline Clearinghouse (www.guideline.gov): sinusitis

In the AHRQ update publication [38,43], the authors also studied whether the duration of antibiotic treatment in acute bacterial rhinosinusitis affects efficacy. There are eight studies retrieved after 1997 that reported data on comparisons of the effect of treatment duration on outcomes. One study that compared 10 days with 5 days of amoxicillin/clavulanate 500 mg three times daily reported a statistically non-significant 27% reduction in clinical failure rate [44]. Studies on telithromycin (10 vs 5 days), gemifloxacin (7 vs 5 days), gatifloxacin (10 vs 5 days) and azithromycin (6 vs 3 days) all showed therapeutic equivalence. In conclusion, the authors found no difference between the shorter and longer duration therapies.

Williams et al. published a randomized control trial of 3 versus 10 days of trimethoprim/sulfamethoxazole for acute maxillary sinusitis and concluded that 3-day treatment was as effective as 10-day treatment at 14 days [45]. This study examined 80 consecutive men from general medical and acute care clinics with sinus symptoms and radiographic evidence of maxillary sinusitis, defined as complete opacity, air-fluid level, or 6 mm or greater of mucosal thickening. The primary outcome was number of days to cure, or improvement by day 14. Groups were comparable at baseline; 77% of patients assigned to 3-day trimethoprim/sulfamethoxazole rated their sinus symptoms as cured or much improved compared with 76% of patients assigned to 10-day trimethoprim/sulfamethoxazole. Median days to cure or much improved were 5.0 and 4.5 days for the 3-day and 10-day groups, respectively ($P = 0.34$). Radiograph scores improved in both groups compared with baseline ($P < 0.001$), but improvement did not differ between groups ($P = $ NS). The 30-day relapse rate and the 60-day recurrence rate did not differ significantly between treatment groups.

In summary, shorter duration therapies can be considered, as the evidence supports that they are equivalent to longer therapy, with less risk of adverse effects. The minimum duration of therapy is not yet defined, and until additional evidence exists, it seems prudent to treat for at least 5–7 days.

Question 6: In patients with rhinosinusitis (population), do nasally inhaled corticosteroids (intervention) improve clinical cure (i.e., resolution of symptoms) and reduce complications (outcomes) compared to standard care (control)?

Search strategy

- Cochrane Library: sinusitis

A Cochrane review recently published examined whether topical intranasal corticosteroids (INCS) are effective in relieving symptoms of acute sinusitis [46]. Four studies [47–50] met the inclusion criteria comparing INCS to placebo. The primary outcome was the proportion of patients with either resolution or improvement of symptoms. Secondary outcomes included any adverse effects. One study was included in the review but not in the meta-analysis, since it was not possible to extract the study data and the study had a high drop-out rate [47]. Using an intention-to-treat analysis, data from the other three trials revealed that 73% of INCS-treated participants compared to 64.4% of controls had resolution or marked improvement of symptoms (NNT = 7). The combined results for 200 μg, 400 μg and 800 μg doses were more likely to have complete relief or improvement compared to placebo (relative risk reduction (RRR) = 1.11; 95% CI: 1.04 to 1.18). A separate meta-analysis on the different doses revealed a statistically significant beneficial effect with 400 μg compared to 200 μg of mometasone furoate nasal spray (MFNS, Nasonex®): RRR = 1.10 (95% CI: 1.02 to 1.18) versus RRR = 1.04 (95% CI: 0.98 to 1.11). One study that used 800 μg MFNS found a statistically significant effect (RRR = 1.21; 95% CI: 1.05 to 1.39) [50]. There was no increase in risk of severe adverse effects even with the higher doses of the therapeutic range, and no statistically significant difference in relapse rate between the groups was found.

In summary, this review supports the rationale of adding INCS to antibiotic therapy for acute episodes of rhinosinusitis and suggests that higher doses may be needed. Their effectiveness as monotherapy remains to be demonstrated.

Question 7: In patients with rhinosinusitis (population), do topical nasal decongestants (intervention) improve clinical cure (i.e., resolution of symptoms) and reduce complications (outcomes) compared to placebo (control)?

Search strategy

- PubMed – clinical queries: sinusitis AND nasal decongestants

The Cochrane review of antibiotics for acute maxillary sinusitis [33] aimed to examine the effects of adjuvant therapy such as topical decongestants; however, they concluded that better data are needed to obtain a definitive answer. The AHRQ also could not perform meta-analysis of ancillary treatment for rhinosinusitis due to different treatments, diagnostic criteria and outcome measurements [41]. Only a few studies were noted with a PubMed clinical queries search.

Nasal decongestant sprays are α-adrenergic agonists that rapidly shrink the vascular tissue of the turbinates and theoretically may relieve nasal obstruction. However, a double-blind study by McCormick et al. [51] failed to demonstrate any benefits of decongestant–antihistamine combinations as an adjunct to antibiotics for acute sinusitis in children. In addition, a recent, randomized, prospective, double-blind study, investigating the effect of either an isotonic mineral salts solution or xylometazoline solution (0.05%) in 66 young children did not demonstrate any significant benefit from topical decongestants [52]. The main outcomes at 14 days of treatment were the degree of mucosal inflammation, nasal patency, general state of health, condition of the middle ear and auditory function as well as an assessment of complaints by the parents. At the end of the study, there was an improvement in both treatment groups with no differences between the treatment groups.

In summary, it is generally accepted that topical decongestants should not be used for longer than 3 days as it is thought to cause rebound vasodilation. Since its effectiveness is also questionable, topical decongestants are presently not recommended for acute rhinosinusitis.

Conclusions

Regarding the patient in our clinical scenario, you agree that a sinus radiograph is not indicated after reviewing the clinical examination. You explain to the patient, after verifying that she is not penicillin allergic, that she may benefit from a 7-day course of amoxicillin which is cheaper and probably as efficacious as levofloxacin, with a decreased risk of bacterial resistance. You advise her that if there is no clinical improvement within 72 hours, she should consult her family doctor who may decide to change to another antibiotic at that time.

Overall, acute rhinosinusitis is a common problem in some EDs. Patients should be examined and a careful history should be used to rule out more malignant causes. In most cases, the treatment will be supportive. In moderate to severe cases, antibiotics may be indicated and, if so, first-line agents such as amoxicillin seem appropriate for short courses. Newer, second-line agents may be best employed for relapse, recent antibiotic use, resistance, sensitivities and high-risk patients; however, much of this evidence is from consensus and expert opinions. Overall, decongestants do not appear effective although the use of nasal topical corticosteroids may be of benefit.

References

1 Infectious rhinosinusitis in adults: classification, etiology and management. International Rhinosinusitis Advisory Board. *Ear Nose Throat J* 1997;**76**:1–22.

2 Benninger MS, Sedory Holzer SE, Lau J. Diagnosis and treatment of uncomplicated acute bacterial rhinosinusitis: summary of the Agency for Health Care Policy and Research evidence-based report. *Otolaryngol Head Neck Surg* 2000;**122**:1–7.

3 Schappert SM. National Ambulatory Medical Care Survey: 1992 summary. *Adv Data* 1994;**253**:1–20.

4 Gwaltney JM, Jr., Phillips CD, Miller RD, Riker DK. Computed tomographic study of the common cold. *N Engl J Med* 1994;**330**:25–30.

5 Hickner JM, Bartlett JG, Besser RE, Gonzales R, Hoffman JR, Sande MA. Principles of appropriate antibiotic use for acute rhinosinusitis in adults: background. *Ann Intern Med* 2001;**134**:498–505.

6 Gwaltney JM, Jr. Acute community-acquired sinusitis. *Clin Infect Dis* 1996;**23**:1209–23.

7 Anon JB, Jacobs MR, Poole MD, et al. Antimicrobial treatment guidelines for acute bacterial rhinosinusitis. *Otolaryngol Head Neck Surg* 2004;**130**:1–45.

8 Institute for Clinical Systems Integration. Acute sinusitis in adults. *Postgrad Med* 1998;**103**:154–60.

9 DeAlleaume L, Parker S, Reider JM. Clinical inquiries. What findings distinguish acute bacterial sinusitis? *J Fam Pract* 2003;**52**:563–5.

10 Reider JM, Nashelsky J, Neher J. Clinical inquiries. Do imaging studies aid diagnosis of acute sinusitis? *J Fam Pract* 2003;**52**:565–7.

11 Williams JW, Jr., Simel DL. Does this patient have sinusitis? Diagnosing acute sinusitis by history and physical examination. *JAMA* 1993;**270**:1242–6.

12 Berg O, Carenfelt C. Analysis of symptoms and clinical signs in the maxillary sinus empyema. *Acta Otolaryngol* 1988;**105**:343–9.

13 Lindbaek M, Hjortdahl P, Johnsen UL. Use of symptoms, signs, and blood tests to diagnose acute sinus infections in primary care: comparison with computed tomography. *Fam Med* 1996;**28**:183–8.

14 Williams JW, Jr., Simel DL, Roberts L, Samsa GP. Clinical evaluation for sinusitis. Making the diagnosis by history and physical examination. *Ann Intern Med* 1992;**117**:705–10.

15 Low DE, Desrosiers M, McSherry J, et al. A practical guide for the diagnosis and treatment of acute sinusitis. *Can Med Assoc J* 1997;**156**(Suppl 6):S1–14.

16 Kish MA. Guide to development of practice guidelines. *Clin Infect Dis* 2001;**32**:851–4.

17 Snow V, Mottur-Pilson C, Hickner JM. Principles of appropriate antibiotic use for acute sinusitis in adults. *Ann Intern Med* 2001;**134**:495–7.

18 Varonen H, Makela M, Savolainen S, Laara E, Hilden J. Comparison of ultrasound, radiography, and clinical examination in the diagnosis of acute maxillary sinusitis: a systematic review. *J Clin Epidemiol* 2000;**53**:940–48.

19 Engels EA, Terrin N, Barza M, Lau J. Meta-analysis of diagnostic tests for acute sinusitis. *J Clin Epidemiol* 2000;**53**:852–62.

20 McNeill RA. Comparison of the findings on transillumination, X-ray and lavage of the maxillary sinus. *J Laryngol Otol* 1963;**77**:1009–13.

21 Revonta M. Ultrasound in the diagnosis of maxillary and frontal sinusitis. *Acta Otolaryngol Suppl* 1980;**370**:1–55.

22 Kuusela T, Kurri J, Sirola R. Ultrasound in the diagnosis of paranasal sinusitis of conscripts: comparison of results of ultrasonography, roentgen examination, and puncture and irrigation. *Ann Med Milit Fenn* 1982;**57**:138.

23 van Buchem FL, Peeters M, Beaumont J. Acute maxillary sinusitis in general practice: the relation between clinical picture and objective findings. *Eur J Gen Pract* 1995;**1**:155–60.

24 Savolainen S, Pietola M, Kiukaanniemi H, Lappalainen E, Salminen M, Mikkonen P. An ultrasound device in the diagnosis of acute maxillary sinusitis. *Acta Otolaryngol Suppl* 1997;**529**:148–52.

25 Laine K, Maatta T, Varonen H, Makela M. Diagnosing acute maxillary sinusitis in primary care: a comparison of ultrasound, clinical examination and radiography. *Rhinology* 1998;**36**:2–6.

26 Berg O, Carenfelt C. Etiological diagnosis in sinusitis: ultrasonography as clinical complement. *Laryngoscope* 1985;**95**(7 Pt 1):851–3.

27 Moses LE, Shapiro D, Littenberg B. Combining independent studies of a diagnostic test into a summary ROC curve: data-analytic approaches and some additional considerations. *Stat Med* 1993;**12**:1293–316.

28 van Buchem FL, Knottnerus JA, Schrijnemaekers VJJ, Peeters MF. Primary-care-based randomised placebo-controlled trial of antibiotic treatment in acute maxillary sinusitis. *Lancet* 1997;**349**:683–7.

29 Rohr AS, Spector SL, Siegel SC, Katz RM, Rachelefsky GS. Correlation between A-mode ultrasound and radiography in the diagnosis of maxillary sinusitis. *J Allergy Clin Immunol* 1986;**78**(1 Pt 1):58–61.

30 Jensen C, von Sydow C. Radiography and ultrasonography in paranasal sinusitis. *Acta Radiol* 1987;**28**:31–4.

31 Axelsson A, Runze U. Symptoms and signs of acute maxillary sinusitis. *ORL J Otorhinolaryngol Relat Spec* 1976;**38**:298–308.

32 Jannert M, Andreasson L, Helin I, Pettersson H. Acute sinusitis in children – symptoms, clinical findings and bacteriology related to initial radiologic appearance. *Int J Pediatr Otorhinolaryngol* 1982;**4**:139–48.

33 Williams JW, Jr., Aguilar C, Cornell J, et al. Antibiotics for acute maxillary sinusitis. *Cochrane Database Syst Rev* 2003;**2**:CD000243 (doi: 10.1002/14651858.CD000243).

34 Lindbaek M, Hjortdahl P, Johnsen UL. Randomised, double blind, placebo controlled trial of penicillin V and amoxycillin in treatment of acute sinus infections in adults. *BMJ* (clinical research edn.) 1996;**313**: 325–9.

35 Axelsson A, Chidekel N, Grebelius N, Jensen C. Treatment of acute maxillary sinusitis. A comparison of four different methods. *Acta Otolaryngol* 1970;**70**:71–6.

36 Tang A, Frazee B. Evidence-based emergency medicine/systematic review abstract: antibiotic treatment for acute maxillary sinusitis. *Ann Emerg Med* 2003;**42**:705–8.

37 Merenstein D, Whittaker C, Chadwell T, Wegner B, D'Amico F. Are antibiotics beneficial for patients with sinusitis complaints? A randomized double-blind clinical trial. *J Fam Pract* 2005;**54**:144–51.

38 Ip S, Fu L, Balk E, Chew P, Devine D, Lau J. Update on acute bacterial rhinosinusitis. *Evid Rep Technol Assess (Summ)* 2005;**124**:1–3.

39 de Bock GH, Dekker FW, Stolk J, Springer MP, Kievit J, van Houwelingen JC. Antimicrobial treatment in acute maxillary sinusitis: a meta-analysis. *J Clin Epidemiol* 1997;**50**:881–90.

40 de Ferranti SD, Ioannidis JP, Lau J, Anninger WV, Barza M. Are amoxycillin and folate inhibitors as effective as other antibiotics for acute sinusitis? A meta-analysis. *BMJ* 1998;**317**:632–7.

41 Agency for Health Care Policy and Research. *Diagnosis and Treatment of Acute Bacterial Rhinosinusitis: Summary.* Evidence Report/Technology Assessment No. 9 (AHCPR Publication No. 99-E016). Agency for Health Care and Policy Research, Rockville, 1999. Available at http://www.ahrq.gov/clinic/epcsums/sinussum.htm.

42 Willett LR. Review: diagnostic tests for bacterial rhinosinusitis have moderate accuracy; antibiotics reduce clinical failures (Diagnosis). *ACP J Club* 2000;**133**:31.

43 Agency for Health Care Policy and Quality. Update on acute bacterial rhinosinusitis (Structured abstract). Agency for Health Care Policy and Quality, Rockville, 2005. Available at http://www.ahrq.gov/clinic/tp/rhinouptp.htm.

44 Gehanno P, Beauvillain C, Bobin S, et al. Short therapy with amoxicillin-clavulanate and corticosteroids in acute sinusitis: results of a multicentre study in adults. *Scand J Infect Dis* 2000;**32**:679–84.

45 Williams JW, Jr., Holleman DR, Jr., Samsa GP, Simel DL. Randomized controlled trial of 3 vs 10 days of trimethoprim/sulfamethoxazole for acute maxillary sinusitis. *JAMA* 1995;**273**:1015–21.

46 Zalmanovici A, Yaphe J. Steroids for acute sinusitis. *Cochrane Database Syst Rev* 2007;**2**:CD005149.

47 Barlan IB, Erkan E, Bakir M, Berrak S, Basaran MM. Intranasal budesonide spray as an adjunct to oral antibiotic therapy for acute sinusitis in children. *Ann Allergy Asthma Immunol* 1997;**78**:598–601.

48 Dolor RJ, Witsell DL, Hellkamp AS, Williams JW, Jr., Califf RM, Simel DL. Comparison of cefuroxime with or without intranasal fluticasone for the

treatment of rhinosinusitis. The CAFFS Trial: a randomized controlled trial. *JAMA* 2001;**286**:3097–105.

49 Meltzer EO, Bachert C, Staudinger H. Treating acute rhinosinusitis: comparing efficacy and safety of mometasone furoate nasal spray, amoxicillin, and placebo. *J Allergy Clin. Immunol* 2005;**116**:1289–95.

50 Nayak AS, Settipane GA, Pedinoff A, et al. Effective dose range of mometasone furoate nasal spray in the treatment of acute rhinosinusitis. *Ann Allergy Asthma Immunol* 2002;**89**:271–8.

51 McCormick DP, John SD, Swischuk LE, Uchida T. A double-blind, placebo-controlled trial of decongestant-antihistamine for the treatment of sinusitis in children. *Clin Pediatr (Phila)* 1996;**35**:457–60.

52 Michel O, Essers S, Heppt WJ, Johannssen V, Reuter W, Hommel G. The value of Ems Mineral Salts in the treatment of rhinosinusitis in children. Prospective study on the efficacy of mineral salts versus xylometazoline in the topical nasal treatment of children. *Int J Pediatr Otorhinolaryngol* 2005;**69**:1359–65.

53 Conjunctivitis

Nicola E. Schiebel

Department of Emergency Medicine, Mayo Clinic, Rochester, USA

Case scenario

A 24-year-old woman presents to the emergency department (ED) with a 1-day history of bilateral eye redness and discharge. She works as an elementary school teacher and several of her pupils have had "pink eye" over the past 2 weeks. She reports experiencing some rhinorhea and a mild sore throat for 2 days. She denies a history of allergies. She states her eyes feel slightly irritated, but are not particularly painful, watery or itchy. She has not noticed any visual acuity problems, except when the discharge is heavy. She reports that her vision clears immediately if she washes away the discharge with a warm wash cloth. Both eyes were matted shut on the morning of presentation. She did not notice that sunlight was bothersome on her drive into the ED. She denies contact lens use, and has never had any eye disease. She states that she is simply here to get antibiotics so her principal will allow her back to work.

On examination her conjunctiva are diffusely erythematous and she has a mucopurulent discharge bilaterally with some crusting on her upper lids. Her visual acuity is 20/20 bilaterally; pupils are equal and react to light. She has nasal congestion and a clear nasal discharge. The remainder of her physical exam is normal. You diagnose her with infective conjunctivitis and prescribe her ciprofloxacin eye drops every 2 hours while awake and provide her with a note to return to work. You also caution her that she must wash her hands frequently and after every time she touches her eyes to prevent spread at school. The medical student working with you asks you if you think the infection is really bacterial and if so do topical antibiotics really help clear the infection or reduce the risk of transmission to her students?

Evidence-based Emergency Medicine. Edited by Brian H. Rowe
© 2009 Blackwell Publishing, ISBN: 978-1-4051-6143-5.

Background

"Red eye" is a common ophthalmological complaint seen in the ED. While infective conjunctivitis is often the final diagnosis, emergency physicians must be careful not to miss such serious ocular conditions as iritis/uviitis, keratitis, corneal foreign bodies, corneal herpes, corneal ulcers and acute-angle closure glaucoma. Other less serious causes of a red eye include allergic conditions, hordeolum (sty), blepharitis and minor trauma.

Differentiation of bacterial from viral conjunctivitis requires microbiological culture, which is not practical in ED due to both diagnostic delay and cost. There has also been a basic presumption that any bacterial infection requires antibiotic therapy, no matter how benign the natural course of the infection might be. As a result, treatment of all presumed infective conjunctivitis with broad-spectrum topical antibiotics is the practice recommended by standard emergency medicine textbooks [1,2] and is frequently an expectation in the community.

In recent years, however, the routine immediate use of antibiotics for common infections seen in the ED/primary care has been challenged [3]. Systematic reviews of randomized controlled trials have questioned the effectiveness and cost of routine antibiotic use for such common acute problems as otitis media [4] and sore throat [5]. The proportion of patients treated with antibiotics for a viral conjunctivitis in the ED is unknown, but this proportion could be 50% or more based on estimates from primary care [6,7]. It seems reasonable, therefore, to question the routine use of antibiotics for all cases of conjunctivitis and to look to evidence-based medicine to provide guidance on better diagnosis and treatment of a very common and largely benign infection.

Clinical questions

In order to facilitate your search for the best evidence to guide patient management, you should structure your questions as recommended in Chapter 1.

1 In adults with red eye (population), can historical and/or physical findings (exposure) differentiate conjunctivitis from other ocular emergencies (outcome)?

2 In adults with infective conjunctivitis (population), what are the sensitivity and specificity (diagnostic test characteristics) of clinical signs and symptoms (tests) for detecting a bacterial conjunctivitis or positive bacterial culture (outcomes)?

3 In adults with suspected bacterial conjunctivitis (population), does the use of broad-spectrum topical antibiotics (exposure) result in a faster rate of clinical improvement (outcome) compared to no treatment or conservative treatment (control)?

4 In adults with suspected bacterial conjunctivitis (population), does the use of broad-spectrum topical antibiotics (exposure) result in a faster rate of microbiological cure (outcome) compared to no treatment or conservative treatment (control)?

5 In adults with suspected bacterial conjunctivitis (population), does the use of broad-spectrum topical antibiotics (treatment) reduce serious outcomes (outcome) compared to no treatment or conservative treatment (control)?

6 In adults with suspected bacterial conjunctivitis (population), does treatment with broad-spectrum topical antibiotics (treatment) result in common and/or serious side-effects (outcome) compared to no treatment or conservative treatment (control)?

7 In adults with suspected bacterial conjunctivitis (population), does the delayed use of broad-spectrum topical antibiotics (exposure) result in less antibiotic use (outcome)?

General search strategy

For therapeutic questions, you begin addressing these questions by searching for systematic reviews and meta-analysis in the common electronic databases such as the Cochrane Library, MEDLINE and EMBASE. When a systematic review is identified you also search MEDLINE and EMBASE to identify randomized controlled trials that became available after the publication date of the systematic review. When no systematic review or meta-analysis can be identified you broaden your search to include randomized controlled trials. For diagnostic test articles, you search for systematic reviews and observational studies that use the terms sensitivity and specificity or likelihood ratios. Conjunctivitis is its own medical subject heading (MeSH) term, so the subject topic is less complex than other chapters in this book.

Critical review of the literature

Question 1: In adults with red eye (population), can historical and/or physical findings (exposure) differentiate conjunctivitis from other ocular emergencies (outcome)?

Table 53.1 Historical and physical eye exam features suggestive of serious pathology.

History	Physical exam
• History of decrease in visual acuity	• Decrease in visual acuity (on exam)
• Pain (anything more than minor irritation, itchiness, or grittiness)	• Careful examination for foreign body including the upper and lower lids (evert upper lid)
• Photophobia	• Evidence of significant watery discharge
• Profuse watery discharge	• Ciliary redness
• Contact lens use (even occasionally)	
• Eye trauma, or possible foreign body, or acute onset of symptoms (possible foreign body)	
• History of eye surgery	
• Pre-existing symptoms for more than 7 days	

Search strategy

• MEDLINE: conjunctivitis AND signs and symptoms

A search strategy for the Cochrane Library identified no systematic reviews addressing the question outlined above. Similarly, a MEDLINE search did not identify any systematic reviews or prospective cohort studies directly addressing this question. A search for articles evaluating signs and symptoms of acute infective conjunctivitis led to a follow-up randomized controlled trial with some outcome data related to history and physical exam findings for infective conjunctivitis [8]. When combined with textbook guidelines [9], this provides limited indirect evidence that helps to create weak consensus-driven evidence.

Assessment of the acutely red eye requires that serious sight-threatening ocular emergencies be ruled out before infective conjunctivitis can be diagnosed. In a randomized controlled trial evaluating fusidic acid for infective conjunctivitis, patients with red eye were excluded if they had the following: acute loss of vision, wore contact lenses, had any eye trauma, history of eye surgery, ciliary redness and pre-existing symptoms for longer than 7 days [8]. No clinically serious outcomes occurred in any of the patients included in this trial, suggesting that their enrollment criteria successfully excluded serious ocular conditions such as iritis/uviitis, keratitis, corneal foreign bodies or ulcers, and acute-angle closure glaucoma. Emergency medicine textbooks suggest similar criteria be assessed when evaluating an acutely red eye [9]. While more research would be helpful, it seems unlikely to be performed, and the prudent approach by the emergency medicine physician should include a search for the historical and physical exam features listed in Table 53.1. If any of these features are present more serious pathology may be present and examination needs to also include a careful slit lamp and fundoscopic examination. This exam must emphasize a careful search for anterior chamber cells and foreign bodies, fluoroscein staining of the cornea and intraocular pressure measurements. Most importantly, the diagnosis of infective conjunctivitis should only be made once serious ocular emergencies are ruled out.

Question 2: In adults with infective conjunctivitis (population), what is the sensitivity and specificity (diagnostic test characteristics) of clinical signs and symptoms (tests) for detecting a bacterial conjunctivitis or positive bacterial culture (outcomes)?

Search strategy

- MEDLINE: conjunctivitis AND signs and symptoms

A search of the Cochrane Library identified no systematic reviews addressing the question outlined above. A MEDLINE search identified one systematic review performed in 2002 regarding the diagnostic impact of signs and symptoms in acute infectious conjunctivitis [10]. The authors identified studies from PubMed and EMBASE using search strategies devised for studies on diagnostic accuracy. CINAHL and the Cochrane Central Register of Controlled Trials were also searched for relevant diagnostic studies. They also manually searched reference lists of relevant studies identified and of the guideline on red eye from the Dutch College of General Practitioners for additional studies. Finally, they screened the bibliographies of commonly used textbooks. Inclusion criteria required that studies compared signs, symptoms or both with the outcome of bacterial cultures. Studies in neonates, post-operative (eye) patients or trachoma were excluded.

Following screening of 6827 references, only one study that met inclusion criteria was identified. After critical appraisal by two independent reviewers using the QUADAS instrument, however, this study was felt to be methodologically unsound. As a result, the authors were unable to find any methodologically sound evidence for the diagnostic usefulness of clinical signs or symptoms in distinguishing bacterial from viral conjunctivitis [10]. Further MEDLINE search identified one article relevant to this question [6]. Clearly, this is an area where evidence is sparse.

The basic premise of treating acute conjunctivitis is that a significant proportion of patients treated will have a bacterial etiology. Although general ophthalmological and emergency medicine textbooks list signs and symptoms that allegedly make the probability of bacterial infection more likely, these criteria are not based on valid evidence [10]. To date, limited research has been performed to evaluate diagnostic signs and symptoms.

A multi-centered cohort study of 177 adult patients evaluated several historical factors as well as specific signs and symptoms frequently cited in ophthalmological textbooks as predictors of positive bacterial culture [6]. Patients were included if they presented with a red eye and either (muco)purulent discharge or sticking of the eyelids. Historical factors assessed included a history of hay fever, conjunctivitis or allergic conjunctivitis, and a history of attempts to self-treat by cleaning eyes with water. Symptoms evaluated were any sensation of itching, foreign body sensation, burning and glued eyes in the morning. Physical findings included the pattern of redness (peripheral, whole conjunctiva or conjunctival and pericorneal), periorbital edema, type of secretion (none, water, mucous or purulent) and whether there was bilateral involvement. Exclusion criteria included factors that might indicate more serious etiology for the red eye: acute loss of vision, wearing of contact lenses, eye trauma, history of eye surgery, ciliary redness and pre-existing symptoms for longer than 7 days. The overall prevalence of a positive bacterial culture was 32%. Logistic regression analysis identified three determinants with good diagnostic discrimination: early morning glued eye(s), self-reported history of conjunctivitis and itch. A positive history of eyes being glued shut increased the likelihood of positive culture, whereas the other factors decreased it. Based on this analysis, the authors assigned the following clinical scores: 5 for two glued eyes, 2 for one glued eye, −1 for itching and −2 for a history of conjunctivitis.

The authors calculated the probability of positive culture based on these clinical scores. A clinical score of +5 would increase predicted probability of a positive culture from 32% to 77%. In contrast, a score of −3 would reduce predicted probability to 4%. With a cutoff of +2 for prescribing antibiotics, the authors calculated that prescriptions for antibiotics would be reduced from 80% to 40% for their study population. In this study population this would mean 67% (95% CI: 54% to 79%) of patients with a positive culture would be correctly treated (sensitivity) and 73% (95% CI: 65% to 80%) of patients correctly not treated (specificity). These results have not yet been validated in a new cohort, so caution is warranted. This study also does not address the question of whether or not it is safe to leave some patients with bacterial infection untreated (Question 4) or how many patients might be harmed by unnecessary prescriptions (Question 5).

From a clinical perspective, this study suggests that bacterial infection may be predictable on the basis of some common clinical signs and symptoms. It does appear, however, that many of the signs and symptoms commonly cited in textbooks may not be useful for discriminating between viral and bacterial etiologies. Independent validation of these criteria, combined with information on outcomes from antibiotic therapy could lead to significant reductions in antibiotic use for infective conjunctivitis.

Question 3: In adults with suspected bacterial conjunctivitis (population), does the use of broad-spectrum topical antibiotics (exposure) result in a faster rate of clinical improvement (outcome) compared to no treatment or conservative treatment (control)?
Question 4: In adults with suspected bacterial conjunctivitis (population), does the use of broad-spectrum topical antibiotics (exposure) result in a faster rate of microbiological cure (outcome) compared to no treatment or conservative treatment (control)?

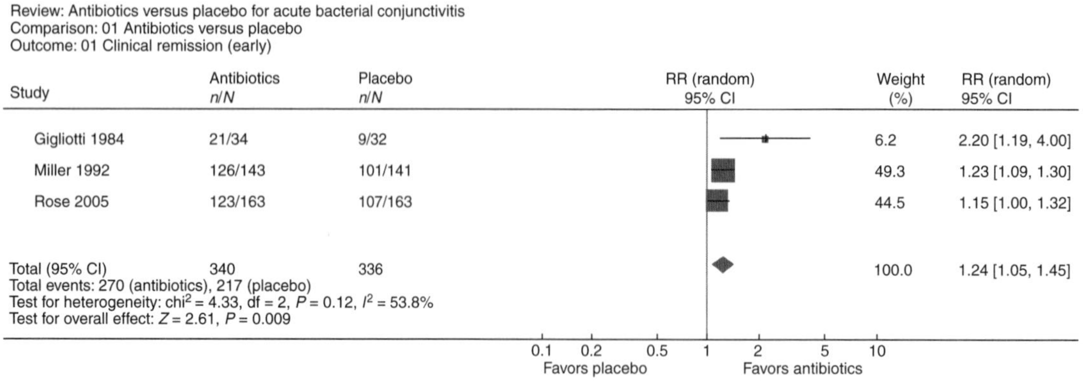

Review: Antibiotics versus placebo for acute bacterial conjunctivitis
Comparison: 01 Antibiotics versus placebo
Outcome: 01 Clinical remission (early)

Study	Antibiotics n/N	Placebo n/N	RR (random) 95% CI	Weight (%)	RR (random) 95% CI
Gigliotti 1984	21/34	9/32		6.2	2.20 [1.19, 4.00]
Miller 1992	126/143	101/141		49.3	1.23 [1.09, 1.30]
Rose 2005	123/163	107/163		44.5	1.15 [1.00, 1.32]
Total (95% CI)	340	336		100.0	1.24 [1.05, 1.45]

Total events: 270 (antibiotics), 217 (placebo)
Test for heterogeneity: chi^2 = 4.33, df = 2, P = 0.12, I^2 = 53.8%
Test for overall effect: Z = 2.61, P = 0.009

0.1 0.2 0.5 1 2 5 10
Favors placebo   Favors antibiotics

Figure 53.1 Comparison of early (days 2–5) clinical improvement rates in patients with suspected bacterial conjunctivitis treated with topical antibiotics or placebo. (Reproduced with permission from Sheikh et al. [11], © Cochrane Database, Wiley.)

Search strategy

• Cochrane Library: bacterial conjunctivitis AND antibiotics

A Cochrane Library systematic review of five trials involving 1034 subjects suggests that acute bacterial conjunctivitis is a self-limiting infection with clinical cure or significant improvement occurring by days 2–5 in 65% (95% CI: 59% to 70%) of the placebo group [11]. Meta-analysis demonstrated, however, that broad-spectrum topical antibiotics lead to slightly faster rates of both clinical improvement and microbiological cure in patients with suspected bacterial conjunctivitis. Treatment with antibiotics provided the best results for early (days 2–5) clinical improvement (RR = 1.24; 95% CI: 1.05 to 1.45) (Fig. 53.1) and microbiological remission (RR = 1.77; 95% CI: 1.23 to 2.54) (Fig. 53.2). The benefit was less impressive for late remission (days 7–10) clinical (RR = 1.11; 95% CI: 1.02 to 1.21) (Fig. 53.3) and microbiological remission (RR = 1.56; 95% CI: 1.17 to 2.09) (Fig. 53.4). The broad-spectrum topical antibiotics that increased the rate of clinical and microbiological cure in patients with suspected bacterial conjunctivitis included: polymyxin/bacitracin ointment, ciprofloxacin drops, norfloxacin drops, chloramphenicol drops and fusidic acid gel.

Three of the studies enrolled a total of 791 patients based on a clinical diagnosis of bacterial conjunctivitis. The prevalence of positive cultures for the 465 adult participants clinically diagnosed with bacterial conjunctivitis was only 31%, suggesting a high proportion likely had a viral etiology. Two of these studies were performed in community-based settings and three were specialty referral practices. None involved patients from ED-based practices, which limits the validity of generalizing the results to ED practice.

In summary, conjunctivitis appears to be a relatively self-limited infection with a significant number of infections caused by non-bacterial causes. There is weak evidence to conclude that broad-spectrum topical antibiotics lead to better clinical and microbiological cure rates in cases of suspected bacterial conjunctivitis seen in the ED.

Question 5: In adults with suspected bacterial conjunctivitis (population), does the use of broad-spectrum topical antibiotics (treatment) reduce serious outcomes (outcome) compared to no treatment or conservative treatment (control)?

Question 6: In adults with suspected bacterial conjunctivitis (population), does treatment with broad-spectrum topical antibiotics (treatment) result in common and/or serious side-effects (outcome) compared to no treatment or conservative treatment (control)?

Search strategy

• Cochrane Library: bacterial conjunctivitis AND antibiotics AND complications
• MEDLINE: bacterial conjunctivitis AND antibiotics AND adverse events

The same systematic review as discussed above, involving 1034 patients, reported no serious complications even in the placebo group [11]. This suggests that treatment of bacterial conjunctivitis reduces the duration of symptoms, with the best evidence demonstrating only marginal benefit from topical antibiotics for rates of clinical and microbiological remission. None of the studies in this review addressed the overall incidence of antibiotic-induced adverse reactions such as corneal hyperemia, inflammation and punctuate corneal staining.

A MEDLINE search identified one meta-analysis of six phase III randomized clinical trials that addressed the incidence of adverse events with the use of six different topical antibiotics for conjunctivitis [12]. In this analysis lomefloxacin 0.3% was compared to one of five different agents: chloramphenicol 0.5%, gentamicin 0.3%, fusidic acid 1%, tobramycin 0.3% or norfloxacin 0.3%. All adverse events were considered non-serious. A total of 41 adverse events occurred in 561 patients treated with topical antibiotics giving an adverse event rate of 7% (95% CI: 5% to 9%). Of 278 patients evaluated after treatment with lomefloxacin, 18 had an

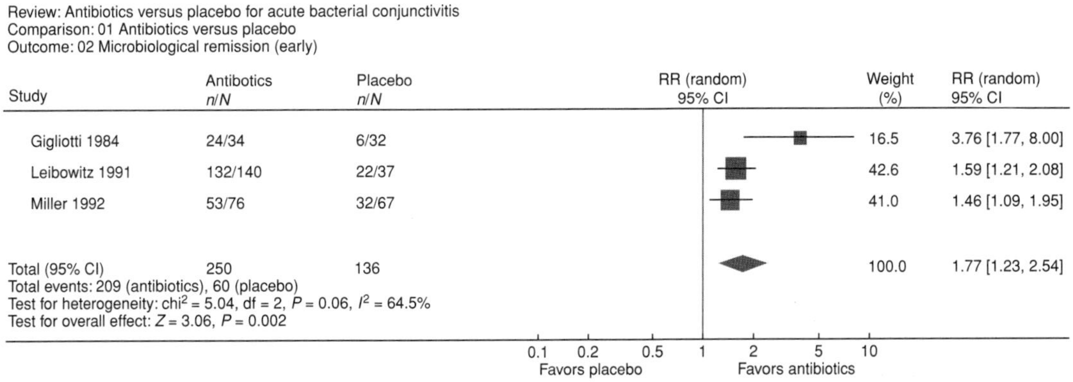

Review: Antibiotics versus placebo for acute bacterial conjunctivitis
Comparison: 01 Antibiotics versus placebo
Outcome: 02 Microbiological remission (early)

Study	Antibiotics n/N	Placebo n/N	RR (random) 95% CI	Weight (%)	RR (random) 95% CI
Gigliotti 1984	24/34	6/32		16.5	3.76 [1.77, 8.00]
Leibowitz 1991	132/140	22/37		42.6	1.59 [1.21, 2.08]
Miller 1992	53/76	32/67		41.0	1.46 [1.09, 1.95]
Total (95% CI)	250	136		100.0	1.77 [1.23, 2.54]

Total events: 209 (antibiotics), 60 (placebo)
Test for heterogeneity: chi^2 = 5.04, df = 2, P = 0.06, I^2 = 64.5%
Test for overall effect: Z = 3.06, P = 0.002

0.1 0.2 0.5 1 2 5 10
Favors placebo   Favors antibiotics

Figure 53.2 Comparison of early (days 2–5) microbiological remission rates in patients with suspected bacterial conjunctivitis treated with topical antibiotics or placebo. (Reproduced with permission from Sheikh et al. [11], © Cochrane Database, Wiley.)

adverse event (6%; 95% CI: 4% to 9%). Twenty-three of the 283 patients in the combined control group suffered an adverse event (8%; 95% CI: 5% to 11%). No one agent in the combined control group appeared to have a significantly higher rate of adverse events than the others.

In summary, given this reported frequency of adverse events, the marginal clinical benefits of topical antibiotics may well be significantly offset by incidents of adverse drug reactions. This is particularly concerning if 70% of patients treated do not have a bacterial etiology for their symptoms.

Question 7: In adults with suspected bacterial conjunctivitis (population), does the delayed use of broad-spectrum topical antibiotics (exposure) result in less antibiotic use (outcome)?

Search strategy

- Cochrane Library: delayed antibiotics AND conjunctivitis
- MEDLINE: delayed antibiotics AND conjunctivitis

Delayed prescribing strategies have become an accepted approach to management of acute respiratory infections such as otitis media [4,13] and sore throat [3,5]. This approach involves providing the patient with an antibiotic prescription and instructions not to fill it unless symptoms do not resolve after 2–3 days. Education as to the usually self-limited nature of their condition accompanies this approach. No systematic reviews could be identified in the Cochrane database on delayed antibiotics for conjunctivitis. The MEDLINE search identified one article relevant to this question.

One multi-centered, randomized controlled trial was identified from the MEDLINE search. In this study involving 30 primary care practices, three different management strategies were evaluated in 307 patients aged 1 year or more presenting with acute infective conjunctivitis [7]. Patients were randomized to receive one of three antibiotic prescribing strategies – immediate antibiotics (chloramphenicol eye drops; n = 104), no antibiotics (n = 94) or delayed antibiotics (n = 109) and the overall incidence of positive bacterial culture was 50%. Antibiotic use was 99% in the immediate antibiotic group, 53% in the delayed group and 30% in the control group. Comparing antibiotic use, the immediate antibiotic group

Review: Antibiotics versus placebo for acute bacterial conjunctivitis
Comparison: 01 Antibiotics versus placebo
Outcome: 03 Clinical remission (late)

Study	Antibiotics n/N	Placebo n/N	RR (random) 95% CI	Weight (%)	RR (random) 95% CI
Gigliotti 1984	31/34	23/32		13.3	1.27 [1.00, 1.61]
Rietveld 2005	45/73	53/90		12.3	1.05 [0.82, 1.34]
Rose 2005	140/163	128/163		74.5	1.09 [0.99, 1.21]
Total (95% CI)	270	285		100.0	1.11 [1.02, 1.21]

Total events: 216 (antibiotics), 204 (placebo)
Test for heterogeneity: chi^2 = 1.49, df = 2, P = 0.47, I^2 = 0.0%
Test for overall effect: Z = 2.32, P = 0.02

0.1 0.2 0.5 1 2 5 10
Favors placebo   Favors antibiotics

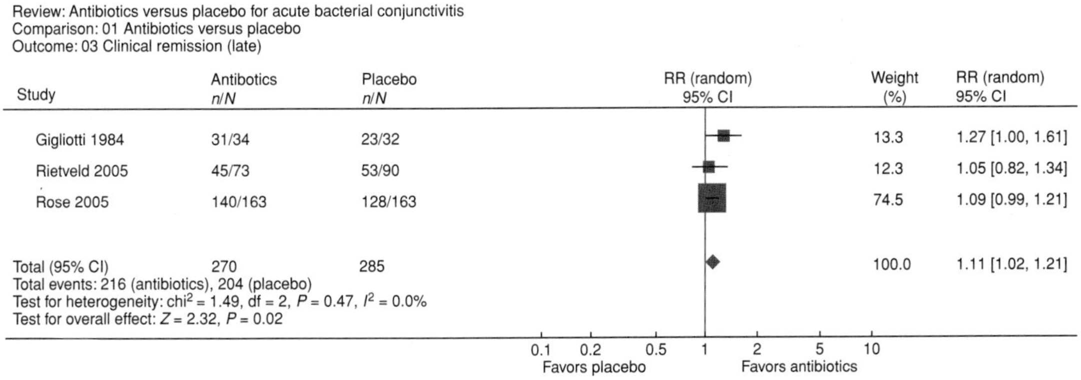

Figure 53.3 Comparison of late (days 7–10) clinical improvement rates in patients with suspected bacterial conjunctivitis treated with topical antibiotics or placebo. (Reproduced with permission from Sheikh et al. [11], © Cochrane Database, Wiley.)

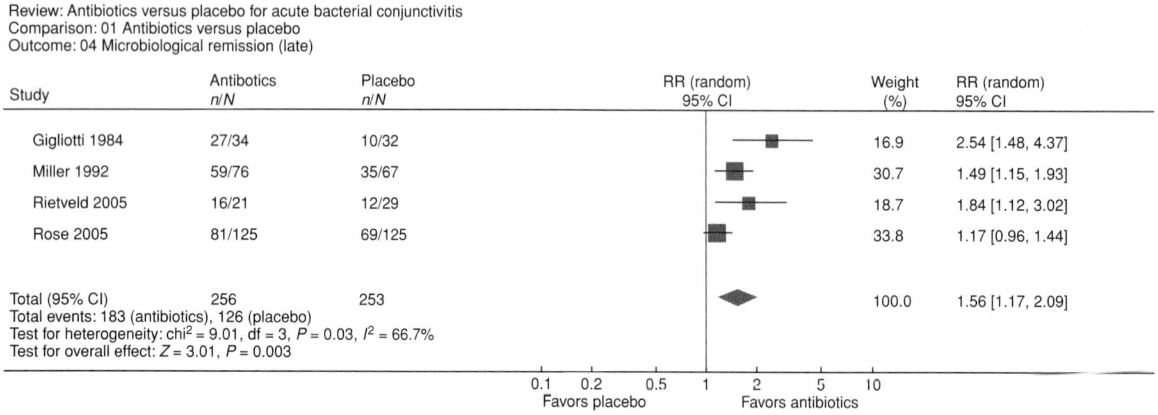

Review: Antibiotics versus placebo for acute bacterial conjunctivitis
Comparison: 01 Antibiotics versus placebo
Outcome: 04 Microbiological remission (late)

Study	Antibotics n/N	Placebo n/N	RR (random) 95% CI	Weight (%)	RR (random) 95% CI
Gigliotti 1984	27/34	10/32		16.9	2.54 [1.48, 4.37]
Miller 1992	59/76	35/67		30.7	1.49 [1.15, 1.93]
Rietveld 2005	16/21	12/29		18.7	1.84 [1.12, 3.02]
Rose 2005	81/125	69/125		33.8	1.17 [0.96, 1.44]
Total (95% CI)	256	253		100.0	1.56 [1.17, 2.09]

Total events: 183 (antibiotics), 126 (placebo)
Test for heterogeneity: chi^2 = 9.01, df = 3, P = 0.03, I^2 = 66.7%
Test for overall effect: Z = 3.01, P = 0.003

0.1 0.2 0.5 1 2 5 10
Favors placebo   Favors antibiotics

Figure 53.4 Comparison of late (days 7–10) microbiological remission rates in patients with suspected bacterial conjunctivitis treated with topical antibiotics or placebo. (Reproduced with permission from Sheikh et al. [11], © Cochrane Database, Wiley.)

versus the no antibiotic group demonstrated an odds ratio of 185.4 (95% CI: 23.9 to 1439.2) whereas for delayed antibiotics versus no antibiotics the odds ratio for antibiotic use was 2.9 (95% CI: 1.4 to 5.7). Average severity of symptoms scored during the first 3 days did not differ significantly between the groups. However, the duration of moderate symptoms was slightly less with antibiotics: no antibiotics group, 4.8 days; immediate antibiotics group, 3.3 days (RR = 0.7; 95% CI: 0.6 to 0.8); and delayed antibiotics group, 3.9 days (RR = 0.8; 95% CI: 0.7 to 0.9).

The management approach did have a significant effect on patients' perceptions of antibiotic effectiveness and perception of need for medical care of this condition. The immediate antibiotic group was more likely than controls to believe that antibiotics were beneficial (OR = 2.4; 95% CI: 1.1 to 5.0) and more likely to state their intention to re-attend for eye infections (OR = 3.2; 95% CI: 1.6 to 6.4). The perceptions of those patients in the delayed antibiotic group were not significantly different from those in the control group.

The only serious outcome was an orbital cellulitis that occurred in the immediate antibiotic group and required admission to hospital 11 days after recruitment. This study provides evidence supporting a more limited approach to antibiotic prescribing for infective conjunctivitis, suggesting that a delayed antibiotic approach may reduce antibiotic use and re-attendance for simple eye infections without significantly changing clinical outcomes. However, none of the patients were enrolled from the ED, which limits the generalizability of these results to ED practice.

Conclusions

The patient mentioned above was treated empirically with antibiotics and by day 4 her eye redness and discharge had almost completely resolved. Best available evidence suggests the probability of a bacterial etiology would have been less than 50%, and at most the ciprofloxacin drops may have shortened the duration of symptoms by a few days.

Another reasonable approach to this patient's presentation would have been to adopt a delayed antibiotic treatment plan. With this approach the patient is provided with a prescription and advice to wait 2–3 days to see if symptoms start to resolve on their own. If the eye symptoms do not resolve, the patient then fills the prescription for a topical antibiotic. This approach not only appears to reduce the use of antibiotics for this relatively benign condition, it also appears to reduce the likelihood of patients re-attending for eye infections.

Overall, emergency physicians will be faced with many patients complaining of red eye symptoms in the ED. A good history and physical examination as well as a thorough eye examination using appropriate modalities are important to exclude other etiologies. Apart from antibiotics, many non-traditional treatments are available (e.g., frequent washing, alternative medical treatments, etc.); many of these remain untested or lack sufficient evidence to be included in this chapter. The use of antibiotics is recommended to reduce symptom duration in patients with reasonable features to suggest bacterial infection.

References

1 Brunette D. Ophthalmology. In: Marx JA, Hockberger RS, Walls RM, eds. *Rosen's Emergency Medicine: Concepts and clinical practice*, 6th edn. Mosby, St. Louis, 2006:1044–65.

2 Porter R. Acute eye infections. In: Harwood-Nuss A, ed. *The Clinical Practice of Emergency Medicine*, 3rd edn. Lippincott Williams & Wilkins, Philadelphia, 2001:47–9.

3 Spurling GK, Del Mar CB, Pooley L, Foxlee R. Delayed antibiotics for symptoms and complications of respiratory infections. *Cochrane Database Syst Rev* 2004;**4**:CD004417.

4 Glasziou PP, Del Mar CB, Sanders SL, Hayem M. Antibiotics for acute otitis media in children. *Cochrane Database Syst Rev* 2004;**1**:CD000219.

5 Del Mar CB, Glasziou PP, Spinks AB. Antibiotics for sore throat. *Cochrane Database Syst Rev* 2006;**4**:CD000023.

6 Rietveld RP, ter Riet G, Bindels PJ, Sloos JH, van Weert HC. Predicting bacterial cause in infectious conjunctivitis: cohort study on informativeness of combinations of signs and symptoms. *BMJ* 2004;**329**(7459):206–10.

7 Everitt HA, Little PS, Smith PW. A randomised controlled trial of management strategies for acute infective conjunctivitis in general practice. *BMJ* 2006;**333**(7563):321.

8 Rietveld RP, ter Riet G, Bindels PJ, Bink D, Sloos JH, van Weert HC. The treatment of acute infectious conjunctivitis with fusidic acid: a randomised controlled trial. *Br J Gen Pract* 2005;**55**(521):924–30.

9 Wightman J, Hamilton G. Red and painful eye. In: Marx JA, Hockberger RS, Walls RM, eds. *Rosen's Emergency Medicine: Concepts and clinical practice*, 6th edn. Mosby, St. Louis, 2006:283–97.

10 Rietveld RP, van Weert HC, ter Riet G, Bindels PJ. Diagnostic impact of signs and symptoms in acute infectious conjunctivitis: systematic literature search. *BMJ* 2003;**327**(7418):789.

11 Sheikh A, Hurwitz B. Antibiotics versus placebo for acute bacterial conjunctivitis. *Cochrane Database Syst Rev* 2006;**2**:CD001211.

12 Jauch A, Fsadni M, Gamba G. Meta-analysis of six clinical phase III studies comparing lomefloxacin 0.3% eye drops twice daily to five standard antibiotics in patients with acute bacterial conjunctivitis. *Graefes Arch Clin Exp Ophthalmol* 1999;**237**(9):705–13.

13 Little P, Gould C, Williamson I, Moore M, Warner G, Dunleavey J. Pragmatic randomised controlled trial of two prescribing strategies for childhood acute otitis media. *BMJ* 2001;**322**(7282):336–42.

9 Minor Procedures

54 Procedural Sedation and Analgesia

David W. Messenger[1] & Marco L. A. Sivilotti[2]

[1] Department of Emergency Medicine, Queen's University, Kingston, Canada
[2] Departments of Emergency Medicine *and* Pharmacology and Toxicology, Queen's University, Kingston *and* Ontario Poison Centre, Toronto, Canada

Clinical scenario

A healthy 28-year-old soccer player presented to the emergency department (ED) after falling onto his outstretched arm. The patient denied taking any regular medications, had no allergies, and last ate 3 hours prior to arrival. At triage, his vital signs were a pulse of 60 beats/min, temperature 37.0°C (oral), respiratory rate 12 breaths/min, blood pressure 120/70 mmHg (left arm) and pulse oximetry of 98% on room air. The distal radius was swollen, deformed and tender, but the skin and neurovascular status were both intact. No other injuries were identified. Plain radiographs of the wrist demonstrated a metaphyseal fracture of the distal radius with dorsal angulation and shortening. He consented to a closed reduction of the fracture in the ED.

A 52-year-old male presented to the ED after awaking with proctalgia after drinking heavily at a party. The patient denied taking any regular medications, had no allergies and had not eaten in 24 hours. At triage, his vital signs were a pulse of 120 beats/min, temperature 37.5°C (oral), respiratory rate 20 breaths/min, blood pressure 150/90 mmHg (left arm) and pulse oximetry (SaO_2) of 92% on room air. Abdominal examination was benign; however, rectal examination revealed a foreign body in the rectum. Abdominal films identified the foreign body to be a screwdriver. He consented to a consultation with general surgery.

Background

A large and growing number of procedures that previously required consultation or admission to the hospital have become the domain of emergency physicians. Examples include cardioversion of stable atrial fibrillation, reduction of limb fractures and joint dislocations, incision and drainage of abscesses, repair of complex

lacerations and removal of foreign bodies. The main reasons for this shift are the lack of available operating rooms or inpatient beds, and the evolving skill set of emergency physicians including the use of procedural sedation and analgesia (PSA).

Procedural sedation and analgesia has therefore become a core skill for emergency physicians. Using potent sedative or dissociative agents, with or without adjunct analgesics, the goal of PSA is to allow patients to better tolerate painful or unpleasant procedures while maintaining spontaneous breathing and protective airway reflexes [1]. In addition to the self-evident improvement in pain relief and operating conditions, PSA allows timely access to definitive care despite increasingly restricted access to operating rooms for ED patients with less serious conditions.

Numerous pharmacological agents are available for PSA, including benzodiazepines, barbiturates, opioids, propofol, etomidate and ketamine. Once restricted to the operating room, these agents have joined the pharmacological arsenal of the emergency physician, paralleling the recognized expertise of emergency physicians in airway management and resuscitation [1,2].

Patient suitability for ED PSA is usually determined by individual physician preference and experience, and little published evidence is available to provide exclusion criteria for sedation in the ED. Most research in ED PSA has included generally healthy patients, most commonly identified using the American Society of Anesthesiologists (ASA) physical status classification system (Table 54.1). ASA class I or II patients are usually considered acceptable for ED PSA [2], while only limited data are available on the safety of sedating more critically ill patients [3]. Published guidelines also suggest that patients with difficult airway anatomy, those at high risk for vomiting and aspiration, and those with underlying cardiopulmonary disease may be at higher risk for complications during ED PSA [1,2].

The continuum of sedation is generally classified into ordered levels of depth (Table 54.2) [4]. Used alone or in combinations for ED PSA, the various agents depress consciousness in a drug- and dose-dependent manner. Agents differ in times of onset and offset, potency, safety margin, familiarity and costs, as well as unique national or local restrictions on availability. Unique to ketamine

Evidence-based Emergency Medicine. Edited by Brian H. Rowe
© 2009 Blackwell Publishing, ISBN: 978-1-4051-6143-5.

Table 54.1 American Society of Anesthesiologists (ASA) physical status classification.

ASA class I	Healthy
ASA class II	Mild systemic disease without functional limitation
ASA class III	Severe systemic disease with definite functional limitation
ASA class IV	Severe systemic disease with a constant threat to life

is the distinct state of dissociative sedation in which patients enter a trance-like cataleptic state of profound analgesia and amnesia despite maintaining protective airway reflexes, spontaneous respirations and cardiopulmonary stability [5].

As PSA has become more widely practiced by non-anesthesiologists, important questions have arisen regarding appropriate patient and drug selection, duration of pre-procedure fasting and required patient monitoring and supportive measures, among others [1]. This chapter explores ED PSA in further detail; however, readers are directed to individual chapters that deal with the underlying conditions (e.g., fractures and dislocations: see Chapters 31 and 34; abscess drainage: see Chapter 56; electrical cardioversion: see Chapters 20 and 21; and the repair of lacerations: see Chapter 55).

Clinical questions

In order to address the issues of most relevance to your patient and to help in searching the literature for the evidence regarding these issues, you structure your clinical questions as recommended in Chapter 1.

1 In ED patients who undergo procedural sedation and analgesia (population), is pre-procedure fasting (intervention) associated with a reduction in adverse respiratory events (outcome)?

2 In ED patients who undergo procedural sedation and analgesia (population), does the routine administration of supplemental oxygen (intervention) reduce the incidence of adverse respiratory events (outcome) compared to breathing room air (control)?

3 In ED patients who undergo procedural sedation and analgesia (population), does the addition of capnography to standard monitoring (intervention) allow for earlier detection of adverse respiratory events (outcome)?

4 In ED patients who undergo procedural sedation and analgesia (population), does etomidate (intervention) allow for more rapid,

safe and successful procedures (outcomes) than other short-acting or comparison agents (control)?

5 In ED patients who undergo procedural sedation and analgesia (population), does propofol (intervention) allow for more rapid, safe and successful procedures (outcomes) than other short-acting or comparison agents (control)?

6 In ED patients who undergo procedural sedation and analgesia (population), does ketamine (intervention) allow for more rapid, safe and successful procedures (outcomes) than other short-acting or comparison agents (control)?

General search strategy

This topic is poorly covered by traditional medical subject heading language. You begin to address the topic of ED procedural sedation and analgesia by searching for evidence in the common electronic databases such as MEDLINE and EMBASE, looking specifically for systematic reviews and randomized controlled trials (RCTs), and using the following core search:

• MEDLINE and EMBASE: (*explode* conscious sedation [MeSH] OR *explode* hypnotics and sedatives [MeSH] OR *explode* anesthetics, general [MeSH] OR procedural sedation [keyword]) AND (emergency medicine [MeSH] OR emergency service, hospital [MeSH] OR emergency department [keyword]).

In addition, access to relevant, updated, evidence-based clinical practice guidelines (CPGs) on PSA are reviewed to determine the consensus rating of areas lacking evidence.

Critical review of the literature

Question 1: In ED patients who undergo ED procedural sedation and analgesia (population), is pre-procedure fasting (intervention) associated with a reduction in adverse respiratory events (outcome)?

Search strategy

• MEDLINE: standard search outlined above AND (*explode* fasting [MeSH] OR *explode* respiratory aspiration [MeSH] OR *explode* pneumonia [MeSH])

Table 54.2 Terminology of procedural sedation and analgesia.

Sedation depth	Response to verbal command	Response to tactile stimulus	Spontaneous breathing	Airway protection
Minimal	Responds	Responds	Maintained	Maintained
Moderate	Purposeful response	Purposeful response to light stimulus	Adequate	Maintained
Deep	No purposeful response	Purposeful response to repeated/ painful stimuli only	May be impaired	May be impaired
General anesthesia	No response	No response	Often impaired	Often impaired

Table 54.3 Prospective studies of pre-sedation fasting and frequency of adverse events.

Study	Number of patients	Age group	Most common procedures	Most common drug regimens	Major findings	Limitations
Agrawal, et al. [6]	1014	Pediatric patients (median age 5.4 years)	Orthopedic procedures (40%) Diagnostic imaging (25%) Laceration repair (17%)	IV/IM ketamine ± midazolam (46.7%) Midazolam/fentanyl (23.2%) Chloral hydrate (12.3%) Pentobarbital (11.8%)	Aspiration in 0/1014 Oxygen desaturation <90% in 32/1014 patients Emesis in 15/1014 patients Apnea in 13/1014 patients No difference in fasting duration between patients with and without adverse events during sedation (7.3 hours (IQR = 5.9 to 9.4 hours) vs 6.8 hours (IQR = 4.8 to 9.4 hours) for solids)	Relatively long fasting durations in study patients (median 5 hours)
Treston [7]	272	Pediatric patients (1–12 years)	Laceration repair (49.6%) Fracture reduction (27.9%)	IV ketamine (average dose 1.25 mg/kg)	Vomiting in 36/257 patients with documented fasting times Trend towards increased incidence of vomiting with increased fasting durations (>3 hours = 15.7%; 2–3 hours = 14%; 1 hour = 6.6%)	Incidence of adverse events other than vomiting not reported
Roback, et al. [8]	2085	Pediatric patients (median age 6.7 years)	Fracture reduction (56.3%) Laceration repair (18.3%)	Ketamine (63%) Midazolam/Ketamine (12.8%) Midazolam/Fentanyl (12.1%)	172/2085 patients had an adverse respiratory event (apnea, laryngospasm, desaturation <90%) No difference in adverse events or vomiting between patients fasted for 0–2 hours (12.0%), 2–4 hours (16.4%), 4–6 hours (14.0%), 6–8 hours (14.6%) or >8 hours (14.5%)	Pre-procedure fasting duration was not reported in 530/2085 study subjects
Babl, et al. [9]	220	Pediatric patients (14 months to 17 years)	Orthopedic procedures (44.6%) Laceration repair (21.4%) Vascular access (18.2%)	Inhaled nitrous oxide (100%)	Emesis in 15/220 in ED Nausea in 4/220 in ED Dizziness in 10/220 in ED No difference in emesis rates between patients who were fasted according to AAP/ASA fasting guidelines and those who were not (6.3% (95% CI: 1.8% to 15.5%) vs 7.1% (95% CI: 3.6% to 12.3%)) No difference in median fasting duration of patients with and without emesis (4.2 hours (IQR = 2.92 to 6.2 hours) vs 4.4 hours (IQR = 3.0 to 6.6 hours) for solids)	Only examined inhaled nitrous oxide; difficult to apply results to subjects sedated with more common parenteral medications

AAP, American Academy of Pediatrics; ASA, American Society of Anesthesiologists; CI: confidence interval; IQR, inter-quartile range.

The above search identified 26 English articles from MEDLINE and 80 articles from EMBASE. Additional articles were identified through references listed in the articles obtained. There are no RCTs that have evaluated the impact of pre-procedure fasting on the frequency of adverse respiratory events during ED PSA. Four prospective case series in children examined the frequency of adverse events during ED PSA in relation to the duration of pre-procedure fasting (Table 54.3) [6–9]. None of these studies demonstrated fewer adverse respiratory events or emesis in patients with longer pre-procedure fasting durations. In fact, Treston demonstrated a trend towards increased vomiting in patients with increased duration of fasting [7]; however, this finding was most likely secondary to selection bias.

No studies examined the association between pre-procedure fasting duration and adverse events in adult ED patients. A single case report describes pulmonary aspiration as a complication of ED PSA [10]. Thus, there is a paucity of evidence specific to emergency medicine to allow for a clear, evidenced-based approach to pre-procedure fasting in this setting. The most recent American College of Emergency Physicians clinical policy for PSA does not recommend a specific minimum fasting period prior to the administration of PSA because of the lack of evidence [1]. Existing guidelines are derived largely from retrospective anesthesiology studies, which may have limited relevance to the unique population and environment of the ED. Identified predictors of aspiration risk from operative anesthesia include airway abnormalities,

Table 54.4 Recommended maximum sedation depth based on pre-procedure fasting duration, patient risk and procedure urgency.* (Adapted from Green et al. [12].)

Oral intake in preceding 3 hours	Maximum depth of sedation in higher risk patients	Maximum depth of sedation in standard risk patients
None	Any sedation depth	Any sedation depth
Clear fluids	Brief deep sedation for urgent procedures only	All levels of sedation for urgent procedures
	Extended moderate sedation acceptable for semi-urgent procedures	Brief deep sedation for semi-urgent procedures
		Extended moderate sedation acceptable for non-urgent procedures
Light snack	Dissociative or short-duration moderate sedation for urgent procedures only	Brief deep sedation for urgent procedures only
		Dissociative or short-duration moderate sedation for semi-urgent procedures
Heavier snack or meal	Dissociative or short-duration moderate sedation for urgent procedures only	Extended moderate sedation for urgent procedures only

*All levels of sedation are acceptable for emergent procedures regardless of oral intake in preceding 3 hours. Minimal sedation is always acceptable regardless of recent oral intake.

advanced age, greater underlying illness and factors predisposing to esophageal reflux [11].

A consensus-based clinical practice advisory has recently been published by a group of ED PSA researchers [12]. This guideline recommends a stepwise approach to patient assessment prior to ED PSA (Table 54.4). The factors to be considered are as follows: (i) the presence of risk factors for aspiration or difficult ventilation including extremes of age; (ii) timing and nature of oral intake in the prior 3 hours (nothing, clear liquids only, light snack or heavy meal); (iii) the urgency of the proposed procedure; and (iv) the anticipated depth and duration of PSA. The authors then propose prudent limits of targeted depth and length of ED PSA based on this risk assessment.

In summary, pre-procedural fasting has not been shown to influence the incidence of adverse events during ED PSA. Experts concur that pre-procedural fasting state, both in terms of duration and type of intake, be balanced against the patient's underlying risk factors, as well as the urgency and anticipated depth and duration of sedation.

Question 2: In ED patients who undergo procedural sedation and analgesia (population), does the routine administration of supplemental oxygen (intervention) reduce the incidence of adverse respiratory events (outcome) compared to breathing room air (control)?

Search strategy

- MEDLINE: standard search outlined above AND (*explode* oxygen [MeSH] OR *explode* oxygen inhalation therapy [MeSH] OR supplemental oxygen [keyword])

The above search identified 26 English articles from MEDLINE and 68 articles from EMBASE. Additional articles were identified through references listed in the articles obtained. A single RCT studied the impact of supplemental oxygen administration

(2 L/min via nasal cannula) on respiratory depression during ED PSA with fentanyl and midazolam [13]. In this blinded study of 80 adult and pediatric patients, the frequency of respiratory depression was similar between those subjects who received oxygen (45.5%) and those administered room air (52.8%) (observed difference = −7.3%; 95% CI: −27.8% to 14.1%). However, this study was only powered to detect a 20% difference in hypoxic events. Moreover, subjects were not sedated to a pre-specified level of responsiveness (Ramsay scores ranged between 2 and 5). The relevance of these observations to deeply sedated patients, in whom respiratory depression is more likely, is therefore unclear.

A small number of trials have reported rates of adverse events in patients who received supplemental oxygen compared to those who did not, though none of these investigations was specifically designed to address the utility of supplemental oxygen, and oxygen administration was neither blinded nor randomized [14–16]. These studies report conflicting results, with observed hypoxemia rates ranging from 8.5% to 14.9% among patients administered oxygen versus 4.8% to 22.2% among patients breathing room air.

Supplemental oxygen administration is generally assumed to be harmless, and to reduce the frequency of hypoxemia; however, routine administration may mask the early detection of respiratory depression during ED PSA [17,18]. As such, oxygen may not be a risk-free intervention. Although capnography may provide an alternate means of identifying respiratory depression in patients receiving supplemental oxygen [19] (see Question 3), this technology remains unfamiliar or unavailable to many emergency physicians.

Published practice guidelines vary in their recommendations for supplemental oxygen administration, reflecting the scarce evidence. The ASA recommends routine supplemental oxygen administration to all patients who undergo deep sedation [20], while both the American College of Emergency Physicians and Canadian Association of Emergency Physicians acknowledge that the administration of oxygen may delay the recognition of hypoventilation and make no specific recommendation for its use [1,2].

In summary, the available studies do not demonstrate that supplemental oxygen reduces adverse respiratory events during ED PSA. No consensus exists among experts on best practice in this regard. Routine supplemental oxygen administration could delay the onset of hypoxemia and the recognition of hypoventilation in sedated patients, though the clinical significance of this delay remains unanswered.

Question 3: In ED patients who undergo ED procedural sedation and analgesia (population), does the addition of capnography to standard monitoring (intervention) allow for earlier detection of adverse respiratory events (outcome)?

Search strategy

- MEDLINE: standard search outlined above AND (*explode* capnography [MeSH] OR *explode* carbon dioxide [MeSH] OR end-tidal carbon dioxide [keyword] OR end-tidal CO$_2$ [keyword])

The above search identified 19 English articles from MEDLINE and 35 articles from EMBASE. Additional articles were identified through references listed in the articles obtained. No prospective ED trial has randomized patients to end-tidal carbon dioxide (ETCO$_2$) monitoring versus no ETCO$_2$ monitoring; however, several cohort studies suggest that capnography helps detect respiratory depression during ED PSA [13–16,21–23].

In a series of studies of different PSA agents by Miner and colleagues, abnormalities in capnography were common and were frequently associated with other acute respiratory events during sedation [14–16]. These investigators have proposed an outcome measure of "subclinical respiratory depression" for ED PSA research, defined as any one of: oxygen desaturation <90%, ETCO$_2$ >50 mmHg, change in ETCO$_2$ value of ±10 mmHg, or loss of waveform on the capnograph. In a prospective case series of 60 patients undergoing ED PSA, Burton and colleagues examined the relationship between abnormal ETCO$_2$ findings and acute respiratory events [22]. Overall, 36 patients (60%) in this study had abnormal ETCO$_2$ findings (absolute change from baseline of ±10 mmHg or ETCO$_2$ level ≤30 mmHg or ≥50 mmHg). Of these, 16 had no other acute respiratory events or interventions. Of the 20 patients who had a documented acute respiratory event, 14 (70%) had abnormal ETCO$_2$ findings that preceded their event, most often an ETCO$_2$ value of ≤30 mmHg. Unfortunately, these studies each included patients who were breathing room air or supplemental oxygen, making it difficult to generalize the findings.

In a prospective case series of propofol sedation for children breathing supplemental oxygen, capnography detected all observed episodes of apnea (5/125 subjects) prior to clinical examination or pulse oximetry. Capnography was also the first indicator of airway obstruction in six of 10 occurrences, suggesting that its use might allow for detection of respiratory impairment earlier than standard monitoring practices [23]. In a randomized trial

investigating the effect of supplemental oxygen administration in 80 adult patients during ED PSA, sedating physicians blinded to capnography measurements failed to recognize all 28 patients who met pre-specified capnography criteria for respiratory depression, but who did not develop hypoxemia [13]. Additionally, capnography abnormalities indicative of respiratory depression persisted longer in patients who received supplemental oxygen, providing limited support to the theory that oxygen administration can obscure subtle respiratory depression.

During a randomized controlled ED trial of adjunct analgesic agents for propofol PSA, ETCO$_2$ data were prospectively collected from 63 adult patients breathing room air [24]. Of the 36 patients who developed oxygen desaturation, only 21 (58%) had abnormalities in capnography (ETCO$_2$ >50 mmHg, change in ETCO$_2$ from baseline of ±10 mmHg or more, or loss of the waveform). However, these abnormalities preceded oxygen desaturation in only two cases, and usually lagged behind desaturation (median time difference: 2 minutes 4 seconds; inter-quartile range (IQR): 0 minutes 1 second to 5 minutes 55 seconds). These data suggest that for patients breathing room air, these capnography thresholds are unlikely to signal respiratory depression earlier than standard pulse oximetry monitoring.

In summary, the available evidence suggests that capnography frequently identifies otherwise occult signs of altered respiration during ED PSA. Capnography may detect respiratory depression earlier than standard patient monitoring, particularly in patients who are administered supplemental oxygen. Further study is needed to address the clinical significance of capnography changes not associated with adverse respiratory events, the capnography threshold or changes in wave morphology that predict a need for airway/breathing interventions, and, most importantly, whether the use of capnography reduces the incidence of hypoxemia and other adverse respiratory events during ED PSA [25].

Question 4: In ED patients who undergo ED procedural sedation and analgesia (population), does etomidate (intervention) allow for more rapid, safe and successful procedures (outcomes) than other short-acting or comparison agents (control)?

Search strategy

- MEDLINE, EMBASE and Cochrane: etomidate AND emergency department. Limited to RCTs and systematic reviews

The search above identified one systematic review examining the use of etomidate for PSA in the ED published in 2004 [26]. In addition, the Canadian Agency for Drugs and Technologies in Health (CADTH) recently commissioned a health technology assessment on the safety and efficacy of short-acting agents used for PSA in the ED [27]. This assessment represents a comprehensive search of the published and gray literature, and will be summarized in response to Questions 4 through 6 below. In all, 1794 potential citations were identified regarding short-acting PSA agents. Further screening identified nine RCTs overall, four of which evaluated etomidate. Three RCTs compared etomidate with midazolam, and two compared etomidate with propofol, including one three-arm study of etomidate versus propofol versus midazolam. Seven additional case series were identified that provided evidence on safety outcomes for etomidate and were included in this review. Overall, a total of 489 patients (157 patients enrolled in RCTs and 332 enrolled in observational studies) informed the findings of this review.

Overall, etomidate was found to be slightly less effective than propofol in terms of procedural success (RR = 1.09; 95% CI: 1.01 to 1.17 in favor of propofol) and had no difference in duration of procedure (weighted mean difference (WMD) = −0.73 minutes; 95% CI: −2.13 to 0.68). Etomidate was as effective as midazolam in terms of procedural success (RR = 1.08; 95% CI: 0.91 to 1.28); however, it required less patient monitoring time than midazolam (WMD = −14.16 minutes; 95% CI, −19.28 to −9.04). The safety analysis suggested higher rates of total adverse effects (27.2%; 95% CI: 23.4% to 31.3%) for etomidate than other rapid acting agents (10–15%) and higher than standard care comparators, such as benzodiazepines and/or narcotics (17.3%; 95% CI: 12.4% to 23.7%). These side-effects rarely resulted in hospitalization and were predominantly self-limiting. The main side-effects encountered were airway issues (e.g., composite measure of respiratory events/depression = 29.2%; 95% CI: 23.3% to 36%) and myoclonus (14.6%; 95% CI: 11.1% to 19%). Emesis (1.1%; 95% CI: 0.5% to 2.5%) and hypotension (3.2%; 95% CI: 2.0% to 5.2%) were uncommon.

In summary, etomidate is a relatively effective short-acting PSA agent. However, clinically important side-effects from this agent include myoclonus and respiratory depression. These side-effects coupled with concerns regarding adrenal suppression and the availability of other agents with equal or better efficacy argue against the routine use of etomidate for procedural sedation [28].

Question 5: In ED patients who undergo ED procedural sedation and analgesia (population), does propofol (intervention) allow for more rapid, safe and successful procedures (outcomes) than other short-acting or comparison agents (control)?

Search strategy

- MEDLINE, EMBASE and Cochrane: propofol AND emergency department. Limited to RCTs and systematic reviews

The search above identified one systematic review examining the use of propofol for PSA in the ED [29]. The recent CADTH report cited above [27] identified seven RCTs involving propofol. Three of these compared propofol with midazolam, two compared propofol with etomidate, one compared propofol with ketofol, one compared propofol alone with propofol and alfentanil, and one

compared propofol with methohexital. One of the studies was a three-arm study of etomidate versus propofol versus midazolam. Overall, 25 additional case series studies were identified that provided evidence on safety outcomes for propofol and were included in this review. These summary results arise from a total of 7388 patients (343 patients enrolled in RCTs and 7045 patients enrolled in observational studies).

From this review, propofol was as effective as other agents in terms of both procedural success and procedure times, with a higher success rate than etomidate (see above). The use of propofol resulted in a shorter procedure time when compared to midazolam or to propofol plus alfentanil (WMD = −10.29 minutes; 95% CI: −16.17 to −4.42). The side-effects profile for all studies included in the safety analysis suggested lower rates of total adverse effects (10%; 95% CI: 9.4% to 10.7%) for propofol than other rapid-acting agents (12–27%) and lower than standard care comparators (17.3%; 95% CI: 12.4% to 23.7%). The main side-effects identified for this agent were airway issues (e.g., composite measure of respiratory events/depression = 27.7%; 95% CI: 26.6% to 33%). Emesis (0.4%; 95% CI: 0.2% to 0.9%) and hypotension (3.1%; 95% CI: 2.8% to 3.6%) were uncommon.

From this review, propofol was at least as effective as other fast-acting agents and appears to safer based on the reported experience.

Question 6: In ED patients who undergo ED procedural sedation and analgesia (population), does ketamine (intervention) allow for more rapid, safe and successful procedures (outcomes) than other short-acting or comparison agents (control)?

Search strategy

- MEDLINE, EMBASE and Cochrane: ketamine AND emergency department. Limited to RCTs and systematic reviews

Based on the CADTH report cited above [27], no RCTs were found that evaluated ketamine as sole agent in adults. Overall, five case series studies were identified that provided evidence on safety outcomes for ketamine and were included in this review. Overall, only 148 patients have been reported in observational studies of ketamine as a PSA agent in adults.

The side-effects profile for all studies included in the safety analysis suggested low rates of total adverse effects (12.2%; 95% CI: 7.8% to 18.4%) for ketamine compared to other rapid-acting agents (10–27%) and to standard care comparators (17.3%; 95% CI: 12.4% to 23.7%). The main side-effects identified for this agent were emergence phenomena (7.4%; 95% CI: 4.2% to 12.8%) and emesis (5.2%; 95% CI: 2.2% to 11.6%). Airway issues (e.g., composite measure of respiratory events/depression = 4.2%; 95% CI: 1.6% to 10.2%) and hypotension (0%; 95% CI: 0.0% to 2.7%) were uncommon.

Overall, the evidence upon which ED decisions regarding ketofol can be based arises from 156 patients (32 in RCTs and 124 in observational studies) [27]. One unpublished RCT has compared ketamine 0.3 mg/kg to fentanyl 1.5 μg/kg for procedural sedation in adults given propofol [30]. This study reported a substantial reduction in the composite primary outcome of adverse events with the ketamine–propofol combination compared to fentanyl–propofol, largely due to less frequent oxygen desaturation on room air (crude odds ratio = 5.1; 95% CI: 1.9 to 13.6 for fentanyl subjects experiencing a more severe adverse event than ketamine subjects). No statistically significant differences in procedure time were shown (WMD = 3.30 minutes; 95% CI: −0.70 to 7.30).

In summary, ketamine is a very safe and effective short-acting PSA agent that is used often in children, but increasingly in adults undergoing complex or painful procedures. The main side-effect is emergence reaction; however, overall, the incidence of adverse events using this agent is low. Because of its analgesic properties even at low doses, combining ketamine with propofol appears to be both rational and safer than an opioid–propofol combination. Emergency physicians should become familiar with and balance the efficacy and side-effect profile of ketamine either alone or in combination with propofol.

Conclusions

In the first scenario, you decided to reduce the distal radius fracture using PSA with propofol and fentanyl. Supplemental oxygen was administered at 2 L/min by nasal cannula, and a cardiac monitor, pulse oximeter and capnograph were applied for continuous monitoring. After 50 μg of fentanyl and 1.0 mg/kg of propofol IV, the patient reached a state of deep sedation. A loss of capnograph waveform was rapidly corrected with repositioning of the patient's airway and traction on the fracture. No hypoxemia developed. The fracture was successfully reduced and immobilized, and the patient recovered uneventfully. He was discharged home from the ED with standard post-PSA discharge instructions, and outpatient orthopedic follow-up was arranged.

In the second scenario, the general surgeon requested assistance with using PSA to remove the foreign body in the ED. Following a careful assessment of the patient and pre-oxygenation at 2 L/min, PSA was completed using a 0.3 mg/kg ketamine bolus followed by 0.8 mg/kg of propofol titrated IV over 4 minutes, and the patient became unresponsive to painful stimulation. During the 10-minute procedure, an additional 0.4 mg/kg of propofol was administered. Mild hypotension developed following removal of the foreign body but responded to a bolus of 500 cm³ normal saline. Recovery was otherwise uneventful. He was discharged home from the ED with standard post-PSA discharge instructions, and outpatient follow-up was arranged with the general surgeon.

Emergency physicians must frequently perform unpleasant or painful procedures to treat illnesses and injuries. Procedural sedation and analgesia facilitate these procedures by minimizing patient discomfort and anxiety, and improving operating conditions. Despite this, a growing body of published research on ED PSA has lagged behind the widespread adoption of this practice. Few randomized trials exist to answer key questions about best practice, including pre-procedure patient preparation, intra-procedure monitoring and supportive care, discharge readiness and choice of pharmacological agents. Nevertheless, the reported experiences from a number of cohort studies demonstrate that PSA can be safely performed in the ED, and that clinically important adverse events are rare. Rather than adopting an arbitrary fasting interval as a rigid prerequisite for PSA, physicians should balance fasting duration, type of intake and patient-specific risk factors against the urgency and anticipated depth and duration of sedation. The use of supplemental oxygen may not be risk-free, as it can delay recognition of respiratory depression. On the other hand, technologies such as capnography may serve to enhance patient safety during ED PSA. Finally, agents such as propofol, etomidate and ketamine can be used successfully in the ED, either alone or in combination. Physicians must be aware, however, of the risks, benefits and interactions of the drugs they employ and be prepared to intervene if hypotension, airway issues or other adverse events occur.

References

1 Godwin SA, Caro DA, Wolf SJ, et al. Clinical policy: procedural sedation and analgesia in the emergency department. *Ann Emerg Med* 2005;**45**(2):177–96.

2 Innes G, Murphy M, Nijssen-Jordan C, Ducharme J, Drummond A. Procedural sedation and analgesia in the emergency department. Canadian consensus guidelines. *J Emerg Med* 1999;**17**(1):145–56.

3 Miner JR, Martel ML, Meyer M, Reardon R, Biros MH. Procedural sedation of critically ill patients in the emergency department. *Acad Emerg Med* 2005;**12**(2):124–8.

4 Joint Council for the Accreditation of Healthcare Organizations. *Comprehensive Accreditation Manual for Hospitals, the Official Handbook.* JCAHO Publication, Chicago, 2004.

5 Green SM, Krauss B. The semantics of ketamine. *Acad Emerg Med* 2000;**36**:480–82.

6 Agrawal D, Manzi SF, Gupta R, Krauss B. Preprocedural fasting state and adverse events in children undergoing procedural sedation and analgesia in a pediatric emergency department. *Acad Emerg Med* 2003;**42**(5):636–46.

7 Treston G. Prolonged pre-procedure fasting time is unnecessary when using titrated intravenous ketamine for paediatric procedural sedation. *Emerg Med Australasia* 2004;**16**(2):145–50.

8 Roback MG, Bajaj L, Wathen JE, Bothner J. Preprocedural fasting and adverse events in procedural sedation and analgesia in a pediatric emergency department: are they related? *Ann Emerg Med* 2004;**44**(5):454–9.

9 Babl FE, Puspitadewi A, Barnett P, Oakley E, Spicer M. Pre-procedural fasting state and adverse events in children receiving nitrous oxide for procedural sedation and analgesia. *Pediatr Emerg Care* 2005;**21**(11):736–43.

10 Cheung KW, Watson M-L, Field S, Campbell SG. Aspiration pneumonitis requiring intubation after procedural sedation and analgesia: a case report. *Ann Emerg Med* 2007;**49**(4):462–4.

11 Green SM, Krauss B. Pulmonary aspiration risk during emergency department procedural sedation – an examination of the role of fasting and sedation depth. *Acad Emerg Med* 2002;**9**(1):35–42.

12 Green SM, Roback MG, Miner JR, Burton JH, Krauss B. Fasting and emergency department procedural sedation and analgesia: a consensus-based clinical practice advisory. *Ann Emerg Med* 2007;**49**(4):454–61.

13 Deitch K, Chudnofsky CR, Dominici P. The utility of supplemental oxygen during emergency department procedural sedation and analgesia with midazolam and fentanyl: a randomized, controlled trial. *Ann Emerg Med* 2007;**49**(1):1–8.

14 Miner JR, Heegaard W, Plummer D. End-tidal carbon dioxide monitoring during procedural sedation. *Acad Emerg Med* 2002;**9**(4):275–80.

15 Miner JR, Biros MH, Heegaard W, Plummer D. Bispectral electroencephalographic analysis of patients undergoing procedural sedation in the emergency department. *Acad Emerg Med* 2003;**10**(6):638–43.

16 Miner JR, Biros M, Krieg S, Johnson C, Heegaard W, Plummer D. Randomized clinical trial of propofol versus methohexital for procedural sedation during fracture and dislocation reduction in the emergency department. *Acad Emerg Med* 2003;**10**(9):931–7.

17 Fu ES, Downs JB, Schweiger JW, Miguel RV, Smith RA. Supplemental oxygen impairs detection of hypoventilation by pulse oximetry. *Chest* 2004;**126**(5):1552–8.

18 Stemp LI, Ramsay MA. Pulse oximetry in the detection of hypercapnia. *Am J Emerg Med* 2006;**24**(1):136–7.

19 Green SM. Research advances in procedural sedation and analgesia. *Ann Emerg Med* 2007;**49**(1):31–6.

20 American Society of Anesthesiologists. Practice guidelines for sedation and analgesia by non-anesthesiologists. *Anesthesiology* 2002;**96**(4):1004–17.

21 Yldzdas D, Yapcoglu H, Ylmaz HL. The value of capnography during sedation or sedation/analgesia in pediatric minor procedures. *Pediatr Emerg Care* 2004;**20**(3):162–5.

22 Burton JH, Harrah JD, Germann CA, Dillon DC. Does end-tidal carbon dioxide monitoring detect respiratory events prior to current sedation monitoring practices? *Acad Emerg Med* 2006;**13**(5):500–504.

23 Anderson JL, Junkins E, Pribble C, Guenther E. Capnography and depth of sedation during propofol sedation in children. *Ann Emerg Med* 2007;**49**(1):9–13.

24 Messenger DW, Sivilotti MLA, van Vlymen J, Dungey PE, Murray HE. Which alarms first during procedural sedation: the pulse oximeter or the capnograph? (Abstract). *Can J Emerg Med* 2007;**9**(3):186.

25 Krauss B, Hess DR. Capnography for procedural sedation and analgesia in the emergency department. *Ann Emerg Med* 2007;**50**(2):172–81.

26 Falk J, Zed PJ. Etomidate for procedural sedation in the emergency department. *Ann Pharmacother* 2004;**38**:1272–7.

27 Bond K, Karkhaneh M, Spooner C, et al. *Short-acting Procedural Sedation Agents in Canadian Emergency Departments (Technology overview).* Canadian Agency for Drugs and Technologies in Health, Ottawa, 2008.

28 Green SM. Research advances in procedural sedation and analgesia. *Ann Emerg Med* 2007;**49**(1):31–6.

29 Wilbur K, Zed PJ. Is propofol an optimal agent for procedural sedation and rapid sequence intubation in the emergency department? *Can J Emerg Med* 2001;**3**(4):302–10.

30 Messenger DW, Murray HE, Dungey PE, Van Vlymen J, Sivilotti MLA. Low-dose ketamine versus fentanyl as adjunct analgesic to procedural sedation with propofol: a randomized, clinical trial. *Can J Emerg Med* 2007;**9**(3):183.

55 Wound Repair

Helen Ouyang[1] & James Quinn[2]

[1]Department of Emergency Medicine, Brigham and Women's Hospital *and* Massachusetts General Hospital, Boston, USA
[2]Division of Emergency Medicine, Stanford University, Stanford, USA

Case scenario

A 20-year-old man arrived in the emergency department (ED) after being bitten on his hand by a stray dog 2 hours prior to presentation. There were two lacerations, each approximately 2 cm long, on the dorsal side of his right hand. The patient had cleaned out the wound with hydrogen peroxide and wrapped his hand loosely with gauze on the way to the hospital. The patient did not think there were any retained foreign bodies. The incident was not witnessed.

The physical examination revealed two bite wounds, 1 cm apart and each approximately 2 cm long, on the dorsal side of his right hand located equidistant between the metacarpophalangeal joint of his first finger and the radial carpal bone. There was no evidence of any foreign bodies in the wound. The wound site was wrapped in clean, bloody gauze and was not acutely bleeding at the time of presentation. The patient was in obvious pain. The necessary nerve and motor function tests were all normal. The remainder of the physical examination was normal. A plain radiograph of the hand confirmed the absence of radio-opaque foreign bodies. The patient had been fully immunized and had never had any medical problems prior to this. He also denied any drug allergies and was not on any medications.

While you provided appropriate oral analgesics and a tetanus shot, the patient expressed concern about infection. The intern with you asked about possibly using adhesives rather than sutures because of the patient's present discomfort. The medical student with you asked if it is even necessary to close the wound because she heard in lecture that all dog-bite wounds should be left open.

Background

Traumatic wounds are common presentations in the ED, accounting for 7.27 million visits per year in the USA, which is equivalent

Evidence-based Emergency Medicine. Edited by Brian H. Rowe
© 2009 Blackwell Publishing, ISBN: 978-1-4051-6143-5.

to roughly 9% of all injury-related ED presentations [1]. The main goals of wound management are to avoid infection, preserve prior motor and nerve functions, and to achieve the optimal cosmetic outcome. In the ED, the most common patient population to present with open wounds is that of young men [2]. Anatomically, upper extremity lacerations present most frequently (35%), followed by the face (28%), trunk (14.5%), lower extremity (12.5%) and head and neck (10%) [3]. More than 50% of all lacerations are caused by blunt injury, and the majority of the rest are caused by sharp objects [4,5]. Mammalian bites make up 5% of total traumatic wounds presenting to the ED and account for 1% of all ED visits [2]. The vast majority of these bite wounds are from dogs [6].

Emergency physicians should develop an organized approach to the diagnosis and treatment of wounds. A history, physical examination (including assessing neurovascular integrity and bone/joint involvement) and decisions regarding closure are critical to the success of the management plan. Given the high prevalence of lacerations and variety of treatment options and practice patterns, a review of the evidence including new wound closure methods, as well as controversies surrounding the treatment of mammalian bites, are outlined.

Clinical questions

1 In adults with a new wound from a dog bite (population), does healing by secondary intention (intervention) result in a decreased rate of infection (outcome) compared to primary closure (control)?

2 In adults with traumatic lacerations (population), does the use of tissue adhesives (intervention) result in similar healing (outcome) compared to traditional wound closure methods (control)?

3 In adult patients presenting with traumatic lacerations (population), does irrigating with tap water (intervention) result in similar rates of infection and healing (outcome) compared with other irrigation solutions or none at all (control)?

4 In adults presenting to the ED with a traumatic laceration (population), does using clean non-sterile gloves (intervention) versus sterile gloves (control) result in similar infection rates (outcome)?

5 In adults presenting to the ED with a traumatic laceration (population), are topical anesthetics (intervention) efficacious and safe (outcome) compared to traditional injected anesthetics (control)?

6 In adults presenting to the ED with a traumatic laceration (population), does the use of warmed anesthetic (intervention) minimize injection pain (outcome) compared to anesthetic at room temperature (control)?

7 In adults presenting to the ED with a traumatic laceration (population), does the use of anesthetic with bicarbonate (intervention) minimize injection pain without increasing infection rates (outcome) compared to anesthetic without bicarbonate (control)?

8 In adults presenting to the ED with a traumatic laceration (population), does the use of topical antibiotic ointment (intervention) minimize infection rates and maximize cosmetic outcome (outcomes) compared to no antibiotic (control)?

9 In adult patients with dog-bite wounds (population), does the use of prophylactic antibiotics (intervention) prevent wound infection (outcome) compared to standard wound cleaning alone (control)?

General search strategy

You begin to address these questions by searching for evidence in the common electronic databases such as the Cochrane Library and MEDLINE looking specifically for systematic reviews and meta-analyses. The Cochrane Database of Systematic Reviews includes high-quality systematic review evidence on the treatment of traumatic lacerations. You also search the Cochrane Central Register of Controlled Trials (CENTRAL) and MEDLINE to identify randomized controlled trials that became available after the publication date of the systematic review or, if no systematic reviews were identified, to locate high-quality randomized controlled trials or observational studies that directly address the clinical question. In addition, access to relevant, updated, evidence-based clinical practice guidelines (CPGs) is used to determine the consensus rating of areas lacking evidence.

Critical review of the literature:

Question 1: In adults with a new wound from a dog bite (population), does healing by secondary intention (intervention) result in a decreased rate of infection (outcome) compared to primary closure (control)?

Search strategy

- MEDLINE: (primary closure AND mammalian bites) OR (primary closure AND dog bites)

There has been ongoing controversy surrounding the question of primary closure of mammalian bites, specifically those from canines. Physicians often have reservations about primarily closing wounds due to the possibility of a higher rate of infection, though if no infection develops, closing the wound would be expected to result in a better cosmetic outcome. Since no official guidelines exist, practitioners must rely on their clinical judgment. Some authors recommend that bite wounds to the hand should be left open, while those afflicted at other anatomic sites may be treated by primary closure after thorough cleansing [7].

Because dog bites are most common, the majority of studies regarding mammalian bites enrolled lacerations caused by canines. Although the search strategy failed to identify any high-quality systematic reviews that would allow definitive conclusions, there have been three studies in the ED setting that may help elucidate some of these issues.

We identified one controlled trial that randomized ED patients with dog bites to either primary closure or leaving the wound open [8]. A total of 169 dog-bite lacerations were included, with 77 left open and 92 sutured [8]. The lacerations were surgically debrided and irrigated; however, no prophylactic antibiotics were provided. Infection developed in 7.8% of wounds treated by leaving the wound open and 7.6% of sutured wounds (RR = 1.02; 95% CI: 0.36 to 2.92). The investigators noted that more wound infections occurred in the hand compared to other anatomic locations, in both the control and intervention groups ($P < 0.01$). In the subgroup analysis including only hand wounds, more became infected in the group whose wounds were closed primarily (17%) compared to those left open (9%) [8].

A prospective, observational cohort study enrolled 145 consecutive mammalian-bite patients (88 dog bites) treated with primary closure; 87% received high-pressure irrigation and 81% were discharged with oral antibiotics. At the time of suture removal, eight of the 145 patients developed infection (5.5%; 95% CI: 1.8% to 9.2%); four of these infections were located on the head and four were located on the upper extremity. The authors concluded that an infection rate of 5.5% is acceptable if cosmesis is a priority [9].

Finally, when considering hand lacerations in general, one should consider that the results of one randomized controlled trial comparing 2 cm hand lacerations closed with sutures compared to those treated conservatively with a bandage had similar cosmetic and functional outcomes, indicating that allowing small hand wounds to heal by secondary intention is an acceptable practice [10].

In summary, based on the limited evidence available, it is reasonable to conclude that physicians should consider avoiding primary closure of mammalian bite wounds of the hand whenever possible. If cosmetic outcome is important to the patient and the wound does not involve the hand, it may be desirable to close primarily or consider delayed closure.

Question 2: In adults with traumatic lacerations (population), does the use of tissue adhesives (intervention) result in similar healing (outcome) compared to traditional wound closure methods (control)?

Search strategy

- Cochrane Library: traumatic lacerations AND tissue adhesives
- MEDLINE: tissue adhesives AND standard wound closure

Tissue adhesives have been available and used for years to effectively close traumatic lacerations, and many studies have tried to determine how they compare to traditional wound closure methods. A Cochrane systematic review was identified that included 10 randomized controlled trials involving 1053 lacerations. These studies compared tissue adhesives to traditional wound closure methods, and used cosmesis as the primary outcome. There were no differences between tissue adhesives and traditional wound closure methods for cosmesis outcomes. The authors concluded that tissue adhesives are comparable to sutures, staples or tape for closure of simple lacerations and may be a better alternative as a pain-free method that requires no follow-up for removal [11]. Cosmetic outcome studies generally use either the cosmetic visual analog scale (CVAS) or the wound evaluation score (WES). Research has shown that early cosmesis scores at 7–14 days correlate poorly with late scores at 6–9 months [12,13]; however, no significant difference was found in short- or long-term outcomes using either of these scoring systems. Besides cosmetic outcome, complications such as dehiscence, induration, erythema, discharge and the need for delayed closure are all important secondary outcomes (Fig. 55.1). Tissue adhesives result in a slightly higher baseline risk of dehiscence (risk difference = 0.02; 95% CI: 0.0 to 0.05) with a lower risk of erythema (risk difference = −0.10; 95% CI: −0.19 to 0.0).

A meta-analysis published in 2004 compared 2-octylcyanoacrylate (OCA) tissue adhesive with standard wound closure and reached similar conclusions [14]. Cosmetic outcomes were equivalent with both techniques and the overall dehiscence rate was 0.9% with OCA compared to 0.3% with standard wound closure [14].

A study of patient priorities in traumatic lacerations showed that avoidance of infection, normal function, cosmetic outcome and least painful repair are the most important to patients [15,16]. In fact, there have been two studies that allowed the patient to rate their own scars rather than, or in addition to, an independent evaluator like a plastic surgeon [17,18]. In the first study, the investigators found that cosmetic outcomes of wounds treated with OCA were the same as with standard techniques using a patient-based

rating system (83.8 ± 19.4 mm vs 82.5 ± 17.6 mm, $P = 0.72$), which was congruent with physician ratings [17]. In the other study, 25 women underwent bilateral breast surgery in which one breast was closed with sutures and the other with OCA; 24 of the women (95%) felt the side closed with the tissue adhesive had a better cosmetic outcome and preferred it to sutures [18]. Tissue adhesives also have the added advantage of providing an antimicrobial dressing and can be used as a dressing to cover sutures and reinforce wounds closed with adjuncts such as surgical tapes [19]. Care must be taken in using adhesives alone in high-tension wounds.

In summary, based on the available evidence, patients who are ideal candidates for tissue adhesives are those who present with simple, low-tension lacerations. They should especially be considered in those patients who are to not likely return for follow-up for suture removal or who cannot tolerate the pain of traditional sutures.

Question 3: In adult patients presenting with traumatic lacerations (population), does irrigating with tap water (intervention) result in similar rates of infection and healing (outcome) compared with other irrigation solutions or none at all (control)?

Search strategy

- Cochrane Library and MEDLINE: wounds AND irrigation

While sterile normal saline is commonly used in the ED for irrigation, it has been questioned whether tap water is equally effective compared to normal saline. Traditionally, sterile normal saline was preferred due to its isotonicity, which is thought to not interfere with the body's normal healing process [20,21]. A Cochrane systematic review assessing the effectiveness of tap water cleansing included three controlled trials involving 1162 patients (Fig. 55.2) [22]. The pooled results failed to identify a clinically important or statistically significant difference in the rates of infection (RR = 1.07; 95% CI: 0.43 to 2.64); however, the single trial including adult patients reported lower infection rates in wounds cleaned with tap water compared with normal saline (RR = 0.55; 95% CI: 0.31 to 0.97) [23]. It is important to note, however, that the two solutions were administered at different temperatures – the tap water at 37°C and the normal saline at room temperature and no control for volume or pressure was reported [22]. The other two trials measured infection rates in children and the pooled results demonstrate no statistically significant difference in using the two solutions [22,24,25].

A large, multi-center, prospective study conducted among three different hospitals compared infection rates of wounds irrigated with normal saline compared to tap water. The infection rates between the two different solutions were equivalent; 12 (4%) of the 300 subjects in the tap water group had wound infections

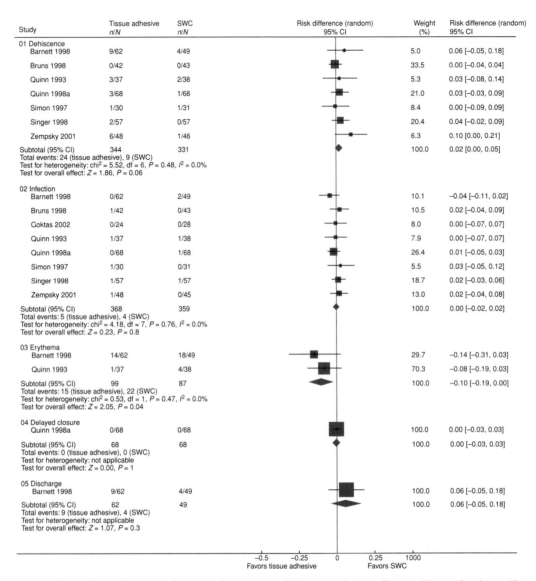

Study	Tissue adhesive n/N	SWC n/N	Risk difference (random) 95% CI	Weight (%)	Risk difference (random) 95% CI
01 Dehiscence					
Barnett 1998	9/62	4/49		5.0	0.06 [−0.05, 0.18]
Bruns 1998	0/42	0/43		33.5	0.00 [−0.04, 0.04]
Quinn 1993	3/37	2/38		5.3	0.03 [−0.08, 0.14]
Quinn 1998a	3/68	1/68		21.0	0.03 [−0.03, 0.09]
Simon 1997	1/30	1/31		8.4	0.00 [−0.09, 0.09]
Singer 1998	2/57	0/57		20.4	0.04 [−0.02, 0.09]
Zempsky 2001	6/48	1/46		6.3	0.10 [0.00, 0.21]
Subtotal (95% CI)	344	331		100.0	0.02 [0.00, 0.05]
Total events: 24 (tissue adhesive), 9 (SWC)					
Test for heterogeneity: chi² = 5.52, df = 6, P = 0.48, I² = 0.0%					
Test for overall effect: Z = 1.86, P = 0.06					
02 Infection					
Barnett 1998	0/62	2/49		10.1	−0.04 [−0.11, 0.02]
Bruns 1998	1/42	0/43		10.5	0.02 [−0.04, 0.09]
Goktas 2002	0/24	0/28		8.0	0.00 [−0.07, 0.07]
Quinn 1993	1/37	1/38		7.9	0.00 [−0.07, 0.07]
Quinn 1998a	0/68	1/68		26.4	0.01 [−0.05, 0.03]
Simon 1997	1/30	0/31		5.5	0.03 [−0.05, 0.12]
Singer 1998	1/57	1/57		18.7	0.02 [−0.03, 0.06]
Zempsky 2001	1/48	0/45		13.0	0.02 [−0.04, 0.08]
Subtotal (95% CI)	368	359		100.0	0.00 [−0.02, 0.02]
Total events: 5 (tissue adhesive), 4 (SWC)					
Test for heterogeneity: chi² = 4.18, df = 7, P = 0.76, I² = 0.0%					
Test for overall effect: Z = 0.23, P = 0.8					
03 Erythema					
Barnett 1998	14/62	18/49		29.7	−0.14 [−0.31, 0.03]
Quinn 1993	1/37	4/38		70.3	−0.08 [−0.19, 0.03]
Subtotal (95% CI)	99	87		100.0	−0.10 [−0.19, 0.00]
Total events: 15 (tissue adhesive), 22 (SWC)					
Test for heterogeneity: chi² = 0.53, df = 1, P = 0.47, I² = 0.0%					
Test for overall effect: Z = 2.05, P = 0.04					
04 Delayed closure					
Quinn 1998a	0/68	0/68		100.0	0.00 [−0.03, 0.03]
Subtotal (95% CI)	68	68		100.0	0.00 [−0.03, 0.03]
Total events: 0 (tissue adhesive), 0 (SWC)					
Test for heterogeneity: not applicable					
Test for overall effect: Z = 0.00, P = 1					
05 Discharge					
Barnett 1998	9/62	4/49		100.0	0.06 [−0.05, 0.18]
Subtotal (95% CI)	62	49		100.0	0.06 [−0.05, 0.18]
Total events: 9 (tissue adhesive), 4 (SWC)					
Test for heterogeneity: not applicable					
Test for overall effect: Z = 1.07, P = 0.3					

−0.5 −0.25 0 0.25 1000
Favors tissue adhesive   Favors SWC

Figure 55.1 Comparison of tissue adhesives for traumatic lacerations, showing increased dehiscence with tissue adhesive and increased erythema with standard wound closure (SWC). (Reproduced with permission from Farion et al. [11], © Wiley.)

compared with 11 (3.3%) of the 334 subjects in the saline group (RR = 1.21; 95% CI: 0.5 to 2.7) [26].

In summary, tap water appears to be a viable, cost-effective alternative to sterile normal saline for wound irrigation in the ED. Despite the fact that the published trials have inconsistent methods (e.g., differences in temperature, volume and irrigation pressure) there appears to be no benefit to sterile saline over clean tap water.

Question 4: In adults presenting to the ED with a traumatic laceration (population), does using clean non-sterile gloves (intervention) versus sterile gloves (control) result in similar infection rates (outcome)?

Search strategy

- MEDLINE: sterile gloves

In North America, sterile techniques such as the routine use of sterile gloves have been adopted from standard surgical practice and applied to the management of lacerations in the ED. The search strategy above identified one prospective randomized study [27] that challenges previously published recommendations for using sterile gloves in the ED setting [28]. This tri-center study enrolled 816 patients presenting to the ED with uncomplicated lacerations; those who had pre-existing risk factors for wound infection or

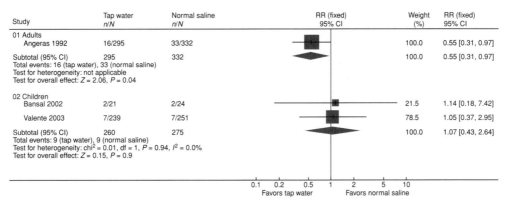

Study	Tap water n/N	Normal saline n/N	RR (fixed) 95% CI	Weight (%)	RR (fixed) 95% CI
01 Adults					
Angeras 1992	16/295	33/332		100.0	0.55 [0.31, 0.97]
Subtotal (95% CI)	295	332		100.0	0.55 [0.31, 0.97]
Total events: 16 (tap water), 33 (normal saline)					
Test for heterogeneity: not applicable					
Test for overall effect: Z = 2.06, P = 0.04					
02 Children					
Bansal 2002	2/21	2/24		21.5	1.14 [0.18, 7.42]
Valente 2003	7/239	7/251		78.5	1.05 [0.37, 2.95]
Subtotal (95% CI)	260	275		100.0	1.07 [0.43, 2.64]
Total events: 9 (tap water), 9 (normal saline)					
Test for heterogeneity: chi² = 0.01, df = 1, P = 0.94, I² = 0.0%					
Test for overall effect: Z = 0.15, P = 0.9					

0.1   0.2   0.5   1   2   5   10
Favors tap water   Favors normal saline

Figure 55.2 Comparison of infection rates in wounds cleaned with tap water compared to normal saline. (Reproduced with permission from Fernandez et al. [22], © Wiley.)

who were determined to require prophylactic antibiotics (e.g., bites, contaminated wounds) were excluded. A block randomization scheme based on anatomic site of the laceration was used and follow-up at the time of suture removal was successful in 96% of those who were randomized. There was no difference between the two treatment options (RR = 1.37; 95% CI: 0.75 to 2.52); the observed infection rate was 6.1% among those randomized to sterile gloves compared to 4.4% among those randomized to clean gloves [27].

In summary, this multi-center, prospective, single-blinded, randomized trial suggests that the use of non-sterile clean gloves for treating simple lacerations in a patient with no pre-existing risk factors is acceptable. In the USA, the estimated cost for clean gloves is $0.10 per pair versus $0.70 for sterile gloves, indicating relative cost savings and convenience.

Question 5: In adults presenting to the ED with a traumatic laceration (population), are topical anesthetics (intervention) efficacious and safe (outcome) compared to traditional injected anesthetics (control)?

Search strategy

• MEDLINE: topical anesthetics

Pain control during the repair of traumatic lacerations is conventionally performed through local anesthetic infiltration, which causes additional pain for patients already in discomfort and distress [29]. This often makes repair difficult for the physician, especially for pediatric patients. The first report of successful topical anesthetic use for laceration repair was published in 1980 [30], but since then questions have been raised regarding its effectiveness for pain control, time to anesthetic effect, and adverse events related to topical mixtures containing cocaine.

One systematic review of randomized controlled trials was identified, which included 25 trials and involved 2096 subjects [31].

The primary outcome was efficacy of analgesia measured by patients' self-reports of pain intensity. The authors compared the efficacy of each topical anesthetic with traditional injected local anesthetic. In addition, they compared the efficacy of each topical amide or ester local anesthetic with an eutectic mixture of local anesthetics (EMLA), which consists of prilocaine and lidocaine, and was the first commercially available and most frequently used topical anesthetic [32,33]. Due to both statistical and clinical heterogeneity among trials, the investigators determined that it was inappropriate to pool results. Clinical heterogeneity included anatomic location, depth of dermal instrumentation and selection of various patient populations. Not surprisingly, the results were also inconsistent – half of the studies favored EMLA with regard to anesthetic efficacy, whereas the other half favored infiltrated local anesthetic [31]. Besides the efficacy of EMLA compared to traditional anesthetics, the authors also reviewed trials comparing topical amide and ester anesthetics with EMLA. Despite the pooled results that topical tetracaine and liposomal lidocaine both provided greater anesthesia than EMLA based on a 100 mm visual analog scale (VAS) (weighted mean difference (WMD) = −8.1 and −10.9 mm, respectively), these differences are likely not clinically important [31]. Since liposomal lidocaine does provide a more rapid onset than EMLA (30 vs 60 minutes) [34], it may be a preferred option considering the time constraints of the ED.

Because the delayed onset of anesthesia for topical analgesics currently cannot be circumvented, some studies have been conducted on pre-treating lacerations at triage with topical anesthesia, especially in pediatric patients or less pain-tolerant patients. This algorithm was initially studied by Singer and Stark in their trial of pre-treating lacerations with LET (lidocaine, epinephrine, tetracaine) by triage nurses. The patients in the LET group were more frequently anesthesized (RR = 3.18; 95% CI: 1.01 to 9.98) and experienced less pain from subsequent lidocaine injection (22 vs 44 mm on VAS, P = 0.02) [35]. One prospective, randomized, double-blinded, controlled trial in a pediatric ED in Australia found that those pre-treated with topical anesthesia reduced median treatment time by 31 minutes versus placebo (95% CI: 15 to

47 minutes). In this trial, those treated with topical anesthesia did not have further treatment with topical or infiltrated anesthesia after triage [36].

Concern has also been raised about the content of cocaine in some topical anesthetic mixtures, especially when one study found that the standard application of TAC (tetracaine, adrenaline, cocaine) solution results in a measurable, albeit low, cocaine level in 75% of children [37]. In one prospective, randomized, double-blinded trial, no statistically significant difference was demonstrated in the effectiveness of tetraphen (non-cocaine topical anesthetic) compared to TAC [38]. It appears that 4% or 5% lidocaine, bupivanor and tetraphen have similar effectiveness to TAC [39]. In addition, a study comparing TLE (topical lidocaine and epinephrine) with TAC found them to be equivalent in efficacy, 2.66 mm versus 3.29 mm, respectively ($P = 0.33$). Furthermore, the cost of TAC is US\$27 versus \$0.80 for TLE, which would have saved this study hospital nearly \$60,000 in annual costs if TLE was used instead of TAC [40].

In summary, current topical anesthetic mixtures appear to be as effective as traditional infiltrated lidocaine in vascular areas of the body and the questionable safety of cocaine may be less of an issue as newer cocaine-free agents appear to be of equivalent efficacy. Although some of the studies were conducted primarily in the pediatric population, there is no plausible reason to believe that the results in adult populations would be different. By using topical, cocaine-free anesthesia at triage, both time and money can be saved, with a quicker reduction of time to pain control and as an adjunct if infiltration is needed.

Question 6: In adults presenting to the ED with a traumatic laceration (population), does the use of warmed anesthetic (intervention) minimize injection pain (outcome) compared to anesthetic at room temperature (control)?

Search strategy

- MEDLINE: (warmed AND local anesthetic) OR (temperature AND local anesthetic)

Various techniques have been investigated to minimize the pain upon injection of anesthetics, including warming the anesthetic solution as opposed to using it at conventional room temperature. In one double-blind, randomized controlled study of 26 subjects, each patient was injected with solutions at both temperatures of 40 and 21°C. The mean difference in pain score between the room temperature and warmed solutions was 15 mm on a 100 mm VAS, which was statistically significant; however, of the 21 subjects who found the warmed solution less painful, only about half (11) thought the reduction of pain was clinically important [41]. In another double-blind, randomized controlled study of 157 patients, each subject was injected with local anesthetic at either 21 or 37°C. Using a VAS to assess pain, the authors concluded that there was

no significant difference in the level of pain experienced by the two groups [42].

In another study, 136 patients were assigned to receive anesthetic solutions at four increasing temperatures: 10, 18, 37 and 42°C. The authors concluded that warming the anesthetic solution significantly reduced pain, especially at 42°C. In another randomized, double-blind, controlled study limited to digital nerve blocks on 20 subjects, those who were randomly assigned to the 42°C injection experienced a statistically significant decrease in pain of 10.5 mm on the VAS [43]. Yet in another randomized, double-blind, crossover study, 20 subjects reported that room temperature buffered lidocaine was more painful, while 17 reported that the 37°C solution was more painful ($P = 0.74$). The median pain score increase of 5 mm on the 100 mm VAS favoring warm lidocaine was not statistically significant ($P = 0.42$) [44].

The evidence is disparate regarding whether warming anesthetic solution reduces pain of local infiltration; however, there does appear to be a dose response to increasing temperature. While it appears that increasing the temperature of the local anesthetic over 40°C reduces pain more, one must also bear in mind that even warmed lidocaine that is maintained at 43°C drops to approximately 37°C after drawing up in a syringe and injecting within 20–30 seconds [45]. In addition, review of the literature suggests that a difference in the 100 mm pain VAS only becomes clinically significant at or greater than 10 mm [46–48]. Many of the studies failed to reach this clinically important threshold. In summary, it seems reasonable to conclude that the time and cost needed to heat these anesthetic solutions prior to infiltration may outweigh the clinical benefits.

Question 7: In adults presenting to the ED with a traumatic laceration (population), does the use of anesthetic with bicarbonate (intervention) minimize injection pain without increasing infection rates (outcome) compared to anesthetic without bicarbonate?

Search strategy

- MEDLINE: (buffer AND local anesthetic) OR (bicarbonate AND local anesthetic)

In addition to heating lidocaine to minimize pain upon infiltration of local anesthesia, practitioners have considered buffering the solution to reduce the pain of injection. Several authors have suggested that the buffering of local anesthetics decreases pain upon infiltration [49,50]. Yet, because buffering decreases the shelf life of anesthetics, as well as increasing time and inconvenience, it is uncertain whether the benefit gained from pain reduction is effective enough to incorporate buffering into routine ED practice.

In a double-blind, paired clinical study in which 60 subjects each received both buffered and plain lidocaine solution, the pain score was 5.2 mm higher for the plain solution, which was neither statistically or clinically significant [51]. Similarly, in another randomized, double-blind, paired study, 30 subjects were each infiltrated with both plain and buffered diphenhydramine. The difference in pain scores was only 4.7 mm, and was not statistically significant [52].

One double-blind, prospective study of 62 subjects in which each volunteer was injected with both buffered and unbuffered bupivicaine concluded that the mean pain score for the buffered agent was 8 mm lower than the unbuffered one, which did reach statistical significance [53]. In another randomized, double-blind study of 25 volunteers, each subject was injected with plain and buffered lidocaine, lidocaine with epinephrine, and mepivacaine. While the buffered solutions were all statistically significantly less painful, the largest mean difference in VAS was 5.1 mm [54]. Once again, it is important to keep in mind that multiple studies have shown that a pain score difference has to be at least 10 mm on the VAS to be clinically significant.

Past studies have also suggested that both warming and buffering local anesthetic infiltration may have a synergistic effect [55]. In one randomized, double-blind clinical trial, four different test solutions were included: plain lidocaine, warmed lidocaine, buffered lidocaine, and both warmed and buffered lidocaine [56]. The pain score on the VAS was lowest for the combined warmed and buffered lidocaine, averaging about 15 mm less than the room temperature plain lidocaine, leaving the authors to conclude that warming and buffering lidocaine in combination has the greatest clinical effect.

In summary, buffering of local anesthetics to minimize the pain of infiltration appears to provide minimal benefit. While the combination of both warming and buffering may provide slightly more relief, the decrease in pain with infiltration is still small. Given the time and cost of such preparations and lack of important clinical benefit, it is not recommended that they be routinely used in the ED.

Question 8: In adults presenting to the ED with a traumatic laceration (population), does the use of topical antibiotic ointment (intervention) minimize infection rates and maximize cosmetic outcome (outcomes) compared to no antibiotic (control)?

Search strategy

- MEDLINE: topical antibiotics AND wounds

A prospective, randomized, double-blind, placebo-controlled study was undertaken to evaluate the effectiveness of topical antibiotics versus a petrolatum control, as well as to compare the different infection rates among different antibiotics, namely topical bacitracin zinc, neomycin sulfate, polymyxin B sulfate combination (triple antibiotic ointment) and silver sulfadiazine. The results demonstrated that the wound infection rates for the topical antibiotics groups were lower than the petrolatum control: bacitracin 6/109 (5.5%), triple antibiotic 5/110 (4.5%), silver sulfadiazine 12/99 (12.1%) and petrolatum 19/108 (17.6%) [57].

Another study conducted among post-operative ambulatory surgery patients compared bacitracin ointment to petrolatum and found no significant difference in the rates of infection (relative difference = 1.1%; 95% CI: −0.4 to 2.7%). It must be emphasized, however, that this study was conducted among post-operative surgical wounds and not on traumatic lacerations.

Given the results of the trial conducted in the ED setting, topical antibiotics on traumatic wounds are recommended [57]. However, the duration of treatment has not been clarified in any clinical trials. Animal studies have suggested that basal cell migration, which is facilitated by a moist environment, is complete at 24–48 hours, thus essentially preventing surface contamination of wounds and thereby justifying the rationale for the use of topical antibiotics for only 48 hours [58]. Topical antibiotic ointments should not be applied on tissue adhesives as they may result in dehiscence [5].

Question 9: In adult patients with dog-bite wounds (population), does the use of prophylactic antibiotics (intervention) prevent wound infection (outcome) compared to standard wound cleaning alone (control)?

Search strategy

- Cochrane Library: antibiotics AND mammalian bites
- MEDLINE: bites AND antibiotics

The use of prophylactic antibiotics in dog bites has been an area of intense debate and research. In the past, clinicians have favored prophylactic antibiotics despite the paucity of randomized clinical trials and the problems related to various outcome measures for infection [59]. A Cochrane systematic review which addressed the use of prophylactic antibiotics in mammalian bites included eight randomized, or quasi-randomized, controlled trials that compared the use of antibiotics within 24 hours of injury to either placebo or no intervention; six of these trials were focused exclusively on dog bites [60]. The pooled results failed to identify a difference in the proportion of infections with the use of prophylactic antibiotics for dog bites (OR = 0.74; 95% CI: 0.30 to 1.85) compared to placebo. A subgroup analysis of hand bites demonstrated a significant reduction in the rate of infection among those treated with antibiotics (OR = 0.10; 95% CI: 0.01 to 0.86); however, the subgroup analysis was strongly influenced by one study with a very high baseline infection rate (47%) (Fig. 55.3). The authors of the Cochrane review concluded that prophylactic antibiotics should be strongly considered for hand bites.

A cost–benefit analysis of this topic concluded that treating all dog bites with prophylactic antibiotics was cost beneficial if the risk of wound infection is greater than 5% [61]. However, a clear definition of high-risk bite wounds is not available in the literature and sutured bite wounds on any location appear to be high risk. The risk of infection in hand wounds is inconsistent, although it appears to be greater than 5%.

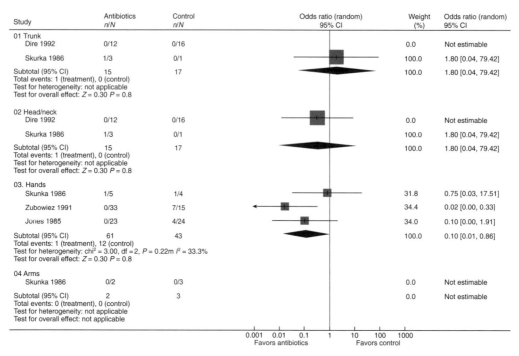

Study	Antibiotics n/N	Control n/N	Odds ratio (random) 95% CI	Weight (%)	Odds ratio (random) 95% CI
01 Trunk					
Dire 1992	0/12	0/16		0.0	Not estimable
Skurka 1986	1/3	0/1		100.0	1.80 [0.04, 79.42]
Subtotal (95% CI)	15	17		100.0	1.80 [0.04, 79.42]
Total events: 1 (treatment), 0 (control)					
Test for heterogeneity: not applicable					
Test for overall effect: $Z = 0.30$ $P = 0.8$					
02 Head/neck					
Dire 1992	0/12	0/16		0.0	Not estimable
Skurka 1986	1/3	0/1		100.0	1.80 [0.04, 79.42]
Subtotal (95% CI)	15	17		100.0	1.80 [0.04, 79.42]
Total events: 1 (treatment), 0 (control)					
Test for heterogeneity: not applicable					
Test for overall effect: $Z = 0.30$ $P = 0.8$					
03. Hands					
Skunka 1986	1/5	1/4		31.8	0.75 [0.03, 17.51]
Zubowiez 1991	0/33	7/15		34.4	0.02 [0.00, 0.33]
Jones 1985	0/23	4/24		34.0	0.10 [0.00, 1.91]
Subtotal (95% CI)	61	43		100.0	0.10 [0.01, 0.86]
Total events: 1 (treatment), 12 (control)					
Test for heterogeneity: chi² = 3.00, df = 2, $P = 0.22$m I² = 33.3%					
Test for overall effect: $Z = 0.30$ $P = 0.8$					
04 Arms					
Skunka 1986	0/2	0/3		0.0	Not estimable
Subtotal (95% CI)	2	3		0.0	Not estimable
Total events: 0 (treatment), 0 (control)					
Test for heterogeneity: not applicable					
Test for overall effect: not applicable					

0.001 0.01 0.1 1 10 100 1000
Favors antibiotics   Favors control

Figure 55.3 Comparison of mammalian bite infection rates with prophylactic antibiotics. (Reproduced with permission from Medeiros & Saconato [60], © Wiley.)

The selection of prophylactic antibiotic to prescribe has also been investigated. One multi-center, prospective study examined infected wounds from either dog or cat bites and found that *Pasteurella* species, particularly *Pasteurella canis*, were the most common pathogens and were isolated from half of all infected dog bites. Other species commonly isolated included streptococci, staphylococci, *Moraxella*, *Neisseria* and anaerobes [62]. Although there is a lack of strong evidence to support any particular antibiotic choice, these findings provide biological plausibility supporting the use of a β-lactam antibiotic-like amoxicillin combined with a β-lactamase inhibitor (amoxicillin/clavulanic acid) [63].

In summary, prophylactic antibiotics should be strongly considered in dog bites at high risk of infection. To date, these appear to be primarily dog bites to the hand. Wounds that are sutured may also be at higher risk; however, further research is needed to determine reliable clinical predictors of infection. If antibiotics are used, a reasonable choice would be a β-lactam combined with a β-lactamase inhibitor. For simple lacerations, there is no benefit to the routine use of systemic prophylactic antibiotics because the baseline infection rate in simple lacerations is low [5,64].

and he was prescribed amoxicillin/clavulinic acid. Since the intern expressed concern regarding the patient's discomfort, topical anesthetics could have been considered and applied at triage. Buffering or warming injectable lidocaine or bupivcaine may have provided a very small benefit in terms of pain at the injections site. Irrigation with normal saline was reasonable since his wound was more complicated than a simple laceration and data on tap water in complex wounds is unclear. For the same reason, use of sterile gloves was appropriate given that the trial reviewed did not include patients who had more complex injuries like bites or patients discharged with antibiotics.

Had this been a simple laceration, his wound may have been irrigated with tap water and closed with sutures using clean, nonsterile gloves. For animal bites, especially involving the hand, there is evidence to support conservative treatment using a gauze bandage with antibiotic ointment. Wound closure with tissue adhesives is primarily reserved for low-tension areas such as the face and there is a lack of research to support its use in animal bites. The evidence supports the use of systemic antibiotics in this patient with a dog bite to the hand; however, antibiotics are not indicated for routine simple lacerations.

Conclusions

The patient in this case scenario had his hand infiltrated with lidocaine, the wound was irrigated with normal saline and explored using sterile gloves, and left open for secondary closure,

Conflicts of interest

None were declared by Dr. Ouyang. Dr. Quinn is a consultant for Chemence Medical Products Incorporated, the maker of tissue adhesives, and Ethicon Inc. He has also received speaking fees from Ethicon Inc., the makers of tissue adhesives and sutures.

References

1 McCaig LF, Ly N. National Hospital Ambulatory Medical Care Survey: 2000 emergency department summary. Advance Data from Vital and Health Statistics, No 326, April 22, 2002. Available at http://www.cdc.gov/nchs/data/ad/ad326.pdf (accessed Dec 20, 2006).

2 Hollander JE, Singer AJ, Valentine S, Henry MC. Wound registry: development and validation. *Ann Emerg Med* 1995;**25**:675–85.

3 Singer AJ, Thode HC, Jr., Hollander JE. National trends in ED lacerations between 1992 and 2002. *Am J Emerg Med* 2006;**24**:183–8.

4 Edlich RF, Rodeheaver GT, Morgan RF, Berman DE, Thacker JG. Principles of emergency wound management. *Ann Emerg Med* 1988;**17**:1284–302.

5 Hollander JE, Singer AJ. State of the art laceration management. *Ann Emerg Med* 1999;**34**:356–67.

6 Goldstein EJC. Bite wounds and infection. *Clin Infect Dis* 1992;**14**: 633–40.

7 Garbutt F, Jenner R. Best evidence topic report. Wound closure in animal bites. *Emerg Med J* 2004;**21**:589–90.

8 Maimaris C, Quinton DN. Dog-bite lacerations: a controlled trial of primary wound closure. *Arch Emerg Med* 1988;**5**:156–61.

9 Chen E, Hornig S, Shepherd SM, Hollander JE. Primary closure of mammalian bites. *Acad Emerg Med* 2000;**8**:157–61.

10 Quinn J, Cummings S, Callaham M, Sellers K. Suturing versus conservative management of lacerations for the hand: randomised controlled trial. *BMJ* 2002;**10**: 325:299.

11 Farion K, Osmond MH, Hartling L, et al. Tissue adhesives for traumatic lacerations in children and adults. *Cochrane Database Syst Rev* 2002;**3**:CD003326.

12 Hollander JE, Blasko B, Singer AJ, Valentine S, Thode HC, Jr., Henry MC. Poor correlation of short- and long-term cosmetic appearance of repaired lacerations. *Acad Emerg Med* 1995;**12**:983–7.

13 Quinn J, Wells G, Sutcliffe T, et al. Tissue adhesive versus suture wound repair at 1 year: randomized clinical trial correlating early, 3-month, and 1-year cosmetic outcome. *Ann Emerg Med* 1998;**32**:645–9.

14 Singer AJ, Thode HC, Jr. A review of the literature on octylcyanoacrylate tissue adhesive. *Am J Surg* 2004;**187**:238–48.

15 Quinn JV. Clinical wound evaluation. *Acad Emerg Med* 1996;**3**:298–9.

16 Singer AJ, Mach C, Thode HC, Jr., Hemachandra S, Shofer FS, Hollander JE. Patient priorities with traumatic lacerations. *Am J Emerg Med* 2000;**18**:683–6.

17 Singer AJ, Hollander JE, Valentine SM, Turque TW, McCuskey CF, Quinn JV. Prospective, randomized, controlled trial of tissue adhesive (2-octylcyanoacrylate) vs standard wound closure techniques for laceration repair. Stony Brook Octylcyanoacrylate Study Group. *Acad Emerg Med* 1998;**5**:94–9.

18 Bazell GM, Boschert MT, Concannon MJ, Puckett CL. Reduction mammoplasty incision closure with octyl-2-cyanoacrylate (Abstract). *South Med J* 2000;**3**(Suppl):79S–80S.

19 Bhende S, Rothenburger S, Spangler DJ, Dito M. In vitro assessment of microbial barrier properties of Dermabond topical skin adhesives. *Surg Infect* 2002;**3**:251–7.

20 Lawrence JC. Wound irrigation. *J Wound Care* 1997;**6**:23–6.

21 Philips D, Davey C. Wound cleansing versus wound disinfection: a challenging dilemma. *Perspectives* 1997;**21**:15–16.

22 Fernandez R, Griffiths R, Ussia C. Water for wound cleansing. *Cochrane Database Syst Rev* 2002;**4**:CD003861.

23 Angeras MH, Brandberg A, Falk A, Seeman T. Comparison between sterile saline and tap water for the cleaning of acute traumatic soft tissue wounds. *Eur J Surg* 1992;**158**:347–50.

24 Bansal BC, Wiebe RA, Perkins SD, Abramo TJ. Tap water for irrigation of lacerations. *Am J Emerg Med* 2002;**20**:469–72.

25 Valente JH, Forti RJ, Freundlich LF, Zandieh SO, Crain EF. Wound irrigation in children: saline solution or tap water? *Ann Emerg Med* 2003;**41**:609–16.

26 Moscati RM, Mayrose J, Reardon RF, Janicke DM, Jehle DV. A multicenter comparison of tap water versus sterile saline for wound irrigation. *Acad Emerg Med* 2007;**14**:404–9.

27 Perelman VS, Francis GJ, Rutledge T, Foote J, Martino F, Dranitsaris G. Sterile versus nonsterile gloves for repair of uncomplicated lacerations in the emergency department: a randomized controlled trial. *Ann Emerg Med* 2004;**43**:362–70.

28 Singer AJ, Hollander JE, Quinn JV. Evaluation and management of traumatic lacerations. *N Engl J Med* 1997;**337**:1142–9.

29 Kundu S, Achar S. Principles of office anesthesia: part II. Topical anesthesia. *Am Fam Phys* 2002;**66**:99–102.

30 Pryor GJ, Kilpatrick WR, Opp DR. Local anesthesia in minor laceration: topical TAC vs lidocaine infiltration. *Ann Emerg Med* 1980;**9**:568–71.

31 Eidelman A, Weiss JM, Lau J, Carr DB. Topical anesthetics for dermal instrumentation: a systematic review of randomized, controlled trials. *Ann Emerg Med* 2005;**46**:343–51.

32 Van Kan HJ, Egberts AC, Rijnvos WP, ter Pelkwijk NJ, Lenderink AW. Tetracaine versus lidocaine-prilocaine for preventing venipuncture-induced pain in children. *Am J Health Syst Pharmacol* 1997;**54**:388–92.

33 Gajraj NM, Pennant JH, Watcha MF. Eutectic mixture of local anesthetics (EMLA) cream. *Anesth Analg* 1994;**78**:574–83.

34 Eichenfeld LF, Funk A, Fallon-Friedlander S, Cunningham BB. A clinical study to evaluate the efficacy of ELA-Max (4% liposomal lidocaine) as compared with eutetic mixture of local anesthetics cream for pain reduction of venipuncture in children. *Pediatrics* 2002;**109**:1093–9.

35 Singer AJ, Stark MJ. Pretreatment of lacerations with lidocaine, epinephrine, and tetracaine at triage: a randomized double-blind trial. *Acad Emerg Med* 2000;**7**:751–6.

36 Priestley S, Kelly A, Chow L, Powell C, Williams A. Application of topical local anesthetic at triage reduces treatment time for children with lacerations: a randomized controlled trial. *Ann Emerg Med* 2003;**42**:34–40.

37 Terndrup TE, Walls HC, Mariani PJ, Gavula DP, Madden CM, Cantor RM. Plasma cocaine and tetracaine levels following application of topical anesthesia in children. *Ann Emerg Med* 1992;**21**:162–6.

38 Smith, GA, Strausbaugh SD, Harbeck-Weber C, Cohen DM, Shields BJ, Powers JD. New non-cocaine-containing topical anesthetics compared with tetracaine-adrenaline-cocaine during repair of lacerations. *Pediatrics* 1997;**100**:825–30.

39 Bush S. Is cocaine needed in topical anaesthesia? *Emerg Med J* 2002;**19**:418–22.

40 Blackburn PA, Butler KH, Hughes MJ, Clark MR, Riker RL. Comparison of tetracaine-adrenaline-cocaine (TAC) with topical lidocaine-epinephrine (TLE): efficacy and cost. *Am J Emerg Med* 1995;**13**:315–17.

41 Fialkov JA, McDougall EP. Warmed local anesthetic reduces pain of in-filtration. *Ann Plast Surg* 1996;**36**:11–13.

42 Dalton AM, Sharma A, Redwood M, Wadsworth J, Touquet R. Does the warming of local anaesthetic reduce the pain of its injection? *Arch Emerg Med* 1989;**6**:247–50.

43 Waldbillig DK, Quinn JV, Stiell IG, Wells GA. Randomized double-blind controlled trial comparing room-temperature and heated lidocaine for digital nerve blocks. *Ann Emerg Med* 1995;**26**:677–81.

44 Martin S, Jones JS, Wynn BN. Does warming local anesthetic reduce the pain of subcutaneous injection? *Am J Emerg Med* 1996;**14**:10–14.

45 Davidson JAH, Boom SJ. Warming lignocaine to reduce pain associated with injection. *BMJ* 1992;**305**:617–18.

46 Powell CV, Kelly AM, Williams A. Determining the minimum clinically significant difference in visual analogue pain score for children. *Ann Emerg Med* 2001;**37**:28–31.

47 Todd KH, Funk KG, Funk JP, Bonacci R. Clinical significance of reported changes in pain severity. *Ann Emerg Med* 1996;**27**:485–9.

48 Gallagher EJ, Bijur PE, Latimer C, Silver W. Reliability and validity of a visual analog scale for acute abdominal pain in the ED. *Am J Emerg Med* 2002;**20**:287–90.

49 Orlinsky M, Hudson C, Chan L, DesLauriers R. Pain comparison of unbuffered versus buffered lidocaine in local wound infiltration. *J Emerg Med* 1992;**10**:411–15.

50 Bancroft JW, Benenati JF, Becker GJ, Katzen BT. Neutralized lidocaine: use in pain reduction in local anesthesia. *J Vasc Interv Radiol* 1992;**3**:107–9.

51 Burns CA, Ferris G, Feng C, Cooper JZ, Brown MD. Decreasing the pain of local anesthesia: a prospective, double-blind comparison of buffered, premixed 1% lidocaine with epinephrine versus 1% lidocaine freshly mixed with lidocaine. *J Am Acad Dermatol* 2006;**54**:128–31.

52 Singer AJ, Hollander JE. Infiltration pain and local anesthetic effects of buffered vs plain 1% diphenhydramine. *Acad Emerg Med* 1995;**2**:884–8.

53 Cheney PR, Molzen G, Tandberg D. The effect of pH buffering on reducing the pain associated with subcutaneous infiltration of bupivicaine. *Am J Emerg Med* 1991; **9**:147–8.

54 Christoph RA, Buchanan L, Begalla K, Schwartz S. Pain reduction in local anesthetic administration through pH buffering. *Ann Emerg Med* 1988;**17**:117–20.

55 Mader TJ, Playe SJ, Garb JL. Reducing the pain of local anesthetic infiltration: warming and buffering have a synergistic effect. *Ann Emerg Med* 1994;**23**:550–54.

56 Colaric KB, Overton DT, Moore K. Pain reduction in lidocaine administration through buffering and warming. *Am J Emerg Med* 1998;**16**:353–8.

57 Dire DJ, Coppola M, Dwyer DA, Lorette JJ, Karr JL. Prospective evaluation of topical antibiotics for preventing infections in uncomplicated soft-tissue wounds repaired in the ED. *Acad Emerg Med* 1995;**2**:4–10.

58 Edlich RF, Smith QT, Edgerton MT. Resistance of the surgical wound to antimicrobial prophylaxis and its mechanisms of development. *Am J Surg* 1973;**126**:583–91.

59 Callaham M. Prophylactic antibiotics in dog bite wounds: nipping at the heels of progress. *Ann Emerg Med* 1994;**23**:577–9.

60 Medeiros I, Saconato H. Antibiotic prophylaxis for mammalian bites. *Cochrane Database Syst Rev* 2001;**2**:CD001738.

61 Quinn J, Gilbreath A, Strahs M. Prophylactic antibiotics for dog bites: a cost–benefit approach. *Acad Emerg Med* 2002;**9**:397–8.

62 Talan DA, Citron DM, Abrahamian FM, Moran GJ, Goldstein EJC. Bacteriologic analysis of infected dog and cat bites. *N Engl J Med* 1999;**340**:85–92.

63 Fleisher, GR. The management of bite wounds. *N Engl J Med* 1999;**340**:138–40.

64 Cummings P, Del Beccaro MA. Antibiotics to prevent infection of simple wounds: a meta-analysis of randomized studies. *Am J Emerg Med* 1995;**13**:396–400.

56 Soft Tissue Abscess

Heather Murray

Departments of Emergency Medicine *and* Community Health and Epidemiology, Queen's University, Kingston, Canada

Clinical scenario

A 32-year-old male presented to the emergency department (ED) complaining of a painful swelling in the right antecubital fossa for approximately 3 days. He was known to be an intravenous drug user (IVDU), and admitted to recent use of the right antecubital fossa as an injection site. He acknowledged being positive for hepatitis B and C; however, he had recently tested negative for human immunodeficiency virus (HIV). He reported a previous episode of bacterial endocarditis a few years previously requiring several weeks of intravenous antibiotic treatment. He was homeless and was employed as a casual laborer, but had not been able to work since the swelling developed.

He appeared uncomfortable, with the following vital signs: pulse 110 beats/min, blood pressure 130/85 mmHg, respiratory rate 16 breaths/min and oral temperature 37.5°C. Examination of his right antecubital fossa revealed a large (10 cm diameter) exquisitely tender fluctuant mass with approximately 3 cm of surrounding erythema.

Background

Soft tissue abscess is a common emergency presentation for patients with a wide range of circumstances and co-morbidities. However, the inclusion of abscesses in clinical trials with other skin and soft tissue infections (SSTIs) such as cellulitis, the lack of a distinct medical subject heading (MeSH) for soft tissue abscess, and a general lack of published research in this area have made evidence difficult to find and evidence-based treatment recommendations challenging to develop.

The bacteriological cause of cutaneous abscesses is dependent on the anatomic region of the abscess. One study examined wound culture results in 78 patients with skin and soft tissue abscesses [1].

Evidence-based Emergency Medicine. Edited by Brian H. Rowe
© 2009 Blackwell Publishing, ISBN: 978-1-4051-6143-5.

Forty-two percent of cultured abscesses grew aerobes exclusively, 28% grew anaerobes exclusively and 27% grew a mixture of aerobes and anaerobes. *Staphylococcus* and *Streptococcus* species were the predominant aerobic organisms, isolated from the head/neck, extremities and axillary regions. The predominant anaerobic organisms were *Peptococcus* and *Bacteroides*, which were primarily isolated from the anogenital regions. One later study compared the bacteriology of cutaneous abscesses in patients with a history of intravenous drug abuse to abscesses in non-IV drug-abusing patients [2]. The results of this small study (86 IVDU patients vs 75 non-IVDU patients) showed substantial overlap in the type and number of pathogens cultured, although there was a higher percentage of anaerobic oral flora grown in cultures from the IV drug abusers [2].

One recent and notable change in the spectrum of pathogens causing soft tissue abscess is the emergence of resistant organisms, mainly in the form of methicillin-resistant *Staphylococcus aureus* (MRSA). Recently, community-acquired MRSA (CA-MRSA) has emerged as a prominent pathogen causing purulent SSTIs, particularly skin and soft tissue abscesses [3–5]. Although the vast majority of the skin infections caused by CA-MRSA are superficial and easily treated, there have been concerning clusters of invasive infections in previously healthy hosts, with fulminant multi-focal sepsis and necrotizing pneumonias [6].

Many risk factors for CA-MRSA have been identified and include children, competitive athletes, soldiers, indigenous people, prisoners, intravenous drug users and homosexual men [7]. Recent Canadian guidelines for the identification and management of MRSA suggest that CA-MRSA should be suspected in patients with SSTIs in areas where 10–15% of community isolates of *S. aureus* are methicillin resistant, in severe infections compatible with *S. aureus* (i.e., sepsis, necrotizing fasciitis), when risk factors for CA-MRSA are present, and where there has been a poor response to β-lactam therapy in patients with presumed staphylococcal infection [5]. However, the identification of risk factors for CA-MRSA was not helpful in a recent US prospective cohort study, where most patients without CA-MRSA had at least one risk factor, while nearly half of those with positive CA-MRSA cultures had no identifiable risk factors [3]. Clearly, the emergence of these infections in EDs represents a potentially devastating problem, although the full implications are not yet clear. Structured reporting and surveillance of SSTI pathogens may be an important start towards defining their impact [8,9].

Clinical questions

In order to address the issues of most relevance to your patient and to help in searching the literature for the evidence regarding these issues, you structure your clinical questions as recommended in Chapter 1.

1 In ED patients with suspected abscesses (population), does ED-based soft tissue ultrasound imaging (intervention) improve abscess detection and change management (outcomes) compared to standard care clinical examination (control)?

2 In ED patients with proven abscesses (population), do systemic antibiotics (intervention) reduce time to infection clearance, pain and swelling (outcome) compared to standard care with incision and drainage (control)?

3 In ED patients with proven abscesses (population), does the outcome (prognosis) of abscesses caused by CA-MRSA (exposure) differ from those not caused by CA-MRSA (unexposed)?

4 In ED patients with proven abscesses (population), are there evidence-based criteria that are sensitive and specific (test characteristics) for identifying patients who require antibiotic pretreatment for the prevention of bacterial endocarditis (outcome) prior to abscess drainage (exposure)?

5 In ED patients with proven recurrent abscesses of non-intravenous-drug-using etiology (population), does long-term antibiotic treatment (intervention) reduce future recurrence (outcome) compared to routine ED care?

General search strategy

You begin to address the topic of abscess by searching for evidence in the common electronic databases such as MEDLINE and EMBASE looking specifically for systematic reviews and randomized controlled trials. This topic is not covered by a large body of evidence; consequently, only one meta-analysis has been published on abscess drainage, and no Cochrane reviews were identified for the questions above. Finally, access to relevant, updated, evidence-based clinical practice guidelines (CPGs) on abscess and cellulitis are accessed to determine the consensus rating of areas lacking evidence.

Critical review of the literature

Question 1: In ED patients with suspected abscesses (population), does ED-based soft tissue ultrasound imaging (intervention) improve abscess detection and change management (outcomes) compared to standard care clinical examination (control)?

Search strategy

- MEDLINE and Cochrane Library: *explode* soft tissue infection (skin and soft tissue infection, cutaneous abscess, soft tissue abscess, SSTI [mp and text words combined]) AND (portable ultrasound OR ultraso$.mp)

Accurate and early identification of patients with SSTI requiring incision and drainage is critical in order to both expedite appropriate treatment and to prevent invasive therapy for patients without abscess. Since the typical appearance of fluctuance, erythema and localized pain may not always be present, other imaging modalities (e.g., bedside ultrasound) and techniques (e.g., needle aspiration) are emerging as diagnostic modalities in this area. One recent study reporting the use of soft tissue ultrasound by emergency physicians trained in bedside ultrasound demonstrated an improvement in diagnostic accuracy when ultrasonography was used to identify fluid collections. Ten of 59 patients deemed not to have abscess by physical exam had fluid seen on ultrasound, with eight of the 10 patients showing frank pus at incision and drainage [10]. This finding was repeated in a second study which showed that the use of bedside ultrasound led to management changes in 56% of ED patients assessed for cellulitis [11]. This second study also suggested that ED-based sonography was useful in the detection of subcutaneous fluid across all ranges of pre-test probability for abscess (suggesting that ED physicians may have limited accuracy in the detection of subcutaneous fluid in patients with presumed cellulitis) [11]. Both these studies are preliminary, without comparator groups and without evidence that the addition of bedside ultrasound and the resultant interventions changed patient outcomes.

In summary, there is a paucity of evidence to support the use of bedside ultrasound in the identification of subcutaneous abscess. Clearly it is a modality under development and readers should search for additional evidence in the future.

Question 2: In ED patients with proven abscesses (population), do systemic antibiotics (intervention) reduce time to infection clearance, pain and swelling (outcomes) compared to standard care with incision and drainage (control)?

Search strategy

- MEDLINE and Cochrane Library: *explode* soft tissue infection (skin and soft tissue infection, cutaneous abscess, soft tissue abscess, SSTI [mp and text words combined]) AND incision and drainage [text word]. Limited to clinical trial (publication type)

It is generally accepted that treatment of skin and soft tissue abscess requires incision and drainage of localized purulent collections. However, there exists some overlap between the discrete conditions of cellulitis (or erysipelas) and subcutaneous abscess. Some abscesses are complicated by surrounding signs of cellulitis, occasionally developing regional and even systemic spread. Conversely, some episodes of cellulitis may develop the enzymatic liquefaction and necrosis that leads to localized abscesses.

A 1992 consensus document from the Infectious Diseases Society of America (IDSA) and United States Food and Drug Administration (FDA) recommended that patients harboring abscesses with noticeable surrounding areas of erythema or systemic symptoms of infection be eligible for inclusion in clinical trials of antibiotic therapy, following incision and drainage [12]. Although many of the clinical trials of antibiotics for skin and soft tissue infections have subsequently included abscess in their eligibility criteria, none of them are designed with placebo controls (considered unethical for infectious disease research). As a result, there is very little published evidence to guide the treatment of this very common entity.

One recent systematic review has specifically examined this issue [13]. A search spanning 30 years identified only five relevant studies and one abstract. Three of these studies were randomized controlled trials, one of which lacked a placebo group and was not blinded [14]. The two remaining randomized controlled trials both demonstrated high cure rates (>90%) and similar outcomes in the groups receiving adjuvant antibiotics or placebo therapy [15,16]. Several limitations were noted in both studies, including very small sample sizes and the lack of a pre-specified definition for abscess [13]. The most significant issue raised in the systematic review was the fact that associated cellulitis was not specifically addressed in any of the studies. There is also no mention of whether any of the studies included patients with systemic signs of infection such as fever and the impact of these signs on abscess resolution. Only one of the studies included patients with relevant co-morbidities. The systematic review concludes that evidence is "lacking and sorely needed" to properly address the issue of adjuvant antibiotics in the treatment of cutaneous abscesses [13].

In summary, high cure rates have been observed in two small clinical trials of patients with cutaneous abscesses treated using incision and drainage with and without adjuvant antibiotics. One published expert consensus guideline recommends that patients with systemic signs of infection, such as high fever or extensive surrounding erythema, receive adjuvant broad-spectrum antibiotics [17]. There are no evidence-based recommendations for deciding which patients (if any) require adjuvant antibiotics after adequate incision and drainage.

Question 3: In ED patients with proven abscesses (population), does the outcome (prognosis) of abscesses caused by CA-MRSA (exposure) differ from those not caused by CA-MRSA (unexposed)?

Search strategy

- MEDLINE and Cochrane Library: *explode* soft tissue infection (skin and soft tissue infection, cutaneous abscess, soft tissue abscess, SSTI [mp and text words combined]) AND (CA-MRSA OR community-acquired methicillin resistant Staph$ aureus [mp and text word])

The majority of soft tissue abscesses are caused by *Staphylococcus aureus* alone (~25%) or by a combination of *S. aureus* with other indigenous skin flora and microorganisms colonizing regional mucous membranes [17]. The arrival of MRSA as a pathogen has translated into a shift in the type of infections observed. There have been many case reports and small case series of fulminant bacteremia in previously healthy patients caused by CA-MRSA, usually from the strains carrying PVL (Panton–Valentine leukocidin) genes [18–23]. Given the increasing prevalence of CA-MRSA as a causative agent in skin and skin structure infections, early identification of patients at risk of fulminant infection would be of great value.

One prospective, observational study reviewed 69 children presenting to a single pediatric urban center with skin and soft tissue abscesses whose wounds subsequently grew CA-MRSA after incision and drainage [24]. No information is presented on the number of CA-MRSA-positive cultures seen during the study period, nor on the number of excluded patients (exclusion criteria were absence, non-functioning telephone number or "inadequate documentation on the initial evaluation") [24]. All children were treated with antibiotic therapy prior to culture results, the vast majority (93%) were initially treated with an "ineffective" antibiotic (one to which the cultured CA-MRSA had demonstrated resistance). No information on the rate of polymicrobial infection is presented. Subsequent treatment was variable and not protocol driven, with considerable heterogeneity of antibiotic choice and change rate, timing of follow-up assessments and outcomes. A small number of the "inappropriately treated" patients (4/62) were admitted, presumably due to failure to improve or clinical worsening, as was one of the five patients treated with an "appropriate" antibiotic. No patients in the study group had septicemia. Multivariate analysis identified an initial abscess size of >5 cm to be associated with subsequent admission, but inappropriate antibiotic choice was not associated with admission risk. The authors conclude that skin and soft tissue abscesses caused by CA-MRSA can be effectively "managed with therapeutic drainage, without adjuvant antibiotics, if the infected site has a diameter of <5 cm" [24].

A larger, more rigorous epidemiological survey of CA-MRSA isolates also failed to demonstrate an association between treatment with antibiotics inactive against CA-MRSA and poor outcomes in 453 patients with SSTIs caused by CA-MRSA [25]. This study used structured surveillance data over a 2-year period with strict case definition requirements to identify 1647 infections caused by CA-MRSA within three US geographic communities (Baltimore, Atlanta, Minnesota). Of note, 103 (6%) of the identified infections were noted to be invasive. Subgroup analysis of 453 patients with CA-MRSA SSTIs who received antibiotic therapy at the time of initial presentation (including 196 patients with abscesses who initially had incision and drainage performed) failed to show any association between initial antibiotic choice and any of the following outcomes: unplanned follow-up with health care provider, requirement for incision and drainage at follow-up or subsequent change in antibiotics. The authors concluded

"Our data suggest that patients with community-associated MRSA skin or soft-tissue disease who initially receive inactive antimicrobial therapy have outcomes similar to those among patients who are treated with antimicrobial agents to which the organism is susceptible in vitro [25]."

One randomized controlled trial compared oral antibiotics with placebo after incision and drainage at an inner city hospital with a high prevalence of MRSA [16]. One hundred and sixty-six patients, including many patients with significant co-morbidities, such as hepatitis, HIV and diabetes, were randomized to cephalexin or placebo. Fifty-two percent of the cultured wounds grew MRSA isolates. There was no difference in the rates of cure and symptom resolution in the two groups (cephalexin 86% vs placebo 93%), even when the subgroup of MRSA-positive infections was examined.

Overall, no evidence currently exists to suggest that abscesses caused by CA-MRSA have a different prognosis from those caused by methicillin-susceptible isolates. The published studies discussed demonstrate two interesting findings. Firstly, rates of antibiotic coverage in presumably uncomplicated abscesses are very high, despite a lack of evidence to support the routine use of prophylactic antibiotics after adequate incision and drainage has been performed. It is not clear if this represents a general practice pattern of antibiotic over-treatment for abscesses or selection bias within the trials (such as a higher rate of associated cellulitis or systemic symptoms in the patients studied). Secondly, the addition of antibiotics inactive against CA-MRSA appeared to have no association with future adverse outcomes in either study. It seems plausible that treatment with antibiotics inactive against CA-MRSA is comparable to no antibiotic treatment, but it is still a leap of faith. A welcome addition to the literature would be a clinical trial that treated abscesses with incision and drainage, prospectively followed patients until clinical cure, and then compared outcomes in CA-MRSA-positive patients with those of the control group.

In summary, SSTIs caused by MRSA in general, and CA-MRSA specifically, are an increasingly common problem for emergency physicians. Given the spectre of rare and unpredictable fulminant infection caused by CA-MRSA, it seems unlikely that practice patterns will shift away from routine antibiotic use. Once again, this is an area of emerging evidence and it is important for ED physicians to re-examine this literature over the next several years.

Question 4: In ED patients with proven abscesses (population), are there evidence-based criteria that are sensitive and specific (test characteristics) for identifying patients who require antibiotic pre-treatment for the prevention of bacterial endocarditis (outcome) prior to abscess drainage (exposure)?

Search strategy

- MEDLINE and Cochrane Library: *explode* soft tissue infection (skin and soft tissue infection, cutaneous abscess, soft tissue abscess, SSTI

[mp and text words combined]) AND bacterial or infective endocarditis [mp and text word] AND prevention, antibiotic prophylaxis, prophylaxis

The American Heart Association (AHA) has recently published updated consensus-based guidelines for the prevention of infective endocarditis (IE) using prophylactic antibiotics [26]. This guideline recommends limiting the use of prophylactic antibiotics prior to performing procedures on infected skin, skin structures and musculoskeletal tissue to patients with "underlying cardiac conditions associated with the highest risk of adverse outcome" (Table 56.1). This recommendation is classified as a IIb recommendation, level C evidence, which the working group defines as an opinion-based recommendation (e.g., usefulness/efficacy is less well established).

This list has been substantially shortened from the 1997 guidelines where patients were stratified into high- and moderate-risk for acquiring IE, and antibiotic prophylaxis was recommended for all of these patients prior to incision and drainage of abscesses, or any other procedure on infected skin, skin structure or musculoskeletal tissue [27]. Patients previously described as moderate-risk (e.g., previous rheumatic heart disease, acquired valvular disease including mitral valve prolapse, congenital heart disease other than the conditions listed in Table 56.1, and hypertrophic cardiomyopathy) have been removed from the list of recommended prophylactic therapy [26].

The prophylactic regimen recommended consists of an agent active against *Staphylococcus* and β-hemolytic streptococci such as an anti-staphylococcal penicillin or cephalosporin, administered by mouth or parenterally, 30–60 minutes prior to the procedure. Vancomycin or clindamycin are listed as alternate agents where allergy or intolerance is a concern, or where there is suspicion of methicillin-resistant staphylococcal infection [26].

These guidelines represent a notable change from the previous 1997 guidelines [27] by restricting prophylaxis to those patients with a high risk of *adverse outcome* from IE, and not for those with a higher risk of acquiring IE. This decision was made by consensus, and the report credits an increasing number of publications questioning the effectiveness of routine antibiotic prophylaxis in preventing the development of IE, particularly in the setting of dental procedures.

A 2006 Cochrane systematic review concluded that there was no evidence to support or reject the use of prophylactic penicillin

Table 56.1 Conditions deemed to warrant infective endocarditis prophylaxis [26].

Prosthetic cardiac valve
Previous episode of infective endocarditis
Congenital heart disease (CHD) in the following circumstances:
- Unrepaired cyanotic CHD including palliative shunts and conduits
- CHD repaired with prosthetic material or device (during the first 6 months after repair, since endothelization occurs within 6 months of procedure)
- Repaired CHD with residual defects near or at the site of prosthetic material
Cardiac transplantation recipients with acquired valvulopathy

in order to prevent IE following invasive dental procedures [28]. Even in the latest 1997 AHA guidelines [27], emphasis was placed on the fact that most cases of bacterial endocarditis are not attributable to a recent invasive procedure, and this sentiment is carried further in the 2007 guidelines. These new AHA guidelines state "no published data demonstrate convincingly that the administration of prophylactic antibiotics prevents IE associated with a bacteremia from an invasive procedure". The increasing frequency of antimicrobial resistance, the risk of adverse events from antibiotic administration and the relatively low incidence of IE in North America (5–7 cases per 100,000 person-years) [29] have strengthened the case for limiting the use of antimicrobial prophylaxis to patients at high risk of mortality from IE.

How common are bacteremic episodes after incision and drainage of soft tissue abscess? One small prospective study from 1997 has examined this question [30]. Fifty afebrile patients with cutaneous, non-draining, purulent abscesses underwent blood cultures before and 2 and 10 minutes after incision and drainage procedures were performed. Thirteen of the 50 patients admitted to previous intravenous drug abuse. None of the 50 pre-procedure or 100 post-procedure blood cultures in any of the 50 subjects were positive. Despite this negative result, many routine daily activities such as brushing teeth or chewing food have been shown to cause small, transient episodes of bacteremia [31,32]. The magnitude and duration of bacteremia from tissue trauma is generally believed to be a function of the degree of trauma, density of microbial colonization and degree of infection or inflammation in the tissues, although this is a theoretical construct [26]. It is hard not to endorse an increased risk of bacteremia from incision and drainage procedures, given the degree of invasion, inflammation and bacterial colonization of skin and soft tissue abscesses. The absence of evidence of bacteremia from this one small study does not translate into absence of risk.

In summary, without evidence to support withholding prophylactic antibiotics in high-risk individuals, the current best practice is to follow the expert opinion-based 2007 AHA guidelines for the prevention of infective endocarditis in individuals at high risk of poor outcomes from IE (see Table 56.1).

Question 5: In ED patients with proven recurrent abscesses of non-intravenous-drug-using etiology (population), does long-term antibiotic treatment (intervention) reduce future recurrence (outcome) compared to routine ED care (comparator)?

Search strategy

- MEDLINE and Cochrane Library: *explode* soft tissue infection (skin and soft tissue infection, cutaneous abscess, soft tissue abscess, furuncle, furunculosis, carbuncle, SSTI [mp and text words combined]) AND prevention, antibiotic prophylaxis, prophylaxis

Recurrent abscesses caused by staphylococcal infection in otherwise healthy hosts are thought to be attributed at least in part by chronic colonization of the skin or nasal passages with staphylococcal organisms [17]. There may be some clinical overlap between the terms soft tissue abscess, furuncle (a small purulent infection of the hair follicle base) and carbuncle (coalescence of several furuncles); however, furunculosis is the term generally used to describe patients with recurrent furuncles. Furuncles are small enough that incision and drainage may not be required, and treatment of furunculosis has been focused on antibiotic therapy.

Eradication of the nasal carriage has been studied in one small randomized trial of 34 immunocompetent patients with proven nasal colonization and "recurrent skin infections" [33]. In this double-blinded, placebo-controlled trial, patients applied nasal mupirocin ointment or placebo to their nasal mucosa for a 5-day period at the beginning of every month over a 1-year study period. Application of the mupirocin ointment was shown to decrease both the number of positive nasal cultures (22 vs 83, $P < 0.001$) and the number of recorded skin infections (26 vs 62, $P < 0.002$) when compared to the placebo group.

Two small clinical trials have examined the issue of systemic antibiotics in the prevention of recurrent staphylococcal infections. The first was a double-blinded, placebo-controlled trial of low-dose clindamycin (150 mg as a daily oral dose) for 3 months in 22 patients with a history of three or more skin abscesses caused by *Staphylococcus aureus* [34]. The authors report that the rate of recurrent abscess during the treatment period was significantly lower in the treatment group (2/11 clindamycin vs 7/11 placebo). However the very small sample size impairs the power of this study, and in fact calculated confidence intervals for these data overlap (treatment event rate = 18%, 95% CI: 5% to 47%; placebo event rate = 64%, 95% CI: 35% to 85%).

The second trial, published in 2007, was a prospective cohort study of low-dose azithromycin suppressive therapy in 24 patients with a history of three or more episodes of furuncles caused by MRSA [35]. After initial curative therapy with oral azithromycin (500 mg/day for 3 days), all patients received a weekly dose of azithromycin 500 mg for a 12-week period. Additional daily use of an antibacterial skin wash was also prescribed. No mention is made of incision and drainage in any of the patients. Two patients were classified as treatment failures (any recurrence of furuncles) over the 3-month study period. One additional patient developed a furuncle during a 3-month follow-up period, and was considered to have relapsed. Since all enrolled patients suffered at least three furuncles in the 6-month period leading up to the trial, a cure rate of 92% (95% CI: 74% to 98%) was assumed to be substantially better than expected. In the absence of a comparator group, however, the absolute improvement in lesion development remains unknown, as does the relative impact of a daily antibacterial skin wash.

In summary, there is minimal evidence to evaluate the effectiveness of topical or systemic antibiotics in the prevention of recurrent skin abscesses. Topical mupirocin decreases nasal carriage rates and episodes of skin infection in patients with nasal staphylococcal colonization. Two under-powered studies of patients with recurrent furuncles suggested that oral antibiotics administered in a low-dose suppressive regimen may decrease the frequency of infections; however, this evidence should be considered preliminary and not conclusive.

Conclusions

Your patient required incision and drainage, which produced a large amount of purulent material; you sent a swab of the wound for culture and sensitivity given his increased risk for both CA-MRSA and polymicrobial infection. Since he reported a previous episode of bacterial endocarditis, and was thus at high risk for complications from bacterial endocarditis, you elected to pre-treat him with oral clindamycin 30 minutes before the procedure. You were also concerned about his signs of systemic infection (low-grade fever, tachycardia and surrounding erythema). After packing his wound with gauze, you provided him with a prescription for a short course of oral clindamycin and arranged for him to be seen the following day for packing removal and re-evaluation.

Changing bacterial pathogens and a paucity of good-quality evidence renders decision making difficult for the adjuvant care of patients with soft tissue abscess. Incision and drainage of purulent collections remains the mainstay of treatment. Bedside ultrasound, although currently unproven to affect clinical outcomes, is emerging as a diagnostic aid for focal fluid collections. There is no evidence to support withholding or administering adjuvant antibiotic therapy for patients with soft tissue abscess. Most practitioners will administer antibiotics for patients with substantial surrounding erythema, lymphangitis or systemic symptoms such as fever and nausea, but the risk and/or benefit from this strategy, as well as the optimal duration and route of administration is unknown. CA-MRSA is an emerging pathogen for purulent skin and soft tissue infections, and the next few years will likely see the implementation of structured surveillance programs and changing empirical antibiotic regimens. Recommendations for the administration of prophylactic antibiotics for the prevention of infective endocarditis before abscess incision and drainage have recently been reworked, and prophylaxis is now recommended only for those patients with a high risk of adverse outcome from bacterial endocarditis (see Table 56.1). Patients with recurrent skin and soft tissue abscesses should have nasal swabs to assess nasal colonization with staphylococcal species. Eradication of the carrier state with topical mupirocin may decrease the frequency of recurrent abscesses.

Conflicts of interest

None were reported.

References

1 Llera JL, Levy RC, Staneck JL. Cutaneous abscesses: natural history and management in an outpatient facility. *J Emerg Med* 1984;**1**(6):489–93.

2 Summanen PH, Talan DA, Strong C, et al. Bacteriology of skin and soft-tissue infections: comparison of infections in intravenous drug users and individuals with no history of intravenous drug use. *Clin Infect Dis* 1995;**20**(Suppl):82.

3 Moran GJ, Krishnadasan A, Gorwitz RJ, et al. Methicillin-resistant *S. aureus* infections among patients in the emergency department. *N Engl J Med* 2006;**355**(7):666–74.

4 Gilbert M, MacDonald J, Gregson D, et al. Outbreak in Alberta of community-acquired (USA300) methicillin-resistant *Staphylococcus aureus* in people with a history of drug use, homelessness or incarceration. *Can Med Assoc J* 2006;**175**(2):149–54.

5 Morrison MA, Hageman JC, Klevens RM. Case definition for community-associated methicillin-resistant *Staphylococcus aureus. J Hosp Infect* 2006;**62**(2):241.

6 Maltezou HC, Giamarellou H. Community-acquired methicillin-resistant *Staphylococcus aureus* infections (Review). *Int J Antimicrob Agents* 2006;**27**(2):87–96.

7 Kowalski TJ, Berbari EF, Osmon DR. Epidemiology, treatment, and prevention of community-acquired methicillin-resistant *Staphylococcus aureus* infections (Review). *Mayo Clin Proc* 2005;**80**(9):1201–7, quiz 1208.

8 Allen UD. Public health implications of MRSA in Canada (Comment). *Can Med Assoc J* 2006;**175**(2):161.

9 Nicolle L. Community-acquired MRSA: a practitioner's guide. *Can Med Assoc J* 2006;**175**(2):145.

10 Squire BT, Fox JC, Anderson C. ABSCESS: applied bedside sonography for convenient evaluation of superficial soft tissue infections. *Acad Emerg Med* 2005;**12**(7):601–6.

11 Tayal VS, Hasan N, Norton HJ, Tomaszewski CA. The effect of soft-tissue ultrasound on the management of cellulitis in the emergency department. *Acad Emerg Med* 2006;**13**(4):384–8.

12 Calandra GB, Norden C, Nelson JD, Mader JT. Evaluation of new anti-infective drugs for the treatment of selected infections of the skin and skin structure. Infectious Diseases Society of America and the Food and Drug Administration. *Clin Infect Dis* 1992;**15**(Suppl 1):S148–54.

13 Hankin A, Everett WW. Are antibiotics necessary after incision and drainage of a cutaneous abscess? (Review). *Ann Emerg Med* 2007;**50**(1):49–51.

14 Macfie J, Harvey J. The treatment of acute superficial abscesses: a prospective clinical trial. *Br J Surg* 1977;**64**(4):264–6.

15 Llera JL, Levy RC. Treatment of cutaneous abscess: a double-blind clinical study. *Ann Emerg Med* 1985;**14**(1):15–19.

16 Rajendran PM, Young D, Maurer T, Chambers H, Perdreau-Remington F, Ro P, Harris H. Randomized, double-blind, placebo-controlled trial of cephalexin for treatment of uncomplicated skin abscesses in a population at risk for community-acquired methicillin-resistant *Staphylococcus aureus* infection. *Antimicrob Agents Chemother.* 2007;**51**(11):4044–4048

17 Stevens DL, Bisno AL, Chambers HF, et al. Practice guidelines for the diagnosis and management of skin and soft-tissue infections. *Clin Infect Dis* 2005;**41**(10):1373–406 (erratum in *Clin Infect Dis* 2006;**42**(8):1219, note dosage error in text).

18 Centers for Disease Control and Prevention. Four pediatric deaths from community-acquired methicillin-resistant *Staphylococcus aureus* – Minnesota and North Dakota, 1997–1999. *JAMA* 1999;**282**(12):1123–5.

19 Mongkolrattanothai K, Boyle S, Kahana MD, Daum RS. Severe *Staphylococcus aureus* infections caused by clonally related community-acquired methicillin-susceptible and methicillin-resistant isolates. *Clin Infect Dis* 2003;**37**(8):1050–58.

20 Francis JS, Doherty MC, Lopatin U, et al. Severe community-onset pneumonia in healthy adults caused by methicillin-resistant *Staphylococcus aureus* carrying the Panton-Valentine leukocidin genes [see comment]. *Clin Infect Dis* 2005;**40**(1):100–7.

21 Bahrain M, Vasiliades M, Wolff M, Younus F. Five cases of bacterial endocarditis after furunculosis and the ongoing saga of community-acquired methicillin-resistant *Staphylococcus aureus* infections. *Scand J Infect Dis* 2006;**38**(8):702–7.

22 Gonzalez BE, Martinez-Aguilar G, Hulten KG, et al. Severe staphylococcal sepsis in adolescents in the era of community-acquired methicillin-resistant *Staphylococcus aureus*. *Pediatrics* 2005;**115**(3):642–8.

23 Boussaud V, Parrot A, Mayaud C, et al. Life-threatening hemoptysis in adults with community-acquired pneumonia due to Panton-Valentine leukocidin-secreting *Staphylococcus aureus*. *Intensive Care Med* 2003;**29**(10):1840–43.

24 Lee MC, Rios AM, Aten MF, et al. Management and outcome of children with skin and soft tissue abscesses caused by community-acquired methicillin-resistant *Staphylococcus aureus*. *Pediatr Infect Dis J* 2004;**23**(2):123–7.

25 Fridkin SK, Hageman JC, Morrison M, et al. Methicillin-resistant *Staphylococcus aureus* disease in three communities. *N Engl J Med* 2005;**352**(14):1436–44 (erratum in *N Engl J Med* 2005;**352**(22):2362).

26 Wilson W, Taubert KA, Gewitz M, et al. Prevention of infective endocarditis. Guidelines from the American Heart Association. A guideline from the American Heart Association Rheumatic Fever, Endocarditis, and Kawasaki Disease Committee, Council on Cardiovascular Disease in the Young, and the Council on Clinical Cardiology, Council on Cardiovascular Surgery and Anesthesia, and the Quality of Care and Outcomes Research Interdisciplinary Working Group. *Circulation* 2007;**116**(15):1736–54.

27 Dajani AS, Taubert KA, Wilson W, et al. Prevention of bacterial endocarditis. Recommendations by the American Heart Association (Review). *JAMA* 1997;**277**(22):1794–801.

28 Oliver R, Roberts GJ, Hooper L. Penicillins for the prophylaxis of bacterial endocarditis in dentistry (Systematic review). *Cochrane Database Syst Rev* 2004;**2**:CD003813 (doi: 10.1002/14651858.CD003813.pub2).

29 Tleyjeh IM, Steckelberg JM, Murad HS, et al. Temporal trends in infective endocarditis: a population-based study in Olmsted County, Minnesota. *JAMA* 2005;**293**(24):3022–8.

30 Bobrow BJ, Pollack CV, Jr., Gamble S, Seligson RA. Incision and drainage of cutaneous abscesses is not associated with bacteremia in afebrile adults. *Ann Emerg Med* 1997;**29**(3):404–8.

31 Seymour RA. Dentistry and the medically compromised patient (Review). *Surgeon J Roy Coll Surgeons Edinburgh Ireland* 2003;**1**(4):207–14.

32 Roberts GJ. Dentists are innocent! "Everyday" bacteremia is the real culprit: a review and assessment of the evidence that dental surgical procedures are a principal cause of bacterial endocarditis in children (Review). *Pediatr Cardiol* 1999;**20**(5):317–25.

33 Raz R, Miron D, Colodner R, Staler Z, Samara Z, Keness Y. A 1-year trial of nasal mupirocin in the prevention of recurrent staphylococcal nasal colonization and skin infection. *Arch Intern Med* 1996;**156**(10):1109–12.

34 Klempner MS, Styrt B. Prevention of recurrent staphylococcal skin infections with low-dose oral clindamycin therapy. *JAMA* 1988;**260**(18):2682–5.

35 Aminzadeh A, Demircay Z, Ocak K, Soyletir G. Prevention of chronic furunculosis with low-dose azithromycin. *J Dermatol Treat* 2007;**18**(2):105–8.

57 Ultrasound Use: Three Select Applications

Srikar Adhikari[1] & Michael Blaivas[2]

[1]Department of Emergency Medicine, University of Nebraska, Omaha, USA
[2]Department of Internal Medicine, Northside Hospital Forsyth, Cumming USA

Clinical scenario

A 70-year-old man with a history of hypertension, hypercholesterolemia and smoking was driving unrestrained with his 15-year-old grand-daughter. He suddenly complained of severe back and abdominal pain, passed out and crashed into an oncoming car at moderate speed. His grand-daughter was restrained and appeared to be uninjured in the accident as she was able to exit the car and attend to her grandfather. On arrival of emergency medical services (EMS), the patient was slightly confused and complained of diffuse abdominal and back pain. On arrival to the emergency department (ED), his Glasgow Coma Score was 14 and initial vital signs were blood pressure 80/56 mmHg, pulse 125/min, respiration 24 breaths/min, temperature 36.4°C (oral) and pulse oximetry 99% (on room air). He was placed on supplemental oxygen, an 18 gg IV catheter was initiated and 1 L of normal saline was hung; however, there was difficulty obtaining better vascular access.

The patient responded poorly to the initial fluid bolus with repeat vital signs of blood pressure 95/62 mmHg, pulse 100 beats/min and respiration 22 breaths/min. A four-view FAST (focused assessment with sonography for trauma) examination of the patient demonstrated free fluid in Morison's pouch. The trauma surgeon on call was paged immediately and the results were discussed; you also mention a 5.1 cm abdominal aortic aneurysm (AAA) found on sonography. When you described this finding to the trauma surgeon, she requested that vascular surgery be consulted and to obtain central access above the chest. She also suggested obtaining an abdominal computerized tomography (CT) scan while she and the vascular surgeon travel to the hospital. Based on the patient's condition and the ultrasound findings, you were uncomfortable with the idea of having the patient transported downstairs to the radiology department for further imaging and wondered if the patient should go directly to the operating room instead.

Background

Emergency department ultrasound

Ultrasound use in the traditional imaging setting dates back decades and did not find broad application in imaging laboratories until legible and interpretable images were produced in a variety of examinations in the late 1970s. By the middle of the next decade, emergency physicians and other clinicians was beginning to utilize ultrasound for critical applications when service was lacking. In time, a well-accepted list of applications were established in emergency ultrasound focusing on emergent and critical conditions such as AAA detection or abdominal trauma evaluation.

With the development of compact ultrasound machines, sometimes specifically designed for the clinical setting, clinical ultrasound expanded tremendously with the creation of a variety of protocols and clinician-specific applications. Examples of such developments include ultrasound-guided vascular access in critically ill patients and the utilization of ultrasound for directing resuscitative efforts in medical and surgical patients. With the recognition of clinical ultrasound by traditional imaging societies, the acceptance of clinical ultrasound is likely to increase. Moreover, formal adoption of ultrasound education into clinical specialty residency training (e.g., emergency medicine, anesthesiology, surgery), potential adoption by other specialties (e.g., internal medicine), and the adaptation of ultrasound education into several medical school curricula means the future of clinical ultrasound is likely to expand further.

Central venous access

Central venous catheter (CVC) insertion is common in the United States, with more than 5 million central venous catheters placed annually [1,2]. The procedure is, however, not without the potential for significant complications. Associated iatrogenic complications include arterial puncture, hematoma, airway loss from expanding carotid hematoma, pneumothorax, hemothorax and air embolus. Complication rates have been reported to be as high as 10% and unsuccessful cannulation may occur in up to 20% of cases [3,4]. CVC insertion has traditionally been performed using anatomic landmarks as a guide to the position of the central veins; however, in some patients these landmarks may be distorted, and anatomic variations in the positions of the vessels may prevent cannulation [5].

Central venous catheterization is a common and essential procedure in the ED. In the emergent situation, central venous cannulation with poorly defined landmarks frequently involves multiple needle punctures to locate the vein. The incidence of complications increases when multiple needle passes are required for catheterization [6–10]. The risk of mechanical complications increases six-fold after three needle passes [3,11].

The use of ultrasound guidance for central venous cannulation has been endorsed by several medical societies and the Agency for Healthcare Research and Quality (AHRQ) listed the use of real-time ultrasound guidance for central venous catheterization as one of the 11 practices to improve patient care [12]. Similarly, the National Institute for Health and Clinical Excellence (NICE) in Great Britain recommends real-time ultrasound guidance for central venous catheter placement [13].

Blunt abdominal trauma

Trauma is the leading cause of death in people younger than 45 years, and EDs in most countries deal with most of these severe cases. Moreover, more than 38 million people are seen in EDs for trauma annually [14]. On average, deaths from trauma result in 40 years of life lost and 18 years of productive life lost [15]. The annual cost of treating trauma patients in the United States is more than $100 billion [16].

The prevalence of blunt abdominal injury among trauma admissions reported in the international literature ranges from 6% to 65% [17]. The evaluation of blunt abdominal trauma remains a challenge for the trauma team, especially when there is a multiple trauma situation. The signs and symptoms that indicate the presence of an intra-abdominal injury are notoriously unreliable. In an autopsy study, 43% of abdominal injuries were missed during the primary survey in the ED [18].

The goal of the clinician is to identify patients who will benefit from operative intervention as quickly as possible. For years, diagnostic peritoneal lavage (DPL) remained the standard initial diagnostic tool. Although DPL is very sensitive, it has a high false-positive rate leading to unnecessary laparotomy [19–21]. In the past decade, CT scanning has become the standard imaging modality in the assessment of trauma patients [22–24]. However, the utility of CT scanning may be limited in hemodynamically unstable patients since monitoring and resuscitation is difficult in a typical CT suite. Moreover, CT may not be readily available in rural areas and low-volume EDs.

In summary, emergency physicians have begun to increasingly utilize bedside ultrasound in the initial evaluation of the trauma victim. Several studies have validated the ability of emergency physicians with proper training to perform the FAST examination. The bedside ultrasound examination is a rapid, non-invasive,

repeatable and inexpensive tool. FAST examination is primarily performed to detect the presence of free fluid as an indicator of organ injury [25]. Emergency physicians should recognize, however, that the prevalence of intra-abdominal organ injury without accompanying free fluid ranges from 5% to 37% [26].

Clinical questions

In order to address the issues of most relevance to bedside ultrasound and to help in searching the literature for the evidence regarding these, you structure your questions as recommended in Chapter 1.

1 In ED patients requiring central venous access (population), does ultrasound guidance (intervention) reduce the number of attempts, time to insertion and complication rate (outcomes) compared to landmark techniques (control)?

2 In ED patients suspected of having AAA (population), what are the likelihood ratios (diagnostic test characteristics) of bedside ultrasound performed by emergency physicians (test) for the diagnosis of AAA (outcome)?

3 In ED patients with AAA (population), does bedside ultrasound (intervention) decrease the time to operative repair and reduce morbidity and mortality (outcomes) compared to traditional imaging modalities and pathways (control)?

4 In hemodynamically stable ED patients with blunt abdominal trauma (population), what are the likelihood ratios (diagnostic test characteristics) of the FAST examination performed by emergency physicians (test) for the diagnosis of hemoperitoneum (outcome)?

5 In ED patients with blunt abdominal trauma (population), can the quantity of intraperitoneal free fluid on the FAST examination, alone or in combination with vital signs (intervention), predict the need for exploratory laparotomy (outcome)?

6 In ED patients with blunt abdominal trauma (population), does the use of the FAST examination within a trauma algorithm (intervention) reduce mortality, abdominal computerized tomography scan utilization, diagnostic peritoneal lavage and laparotomy rates (outcomes) compared with algorithms that do not include the FAST examination (control)?

7 In ED patients with torso trauma (population), does the use of the FAST examination (intervention) decrease time to operative intervention and length of hospital stay (outcomes)?

General search strategy

You begin to address these questions by searching for evidence in the common electronic databases such as the Cochrane Library, MEDLINE and EMBASE looking specifically for systematic reviews and meta-analyses. You also search the Cochrane Central Register of Controlled Trials (CENTRAL) and MEDLINE to identify randomized controlled trials that became available after the publication date of the systematic review or, if no systematic reviews were identified, to locate high-quality randomized controlled trials that directly address the clinical question. In addition, access to relevant, updated, evidence-based clinical practice guidelines (CPGs) on bedside ultrasound, abdominal aortic aneurysm, central venous catheterization, blunt abdominal trauma and FAST examination are obtained to determine the consensus rating of areas lacking evidence.

Searching for evidence synthesis: primary search strategy

- MEDLINE and EMBASE: (ultrasonography OR ultrasound OR sonography) AND (systematic review OR meta-analysis OR meta-analysis) AND topic

Critical review of the literature

Question 1: In ED patients requiring central venous access (population), does ultrasound guidance (intervention) reduce the number of attempts, time to insertion and complication rate (outcomes) compared to landmark techniques (control)?

Search strategy

- Cochrane Library, MEDLINE and EMBASE: (catheterization OR central venous OR central venous catheter OR central line) AND (ultrasonography OR ultrasound) AND emergency

Our search yielded two systematic reviews (with strict inclusion criteria) and three primary studies that directly addressed the clinical question. Randolph et al. [27] reviewed eight studies of ultrasound in comparison to the landmark technique for central line insertion. Studies were included in this meta-analysis if they were randomized clinical trials, evaluated real-time ultrasound, and reported on specified outcomes including complication rate, success rate, number of attempts and time to insertion. This meta-analysis concluded that ultrasound guidance reduced the failure rate for both internal jugular and subclavian CVC insertion (RR = 0.32; 95% CI: 0.18 to 0.55). There was also a reduction in the complication rate (RR = 0.22; 95% CI: 0.10 to 0.45) and in the number of attempts required for successful catheter placement (RR = 0.60; 95% CI: 0.45 to 0.79). Most of these studies included ultrasound operators with minimal experience; however, no studies were performed in the ED.

The meta-analysis performed by Hind et al. [28] included 18 trials ($N = 1646$) assessing either Doppler or 2D ultrasound-guided central line placement compared to the anatomic landmark method in a broad range of clinical settings. Two studies were performed in the ED setting, seven in intensive care units and the remainder in elective-type scenarios. Only four studies were clearly performed by non-anesthesiologists. This review provided the foundation for the NICE guidelines [13] published in 2002; the authors searched 15 bibliographic databases until October 2001, as part of the NICE guideline development process. This meta-analysis showed that 2-D ultrasound guidance for internal jugular vein cannulation was associated with a lower failure rate both overall (RR = 0.14; 95% CI: 0.06 to 0.33) and on the first attempt (RR = 0.59; 95% CI: 0.39 to 0.88). Similarly, the risk of failure was lower using ultrasound guidance for subclavian and femoral vein catheterization in adults (RR = 0.14, 95% CI: 0.04 to 0.57 and RR = 0.29, 95% CI: 0.07 to 1.21, respectively). Overall, the complication rate was 5/296 (1.7%) using 2D ultrasound and 68/312 (22%) using the landmark method (OR = 0.14; 95% CI: 0.06 to 0.33). Using a 2D ultrasound probe, it was 69 seconds (95% CI: 46 to 92 seconds) faster to insert a CVC.

In a prospective randomized study, the performance of emergency medicine residents inserting CVCs both with and without ultrasound guidance in adult ED patients was assessed [29]. Prior to the study, the residents had no experience obtaining central access via ultrasound guidance. These residents had received two 1-hour lectures on ultrasound use as preparation for the study. One hundred and twenty-two consecutive ED patients requiring CVC access over a 6-month period were enrolled and randomized according to the date of presentation. The primary outcome was not defined at the outset of the study and no power calculation was performed. They found ultrasound guidance led to a statistically significant decrease in the time required for CVC insertion (time from needle touching skin to successful flashback): 463 seconds (± 627 seconds) for the landmark method versus 93 seconds (± 176 seconds) in the ultrasound group. Of note, the skin to blood time did not include equipment set-up or time required to perform the initial ultrasound examination. The total number of attempts was also reduced using ultrasound guidance: 1.55 attempts (± 1) in the ultrasound group versus 3.54 attempts (± 2.7) in the landmark group ($P < 0.0001$). There was no significant difference in complication rates: 14% for the landmark method and 12% for ultrasound guidance.

Milling et al. [30] performed a randomized controlled trial to determine whether static and/or dynamic ultrasound-guided internal jugular CVC placement is superior to the traditional landmark technique as measured by overall success rate, first-pass success, number of attempts, time to cannulation and complication rate. The trial enrolled a convenience sample of 201 ED and medical intensive care unit (MICU) patients over a 6-month period. The results indicate that entering the vein on first pass was better using ultrasound guidance when compared to the standard landmark method for static vein location (OR = 3.4; 95% CI: 1.6 to 7.2) and using dynamic guidance (OR = 5.8; 95% CI: 2.7 to 13). There was also reduction in the mean number of attempts required to enter the vein for dynamic ultrasound (2.3; 95% CI: 1.6 to 3.0) and static ultrasound (2.9; 95% CI: 2.3 to 3.5) when compared to the landmark technique (5.2; 95% CI: 4.1 to 6.3). The mean total time to cannulation was reduced using ultrasound guidance: dynamic ultrasound was 109 seconds (95% CI: 47 to 171), static ultrasound was 126 seconds (95% CI: 89 to 163), and the landmark technique was 250 seconds (95% CI: 184 to 316). Although there is the potential for selection bias given the convenience sampling method, this study suggests that dynamic ultrasound guided internal jugular cannulation is substantially better than either static or landmark techniques.

In another randomized controlled trial, internal jugular vein cannulation under ultrasound guidance was compared with the landmark technique [31]. Investigators enrolled 130 adult ED patients who required central venous access. The percentage of patients in whom internal jugular vein catheterization was successful, both within three attempts (94% vs 78%) and on the first attempt (77% vs 55%), was higher in the ultrasound group than in the landmark group. There was essentially no clinically important difference in the time for insertion between the two methods. The mean time from the beginning of the procedure (not including ultrasound equipment preparation) to establishing a working central line was 281 seconds (median 198 seconds) in the ultrasound group and 271 seconds (median 180 seconds) in the landmark group (difference in means = 10 seconds; 95% CI: −118 to 98). The complication rate was lower in the ultrasound group compared to landmark group (4.6% vs 17%).

In summary, the existing literature provides strong evidence that ultrasound-guided CVC placement significantly reduces the number of attempts at insertion, the number of catheter placement failures and the complications during catheter placement. Given the consistent results in different patient settings and among operators with different experience levels, these conclusions also appear to have external validity.

Question 2: In ED patients suspected of having AAA (population), what are the likelihood ratios (diagnostic test characteristics) of bedside ultrasound performed by emergency physicians (test) for the diagnosis of AAA (outcome)?

Search strategy

- Cochrane Library, MEDLINE and EMBASE: abdominal aortic aneurysm AND (ultrasonography OR ultrasound) AND emergency

With an aging population in industrialized countries, the incidence of AAA is increasing [32]. As many as 5–10% of men aged 65–79 years have an AAA [33]. Delay in diagnosis of an AAA can be life-threatening, whereas early recognition and surgical intervention can reduce morbidity and mortality. Of those who survive to the operating room and undergo emergency surgery for ruptured AAA, 50% die prior to discharge; however, the 30-day operative mortality for an elective surgical repair of AAA is only 5% [34–39]. The classic triad of hypotension, back pain and pulsatile abdominal mass is present in only 50% of patients presenting with ruptured AAA [40]. In a study by Fink et al., the sensitivity and specificity of detecting an AAA by physical examination were 68% and 75%, respectively [41]. A meta-analysis by Lederle and Simel also suggested that physical examination is not adequate to exclude the diagnosis of AAA [42]. Additionally, over 75% of patients with an AAA are unaware that they have this condition [43,44].

Several studies have demonstrated that the sensitivity of ultrasound for detecting AAA is 100% and that ultrasound is accurate for determining the size of the aorta [45–48]. One of the few limitations of bedside ultrasound in the ED is the unprepared bowel, and one study suggested that up to 8% of all patients may have incomplete visualization of the aorta [49]. In a study conducted among a convenience sample of patients older than 50 years with abdominal pain/back pain, the aorta was visualized in 66 of 68 patients [48]. In a prospective ED study, 114 patients suspected of having an AAA were enrolled over a 2-year period [50]. Ultrasound performed by emergency medicine faculty and senior residents was 100% sensitive and 96% specific for AAA using operative findings or advanced imaging interpreted by a radiologist as the reference standard. Another study examined 238 patients suspected of AAA with at least one of the following: abdominal, back, flank or chest pain, or hypotension [51]. The investigators reported a sensitivity of 94% and specificity of 100% for AAA. In a prospective cohort study conducted by Dent et al., all 120 ED patients who underwent an abdominal aortic ultrasound by an emergency physician during a 1-year period were included. In the hands of emergency physicians, ultrasound had a sensitivity of 96.3% (95% CI: 81.0% to 99.9%) and a specificity of 100% (95% CI: 91.8% to 100%) for AAA [52].

Unfortunately, all of these studies reported either perfect sensitivity or perfect specificity thus precluding calculation of likelihood ratios. Although all of the studies identified in our search had small sample sizes and may be prone to some degree of selection bias, the data suggest that emergency physicians can accurately detect AAA with bedside ultrasound.

Question 3: In ED patients with AAA (population), does bedside ultrasound (intervention) decrease the time to operative repair and reduce morbidity and mortality (outcomes) compared to traditional imaging modalities and pathways (control)?

Search strategy

- Cochrane Library, MEDLINE and EMBASE: abdominal aortic aneurysm AND (ultrasonography OR ultrasound) AND emergency

Our search revealed only one before/after type study, in abstract form. Plummer et al. demonstrated decreased time to diagnosis in patients with ruptured AAAs when ED bedside ultrasound was used (5.4 minutes) compared with traditional imaging modalities (83 minutes) [53]. The authors compared two groups of patients prior to and after the introduction of emergency ultrasound. There were no baseline differences between the groups. In this study, the time to disposition for patients requiring surgical intervention decreased from 90 to 12 minutes.

In summary, although this time difference would intuitively appear to be clinically significant, there is insufficient evidence at this time to suggest that ED bedside ultrasound improves patient-important outcomes such as mortality.

Question 4: In hemodynamically stable ED patients with blunt abdominal trauma (population), what are the likelihood ratios (diagnostic test characteristics) of the FAST examination performed by emergency physicians (test) for the diagnosis of hemoperitoneum (outcome)?

Search strategy

- Cochrane Library, MEDLINE and EMBASE: abdominal trauma AND focused AND (ultrasonography OR ultrasound OR FAST)

We identified two prospective cohort studies, one retrospective study and one systematic review that addressed the clinical question. In a prospective cohort study performed by Rozycki et al. [54], 1197 hemodynamically stable patients with suspected blunt abdominal trauma were enrolled and FAST examinations were performed. Patients with a positive ultrasound examination for hemoperitoneum underwent a CT scan (if they were hemodynamically stable) or immediate celiotomy (if they were hemodynamically unstable). The investigators reported an ultrasound sensitivity of 75% and specificity of 99.8% for detecting hemoperitoenum when compared to CT or DPL results (positive likelihood ratio (+LR) = 300; negative likelihood ratio (–LR) = 0.17). Miller et al. prospectively enrolled 372 hemodynamically stable patients with suspected blunt abdominal injury [55]. A protocol for evaluating hemodynamically stable trauma patients with suspected blunt abdominal injury was implemented using a FAST examination as a screening tool and a CT scan of the abdomen and pelvis as a confirmatory study. The FAST scan sensitivity was 42% and specificity was 98% (+LR = 21; –LR = 0.6).

Lee et al. retrospectively reviewed data entered in a trauma registry database and correlated them with medical records, radiology reports and surgical laparotomy reports [56]. Overall, 3907 hemodynamically stable patients with suspected blunt abdominal injury were included and the investigators reported a sensitivity of 85% and specificity of 96% for hemoperitoneum (+LR = 21; –LR = 0.15). Stengel et al. conducted a systematic review and meta-analysis of prospective clinical trials of ultrasonography for blunt abdominal trauma [57]. Publications were retrieved by structured searching among databases, review articles and major text-books. Thirty trials enrolling 9047 patients were included in the final analysis. The review concluded that ultrasound has an excellent specificity but rather low sensitivity (below 90%) regardless of the chosen endpoint (that is, free fluid or organ injury).

In summary, ultrasound for the detection of hemoperitoneum has good specificity but is not very sensitive. In other words, with positive FAST ultrasound results, emergency physicians can be reasonably confident that blunt abdominal injury is present; however, negative results cannot rule out such injury.

Question 5: In ED patients with blunt abdominal trauma (population), can the quantity of intraperitoneal free fluid on the FAST examination, alone or in combination with vital signs (intervention), predict the need for exploratory laparotomy (outcome)?

Search strategy

- Cochrane Library, MEDLINE and EMBASE: abdominal trauma AND focused AND (ultrasonography OR ultrasound OR FAST)

Ma et al. conducted a prospective study to determine whether the quantity of free intraperitoneal fluid on the FAST examination, alone or in combination with vital signs, improved sensitivity in predicting the need for operative intervention in patients with blunt abdominal trauma [58]. This study was conducted at two level I trauma centers where a convenience sample of 270 patients presented with major blunt abdominal trauma over a 2-year period. The FAST exam was performed and interpreted by emergency physicians, who focused primarily on the presence and amount of free fluid, rather than evidence of solid organ injury. Combined intraperitoneal free fluid levels in five intraperitoneal areas were measured and defined as small (<1.0 cm), moderate (>1.0 cm, <3.0 cm) or large (>3.0 cm). Of the 270 patients enrolled, 33 (12%) had positive FAST findings. Of the 18 patients with a large fluid accumulation, 16 underwent exploratory laparotomy (sensitivity = 89%; 95% CI: 72% to 97%) and the eight patients with unstable vital signs underwent exploratory laparotomy (sensitivity = 100%; 95% CI: 94% to 100%). Of the 10 patients with a moderate fluid accumulation, six underwent exploratory laparotomy (sensitivity = 60%; 95% CI: 43% to 79%) and four of the six patients with unstable vital signs underwent exploratory laparotomy (sensitivity = 67%; 95% CI: 39% to 84%). The convenience sampling in this study may have introduced selection bias. Also, those who had negative FAST scans often received no confirmatory study to verify a true negative (verification bias).

In summary, our search identified only one prospective study attempting to quantify if the amount of free fluid predicted the need for operative intervention. A large intraperitoneal free fluid accumulation (>3 cm) on ultrasound in combination with unstable vital signs appears to be sensitive for determining the need for exploratory laparotomy in patients presenting with blunt abdominal trauma.

Question 6: In ED patients with blunt abdominal trauma (population), does the use of the FAST examination within a trauma algorithm (intervention) reduce mortality, abdominal computerized tomography scan utilization, diagnostic peritoneal lavage and laparotomy rates (outcomes) compared with algorithms that do not include the FAST examination (control)?

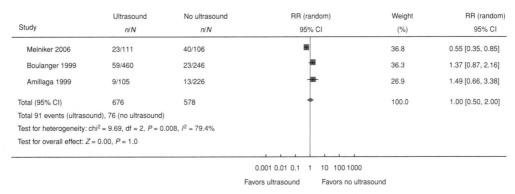

Study	Ultrasound *n*/*N*	No ultrasound *n*/*N*	RR (random) 95% CI	Weight (%)	RR (random) 95% CI
Melniker 2006	23/111	40/106		36.8	0.55 [0.35, 0.85]
Boulanger 1999	59/460	23/246		36.3	1.37 [0.87, 2.16]
Amillaga 1999	9/105	13/226		26.9	1.49 [0.66, 3.38]
Total (95% CI)	676	578		100.0	1.00 [0.50, 2.00]

Total 91 events (ultrasound), 76 (no ultrasound)
Test for heterogeneity: chi^2 = 9.69, df = 2, P = 0.008, I^2 = 79.4%
Test for overall effect: Z = 0.00, P = 1.0

0.001 0.01 0.1 1 10 100 1000
Favors ultrasound   Favors no ultrasound

Figure 57.1 A Forest plot of mortality and risk of mortality following emergency ultrasound-based algorithms for diagnosing blunt abdominal trauma.

Search strategy

- Cochrane Library, MEDLINE and EMBASE: abdominal trauma AND focused AND (ultrasonography OR ultrasound OR FAST)

Stengel et al. performed a Cochrane systematic review to assess the efficiency and effectiveness of trauma algorithms that include ultrasound examination in patients with suspected blunt abdominal injury [59]. The authors searched MEDLINE, EMBASE, CENTRAL, controlled trial registers and other specified resources for randomized controlled trials and quasi-randomized trials. Outcome measures included mortality, utilization of CT and DPL, and laparotomy rates. Only two randomized controlled trials and two quasi-randomized trials met the inclusion criteria, involving a total of 1037 patients. There was significant clinical and statistical heterogeneity among the studies included in this review. There was no evidence of a mortality difference between the two groups (Fig. 57.1). There was a trend toward reduced utilization of CT with ultrasound-based algorithms; however, this trend did not reach statistical significance. No differences were noted in the DPL and laparotomy rates.

In summary, there remains insufficient evidence to justify the routine use of ultrasound-based algorithms in patients with suspected blunt abdominal trauma.

Question 7: In ED patients with torso trauma (population), does use of the FAST examination (intervention) decrease time to operative intervention and length of hospital stay (outcomes)?

Search strategy

- Cochrane Library, MEDLINE and EMBASE: abdominal trauma AND focused AND (ultrasonography OR ultrasound OR FAST)

Melniker et al. conducted a randomized controlled clinical trial assessing whether point-of-care limited ultrasonography (PLUS)

compared to usual care (control group) among patients presenting to the ED with suspected torso injury decreased time to operative care [60]. The primary outcome was the time from ED arrival to operative care; secondary outcomes were average hospital stay, utilization of CT scan, complications and total charges. The study was conducted in two level 1 trauma centers over a 6-month period and 262 patients were enrolled. The time from ED arrival to operative care was on average 57 minutes (median = 60 minutes; inter-quartile range (IQR) = 41 to 70 minutes) for the PLUS group and 166 minutes (median = 157 minutes; IQR = 90 to 78 minutes) for the control group. Time to operative care was 64% shorter for the PLUS group compared to control patients. The PLUS group underwent fewer CT scans (OR = 0.16; 95% CI: 0.07 to 0.32), spent 27% fewer days in the hospital, had fewer complications (OR = 0.27; 95% CI: 0.11 to 0.67) and were charged 35% less compared to the control group.

In summary, this study demonstrated that FAST in patients with suspected torso trauma can decrease time to operative care, with a decrease in resource utilization.

Conclusions

In the situation described above, you decided to keep the patient in the ED and proceed with placing an internal jugular cordis introducer sheath under ultrasound guidance for high-volume resuscitation. The patient remained hypotensive despite aggressive resuscitation. After the trauma surgeon and vascular surgeon arrive at the ED, your repeat bedside ultrasound examination revealed a large amount of free fluid in Morison's pouch and an AAA. The surgeons decided to take the patient to the operating room from the ED. The two surgeons explored the patient's abdomen jointly and a ruptured spleen was discovered with ongoing bleeding that was initially packed while the remaining abdominal organs were evaluated. The vascular surgeon made the decision to repair the AAA when it became evident that intra-abdominal injury was limited to the spleen. During the successful AAA repair, splenic hemorrhage resumed resulting in significant blood loss, removal of the spleen and multiple transfusions. The patient survived the operating suite, had a protracted course in the surgical intensive care unit, developed multiple infections and required ongoing blood replacement. Post-operative CT scanning and evaluation of the abdominal aorta during surgery revealed a rupture that was contained retroperitoneally. Ultimately, it is hypothesized that the AAA rupture led to a drop in blood pressure and syncope, which then resulted in a motor vehicle crash and secondary injuries.

Overall, bedside ultrasonography in the ED setting is becoming routine. While it is evident by this review that further prospective, controlled studies are needed, it is clear that evidence of benefit and improved outcome does exist. A practical difficulty that is often a shocking surprise to novice ultrasound investigators is the frequent unwillingness of clinical sonologists to engage in randomized studies that would mandate a non-ultrasound use arm in critically ill patients. Sonologists often grow dependent on the technology and are reluctant to part with it in critical situations. However, much work remains to be performed and with proper planning, studies should be able to evaluate ultrasound impact on outcome and efficiency without compromising patient care or individual clinicians' dependence on the technology. Now that ultrasound is being integrated into residency and medical school education, such outcome studies are not only more important but data may be more easily gathered as larger numbers of patients undergo point-of-care ultrasound examinations in a variety of clinical settings. Future updates of this text promise further clarity in this field.

References

1 McGee DC, Gould MK. Preventing complications of central venous catheterization. *N Engl J Med* 2003;**348**:1123–1133.

2 Mermel LA, Farr BM, Sherertz RJ, et al. Guidelines for the management of intravascular catheter-related infections. *Clin Infect Dis* 2001;**32**:1249–72.

3 Mansfield PF, Hohn DC, Fornage BD, Gregurich MA, Ota DM. Complications and failures of subclavian-vein catheterization. *N Engl J Med* 1994;**331**:1735–8.

4 Sznajder JI, Zveibil FR, Bitterman H, Weiner P, Bursztein S. Central vein catheterization. Failure and complication rates by three percutaneous approaches. *Arch Intern Med* 1986;**146**:259–61.

5 Denys B, Uretsky B, Reddy P. Ultrasound-assisted cannulation of the internal jugular vein. *Circulation* 1993;**87**:1557–62.

6 Conz PA, Dissegna D, Rodighiero MP, et al. Cannulation of the internal jugular vein: comparison of the classic Seldinger technique and an ultrasound guided method. *J Nephrol* 1997;**10**:311–13.

7 Lee W, Leduc L, Cotton DB. Ultrasonographic guidance for central venous access during pregnancy. *Am J Obstet Gynecol* 1989;**161**:1012–13.

8 Trottier SJ, Veremakis C, O'Brien J, et al. Femoral deep vein thrombosis associated with central venous catheterization: results from a prospective, randomized trial. *Crit Care Med* 1995;**23**:52–9.

9 Bagwell CE, Salzberg AM, Sonnino RE, et al. Potentially lethal complications of central venous catheter placement. *J Pediatr Surg* 2000;**35**:709–13.

10 Meredith JW, Young JS, O'Neil EA, et al. Femoral catheters and deep venous thrombosis: a prospective evaluation with venous duplex sonography. *J Trauma* 1993;**35**:187–90.

11 Feller-Kopman D. Ultrasound-guided central venous catheter placement: the new standard of care? *Crit Care Med* 2005;**33**:1875–7.

12 Agency for Healthcare Research and Quality. Making health care safer: a critical analysis of patient safety practices (Summary). *Evid Rep Technol Assess* 2001;**43**:i–x, 1–668.

13 National Institute for Clinical Excellence. *Guidance on the Use of Ultrasound Locating Devices for Placing Central Venous Catheters.* Technology Appraisal Guidance No. 49. National Institute for Clinical Excellence, London, 2002, www.nice.org.uk.

14 American Hospital Association. *Policy Forum (Trendwatch).* Available at http://www.ahapolicyforum.org/ahapolicyforum/trendwatch/twmarch2001.html (accessed August 11, 2001).

15 Shackford SR, Mackersie RC, Holbrook TL, et al. The epidemiology of traumatic death: a population-based analysis. *Arch Surg* 1993;**128**:571–5.

16 O'Keefe GE, Maier RV, Diehr P, et al. The complications of trauma and their associated costs in a level I trauma center. *Arch Surg* 1997;**132**:920–24.

17 Stengel D, Bauwens K, Keh D, et al. Emergency ultrasound for blunt abdominal trauma – meta-analysis update 2003. *Zentralbl Chir* 2003;**128**:1027–37.

18 Hodgson NF, Stewart TC, Girotti MJ. Autopsies and death certification in deaths due to blunt trauma: what are we missing? *Can J Surg* 2000;**43**:130–36.

19 Hodgson NF, Stewart TC, Girotti MJ. Open or closed diagnostic peritoneal lavage for abdominal trauma? *J Trauma* 2000;**6**:1091–5.

20 Amoroso TA. Evaluation of the patient with blunt abdominal trauma an evidence-based approach. *Emerg Med Clin North Am* 1999;**17**:63–75.

21 EAST Practice Management Guidelines Work Group. *Practice Management Guidelines for the Evaluation of Blunt Abdominal Trauma, 2001.* Available at http://www.east.org (accessed February 27, 2003).

22 Jhirad R, Boone D. Computed tomography for evaluating blunt abdominal trauma in the low-volume nondesignated trauma center: the procedure of choice? *J Trauma* 1998;**45**:64–8.

23 Linsenmaier U, Krotz M, Häuser H, et al. Whole-body computed tomography in polytrauma: techniques and management. *Eur Radiol* 2002;**12**:1728–40.

24 Livingston DH, Lavery RF, Passanante MR, et al. Admission or observation is not necessary after a negative computed tomographic scan in patients with suspected blunt abdominal trauma. *J Trauma* 1998;**44**:273–82.

25 Scalea TM, Rodriguez A, Chiu WC, et al. Focused assessment with sonography for trauma (FAST): results from an international consensus conference. *J Trauma* 1999;**46**:466–72.

26 Yoshii H, Sato M, Yamamoto S, et al. Usefulness and limitations of ultrasonography in the initial evaluation of blunt abdominal trauma. *J Trauma* 1998;**45**:45–50.

27 Randolph AG, Cook DJ, Gonzales CA, et al. Ultrasound guidance for placement of central venous catheters: a meta-analysis of the literature. *Crit Care Med* 1996;**24**:2053–8.

28 Hind D, Calvert N, McWilliams R, Davidson A, Paisley S, Beverley C, Thomas S. Ultrasonic locating devices for central venous cannulation: meta-analysis. *BMJ* 2003;**327**:361–4.

29 Miller AH, Roth BA, Mills TJ, et al. Ultrasound guidance versus the landmark technique for the placement of central venous catheters in the emergency department. *Acad Emerg Med* 2002;**9**:800–805.

30 Milling TJ, Jr., Rose J, Briggs WM, et al. Randomized, controlled clinical trial of point-of-care limited ultrasonography assistance of central venous cannulation: the Third Sonography Outcomes Assessment Program (SOAP-3) Trial. *Crit Care Med* 2005;**33**:1764–9.

31 Leung J, Duffy M, Finckh A. Real-time ultrasonographically-guided internal jugular vein catheterization in the emergency department increases success rates and reduces complications: a randomized, prospective study. *Ann Emerg Med* 2006;**48**:540–47.

32 Rose WM, III Ernst CB. Abdominal aortic aneurysm. *Compr Ther* 1995;**21**:339–43.

33 Vardulaki KA, Prevost TC, Walker NM, et al. Incidence among men of asymptomatic abdominal aortic aneurysms: estimates from 500 screen detected cases. *J Med Screen* 1999;**6**:50–54.

34 Ernst CB. Abdominal aortic aneurysm. *N Engl J Med* 1993;**328**:1167–72.

35 Johansson G, Swedenborg J. Ruptured abdominal aortic aneurysms: a study of incidence and mortality. *Br J Surg* 1986;**73**:101–3.

36 Greenhalgh RM. Prognosis of abdominal aortic aneurysm. *BMJ* 1990;**301**:136.

37 Basnyat PS, Biffin AH, Moseley LG, Hedges AR, Lewis MH. Mortality from ruptured aortic aneurysm in Wales. *Br J Surg* 1999;**86**:765–70.

38 Johnston KW. Ruptured aortic aneurysm: six year follow up results of a multi-center prospective study. Canadian Society for Vascular Surgery Aneurysm Study Group. *J Vasc Surg* 1994;**19**:888–900.

39 Cosford PA, Leng GC. Screening for abdominal aortic aneurysm. *Cochrane Database Syst Rev* 2007;**2**:CD002945.

40 Rohrer MJ, Cutler BS, Wheeler HB. Long-term survival and quality of life following ruptured abdominal aneurysm. *Arch Surg* 1988;**123**:1213–17.

41 Fink HA, Lederle FA, Roth CS, Bowles CA, Nelson DB, Haas MA. The accuracy of physical examination to detect abdominal aortic aneurysm. *Arch Intern Med* 2000;**160**:833–6.

42 Lederle FA, Simel DL. The rational clinical examination. Does this patient have an abdominal aortic aneurysm. *JAMA* 1999;**281**:77–82.

43 Marston WA, Ahlquist R, Johnson G, Jr., Meyer AA. Misdiagnosis of ruptured abdominal aortic aneurysms. *J Vasc Surg* 1992;**16**:17–22.

44 Barkin AZ, Rosen CL. Ultrasound detection of abdominal aortic aneurysm. *Emerg Med Clin North Am* 2004;**22**:675–82.

45 LaRoy LL, Cormier PJ, Matalon TA, Patel SK, Turner DA, Silver B. Imaging of abdominal aortic aneurysms. *Am J Roentgenol* 1989;**152**:785–92.

46 Maloney JD, Pairolero PC, Smith SF, Hattery RR, Brakke DM, Spittell JA, Jr. Ultrasound evaluation of abdominal aortic aneurysms. *Circulation* 1977;**56**:II80–85.

47 Schlager D, Lazzareschi G, Whitten D, Sanders AB. A prospective study of ultrasonography in the ED by emergency physicians. *Am J Emerg Med* 1994;**12**:185–9.

48 Kuhn M, Bonnin RLL, Davey MJ, Rowland JL, Langlois SLP. Emergency department ultrasound scanning for abdominal aortic aneurysm: accessible, accurate and advantageous. *Ann Emerg Med* 2000;**36**:219–23.

49 Blaivas M, Theodoro D. Frequency of incomplete abdominal aorta visualization by emergency department bedside ultrasound. *Acad Emerg Med* 2004;**11**:103–5.

50 Tayal V, Graf C, Gibbs M. Prospective study of accuracy and outcome of emergency department ultrasound for abdominal aortic aneurysm over two years. *Acad Emerg Med* 2003;**10**:867–71.

51 Constantino T, Bruno E, Handly N, et al. Accuracy of emergency medicine ultrasound in the evaluation of abdominal aortic aneurysm. *J Emerg Med* 2005;**29**:455–60.

52 Dent B, Kendall RJ, Boyle AA, Atkinson PR. Emergency ultrasound of the abdominal aorta by UK emergency physicians: a prospective cohort study. *Emerg Med J* 2007;**24**:547–9.

53 Plummer D, Clinton J, Matthew B. Emergency department ultrasound improves time to diagnosis and survival in ruptured abdominal aortic aneurysm. *Acad Emerg Med* 1998;**5**:417.

54 Rozycki GS, Ballard RB, Feliciano DV, Schmidt JA, Pennington SD. Surgeon-performed ultrasound for the assessment of truncal injuries: lessons learned from 1540 patients. *Ann Surg* 1998;**228**:557–67.

55 Miller MT, Pasquale MD, Bromberg WJ, Wasser TE, Cox J. Not so fast. *J Trauma* 2003;**54**:52–9.

56 Lee BC, Ormsby EL, McGahan JP, Melendres GM, Richards JR. The utility of sonography for the triage of blunt abdominal trauma patients to exploratory laparotomy. *Am J Roentgenol* 2007;**188**:415–21.

57 Stengel D, Bauwens K, Sehouli J, et al. Systematic review and meta-analysis of emergency ultrasonography for blunt abdominal trauma. *Br J Surg* 2001;**88**(7):901–12.

58 Ma OJ, Kefer MP, Stevison KF, Mateer JR. Operative versus non-operative management of blunt abdominal trauma: role of ultrasound-measured intraperitoneal fluid levels. *Am J Emerg Med* 2001;**19**:284–6.

59 Stengel D, Bauwens K, Sehouli J, et al. *Emergency Ultrasound-based Algorithms for Diagnosing Blunt Abdominal Trauma.* Cochrane Library, Wiley, London, 2005:1–20.

60 Melniker LA, Leibner E, McKenney M, Lopez P, Briggs W, Mancuso C. Randomized controlled clinical trial of point-of-care, limited ultrasonography for trauma in the emergency department: the First Sonography Outcomes Assessment Program Trial. *Ann Emerg Med* 2006;**48**:227–35.

10 Public Health

58 Injury Prevention

Mary Patrica McKay[1] & Liesl A. Curtis[2]

[1]Department of Emergency Medicine, George Washington University, Washington DC, USA
[2]Department of Emergency Medicine, Georgetown University, Washington DC, USA

Clinical scenarios

A 115 pound (52 kg), 20-year-old female college student comes to the emergency department (ED) asking for the morning after pill. She believes she had unintentional sex the previous night, although she cannot recall events. After some questioning, she recalls having about 10 mixed drinks at a party and awoke this morning naked in bed with a fellow student she had met earlier in the evening. She recalled being interested in having sex with him but could not recall the nature of events. He told her they had had intercourse but neither could remember using a condom. She just wants the morning after pill.

A 74-year-old man presents to the ED after falling. There is no concern for syncope; the patient is clear that he tripped over a rug in his home when getting up to use the bathroom. His medications include Flomax and atenolol, and he was recently prescribed trazodone for trouble sleeping. He struck his head on the edge of a piece of furniture while falling and presents with a scalp laceration requiring sutures. While the sutures are being placed, his wife wants to know what they can do to prevent him from falling again (she is afraid of a more severe injury), and wonders if the new medication had anything to do with him falling this time.

Background

More than one-third of all ED visits are for the treatment of an injury [1]. Many of these injuries are preventable through behavior changes (not drinking and driving), correct use of protective equipment (bicycle helmet use) or environmental improvements (installing childproof latches and electric socket covers). The primary goal of ED treatment is and should be appropriate care for the patient's injury. However, being treated for an injury in the

Evidence-based Emergency Medicine. Edited by Brian H. Rowe
© 2009 Blackwell Publishing, ISBN: 978-1-4051-6143-5.

ED appears to present a unique opportunity for injury prevention – a "teachable moment". Speaking to the patient about the cause of the injury and ways the injury could have been prevented offers an opportunity to prevent the recurrence of the injury (tertiary prevention) or to address underlying causes of injury such as substance use.

Behavioral change is not generally an instantaneous event. Instead, individuals go through a process of change, which includes considering the new behavior, planning on/for it, performing it and finally automating or maintaining it. The transtheoretical (stages of change) model contains the following stages: pre-contemplation (benefits of lifestyle change are not being considered), contemplation (starting to consider change but not yet begun to act on this intention), preparation (ready to change the behavior and preparing to act), action (making the initial steps toward behavior change) and maintenance (maintaining behavior change while often experiencing relapses) [2].

There are many theories and models on how this behavior change occurs [3–7], most of which overlap significantly. In each of these models, education appears to be critical to starting the process – the individual must know about the alternative behavior and begin to understand that it is "good" or desirable in some way. The importance of the behavior then must become personalized and internalized. For an individual to perform injury prevention or safety behaviors, they have to perceive themselves as "at risk" for negative consequences and anticipate that the safety behavior will prevent these consequences. They must also believe they have the requisite skills and resources to carry out the new behavior. Social norms also play a large role in safety behaviors; if the behavior is "normal" or "acceptable" behavior in the individual's social group, they are much more likely to perform it.

Variously described as "behavior change counseling" and "motivational interviewing" or "negotiated interviewing", much research has centered on effective methods to help patients move through the stages of change to initiate a desired health or safety behavior, or to eliminate an unsafe/unhealthy behavior [8,9]. Rather than confronting the patient, motivational interviewing utilizes "reflective listening" (reflecting back to the patient their reasons for not performing the safety behavior, e.g., "It sounds like you're saying that you drink to relax with friends, but end up going too far and then driving your car"). The goal is to help patients think about and express their personal motivations for and against change and help them understand how their behavior reflects their lives and values. Educational information about the risk of injury and/or health and safety benefits of the behavior, as well as norms for the behavior, are presented neutrally only after the practitioner has elicited the patient's point of view. The decision for change is initiated by the patient and supported by the practitioner. This method has been reported to be effective when dealing with alcohol overuse syndromes [10,11].

A single interaction in the ED is unlikely to motivate someone unready to change through all the stages to routinely perform a safety behavior. Thus, it is unlikely that any ED-based intervention will, for example, convert an individual into a routine belt-user if he or she a priori believes that seat belts cause harm by preventing the user's escape from a burning vehicle. However, intervention in the ED may move the person from pre-contemplation to contemplation and then other social and environmental events may later push them to ultimately change their behavior.

Injury prevention experts focus on a combination of education, enforcement, economic incentive, empowerment and engineering to motivate individuals through the stages of change. In order to effectively change behavior, the message needs to be "sticky" (meaningful to the individual) and a person needs to hear it in more than one context and likely from more than one person [12]. Because of the "white coat effect", emergency physicians are particularly effective as deliverers of health and safety messages. For example, if the visit is the result of an injury it may be a particularly opportune context in which to deliver an injury prevention message (providing education and empowerment). If a patient receives the same message from friends and family, sees the behavior being routinely performed in TV programs and movies, and if there are negative consequences from failure to perform the behavior (e.g., a traffic ticket), the person is more likely to move through the stages of change to perform and maintain the desired behavior.

Each patient is already at a particular stage at the time they present to the ED, and even with an effective intervention, an individual may only move from considering the change to planning on changes rather than actually acting upon the change [13]. This makes injury prevention interventions aimed at safety behaviors complex to study. The optimal outcome of a successful intervention is a decrease in injury occurrence, morbidity or mortality. An alternative outcome is objective evidence of increased safety behavior performance (e.g., observed motorcycle helmet use). For some behaviors such as alcohol use, researchers have had to rely on subjects' self-report of the behavior and compare this to a control group's self-report. Finally, some interventions may successfully advance patients to a further stage of change without affecting their behavior or risk of injury in the near future.

Therefore, in writing this chapter we accepted changes in intention and self-report of behavior changes, as well as objectively measured behaviors, as acceptable outcomes in the studies we chose. For each topic, we sought to identify interventions tested in the ED. When those were lacking, we reviewed interventions that would readily transfer to the practice environment in emergency medicine.

Foci for this chapter

The most prevalent, serious types of injury or injury risk factors were chosen as foci for this chapter:
- Alcohol: the relative risk of having an injury requiring an ED visit is 3.97 for the first 6 hours after drinking compared with non-drinking periods [14]. Based on data from the National Hospital Ambulatory Medical Care Survey, researchers estimate there are 7.6 million visits (7.9% of all ED visits) to EDs in the USA for diseases and injuries directly related to alcohol use each year [15].
- Falls: there were 7.9 million ED visits in the USA for fall-related injuries in 2005 [16], and falls among older adults alone account for an estimated US$8 billion in acute care charges annually [17].
- Intimate partner violence: although perhaps not quite as frequent as originally believed, intimate partner violence is an issue for many ED patients in North America, with prevalence as high as 20% [18,19].
- Safety belts: although safety belt use reached 82% in the USA in 2005 [20], 52% of more than 31,000 fatally injured vehicle occupants in 2005 were unrestrained at the time of the crash [21].
- Firearms: firearms caused 29,569 fatalities and nearly 70,000 injuries in 2004 in the USA [22].

Clinical questions

1 For ED patients (population), what ED-based interventions (intervention) effectively change patients' drinking behavior and/or risk of injury (outcome) from alcohol use?

2 In older adults (population), what ED-based interventions (intervention) decrease falls (outcome)?

3 For intimate partner violence victims identified in the ED (population), what ED-based interventions (intervention) decrease injury (outcome)?

4 For adult patients in the ED (population), what interventions (intervention) increase the use of safety belts in vehicles (outcomes)?

5 For adults who present to the ED (population), what strategies or programs (intervention) have been proven to decrease the risk of firearm injury (outcome)?

General search strategy

For each question, the Cochrane database was searched and MEDLINE was searched using PubMed with limits set to "published in the last 10 years", "clinical trial", "English" and "adults 19+". For safety belts, firearms and helmets, trials carried out in countries other than the USA were disregarded as many issues related to injury prevention are tied directly to country-specific legislation. For each question, an identifier and its variations were used as search strings (e.g., "seat belts" and "safety belts"). The "related articles" button was used sequentially to follow relevant articles after all hits had been reviewed or there were at least 40 consecutive irrelevant papers.

Of note, "emergency department" and its variations were used to perform the initial search but removed if there were less than three trials carried out in the ED.

Critical review of the literature

Question 1: For ED patients (population), what ED-based interventions (intervention) effectively change patients' drinking behavior and/or risk of injury (outcome) from alcohol use?

Search strategy

- Cochrane: alcohol
- MEDLINE: alcohol AND injury prevention[bend]

Acute alcohol intoxication is associated with an increased risk of death from drowning, falls, motor vehicle crashes (for occupants and pedestrians), suicide and homicide [23]. Intoxication is also associated with other risky behaviors, such as unplanned sexual contacts, multiple sexual contacts and illicit drug use [24]. Chronic alcohol ingestion is associated with cirrhosis, pancreatitis, and renal, esophageal and head and neck cancers, as well as gastritis, alcohol withdrawal syndromes, cardiomyopathy and various neuropathies [25]. About 10–12% of the US population has an alcohol use disorder [26] and approximately 4% are dependent on alcohol [27].

Alcohol is a global health issue. The World Health Organization estimated the per capita alcohol consumption for people over age 15 years in 2003 using alcohol sales and population data. Uganda tops the chart at 19.47 L of pure alcohol per capita. Among English-speaking countries, Ireland ranks number four at 14.45 L of alcohol consumed per capita, the UK is number 22 (10.39 L), New Zealand is number 27 (9.79 L), Australia is number 35 (9.19 L), the USA is number 41 (8.51 L) and Canada is number 43 (8.26 L) [28]. In a survey of Canadians aged over 15 who consume alcohol, 22.6% exceeded low-risk limits on alcohol consumption (three drinks for women, four for men) at least once in the previous year and 17% of the same group scored in the "at risk" or higher range on the AUDIT screen (see below for an explanation of this screening tool) [29]. Alcohol is estimated to account for 2.4% of deaths among the Canadian population aged less than 69 years [30].

In some US EDs, the proportion of ambulance patients abusing alcohol may be as high as 24% [31]. Eleven percent of unintentional injuries and nearly 50% of intentional injuries are temporally related to alcohol use. In fact, nearly 50% of admitted

---

Box 58.1 NIAAA pre-screening questions.

1. Do you sometimes drink beer, wine or other alcoholic beverages? (If "no", screening is complete.)
2. How many times in the last year have you had more than (four for men, three for women) drinks in a day?
(If the answer is anything other than "none", the patient is at risk for an alcohol use disorder and further investigation is warranted.)

---

adult trauma patients are acutely intoxicated, heavy alcohol users, or both. These patients are at more than twice the risk for readmission for new trauma within 28 months [32]. Interventions that successfully decrease the incidence of binge drinking and/or the prevalence of chronic drinking will significantly reduce the health burden caused by alcohol.

Attempts at intervention should be based on routine screening for alcohol abuse because patients may not be acutely intoxicated and may not appear to have a problem at the time they are evaluated in the ED. The National Institute for Alcohol Abuse and Alcoholism (NIAAA) currently recommends screening by combining questions about the quantity and frequency of drinking (Box 58.1) with CAGE questions (Box 58.2) or the AUDIT survey (Box 58.3). For quantity and frequency, more than 14 drinks per week or four drinks per occasion for men and seven drinks per week or three drinks per occasion for women indicates concerning levels of alcohol use. Patients who report alcohol overuse or negative consequences of their drinking are candidates for intervention.

One Cochrane review was found regarding intervention for problem drinkers. This review, last updated in 2004, concludes that screening and intervening for alcohol overuse and dependence syndromes, particularly brief counseling, appear to reduce injuries (RR = 0.65; 95% CI: 0.21 to 2.00) and their antecedents but suggests larger trials are needed to document the reduction in actual injuries [33]. This review included studies with widely

---

Box 58.2 CAGE questions.

Cut: Ever felt you ought to cut down on your drinking?

Annoyed: Have people annoyed you by criticizing your drinking?

Guilt: Ever felt bad or guilty about your drinking?

Eye opener: Ever had an eye opener to steady nerves in the a.m.?

Interpretation:
 2 "yes" answers = strong indication for alcoholism
 3 "yes" answers = alcoholism confirmed

Box 58.3 AUDIT survey.

(Score of answer contained in parentheses)

1. How often do you have a drink containing alcohol?

    (0) never (1) monthly or less (2) 2–4 times/month (3) 2–3 times/week (4) 4 or more times/week

2. How many drinks containing alcohol do you have on a typical day when you are drinking? [number of standard drinks]

    (0) 1–2 (1) 3–4 (2) 5–6 (3) 7–9 (4) 10 or more

3. How often do you have six or more drinks on one occasion?

    (0) never (1) less than monthly (2) monthly (3) weekly (4) daily or almost daily

4. How often during the last year have you found that you were not able to stop drinking once you had started?

    (0) never (1) less than monthly (2) monthly (3) weekly (4) daily or almost daily

5. How often during the last year have you failed to do what was normally expected from you because of drinking?

    (0) never (1) less than monthly (2) monthly (3) weekly (4) daily or almost daily

6. How often during the last year have you needed a first drink in the morning to get yourself going after a heavy drinking session?

    (0) never (1) less than monthly (2) monthly (3) weekly (4) daily or almost daily

7. How often during the last year have you had a feeling of guilt or remorse after drinking?

    (0) never (1) less than monthly (2) monthly (3) weekly (4) daily or almost daily

8. How often during the last year have you been unable to remember what happened the night before because you had been drinking?

    (0) never (1) less than monthly (2) monthly (3) weekly (4) daily or almost daily

9. Have you or someone else been injured as a result of your drinking?

    (0) No (2) Yes, but not in the last year (4) Yes, during the last year

10. Has a relative or friend or doctor or other health worker been concerned about your drinking or suggested you cut down?

    (0) No (2) Yes, but not in the last year (4) Yes, during the last year

    Score of 8 or greater means there is an issue
    Score of 11 or greater is consistent with dependence

divergent patient populations as well as widely varying interventions; only one was performed using injured ED patients. The take home point of this review for emergency physicians is that there appear to be some beneficial effects of interventions of various sorts.

Patients in the ED for illness or injuries related to alcohol may be in the midst of a particularly "teachable moment" with regard to alcohol consumption [34], and may be accepting of counseling for alcohol use while in the ED [35]. Based on a systematic review conducted in 2002, brief interventions or "negotiated interviews" are effective in reducing drinking and injury recidivism over the following 12 months [36]. All of the included trials conducted in whole or in part in the ED showed a positive effect of the intervention. Other clinical intervention trials in the ED show a decrease in alcohol consumption primarily for binge or "at risk" drinkers rather than those who are already dependent, and the benefit lasts at least 12 months [37].

The details of an optimal, brief ED intervention are still unclear. Recently comparisons have been made between negotiated interviewing and tailored advice or combinations of the two. Tailored advice is aimed specifically at the demographic characteristics of the patients and for their reported drinking behaviors. Among college binge drinkers, tailored advice alone was at least as good as negotiated interviewing [38], and among ED patients, computerized tailored advice combined with an interview further decreased reported drinking at 12 months [39].

There is now enough evidence supporting the effectiveness of screening and brief intervention among admitted trauma patients that the American College of Surgeons Committee on Trauma (COT) has added a requirement that level I or II trauma centers perform and document screening and intervention in order to be verified as such by the COT [40].

In summary, there is good evidence to support screening and brief intervention (with or without tailored advice) in the ED. However, many ED physicians are not currently trained in the method for such an intervention. In order to be willing to screen and intervene, physicians must be comfortable with the technique. This appears to take some practice; a 1-hour lecture may be insufficient [41]. A 4-hour interactive training program on screening and intervention was successful at increasing emergency medicine residents' attempts to intervene with patients in the ED [42]. Recent publications and information available from the American College of Emergency Physicians (ACEP, at http://www.acep.org/webportal/PracticeResources/issues/pubhlth/alcscreen/) and the NIAAA (clinicians' guide at http://pubs.niaaa.nih.gov/publications/Practitioner/CliniciansGuide2005/guide.pdf) can provide further information on how to carry out this intervention and provide patients with appropriate local referrals.

Question 2: In older adults (population), what ED-based interventions (intervention) decrease falls (outcome)?

Search strategy

- Cochrane and MEDLINE: (falls AND emergency department) OR (fall AND prevention AND intervention AND emergency department). Studies performed in English-speaking countries other than the USA were included

Falls and fall-related injuries are a common and serious cause of morbidity and mortality in elderly patients. In a 1-year period, 28–35% of people older than 65 years in the UK reported falling [43]. In Thailand the prevalence of falls among older adults is 19.8% [44] and in Singapore it is 19.3% [45]. In 2005, there were more than 1.8 million fall-related injuries and nearly 15,000 fall-related fatalities among people aged 65 and older in the United States [46]. In fact, in the USA, falls are the most common mechanism of non-fatal injuries resulting in ED visits for people over 65 years [47]. Falls among older individuals may require hospital admission. In Brisbane, Australia, 84% of injury admissions among patients older than 65 years were for fall-related injuries [48].

Both intrinsic and extrinsic causes contribute to the increased risk of falling for older adults. Intrinsic causes include weakness, balance problems, decreased vision and cognitive impairment. Extrinsic factors include polypharmacy and environmental issues such as poor lighting, loose carpets and absent hand rails. Compared to younger people, elderly patients are both more likely to fall and to have an injury from the fall due to underlying medical problems (e.g., osteoporosis, slower reflexes, anticoagulant therapy). Approximately 35–40% of community-dwelling patients over 65 years fall each year and about 5–10% of these falls result in injuries requiring medical care, about half of which are fractures [49]. Fall-related injuries account for 6% of medical expenses in this age group [50].

Eighty-two percent of older patients who have fallen are discharged home after evaluation in the ED [2]. However, having one fall identifies individuals at increased risk for falling. Recurrent fallers are at a higher risk of early admission to a nursing care facility and premature death [51]. This highlights a need and potential opportunity for intervention in the ED.

The American Geriatrics Society, British Geriatrics Society and the American Academy of Orthopedics convened a panel and performed a systematic review in 2001 [52]. Their recommendations emphasize the need for a multi-factorial approach for the outpatient approach to elderly patients with a fall. Specific recommendations included exercise and balance training (class B), environmental modification (class B), medication reassessment for patients on four or more medications or any psychotropic medication (class C) and behavioral and educational programs (class B). Of note, educational programs have not been shown to work in isolation [53].

The Cochrane review [54] (last updated in 2003), which included 62 trials involving 21,668 people, found the following interventions likely to be beneficial:

1 A multi-disciplinary, multi-factorial, health/environmental risk factor screening/intervention program either in the community – both for an unselected population of older people (four trials, 1651 participants: pooled RR = 0.73; 95% CI: 0.63 to 0.85) and for a population of older people with a history of falling or selected because of known risk factors (five trials, 1176 participants: pooled RR = 0.86; 95% CI: 0.76 to 0.98) – or in residential care facilities (one trial,

439 participants: cluster-adjusted incidence rate ratio = 0.60; 95% CI: 0.50 to 0.73).

2 A program of muscle strengthening and balance retraining, individually prescribed at home by a trained health professional (three trials, 566 participants: pooled RR = 0.80: 95% CI: 0.66 to 0.98).

3 Home hazard assessment and modification that is professionally prescribed for older people with a history of falling (three trials, 374 participants: RR = 0.66; 95% CI: 0.54 to 0.81).

4 Withdrawal of psychotropic medication (one trial, 93 participants: relative hazard = 0.34; 95% CI: 0.16 to 0.74).

5 Cardiac pacing for patients with cardio-inhibitory carotid sinus hypersensitivity (one trial, 175 participants: weighted mean difference = –5.20; 95% CI: –9.40 to –1.00).

6 A 15-week tai chi group exercise intervention (one trial, 200 participants: risk ratio = 0.51; 95% CI: 0.36 to 0.73).

Subsequent to the Cochrane review, Chang et al. published a meta-analysis in 2004 and concluded that a multi-factorial falls risk assessment and management program was the most effective component in fall prevention. The risk for falling decreased by 18% and the average number of falls was reduced by 43% when interventions that used multi-dimensional risk assessment and risk reduction were analyzed as a group [55]. Irvin et al. systematically reviewed preventive interventions with "potential applicability" in the ED, including geriatric falls, and although they found no ED-based studies, concluded that multi-dimensional programs prevent falls and fractures (class B) [56].

However, a multi-disciplinary, multi-factorial approach to elders with falls may not be readily accomplished from the ED. In a 2005 study by Donaldson et al., only 32% of older adults reported seeing their primary care doctor after an ED visit for a fall and 18% reported another fall since their index event [57]. Simply instituting ED practice guidelines that included a fall-related after care instruction sheet had no effect on falls, although it did raise physician awareness and increased the number of patients they diagnosed with falls due to loss of consciousness, stroke, transient ischemic attack (TIA) or seizures [58,59]. Some of the difficulty with these interventions may come from those patients who are reluctant to exercise, cease psychotropic medication or have a home safety assessment. However, 52% of patients reported considering falls prevention after a fall, again highlighting the teachable moment in the ED and the process of moving through stages of change [60].

From the ED perspective, the emphasis needs to be on the recognition of elders as having a high risk for further falls and the ED intervention needs to include detailed after care instructions. Communicating with a patient's primary care physician and family members about the patient's fall risk can facilitate the appropriate follow-up. Optimally, emergency physicians could refer patients discharged after a fall or with multiple fall risk factors directly to an outpatient falls prevention team. While this may not be available in many communities, when it is available ED physicians can and do utilize it [61].

Question 3: For intimate partner violence victims identified in the ED (population), what ED-based interventions (intervention) decrease injury (outcome)?

Search strategy

- Cochrane and MEDLINE: (intimate partner violence OR domestic violence) AND emergency department AND (prevention OR screening). Studies performed in English-speaking countries other than the USA were included in the Cochrane search

The Cochrane Library was searched. A systematic review entitled "Domestic violence screening and intervention programmes for adults with dental or facial injury" was found [62]. Additionally, a promising review entitled "Advocacy interventions to reduce or eliminate violence and promote the physical and psychosocial well-being of women who experience intimate partner abuse" is in protocol stage [63].

Intimate partner violence (IPV) focuses on violence between two adult partners and is a subset of domestic violence and family violence. IPV may be physical, sexual, emotional, financial, or a combination of these. This abuse is intentional and is perpetrated to maintain power and control over the victim. IPV can occur in any intimate relationship including current and former relationships and heterosexual and same-sex relationships. Perpetrators and victims can be of any gender, age, socio-economic group, race or religious background.

Among couples living together, and using both partners' reports, rates of IPV in the USA are 5–14% for male-to-female violence, 6–18% for female-to-male partner violence, and 8–21% for any partner-to-partner violence [64]. In the ED, up to 7% of female patients presenting to the ED have an IPV event as the reason for the visit; 14–22% of all female ED patients have experienced IPV in the previous year and the lifetime prevalence is 54% [65]. (Few studies included screening men for IPV in the ED.) A global review of population-based studies from 1982 to 1999 looked at the proportion of women ever physically assaulted by an intimate male partner with the following results: Africa (13–45%), Latin America and the Caribbean (13–69%), North America (Canada 27–29%; USA 22%), Asia and the western Pacific region (10–67%), Europe (14–58%) and the eastern Mediterranean region (34%) [66]. Additionally, a World Health Organization survey study in 10 countries between 2000 and 2003 found 15–71% of "ever partnered" women reported experiencing intimate partner violence at some point in their life [67].

By its nature, IPV is undesirable. Ideally, violence prevention efforts by emergency physicians would be targeted at identifying individuals likely to be perpetrators and would be successful in preventing the behavior. We found no studies in any health environment that studied IPV perpetrators; all are focused on past or current IPV victims. The initial step is to screen for IPV victimization with the idea that "screening will lead to an increased identification of women who are experiencing violence, lead to ap-propriate interventions and support, and ultimately decrease exposure to violence and its detrimental health consequences, both physical and psychological" [68].

A number of meta-analyses and systematic reviews [62,63,65,69] suggest there are effective methods for IPV screening and that screening programs generally increase rates of IPV victim identification. Several instruments [69,70] have been developed for screening and have demonstrated internal consistency, but none have been "evaluated against measurable violence or health outcomes". Referrals to community resources, shelters, social workers and police often increase when abused women are actively identified, but the studies were not designed to show improvement in violence or health outcomes. We found no studies describing interventions that are effective at decreasing the likelihood of future victimization or in improving any other measured health outcome. As a result, no systematic review or meta-analysis found evidence to support routine screening.

Although current evidence does not support routinely screening ED patients for IPV, IPV is a pervasive problem that crosses all socio-economic lines and future research needs to focus on developing effective interventions. In the day-to-day practice of emergency medicine, ED physicians must be prepared to discuss IPV with patients and offer appropriate referral to law enforcement and/or local social services.

Question 4: For adult patients in the ED (population), what interventions (intervention) increase the use of safety belts in vehicles (outcomes)?

Search strategy

- Cochrane and MEDLINE: seat belt OR safety belt

No Cochrane information and no systematic reviews were found. Only three studies were found, two focusing on teens and young adults; one on pregnant women. Only one study performed the intervention in a pediatric ED.

Safety belts reduce the risk of serious injury by 45–86% [71,72]. However, safety belts are active restraints and require specific behavior from the vehicle occupant. Safety belt legislation is particularly effective at increasing belt use. Safety belt use was first mandated in Victoria, Australia in 1970; belt use there has been sustained above 95% in the front of the vehicle for more than a decade [73]. Belt use in the UK reached a level of 95% after the introduction of mandatory safety belt use legislation (from 37%). In Canada, where belt use is mandatory throughout the vehicle, front occupant use was 90.5% in 2005 [74]. For comparison, belt use in front seating locations in the United States was 80.5% in 2005 [75], with 25 states and the District of Columbia having primary safety belt legislation and higher belt use rates. In all of these countries, the proportion of fatally injured persons who were unbelted at the time of the crash is more than 30%, partly because those who are unbelted are significantly more likely to die.

Two types of interventions regarding adult safety belt use have been studied in different settings and populations: motivational interviewing (behavior change counseling) and simple education. Adolescents and younger adults were the focus of two studies using interviewing, likely because the crash fatality rate is highest in this age group and restraint use is the lowest [76]. Physicians performed this brief interviewing intervention during a routine office visit for 11–24-year-olds, but there was no increased effect on self-report of belt use [77]. An earlier study, performed in a pediatric ED, studied 12–20-year-olds who presented with an injury from any cause. After self-reporting various risk behaviors, a trained study interventionist performed brief behavior change counseling aimed at one reported risk behavior per participant. This study found a significantly higher increase in the report of belt use at 6 months' post intervention [78]. However, this finding may not generalize to older adults, or to situations where the intervention is less standardized (e.g., performed by physicians rather than a trained interventionist).

The second type of intervention is educational and is perhaps better suited to adjusting/improving a safety behavior once already present. In a study of pregnant women, the subjects reported increasing their use of safety belts when pregnant (compared to pre-pregnancy), but frequently reported malpositioning the belts [79]. The tested intervention was primarily aimed at educating Medicaid or indigent pregnant patients attending a prenatal clinic to correctly locate the straps over the gravid abdomen (the lap portion should be pushed under the "bump" to lie on the anterior pelvic bones; the shoulder harness should lie between the breasts). The intervention consisted of printed materials and brief training for staff to discuss the issue with patients. The intervention significantly increased self-report of correct belt use [80]. This purely educational intervention is readily transferable to the ED and educational materials could be presented visually with posters in the waiting area.

In summary, there is early evidence that simple interventions in health care settings and in the ED can increase belt use in high-risk groups such as adolescents and pregnant women. While more research is required to prove this finding generalizes to all adults, emergency physicians should discuss proper belt use with adult patients, particularly if they present for injuries related to a motor vehicle crash.

Question 5: For adults who present to the ED (population), what strategies or programs (intervention) have been proven to decrease the risk of firearm injury (outcome)?

Search strategy

- MEDLINE: firearm AND gun

No Cochrane reviews were identified. No controlled trials of interventions aimed primarily at adult injury prevention were identified in any practice location.

Firearm injuries represent a significant health issue. Annually, intentional and unintentional firearm injury accounts for nearly 30,000 fatalities (10.1 deaths/100,000 persons) and 70,000 ED visits in the USA [22]. Firearm ownership is widespread in the USA. In 2004, nearly half of American men and 11% of women reported owning a gun, totaling more than 38% of all US households; 16% of adults reported owning at least one handgun [81]. In Canada, where 17% of households reported owning a gun in 2000 [82], there were 816 firearm-related fatalities in 2002 (approximately 2.6 deaths/100,000 persons) [83]. In Australia, approximately 5.2% of adults were licensed firearm owners in 2001 (the rate of illegal ownership is unknown) [84], and there were 333 fatalities related to firearms in the same year (1.8 deaths /100,000 persons) [85]. In both Canada and Australia, the large majority of firearm fatalities are suicide; in the USA nearly 40% are homicide.

In many homes, the safety of gun storage is questionable. In 2002, 4.3% of US households reported they had loaded and unlocked firearms in the home; a child less than 18 years old was living in more than half the homes with loaded, unlocked guns (2.5% of all US households) [86]. Homes with adolescent children are more likely to have loaded, unlocked guns than those with younger ones [87]. The presence of a firearm in a home is associated with significantly increased risk of both homicide and suicide [88–90] and the presence of a loaded, unlocked firearm is associated with an increased risk of unintentional firearm injury [91].

A large majority of surveyed surgeons, internists and pediatricians believe firearm violence is a major public health issue, and that physicians should be involved in firearm injury prevention, but less than a third make firearms safety part of routine patient care [92,93]. However, office-based intervention by physicians regarding safe firearm storage practices improves patients' reports of firearm storage behavior [94].

Individuals at increased risk of both intentional and unintentional firearm injury often present to the ED before the injury. In one study, persons who were ultimately the victim or convicted perpetrator of homicide were more likely than matched controls to have had ED visits for any reason and much more likely to have visits related to assault, firearm injury or substance abuse in the 3 years preceding the homicide [95]. Individuals with ED visits for mental health issues may be at particular risk of completing a suicide when a gun is available [96].

In the ED, a parental intervention for suicide risk reduction for adolescents with mental health complaints resulted in improved firearm storage safety (38%) or removal of the firearm (25%) from the home [97]. However, there is only poor agreement between adult partners on the number and type of firearms present in the homes of children visiting a pediatric ED – making accurate risk reduction potentially difficult [98].

The dearth of good evidence on this topic highlights the need for improved research into methods of prevention of firearm injury, particularly using objective outcomes such as actual injuries rather than self-report of gun storage practices. However, the US Congress has limited federal funding for gun-related research, stating in a recent (fiscal year 2006) appropriations bill:

> Provided further, That none of the funds made available for injury prevention and control at the Centers for Disease Control and Prevention may be used, in whole or in part, to advocate or promote gun control [99]

In effect, the Centers for Disease Control and Prevention (CDC) may continue to perform data collection and dissemination but not perform any intervention aimed at gun control in order to reduce the morbidity and mortality related to guns.

In summary, there is little current evidence to support an ED-based intervention to reduce adults' risk of firearms injury. However, discussing safe firearm storage practices (i.e., unloaded and locked) with individuals at high risk – particularly patients with mental illness, substance abuse or injuries due to interpersonal violence – can be carried out readily in the ED and may reduce the risk of firearm-related injury. Targeting family members, particularly parents of adolescents and young adults, may increase the effect.

Conclusions

In the scenario given above, in addition to appropriate post-exposure prophylaxis for both pregnancy and sexually transmitted diseases, the ED physician screened the patient for alcohol use disorder. The patient reported routinely drinking more than three drinks during one drinking episode, although she "only drank on the weekends". She scored 2/4 CAGE questions, indicating a drinking disorder. In a non-threatening way, the ED physician performed a brief intervention that included discussing social norms with her (less than three drinks on any occasion and less than seven in 1 week for women). Before leaving, the patient contracted to cut down on her binge drinking with the ED physician. She followed up with student health and did not return to the ED during the rest of her college career.

For the second patient, the new medication, because it does cause drowsiness, may well have contributed to the fall. The risks and benefits of the medication were discussed with the patient and his wife, and he chose not to continue taking it. The ED physician also discussed increasing physical activity, particularly walking and balancing exercises, and recommended the couple check with their local senior center. The next week they did so, and began to take an exercise class that included walking, stretching and balance exercises. They also reviewed the risk areas in their home and asked their son-in-law to install grab bars in the bathroom. Neither of them fell again.

Conflicts of interest

Neither author has any conflicts of interest.

References

1 McCaig LF, Burt CW. National Hospital Ambulatory Medical Care Survey: 2003, emergency department summary. *Adv Data Vital Health Stat* 2005;**358**:1–38.

2 Prochaska JO, DiClemente CC. Stages and processes of self-change of smoking: toward an integrative model of change. *J Consult Clin Psychol* 1983;**51**:390–95.

3 Ajzen I, Fishbein M. *Understanding Attitudes and Predicting Social Behavior*. Prentice-Hall, Englewood Cliffs, 1980.

4 Fishbein M. Theory of reasoned action: some applications and implications. In: Howe H & Page M, eds. *Nebraska Symposium on Motivation, 1979*. University of Nebraska Press, Lincoln, 1980:65–116.

5 Becker MF. The Health Belief Model and sick-role behavior. *Health Ed Monogr* 1974;**2**:409–19.

6 Bandura A. *Social Foundations of Thought and Action*. Prentice-Hall, Englewood Cliffs, 1986.

7 Bandura A. *Social Learning Theory*. Prentice-Hall, Englewood Cliffs, 1989.

8 Miller WR, Rollnick S. *Motivational Interviewing: Preparing people to change addictive behavior*. Guilford Press, New York, 1991.

9 Miller WR. Motivational interviewing with problem drinkers. *Behav Psychother* 1983;**11**:147–72.

10 Burke BL, Arkowitz H, Menchola M. The efficacy of motivational interviewing: a meta-analysis of controlled clinical trials. *J Consult Clin Psychol* 2003;**71**:843–61.

11 Dunn C, Deroo L, Rivara F. The use of brief interventions adapted from motivational interviewing across behavioral domains: a systematic review. *Addiction* 2001;**96**:1725–42.

12 Gladwell M. *The Tipping Point: How little things make a big difference*. Little, Brown and Company, New York, 2000.

13 Leontieva L, Horn K, Haque A, Kelmkamp J, Ehrlich P, Williams, J. Readiness to change problematic drinking assessed in the emergency department as a predictor of change. *J Crit Care* 2005;**20**(3):251–6.

14 Borges G, Cherpitel CJ, Mondragon L, Poznyak V, Peden M, Gutierrez I. Episodic alcohol use and risk of nonfatal injury. *Am J Epidemiol* 2004;**159**(6):565–71.

15 McDonald AJ, III, Wang N, Camargo CA, Jr. US emergency department visits for alcohol-related diseases and injuries between 1992 and 2000. *Arch Intern Med* 2004;**164**(5):531–7.

16 Centers for Disease Control, National Center for Injury Prevention and Control. Web Based Injury Statistics Query and Reporting System (WISQARS), queried using "falls". Available at http://webappa.cdc.gov/sasweb/ncipc/nfirates2001.html (accessed March 21, 2007).

17 Roudsari BS, Ebel BE, Corso PS, Molinari NA, Koepsell TD. The acute medical care costs of fall-related injuries among the U.S. older adults. *Injury* 2005;**36**(11):1316–22.

18 Abbott J, Johnson R, Koziol-McLain J, Lowenstein SR. Domestic violence against women. Incidence and prevalence in an emergency department population. *JAMA* 1995;**273**(22):1763–7.

19 Cox J, Bota GW, Carter M, Bretzlaff-Michaud JA, Sahai V, Rowe BH. Domestic violence. Incidence and prevalence in a northern emergency department. *Can Fam Physician* 2004;**50**:90–97.

20 National Highway Traffic Safety Administration. Traffic Safety Facts. Research note. DOT HS 809 970. Safety belt use in 2005 – use in states and territories. Available at http://www-nrd.nhtsa.dot.gov/Pubs/809970.PDF (accessed March 20, 2005).

21 National Highway Traffic Safety Administration. Traffic Safety Facts, 2004 data. Occupant protection. Available at http://www-nrd.nhtsa.dot. gov/pdf/nrd-30/NCSA/TSF2004/809909.pdf (accessed March 20, 2007).

22 Centers for Disease Control, National Center for Injury Prevention and Control. Web Based Injury Statistics Query and Reporting System (WISQARS), queried using "firearm". Available at http://webappa.cdc. gov/sasweb/ncipc/nfirates2001.html (accessed March 21, 2007).

23 Centers for Disease Control. Alcohol-attributable deaths and years of potential life lost – United States, 2001. *MMWR* 2004;**53**(37):866–70. Available at http://www.cdc.gov/mmwr/preview/mmwrhtml/ mm5337a2.htm#tab (accessed April 9, 2007).

24 Wingood GM, DiClemente RJ. The influence of psychosocial factors, alcohol, drug use on African-American women's high-risk sexual behavior. *Am J Prev Med* 1998;**15**:54–9.

25 Centers for Disease Control. Alcohol-Attributable Deaths Report, United States 2001. Available at http://apps.nccd.cdc.gov/ ardi/Report.aspx?T=AAM&P=9d3057a6-5cda-416d-ba10-41e7b8ebd 521&R=c22869f8-a1d3-48a8-8095-9142c6de5baf&M=1d04dc84-f775-4032-9ab3-75bc10221b2b (accessed March 25, 2007).

26 Moore MH, Gerstein DR, eds. *Alcohol and Public Policy: Beyond the shadow of prohibition.* National Academy Press, Washington, 1981.

27 American Psychiatric Association. *DSM-IV: Diagnostic and Statistical Manual of Mental Disorder,* 4th edn. American Psychiatric Association, Washington, 1994.

28 World Health Organization. Global Status Report on Alcohol 2004. Available at http://www.who.int/substance_abuse/publications/global_status_ report_2004_overview.pdf. (accessed May 15, 2007).

29 Canadian Centre on Substance Abuse. Canadian Addiction Survey 2005. Available at http://www.ccsa.ca/NR/rdonlyres/6806130B-C314-4C96-95CC-075D14CD83DE/0/ccsa0040282005.pdf (accessed May 15, 2007).

30 Rehm J, Giesbrecht N, Patra J, Roerecke M. Estimating chronic disease deaths and hospitalizations due to alcohol use in Canada 2002: implications for policy and preventions strategies. *Prev Chronic Dis* (online). Available at http://www.cdc.gov/pcd/issues/2006/oct/05_0009.htm (accessed June 9, 2008).

31 Whiteman PJ, Hoffman RS, Goldfrank LR. Alcoholism in the emergency department: an epidemiologic study. *Acad Emerg Med* 2000;**7**(1):14–20.

32 Rivara FP, Jurkovich GJ, Gurney JG, et al. The magnitude of acute and chronic alcohol abuse in trauma patients. *Arch Surg* 1993;**128**:907–12.

33 Dinh-Zarr R, Goss C, Heitman E, Roberts I, DiGuiseppi C. Interventions for preventing injuries in problem drinkers. *Cochrane Database Syst Rev* 2004;**3**:CD001857 (doi: 10.1002/14651858.CD001857.pub2).

34 Longabaugh R, Minugh PA, Nirenberg TD, Clifford PR, Becker B, Woolard R. Injury as a motivator to reduce drinking. *Acad Emerg Med* 1995;**2**(9):817–25.

35 Hungerford DW, Pollock DA, Todd KH. Acceptability of emergency department based screening and brief intervention for alcohol problems. *Acad Emerg Med* 2005;**7**(12):1383–92.

36 D'Onofrio G, Degutis LC. Preventive care in the emergency department: screening and brief intervention for alcohol problems in the emergency department: a systematic review. *Acad Emerg Med* 2002;**9**(6):627–38.

37 Bazargan-Hejazi S, Bing E, Bazargan M, et al. Evaluation of a brief intervention in an inner-city emergency department. *Ann Emerg Med* 2005;**46**(1):67–76.

38 Juarez P, Walters ST, Daugherty M, Radi C. A randomized trial of motivational interviewing and feedback with heavy drinking college students. *J Drug Ed* 2006;**36**(3):233–45.

39 Blow FC, Barry KL, Walton MA, et al. The efficacy of two brief intervention strategies among injured, at-risk drinkers in the emergency department: impact of tailored messaging and brief advice. *J Stud Alcohol* 2006;**67**(4):568–78.

40 American College of Surgeons, Committee on Trauma. *Resources for Optimal Care of the Injured Patient.* American College of Surgeons, 2006.

41 Saitz R, Sullivan LM, Samet JH. Training community based clinicians in screening and brief intervention for substance abuse problems: translating evidence into practice. *Subst Abuse* 2000;**21**:21–31.

42 D'Onofrio G, Nadel ES, Degutis LC, et al. Improving emergency medicine residents' approach to patients with alcohol problems: a controlled educational trial. *Ann Emerg Med* 2002;**40**(1):50–62.

43 Masud T, Morris RO. Epidemiology of falls. *Age Ageing* 2001;**30**(S4):3–7.

44 Assantachai P, Praditsuwan R, Chatthanawaree W, et al. Risk factors for falls in the Thai elderly in an urban community. *J Med Assoc Thai* 2003;**86**(2):124–30.

45 Chu LW, Chi I, Chiu AY. Incidence and predictors of falls in the Chinese elderly. *Ann Acad Med Singapore* 2005;**34**(1):60–72.

46 National Center for Injury Prevention and Control. Web-based Injury Statistics Query and Reporting System (WISQARS), queries using "age 65+ and unintentional falls". Available at http://webappa.cdc. gov/sasweb/ncipc/mortrate.html (accessed March 23, 2007).

47 Kocher KE, Dellinger AM. Public health and aging: nonfatal injuries among older adults treated in hospital emergency departments – United States, 2001. *MMWR* 2003;**52**(42):1019–22.

48 Peel NM, Kassulke DJ, McClure RF. Population based study of hospitalised fall related injuries in older people. *Injury Prev* 2002;**8**: 280–83.

49 Baraff LJ, Lee TJ, Kader S, et al. Effect of a practice guideline on the process of emergency department care of falls in elder patients. *Acad Emerg Med* 1999;**6**:1216–23.

50 Davison J, Bond J, Dawson P, et al. Patients with recurrent falls attending accident & emergency benefit from multifactorial intervention – a randomized controlled trial. *Age Ageing* 2005;**34**:162–8.

51 Russell MA, Hill KD, Blackberry I, et al. Falls risk and functional decline in older fallers discharged directly from emergency departments. *J Gerontol A Biol Sci Med Sci* 2006;**61**(10):1090–95.

52 American Geriatrics Society, British Geriatrics Society, American Academy of Orthopaedic Surgeons Panel on Falls Prevention. Guideline for the prevention of falls in older persons. *J Am Geriatr Soc* 2001;**49**:664–72.

53 Rucker D, Rowe BH, Johnson JA, et al. Educational intervention to reduce falls and fear of falling in patients after fragility fracture: results of a controlled pilot study. *Prev Med* 2006;**42**(4):316–19.

54 Gillespi LD, Gillespie WJ, Robertson MC, et al. Interventions for preventing falls in elderly people. *Cochrane Database Syst Rev* 2003;**4**:CD000 340.

55 Chang JT, Morton SC, Rubenstein LZ, et al. Interventions for the prevention of falls in older adults: systematic review and meta-analysis of randomized clinical trials. *BMJ* 2004;**328**(7441):680.

56 Irvin CB, Wyer PC, Gerson LW, et al. Preventive care in the emergency department, Part ii: Clinical preventive services – an emergency medicine evidence-based review. *Acad Emerg Med* 2000;**7**:1042–54.

57 Donaldson MG, Khan KM, Davis JC, et al. Emergency department fall-related presentations do not trigger fall risk assessment: a gap in

care of high-risk outpatient fallers. *Arch Gerontol Geriatr* 2005;**41**(3): 311–17.

58 Baraff LJ, Lee TJ, Kader S, et al. Effect of a practice guideline on the process of emergency department care of falls in elder patients. *Acad Emerg Med* 1999;**6**:1216–23.

59 Baraff JL, Lee TJ, Kader S, et al. Effect of a practice guideline for emergency department care of falls in elder patients on subsequent falls and hospitalizations for injuries. *Acad Emerg Med* 1999;**6**:1224–31.

60 Whitehead CH, Wundke R, Crotty M. Attitudes to falls and injury prevention: what are the barriers to implementing falls prevention strategies? *Clin Rehab* 2006;**20**:536–42.

61 Fortinsky RH, Iannuzzi-Sucich M, Baker DI, et al. Fall-risk assessment and management in clinical practice: views from healthcare providers. *J Am Geriatr Soc* 2004;**52**:1522–6.

62 Coulthard P, Yong S, Adamson L, et al. Domestic violence screening and intervention programmes for adults with dental or facial injury. *Cochrane Database Syst Rev* 2004;**2**:CD004486 (doi: 10.1002/14651858. CD004486.pub2).

63 Ramsey J, Feder G, Rivas C, et al. Advocacy interventions to reduce or eliminate violence and promote the physical and psychosocial well-being of women who experience intimate partner abuse (Protocol). *Cochrane Database Syst Rev* 2005;**1**:CD005043.

64 Schafer J, Caetano R, Clark CL. Rates of intimate partner violence in the United States. *AmJ Public Health* 1998;**88**(11):1702–4.

65 Anglin D, Sachs C. Preventive care in the emergency department: screening for domestic violence in the emergency department. *Acad Emerg Med* 2003;**10**:1118–27.

66 Heise L, Gracia-Moreno C. Violence by intimate partners. In: Krug EG, Dahlberg LL, Mercy JA, Zwi AB, Lozano R, eds. *World Report on Violence and Health.* World Health Organization, Geneva, 2002:87–121.

67 Garcia-Moreno C, Jansen HAFM, Ellsberg M, et al. Prevalence of intimate partner violence: findings from the WHO multi-country study on women's health and domestic violence. *Lancet* 2006;**368**:1260–69.

68 Ramsay J, Richardson J, Carter YH, et al. Should health professionals screen women for domestic violence? (Systematic review) *BMJ* 2002;**325**:314.

69 Nelson HD, Nygren P, McInerney Y, et al. Screening women and elderly adults for family and intimate partner violence: a review of the evidence for the U.S. Preventive Services Task Force. *Ann Intern Med* 2004;**140**:387–96.

70 Rhodes KV, Drum M, Anliker E, et al. Lowering the threshold for discussions of domestic violence. *Arch Intern Med* 2006;**166**:1107–14.

71 Kahane, CJ. *Fatality Reduction by Safety Belts for Front Seat Occupants of Cars and Light Trucks. Updated and expanded based on 1986–1999 FARS data.* DOT HS 809 199. US Department of Transportation, Washington, 2000.

72 Rivara, FP, Koepsell, TD, Grossman, DC, Mock, C. Effectiveness of automatic shoulder belt systems in motor vehicle crashes. *JAMA* 2000;**283**(21):2826–8.

73 Australian Transport Safety Bureau. CR 215: Benefits of Retrofitting Seat Belt Reminder Systems to Australian Passenger Vehicles. Australian Transport Safety Bureau, 2004. Available at http://www.atsb.gov.au /publications/2004/Belt_Analysis_9.aspx (accessed May 16, 2007).

74 Transport Canada. Transport Canada's Surveys of Seat Belt Use in Canada, 2004–2005. Available at http://www.tc.gc.ca/roadsafety/tp2436/rs200601/menu.htm#HIGHLIGHTS (accessed May 15, 2007).

75 National Highway Traffic Safety Administration. Traffic Safety Facts, 2005 Data. Occupant protection. Available at http://www-nrd.nhtsa.dot.gov/Pubs/810621.PDF (accessed May 15, 2007).

76 National Highway Traffic Safety Administration. Safety Belts and Older Teens, 2005 Report. Available at http://www.nhtsa.dot.gov/people/injury/NewDriver/beltsandTeenfacts/images/SafetyBeltsandTeens.pdf (accessed March 19, 2007).

77 Leverence RR, Martinez M, Whisler S, et al. Does office-based counseling of adolescents and young adults improve self-reported safety habits? A randomized controlled effectiveness trial. *J Adolesc Health* 2005;**36**(6):523–8.

78 Johnston BD, Rivara FP, Droesch RM, Dunn C, Copass MK. Behavior change counseling in the emergency department to reduce injury risk: a randomized, controlled trial. *Pediatrics* 2002;**110**(2 Pt 1):267–74.

79 Tyroch AH, Kaups KL, Rohan J, Song S, Beingesser K. Pregnant women and car restraints: beliefs and practices. *J Trauma* 1999;**46**(2):241–5.

80 McGwin G, Jr., Willey P, Ware A, Kohler C, Kirby T, Rue LW, III. A focused educational intervention can promote the proper application of seat belts during pregnancy. *J Trauma* 2004;**56**(5):1016–21.

81 Hepburn L, Miller M, Azrael D, Hemenway D. The US gun stock: results from the 2004 national firearms survey. *Injury Prev* 2007;**13**:15–19.

82 The Canadian Firearms Centre. Fall 2000 Estimate of Firearms Ownership. Available at http://www.cfc-cafc.gc.ca/media/news_releases/2001/survey2001_e.pdf (accessed May 16, 2007).

83 Wilkins K. Deaths involving firearms. *Health Rep* 2005;**16**(4):36–43. Available at http://www.statcan.ca/english/ads/82-003-XPE/pdf/16-4-04.pdf (accessed May 17, 2007).

84 Sporting Shooters Association of Australia. Firearm Licensees. Available at http://www.ssaa.org.au/newssaa/political%20archive/graphs/ LicenseesRegisteredFirearms.jpg (accessed May 16, 2007).

85 Kreisfeld R. NISU Briefing. Firearm deaths and hospitalizations in Australia. Available at http://www.nisu.flinders.edu.au/briefs/firearm_deaths_2005.pdf (accessed May 15, 2007).

86 Okoro CA, Nelson DE, Mercy JA, Balluz LS, Crosby AE, Mokdad AH. Prevalence of household firearms and firearm-storage practices in the 50 states and the District of Columbia: findings from the Behavioral Risk Factor Surveillance System, 2002. *Pediatrics* 2005;**116**(3):e370–76.

87 Johnson RM, Miller M, Vriniotis M, Azrael D, Hemenway D. Are household firearms stored less safely in homes with adolescents? Analysis of a national random sample of parents. *Arch Pediatr Adolesc Med* 2006;**160**(8):788–92.

88 Dahlberg LL, Ikeda RM, Kresnow MJ. Guns in the home and risk of a violent death in the home: findings from a national study. *Am J Epidemiol* 2004;**160**(10):929–36.

89 Kung HC, Pearson JL, Wei R. Substance use, firearm availability, depressive symptoms, and mental health service utilization among white and African American suicide decedents aged 15 to 64 years. *Ann Epidemiol* 2005;**15**(8):614–21.

90 Kellermann AL, Somes G, Rivara FP, Lee RK, Banton JG. Injuries and deaths due to firearms in the home. *J Trauma* 1998;**45**(2):263–7.

91 Miller M, Azrael D, Hemenway D, Vriniotis M. Firearm storage practices and rate of unintentional firearm deaths in the United States. *Accid Anal Prev* 2005;**37**:661–7.

92 American Academy of Pediatrics Division of Health Policy Research Periodic Survey of Fellows. Executive Summary. Available at http://www.aap.org/research/periodicsurvey/ps47exs.htm (accessed March 20, 2007).

93 Cassel CK, Nelson EA, Smith TW, Schwab CW, Barlow B, Gary NE. Internists' and surgeons' attitudes toward guns and firearm injury prevention. *Ann Intern Med* 1998;**128**(3):224–30.

94 Albright TL, Bruge Sk. Improving firearm storage habits: impact of brief office counseling by family physicians. *J Am Board Fam Pract* 2003;**16**:40–46.

95 Crandall CS, Jost PF, Broidy LM, Daday G, Sklar DP. Previous emergency department use among homicide victims and offenders: a case–control study. *Ann Emerg Med* 2004;**44**(6):646–55.

96 Shen X, Hackworth J, McCabe H, Lovett L, Aumage J, O'Neil J, Bull M. Characteristics of suicide from 1998–2001 in a metropolitan area. *Death Stud* 2006;**30**(9):859–71.

97 Kruesi MJ, Grossman J, Pennington JM, Woodward PJ, Duda D, Hirsch JG. Suicide and violence prevention: parent education in the emergency department. *J Am Acad Child Adolesc Psychiatry* 1999;**38**(3):250–55.

98 Coyne-Beasley T, Baccaglini L, Johnson RM, Webster B, Wiebe DJ. Do partners with children know about firearms in their home? Evidence of a gender gap and implications for practitioners. *Pediatrics* 2005;**115**(6):e662–7.

99 House Report 108-792 – Making appropriations for foreign operations, export financing, and related programs for the fiscal year ending September 30, 2005, and for other purposes. Available at http://thomas. loc.gov/cgi-bin/cpquery/?&sid=cp108ose4T&refer=&r_n=hr792.108& db_id=108&item=&sel=TOC_1050582& (accessed March 22, 2007).

59 Intimate Partner Violence

Debra Houry

Center for Injury Control, Department of Emergency Medicine, Emory University College of Medicine, Emory University, Atlanta, USA

Clinical scenario

A 20-year-old woman presents to the emergency department (ED) after falling down several stairs and hitting her head in the doorway. She had no loss of consciousness and denies trauma elsewhere. On physical exam, the triage nurse notes a large periorbital ecchymosis and several old bruises on the patient's arms and neck. Vital signs are temperature 37°C, pulse 70 beats/min, blood pressure 110/60 mmHg and respiration 16 breaths/min.

She is accompanied by her husband, a 25-year-old male who refuses to leave during the examination. You suspect that she received her injuries from him and that she is an intimate partner violence (IPV) victim. You are unsure what the most likely findings are on physical exam and other risk factors for IPV. You would like to ask her about IPV, but are unsure if screening is effective. Finally, you would like to know what interventions are effective for IPV and what your legal obligations are.

Background

Intimate partner violence is also referred to as "domestic violence", sexual assault, spousal abuse, family violence, and other terms. IPV is the new and accepted term to describe victimization between an individual and their partner. Since partnerships can be of many kinds, and marriage arrangements are not necessary, the use of spousal and marital terms are no longer in vogue. Moreover, since partners may be same sex or opposite sex, IPV may occur in both heterosexual and homosexual relationships. Finally, while male IPV does exist, it is most commonly observed in women. During the remainder of this chapter, the use of the term IPV will relate to women being victimized by a male partner in a relationship.

Evidence-based Emergency Medicine. Edited by Brian H. Rowe
© 2009 Blackwell Publishing, ISBN: 978-1-4051-6143-5.

Each year, nearly 5.3 million intimate partner victimizations occur among women aged 18 and older in the USA [1]. This violence results in approximately 2 million injuries and 1300 deaths [1]. A population-based study revealed that 29% of women in the United States have experienced physical, sexual or psychological IPV in their lifetime [2]. In addition, many victims of IPV present to EDs with injuries or for treatment of medical and/or psychological complaints that are directly related to IPV [3]. Abbott and colleagues reported that 54% of the female ED patients they surveyed had been a victim of IPV at some point in their lifetime [3]. Houry et al. found that 36% of female ED patients who were in a relationship in the past year disclosed that they were victims of IPV [4]. Dearwater et al. found female patients who presented to the ED with non-traumatic complaints had a rate of IPV of ~2%. The lifetime prevalence of IPV was much higher (37%) and closer to that reported by others [5]. In Canada, similar incidence (~2%) and lifetime prevalence (~50%) data have been reported in patients presenting to the ED with non-traumatic complaints [6]. Other countries where this research has been completed report similar findings [7,8].

Clinical questions

1 In women who present to the ED (population), is screening for intimate partner violence (intervention) effective at reducing future violence and injury (outcome)?

2 In women who present to the ED with possible intimate partner violence (population), what physical exam findings (exposure) are most sensitive and specific (diagnostic test characteristics) for intimate partner violence?

3 In women who present to the ED with possible intimate partner violence (population), what history or risk factors (exposure) should make clinicians consider intimate partner violence (outcome)?

4 In women who present to the ED with intimate partner violence (population), what interventions (interventions) are most effective in reducing future injury and death (outcomes)?

5 In IPV perpetrators (population), are any treatments (interventions) effective in reducing future injury and death (outcomes) in their partners?

6 In women who present to the ED with intimate partner violence (population), what steps are mandated by the law (exposures) to eliminate future injury and death (outcomes)?

General search strategy

You start your search by using database searches in Cochrane, MEDLINE and EMBASE. You know that not many randomized trials have been conducted for intimate partner violence so you start with a very broad search using the term "domestic violence". Your first search of the Cochrane Library for domestic violence yields only one systematic review. You expand your search with MEDLINE and EMBASE and find six additional relevant systematic reviews and meta-analyses.

Searching for evidence synthesis:

- Cochrane Library: domestic violence
- MEDLINE: domestic violence AND MEDLINE English articles AND EBM reviews
- EMBASE: domestic violence AND English articles AND adult and reviews

Question 1: In women who present to the ED (population), is screening for intimate partner violence (intervention) effective at reducing future violence and injury (outcome)?

Search strategy

- Cochrane Library: domestic violence
- MEDLINE: domestic violence AND MEDLINE English articles AND EBM reviews

There is variation in many countries with respect to recommendations for routine screening for IPV. Currently, the Joint Commission on Accreditation of Healthcare Organizations (JCAHO) requires US hospitals to have policies and protocols in place to identify and refer victims of IPV. In addition, many medical organizations such as the American Medical Association recommend screening for IPV [9]. Conversely, the Canadian, British and Australasian emergency physician associations do not have a formal policy on IPV screening.

This policy and practice variation reflects the current level of evidence available to guide action. For example, the US Preventive Services Task Force (USPSTF) found insufficient evidence to recommend for or against routine screening of women for IPV and gave it an "I" (insufficient evidence) recommendation [10]. A total of 806 abstracts were initially reviewed, 14 met inclusion criteria, but no study actually evaluated screening using abuse out-

comes. Thus, the USPSTF concluded that the research regarding screening did not look at effectiveness, was of poor quality or was conflicting. Their conclusion was that the balance of benefits and harms could not be determined.

In addition, one Cochrane review was identified on domestic violence [11]. This review did not find any eligible randomized controlled trials (RCTs) and found no evidence to support or refute screening for domestic violence in adults with dental or facial injury. Screening tools to detect domestic violence exist but prospective validation is lacking and no RCTs have specifically evaluated their effectiveness for patients presenting with facial and/or dental injuries.

Anglin and Sachs systematically reviewed 339 articles pertaining to IPV [12]. They also found that there was no research on screening outcomes for IPV; however, they did report that screening was feasible in an ED. Another systematic review [13] concluded that screening in health care settings cannot be justified at this time; however, the same review also found that the majority of female patients found screening for IPV acceptable.

Some preliminary research presented at the 2007 National Conference on Healthcare and Domestic Violence demonstrated that screening for IPV was both safe and effective [14]. Over 3000 men and women were prospectively screened for IPV in an ED waiting room and IPV victims were followed up to 3 months after screening. The authors found no increase in violence after screening and also reported that many IPV victims had contacted resources and developed safety plans. In addition, a prospective cohort study revealed that women who screened positive for IPV were 11.3 times more likely to experience physical violence and 7.3 times more likely to experience verbal aggression at 4-month follow-up than women who had not screened positive for IPV at their index ED visit [15].

In summary, while screening of patients appears safe and well accepted by patients in the ED, there has not been enough research to definitively recommend for or against screening. In the USA, the JCAHO and many medical organizations do recommend screening for IPV. EDs have high prevalence rates of undetected IPV, thus screening may be useful in this medical setting. The persisting questions are how this is operationalized, the tool(s) to complete this, and the effectiveness of the intervention (i.e., what interventions will reduce future violence).

Question 2: In women who present to the ED with possible intimate partner violence (population), what physical examination findings (exposure) are most sensitive and specific (diagnostic test characteristics) for intimate partner violence?

Search strategy

- MEDLINE: domestic violence AND injury AND emergency department

With any victim of abuse, whether it be partner violence, child maltreatment, or elder abuse, it is important to look for injuries in multiple stages of healing, defensive injuries and injuries not consistent with the story.

Your search for meta-analyses, systematic reviews or RCTs yields no papers. However, your MEDLINE search results in 198 papers and, of these, the majority are cross-sectional studies or retrospective reviews. Several injury patterns have been reported in literature. Maxillofacial injuries in IPV victims were noted in a retrospective review, and one-third of IPV victims with injuries had facial fractures [16]. A cross-sectional study reported that IPV victims were 7.5 times more likely to have head, neck and facial injuries than other trauma patients ($P < 0.001$) [17]. Spedding et al. conducted a retrospective review and found that head, arm and abdominal injuries were significantly associated with IPV, particularly when multiple injuries were present [18]. Finally, Muelleman et al. conducted a multi-center, cross-sectional study and concluded that battered women were more likely to be injured in the head, face, neck, thorax and abdomen than women injured by other mechanisms [19]. Thus, IPV should be considered in women with maxillofacial injuries as well as injuries to the "center" of the body (neck, thorax, abdomen).

Question 3: In women who present to the ED with possible intimate partner violence (population), what history or risk factors (exposure) should make clinicians consider intimate partner violence (outcome)?

Search strategy

- MEDLINE: (domestic violence AND identification AND emergency department) OR (domestic violence AND risk factors AND emergency department)

Anyone can be a victim of IPV: IPV crosses ethnic, socio-economic, educational and gender boundaries. Certain risk factors and associations with IPV victimization have been reported in the literature. Again your search for meta-analyses or RCTs does not yield any papers; however, your MEDLINE search results in 59 research studies with "identification" and 88 papers with the "risk factors". Several of these studies are prospective cohort or cross-sectional studies.

Grisso et al. found that in a cohort of female ED patients, low median income, a high rate of change of residence and poor education were independently associated with the risk of violent injuries [20]. In addition, a cross-sectional study revealed that younger age ($OR = 2.2$), children younger than 18 years living in the home ($OR = 2.0$) and ending a relationship within the past year ($OR = 7.0$) were correlated with IPV [5].

Alcohol and drug abuse have also been associated with IPV. El-Bassel and colleagues conducted face-to-face interviews with women at an inner city ED and found that a higher proportion of abused women reported a history of regular crack, cocaine or

heroin use than non-abused women. In addition, participants who were physically abused by their partner during the past were more likely than non-abused women to report higher scores on the alcohol use disorders identification test (4.9 vs 2.4) and the drug abuse severity test (3.0 vs 1.3) [21]. Grisso led a case–control study and concurred that women's use of illicit drugs and alcohol abuse were factors associated with violence [20].

In addition, the presence of mental health symptoms has been associated with IPV victimization [4]. A cohort study of African-American female ED patients reported that depressive symptoms, symptoms of post-traumatic stress disorder (PTSD) and suicidality were positively correlated with physical, sexual and emotional IPV. An additional effect was also noted. Mental health symptoms increased significantly with amount of abuse: depression ($OR = 5.9$ for three types of abuse), PTSD ($OR = 9.4$ for three types) and suicidality ($OR = 17.5$ for three types).

The majority of studies, until recent years, have focused on females. Thus, much of the research on male victims has not been collected using validated tools for males. No RCTs or systematic reviews researching male victims of IPV were identified in the MEDLINE search. A cross-sectional study reported that male IPV victims were more likely to be younger, single, African-American and uninsured than male ED patients who did not experience IPV by a female partner [22]. A case–control study concluded that male IPV victims who sought treatment in the ED have higher rates of IPV perpetration arrests (51% vs 22%) and non-aggravated assaults (44% vs 20%) compared to male ED patients matched by age, race and date of visit [23].

Since most research on risk factors and associations with IPV is not high quality, the evidenced-based approach is problematic. This is particularly true for male victims. Overall, emergency physicians should understand some of the common timings and injury patterns for IPV; however, the safest approach is to maintain a very high index of suspicion for this presentation.

Question 4: In women who present to the ED with intimate partner violence (population), what interventions (interventions) are most effective in reducing future injury and death (outcomes)?

Search strategy

- Cochrane Library: domestic violence
- MEDLINE: domestic violence AND MEDLINE English articles AND EBM reviews

Critics of IPV screening state that without an effective intervention, why identify victims? Wathen and MacMillan conducted a systematic review of interventions for IPV and concluded that in most studies the effectiveness of interventions was unclear [24]. Of 22 studies that met inclusion criteria, only one intervention was conducted in the ED. This New Zealand project studied the effectiveness of a protocol on identifying victims of IPV, improving documentation and increasing referrals [25]. Unfortunately, the initial improvements were not sustained at 1-year follow-up. Davis and Taylor tested public intervention programs addressing primary and secondary prevention of IPV [26]. Primary prevention using public education did not reduce frequency of new violence or severity of violence incurred by IPV victims. In the secondary prevention arm, the only difference was that abused individuals in the intervention called the police more frequently. As Wathen and MacMillan point out, no studies have looked at the harm associated with the use of screening tools or with the intervention itself [24]. They also conclude that research on interventions is still in the early stages and the benefits of interventions are unclear.

Another systematic review screened 667 citations and only found two that met inclusion criteria [12]. One of the studies demonstrated less violence on a questionnaire among the intervention group (three counseling sessions during prenatal care) 12 months later [27]. The authors of the review conclude that very few intervention studies have been conducted and that the outcomes have been based on questionnaires and not episodes of violence [10]. In addition, one Cochrane review was identified on domestic violence [11]. This review did not find any eligible RCTs on interventions and stated that there was a lack of evidence that intervention programs are effective at reducing the frequency of physical assaults and at reducing the severity of facial injuries in IPV victims [11].

Ramsay and colleagues [13] also concluded that not enough high-quality studies on interventions had been conducted. They reviewed six intervention studies and found that these papers had inconsistent results and used weak study designs. Anglin and Sachs [12] identified an additional intervention study by Muelleman and Geighny [28] in their systematic review. Muelleman and Geighny implemented an ED-based advocacy system and reported that IPV victims in the intervention were more likely to use a shelter or counseling services within 1 year compared to the control group. There was no difference, however, in calls to police or ED visits for IPV, and no measures of health status or decreasing the incidence of violence were measured. In summary, the evidence does not suggest a long-term improvement for IPV victims after ED interventions; however, very few intervention studies have been conducted.

Question 5: In IPV perpetrators (population), are any treatments (interventions) effective in reducing future injury and death (outcomes) in their partners?

Search strategy

- MEDLINE: domestic violence AND MEDLINE English articles AND EBM reviews

Primary prevention for IPV victims includes treating perpetrators so that they do not inflict further violence on their partners. Recently, the Centers for Disease Control and Prevention emphasized

research on primary prevention for IPV [29]. Babcock and colleagues conducted a meta-analysis of 22 experimental and quasi-experimental studies evaluating treatment for IPV perpetrators [30]. They reported that interventions had little impact on reducing recidivism rates beyond the effect of being arrested. One of the randomized studies looked at batterers on probation assigned to a psycho-educational program versus no treatment and found no differences between the groups based on police records or victim reports [31]. However, this study had very high attrition rates, low follow-up rates and uneven assignment of groups. Another study of US Navy personnel compared cognitive-behavioral treatment with couples therapy and a no treatment control [32]. Neither intervention was significantly different from the control group in recidivism rates based on victim reports, although participants were not mandated to participate in treatment, which could have led to self-selection bias.

Wathen and Macmillan also reviewed interventions for batterers in their systematic review [24]. The authors identified only two RCTs with quality ratings of fair or good. Dunford's study was summarized above and was rated as "good" [32]. The additional "fair" study was a quasi-randomized, uncontrolled trial that found no differences in recidivism rates based on victims' reports and arrests [33]. However, this study did not have a control group, was not blinded and had moderate attrition rates.

In summary, there is no conclusive evidence on the effectiveness of batterer intervention programs, and the safety of victims cannot be assumed through these interventions.

Question 6: In women who present to the ED with intimate partner violence (population), what steps are mandated by the law (exposures) to eliminate future injury and death (outcomes)?

Search strategy

- MEDLINE: domestic violence AND mandatory reporting

Variability in reporting practices exist for emergency physicians. For example, some emergency physicians in the United States may need to report IPV injury cases to authorities. Other countries do not have mandatory reporting laws, although there has been debate in Canada over a mandatory reporting law for gunshot wounds [34]. Currently, 45 states have laws that mandate physician reporting of injuries caused by weapons, crimes or IPV [35]. The type of injury and which agency to report to vary greatly by state.

No RCTs or prospective cohort studies have been conducted on how these laws affect patients. A population-based telephone survey revealed that abused women were less likely to support mandatory reporting compared to non-abused women (59% vs 73%) [36]. Rodriguez and colleagues found that women who had experienced recent physical or sexual abuse (OR = 2.2) or were non-English speaking (OR = 2.1) were more likely to oppose mandatory reporting than women who had never been abused [37]. On the other hand, Houry et al. reported that only 12% of ED patients would be deterred from seeking medical care because of mandatory reporting, with no differences in care seeking between IPV victims and other ED patients [38]. Only one time-trend analysis before and after the mandatory reporting law was enacted in California looked at the effect of the mandatory reporting law [39]. The authors did not find any increases in IPV dispatches to medical facilities 2 years after the implementation of the law. To date, no research has studied the effect of the law on the IPV outcomes for victims. Thus, at this time, no evidence exists to support or refute these mandatory reporting laws.

Conclusions

Armed with this information, you talk with the patient about IPV when her husband leaves the room and she discloses that her husband hit her. You refer her to the hospital social worker for community resources and to develop a safety plan. You tell her that the violence is not her fault and that no one deserves to be abused. Moreover, the potential escalation of violence is a threat to her life. After ensuring her safety and treating her injuries, you discharge her from the ED.

IPV is multifaceted issue. In the USA, emergency physicians are encouraged to screen for IPV based on JCAHO mandates and medical organization recommendations; however, very little evidence exists to recommend for or against screening. In addition, emergency physicians are used to assessing, treating and repairing the presenting problem in ED patients and currently research does not demonstrate any improved outcomes for IPV victims or perpetrators after an intervention. Until we have higher quality evidence to support or refute screening and interventions for IPV, emergency physicians must do what they believe is best for their patients. Most importantly, a heightened index of suspicion, case finding, ensuring a safe environment (if possible) and referral to professional agencies would seem appropriate.

Conflicts of interest

Dr. Houry is supported by research grants through the Centers for Disease Control and Prevention, National Institute of Mental Health and UCB Pharma.

References

1 Centers for Disease Control and Prevention. *Costs of Intimate Partner Violence Against Women in the United States.* US Department of Health and Human Services, CDC, Atlanta, 2003.

2 Coker AL, Davis KE, Arias IA, et al. Physical and mental health effects of intimate partner violence for men and women. *Am J Prev Med* 2002;**23**:260–68.

3 Abbott J, Johnson R, Koziol-McLain J, Lowenstein DR. Domestic violence against women: incidence and prevalence in an emergency department population. *JAMA* 1995;**273**:1763–7.

4 Houry D, Kemball R, Rhodes KV, Kaslow N. Intimate partner violence and mental health symptoms in African American female ED patients. *Am J Emerg Med* 2006;**24**:444–50.

5 Dearwater SR, Coben JH, Campbell JC, et al. Prevalence of intimate partner abuse in women treated at community hospital emergency departments. *JAMA* 1998;**280**:433–8.

6 Cox J, Bota GW, Carter M, Bretzlaff-Michaud JA, Sahai V, Rowe BH. Domestic violence. Incidence and prevalence in a northern emergency department. *Can Fam Physician* 2004;**50**:90–97

7 Luke N, Schuler SR, Mai BT, Vu Thien P, Minh TH. Exploring couple attributes and attitudes and marital violence in Vietnam. *Violence Against Women* 2007;**13**:5–27.

8 Ghazizadeh A. Domestic violence: a cross-sectional study in an Iranian city. *East Mediterr Health J* 2005;**11**:880–87.

9 American Medical Association. Diagnostic and treatment guidelines on domestic violence. *Arch Fam Med* 1992;**1**:39–47.

10 Nelson H, Nygren P, McInerney Y. Screening for Family and Intimate Partner Violence. Systematic Evidence Review No. 28 (prepared by the Oregon Health and Science Evidence-based Practice Center under Contract No. 290-97-0018). Agency for Healthcare Research and Quality, Rockville, 2004.

11 Coulthard P, Yong S, Adamson L, Warburton A, Worthington HV, Esposito M. Domestic violence screening and intervention programmes for adults with dental or facial injury. *Cochrane Database Syst Rev* 2004;**2**:CD004486 (doi: 10.1002/14651858.CD004486.pub2).

12 Anglin D, Sachs C. Screening for domestic violence in the emergency department. *Acad Emerg Med* 2003;**10**:1118–27.

13 Ramsay J, Richardson J, Carter YH, Davidson LL, Feder G. Should health professionals screen for domestic violence? (Systematic review). *BMJ* 2002;35:**325**:314.

14 Houry D, Kaslow N, Kemball RS, et al. Safety and effectiveness of IPV screening in the ED. Presented at the National Conference on Healthcare and Domestic Violence, San Francisco, March 2007.

15 Houry D, Feldhaus K, Peery B, et al. A positive domestic violence screen predicts future domestic violence. *J Interpersonal Violence* 2004;**19**: 955–66.

16 Le BT, Dierks EJ, Ueeck BA, Homer LD, Potter BF. Maxillofacial injuries associated with domestic violence. *J Oral Maxillofac Surg* 2001;**59**: 1277–83.

17 Perciaccante VJ, Ochs HA, Dodson TB. Head, neck, and facial injuries as markers of domestic violence in women. *J Oral Maxillofac Surg* 1999;**57**:760–62.

18 Spedding RL, McWilliams M, McNicholl BP, Dearden CH. Markers for domestic violence in women. *J Accident Emerg Med* 1999;**16**: 400–402.

19 Muelleman RL, Lenaghan PA, Pakieser RA. Battered women: injury locations and types. *Ann Emerg Med* 1996;**28**:486–92.

20 Grisso JA, Schwarz DF, Hirschinger N, et al. Violent injuries among women in an urban area. *N Engl J Med* 1999;**341**:1899–905.

21 El-Bassel N, Gilbert L, Witte S, et al. Intimate partner violence and substance abuse among minority women receiving care from an inner-city emergency department. *Womens Health Issues* 2003;**13**:16–22.

22 Mechem CC, Shofer FS, Reinhard SS, Hornig S, Datner E. History of domestic violence among male patients presenting to an urban emergency department. *Acad Emerg Med* 1999;**6**:786–91.

23 Muelleman RL, Burgess P. Male victims of domestic violence and their history of perpetrating violence. *Acad Emerg Med* 1998;**5**:866–70.

24 Wathen CN, MacMillan HL. Interventions for violence against women: scientific review. *JAMA* 2003;**289**:589–600.

25 Fanslow JL, Norton RN, Robinson EM. One year follow-up of an emergency department protocol for abused women. *Aust NZ J Public Health* 1999;**23**:418–20.

26 Davis RC, Taylor BG. A proactive response to family violence: the results of a randomized experiment. *Criminology* 1997;**35**:307–33.

27 Parker B, McFarlane J, Soeken K, Silva C, Reel S. Testing an intervention to prevent future abuse to pregnant women. *Res Nursing Health* 1999;**22**:59–66.

28 Muelleman RL, Geighny KM. Effects of an emergency department-based advocacy program for battered women on community resource utilization. *Ann Emerg Med* 1999;**11**:62–6.

29 National Center for Injury Prevention and Control. CDC Injury Research Agenda. Centers for Disease Control and Prevention, Atlanta, 2002.

30 Babcock JC, Green CE, Robie C. Does batterers' treatment work? A meta-analytic review of domestic violence treatment. *Clin Psychol Rev* 2004;**23**:1023–53.

31 Feder L, Forde D. A test of the efficacy of court-mandated counseling for convicted misdemeanor violence offenders: results from the Broward experiment. Paper presented at the International Family Violence Research Conference, Durham, NH, USA, July 1999.

32 Dunford FW. The San Diego Navy experiment: an assessment of interventions for men who assault their wives. *J Consult Clin Psychol* 2000;**68**:468–76.

33 Saunders DG. Feminist-cognitive-behavioral and process-psychodynamic treatments for men who batter. *Violence Victims* 1996; **11**:393–41.

34 Ovens H, Morrison H, Drummond A, Borgundvaag B. The case for mandatory reporting of gunshot wounds in the emergency department. Ontario Medical Association Section on Emergency Medicine Position Statement. *Ontario Med Rev* 2003:17–22. Available at www.oma.org/pcomm/omr/nov/03gunshot.

35 Houry D, Sachs CJ, Feldhaus KM, Linden J. Violence-inflicted injuries: reporting laws in the fifty states. *Ann Emerg Med* 2002;**39**:56–60.

36 Sachs CJ, Koziol-McLain J, Glass N, Webster D, Campbell J. A population-based survey assessing support for mandatory domestic violence reporting by health care personnel. *Women Health* 2002;**35**:121–33.

37 Rodriguez MA, McLoughlin E, Nah G, Campbell JC. Mandatory reporting of domestic violence injuries to the police: what do emergency department patients think? *JAMA* 2001;**286**:580–83.

38 Houry D, Feldhaus K, Thorson AC, Abbott J. Mandatory reporting laws do not deter patients from seeking medical care. *Ann Emerg Med* 1999;**34**:336–41.

39 Sachs CJ, Peek C, Baraff LJ, Hasselblad V. Failure of the mandatory domestic violence reporting law to increase medical facility reporting to police. *Ann Emerg Med* 1998;**31**:488–94.

60 Smoking Cessation

Lisa Cabral & Steven L. Bernstein

Albert Einstein College of Medicine, Montefiore Medical Center, Department of Emergency Medicine, New York, USA

Clinical scenario

A 55-year-old female presents to the emergency department (ED) with a 1-day history of shortness of breath and productive cough. On further history, she reports smoking a pack of cigarettes a day and has been smoking for 40 years. Her last cigarette was right before she entered the ED today. On primary assessment she is noted to be in moderate respiratory distress; her respiratory rate is 30 breaths/min and oxygen saturation is 90% while breathing room air. You can smell cigarette smoke on her breath. Physical examination reveals a barrel-shaped chest, poor air movement, diffuse rhonchi and expiratory wheezing throughout both lung fields.

Treatment for chronic obstructive pulmonary disease (COPD) exacerbation is initiated with inhaled albuterol/ipratropium bromide and intravenous methylprednisolone. You ask yourself whether you should advise her to quit smoking or start her on medications to help her quit. You are unsure whether this is the role of the emergency physician, and whether your advice would be effective.

Background

Tobacco use continues to be a major public health concern in developed countries, and a growing public health threat in developing countries. Globally, 1 billion men smoke, as do 250 million women. In developing countries, 50% of men smoke, as do 9% of women. In developed countries, 35% of men and 22% of women smoke [1]. In the USA, tobacco accounts for 430,000 deaths each year [2]. Tobacco use is the single greatest cause of preventable death and disease in the United States [3], where 20.9% of the population smokes [4]. Cigarette smoking has been associated with

Evidence-based Emergency Medicine. Edited by Brian H. Rowe
© 2009 Blackwell Publishing, ISBN: 978-1-4051-6143-5.

lung cancer, cancers of the aerodigestive tract, COPD, pneumonia, coronary artery disease, stroke, peptic ulcer disease, osteoporosis, and numerous other illnesses. Cigarette smoking also has health effects on the non-smoker exposed to second-hand smoke. Environmental tobacco smoke has been found to increase respiratory infections in children and to increase the risk of development of lung cancer and heart disease in adults [5].

In response to the global burden of death and illness caused by smoking, the World Health Organization (WHO) in 2003 adopted the Framework Convention on Tobacco Control [6]. This document, the first public health treaty ever negotiated under WHO's auspices, requires ratifying countries to comply with a set of standards in tobacco control encompassing tobacco product advertising, pricing, packaging, manufacturing and research. As of June 2007, 168 countries have signed the treaty, and 147 have ratified it [7].

Smoking is a leading health indicator of *Healthy People 2010*, a set of health objectives for the USA [8]. Goals within the Healthy People program include reducing tobacco use, increasing smoking cessation attempts and increasing physician counseling on smoking cessation. Treatment of tobacco-related disease is an enormous economic burden costing the US $75 billion in medical costs and $92 billion in lost productivity [2]. By decreasing the numbers of active smokers, smoking cessation interventions are extremely cost-effective [9,10]. These interventions have the potential to reduce progressive lung decline and delay or prevent the onset of costly chronic heart and pulmonary diseases as well as cancer [10].

Tobacco use among ED patients is common, as are tobacco-related illnesses. Evidence suggests that ED patients smoke more than the general population. For example, surveys have shown prevalence rates of adult ED smokers as high as 48% in urban areas [11], and as low as 21% in an affluent suburban ED [12]. A study of 1847 adults with asthma visiting 64 EDs in the USA and Canada found a prevalence rate of tobacco use of 35% [13]. Among children who visit the ED, environmental tobacco smoke exposure is common as well. One single-site study found that 41% of parents of children presenting with asthma or bronchiolitis were smokers [14]. Tobacco use is less common among elderly ED patients, with a prevalence of 9.5% among patients older than 65 years [15].

In a single ED study from the USA, approximately 5% of ED visits and 10% of ED admissions were attributable to tobacco [16]. Clearly smoking is an important health concern in most EDs. This chapter will explore the identification of patients, the issues of documentation and measurement, and possible interventions for smokers in the ED.

Clinical questions

1 Are ED patients (population) interested in quitting smoking (outcome)?
2 In ED patients who smoke cigarettes (population), what is the efficacy of physician advice (intervention) for smoking cessation (outcome) compared to standard care (control)?
3 In ED patients who use tobacco (population), what is the efficacy of prescribing nicotine replacement therapy (intervention) for smoking cessation (outcome) compared to standard care (control)?
4 In ED patients who use tobacco (population), what is the efficacy of prescribing non-nicotine replacement therapy medications (intervention) for smoking cessation (outcome) compared to standard care (control)?
5 In ED patients who use tobacco (population), what is the efficacy of behavioral interventions (intervention) for smoking cessation (outcome) compared to supportive psychotherapy (control)?
6 In the ED setting (population), what kinds of systems changes (intervention) are possible to enhance tobacco control efforts (outcome) compared to simple interventions applied by individual physicians (control)?
7 In patients on nicotine replacement therapy (population), what is the risk for acute myocardial infarction, stroke and death (outcomes) compared to patients who continue to smoke (control)?
8 If our patient (population) continues to smoke (exposure), what is the likelihood she will develop heart disease (outcome)?

General search strategy

You start your search by using database searches in Cochrane and MEDLINE. You know that not many randomized trials have been conducted for smoking cessation in the ED, so you start with a very broad search of the Cochrane Database of Systematic Reviews (CDSR) using the terms "smoking" and "emergency department". Your first search of the Cochrane Library for "smoking" yields 338 systematic reviews, of which 15 remain when combined with "emergency department". None of these 15 reviews, however, directly addresses the issue of smokers in the ED. You expand your search with MEDLINE, restricted to English-language literature, and find 29 additional relevant systematic reviews, meta-analyses and original reports.

Searching for evidence synthesis
- Cochrane Library: emergency department AND smoking
- MEDLINE: emergency department AND smoking AND MEDLINE English articles AND EBM reviews

Question 1: Are ED patients (population) interested in quitting smoking (outcome)?

Search strategy

- MEDLINE: emergency department AND smoking cessation

Emergency department patients who smoke are already interested in quitting, and most have already tried. In fact, most smokers do want to quit. For example, multiple surveys of adult ED patients have shown between 30% and 49% are interested in quitting within the month [17–19]. More than 70% have tried to quit in the 12 months prior to their ED visit, and 34% are interested in an outpatient referral for treatment [20]. Moreover, parents who smoke and have children often are more motivated to quit. For example, among parents and guardians of children in a pediatric ED, 82% want to quit and 76% want to quit within the next month [14].

Smokers with a tobacco-related illness as the cause of their ED visit are slightly more interested in quitting than smokers with a non-tobacco-related visit [21]. This finding has implications for the concept of the "teachable moment"; however, it is unclear whether the difference in interest in quitting cigarettes is clinically significant.

Overall, the evidence suggests that patients are receptive to quitting smoking, regardless of the reason for the ED visit. Moreover, there is no evidence to suggest that efforts to reduce smoking are wasteful.

Question 2: In ED patients who smoke cigarettes (population), what is the efficacy of physician advice (intervention) for smoking cessation (outcome) compared to standard care (control)?

Search strategy

- CDSR (first quarter 2007): smoking AND emergency department
- MEDLINE: physician advice AND smoking cessation

It is estimated that approximately 70% of smokers visit a health care facility every year [10]. A US national survey found that approximately 70% of smokers would quit if urged by their physicians, but only 25% of these smokers reported receiving this advice from their physician [22]. Physicians have a great opportunity to provide cessation counseling to their patients who smoke. A Cochrane database systematic review of 17 trials of brief advice involving over 31,000 patients showed a statistically significant increase in the odds of quitting for patients who received physician advice

[23]. The pooled odds ratio was 1.74 (95% CI: 1.48 to 2.05), suggesting that 40 patients would have to receive smoking cessation advice to result in one additional smoker quitting.

The US Public Health Service and British Thoracic Society issued updated guidelines for tobacco dependence treatment in clinical settings [10,24]. These comprehensive guidelines urge the use of brief clinical interventions in which screening patients for tobacco use is followed by advice to quit. In the US guideline, this is known as the "5 As": **a**sk the patient if he/she smokes, **a**dvise quitting, **a**ssess readiness to quit, **a**ssist with a quit attempt and **a**rrange follow-up. Although not validated in the ED, it is the framework used to design interventions for smoking in health care settings.

Of note, EDs were omitted from the clinical settings discussed in these guidelines, in part because the evidence base addressing the efficacy of ED interventions did not exist at the time the guidelines were drafted.

In summary, while ED interventions to reduce cigarette smoking have been infrequently studied, the weight of evidence from the non-ED setting is strong. Simple interventions applied to smokers can reduce their cigarette consumption.

Question 3: In ED patients who use tobacco (population), what is the efficacy of prescribing nicotine replacement therapy (intervention) for smoking cessation (outcome) compared to standard care (control)?

Search strategy

- CDSR and MEDLINE: nicotine replacement therapy AND smoking cessation

Many studies indicate that most smokers who quit do so without pharmacological intervention [25]. This likely reflects, at least in part, under-use of effective pharmacotherapy. Although most patients wish to reduce or quit smoking, many find this difficult without some form of pharmacological assistance. Nicotine replacement therapy (NRT) is commonly used as a smoking cessation treatment aid. It aids in decreasing nicotine withdrawal symptoms, which is a major barrier to smoking cessation. Currently there are five nicotine replacement products: gum, lozenge, transdermal patch, nasal spray and vapor inhaler. A Cochrane systematic review of 123 studies involving 35,600 participants, largely conducted in primary care or inpatient settings, found that the five forms of NRT were all significantly more effective than placebo in helping smokers quit [26]. The pooled effectiveness measured by abstinence for any form of NRT relative to control (no treatment) was impressive (OR = 1.77; 95% CI: 1.66 to 1.88). For nicotine gum the OR is 1.66 (95% CI: 1.52 to 1.81), for nicotine spray the OR is 2.35 (95% CI: 1.63 to 3.38), for transdermal patch the OR is 1.81 (95% CI: 1.63 to 2.02), for nicotine inhaler the OR is 2.14 (95% CI: 1.44 to 3.18) and for nicotine lozenge the OR is 2.05 (95% CI: 1.62 to 2.59) [26].

The evidence shows NRT should be used in patients who are motivated to quit, have at least moderate nicotine dependence, and who consume at least 10–15 cigarettes a day. The benefit of using nicotine replacement therapy was seen throughout the 6–12-month follow-up period; however, beyond this point there was significant relapse.

These studies have been conducted primarily in primary care settings. There are currently randomized control trials being conducted in ED settings that are investigating the efficacy of NRT for smoking cessation in ED patients.

Table 60.1 reviews the varieties of nicotine replacement products available.

Question 4: In ED patients who use tobacco (population), what is the efficacy of prescribing non-nicotine replacement therapy medications (intervention) for smoking cessation (outcome) compared to standard care (control)?

Search strategy

- CDSR and MEDLINE: (bupropion OR varenicline AND smoking cessation

Bupropion is an atypical antidepressant and is one of many antidepressants that have been studied for smoking cessation. Antidepressants might aid in smoking cessation by relieving the depressive symptoms caused by nicotine withdrawal and may substitute for antidepressant effects of nicotine. A Cochrane systematic review of 19 studies involving over 4000 participants found that bupropion doubles the odds of quitting [27]. The pooled analyses suggest that bupropion is effective in promoting smoking cessation (OR = 2.06; 95% CI: 1.77 to 2.40) [27]. Interestingly, the efficacy of bupropion was independent of a past history of depression. Common side-effects of bupropion use include insomnia, dry mouth and nausea. Bupropion also increases the seizure threshold and is contraindicated in patients with seizure disorder.

Varenicline is a selective nicotinic acetylcholine receptor partial agonist. It stimulates the receptor enough to block symptoms of withdrawal, but prevents nicotine from binding. It was approved by the US Food and Drug Administration and European Commission in 2006. A Cochrane review of five randomized trials of varenicline involving 4924 participants found that varenicline effectively promoted continuous abstinence at 12 months compared to placebo (OR = 3.22; 95% CI: 2.43–4.27) and bupropion (OR = 1.66; 95% CI: 1.28–2.16) [28]. These studies, summarized in Table 60.2, demonstrate that varenicline is an efficacious treatment for smoking cessation. Its novel mechanism of action distinguishes it from nicotine replacement and bupropion. The main side-effect of varenicline is nausea, which is usually mild to moderate and typically abates over time. Table 60.3 summarizes prescribing information for bupropion and varenicline.

Table 60.1 Nicotine replacement products for smoking cessation. (Adapted from US Department of Health and Human Services [10].)

Nicotine replacement therapy	Dosage	Duration	Adverse effects	Advantages	Disadvantages	Availability

Nicotine patch	21 mg/24 hours
	14 mg/24 hours
	7 mg/24 hours
	15 mg/16 hours
		4 weeks,
		  then 2 weeks,
		  then 2 weeks
		8 weeks
			Local skin irritation, insomnia	Provides steady level of nicotine, easy to use	User can not adjust dose for craving	Prescription and OTC

Nicotine gum	1–24 cig/day: 2 mg gum up to 24 pieces/day >25 cig/day: 4 mg gum up to 24 pieces/day	Up to 12 weeks	Mouth soreness, sore jaw, dyspepsia	User controls dose, oral substitute for cigarettes	Can not eat or drink while chewing gum, can damage dental work	OTC
Nicotine lozenge	2 mg or 4 mg Weeks 1–6: 1 lozenge/1–2 hours Weeks 7–9: 1 lozenge/2–4 hours Weeks 10–12: 1 lozenge/4–8 hours	12 weeks	Soreness of the teeth and gums, indigestion, irritated throat	User controls dose, oral substitute for cigarettes	Can not eat or drink while using lozenge	OTC
Nicotine inhaler	6–16 cartridges/day (4 mg/cartridge)	3–6 months	Local irritation of mouth and throat	User controls dose	Frequent puffing needed	Prescription only
Nicotine nasal spray	8–40 doses/day (dose = 0.5 mg/nostril)	3–6 months	Nasal irritation	User controls dose, most rapid delivery of nicotine	Most irritating product to use	Prescription only

cig, cigarettes; OTC, over the counter.

Table 60.2 Summary of randomized clinical trials of varenicline. Compared to control for primary outcome (quitting).

Study	Design	Intervention vs control	Odds ratio (OR)	95% CI
Gonzales et al. [43]	Multi-center, double-blind, placebo-controlled trial	Varenicline (1 mg bid) vs placebo	3.85	2.70 to 5.50
Jorenby et al. [44]	Multi-center, double-blind, placebo-controlled trial	varenicline (1 mg bid) vs placebo	3.85	2.69 to 5.50
Tonstad et al. [45]	Multi-center, double-blind, placebo-controlled trial	Varenicline (1 mg bid) vs placebo	2.48	1.95 to 3.16
Nides et al. [46]	Multi-center, double-blind, placebo-controlled trial	Varenicline (1 mg bid) vs placebo	4.71	2.60 to 8.53

Table 60.3 Non-nicotine pharmacotherapy for smoking cessation. (Adapted from US Department of Health and Human Services [10].)

Pharmacotherapy	Dosage	Duration	Adverse effects	Advantages	Disadvantages	Availability
Sustained-release bupropion	150 mg/day for 3 days, then 150 mg twice a day (begin 1 week pre-quit)	7–12 weeks (up to 6 months)	Insomnia, dry mouth	Easy to use	Increases risk of seizures (<0.1%)	Prescription only
Varenicline	Days 1–3: 0.5 mg once daily Days 4–7: 0.5 mg twice daily Day 8 to end of treatment: 1 mg twice daily (begin 1 week pre-quit)	12 weeks	Nausea, headache, insomnia and abnormal dreams	Easy to use		Prescription only

In summary, numerous efficacious pharmacological treatments exist for smoking cessation. These treatments are well tolerated and have long-term quit rates between 20% and 30%, although many patients require repeated treatment because of the chronic relapsing nature of nicotine addiction.

Question 5: In ED patients who use tobacco (population), what is the efficacy of behavioral interventions (intervention) for smoking cessation (outcome) compared to supportive psychotherapy?

Search strategy

- CDSR: smoking cessation AND behavioral intervention AND emergency department

No systematic reviews or meta-analyses have been published that address this subject. Two randomized trials, one reported in abstract form, assessed the efficacy of a behavioral intervention in helping ED smokers quit. Richman et al. randomized 152 adult patients to receive either: (i) a brief, scripted counseling by the ED attending referring the patient to the hospital's tobacco treatment program, along with a packet of information from the American Heart Association and a two-page pamphlet; or (ii) just the pamphlet [29]. Three-month smoking cessation rates in the intervention and control groups were comparable: 10.9% and 10.4%, respectively. In this study, patients were not offered pharmacotherapy, and it is unclear how attending physicians' adherence to the counseling protocol was assessed. In addition, the behavioral intervention offered was modest – primarily informational in nature – and did not employ techniques such as motivational interviewing, which are known to be efficacious in behavior change [30]. Lastly, this study did not use biochemical verification of smoking status (such as a test for exhaled carbon monoxide or cotinine, a nicotine metabolite).

Bock et al. studied 620 smokers admitted to an ED observation unit with chest pain [31]. All subjects were offered NRT and given brief physician advice to quit. Patients in the intervention arm received a 45-minute motivational interview and two follow-up booster telephone calls. Abstinence rates at 1, 3 and 6 months in the intervention and control arms were, 16.5% versus 10% ($P < 0.05$), 14.3% versus 11.5% ($P = 0.08$) and 11.4% versus 11.8% ($P > 0.05$), respectively. Thus, behavioral interventions may induce short-term abstinence in an ED smoker; however, the duration of the effect may be short lived.

In summary, the evidence base addressing the efficacy of ED-initiated behavioral treatment of nicotine addiction is insufficient to make firm recommendations. Evidence from primary care settings strongly indicates the efficacy of behavioral treatment, which is even greater when combined with pharmacotherapy.

Question 6: In the ED setting (population), what kinds of systems changes (intervention) are possible to enhance tobacco control efforts (outcome) compared to simple interventions applied by individual physicians (control)?

Search strategy

- CDSR and MEDLINE (1996–2007): smoking cessation AND systems

No randomized controlled trials or prospective cohort studies have been conducted in EDs assessing the efficacy of system changes in promoting tobacco screening and intervention. Based on the large body of data obtained in primary care settings, however, and some ED studies, a recent statement addressed the issue of ED systems changes and tobacco control [32].

The American College of Emergency Physicians (ACEP) Smoking Cessation Task Force, composed of representatives of major emergency medicine organizations, published a joint statement for ED-based tobacco control interventions [32]. Recommendations for tobacco control interventions for clinicians include:

1 Ask all patients who visit an ED about tobacco use.

2 Advise all smokers to quit.

3 Refer smokers to a "quitline", for example, in the USA and Canada, the North American Smokers' Quitline (800-QUIT-NOW), or a local smoking cessation center.

4 Consider medication therapy.

Quitlines may offer busy ED providers a particularly useful way to initiate tobacco dependence treatment [33]. A quitline is a toll-free telephone service sponsored by an agency of government or health insurance plan that offers patients individual counseling, referrals to local intensive treatment programs, brochures and other literature, and, in some regions, free nicotine replacement products. In the UK and North America, quitlines are open 7 days a week, and services are typically available in languages other than English. Providers may refer patients to the quitline by means of a fax or electronic referral, and the quitline can proactively call the patient. Quitlines are effective. The California Smokers' Quitline randomized 3282 callers to receive either seven counseling sessions proactively (treatment group) or received some counseling only if the smoker called back (control group) [34]. Both groups received self-help materials. The 1-year abstinence rates for the treatment and control groups were 9.1% and 6.9% ($P < 0.001$), respectively. Abstinence rates for smokers who received any counseling versus those who received none were 7.5% versus 4.1% ($P < 0.001$).

The ACEP task force also recommended: (i) creating a field in the electronic medical record for tobacco use; (ii) installing cessation guidelines on provider personal digital assistants; (iii) facilitating referral to cessation programs; (iv) using health educators for tobacco screening; and (v) running public service videos in the ED waiting area.

Aligning payment incentives may increase the use of cessation services. A Cochrane systematic review found a modest increase in quit rates after systems changes in primary care settings that included reducing patient costs for cessation treatment and offering incentives to providers for identifying and treating smokers [35].

In summary, additional work is needed to assess the efficacy of specific systems changes in promoting tobacco control interventions in the ED. Interventions that facilitate referral to a smokers' quitline may be particularly time efficient and clinically effective.

Question 7: In patients on nicotine replacement therapy (population), what is the risk for acute myocardial infarction, stroke and death (outcomes) compared to patients who continue to smoke (control)?

Search strategy

- CDSR and MEDLINE: nicotine replacement therapy AND acute myocardial infarction, stroke, death

There have been safety concerns regarding the use of nicotine replacement products in the setting of cardiovascular disease arising from case reports of acute myocardial infarction soon after initiation of NRT [36]. There are no Cochrane database systematic reviews for this topic. A MEDLINE search on this topic revealed no high-quality evidence; however, one observational study was identified. This observational study represented a secondary analysis of data collected from 1985 to 2003 as part of the UK's The Health Improvement Network (THIN) project, a longitudinal database of general practice patients [37]. Of 33,247 patients who received NRT, there were 861 who sustained a myocardial infarction, 506 who subsequently had a stroke and 960 deaths. The risk of heart attack or stroke was substantially higher in the 56 days preceding the prescription of NRT than in the 56 days after, suggesting that heart attack or stroke typically triggers an NRT prescription. In this study, there was no excess risk of heart attack or stroke following NRT prescription, suggesting that NRT is safe.

In summary, there is no evidence to suggest that NRT causes heart attacks and the evidence that does exist consists of sporadic case reports. NRT should be considered safe and effective, with few if any absolute contraindications.

Question 8: If our patient (population) continues to smoke (exposure), what is the likelihood she will develop heart disease (outcome)?

Search strategy

- CDSR and MEDLINE: coronary heart disease AND (smoking cessation, pulmonary disease OR smoking cessation, cancer OR smoking cessation)

The 2004 Surgeon General's report *The Health Consequences of Smoking* reaffirms the causal relationship between smoking and many diseases, including cardiovascular disease, pulmonary dis-

ease and cancer [38]. A Cochrane database systematic review of 20 trials showed a substantial reduction in mortality and non-fatal myocardial infarction in those patients who quit smoking. The pooled RR for mortality was 0.64 (95% CI: 0.58 to 0.71); the pooled RR for non-fatal myocardial infarction was 0.68 (95% CI: 0.57 to 0.82) [39].

If our patient continues to smoke she is 2–4 times more likely to develop coronary heart disease than a non-smoker [40], two times more likely to develop a stroke [41], 10 times more likely to die from chronic obstructive lung disease [41] and 13 times more likely to die from lung cancer [38].

Conclusions

After reviewing the preceding information, you ask the patient if she thinks that smoking is contributing to her breathing problems. She says "yes", and she would like to quit. Although she has tried in the past, these efforts have not worked. You tell her that smoking is a chronic relapsing disease, and that smokers typically make multiple quit attempts before finally succeeding. At discharge, in addition to prescriptions for her inhaled β-agonist and corticosteroids [42], you write her a prescription for a 21 mg nicotine patch and give her a brochure referring her to a smokers' quitline.

Tobacco use is common in ED patients, and considerably more prevalent than in the general population. Patients who smoke are more likely to be admitted and use a disproportionate share of ED and hospital resources. Numerous effective treatments for tobacco use exist. Evidence-based treatment approaches include both pharmacotherapy and counseling, with the highest success rates typically involving a combination of these. Nearly all insurance plans cover NRT, and many cover bupropion and varenicline. In the USA, Medicare, some private plans and, in some states, Medicaid, cover counseling. The North American Smokers' Quitline is available at no cost to any smoker in the United States or Canada.

The efficacy of ED-based brief interventions to promote smoking cessation is unclear. Current evidence suggests its feasibility. Randomized trials incorporating behavioral and pharmacological interventions currently in progress will assess the efficacy of ED-based tobacco interventions. If the experience in primary care settings can be generalized to the ED, then it is possible that brief ED-based tobacco control interventions will have a modest but real effect in promoting cessation. Moreover, smoking cessation is a cost-effective intervention.

Conflicts of interest

Dr. Bernstein is supported by research grants from the National Institutes of Health/National Institute on Drug Abuse, the Robert Wood Johnson Foundation and the New York State Department of Health. He has served as an expert witness for the plaintiff in litigation against tobacco companies. Dr. Cabral is supported by an intramural grant from a disparities reduction center at the Albert Einstein College of Medicine, which is funded by the National Institutes of Health/National Center on Minority Health and Health Disparities.

References

1 Mackay J, Eriksen M, Shafey O. *The Tobacco Atlas*, 2nd edn. American Cancer Society, Atlanta, 2006.

2 Centers for Disease Control and Prevention. Annual smoking-attributable mortality, years of potential life lost, and productivity losses – United States, 1997–2001. *MMWR* 2005;**54**:624–8.

3 Centers for Disease Control and Prevention. Cigarette smoking-attributable mortality – United States, 2000. *MMWR* 2003;**52**:842–4.

4 Centers for Disease Control and Prevention. Cigarette smoking among adults – United States, 2004. *MMWR* 2005;**54**:1121–4.

5 US Department of Health and Human Services. *The Health Consequences of Involuntary Exposure to Tobacco Smoke: A report of the Surgeon General.* US Department of Health and Human Services, CDC, National Center for Chronic Disease Prevention and Health Promotion, Office on Smoking and Health, 2006.

6 World Health Organization. WHO Framework Convention on Tobacco Control. World Health Organization, Geneva, 2003.

7 World Health Organization. Tobacco Free Initiative. WHO Framework Convention on Tobacco Control (WHO FCTC), 2007. Available at http://www.who.int/tobacco/framework/en/ (accessed June 21, 2007).

8 US Department of Health and Human Services. *Healthy People 2010: Understanding and improving health*, 2nd edn. US Government Printing Office, Washington, 2000.

9 Cromwell J, Bartosch WJ, Fiore MC, Hasselblad V, Baker T. Cost-effectiveness of the clinical practice recommendations in the AHCPR guideline for smoking cessation. *JAMA* 1997;**278**:1759–66.

10 Fiore MC, Jaen CR, Baker TB, et al. Treating Tobacco Use and Dependence: 2008 update. Clinical Practice Guideline. US Department of Health and Human Services, Public Health Service, Rockville, 2008.

11 Lowenstein SR, Koziol-McLain J, Thompson M, et al. Behavioral risk factors in emergency department patients: a multisite study. *Acad Emerg Med* 1998;**5**:781–7.

12 Richman PB, Dinowitz S, Nashed A, Eskin B, Cody R. Prevalence of smokers and nicotine-addicted patients in a suburban emergncy department. *Acad Emerg Med* 1999;**6**:807–10.

13 Silverman RA, Boudreaux ED, Woodruff PG, Clark S, Camargo CA, Jr. Cigarette smoking among asthmatic adults presenting to 64 emergency departments. *Chest* 2003;**123**:1472–9.

14 Mahabee-Gittens M. Smoking in parents of children with asthma and bronchiolitis in a pediatric emergency department. *Pediatr Emerg Care* 2002;**18**:4–7.

15 Girard DD, Partridge RA, Becker B, Bock B. Alcohol and tobacco use in the elder emergency department patient: assessment of rates and medical care utilization. *Acad Emerg Med* 2004;**11**:378–82.

16 Bernstein SL. The impact of smoking-related illness in the emergency department: an attributable risk model. *Am J Emerg Med* 2002;**20**:161–4.

17 Lowenstein SR, Tomlinson D, Koziol-McLain J, Prochazka A. Smoking habits of emergency department patients: an opportunity for disease prevention. *Acad Emerg Med* 1995;**2**:165–71.

18 Klinkhammer MD, Patten CA, Sadosty AT, Stevens SR, Ebbert JO. Motivation for stopping tobacco use among emergency department patients. *Acad Emerg Med* 2005;**12**:568–71.

19 Boudreaux ED, Baumann BM, Friedman K, Ziedonis DM. Smoking stage of change and interest in an emergency department-based intervention. *Acad Emerg Med* 2005;**12**:211–18.

20 Boudreaux ED, Kim S, Hohrmann JL, Clark S, Camargo CA, Jr. Interest in smoking cessation among emergency department patients. *Health Psychol* 2005;**24**:220–24.

21 Bernstein SL, Cannata M. Nicotine dependence, motivation to quit, and diagnosis in emergency department patients who smoke. *Addict Behav* 2006;**31**:288–97.

22 Janz NK, Becker MH, Kirscht JP, Eraker SA, Billi JE, Woolliscroft JO. Evaluation of a minimal contact smoking cessation intervention in an outpatient setting. *Am J Public Health* 1987;**77**:805–9.

23 Lancaster T, Stead LF. Physician advice for smoking cessation (Cochrane review). *Cochrane Database Syst Rev* 2004;**4**:CD000165.

24 West R, McNeill A, Raw M. Smoking cessation guidelines for health professionals: an update. *Thorax* 2000;**55**:987–99.

25 Doran CM, Valenti L, Robinson M, Britt H, Mattick RP. Smoking status of Australian general practice patients and their attempts to quit. *Addict Behav* 2006;**31**:758–66.

26 Silagy C, Lancaster T, Stead L, Mant D, Fowler G. Nicotine replacement therapy for smoking cessation (Cochrane review). *Cochrane Database Syst Rev* 2004;**3**:CD 000146 (doi: 10.1002/14651858.CD 000146.pub2. 2004).

27 Hughes JR, Stead LF, Lancaster T. Antidepressants for smoking cessation (Cochrane review). *Cochrane Database Syst Rev* 2007;**1**:CD 000031 (doi: 10.1002/14651858.CD000031.pub3. 2007).

28 Cahill K, Stead LF, Lancaster T. Nicotine receptor partial agonists for smoking cessation. *Cochrane Database Syst Rev* 2007;**1**:CD006103 (doi: 10.1002/14651858.CD006103.pub2.2007).

29 Richman PB, Dinowitz S, Nashed A, et al. The emergency department as a potential site for smoking cessation intervention: a randomized, controlled trial. *Acad Emerg Med* 2000;**7**:348–53.

30 Miller WR, Rollnick S. *Motivational Interviewing: Preparing people for change*, 2nd edn. Guilford Press, New York, 2002.

31 Bock B, Partridge RA, Woolard R, Becker BM. Effective smoking cessation intervention for emergency department patients with chest pain (Abstract). *Acad Emerg Med* 2004;**11**:525–6.

32 Bernstein SL, Boudreaux ED, Cydulka RK, et al. Tobacco control interventions in the emergency department: a joint statement of emergency medicine organizations (Executive summary). *Ann Emerg Med* 2006;**48**:417–26.

33 Ossip-Klein DJ, McIntosh S. Quitlines in North America: evidence base and applications. *Am J Med Sci* 2003;**326**:201–5.

34 Zhu SH, Anderson CM, Tedeschi GJ, et al. Evidence of real-world effectiveness of a telephone quitline for smokers. *N Engl J Med* 2002;**347**:1087–93.

35 Kaper J, Wagena E, Severenes J, Schayck CV. Healthcare financing systems for increasing the use of tobacco dependence treatment. *Cochrane Database Syst Rev* 2007;**1**:CD004305.

36 Mathew TP, Herity NA. Acute myocardial infarction soon after nicotine replacement therapy. *Q J Med* 2001;**94**:503–6.

37 Hubbard R, Lewis S, Smith C, et al. Use of nicotine replacement therapy and the risk of acute myocardial infarction, stroke, and death. *Tobacco Control* 2005;**14**:416–21.

38 US Department of Health and Human Services. *The Health Consequences of Smoking: A report of the Surgeon General.* Department of Health and Human Services, CDC, Atlanta, 2004.

39 Critchley J, Capewell S. Smoking cessation for the secondary prevention of coronary heart disease (Review). *Cochrane Database*

Syst Rev 2003;**4**:CD003041 (doi: 10.1002/14651858.CD003041.pub2. 2003).

40 US Department of Health and Human Services. *Reducing the Health Consequences of Smoking: 25 years of progress. A report of the Surgeon General.* US Department of Health and Human Services Publication No. 89-8411. Public Health Service, Office on Smoking and Health, Rockville, 1989.

41 Centers for Disease Control and Prevention. Tobacco use among US racial/ethnic minority groups, African Americans, American Indians and Alaska Natives, Asian Americans and Pacific Islanders, Hispanics: a report of the Surgeon General (Executive summary). *MMWR* 1998;**47**:1–16.

42 Aaron SD, Vandemheen KL, Hebert P, et al. Outpatient oral prednisone after emergency treatment of chronic obstructive pulmonary disease. *N Engl J Med* 2003;**348**:2618–25.

43 Gonzales D, Rennard SI, Nides M, et al. Varenicline, an alpha4beta2 nicotinic acetylcholine receptor partial agonist, vs sustained-release bupropion and placebo for smoking cessation: a randomized controlled trial. *JAMA* 2006;**296**:47–55.

44 Jorenby DE, Hays JT, Rigotti NA, et al. Efficacy of varenicline, an alpha4beta2 nicotinic acteylcholine receptor partial agonist, vs placebo or sustained-release bupropion for smoking cessation: a randomized controlled trial. *JAMA* 2006;**296**:56–63.

45 Tonstad S, Tonnesen P, Hajek P, et al. Effect of maintenance therapy with varenicline on smoking cessation: a randomized controlled trial. *JAMA* 2006;**296**:64–71.

46 Nides M, Oncken C, Gonzales D, et al. Smoking cessation with varenicline, a selective alpha4beta2 nicotinic receptor partial agonist. *Arch Intern Med* 2006;**166**:1561–8.

61 Immunization

Jeremy Hess[1] & Katherine L. Heilpern[2]

[1] Departments of Emergency Medicine *and* Environmental and Occupational Health, Emory University Schools of Medicine and Public Health, Emory University, Atlanta, USA
[2] Department of Emergency Medicine, Emory University School of Medicine, Emory University, Atlanta, USA

Clinical scenario

You are the medical director of a community emergency department (ED), and you are about to leave after an evening shift. You are reflecting on the patients you saw that day and considering, as you often do, some of the ED systems issues that came up in the course of their care. One of your patients, an older but still spry 78-year-old gentleman who came in following a ground level fall, sticks in your mind. As per protocol in your ED, he was asked if he had received the pneumococcal vaccine, and as is often the case, he was unsure. His records were with his primary care provider (PCP). You elected to encourage him to follow up with his PCP instead of giving him the vaccine in the ED, but you are wondering if that was the right decision. You are leaving on time and have a moment, so you decide to exercise your evidence-based medicine skills and see if you can answer the question of whether your ED should empirically vaccinate all eligible elderly patients with the pneumococcal vaccine if they are uncertain of their vaccination status. You formulate your PICO (**p**opulation, **i**ntervention, **c**ontrol and **o**utcome) question, pull up MEDLINE, and start to look for the evidence.

Background

Immunization is the process of artificially inducing immunity to or providing protection from an infectious disease. Immunization can be active or passive: active immunization entails the administration of toxoids, proteins or other vaccine components that induce the body to develop an active immune response, either cell or antibody mediated; passive immunization involves the administration of exogenously developed antibody for a specific pathogen.

We now have a thorough theoretical and empirical knowledge base to guide vaccine development and administration. In general, there are now two major categories of immunization: vaccination with live, usually attenuated, infectious agents to induce immunity, and immunization via inactivated agents or detoxified pathogen components. Vaccines have several components: the immunizing agent (either vaccine, toxoid, immunoglobulin or specific immunoglobulin), the suspending agent, associated preservatives and antibiotics, and adjuvants or compounds that enhance the immune response to the immunogenic component(s) of the vaccine. The immune response engendered by a particular vaccine depends on several variables, including dose, type and concentration of adjuvants, route of administration, and recipient age.

The evidence base for vaccination and, in particular, the risk–benefit assessment of when to administer certain vaccines with significant harmful sequelae, has also evolved significantly since Jenner's day. A large body of evidence supports the efficacy of most vaccines that are part of the routine recommended immunization schedule (Figs. 61.1–61.3) [1]. There are several other infectious diseases for which vaccination is indicated based on clinical conditions (Fig. 61.4) [1], as well as diseases that are preventable through vaccination but not routinely encountered by the majority of the population, so prophylaxis for these diseases is based on anticipated exposure. Uncertainty around whom and when to immunize for most conditions has been well considered, and there is generally a strong evidence base for the above-mentioned immunizations.

For emergency medicine practitioners in the developed world, there is a baseline assumption that the majority of their patients have received recommended childhood immunizations; however readers from other parts of the developing world may not enjoy this level of immunization coverage. These assumptions play into pre-test probabilities when evaluating for a number of different diseases. EM physicians venture into uncertain territory, however, when faced with several common questions regarding immunization and the ED patient. The most common immunization issues the ED physician is likely to face include:

- When to administer routine immunizations for ED patients.
- When to initiate post-exposure immunotherapy and treatment.

Evidence-based Emergency Medicine. Edited by Brian H. Rowe

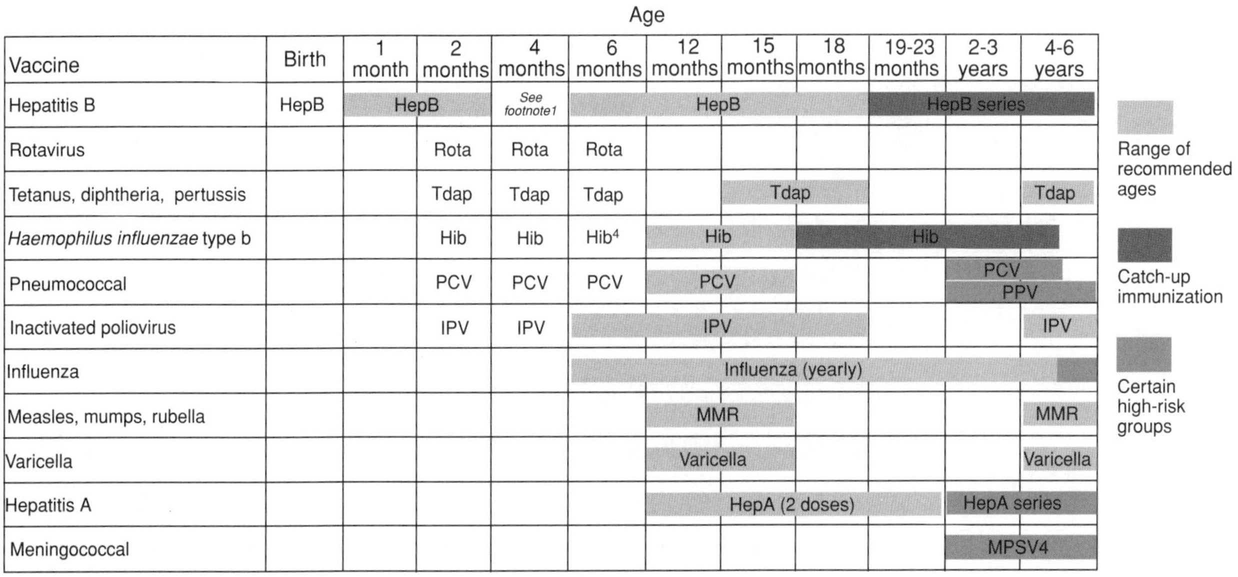

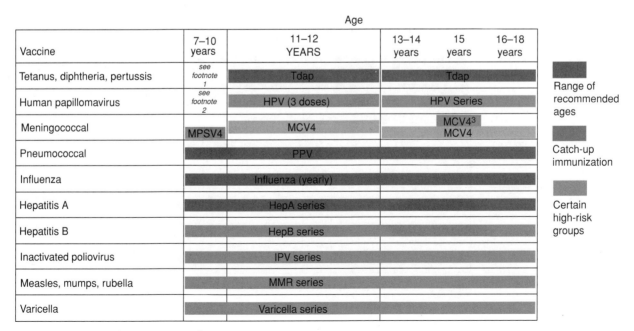

Age

Vaccine	Birth	1 month	2 months	4 months	6 months	12 months	15 months	18 months	19-23 months	2-3 years	4-6 years
Hepatitis B	HepB	HepB		See footnote1	HepB				HepB series		
Rotavirus			Rota	Rota	Rota						
Tetanus, diphtheria, pertussis			Tdap	Tdap	Tdap		Tdap				Tdap
Haemophilus influenzae type b			Hib	Hib	Hib⁴	Hib		Hib			
Pneumococcal			PCV	PCV	PCV	PCV				PCV PPV	
Inactivated poliovirus			IPV	IPV	IPV						IPV
Influenza						Influenza (yearly)					
Measles, mumps, rubella						MMR					MMR
Varicella						Varicella					Varicella
Hepatitis A						HepA (2 doses)				HepA series	
Meningococcal										MPSV4	

Range of recommended ages

Catch-up immunization

Certain high-risk groups

Figure 61.1 Recommended pediatric immunizations for ages 0–6 years.

- How the pediatric immunization schedule affects pre-test probabilities for certain childhood illnesses.
- What role ED immunization should play in the containment of potential outbreaks and, as a corollary, when to give immunoprophylaxis to those who have been potentially exposed to a vaccine-preventable condition.
- The role of immunization in bioterror threats and attacks.
- Complications of vaccine administration.

From the evidence-based medicine perspective, these issues are primarily ones of prognosis, therapy and prevention; the study types that are most helpful in informing practice are prospective cohort studies, randomized clinical trials and retrospective case–control studies. The amount of evidence available to help inform decisions in these areas varies, both by disease and by population. To investigate some of the most salient, we have outlined several evidence-based investigations of important issues the practicing ED physician might face.

Age

Vaccine	7–10 years	11–12 YEARS	13–14 years	15 years	16–18 years
Tetanus, diphtheria, pertussis	see footnote 1	Tdap		Tdap	
Human papillomavirus	see footnote 2	HPV (3 doses)		HPV Series	
Meningococcal	MPSV4	MCV4		MCV4³ MCV4	
Pneumococcal		PPV			
Influenza		Influenza (yearly)			
Hepatitis A		HepA series			
Hepatitis B		HepB series			
Inactivated poliovirus		IPV series			
Measles, mumps, rubella		MMR series			
Varicella		Varicella series			

Range of recommended ages

Catch-up immunization

Certain high-risk groups

Figure 61.2 Recommended pediatric immunizations for ages 7–18 years.

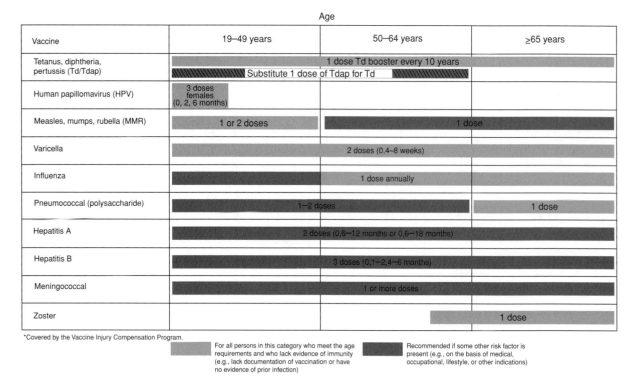

Figure 61.3 Recommended schedule for adult immunizations.

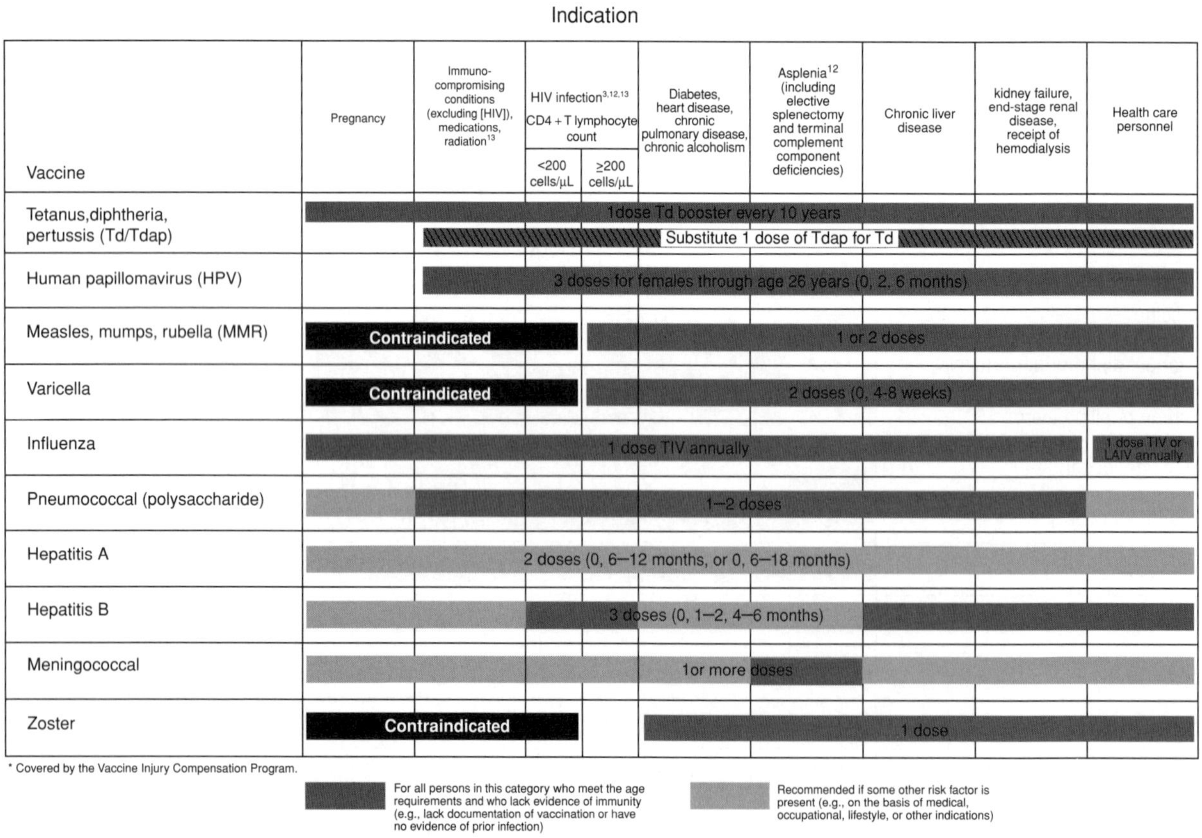

Figure 61.4 Recommended adult immunizations for patients with certain medical conditions. HIV, human immunodeficiency virus.

Clinical questions

In order to address the issues of most relevance to your scenario and to help in searching the literature for the evidence regarding these, you structure your questions as recommended in Chapter 1 using the standard PICO format.

1 For an elderly patient who is up to date on routine tetanus vaccinations and has a contaminated wound sustained 30 hours prior to presentation (population), is administration of tetanus toxoid (intervention) more effective than routine wound therapy without vaccination (control) in reducing the incidence of tetanus infection (outcome)?

2 For an 18-year-old man bitten by a dog that has not yet been captured and quarantined (population), is immediate initiation of active and passive rabies immunization series (intervention) more effective than observation (control) of the animal in reducing the incidence of rabies (outcome), with the caveat that active immunization will be initiated within 7 days if the animal is not successfully quarantined?

3 For all ED patients over 65 years who do not know their pneumococcal vaccination status (population), is empirical pneumococcal vaccine administration (intervention) more effective at reducing the incidence of pneumonia (outcome) than instructing patients to follow up with their PCPs to determine if vaccination is indicated (comparison)?

4 For practicing ED physicians (population), is routine smallpox immunization (intervention) in the absence of an outbreak more effective at containing a potential outbreak (outcome) than vaccination after an outbreak is detected (control)?

5 For frontline responders (population), does routine vaccination for inhalational anthrax (intervention) cause more morbidity (outcome) than outbreak-specific vaccination (control), assuming one anthrax outbreak every 10 years?

6 For the non-immunized household contact (population) of a patient diagnosed with hepatitis A, is active immunization (intervention) as effective at reducing the incidence of clinical infection (outcome) as passive immunization (comparison)?

7 For patients receiving intramuscular injections including vaccinations in the ED (population), what are the most effective strategies (intervention) to reduce pain (outcome)?

General search strategy

Searches to answer PICO questions start with databases, including Cochrane, MEDLINE and EMBASE; the Cochrane databases focus in particular on the evidence pertaining to particular issues of concern. A search using the term "immunization" in the Evidence Based Medicine Reviews Databases (Cochrane Database of Systematic Reviews, American College of Physicians Journal Club, Database of Abstracts of Reviews and Effects and the Cochrane Central Register of Controlled Trials) returns 55 re-

sults, the majority of which are only tangentially relevant to the questions above. Conducting a MEDLINE search on "immunization" yields over 2000 results since 1996 alone. Thus, the search can be narrowed by focusing on particular diseases and outcomes of concern, and by including all the above databases in your search.

Critical review of the literature

Question 1: For an elderly patient who is up to date on routine tetanus vaccinations and has a contaminated wound sustained 30 hours prior to presentation (population), is administration of tetanus toxoid (intervention) more effective than routine wound therapy without vaccination (control) in reducing the incidence of tetanus infection (outcome)?

Search strategy

- MEDLINE: (tetanus AND epidemiology) OR (prevention AND control)

There are no randomized clinical trials or meta-analyses directly relevant to the question above, though there are retrospective analyses and systematic reviews. There was one systematic review of tetanus immunization in women who are pregnant or of childbearing age, examined its effect on lowering the incidence of tetanus in neonates [2], although this deals with a different population. A report on tetanus surveillance in the USA from 1998 to 2000 reveals a very low incidence of tetanus among the general population, with an incidence at 0.16 per 1 million person-years. This incidence has been declining steadily since the introduction of tetanus vaccination in the 1940s.

Retrospectively, those currently most likely to develop tetanus are elderly patients (>65 years) who do not seek prompt care for traumatic injuries, Hispanic patients and elderly diabetics. Case fatality is 18%, with 75% of deaths occurring in patients older than 60 [3]. Clearly, tetanus is a more significant problem in the elderly, those without a clear vaccination history, and those with high-risk conditions leading to immune compromise. Elderly women, in particular, may be at increased risk given that they generally did not get tetanus updates through military service.

Guidelines from the Advisory Committee on Immunization Practice [4] recommend that patients with contaminated wounds (not minor and clean) who have received tetanus toxoid at least three times, receive a booster if their last update was 5 or more years ago. Otherwise, routine wound care is recommended, as more frequent boosters can contribute to the development of vaccine side-effects [4].

In summary, there are no randomized clinical trials applicable to this question; given the severity of the disease and the starkly low incidence, only retrospective data are available, but the evidence base is nevertheless strong. In the scenario, if the patient had a booster less than 5 years ago, then only routine wound care is recommended. Otherwise, routine wound care and tetanus booster are the standard of care.

Question 2: For an 18-year-old man bitten by a dog that has not yet been captured and quarantined (population), is immediate initiation of active and passive rabies immunization series (intervention) more effective than observation (control) of the animal in reducing the incidence of rabies (outcome), with the caveat that active immunization will be initiated within 7 days if the animal is not successfully quarantined?

Search strategy

- MEDLINE: rabies AND (epidemiology OR prevention and control)

The initial search yields over 600 articles but no evidence-based reviews; again there are retrospective studies and systematic reviews. Once patients exposed to rabies have developed symptoms, the disease is almost always fatal; however, extensive field experience with post-exposure care has shown that aggressive post-exposure local wound care coupled with passive and active immunization is uniformly effective at preventing infection [5–7]. Post-exposure treatment is a medical urgency, not a medical emergency, but the decision to treat should not be delayed.

The decision is based on a priori probability of rabies exposure. While rabies prevalence is low in most parts of the developed world, certain regions and animals are more likely to transmit the virus. If the animal is known to be vaccinated against rabies then it is not likely to be rabid. Among dogs, those living on the USA–Mexico border are more likely to be rabid; unprovoked attacks also increase the probability of rabies infection. In general, a provoked bite from a known dog in an area without endemic rabies would suggest a low pre-test probability that the dog is rabid; and, vice versa, an unprovoked bite, or one from a stray or in an endemic area, prompts more concern. From 1980 to 1997, there were 1–2 humans infected by rabid dogs in the USA per year [8], though 16,000–39,000 post-exposure regimens are administered annually [9] for all exposures.

For our scenario of the young adult bitten by a dog not yet quarantined, the default position is passive immunization, and the emergency physician in this case should administer passive vaccination. The vaccine is well tolerated and rabies infection can have devastating consequences. Passive immunization confers immediate immunity that lasts approximately 3 weeks. Administering immunoglobulin only is reasonable if quarantine is anticipated within several days, but if the animal cannot be quickly located, a decision whether to actively immunize should be made in consultation with public health officials within 1–2 days. There

is no specific evidence to guide the decision, only probabilistic reasoning and cost–benefit analysis of the side-effects of the vaccine (generally mild) contrasted with the potential for rabies infection.

Question 3: For all ED patients over 65 years who do not know their pneumococcal vaccination status (population), is empirical pneumococcal vaccine administration (intervention) more effective at reducing the incidence of pneumonia (outcome) than instructing patients to follow up with their PCPs to determine if vaccination is indicated (comparison)?

Search strategy

- MEDLINE: pneumococcal vaccines AND administration AND (dosage OR economics)

There are several evidence-based reviews related to pneumococcal vaccine; while none address your question exactly, several studies and reviews shed light on the question, and one study provides information regarding the efficacy of referring patients to their PCPs for vaccination.

A recent Cochrane review of case–control and prospective studies of pneumococcal vaccine efficacy found no evidence of protection against pneumonia or death, but that there was a protective effect against invasive disease (i.e., bacteremia) [10]. According to this review, the number needed to treat (NNT) invasive bacteremia in the developed world is approximately 20,000; no reliable figures are available for the developing world [10]. A broader search reveals several other studies on the epidemiology of pneumococcal disease and vaccine policy.

Pneumococcal bacteremia is a serious complication of pneumococcal infection, and occurs in 50–83 per 100,000 people over 65 annually in the USA, with an overall annual incidence of more than 50,000 cases with a 19% mortality rate [11]. Vaccination with polyvalent pneumococcal vaccine prevents 56–69% of bacteremia cases [12,13] and has been associated with fewer complications and shorter hospital stays in hospitalized patients with community-acquired pneumonia [14]. Indications for adult vaccination include age 65 years or greater, diabetes mellitus, chronic renal failure, immune suppression, malignancy, cardiovascular disease, chronic lung disease, chronic hepatic disease and hemoglobinopathies [15]. There are several studies focusing on each of these indications and outcomes associated with pneumococcal vaccination; however, the Cochrane review cited above included populations with each of these indications.

A portion of the literature has direct relevance for the question of whether to administer vaccine in the ED. In 1999, it was estimated that only approximately 20–25% of ED patients eligible for pneumococcal vaccination had received the vaccine [16,17], and the ED was identified as an under-utilized venue for pneumococcal vaccination [18]. Moreover, Parramore et al. documented a dramatic difference in public versus private ED patients with vaccination indications, representing a significant disease prevention opportunity for EDs in the public sector [19]. Sack et al. conducted a retrospective analysis of patients with pneumococcal bacteremia seen in their ED who had indications for pneumococcal vaccination, then applied a model to determine the number of infections, deaths and hospital costs that would have resulted from a universal ED pneumococcal vaccination program using both optimistic and pessimistic assumptions [18]. Their findings demonstrated unequivocally that an ED-based pneumococcal vaccination program would save lives and costs, with average cost reductions of $4500–5000 and mortality reductions of up to 70%. This echoed a finding by Sisk et al. that vaccination of the 23 million elderly unvaccinated people in the USA would have resulted in 78,000 years of additional healthy life and saved $194 million [20]. Repeat vaccination is not associated with any increase in medically attended adverse effects compared with a single vaccination in the general adult population [21].

Referring patients for immunization appears to be an ineffective strategy when compared to immunization when a vaccination indication is determined. In an analysis by Manthey et al., a convenience sample of ED patients were reviewed for pneumococcal immunization indications, and, if indicated, referred to their PCPs for vaccination. Approximately 10% followed up, compared with 74% who responded that they would have received the vaccine in the ED if it was available [22]. Pallin et al. reviewed immunization records from 1992 to 2000 and determined that large-scale administration of vaccines in the ED is feasible, though relatively uncommon for vaccines other than tetanus [23], and Kapur and Tenenbein found that ED patients are willing to receive vaccines other than tetanus in the ED [24]. Slobodkin et al. found that pneumococcal immunization in the ED is both necessary and feasible [25].

In summary, since referrals for vaccination are relatively ineffective, patients are willing to receive them in the ED, ED vaccination is feasible, repeat vaccination has no adverse effects, and there is a strong argument for empirical vaccination based on cost–benefit analyses, it appears that empirical vaccination of all eligible patients presenting to the ED is an unqualified boon to patients and society alike. Several papers address systems that can increase coverage rates. Standing orders, including computer-based standing orders, have been effective at increasing coverage [26,27] and are recommended by the National Immunization Program (http://www.cdc.gov/nip/homehcp.htm) [28].

Question 4: For practicing ED physicians (population), is routine smallpox immunization (intervention) in the absence of an outbreak more effective at containing a potential outbreak (outcome) than vaccination after an outbreak is detected (control)?

Search strategy

- MEDLINE: smallpox vaccination AND administration AND (dosage OR history OR adverse effects OR economics)

There is one systematic review relevant to the question, focused on the US experience with smallpox vaccination from 1963 to 1968, as well as several cohort studies on recipients in the 21st century. There are also several discussions of the various issues at play in the decision to vaccinate specific populations. Decisions regarding vaccination policy require evaluation of disease incidence and epidemiology and vaccine characteristics; for live-attenuated vaccines such as smallpox, there are also important considerations related to disease transmission to vulnerable individuals after vaccination [29,30]. There are no large-scale clinical trials evaluating the safety and efficacy of smallpox vaccination of health care personnel in the modern era, with its higher prevalence of immunocompromised individuals. In the vaccine recipient, there are three significant complications: post-vaccinial central nervous disease, progressive vaccinia and eczema vaccinatum. There are data on the incidence of these and other, relatively minor, complications of smallpox immunization derived from vaccination efforts in the 1960s; post-vaccinial encephalitis, the most concerning complication, occurs in 2.9 per million primary vaccinated subjects [31]. In a recent smallpox vaccination campaign in the US military, roughly 3% of primarily vaccinated individuals required sick leave after the immunization. There was one case of encephalitis, and 37 cases of myopericarditis, but no deaths were observed [32].

Epidemiologically, smallpox outbreaks spread slow, and vaccination of potential contacts within 2–3 days of outbreaks effectively eradicated the disease during the final stage of the eradication campaign; outbreaks were generally halted quickly once identified [33]. Mathematical modeling of a bioterrorist event resulting in an epidemic in naive individuals reveals that a combination of isolation of infected individuals and the vaccination of contacts will contain the outbreak within two infective generations, or 4 weeks [34,35]. Current recommendations from the Centers for Disease Control and Prevention (CDC) hold that, in the absence of a smallpox outbreak, only individuals working directly with smallpox in laboratories or potentially through smallpox response teams should be immunized. In the event of an outbreak, individuals with smallpox contact should receive immunization and other personnel may be vaccinated prophylactically as well [36]. These recommendations include that all acute care hospitals identify a team of individuals that will care for suspected smallpox cases, and that these individuals receive pre-event vaccination. Where possible, these teams should include individuals previously immunized against smallpox.

In summary, routine pre-event smallpox vaccination is not current public health policy, though each hospital is encouraged to identify a team of individuals to be immunized that can be called upon in the event of a suspected case.

Question 5: For frontline responders (population), does routine vaccination for inhalational anthrax (intervention) cause more morbidity (outcome) than outbreak-specific vaccination (control), assuming one anthrax outbreak every 10 years?

Search strategy

- MEDLINE: anthrax immunization AND administration AND (dosage OR history OR adverse effects OR economics OR supply and distribution)

Again, there are no evidence-based medicine reviews pertinent to the question. As noted above, decisions regarding vaccination and timing, including vaccination against potential bioterror agents, require the estimation of disease incidence and severity and vaccine characteristics. Different from smallpox, anthrax is a widely available etiological agent, though refinement for use as a weapon requires specialized skills and equipment. There have been intentional outbreaks of inhalational anthrax in the recent past, and several countries are believed to have weaponized anthrax [37]. Nearly all immunologically naive individuals with sufficient inhalational exposure contract the disease, and untreated inhalation anthrax has a nearly 100% mortality [38]. The six-dose vaccine is well tolerated [39–42] and results in immunity levels of 93–100% [43,44], and there is experimental animal evidence that post-exposure prophylaxis with a short course of antibiotics and vaccination prevents infection [45]. The US military elected to vaccinate all personnel who might be exposed to a biological weapons attack while deployed, though there have been legal hurdles related to the experimental nature of the vaccine [46]. With widespread vaccination of the general public, the central issue is cost-effectiveness; studies show that maintaining pre-event vaccination on a population basis would be extremely costly while only offering marginal additional protection compared with post-event vaccination and antibiotic administration, assuming a 1% risk of an anthrax attack on a large US city per year [47]. Vaccinating subsets of the population more likely at risk – soldiers, for instance – may be cost-effective if the calculated risk of an anthrax attack is relatively high or if the cost of vaccination is low. However, emergency response personnel are at only marginally increased risk for an attack, which most likely would be in an isolated location, such as a post office, or widespread in a city, neither of which would increase exposure risk for first responders. The Advisory Committee on Immunization Practices (ACIP) recommendations echo this reasoning [48]:

> Although groups initially considered for preexposure vaccination for bioterrorism preparedness included emergency first responders, federal responders, medical practitioners, and private citizens, vaccination of these groups is not recommended. Recommendations regarding preexposure vaccination should be based on a calculable risk assessment. At present, the target population for a bioterrorist release of *B. anthracis* cannot be predetermined, and the risk of exposure cannot be calculated.
>
> In addition, studies suggest an extremely low risk for exposure related to secondary aerosolization of previously settled *B. anthracis* spores [49,50]. Because of these factors, pre-exposure vaccination for the above groups is not recommended. For the military and other select populations or for groups for which a calculable risk can be assessed, pre-exposure vaccination may be indicated.

Thus, the decision whether to vaccinate is based on the likelihood of exposure in a given population. For most first responders, vaccination is not cost effective, though the calculus differs for other groups with higher exposure risk.

Question 6: For the non-immunized household contact (population) of a patient diagnosed with hepatitis A, is active immunization (intervention) as effective at reducing the incidence of clinical infection (outcome) as passive immunization (comparison)?

Search strategy

- MEDLINE: hepatitis A AND prevention and control AND epidemiology

There is one meta-analysis relevant to the question and one randomized clinical trial. The meta-analysis evaluated the efficacy of post-exposure immunoglobulin administration in reducing the incidence of hepatitis A, and found that effectiveness of post-exposure prophylaxis was 69%, with a relative risk of 0.31 (95% CI: 0.20 to 0.47) [51]. There are no meta-analyses of post-exposure active immunization, but there is a randomized clinical trial of active immunization of household contacts of confirmed hepatitis A cases. In this study, 75 households were immunized and 75 households served as controls. In the immunization group, 2.8% of household contacts developed secondary infections, while 13.3% developed secondary infections in the control group. The efficacy of the vaccine was 79% (95% CI: 7% to 95%), with a NNT of 18 [52]. While the study was under-powered as indicated by the confidence interval around its estimate of effect, it is the only available evidence. A follow-up study in 2005 showed that active immunization of household contacts is indeed feasible, strengthening the rationale for this approach [53] if not the evidence base for active versus passive post-exposure prophylaxis.

In summary, using preliminary evidence, comparison of the efficacy of active versus passive post-exposure prophylaxis suggests that active immunization of household contacts is more effective, but more study is required to confirm or refute the advantage demonstrated in the single case–control study.

Question 7: For children receiving intramuscular injections including vaccinations in the ED (population), what are the most effective strategies (intervention) to reduce pain (outcome)?

Search strategy

- EBM reviews: immunization AND pediatrics AND pain
- MEDLINE: immunization AND pain [keywords]

Needle-related procedures are painful for pediatric patients and provoke anxiety in parents, health care providers and patients who have had similar procedures previously. A wide range of strategies have been deployed for reducing pain from needle-related procedures in children, including cognitive (e.g., cognitive distraction, parent coaching, hypnosis), behavioral (e.g., behavioral distraction, rehearsal) and combined cognitive-behavioral interventions (multiple modalities). Other interventions include sucrose pacifiers and parental holding. An equally wide range of outcome measures, from self-reported pain scales to vital sign measures, have been employed to assess intervention efficacy. There is an evidence-based medicine topic review entitled "Psychological interventions for needle-related procedural pain and distress in children and adolescents" by Uman et al. that discusses all of the relevant literature in a meta-analysis from February 2007 [54]. This review included 28 studies with 1039 combined participants. Several strategies were effective in reducing pain; pain reduction was measured in the review by standardized mean differences (SMDs). Hypnosis, combined cognitive-behavioral interventions and distraction had the highest effect sizes compared with control conditions. For hypnosis, the SMD was −1.47 (95% CI: −2.67 to −0.27), for combined interventions the SMD was −0.88 (95% CI: −1.65 to −0.12) and for distraction the SMD was −0.24 (95% CI: −0.45 to −0.04) [54]. Several other promising strategies have been evaluated but the study designs were not strong enough to be included in the systematic review.

Other reviews of the subject harvested from the MEDLINE search suggest that injection site selection matters: in children less than 18 months, the anterolateral thigh injections are associated with the least pain, while in children older than 3 years, the deltoid is the least painful – though these recommendations do not come with a high level of evidentiary validation [55]. Sucrose administration during injections reduces pain scores in randomized trials [56,57], as does non-nutritive sucking on a pacifier [58] and breastfeeding [59,60]. Topical anesthetics also appear to have a small effect [55].

Generally speaking, there is evidence that many interventions effectively reduce distress related to immunizations; however, many of the most effective strategies for reducing pain from needle-related procedures are also more time consuming. Appropriate planning, particularly in inpatient settings, can dramatically reduce the incidence of pain from needle-related procedures [61].

Conclusions

Returning to our introductory scenario, your search reveals that the evidence strongly supports ED immunization with polyvalent pneumococcal vaccine. Girded with the evidence, the next day you convene your team to implement the new screening and immunization strategy, and contact your information services department to develop standing orders for patients with indications for vaccination. You also decide to prospectively track the number of patients with pneumococcal bacteremia seen in your ED over the next 2 years after the new policy. Two years later you compare the incidence with that for the 2 years prior to your immunization campaign, find a clinically and statistically significant difference, and publish your results, adding to the evidence base yourself.

Immunization has a large base of evidence, particularly regarding efficacy, timing and policy recommendations regarding timing and targeted coverage. Certain immunization-related questions that the emergency medicine practitioner may face do not enjoy a substantial evidence base, though there is clearly abundant literature to help guide clinical decisions on an individual and population basis.

Acknowledgments

The authors would like to thank Drs Rowe and Houry for their invitation to contribute to this volume and their expert editing.

Conflicts of interest

None were reported.

References

1 Centers for Disease Control and Prevention. Available at http://www.cdc.gov/vaccines/recs/schedules/default.htm (accessed November 23, 2007).

2 Demicheli V, Barale A, Rivetti A. Vaccines for women to prevent neonatal tetanus. *Cochrane Database Syst Rev* 2005;4:CD002959 (doi: 10.1002/14651858).

3 Pascual FB, McGinley EL, Zanardi LR, et al. Tetanus surveillance – United States, 1998–2000. *Morbidity & Mortality Weekly Report. Surveillance Summaries.* **52**(3):1–8, 2003 Jun 20.

4 Centers for Disease Control and Prevention. Diphtheria, tetanus, and pertussis: recommendations for vaccine use and other preventive measures: recommendations of the Immunization Practices Advisory Committee (ACIP). *MMWR* 1991;**40**:1–28.

5 Anderson LJ, Sikes RK, Langkop CW, et al. Postexposure trial of a human diploid cell strain rabies vaccine. *J Infect Dis* 1980;**142**:133–8.

6 Bahmanyar M, Fayaz A, Nour-Salehi S, Mohammadi M, Koprowski H. Successful protection of humans exposed to rabies infection.

Postexposure treatment with the new human diploid cell rabies vaccine and antirabies serum. *JAMA* 1976;**236**:2751–4.

7 Hattwick MAW. Human rabies. *Public Health Rev* 1974;**3**:229–74.

8 Noah DL, Drenzek CL, Smith JS, et al. Epidemiology of human rabies in the United States, 1980 to 1996. *Ann Intern Med* 1998;**128**:922–30.

9 Krebs JW, Long-Marin SC, Childs JE. Causes, costs and estimates of rabies postexposure prophylaxis treatments in the United States. *J Public Health Manage Pract* 1998;**4**:57–63.

10 Dear KB, Andrews RR, Holden J, Tatham DP. Vaccines for preventing pneumococcal infection in adults. *Cochrane Database Syst Rev* 2003;**4**:CD000422 (doi: 10.1002/14651858).

11 Plouffe JF, Breiman RF, Facklam RR. Bacteremia with *Streptococcus pneumonia*: implications for therapy and prevention. *JAMA* 1997;**278**:1333–9.

12 Gable CB, Holzer SS, Engelhart L, et al. Pneumococcal vaccine: efficacy and associated cost savings. *JAMA* 1990;**262**:2910–15.

13 Shapiro ED, Berg AT, Austrian R, et al. The protective efficacy of polyvalent pneumococcal polysaccharide vaccine. *N Engl J Med* 1991;**325**:1453–60.

14 Fisman DN, Abrutyn E, Spaude KA, Kim A, Kirchner C, Daley J. Prior pneumococcal vaccination is associated with reduced death, complications, and length of stay among hospitalized adults with community-acquired pneumonia. *Clin Infect Dis* 2006;**42**:1093–101.

15 Centers for Disease Control. Update: pneumococcal polysaccharide vaccine usage – United States. *MMWR* 1984;**33**:273–81.

16 Wrenn K, Zeldin M, Miller O. Influenza and pneumococcal vaccination in the emergency department: is it feasible? *J Gen Intern Med* 1994;**9**:425–9.

17 Rodriguez RM, Baraff LJ. Emergency department immunization of the elderly with pneumococcal and influenza vaccines. *Ann Emerg Med* 1993;**22**:1729–32.

18 Sack SJ, Martin DR, Plouffe JF. An emergency department-based pneumococcal vaccination program could save money and lives. *Ann Emerg Med* 1999;**33**:299–303.

19 Parramore CS, Ratnayak K, Wald M, Heilpern KL. Pneumococcal vaccine: a comparison of coverage and need among private vs. public emergency department populations. *Acad Emerg Med* 1999;**6**:374-b.

20 Sisk JE, Moskowitz AJ, Whang W, et al: Cost-effectiveness of vaccination against pneumococcal bacteremia among elderly people. *JAMA* 1997;**278**:1333–9.

21 Walker FJ, Singleton RJ, Bulkow LR, Strikas RA, Butler JC. Reactions after 3 or more doses of pneumococcal polysaccharide vaccine in adults in Alaska. *Clin Infect Dis* 2005;**40**:1730–35.

22 Manthey DE, Stopyra J, Askew K. Referral of emergency department patients for pneumococcal vaccination. *Acad Emerg Med* 2004;**11**:271–5.

23 Pallin DJ, Muennig PA, Emond JA, Kim S, Camargo CA, Jr. Vaccination practices in US emergency departments, 1992–2000. *Vaccine* 2005;**23**:1048–52.

24 Kapur AK, Tenenbein M. Vaccination of emergency department patients at high risk for influenza. *Acad Emerg Med* 2000;**7**:354–8.

25 Slobodkin D, Kitlas JL, Zielske PG. A test of the feasibility of pneumococcal vaccination in the emergency department. *Acad Emerg Med* 1999;**6**:724–7.

26 Dexter PR, Perkins SM, Maharry KS, Jones K, McDonald CJ. Inpatient computer-based standing orders vs physician reminders to increase influenza and pneumococcal vaccination rates. A randomized trial. *JAMA* 2004;**292**:2366–71.

27 Shefer A, McKibben L, Bardenheimer B, Bratzler D, Roberts H. Characteristics of long-term care facilities associated with standing order programs to deliver influenza and pneumococcal vaccinations to residents in 13 states. *J Am Med Dir Assoc* 2005;**6**:97–104.

28 Centers for Disease Control and Prevention. Public health and aging: influenza vaccination coverage among adults aged ≥ 50 years and pneumococcal vaccination coverage among adults aged ≥ 65 years – United States, 2002. *MMWR* 2003;**52**:987–92.

29 Jefferson T. Bioterrorism and compulsory vaccination. *BMJ* 2004;**329**:524–5.

30 Lane JM, Goldstein J. Evaluation of 21 st century risks of smallpox vaccination and policy options. *Ann Intern Med* 2003;**138**:488–93.

31 Lane JM, Ruben FL, Neff JM, Millar JD. Complications of smallpox vaccinations, 1968: national surveillance in the United States. *N Engl J Med* 1969;**281**:1201–8.

32 Grabenstein JD, Winkenwerder W, Jr. US military smallpox vaccination program experience. *JAMA* 2003;**289**:3278–82.

33 Breman JG, Alecaut AB, Malberg DR, Charter RS, Lane JM. Smallpox in the Republic of Guinea, West Africa. II. Eradication using mobile teams. *Am J Trop Med Hyg* 1977;**26**(4):765–74.

34 Meltzer MI, Damon I, LeDuc JW, Millar JD. Modeling potential responses to smallpox as a bioterrorist weapon. *Emerg Infect Dis* 2001;**7**:959–69.

35 Enserink M. Bioterrorism. How devastating would a smallpox attack really be? *Science* 2002;**296**:1592–5.

36 Wharton M, Strikas RA, Harpaz R, et al. Advisory Committee on Immunization Practices. Healthcare Infection Control Practices Advisory Committee. Recommendations for using smallpox vaccine in a pre-event vaccination program. Supplemental recommendations of the Advisory Committee on Immunization Practices (ACIP) and the Healthcare Infection Control Practices Advisory Committee (HICPAC). *Morbidity & Mortality Weekly Report. Recommendations & Reports. 52 (RR-7):1–16, 2003 Apr 4.*

37 Christopher GW, Cieslak TJ, Pavlin JA, Eitzen EM, Jr. Biological warfare. A historical perspective. *JAMA* 1997;**278**:412–17.

38 Dixon TC, Meselson M, Guillemin J, Hanna PC. Anthrax. *N Engl J Med* 1999;**341**:815–26.

39 Hunter D, Zoutman D, Whitehead J, et al. Health effects of anthrax vaccination in the Canadian forces. *Milit Med* 2004;**169**:833–8.

40 Sulsky SI, Grabenstein JD, Delbos RG. Disability among US Army personnel vaccinated against anthrax. *J Occup Environ Med* 2004;**46**:1065–75.

41 Wells TS, Sato PA, Smith TC, Wang LZ, Reed RJ, Ryan MA. Military hospitalizations among deployed US service members following anthrax vaccination, 1998–2001. *Hum Vaccines* 2006;**2**:54–9.

42 Centers for Disease Control and Prevention. Surveillance for adverse events associated with anthrax vaccination – US Department of Defense, 1998–2000. *MMWR* 2000;**49**:341–5.

43 Friedlander AM, Pittman PR, Parker GW. Anthrax vaccine: evidence for safety and efficacy against inhalational anthrax. *JAMA* 1999;**282**:2104–6.

44 Jefferson T, Demicheli V, Deeks J, Graves P, Pratt M, Rivetti D. Vaccines for preventing anthrax. *Cochrane Database Syst Rev* 2007;**1**:CD000975 (doi: 10.1002/14651858).

45 Vietri NJ, Purcell BK, Lawler JV, et al. Short-course postexposure antibiotic prophylaxis combined with vaccination protects against experimental inhalational anthrax. *Proc Natl Acad Sci USA* 2006;**103**:7813–16.

46 Dyer O. US judge halts compulsory anthrax vaccination for soldiers. *BMJ* 2004;**329**:1062.

47 Fowler RA, Sanders GD, Bravata DM, et al. Cost-effectiveness of defending against bioterrorism: a comparison of vaccination and antibiotic prophylaxis against anthrax. *Ann Intern Med* 2005;**142**:601–10.

48 Centers for Disease Control and Prevention. Use of anthrax vaccine in the United States. *MMWR* 2000;**49**:1–20.

49 Meselson M, Guillemin J, Hugh-Jones M, et al. The Sverdlovsk anthrax outbreak of 1979. *Science* 1994;**266**:1202–7.

50 Centers for Disease Control and Prevention. Bioterrorism alleging use of anthrax and interim guidelines for management – United States, 1998. *MMWR* 1999;**48**:69–74.

51 Bianco E, De Masi S, Mele A, Jefferson T. Effectiveness of immune globulins in preventing infectious hepatitis and hepatitis A: a systematic review. *Dig Liver Dis* 2004;**36**:834–42.

52 Sagliocca L, Amoroso P, Stroffolini T, et al. Efficacy of hepatitis A vaccine in prevention of secondary hepatitis A infection: a randomised trial. *Lancet* 1999;**353**:1136–9.

53 Sagliocca L, Bianco E, Amoroso P, et al. Feasibility of vaccination in preventing secondary cases of hepatitis A virus infection. *Vaccine* 2005;**23**:910–14.

54 Uman LS, Chambers CT, McGrath PJ, Kisely S. Psychological interventions for needle-related procedural pain and distress in children and adolescents. *Cochrane Database Syst Rev* 2006;**4**:CD005179 (doi: 10.1002/14651858).

55 Schechter NL, Zempsky WT, Cohen LL, McGrath PJ, McMurtry CM, Bright NS. Pain reduction during pediatric immunizations: evidence-based review and recommendations. *Pediatrics* 2007;**119**:e1184–98.

56 Lewindon PJ, Harkness L, Lewindon N. Randomised controlled trial of sucrose by mouth for the relief of infant crying after immunisation. *Arch Dis Child* 1998;**78**:453–6.

57 Thyr M, Sundholm A, Teeland L, Rahm VA. Oral glucose as an analgesic to reduce infant distress following immunization at the age of 3, 5 and 12 months. *Acta Paediatr* 2007;**96**:233–6.

58 Blass EM, Watt LB. Suckling and sucrose induced analgesia in human newborns. *Pain* 1999;**83**:611–23.

59 Gray L, Miller LW, Phillipp BL, Blass EM. Breastfeeding is analgesic in healthy newborns. *Pediatrics* 2002;**109**:590–93.

60 Efe E, Ozer ZC. The use of breast-feeding for pain relief during neonatal immunization injections. *Appl Nurs Res* 2007;**20**:10–16.

61 Schechter NL, Blankson V, Pachter LM, Sullivan CM, Costa L. The ouchless place: no pain, children's gain. *Pediatrics* 1997;**99**:890–94.

62 Alcohol and Other Drugs

Barbara M. Kirrane, Linda C. Degutis & Gail D'Onofrio

Section of Emergency Medicine, Yale University, New Haven, USA

SCENARIO 1

Clinical scenario

A 38-year-old woman presented to the emergency department (ED) complaining of back pain after falling from a stool. She stated she lost her balance while reaching for a glass in a cabinet above the kitchen sink. She appeared to be intoxicated, complained of pain in the bilateral lumbar paraspinal region, and had normal vital signs and an otherwise unremarkable exam. Upon further questioning, the patient stated that she drinks 4–5 glasses of wine each evening, as a method to "unwind" after the stress of the work day and "get her through" the evening routine as a single parent, preparing dinner, assisting children with homework and such. She stated that when she goes out with her friends she drinks as many as 7–8 drinks on any one occasion.

Background

Unhealthy alcohol use is a major preventable public health problem affecting all racial, cultural and socio-economic groups. It is a leading cause of morbidity and mortality in the USA [1]. There is substantial evidence from primary care settings that brief intervention with at-risk drinkers reduces alcohol misuse, increases treatment contact and is cost-effective [2]. The World Health Organization ranks alcohol use disorders as the second highest diagnosis for contributing to disease burden in the United States, Canada and Western Europe for the ages of 15–44 years [3]. Given that alcohol contributes to such a high burden of disease world-

wide, and that the ED is often the only point of access to health care for many, it seems prudent to screen and intervene in the ED setting.

Clinical questions

In order to address the issues of most relevance to these types of patients and to help in searching the literature for the evidence regarding these issues, you structure your clinical questions as recommended in Chapter 1.

1 In patients who present to the ED (population), is screening for alcohol (intervention) effective at identifying those at risk for injury and alcohol-related complications (outcome)?

2 In patients who present to the ED with alcohol problems (population), what interventions (interventions) are most effective in reducing future harmful drinking (outcome)?

3 In patients who present to the ED (population), what history or risk factors (exposure) should make clinicians consider alcohol problems (outcome)?

General search strategy

You know that screening for alcohol problems may be important in the ED setting, and that there are a number of screening tools available for identification of alcohol problems and interventions to reduce drinking. General searches include the Cochrane Library due to its focus on systematic reviews of therapeutic options. You also search traditional electronic databases such as MEDLINE for any additional randomized controlled trials published after any of the reviews and for observational studies of screening and test studies. Finally, clinical practice guidelines are searched when evidence is limited.

Evidence-based Emergency Medicine. Edited by Brian H. Rowe
© 2009 Blackwell Publishing, ISBN: 978-1-4051-6143-5.

Critical review of the literature

Question 1: In patients who present to the ED (population), is screening for alcohol (intervention) effective at identifying those at risk for injury and alcohol-related complications (outcome)?

Search strategy

- MEDLINE: questionnaires AND alcoholism, diagnosis AND emergency service, hospital

You are aware that there have been several studies performed in which ED patients have been screened for alcohol problems. Your MEDLINE search identifies 26 citations that describe methods and results of screening ED patients for alcohol problems. The populations studied include the range of patients seen in the ED, and several of the studies describe the consequences of alcohol use in the ED patient population.

The concept of screening for alcohol problems in the ED is attractive since there is an opportunity to intervene to prevent further problems. Alcohol problems are prevalent in the ED population and cover a wide spectrum of misuse or unhealthy drinking [4] ranging from at-risk drinking patterns to dependence. "At risk" or "hazardous" drinking levels are defined as those exceeding the National Institute of Alcohol Abuse and Alcoholism (NIAAA) guidelines for low-risk drinking [5]. Box 62.1 provides information on these guidelines by age and sex. By definition these drinkers are at risk for future medical, social or legal consequences. Patients who are experiencing negative consequences due to their alcohol consumption are considered to be harmful drinkers. Approximately 20% of the population in the United States over the age of 12 are hazardous and harmful drinkers [6] and they represent approximately 17% of patients seen in primary care practices [7], and a significant proportion of ED patients within the United States [8,9] and throughout the world [10–14]. Alcohol dependence levels, as measured by >2 positive responses on the CAGE screening questionnaire, have been reported to be as high as 24–31% in large, inner city ED populations [15,16].

Emergency physicians routinely care for patients with unhealthy drinking patterns. There are an estimated 115 million ED visits each year in the USA, and between 10% and 46% of these visits are known to be associated with alcohol [17,18]. The ED is an ideal setting to screen and intervene as rates of heavy drinkers and alcohol-related problems among both injured and non-injured ED patients are higher than in the general population [19]. Cherpitel found that 17% of ED patients screened were positive for harmful drinking [20], and that in the same metropolitan area, ED patients were 1.5–3 times more likely to report heavy drinking, consequences of drinking or ever having treatment for an alcohol problem, than patients presenting to a primary care clinic

[21]. O'Brien et al. [22] found a higher likelihood of self-reported alcohol and drug use among patients who identified the ED as their regular source of care. A single alcohol-related ED visit has been shown to be an important predictor of continued problem drinking, alcohol-impaired driving and possible premature death [23]. In addition, problem drinkers average almost twice as many injury-related events per year as non-problem drinkers and four times as many hospitalizations for injury [24]. Therefore, it is evident that identifying these patients and intervening at the time of the index visit offers a potential for harm reduction.

Emergency physicians are often faced with a busy ED, conflicting demands and ever-increasing responsibilities. Therefore screening strategies must be brief and effective. Evidence suggests that acute sub-critical injury may be an important motivator to reduce drinking, and thus the time of the ED visit may be a valuable teachable moment [25]. Unfortunately, despite high rates of heavy drinking among both injured and non-injured ED patients, routine screening is often not performed. Because of this, an important opportunity to address alcohol-related problems is missed.

Table 62.1 illustrates the screening tools that are commonly used in various settings [26–31]. Each of the tools has been found to be effective in identifying patients with alcohol problems in a variety of settings. Some tools are easier to use than others, based on either length or complexity of a scoring system. Some tools are more specific for identifying hazardous and harmful drinkers and some are more specific for detecting dependence. A definitive diagnosis of dependence may require further assessment. In the ED setting, practitioners have found that it is easiest to use the three quantity and frequency questions, followed by the CAGE questionnaire, thereby providing information about at-risk drinking (drinking above the NIAAA guidelines for low-risk drinking) as well as the possibility of alcohol dependence as identified by the CAGE questions. The quantity/frequency questions are asked first and include:

1 Do you drink alcohol (beer, wine or distilled spirits)?
2 On an average day when you drink, how much do you drink?
3 How many days per week do you drink?
4 An additional question about binge drinking: What is the highest number of drinks that you have had on any one occasion in the past month?

If the patient answers "no" to the first question (do you drink?), there is no need to ask the others. If the patient meets low-risk criteria there is no reason to go on to the CAGE questions. Asking all the questions requires 15–30 seconds.

In conclusion, screening can be performed in the ED, in a variety of ways and by multiple ED practitioners [32]. This may include physicians, nurses, physician associates, technicians, peer educators [33,34], by face-to-face interviews, self-completed surveys or by kiosk [35]. The prevalence of alcohol problems and the overall burden of disease/injury is a compelling argument for its implementation in all EDs.

Box 62.1 NIAAA guidelines: low-risk drinking and the CAGE questionnaire. (Adapted from US Department of Health and Human Services [5].)

If you drink more than the following amounts you can put yourself at risk for illness and/or injury:

- **Men**   **> 14 drinks per week**   *or*   **> 4 drinks per occasion**
- **Women**   **> 7 drinks per week**   *or*   **> 3 drinks per occasion**
- **Age over 65 > 7 drinks per week**   *or*   **> 3 drinks per occasion**

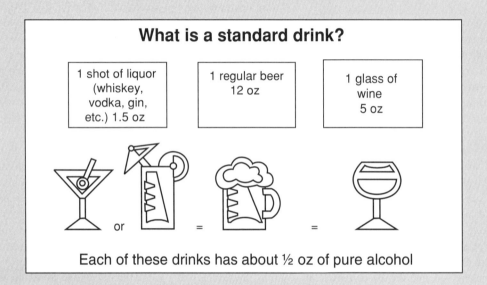

Source: Adapted from U.S. Department of Health and Human Services. National Institutes of Health. National Institute on Alcohol Abuse and Alcoholism. Helping patients with alcohol problems: A health practitioner's guide. Washington, D.C.: Government Printing Office, 2004 (NIH publication no. 04-3769)

CAGE questionnaire

• Have you ever felt that you should cut down on your drinking?
• Have people annoyed you by criticizing your drinking?
• Have you ever felt bad or guilty about your drinking?
• Have you ever had a drink first thing in the morning to steady your nerves or get rid of a hangover?

Table 62.1 Screening tools for alcohol problems (at risk through dependence).

Tool	Number of questions	Population	Comments
CAGE [26]	4	Adults	Easy to use and remember
			Score of >2 is suggestive of dependence
MAST [27]	10	Adults	Long and requires paper prompts
			Requires scoring
AUDIT [28]	12	Adults	Initially developed for hazardous/harmful drinking
			It is suggested that a score of >19 may reflect dependence
			Long, requires paper prompts, complex scoring
TWEAK [29]	5	Adults, especially pregnant women	Initially developed for pregnant women
			No real benefit over CAGE and adds one more question
CRAFFT [30]	6	Adolescents	Developed specifically for adolescents, reflecting harm
RAPS4 [31]	4	Adults	Brief, high sensitivity and performance across demographic subgroups for alcohol dependence
			Much less sensitive to detect hazardous/harmful drinking

Question 2: In patients who present to the ED with alcohol problems (population), what interventions (interventions) are most effective in reducing future harmful drinking (outcome)?

Search strategy

- MEDLINE: brief intervention [text] AND *explode* alcohol AND *explode* emergency service, hospital

You are aware that there have been a number of studies that have examined the efficacy of brief interventions, and that some of these studies have been performed in the ED setting. Your MEDLINE search identifies 4326 citations, eight of which provide information specifically about ED-based trials of brief interventions (BIs).

Brief interventions are counseling sessions ranging from 10 to 45 minutes, typically performed by non-addiction specialists [36]. Evidence suggests BIs are effective in primary care and inpatient trauma settings [37–39]. Gentilello et al. [38] demonstrated that BIs provided to patients admitted to a trauma center were effective in significantly reducing alcohol consumption and decreasing repeat injury hospitalizations in patients who received interventions from a psychologist during their hospitalization after injury.

To date, several randomized controlled studies of BIs in the ED setting have been published in the United States [39–44] and Europe [45–47]. All have concentrated on patients presenting with injuries, either adolescents [42,44] or adults [45,46], rather than general medical illnesses. Most report a positive effect either in harm reduction or alcohol reduction. Table 62.2 describes the studies, including: entry criteria, age group, length of the intervention and whether or not a booster was performed, follow-up times and methods, retention rates and outcomes. There are many challenges in studying the efficacy of BIs in the ED. Several studies report how the assessment may have overwhelmed the intervention and that

both the control and intervention groups decreased their drinking consumption. Also the "control" group most likely received more than usual care. Blow and colleagues studied four interventions for reducing alcohol consumptions and consequences without a control group [48]. Injured patients completed a computerized survey. At-risk drinkers (*n* = 575) were assigned to one of four intervention conditions: (i) tailored alcohol message booklet with brief alcohol advice; (ii) tailored alcohol message booklet only; (iii) generic message booklet with brief alcohol advice; and (iv) generic message booklet only. Each of the intervention groups significantly decreased their alcohol consumption from baseline to 12-month follow-up, with those in the first group significantly decreasing their weekly alcohol consumption by 48.5% ($P < 0.0001$).

In summary, it is evident from this review that the evidence for BI in the ED is mixed. More questions need to be answered in future research. How should the intervention be performed (face-to-face, kiosk/computer, web-based)? What type of personnel should perform the intervention if it is face-to-face (i.e., physician, nurse, health educator)? What subgroups of patients are more receptive to behavioral change? What factors related to the intervention are important (e.g., length, presence of a booster)? What specific components need to be included in the intervention and do these differ with different subgroup characteristics such as age, gender, presence of injury, etc?

Question 3: In patients who present to the ED (population), what history or risk factors (exposure) should make clinicians consider alcohol problems (outcome)?

Search strategy

- MEDLINE: (alcohol abuse.mp OR *explode* alcoholism) AND *explode* emergency service, hospital [MeSH]

Table 62.2 Details of studies examining the effectiveness of brief interventions in patients with alcohol problems.

Study	Study design and size	Population and admission criteria	Intervention	Follow-up times and rates	Outcome	Effect
US studies Monti 1999 [40]	RCT N = 94	Age: 18–19 years Criteria: + BAC or alcohol-related injury	BI: one session (35–40 minutes) No F/U sessions	F/U: 3 months (phone) and 6 months (face-to-face interview) Rate: 93%, 89%	↓in alcohol consumption for both BI and control groups ↓in negative consequences for BI group	Positive effect for harm reduction
Longabaugh et al. [41]	RCT N = 539	Age: ≥ 18 years Criteria: injury not requiring hospitalization and screened positive for harmful and hazardous drinking by AUDIT scores or positive BAC	BI: 40–60 minutes BIB: booster Initial BI and scheduled return visit 7–10 days later	F/U: 1 year Rate: 83%	↓in alcohol consumption for all three groups ↓in negative consequences for BIB group only	Positive effect for harm reduction in BIB
Spirito et al. [42]	RCT N = 152	Age: 13–17 years Criteria: alcohol-related injury by positive BAC or self-report of alcohol use 6 hours prior to injury	BI: 1 (35–45 minutes) SC: 5 minutes	F/U: 3 months (phone) and 6 and 12 months (in person) Rate: 93.4%, 89.5%, 89.5%	↓ in alcohol consumption in both groups ↓in frequency and binging in the BI group when subjects were screened for pre-existing problematic alcohol use	Positive effect for alcohol consumption in pre-existing problematic drinkers
Blow 2004 [43]	RT (no control) N = 575	Age: ≥ 19 years Criteria: at-risk drinkers; injured	BI (4 different groups): 1 Tailored message booklet with brief advice (TM/BA) 2 Tailored message booklet only (TM/NoBA) 3 Generic message booklet with advice (GM/BA) 4 Generic message booklet only (GM/NoBA)	F/U: 3 and 12 months (phone) Rate: > 85% at 3 and 12 months	↓in alcohol consumption in all groups; most significant in group 1	Positive effect for alcohol consumption
Maio et al. [44]	RCT N = 655	Age: 14–18 years Criteria: with minor injury	BI: interactive computer generated	F/U: 3 and 12 months (phone) Rate: 88.5% at 3 and 12 months	↓in alcohol consumption in all groups	
European studies England: Crawford et al. [45]	RCT N = 599	Age: ≥ 18 Criteria: hazardous drinkers; "misusing alcohol"	BI	F/U: 6 and 12 months (phone, in person) Rate: 64.1% at 12 months	↓in alcohol consumption at 6 months No difference at 12 months	Positive effect at 6 months only
Germany: Neumann et al. [46]	RCT N = 1139	Age: ≥ 18 years Criteria: at-risk drinkers with minor injury; positive AUDIT score	BI: computer generated with print-out advice	F/U: 6 months (phone, mail, email) and 12 months (computer, mail) Rate: 63.1% at 6 months; 60% at 12 months	↓in alcohol consumption	Positive effect for alcohol consumption
Spain: Rodriguez-Martos Dauer 2005	RT (no control) N = 85	Age: ≥ 18 years Criteria: alcohol-positive traffic casualty	BI vs minimal intervention	F/U: 3, 6 and 12 months (phone) Rate: 67% at 12 months	↓in alcohol consumption in both groups	Positive/negative effect for alcohol consumption No difference between groups
Non-European studies Australia: Tait et al. [47]	RCT N = 127	Age: 12–19 years Criteria: AOD use	BI	F/U: 4, 8 and 12 months (mode of interview not stated in paper) Rate: 69% at 12 months	↑in enrollment in treatment program ↓in return ED visits for alcohol/drug use	Positive effect for referral and return ED visits

AOD, alcohol and other drugs; BAC, blood alcohol concentration; BI, brief intervention; BIB, brief intervention booster; ED, emergency department; F/U, follow-up; RCT, randomized controlled trial; RT, randomized trial; SC, standard care.

You know that there have been a number of studies related to the prevalence of alcohol problems in ED patients, as well as screening for alcohol problems in ED patients. Your MEDLINE search identified 348 English language references.

Almost any patient who enters the ED may be considered at risk for having an alcohol problem. Reports of alcohol use disorders and alcohol problems in ED patients are extensive. Except for a higher prevalence of alcohol problems in males, there is no one group of patients who can be identified as being more at risk for alcohol problems than other groups. For example, Fleming, et al. found that 13.1% of women and 32.8% of men attending a Swiss ED were at-risk drinkers [49]. In Australia, Roche et al. found similar prevalence rates, and did not identify any differences between ED patients and inpatients [50]. While there are no US studies that specifically identify the epidemiology of alcohol use in ED patients, there are numerous published reports of alcohol use in specific patient populations [51–54].

Overall, based on these reports and on the evidence for long-term consequences of problem alcohol use, recommendations for universal screening for alcohol problems in the ED are supported.

SCENARIO 2

Clinical scenario

A 44-year-old male was brought to the ED with altered mental status after he was found down in the bathroom of a dance club by his room-mate. The room-mate reported that the patient had been drinking alcohol and ingesting an unknown number of prescription pain pills (controlled-release oxycodone) that evening, as he had been doing each weekend night for several months. Recently, however, the room-mate noticed that the patient had been taking larger amounts of these medications. Although they entered the club together several hours earlier, they were separated for most of the evening. The room-mate immediately called 911 when he found the patient on the floor of the bathroom.

On arrival to the ED, the patient was non-verbal and groaning to painful stimuli. His vitals signs were blood pressure 100/70 mmHg; pulse 61 beats/min, respirations 8 breaths/min and temperature 35°C (96°F; axilla). His pulse oximetry was 79% on room air. His pupils were 1 mm bilaterally, breath sounds were clear with symmetric air movement, his bowel sounds were hypoactive and he had a non-tender abdomen. His skin exam was unremarkable, he was moving all extremities and he had symmetric reflexes. An electrocardiogram showed a normal sinus rhythm with normal intervals.

Background

There are approximately 2 million ED visits each year in the USA resulting from exposure to pharmaceutical agents and illicit drugs, such as cocaine and heroin [55]. Of these visits, the great majority

(1.3 million) of exposures stem from misuse or abuse [55]. Additionally, mortality rates attributed to unintentional and intentional drug overdose have increased significantly in recent years [56,57]. While this increase occurred across several categories of drugs, the largest increase was found in the opioid category, including heroin and opioid analgesics. Prescription pain medication sales have steadily increased in the last 15 years for many reasons, including changing philosophies regarding management of pain that lead to a more aggressive approach to pain management, an increase in pharmaceutical company advertising campaigns and increasing ease of availability. While many different modalities and pharmaceutical agents are available for pain management, opioids are frequently first-line agents recommended in clinical guidelines. The euphoric effect created by opioids, however, creates the potential for misuse. In the last several years, there has been increasing misuse of prescription medications among virtually all age groups, with a particular increase in the adolescent age group [58].

Clinical questions

In order to address the issues of most relevance to these types of patients and to help in searching the literature for the evidence regarding these issues, you structure your clinical questions as recommended in Chapter 1.

3 In patients presenting to the ED with a history of intentional drug exposure (population), does a toxicology screen (intervention) aid in clinical management (outcome)?

4 In patients presenting to the ED with a history of intentional drug exposure (population), what are the indications for naloxone (intervention)?

5 In patients with suspected drug overdose (population) who were given naloxone (intervention), what are the complications of this treatment (outcome)?

General search strategy

As with the previous scenario, your search includes database searches in the Cochrane Library and MEDLINE. You know that not many randomized trials have been conducted for naloxone and overdose management so you start with a very broad search of the Cochrane Library.

Critical review of the literature

Question 3: In patients presenting to the ED with a history of intentional drug exposure (population), does a toxicology screen (intervention) aid in clinical management (outcome)?

Your Cochrane Library search is unhelpful; however, the MEDLINE search yields two reviews describing the utility of urine drug screening in the ED. Urine drug of abuse screens are frequently obtained in the acute care setting in patients suspected of drug use. Initially developed as screening tools for the workplace, these screens are frequently immunoassays, which use antibodies to qualitatively detect drugs or their metabolites in the urine. Assays are determined to be positive or negative based on whether the measured substance exceeds a threshold value. Drug of abuse screens have become widely available in acute care clinical laboratories. Specific substances assayed on a drug of abuse screen vary between institutions, but most common assays include amphetamines, cannabinoids, cocaine, opioids and phencyclidine. Though these screens are readily obtainable, the overall contribution to patient management is widely debated.

No systematic reviews have been conducted on this topic. Two clinical trials were identified on independent searches. Montague et al. looked at routine urine drug screens obtained on patients presenting with a diagnosis of deliberate self-poisoning in the ED. Study drug results were not available at the time of patient management. Though, in some cases, screens were positive for unexpected findings for substances not identified in the patients' history, results of urine drug screens would never have changed management as determined by the study chart reviewers [59]. Eisen et al. questioned physicians regarding patient care plans for patients receiving urine drug of abuse testing, and then re-evaluated the answers once test results were known. Specific indications for sending drug screens were not listed; however, the authors excluded patients that had undergone vehicular trauma or sexual assault, two indications where screens may be potentially obtained for legal considerations. The study found that results from screening for drugs of abuse rarely changed management plans, and when so changed, actions were never considered justified by the study's review panel [60].

Clinical care of the poisoned patient centers around providing optimal clinical support, and that in most if not all cases, treatment relies on the collection of good clinical data. Additionally, it is important to note that urine drug screens have several limitations. Qualitative drug screens only detect a small range of drugs; they are not comprehensive screens. Negative drug screens do not exclude all drug exposures and positive screens may represent clinically insignificant concentrations or may be a false result resulting from structural similarity between compounds [61]. The presence of a drug in the body does not necessarily indicate that it contributed to the patient's current clinical presentation, and can potentially mislead the physician to consider that a drug of abuse is responsible for a clinical presentation. For example, the presence of a benzodiazepine in the urine of a patient with altered mental status may lead one to attribute the change in mental status to the benzodiazepine, and then not search for other possibilities, such as infection. Additionally, the presence of a drug may be detected for many days after the exposure [62]. Unexpected positive results found on drug screens seldom change management, and almost never affect outcome [63]. However, some practitioners utilize urine drug screens to increase their confidence in making diagnoses and disposition decisions [64].

Many serum assays, such as acetaminophen, digoxin and lithium, are clinically useful as they define the severity of intoxication and may guide treatment. Specific serum levels should be sent on the basis of clinical suspicion. The general approach to all patients suspected of drug intoxication should include a thorough physical exam, including vital signs and oxygen saturation. Particular attention should be paid to identifying end-organ manifestations for a particular toxidrome. Rapid bedside glucose should be obtained in all patients with an altered mental status. A 12-lead electrocardiogram is a useful tool to identify consequential manifestations of toxic substances. Importantly, a serum acetaminophen level should be sent on every patient presenting with a suicidal ingestion, even if it is not reported as one of the substances that was ingested. Acetaminophen is widely available, both as an individual product and as a combination product. Patients may not recognize the presence of acetaminophen in substances ingested, may consider it benign or may not be completely forthcoming in the history. Additionally, patients with clinically significant acetaminophen concentrations are frequently asymptomatic early after ingestion. There is also a window of time for optimal treatment outcome, as the antidote, *N*-acetylcysteine, is nearly 100% effective if administered within 8 hours of ingestion (see Chapter 28 for further details) [65].

In summary, urine drug screening has many limitations which should be considered when interpreting the results in the acute care clinical setting. Results found on a urine drug screen should never replace good clinical acumen.

Question 4: In patients presenting to the ED with a history of intentional drug exposure (population), what are the indications for naloxone (intervention)?

Few randomized trials have been conducted for naloxone and overdose management so you start with a very broad search. The Cochrane Library and MEDLINE searches described above fail to produce any reviews or randomized trials.

Opioid receptors are located throughout the body and, as a result, exposure to opioids produces clinical effects on several organ systems, including the pulmonary, ophthalmic, gastrointestinal and central nervous systems. However, of the many clinical effects induced by opioid exposure, respiratory depression is by far the most significant and, if severe, may result in death. Therefore, the management of opioid intoxication centers around respiratory support. This may be accomplished by ventilation with a bag valve mask, or, if necessary, endotracheal intubation.

Since the 1960s, an antidote, naloxone, has been available for clinical use, and can reverse opioid-induced respiratory depression, allowing a patient to resume breathing on their own – potentially avoiding the need for further intervention. Naloxone is a non-selective competitive opioid antagonist that inhibits the pharmacological effects of opioids at each receptor. Naloxone may be administered through the intravenous, intramuscular, subcutaneous, intranasal or endotracheal routes. Although naloxone is absorbed orally, it undergoes extensive first-pass metabolism, and thus it has low bioavailability [66]. Naloxone quickly crosses the blood–brain barrier, and clinical effects are seen within minutes [67]. Naloxone has a half-life of 60–90 minutes, with its clinical efficacy lasting for a slightly shorter duration (45–70 minutes), with some variation between individuals resulting from differences in metabolism. Clinical effects reversed by naloxone may return if the duration of effect of the opioid is longer than this time interval, as is the case with methadone and sustained-release oxycodone. Patients exhibiting respiratory depression from a long-acting agent are at risk for recurrent respiratory depression, and must therefore be closely observed. This can be a clinical challenge, as patients will commonly feel back to baseline after naloxone administration, and may desire to leave the ED.

In summary, naloxone is indicated for use in patients who are exhibiting signs of respiratory depression as a result of opioid use. These patients must be closely observed for recurrent respiratory depression due to opioid effects after the administration of naloxone.

Question 5: In patients with suspected drug overdose (population) who were given naloxone (intervention), what are the complications of this treatment (outcome)?

Search strategy

- MEDLINE: naloxone AND adverse effects AND overdose

Your search identified 17 references related to the use of naloxone in overdoses; however, no systematic reviews were identified. Five studies describe adverse effects of naloxone when used in the treatment of opioid overdoses. Naloxone is a relatively safe medication when administered to non-opioid-dependent patients, with side-effects mainly consisting of alterations in mood [68,69]. However, in dependent opioid users, more serious adverse effects may occur. Naloxone may precipitate withdrawal in tolerant individuals,

provoking such symptoms as agitation, vomiting, abdominal pain, diarrhea, diaphoresis and lacrimation. Withdrawal is particularly problematic in a patient who may have another process accounting for their presentation, such as hypoglycemia or a mixed ingestion, and may increase the risk of complications such as aspiration. Naloxone administration is associated rarely with seizures [70] and arrhythmias [71].

Acute lung injury (ALI), characterized as the sudden onset of acute hypoxemic respiratory failure and the presence of bilateral pulmonary infiltrates [72], has been described in patients with heroin overdose, as well as many other opioids, and those receiving treatment with naloxone [73,74]. The etiology of ALI in this patient population has not been clearly elucidated, but several theories include a hypoxia-induced catecholamine surge that results in a stunned myocardium [75] and pressure changes created by inspiring against a closed epiglottis, causing fluid shifts from the pulmonary vasculature into the alveolar spaces [76]. In some cases, ALI is created by the initial hypoxic insult, and was simply unmasked by the naloxone [75]. Generally, patients who developed ALI after naloxone therapy had a significant period of hypoventilation or apnea before treatment with the antidote. Symptoms of ALI generally develop early (within 2–3 hours), but may also develop later [77]. Sources vary as to the recommendation for how long patients at risk for ALI should be monitored, with some recommending up to 24 hours, depending on the clinical severity of the overdose [78].

The efficacy of naloxone in reversing life-threatening symptoms of opioid overdose initially led to widespread recommendations for its use, and it was commonly administered to patients with undifferentiated altered mental status as a method for diagnosing and treating opioid overdose. However, a more narrowed approach may be considered due to the potential for complications in dependent users. A large prospective trial that examined the utility of empirical naloxone administered in the prehospital setting, for patients presenting with altered mental status, found that only a small number of patients (7.6%) demonstrated a positive response to naloxone administration without side-effects. Overall, the strongest predictor of response was a respiratory rate of 12 breaths/min or less [79].

Dosing recommendations vary depending on the source, but in general small doses (0.05 mg) given incrementally are recommended to avoid withdrawal [80]. If respiratory depression reoccurs, repeat boluses should be given, or, alternatively, a continuous infusion may be used, at the dose of two-thirds of the initial dose given per hour [81]. In general, the benefits of naloxone outweigh the potential adverse events.

Conclusions

The physician performed a brief intervention in the ED on the patient in the first clinical scenario. Through this process, the patient made the connection that the unsteadiness that caused her fall from the stool was likely related to alcohol. She responded that she was ready to cut back on her daily consumption of alcohol and create a goal of staying within NIAAA low-risk guidelines of no more than three drinks per night or seven per week. She agreed to follow up with her primary care practitioner.

The second patient was given intravenous fluids and naloxone (0.05 mg × 2 doses), with a subsequent increase in his respiratory rate to 14 breaths/min and pulse oximetry reading to 97% on room air; he became awake and oriented. Forty-five minutes later, it was noticed that his respiratory rate had returned to 8 breaths/min and that he was somnolent with a decreased oxygen saturation of 89%. A second dose of naloxone was given, and the patient was placed on a naloxone infusion. His laboratory work subsequently revealed a normal complete blood count and serum chemistry, and a serum acetaminophen was negative. A urine drug screen was positive for opioids. He was admitted to the hospital, and over the next 12 hours his naloxone infusion was tapered. The next morning he was awake and alert and had a normal physical exam. He was subsequently transferred to an inpatient detoxification unit for further evaluation and treatment.

The misuse of alcohol and other drugs are common presentations to EDs throughout the world and associated with many adverse health effects. Early identification and referral to treatment is beneficial to the individual, family and workplace, and saves health care dollars. It is clear that screening and intervention involve resources, but represent best practice. Questions such as who should perform the screening and intervention (i.e., physicians, nurses, physician extenders or peer educators) and by what method (e.g., face-to-face interview, kiosk, computer, and so forth) all need to be further addressed. Education and referral sources need to be provided. To date the research is promising that such interventions can prevent negative consequences and improve the health of the public.

Conflicts of interest

The authors declare no conflicts of interest in the preparation of this chapter.

References

1 Harwood H. Updating Estimates of the Economic Costs of Alcohol Abuse in the United States: Estimates, Update Methods and Data. Report prepared by the Lewin Group for the National Institute on Alcohol Abuse and Alcoholism, 2000. Based on estimates, analyses, and data reported in Harwood, H.; Fountain, D; and Livermore, G. The Economic Costs of Alcohol and Drug Abuse in the United States 1992. Report prepared for the National Institute on Drug Abuse and the National Institute on Alcohol Abuse and Alcoholism, National Institutes of Health, Department of Health and Human Services. NIH Publication No. 98-4327. Rockville, MD: National Institutes of Health, 1998.

2 Fleming MF, Mundt MP, French MT, Manwell LB, Stauffacher EA, Barry KL. Brief physician advice for problem drinkers: long-term efficacy and benefit-cost analysis. *Alcohol Clin Exp Res* 2002;**26**:36–43.

3 Lopez AD, Mathers CD, Ezzati M, Jamison DT, Murray CJL. *Global Burden of Disease and Risk Factors*. World Health Organization, Geneva, 2006.

4 Saitz R. Clinical practice. Unhealthy alcohol use. *N Engl J Med* 2005;**352**:596–607.

5 US Department of Health and Human Services, National Institutes of Health, National Institute on Alcohol Abuse and Alcoholism. *Helping Patients with Alcohol Problems: A health practitioner's guide.* NIH Publication No. 04-3769. Government Printing Office, Washington, 2004.

6 Secretary of Health and Human Services. *Tenth Special Report to the US Congress on Alcohol and Health.* NIH Publication No. 00-1583. Government Printing Office, Washington, 2000.

7 Manwell LB, Fleming MF, Johnson K, Barry KL. Tobacco, alcohol, and drug use in a primary care sample: 90 day prevalence and associated factors. *J Addict Dis* 1998;**17**:67–81.

8 Cherpitel CJ. Screening for alcohol problems in the emergency department. *Ann Emerg Med* 1995;**26**:158–66.

9 Cherpitel CJ. Alcohol consumption among emergency room patients: comparison of county/community hospitals and an HMO. *J Stud Alcohol* 1993;**54**:432–40.

10 Calle PA, Damen J, De Paepe P, Monsieurs KG, Buylaert WA. A survey on alcohol and illicit drug abuse among emergency department patients. *Acta Clin Belg* 2006;**61**:188–95.

11 Hannon MJ, Luke LC. The burden of alcohol misuse on the emergency department. *Irish Med J* 2006;**99**:118–20.

12 Li Y-M, Tsai S-Y, Hu S-C, Wang C-T. Alcohol-related injuries at an emergency department in Eastern Taiwan. *J Formosa Med Assoc* 2006;**105**:481–8.

13 Soffer D, Zmora O, Klausner JB, et al. Alcohol use among trauma victims admitted to a level I trauma center in Israel. *Israel Med Assoc J* 2006;**8**:98–102.

14 Crawford, MJ, Patton R, Touquet R, et al. Screening and referral for brief intervention of alcohol-misusing patients in an emergency department: a pragmatic randomized controlled trial. *Lancet* 2004;**364**:1334–9.

15 Whiteman PJ, Hoffman RS, Goldfrank LR. Alcoholism in the emergency department: an epidemiologic study. *Acad Emerg Med* 2000;**7**:14–20.

16 Bernstein E, Tracy A, Berstein J, William C. Emergency department detection and referral rates for patients with problem drinking. *Subst Abuse* 2006;**17**:69–76.

17 Cherpitel CJ. Breath analysis and self-report as measures of alcohol-related emergency room admissions. *J Stud Alcohol* 1989;**50**:155–61.

18 Bernstein E, Tracey A, Bernstein J, Williams C. Emergency department detection and referral rates for patients with problem drinking. *Subst Abuse* 1996;**7**:69–76.

19 Cherpitel CJ. Alcohol consumption among emergency room patients: comparison of county/community hospitals and an HMO. *J Stud Alcohol* 1993;**54**:432–40.

20 Cherpitel CJ. Screening for alcohol problems in the emergency department. *Ann Emerg Med* 1995;**26**:158–66.

21 Cherpitel CJ. Drinking patterns and problems: a comparison of primary care with the emergency room. *Subst Abuse* 1999;**20**:85–95.

22 O'Brien GM, Stein MD, Zierler S, Shapiro M, O'Sullivan P, Woolard R. Use of the ED as a regular source of care: associated factors beyond lack of health insurance. *Ann Emerg Med* 1997;**30**:286–91.

23 Davidson P, Koziol-McLain J, Harrison L, Lowenstein SR. Intoxicated ED patients: a 5-year follow-up of morbidity and mortality. *Ann Emerg Med* 1997;**30**:593–7.

24 National Highway Traffic Safety Administration. Current research in alcohol. *Ann Emerg Med* 1997;**30**:817–19.

25 Becker BM, Woolard RH, Longabaugh R, Minugh PA, Nirenberg TD, Clifford PR. Alcohol use among subcritically injured emergency department patients and injury as a motivator to reduce drinking. *Acad Emerg Med* 1995;**2**:784–90.

26 Ewing JA. Detecting alcoholism. The CAGE questionnaire. *JAMA* 1984;**252**:1905–7.

27 Selzer M. The Michigan Alcoholism Screening Test (MAST): the quest for a new diagnostic instrument. *Am J Psychiatry* 1971;**127**:1653–8.

28 Babor T, Ramon de la Fuente J, Saunders J, Grant M. *The Alcohol Use Disorders Identification Test: Guidelines for use in primary health care.* WHO Publication No. 89.4. World Health Organization, Geneva, 1989.

29 Russell M, Martier SS, Sokkol RF, et al. Screening for pregnancy risk-drinking. *Alcohol Clin Exp Res* 1994;**18**:1156–61.

30 Knight J, Sherritt L, Shrier L, et al. Validity of the CRAFFT substance abuse screening test among adolescent clinic patients. *Arch Pediatr Adolesc Med* 2002;**156**:607–14.

31 Cherpitel CJ. A brief screening instrument for problem drinking in the emergency room: the RAPS4. Rapid Alcohol Problems Screen. *J of Stud Alcohol.* 2000;**61**:447–9.

32 D'Onofrio G, Bernstein E, Bernstein J, et al. Patients with alcohol problems in the emergency department. Part 1: Improving detection. *Acad Emerg Med* 1998;**5**:1200–209.

33 Bernstein E, Bernstein J, Levenson S. Project ASSERT: an ED-based intervention to increase access to primary care, preventive services, and the substance abuse treatment system. *Ann Emerg Med* 1997;**30**:181–9.

34 D'Onofrio G, Thomas M, Degutis LC. Project ASSERT: a 5-year evaluation of an emergency department-based screening, brief intervention, and referral to treatment program. *Acad Emerg Med* 2005;**12**(Suppl):60–61.

35 Rhodes KV, Lauderdale DS, Stocking CB, et al. Better health while you wait: a controlled trial of a computer-based intervention for screening and health promotion in the emergency department. *Ann Emerg Med* 2001;**31**;284–91.

36 Miller WR, Rollnick S. *Motivational Interviewing: Preparing people to change addictive behavior*, 2nd edn. Guilford Press, New York, 2002.

37 Fleming MF, Barry KL, Manwell LB, Johnson K, London R. Brief physician advice for problem alcohol drinkers: a randomized controlled trial in community-based primary care practices. *JAMA* 1997;**277**:1039–45.

38 Gentilello LM, Rivara FP, Donovan DM, et al. Alcohol interventions in a trauma center as a means of reducing the risk of injury recurrence. *Ann Surg* 1999;**230**:473–84.

39 D'Onofrio G, Degutis LC. Preventive care in the emergency department: screening and brief intervention for alcohol problems in the emergency department: a systematic review. *Acad Emerg Med* 2002;**9**:627–38.

40 Monti PM, Spirit A, Myers M, Colby SM, Barnett NP, Rohsenow DJ, Woolard R, Lewander W. Brief intervention for harm reduction with alcohol-positive older adolescents in a hospital emergency department. *Journal of Consulting and Clinical Psychology* 1999;**67**:989–994.

41 Longabaugh RH, Woolard RF, Nirenberg TD, et al. Evaluating the effects of a brief motivational intervention for injured drinkers in the emergency department. *J Stud Alcohol* 2001;**62**:806–16.

42 Spirito A, Monti PM, Barnett NP, et al. A randomized clinical trial of a brief motivational intervention for alcohol-positive adolescents treated in an emergency department. *J Pediatr* 2004;**148**:396–402.

43 Blow FC, Barry KL, Walton MA, Maio RF, Chemack ST, Bingham CR, Ignacio RV, Strecher VJ. The efficacy of two brief intervention strategies among injured, at-risk drinkers in the emergency department: Impact of tailored messaging and brief advice. *J Stud Alcohol.* 2006;**67**:568–578.

44 Maio RF, Shope JT, Blow FC, et al. A randomized controlled trial of an emergency department-based interactive computer program to prevent alcohol misuse among injured adolescents. *Ann Emerg Med* 2005;**45**:420–29.

45 Neumann T, Neuner B, Weiss-Gerlach E, et al. The effect of computerized tailored brief advice on at-risk drinking in subcritically injured trauma patients. *J Trauma* 2006;**61**:805–14.

46 Crawford MJ, Patton R, Touquet R, et al. Screening and referral for brief intervention of alcohol-misusing patients in an emergency department: a pragmatic randomised controlled trial. *Lancet* 2004;**364**:1334–9.

47 Tait RJ, Hulse GK, Robertson SI, Sprivulis PC. Emergency department-based intervention with adolescent substance users: 12-month outcomes. *Drug Alcohol Depend* 2005;**79**:359–63.

48 Blow FC, Barry KL, Walton MA, et al. The efficacy of two brief intervention strategies among injured, at-risk drinkers in the emergency department: impact of tailored messaging and brief advice. *J Stud Alcohol* 2006;**67**:568–78.

49 Fleming EA, Gmel G, Bady P, et al. At-risk drinking and drug use among patients seeking care in an emergency department. *J Stud Alcohol* 2007;**68**:28–35.

50 Roche AM, Freeman T, Skinner N. From data to evidence, to action: findings from a systematic review of hospital screening studies for high risk alcohol consumption. *Drug Alcohol Depend* 2006;**83**:1–14.

51 Greene J. Serial inebriate programs: what to do about homeless alcoholics in the emergency department. *Ann Emerg Med* 2007;**49**:791–3.

52 Cunningham WE, Sohler NL, Tobias C, et al. Health services utilization for people with HIV infection: comparison of a population targeted for outreach with the US population in care. *Med Care* 2006;**44**:1038–47.

53 Carballo JJ, Oquendo MA, Garcia-Moreno M, et al. Demographic and clinical features of adolescents and young adults with alcohol-related disorders admitted to the psychiatric emergency room. *Int J Adolesc Med Health* 2006;**18**:87–96.

54 Cherpitel CJ, Bond J, Ye Y. Alcohol and injury: a risk function analysis from the Emergency Room Collaborative Alcohol Analysis Project (ERCAAP). *Eur Addict Res* 2006;**12**:42–52.

55 US Department of Health and Human Services. Drug Abuse Warning Network 2005: National estimates of drug related emergency department visits. Available at www.http://DAWNinfo.samhsa.gov. [Last accessed 3 September 2007].

56 Centers for Disease Control and Prevention. Unintentional poisoning deaths – United States, 1999–2004. *MMWR* 2007;**56**:93–6.

57 Paulozzi LJ, Ryan GW. Opioid analgesics and rates of fatal drug poisonings in the US. *Am J Prev Med* 2006;**31**:506–11.

58 Hertz JA, Knight JR. Prescription drug misuse: a growing national problem. *Adolesc Med* 2006;**17**:751–69.

59 Montague RE, Grace RF, Lewis JH, et al. Urine drug screens in overdose patients do not contribute to immediate clinical management. *Ther Drug Monit* 2001;**23**:47–50.

60 Eisen JS, Sivilotti ML, Boyd DU, et al. Screening urine for drugs of abuse in the emergency department: do test results affect physicians' patient care decisions? *Can J Emerg Med* 2004;**6**:104–11.

61 Belson MG, Simon HK, Sullivan K, et al. The utility of toxicologic analysis in children with suspected ingestions. *Pediatr Emerg Care* 1999;**15**:383–7.

62 Perrone J, De Roos F, Jayaraman S, et al. Drug screening versus history in detection of substance use in ED psychiatric patients. *Am J Emerg Med* 1991;**19**:49–51.

63 Brett AS. Implications of discordance between clinical impression and toxicology analysis in drug overdose. *Arch Intern Med* 1988;**148**:437–41.

64 Wu AHB, McKay C, Broussard LA, et al. National Academy of Clinical Biochemistry Laboratory Medicine Practice Guidelines: recommendations for the use of laboratory tests to support poisoned patients who present to the emergency department. *Clin Chem* 2003;**49**:357–79.

65 Smilkstein MJ, Knapp GL, Kulig KW, et al. Efficacy of oral N-acetylcysteine in the treatment of acetaminophen overdose: analysis of the national multicenter study (1976–1985). *N Engl J Med* 1988;**3190**:1557–62.

66 Sporer KA. Acute heroin overdose. *Ann Intern Med* 1999;**130**:584–90.

67 Chamberlain JM, Klein BL. A comprehensive review of naloxone for the emergency physician. *Am J Emerg Med* 1994;**12**:650–60.

68 Jasinski DR, Martin WR, Haertzen CA. The human pharmacology and abuse potential of N-allylnoroxymorphone (naloxone). *J Pharm Exp Ther* 1967;**157**:420–26.

69 Cohen MR, Cohen RM, Pickar D, et al. Behavioral effects after high dose naloxone administration to normal volunteers. *Lancet* 1981;**2**:1110.

70 Mariani PJ. Seizures associated with low-dose naloxone. *Am J Emerg Med* 1989;**7**:127–9.

71 Cuss FM, Colaco CB, Baron JH. Cardiac arrest after reversal of effects of opiates with naloxone. *BMJ* 1984;**288**:363–4.

72 Rubenfeld GD, Caldwell E, Peabody E, et al. Incidence and outcome of acute lung injury. *N Engl J Med* 2005;**353**:1685–93.

73 Duberstein JL, Kaufman DM. A clinical study of an epidemic of heroin intoxication and heroin induced pulmonary edema. *Am J Med* 1971;**51**:704–14.

74 Sterrett C, Brownfield J, Korn CS, et al. Patterns of presentation in heroin overdose resulting in pulmonary edema. *Am J Emerg Med* 2003;**21**:32–4.

75 Mills CA, Flacke JW, Miller JD, et al. Cardiovascular effects of fentanyl reversal by naloxone at varying arterial carbon dioxide tensions in dogs. *Anesth Analog* 1988;**67**:730–36.

76 Kollef MH, Pluss J. Non-cardiogenic pulmonary edema following upper airway obstruction: 7 cases and a review of the literature. *Medicine (Baltimore)* 1991;**70**:91–8.

77 Cherubin CE. The medical sequel of narcotic addiction. *Ann Intern Med* 1967;**67**:23–33.

78 Nelson LS. Opioids. In: Flomenbaum NF, Howland MAH, Goldfrank LR, Lewin NA, Hoffman RS, Nelson LS, eds. *Goldfrank's Toxicologic Emergencies*, 8th edn. McGraw Hill, New York, 2006:590–613.

79 Hoffman JR, Schriger DL, Luo JS. The empiric use of naloxone in patients with altered mental status: a reappraisal. *Ann Emerg Med* 1991;**20**:246–52.

80 Howland MAH. Opioid antagonists. In: Flomenbaum NE, Howland MAH, Goldfrank LR, Lewin NA, Hoffman RS, Nelson LS, eds. *Goldfrank's Toxicologic Emergencies*, 8th edn. McGraw Hill, New York, 2006:614–19.

81 Goldfrank LR, Weisman RS, Errick JK, et al. A dosing nomogram for continuous infusion intravenous naloxone. *Ann Emerg Med* 1986;**15**:566–70.

63 Elder Abuse

Ralph J. Riviello

Department of Emergency Medicine, Thomas Jefferson University, Philadelphia, USA

Clinical scenario

A 70-year-old woman presented to the emergency department (ED) from the nursing home for evaluation of hematuria and recurrent urinary tract infections. The patient had moderate dementia and other stable chronic medical conditions including diabetes, hypertension and stroke. Her vital signs were stable with a temperature of 37°C (oral), pulse of 72 beats/min, respirations of 18 breaths/min and blood pressure of 142/88 mmHg. On physical exam, the patient was found to have bruises on her inner thigh and external genitalia. The urinalysis was negative except for the presence of sperm. You noticed that the patient is very quiet and withdrawn with her male nurse who accompanied her to the hospital. When you attempt to do a pelvic examination, the patient became increasingly combative and fearful. The pelvic exam revealed vaginal bleeding and a yellowish vaginal discharge.

Your examination led you to suspect that she had been raped and was a victim of elder abuse. At this point, you are unsure about the most common physical findings in elder abuse and what other risk factors are associated with this condition. You would like to ask her about the rape and other forms of elder abuse; however, her dementia precludes you. You wonder if you have missed elder abuse in other patients you have cared for and you are unsure if screening all your elderly patients for abuse would be effective. Finally, you wonder what interventions are effective for elder abuse and if you have any legal requirements regarding the suspected abuse.

Background

Elder abuse is defined by the American Medical Association as, "an act or omission that results in harm or threatened harm to the health or welfare of an elderly person" [1]. "Elderly" is defined differently in the literature; however, it generally refers to people

Evidence-based Emergency Medicine. Edited by Brian H. Rowe
© 2009 Blackwell Publishing, ISBN: 978-1-4051-6143-5.

who are over the age of 65 years; "frail elderly" are people over 65 and frail (e.g., in poor health and susceptible to disease and infirmity) or those over 85 years of age. Elder abuse is seen in all races, ethnic groups, religions, educational backgrounds and socio-economic groups and is a growing problem due to medical and public health advances that prolong adult life. In 2000, there were 420 million people worldwide aged 65 years or older. This number is expected to rise to 974 million by 2030 [2]. In the United States, elders made up about 12% of the population (35.9 million people) in 2003 and will form 20% of the US population in 30 years [2]. In addition, the life expectancy in many developed countries including the United States is at a record high (77.4 years in the USA) [3,4]; life expectancy is even higher in other parts of the world such as Australia (80.6 years), Canada (80.3 years), Japan (81.4 years) and Sweden (80.6 years) [5].

In the USA it is estimated that up to 5% of the community-dwelling elders are victims of abuse [6]; this does not include the 5–10% of elders living in institutions such as nursing homes [7]. Thus, elder abuse can fall under the classification of domestic/interpersonal violence for those living in a community setting or institutional abuse for those in extended care facilities. The exact incidence of elder abuse is not known; however, it is estimated that between 1 and 2 million elderly Americans experience some form of abuse [8]. International prevalence estimates of elder abuse from Canada, Finland, the Netherlands and the United Kingdom range from 4% to 6% [9]. A study from the Republic of Korea [10] found a rate of 6.3% and another from Israel [11] estimated at the rate to be as high as 18.4%.

A 2004 report from the National Center on Elder Abuse found that 8.3 cases of abuse are reported for every 1000 elder Americans [12]. Because studies have found that only one of every 13 or 14 cases of abuse is ever reported [13,14], the true rate of elder abuse is likely even higher. Many reasons have been cited for the lack of reporting, including fear and shame of the abused, physical and mental inability to seek help, and lack of recognition of the abuse by others. In summary, elder abuse is an important international ED and public health concern and emergency physicians need to be aware of this issue.

Clinical questions

1 In elderly patients who are abused (population), what forms of abuse (exposure) should physicians be aware of (outcome)?

2 In elderly patients who present to the ED (population), what history and physical signs (exposure) are most specific (diagnostic test characteristics) for abuse (outcome)?

3 In elderly patients who are abused (population), what risk factors (exposure) may suggest abuse (outcome)?

4 In elderly patients who are abused (population), what risk factors among the abusers (exposure) put them at risk for abuse (outcome)?

5 In elderly patients who present to the ED (population), is screening for abuse (intervention) effective at identifying victims and preventing further abuse (outcomes) compared to case finding (control)?

6 In elderly victims of abuse (population), what interventions (interventions) are most effective in reducing future abuse and death (outcomes) compared to standard care (control)?

7 In elderly victims of abuse who present to the ED (population), what mandatory legal and reporting requirements (exposures) exist to prevent further abuse (outcome)?

General search strategy

You start your search using database searches in Cochrane and MEDLINE. You suspect there have not been many randomized trials for elder abuse. Your first search of the Cochrane Library for elder abuse yields only one review and was more specifically related to domestic violence. You expand your search with MEDLINE and find about 1000 articles; however, no systematic reviews or meta-analyses. Finally, you expand your search with American College of Physicians Physician Information and Education Resource (ACP PIER) and Stat Ref and identify one relevant review.

Searching for evidence synthesis
- Cochrane Library: elder abuse AND maltreatment
- MEDLINE: elder abuse AND MEDLINE English articles AND EBM reviews
- Stat Ref: elder abuse

Critical review of the literature

Question 1: In elderly patients who are abused (population), what forms of abuse (exposure) should physicians be aware of (outcome)?

Search strategy

- Cochrane Library: elder abuse
- MEDLINE: elder abuse AND English articles AND EBM reviews
- MEDLINE: elder abuse AND English articles
- Stat Ref: elder abuse

The American Geriatrics Society has described seven forms of abuse against the elderly: physical, psychological, sexual, financial, neglect, self-neglect and abandonment [15]. Physical abuse includes acts that inflict pain or injury to the victim. Examples include punching, pushing and other physical assaults that might injure the person. Psychological abuse is conduct that results in emotional distress or psychological harm to the victim. Examples include threatening, humiliating and intimidating behaviors. Sexual abuse is sexual contact or exposure without the person's consent, including cases where the person is unable to consent due to cognitive impairment. Financial abuse or exploitation is the unjust, improper or illegal use of another person's resources, property or assets. Neglect is the failure to provide any services necessary to maintain physical and mental health. Self-neglect is failure of the individual to provide essential services for them self due to physical and/or mental inability. In many cases, multiple and concurrent forms of abuse exist [16].

The National Elder Abuse Incidence Study (NEAIS) gathered data on domestic elder abuse through a nationally representative sample of 20 counties [17]. It used reports from the local Adult Protective Services (APS) agency and reports from sentinels (specially trained individuals from community agencies with frequent contact with the elderly). The study found neglect was the most common form of abuse substantiated by the APS (50%), followed by psychological abuse (35%), financial exploitation (30%), physical abuse (26%), abandonment (4%) and sexual abuse (0.3%) [13]. Interestingly, nearly one-half of all abuse cases and two-thirds of neglect cases that are investigated involved some form of self-neglect [18].

In summary, abuse arises from a variety of etiologies and emergency physicians need to be aware of these in order to detect elder abuse.

Question 2: In elderly patients who present to the ED (population), what history and physical signs (exposure) are most sensitive and specific (diagnostic test characteristics) for abuse (outcome)?

Search strategy

- MEDLINE: elder abuse AND (signs and symptoms OR injury)

Extreme and heinous cases of abuse are very easy for physicians to recognize; however, most cases are not that straightforward and many victims are unable to provide an accurate history due to dementia or other medical conditions. Since there is no gold standard test for elder abuse or neglect, one must rely on history and forensic markers. As with any victim of abuse, it is important to look for injuries in multiple stages of healing, defensive injuries and injuries not consistent with the event. In elder abuse victims, age-related physiological changes may make it difficult to distinguish abuse from normal changes. These changes include: capillary fragility, decreased skin collagen, decreased estrogen, vaginal atrophy and drying, osteopenia, incontinence, impaired gait, balance and co-ordination, muscle atrophy, decreased adipose tissue and acquired coagulopathies [7].

Your search for meta-analyses, systematic reviews or randomized controlled trials (RCTs) yields no results; however, your MEDLINE search identifies 50 papers, although the majority are retrospective reviews. In general, most of the evidence for historical features in the following discussion is consensus driven. Some historical clues to abuse include social isolation of the elderly, unexplained transfers of care from other facilities or physicians, delay in seeking treatment after a fall and inconsistent stories. When interviewing a potential abuse victim, start the interview with the patient alone, without the care giver or family present. Be suspicious of the care giver or family member who refuses to leave the patient alone. Try to avoid leading questions and judgmental responses. You should start the interview with general questions about patient safety and move on to specific questions such as who prepares the meals, helps with the medications, helps with activities of daily living, etc.

Several signs may also be suggestive of *physical abuse.* These are outlined in Table 63.1; however, once again, they are largely consensus based rather than evidence based. Suspicious patterns of injury such as lesions in skin folds of the breast, axilla, popliteal fossa and groin may be from abuse. Look for patterned bruises – bruises that retain the shape of an object or that have central clearing [19]. Remember, the age of a bruise cannot be determined by its color [19]. Multiple fractures may suggest abuse or neglect. If there is an established relationship with the elder, look for changes in their behavior, especially if it is sudden. Other subtle clues may include emotional upset or agitation, extreme withdrawal and non-communication or non-responsiveness.

The elderly can be the victims of accidental trauma. These injuries include abrasions and contusions over bony prominences and long bone and vertebral fractures. Worrisome injuries occur in the inner thigh, top of the feet, inner ankle, inner wrists, palms and soles, the ear, posterior neck, mastoid region and the neck [7]. Look for bruises around the wrist, which may indicate improper restraint use. Head trauma is especially prominent in severe physical abuse and carries a high morbidity and mortality. Subdural hemorrhage from inflicted trauma is a common cause of death in elder abuse [7].

Any injury to the face, eye, nose or mouth should be considered suspicious for abuse [7,20–23]. Medical records of 200 victims of interpersonal violence (IPV) found that one-third of IPV victims with injuries had facial fractures [20]. Another cross-sectional study found that IPV victims were 7.5 times more likely to have head, neck and facial injuries than other trauma patients ($P < 0.001$) [21]. In a retrospective review of IPV patients, head, arm and abdominal injuries were significantly associated with IPV, particularly when multiple injuries were present [22]. Finally, a multi-center cross-sectional study concluded that battered women were more likely to be injured in the head, face, neck, thorax and abdomen than women injured by other mechanisms [23]. As with children, elders may sustain inflicted contact burns and scalds.

Table 63.1 Physical findings suggestive of abuse or neglect.

Poor hygiene
Dirty clothing
Dehydration
Severe traumatic injuries:
   Rib fractures
   Intra-abdominal hemorrhage
   Intracerebral hemorrhage
   Fractures
Lack of financial resources for medical care and necessities
Lack of assistive devices:
   Dentures
   Cane or walker
   Eyeglasses
Facial injuries and bruises
Burns
Patterned burns (i.e., cigarettes)
Patterned contusions
Rope or ligature marks (wrists and ankles)
Vaginal injury or bleeding
Sexually transmitted infections
Contusions
   Inner arms and thighs
   Palms, soles
   Ear (pinna)
   Mastoid
   Buttocks
   Multiple and clustered
Unusual alopecia pattern
Decubitus ulcers in non-lumbar/sacral area
Behavioral changes
Unexplained weight loss
Injuries in various stages of healing
Poor dentition

Emergency physicians should look for pattern burns and immersion lines.

Many elder *sexual assault* victims will have anogenital injuries [7]. Most elder sexual assault victims are women and the rape occurs when the woman is by herself [24]. Elderly women are at risk for anogenital injury due to increased vaginal atrophy, vaginal dryness and thinning of the vaginal wall [7]. Signs of sexual assault include bruises of the breasts and/or genital area, unexplained sexually transmitted infections, unexplained vaginal or anal bleeding, torn, stained or bloody underclothing, and the victim's own report of being sexually assaulted or raped [17,25]. Victims may be fearful or aggressive towards male health care workers.

Neglect can be active or passive. In passive neglect the failure on the part of the caretaker is unintentional often because the caretaker is uninformed, misinterprets signs and symptoms of illness, or is distracted by an external stressor [26]. Signs of neglect potentially obvious to health care workers include dehydration, malnutrition, untreated bedsores and poor personal and oral hygiene. Decubitus ulcers can indicate elder neglect. Ulcers located in areas other than the lumbar and sacral areas are suspicious and indicate unusual positioning or improper restraint use for an extended length of time. Other signs of neglect may not be as obvious during a health care interaction. These include hazardous, unsafe, unclean or unsanitary living conditions. Home health workers, social workers or family and friends may detect these forms of neglect.

Financial abuse is often not picked up by health care workers unless the lack of funds or resources adversely affects the ability of the elder to receive care or treatments such as prescriptions.

In summary, signs and symptoms of abuse are often subtle. The emergency physician needs to maintain a high index of suspicion when evaluating elderly patients. Any patient who gives a history of abuse should be believed until proven otherwise. The physician should be suspicious of patients with patterned or unexplained injuries, genital injuries or signs of neglect.

Question 3: In elderly patients who are abused (population), what risk factors (exposure) may suggest abuse (outcome)?

Search strategy

• MEDLINE: elder abuse AND (risk factors OR identification)

Any elderly person can be a victim of elder abuse. Certain risk factors and associations with elder victimization have been reported in the literature. Again your search for meta-analyses or RCTs does not yield any papers; however, your MEDLINE search results in 30 papers with "identification" and 162 papers with "risk factors". Once again, most of these are retrospective reviews, but there are some prospective, survey-based studies that provide useful information and are summarized below.

The NEAIS reviewed over 500,000 cases of elder abuse and neglect [17]. The survey identified the following groups most at risk for elder abuse: women (60–76% of victims), age 80 and older, and physical and mental fragility [13]. Women tended to suffer more psychological abuse (75%) and self-neglect (66%) than male victims. Overall, the oldest elders (age 80 or over) are abused and neglected at rates two to three times that of other elderly persons. Forty-five percent of self-neglecting elders and 52% of neglected elders reported to APS were over 80 years of age. This older group is also disproportionately subjected to physical, emotional and financial abuse. Elders who are unable to care for themselves are at higher risk that those who can care for themselves [17].

In most cases of elder abuse, the elder has some form of dependence on the perpetrator. Strongly associated risk factors of victims include dementia, functional decline and social isolation. A more recent survey of Alzheimer's patients and their primary care givers found that elder abuse victims were not more debilitated than their non-abused peers [27]. Incontinence is also a risk factor. Sometimes provocative actions of the elder put them at risk.

The fear of nursing home placement and fear of retaliation often allows the abuse to continue. Living with other persons tends to put the elder at risk for physical abuse while living alone is shown to increase the risk for financial abuse. Social isolation decreases the likelihood that abuse will be detected and stopped. Institutionalization is seen as a risk factor for elder abuse, although no research exists to truly quantify the risk [28].

In summary, there are several risk factors that put the elder at risk for abuse. These can include advanced age, dementia and dependence on the abuser. The emergency physician should be aware of these risk factors.

Question 4: In elderly patients who are abused (population), what risk factors among the abusers (exposure) put them at risk for abuse (outcome)?

Search strategy

• MEDLINE: elder abuse AND (risk factors OR perpetrators)

Your search reveals no RCTs or meta-analyses; however, your MEDLINE search does reveal several papers on abuser characteristics. The NEIAS has also identified risk factors among perpetrators of elder abuse [17]. These include male gender, younger age and relationship to the victim. The gender distribution of perpetrators is almost equal, but male perpetrators outnumbered females in all forms of abuse except neglect. A family history of using violence during times of stress can be perpetuated when the stressed caretaker abuses the elder [28]. For example, male victims are often abused by their wives and female victims are often abused by their children. In addition, most perpetrators were younger than their victims and the majority was under the age of 60 years. About 90% of abusers are related to their victims, with adult children being the largest category of abusers [17].

Two major risk factors have been identified. A large percentage of abusers have been found to have a history of mental illness or alcohol abuse [26]. In the USA, 44% of male and 14% of female abusers of parents were alcohol dependent [29]. In England, 45% of elder care givers admitted to committing abuse and alcohol consumption was found to be the highest risk factor [30]. A Canadian survey found that severe drinking habits by the abuser lead to harm in 14.6% of elder abuse cases [31].

Mental health disease is also seen among elder abusers. Depression and personality disorders are common among abusers [27,30,32,33]. A history of family violence is another risk factor for perpetration. This is referred to as transgenerational violence [7] as abused spouses may later abuse their abusers, abused children later abuse their parents and own children, thus perpetuating the cycle. Other risk factors among perpetrators include other substance abuse and dependence of the abuser on the victim (for money and housing) [29].

Within institutions, the perpetrator may be a staff member, another resident or a visitor. Poor employee relations, understaffing, inadequate screening and training of employees, mismanagement and staff turnover are all contributing factors [28]. A random sample survey of nursing home staffers in a single US state found that 10% of nurses' aides reported committing at least one act of physical abuse in the preceding year. Another 40% reported committing one act of psychological abuse [34]. Work with demented patients has found that violent acts carried out by a care recipient can trigger reciprocal violence by the care giver [35]. No study has found other specific risk factors unique to institutional abusers.

In summary, while the primary responsibility for care resides with the patient, knowledge of abuser behavior is an important key to detecting elder abuse. For example, physicians should have heightened suspicion for elder abuse if the caretaker exhibits signs or symptoms of mental illness or alcohol abuse, especially if the care giver is a family member, if they live together or when the care giver is dependent upon the elder.

Question 5: In elderly patients who present to the ED (population), is screening for abuse (intervention) effective at identifying victims and preventing further abuse (outcomes) compared to case finding (control)?

Search strategy

- MEDLINE: elder abuse AND screening

The American Medical Association (AMA) [36] and American College of Obstetrics and Gynecology (ACOG) [37] both recommend universal screening to detect abuse victims. The American College of Emergency Physicians (ACEP) does not specify screening in their position paper, but rather states, "emergency physicians have the responsibility to recognize, manage, and report suspected cases of elder abuse" [38]. The AMA suggests that physicians should routinely ask elderly patients direct and specific questions about abuse [36]. Unfortunately, there have been no good studies to support any of these positions. Several other international medical societies and organizations do not have policy statements supporting universal screening for elder abuse or domestic violence. Your search reveals one review and four articles.

The US Preventive Services Task Force (USPSTF) found insufficient evidence to recommend for or against routine screening of women for intimate partner violence or of older adults or their care givers for elder abuse [39–41]. They also found no direct evidence that screening leads to decreased disability or premature death. In addition, they could not find any studies that determined the accuracy of screening tools for identifying family and interpersonal violence among women and older adults. No studies have directly addressed the harms of screening and subsequent interventions for elder abuse.

The USPSTF found very few screening tools for detection of abuse in elders. In addition, none of the instruments have been widely validated [41]. Their review found three of 1045 abstracts that met inclusion criteria for elder abuse and neglect. None of these screening tools were developed or tested in traditional clinical settings. One study used the caregiver abuse screen (CASE) to distinguish abusers from non-abusers [42]. It correlated with the previously validated indicator of abuse and Hwalek–Sengstock elder abuse screening test (HSEAST) but was limited because of its small sample size. The two other studies looked at screening elderly adults. In the first, three groups of elders were studied: abuse victims, those referred to adult protective services but found not to be abused, and non-abused adults from a family practice clinic [43]. They used the HSEAST instrument, which correctly identified 67–74% of cases, and found that scores distinguished abused from not abused ($P < 0.001$). Six of the test items were strongly associated with abuse. The second study used the HSEAST instrument administered to a convenience sample of elders living in public housing in Florida [44]. Scores for abused and non-abused persons were significantly different (mean scores 4.01 vs 3.01, $P = 0.0489$). They also found that a nine-item model performed as well as the traditional 15-item version. The shorter version identified 71.4% of abuse with 17% false-positive and 12% false-negative rates.

The Canadian Task Force on Preventive Health Care (CTFPHC) also determined there was insufficient evidence to include or exclude case finding for elder abuse as part of the periodic health examination, but recommended that physicians be alert for indicators of abuse [45,46]. One concern of screening is the potential harm to the victim after screening as a result of identification. No studies have directly addressed the harms of screening. Some potential harms of screening may include loss of contact with established support systems, psychological distress and escalation of abuse [47].

Despite the lack of evidence supporting screening, physicians should routinely ask elderly patients a few direct questions about abuse because of the prevalence of undetected abuse and the potential usefulness of this information. The previously mentioned screening tools may be used; however, the AMA recommends nine routine screening questions for elder abuse (Table 63.2) [28,36]. As there have been no studies about the safety of screening elders for abuse, physicians should ask about elder abuse without the care giver present and be careful about giving any printed information on abuse to the patient.

Table 63.2 Routine screening questions for elder abuse.

1 Has anyone at home ever hurt you?
2 Has anyone ever touched you without your consent?
3 Has anyone ever made you do things you didn't want to do?
4 Has anyone taken anything that was yours without asking?
5 Has anyone ever scolded or threatened you?
6 Have you ever signed any documents that you didn't understand?
7 Are you afraid of anyone at home?
8 Are you alone a lot?
9 Has anyone ever failed to help you take care of yourself when you needed help?

Question 6: In elderly victims of abuse (population), what interventions (interventions) are most effective in reducing future abuse and death (outcomes) compared to standard care (control)?

Search strategy

- MEDLINE: elder abuse AND (interventions OR treatment OR counseling)

The USPSTF also looked at interventions for elder abuse victims [40,41]. Of 1084 abstracts that were identified by database searches, 72 were further reviewed. None of these studies provided data about effective interventions. According to the task force, some of the papers described individual elder abuse programs, yet none included comparison groups or health outcome measures.

As a physician, the goal of any intervention should be to reduce the risk of future mistreatment by improving the physical, mental and functional capacity of the elderly patient. This helps to decrease the patient's dependence and reduces care givers' stress. Physicians should screen for dementia and depression and treat these conditions when possible. In addition, physicians should use caution when prescribing medications that impact cognitive or functional capacity. The elderly patient and their care giver should be referred to social workers and other appropriate resources such as Meals on Wheels, adult day care, church activities, pastoral visitation, respite care, care-giver training and disease-specific support groups.

If a physician feels a patient is in immediate harm, the patient should be admitted to the hospital until safe living arrangements can be made (Fig. 63.1). In addition, if indicated, physicians should contact local law enforcement agencies. An emergency guardian may need to be appointed. There should be thorough documentation of any physical findings and historical elements provided by the patient. Photographic documentation of injuries is helpful for future police and legal action. Body diagrams should be used to document injuries and wounds. If sexual assault is suspected, a rape kit should be collected by staff with experience.

In summary, very few intervention studies have been conducted. However, physicians should intervene in suspected or identified elder abuse cases and should contact social services or the APS when indicated.

Question 7: In elderly victims of abuse who present to the ED (population), what mandatory legal and reporting requirements (exposures) exist to prevent further abuse (outcome)?

Search strategy

- MEDLINE: elder abuse AND (reporting OR legal requirements)

All 50 states and the District of Columbia have APS laws to establish a system for the reporting and investigation of elder abuse [48]. States vary in the way laws are written and who is covered by them; some define which victims are eligible, age of victim, whether the abuse is civil or criminal, whether reporting is mandatory or voluntary, and who handles the investigation. In many states, the suspicion of abuse is grounds for reporting and often times the reporter remains anonymous. Thirty-seven states mandate health care provider reporting [19]. All states and DC have laws to advocate on behalf of abused residents of long-term facilities. These laws fall under the Long Term Care Ombudsman Program (LTCOP). The ombudsman's phone number is posted in all long-term care institutions. The US model is followed in many developed countries; however, it is not the same case in many other parts of the world. For example, in many countries, no laws for reporting exist.

In the USA, there are varying penalties for failing to report and also various regulations regarding who has reporting responsibility. To date, there have been no known cases of health care providers being convicted for failure to report elder abuse. Some barriers to reporting abuse include: fear of abuse escalation, fear of legal retaliation if the abuse is unfounded, fear of damaging the doctor–patient relationship, inability to identify abuse, lack of health care provider knowledge about elder abuse, and lack of knowledge regarding reporting laws.

Depending on the type of abuse perpetrated, other laws in the jurisdiction of practice may mandate that certain crimes be reported, such as domestic or interpersonal violence, sexual assault and assaults with weapons. Currently, 45 states have laws that mandate physician reporting of these injuries [49]. Physicians, nurses and other health care workers should become familiar with the specific laws of where they practice. Other countries do not have such laws or requirements.

No RCTs have been conducted on the effect of reporting on patient safety and subsequent outcomes. In addition, no studies were conducted specifically looking at elder abuse. Sachs et al. conducted a population-based telephone survey that found abused women were less likely to support mandatory reporting than non-abused women (59% vs 73%) [47]. Rodriguez found that women who were sexually or physically abused (OR = 2.2; 95% CI: 1.6 to 2.9) or who were non-English speaking (OR = 2.1; 95% CI: 1.4 to 3.0), were more likely to oppose mandatory reporting than women who had never been abused [50]. Houry et al. reported that only 12% of ED patients would be deterred from seeking medical care because of mandatory reporting [51]. Thus, there is no evidence to either support or discourage mandatory reporting.

The goal of the emergency physician is to prevent further harm to the patient. If abuse is suspected, the physician should contact their local APS agency and police department if indicated. Knowledge of local laws and procedures is critical; when in doubt contact the appropriate agencies who will further advise the physician regarding duty and options.

One frustration is the conflict between patient safety and autonomy. The patient who has the capacity to make decisions for themselves and chooses to stay in a dangerous environment is a challenge for all members of the health care team. These patients

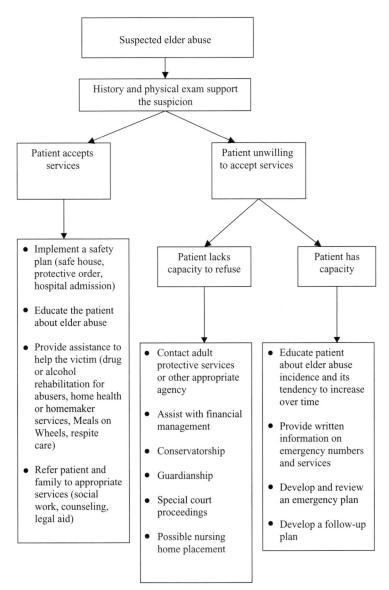

Figure 63.1 Management of the abused elder. (Modified from Lachs & Pillemer [52].)

can decline intervention by the APS. Physicians and health care workers should not be deterred from reporting suspected abuse simply because the patient may refuse intervention.

Conclusions

Armed with this information, in the case described above, you notify the police and APS as well as the ombudsman. A rape kit is collected and standard sexual protocols are followed. For her safety, the patient is admitted to the hospital until she can be moved to a different extended care facility. You later learn from the District Attorney that her rape kit was positive for biological evidence. The DNA was matched to a nurses' aide on the patient's floor and he was arrested.

Elder abuse and neglect is a serious issue. The emergency physician is in a unique position to screen for and to detect elder abuse. Often times the signs of abuse are obvious; at other times they may be subtle. Unfortunately, very little evidence exists to recommend for or against universal screening, despite recommendations of several medical organizations. Moreover, interventions have been poorly studied and emergency physicians are left to institute primary protection as the best measure for reducing further morbidity and mortality. The ultimate goal is to protect the patient from further harm. Physicians should be familiar with their legal requirements and contact the APS in all cases of suspected abuse.

Conflicts of interest

None were reported.

References

1 Council on Scientific Affairs. Elder abuse and neglect. *JAMA* 1987;**257**:966–971.

2 Wan He, Sengupta M, Velkoff VA, DeBarros KA. *US Census Bureau, Current Population Reports, P23-209. 65+ in the United States: 2005.* US Census Bureau, US Government Printing Office, Washington, 2005. Available at http://www.census.gov/prod/2006pubs/p23-209.pdf (accessed January 20, 2006).

3 Collins KA, Presnell SE. Elder homicide: a 20 year study. *Am J Forensic Med Pathol* 2006;**27**:183–7.

4 Kochanek KD, Smith BL. Deaths: preliminary data for 2002. *Natl Vital Stat Rep* 2004;**52**:1–47.

5 US Census Bureau. US Census Bureau International Database. Available at http://www.census.gov/ipc/www/idbnew.html (accessed April 5, 2006).

6 Kurrie S. Elder abuse. *Aust Fam Physician* 2004;**33**:807–12.

7 Collins SA. Elder maltreatment: a review. *Arch Pathol Lab Med* 2006;**130**:1290–96.

8 Shields LB, Hunraker DM, Hunraker JC. Abuse and neglect: a ten-year review of mortality and morbidity in our elders in a large metropolitan area. *J Forensic Sci* 2004;**49**:122–7.

9 Krug EG, Dahlberg LL, Mercy JA, Zwi AB, Lozano R, eds. *World Report on Violence and Health.* World Health Organization, Geneva, 2002.

10 Oh J, Kim HS, Martins D, Kim H. A study of elder abuse in Korea. *Int J Nurs Stud* 2006;**43**:203–14.

11 Siegel-Itzkovich J. A fifth of elderly people in Israel are abused. *BMJ* 2005;**330**:498.

12 Teaster PB, Dugar T, Mendiondo M, Abner E, Cecil K, Otto J. *Abuse of Adults Age 60+: The 2004 Survey of Adult Protective Services – Abuse of adults 60 years of age and older.* National Center on Elder Abuse (NCEA), Washington, 2006. Available at: http://www.elderabusecenter.org/pdf/2-14-06%20FINAL%2060+REPORT.pdf (accessed January 20, 2007).

13 Lett JE. Abuse of the elderly. *J Fla Med Assoc* 1995;**82**:675–8.

14 Fordham H. Elder abuse: diagnosis can often be difficult. *Mich Med* 1992;**91**:30–31.

15 American Geriatrics Society. Position Statement on Elder Mistreatment. Available at http://www.americangeriatrics.org/products/positionpapers/elder_abuse.shtml (accessed January 20, 2007).

16 Collins KA, Bennett AT, Hanzlick R. Elder abuse and neglect. *Arch Intern Med* 2000;**160**:1567–8.

17 National Center on Elder Abuse. National Elder Abuse Incidence Study. American Public Human Services Association, Washington, 1998. Available at http://www.aoa.gov/eldfam/Elder_Rights/Elder_abuse/AbuseReport_full.pdf (accessed January 25, 2007).

18 Kruger RM, Moon CH. Can you spot the signs of elder mistreatment? *Postgrad Med* 1999;**106**:169–83.

19 Liao S, Smith S. Reporting Elder Mistreatment. The Physicians Information and Education Resource (PIER). American College of Physicians, Philadelphia, 2006. Available at http://pier.acponline.org/index.html?hp (accessed February 15, 2007).

20 Le BT, Dierks EJ, Ueeck BA, Homer LD, Potter BF. Maxillofacial injuries associated with domestic violence. *J Oral Maxillofac Surg* 2001;**59**:1277–83.

21 Perciaccante VJ, Ochs HA, Dodson TB. Head, neck, and facial injuries as markers for domestic violence in women. *J Oral Maxillofac Surg* 1999;**57**:760–62.

22 Spedding RL, McWilliams M, McNicholl BP, Dearden CH. Markers for domestic violence in women. *J Accid Emerg Med* 1999;**16**:400–402.

23 Muelleman RL, Lenaghan PA, Pakieser RA. Battered women injury locations and types. *Ann Emerg Med* 1996;**28**:486–92.

24 Teaster PB, Roberto KA. Sexual abuse of older adults: APS cases and outcomes. *Gerontologist* 2004;**44**:788–96.

25 Sillman JS. Elder Abuse. Up to Date. Available at www.uptodate.com (accessed February 15, 2007).

26 Lach MS, Pillemer K. Elder abuse. *Lancet* 2004;**364**:1263–72.

27 Paveza GJ, Cohen D, Eisdorfer C, et al. Severe family violence and Alzheimer's disease: prevalence and risk factors. *Gerontologist* 1992;**32**:493–7.

28 Levine JM. Elder neglect and abuse: a primer for primary physicians. *Geriatrics* 2003;**58**:37–40, 42–44.

29 Greenberg JR, McKibben M, Raymond JA. Dependent adult children and elder abuse. *J Elder Abuse Neglect* 1990;**2**:73.

30 Homer AC, Gilleard C. Abuse of elderly people by their carers. BMJ 1990;**301**:1359.

31 Pittaway E, Gallagher E. *A Guide to Enhancing Services for Abused Older Canadians.* Health Canada, Ottawa, 1995.

32 Reay AM, Browne KD. Risk factor characteristics in carers who physically abuse or neglect their elderly dependents. *Aging Ment Health* 2001;**5**:56–62.

33 Williamson GM, Shaffer DR. Relationship quality and potentially harmful behaviors by spousal caregivers: how we were then, how we are now. *Psychol Aging* 2001;**16**:217–26.

34 Pillemer K, Moore DW. Abuse of patients in nursing homes: findings from a survey of staff. *Gerontologist* 1989;**29**:314–20.

35 Pillemer KA, Suitor JJ. Violence and violent feelings: what causes them among family caregivers? *J Gerontol* 1992;**47**:S165–72.

36 Aravanis S, Adelman R, Breachman R. *Diagnostic and Treatment Guidelines on Elder Abuse and Neglect.* American Medical Association, Chicago, 1992.

37 American College Obstetricians and Gynecologists. *Guidelines for Women's Health Care*, 2nd edn. American College Obstetricians and Gynecologists, Washington, 2002.

38 American College of Emergency Physicians. Management of Elder Abuse and Neglect. American College of Emergency Physicians, Dallas, 2001. Available at http://www.acep.org/webportal/PracticeResources/PolicyStatements/violabuse/ManagementofElderAbuseandNeglect.htm (accessed February 15, 2007).

39 US Preventive Services Task Force. *Guide to Clinical Preventive Services*, 2nd edn. Williams and Wilkins, Baltimore, 1996.

40 US Preventive Services Task Force. Screening for family and intimate partner violence: recommendation statement. *Ann Intern Med* 2004;**140**:382–6.

41 Nelson HD, Nygren P, McInerney Y, Klein J. Screening women and elder adults for family and intimate partner violence: a review of the evidence for the US Preventive Services Task Force. *Ann Intern Med* 2004;**140**:387–96.

42 Reis M, Nahmiash D. Validation of the Caregiver Abuse Screen (CASE). *Can J Aging* 1995;**14**:45–60.

43 Neale AV, Hwalek MA, Scott RO, Sengstock MC, Stahl C. Validation of the Hwalek–Sengstock Elder Abuse Screening Test. *J Appl Gerontol* 1991;**10**:406–18.

44 Moody LE, Voss A, Lengacher CA. Assessing abuse among the elderly living in public housing. *J Nurs Meas* 2000;**8**:61–70.

45 Wathen CN, MacMillan HL. Prevention of violence against women: recommendation statement from the Canadian Task Force on Preventive Health Care. *Can Med Assoc J* 2003;**169**:582–4.

46 Coulthard P, Yong S, Adamson L, Warburton A, Worthington HV, Esposito M. Domestic violence screening and intervention programmes for adults with dental or facial injury. *Cochrane Database Syst Rev* 2004;**2**:CD004486 (doi: 10.1002/14651858.CD004486.pub2).

47 Sachs CJ, Koziol-McLain J, Glass N, Webster D, Campbell J. A population-based survey assessing support for mandatory domestic violence reporting by healthcare professionals. *Women Health* 2002;**35**:121–33.

48 American Bar Association Commission on Law and Aging. *Information about Laws Related to Elder Abuse.* National Center on Elder Abuse, Washington, 2005. Available at http://www.elderabusecenter.org/pdf/publication/InformationAboutLawsRelatedtoElderAbuse.pdf (accessed February 20, 2007).

49 Houry D, Sachs CJ, Feldhaus KM, Linden J. Violence-inflicted injuries: reporting laws in the fifty states. *Ann Emerg Med* 2002;**39**:56–60.

50 Rodriguez MA, Wallace SP, Woolf NH, et al. Mandatory reporting elder abuse: between a rock and a hard place. *Ann Fam Med* 2006;**4**(5): 403–9.

51 Houry D, Feldhaus K, Thorson AC, Abbott J. Mandatory reporting laws do not deter patients from seeking medical care. *Ann Emerg Med* 1999;**34**:336–41.

52 Lachs MS, Pillemer K. Abuse and neglect of elderly persons. *N Engl J Med* 1995;**332**:437–43.

Index

Index

Index

Index

Index